FIFTH EDITION

COMMUNITY HEALTH NURSING
A CANADIAN PERSPECTIVE

LYNNETTE LEESEBERG **STAMLER**

University of Nebraska Medical Center

LUCIA **YIU**

University of Windsor

ALIYAH **DOSANI**

Mount Royal University

JOSEPHINE **ETOWA**

University of Ottawa

CHERYL **VAN DAALEN-SMITH**

York University

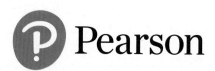

Pearson Canada Inc., 26 Prince Andrew Place, North York, Ontario M3C 2H4.

9780134837888

1 20

Library and Archives Canada Cataloguing in Publication

Title: Community health nursing : a Canadian perspective / [edited by] Lynnette Leeseberg Stamler, University of Nebraska Medical Center, Lucia Yiu, University of Windsor, Aliyah Dosani, Mount Royal University, Josephine Etowa, University of Ottawa, CheryL van Daalen-Smith, York University.
Other titles: Community health nursing (Toronto, Ont.).
Names: Stamler, Lynnette Leeseberg, 1952- editor. | Yiu, Lucia, 1951- editor. | Dosani, Aliyah, editor. | Etowa, Josephine B., 1965- editor. | Van Daalen-Smith, Cheryl, 1962- editor.
Description: Fifth edition. | Includes index.
Identifiers: Canadiana 20190049928 | ISBN 9780134837888 (softcover)
Subjects: LCSH: Community health nursing—Canada—Textbooks. | LCGFT: Textbooks.
Classification: LCC RT98 .C644 2019 | DDC 610.73/430971—dc23

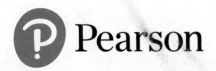

Brief Contents

Contents

List of Canadian Research Boxes

Preface

We would like to begin by thanking students, instructors and professors, and community health nurses (CHNs) who welcomed the first four editions and provided excellent and insightful feedback for this fifth edition. This textbook has been useful not only at multiple levels within undergraduate nursing programs across the country but also in preparation for the Canadian Nurses Association certification examination in community health. To know that each of our previous editions was informative and easy to read yet encouraged learners' thinking made developing this new edition even more meaningful.

Our community health nursing context in Canada is unique. We believe there are historical, political, legislative, cultural, and social influences that shape the health of Canadians. They have moulded the evolution of Canada as a society, our definitions of health, interactions with various health professionals, and our expectations relative to health care delivery. CHNs are both a product of those influences and an influence themselves. Community health nursing has evolved differently in Canada than in other countries. We believe that as practitioners in community health nursing, we must understand these influences to better prepare ourselves to help shape community health nursing and, ultimately, the health of all in Canada.

OUR APPROACH

Over time there has been much discourse on the scope and practice of community health nursing. Historically, "community health nursing" was used to describe all nursing outside the hospital setting. In this textbook, community health nursing is defined as a specialty in nursing that encompasses a number of sub-specialties and a variety of practice areas, including home health nursing and public health nursing.

The community client may be an individual, family, community, system, or population, but care is rendered with an eye to the health of the population. The setting may be a home, institution, community, or agency serving the population. The common academic preparation is the basic baccalaureate education leading to the designation Registered Nurse. The employer may be an individual, family, community, government, non-governmental, or not-for-profit agency. When our chapter authors address a specific health issue or a particular population or aggregate in this textbook, each is speaking through the lens of her or his experience and/or research about a segment within the larger whole of community health nursing.

We believe community health nursing functions within a multiplicity of theories and understandings. Some theories are common to all facets of the nursing profession, such as ethical treatment of clients, family assessment, or the meaning of health. In some cases, nursing drove the development of the theory; in others, we have used the work of theorists in other disciplines. This textbook reflects that multiplicity, and the authors have described how the theories relate to community health nursing.

Community Health Nursing: A Canadian Perspective, Fifth Edition, has been written with the undergraduate student in mind. The work on this edition is in response to the needs expressed by faculty and students for a broad, comprehensive, and yet concise textbook providing an overview of community health nursing. Each topic is written with the understanding that this will be the student's first foray into the community health nursing arena. We have chosen to incorporate the individual, family, community, system, and population as client perspectives throughout the text.

NEW TO THE FIFTH EDITION

The new edition brings many changes. Aliyah Dosani, PhD, RN, has assumed the much-appreciated role of Lead Editor. Another important change is the wonderful addition of Josephine Etowa, PhD, RN, Loyer-DaSilva Research Chair in Public Health Nursing, and Cheryl van Daalen-Smith, PhD, RN, as co-editors. Together, their diverse expertise brings critical analyses and fresh ideas to this textbook.

The fifth edition's most prominent two new features are (1) its intentional focus on social justice and health equity, and (2) the deliberate incorporation of Indigenous content in virtually every chapter. In acknowledgement of the Truth and Reconciliation Commission of Canada, the recent Memorandum of Understanding between the Community Health Nurses of Canada (CHNC) and the Canadian Indigenous Nurses Association (CINA), and nursing's obligation to include Indigenous content and ways of knowing into our curriculum, this edition reflects our concerted effort to involve Indigenous consultants and contributors. These are historic moments in our time. As such, Chapter 22 will assist professors and students to better understand the position of First Nation, Inuit, and Métis peoples in Canada, their strengths and ways of knowing, as well as to appropriately contextualize health issues facing various Indigenous populations. As CHNs are keenly aware of the health impacts of social injustice and health inequity, each chapter specifically addresses key areas of advocacy for the CHN. Canadian Research boxes and Case Studies throughout the text have been thoroughly updated, with many focusing on health equity. We have added "Yes, But Why?" boxes to demonstrate how CHNs can address various social justice and health equity issues from an upstream and critical lens. Furthermore, we have identified which Community Health Nursing Standards of Practice our proposed actionable interventions align with. We've paid particular attention to language, ensuring its use is both political and exacting. And lastly, in keeping with the critical focus of this new edition, we have ensured that our contributors represent the vast diversity inherent in the Canadian population.

As is appropriate to the pace of change in community health and community health nursing, we have made extensive updates to various chapters, with new content, statistics, and Canadian research. As such, you will observe that the titles of some chapters have been updated to reflect this new direction of content. We made further emphasis on the importance of application of theory to practice; we addressed the growing needs of our community clients. You will see that a number of chapters look completely different from previous versions. In addition, you will notice we have included five levels of prevention—primordial, primary, secondary, tertiary, and quaternary—as they related to various topics throughout the textbook.

ABOUT THE CONTRIBUTORS

This fifth edition brings new and former authors to the textbook. As before, some hold academic positions, some are in management or policy positions, and others are front-line practitioners. All came with a commitment to share their work with the readers as they contribute to this Canadian community health nursing text, and this further demonstrates the cyclical nature of theory and practice. Each brings expertise and knowledge to a particular chapter and topic. Each has presented the various historical, geographical, social, political, and theoretical perspectives that assist in explaining and describing community nursing practice. You will find a list of the contributors, their affiliations, and the chapters they authored following the preface. To provide context regarding the varied experience and expertise of our contributors, we have also provided a short biographical sketch of each contributor immediately following the chapter(s) they wrote.

CHAPTER ORGANIZATION

The chapters in *Community Health Nursing: A Canadian Perspective* are organized into five parts:

Part I: The Context of Community Health Nursing in Canada
Part II: Foundations and Tools for Community Health Nursing Practice
Part III: Nursing Care of Selected Populations
Part IV: Selected Community Health Issues
Part V: Looking Ahead

Part I: The Context of Community Health Nursing in Canada introduces students to the general topic area. **Chapter 1: The History of Community Health Nursing in Canada** presents an historical perspective on Canadian community health nursing so students may be enlightened by lessons from the past. In this edition, a timeline is the organizing frame for the chapter. **Chapter 2: Policy, Politics, and Power in Health Care** presents the administration of community health from legislative, cultural, and political perspectives. The impact of policy, politics, and power on health equity and community health nursing practice, and the need for strong community health nursing leadership, have been highlighted. **Chapter 3: Nursing Roles, Functions, and Practice Settings** introduces the readers to the professional practice model, standards of practice, and the Blueprint for Action or national framework and action plan for CHNs. **Chapter 4: Public Health Nursing** and **Chapter 5: Home Health Nursing in Canada** speak to these two specific practice contexts and have been updated accordingly. Part 1 ends with **Chapter 6: Advocacy, Ethical, and Legal Considerations**, the authors of which have used the Canadian Community Health Nursing Standards of Practice (found in Appendix A) to frame a discussion on legal and ethical issues for CHNs. The chapters in Part I form the foundation for community health nursing practice for the subsequent parts of the textbook.

Part II: Foundations and Tools for Community Health Nursing Practice builds the base upon which the sub-specialties rest. **Chapter 7: Theoretical Foundations of Community Health Nursing** outlines several current theories students can use to guide their community health nursing practice. **Chapter 8: Health Promotion** has been consolidated and re-worked and provides an introduction to health promotion and community health nursing work, including harm reduction and social marketing approaches. **Chapter 9: Race, Culture, and Health** examines the different meanings of culture, and ethnic and racial diversity, and highlights how CHNs can continue to deepen their understandings of societal power and privilege, and move forward with anti-racist, anti-oppressive practice. **Chapter 10: Evidence-Informed Decision Making in Community Health Nursing** discusses the importance of incorporating a system to appraise evidence and how to apply this to community health nursing practice. **Chapter 11: Epidemiology** describes the science of epidemiology and how it can inform community health nursing practice. **Chapter 12: Communicable Diseases** describes concepts related to communicable disease and includes the updated Public Health Agency of Canada Guidelines for Infection Prevention and Control. **Chapter 13: Community Nursing Process** provides an overview of the community health nursing process, including community assessment, selected community health practice models, population health promotion, community development, and community participatory tools. In **Chapter 14: Community Health Planning, Monitoring, and Evaluation**, the authors examine specifics around planning, monitoring, and evaluating community health programs, with additional information on the logic model and Gantt charts. This portion of the textbook concludes with **Chapter 15: Digital Health**. Here you will find a discussion of digital health information and how it contributes to community nursing practice. In this edition additional discussion of social media has been included, as well as the most recent digital health competencies. We believe the topics in Parts I and II are essential for an understanding of community health nursing.

Parts III and IV, composed of focus chapters, examine groups and issues that make the picture of community health nursing more complete. In **Part III**, the spotlight is on **Nursing Care of Selected Populations**, which we have deliberately focused on working toward health equity rather than challenges. **Chapter 16: Maternal, Newborn, and Child Health** examines population health promotion approaches with socioenvironmental perspectives on enhancing maternal, newborn, and child health. **Chapter 17: School Health** provides critical conceptualizations of children, childhood, and children's rights. Pressing health challenges and inequities encountered in the school-aged population are explored through a lens of the social determinants of health. In addition to comprehensive school health, a framework for Indigenous school health is presented. The need for an expanded health-promotion role for the public health nurse in schools is highlighted in keeping with a child-centred, rights-based approach. **Chapter 18: Family Health** provides an overview of the social and cultural context family health. **Chapter 19: Gender and Community Health** focuses on applying gender-based analysis to community health nursing practice. Societal causes of gender-based inequities are discussed. **Chapter 20: Lesbian, Gay, Bisexual, Transgender, Queer, and Two Spirit Clients** gives further explanation about the genetic and social influences on sexual orientation and gender identity development. **Chapter 21: Older Adult Health** highlights the role and competencies of CHNs in relation to key issues that affect the health of older persons. The broader social, cultural, and political contexts that shape the well-being of older persons, with an emphasis on equity in health and health care using a social justice lens, are emphasized. **Chapter 22: Indigenous Health** presents and contextualizes the historical and current influences on the health of First Nation, Inuit, and Métis populations in Canada. Indigenous ways of knowing and being, First Nation-specific health care, and cultural safety and humility are discussed. The chapter has been gifted with a traditional perspective from an Elder. **Chapter 23: Community Mental Health** now provides a trauma-informed discussion of emotional distress and invites the reader to apply this to mental health promotion in Canada. The chapter explores critical sociopolitical issues that impact the mental health and well-being of various populations. Specific emphasis is placed on marginalization and mental health while discussing various Indigenous, gender variant, LGBTQ2S, refugee and immigrant, and veteran populations.

Chapter 24: Rural and Remote Health explores the large portion of Canada's population who live in rural settings and the sub-specialty of rural and remote community health nursing. One of the highlights of this edition is the section of "a day in the life" of a rural nurse. **Chapter 25: Chronic Care, Long-Term Care, and Palliative Care** examines issues for those community clients who receive extended or end-of-life care in the community. **Chapter 26: Correctional Health** now reflects a rights-based analysis of people who are incarcerated while exploring the barriers to correctional nurses' full scope of practice within a controlled environment. Highlighted in this edition are working with youth, looking at alternative measures and restorative justice, prisoners' rights movements, and trauma-informed nursing care in a correctional facility. **Chapter 27: Ecological Determinants of Health and Environmental Health Inequities** includes discussion of environmental inequities as well as the nurse's role in assessment and prevention.

In contrast, **Part IV** focuses on **Selected Community Health Issues** that may apply to a variety of populations. Each chapter concentrates on one of five specific issues. In this edition, **Chapter 28: Violence and Health** highlights the links between violence in societies and the social determinants of health and presents an innovative new model from which CHNs may practice. In **Chapter 29: Poverty, Homelessness, and Food Insecurity**, a wide-sweeping structural analysis is provided, ensuring that advocacy efforts focus on the real causes of these issues. Retitled **Chapter 30: Substance Use** looks at licit as well as illicit drug use in Canada. In this edition, information is presented about structural inequities related to substance use, and the debate around harm reduction is enhanced. **Chapter 31: Sexually Transmitted and Blood-Borne Infections** presents the variety of infections as well as how public policy in Canada has been developed around these illnesses. Social marketing as a prevention strategy is highlighted. **Chapter 32: Emergency Preparedness and Disaster Nursing** provides an overview of the role of CHNs in community emergency preparedness planning and disaster situations. Competencies for emergency preparedness for community health nursing are highlighted.

The final section, **Part V: Looking Ahead**, contains **Chapter 33: Global Health**. In this edition, new foci of globalization and global heath alert the learner to the wider picture. The text concludes with a brief look at where the field of community health nursing is headed and the coming opportunities available to decrease inequities by using a critical approach to community health nursing in **Chapter 34: Critical Community Health Nursing: An Imperative**.

Through the text, you will notice some concepts and items are mentioned in several of the chapters, reflecting their thematic presence in critical community health nursing practice. Most obvious, many of the chapters include an intentional focus on social justice and health equity. You will note that each author presents how these topics apply to different situations, depending on the chapter topic. We anticipate that students, instructors and professors, and community health nurses in practice will see this not as redundancy but rather as an example of multiple perspectives and how and why a multiplicity of knowledge and practice exists in community health nursing.

A Note on Appendices

As in previous editions, we have included the recently revised Canadian Community Health Nursing Standards of Practice, as shown in Appendix A (revised March 2019). This document explicitly reflects the current practice standards for Canadian community health nurses. In several chapters, contributors have made reference to the standards to enhance the discussion.

Appendices B and C are the discipline-specific competencies. Appendix B is the Public Health Nursing Discipline Specific Competencies published by the Community Health Nurses of Canada (CHNC) in 2009. They were developed using several source documents and a Delphi process to arrive at consensus. Appendix C contains the Home Health Nursing Competencies. They were developed by the CHNC in partnership with the CHNC Certification, Standards and Competencies Committee and Advisory Group.

Chapter Features

A special effort has been made with this textbook to incorporate features that will facilitate learning and enhance an understanding of community health nursing in Canada.

- **Learning Outcomes** outline what will be learned within each chapter.
- **NEW! Yes, But Why?** boxes explore how CHNs can address various issues from an upstream and critical lens. Each box ends with a list of the CHNC standards that have been addressed.

YES, BUT WHY?

Health in All Policies (HiAP): A Tool for Population Health

What?

In Canada, broad sectors of public policy and legislation such as education policy; transportation, including highways and roads; environment; communication; natural resources; income security; and foreign trade are developed with little or no consideration for their population health implications. A policy with negative consequences for the health of the

- **Canadian Research** boxes present specific studies from the literature or the authors' knowledge to illustrate or augment the material covered in the chapter. Either the researchers themselves are nurses, or we have chosen Canadian health research that community health nurses can use in their practice. Each Research Box is followed by a few Discussion Questions to assist students in using the results.

CANADIAN RESEARCH 2.1

Workforce diversity as a critical enabler for IENs' integration and health equity work (Ramji & Etowa, 2018)

Immigrants are a substantial part of the labour markets in most Western countries. In 2012, about 7% of the 365 422 nurses in Canada had graduated from an international nursing program (CIHI, 2012). In Ontario, Canada's largest province, IENs made up over 12% of the nursing workforce that year (CIHI, 2012). The growing

- **Case Studies** illustrate a practice application of the information presented in the chapter, followed by Discussion Questions.

CASE STUDY

Alcohol is a widely used psychoactive substance in communities across Canada. Dependence on alcohol and its associated harms create public health and other societal problems. Vodina is an 18-year-old boy who lives with his mother in a two-bedroom public housing apartment in an Ottawa neighbourhood. His mother is unmarried and unemployed. They live on welfare assistance, which is barely adequate to cover food, rent, and transportation. They often visit the food bank to make ends meet. To supplement the family income, Vodina, who has not yet completed high school, has been doing odd jobs around their neighbourhood. However, his mother notices he does not

- **Key Terms** are boldfaced where they are introduced and defined in the body of the text. For convenience, the key terms are listed alphabetically at the end of each chapter.

KEY TERMS

accessible   (p. 19)
Canada Health Act   (p. 19)
comprehensive   (p. 19)
determinants of health   (p. 20)
health equity   (p. 25)
health inequity   (p. 25)
health promotion   (p. 20)
home care   (p. 24)
leadership   (p. 28)
medicare   (p. 19)
policy   (p. 25)

- **Study Questions** test students' knowledge of the facts and concepts in the chapter. Answers to the study questions are included in the eText.

STUDY QUESTIONS

1. Identify the origins of medicare in Canada, and summarize the laws that created the present Canadian health care system. What is considered to be phase two of the implementation of medicare?

2. Discuss the events that led to and necessitated passage of the Canada Health Act.

3. What role did organized nursing play in the passage of the Canada Health Act?

4. Discuss the federal and provincial responsibilities for health according to the Canada Health Act.

5. Contrast the funding mechanisms for public health and

■ **Individual** and **Group Critical-Thinking Exercises** challenge students to reflect on the content of the chapter and apply it in different situations.

INDIVIDUAL CRITICAL-THINKING EXERCISES

1. List your core values for health care in Canada. How do your values compare with the values reflected in the five key funding criteria described in the Canada Health Act?

2. How would your life be different if health care in this country was provided based on ability to pay rather than need?

■ **References** cited in the chapter are presented in APA format.

ACKNOWLEDGMENTS

In the creation of a textbook such as this, there are so many people to thank. First, we need to thank Lynnette Leeseburg Stamler and Lucia Yiu for graciously passing this torch to us to keep alive as they transition into retirement. They have offered us much inspiration during the first four editions of the textbook, and we'll honour their vision and keep this legacy alive. Second, thanks to the students and colleagues for encouraging us to take the fifth edition to a new critical level. As this edition began to take shape, we were thankful for the many authors who once again agreed to contribute to the textbook or suggested others who had the expertise we required. Many of our authors took time from other projects to add their knowledge to the textbook, making this project a priority. We are humbled and privileged to be able to work with our colleagues in both academia and front-line practice who have shared their infinite wisdom, knowledge, and expertise with us all. We thank them for their tireless efforts in helping us to shape and bring to you a critical community health nursing lens to the fifth edition of this textbook.

We are grateful to the talented team at Pearson Canada. Cathleen Sullivan and Joanne Sutherland guided us through the whole process of development of this edition. We give our humble thanks to Suzanne Keeptwo, our Indigenous consultant, who took the time to read the Indigenous content in every chapter and advised us regarding our use of language. Susan Johnson provided expertise, ideas, and support, which were invaluable in moving through production. The reviewers, who were nameless to us at the time, contributed significant time and effort in assisting us to make this text strong and representative of Canadian community health nursing. Their names are listed following this section.

Each of us had particular friends and family members who were supportive as we moved through the process of completing a major textbook. We are grateful to all of you. Finally, as teachers, we thank our students, who were guiding forces as we shaped the fifth edition of this textbook.

Many nurses across the country have contributed countless hours to portray community health nursing with passion and pride. We are very excited with this new edition. We hope teachers and learners will also be excited as they continue to learn, explore, and discuss community health nursing as a distinct specialty in Canadian nursing.

Drs. Aliyah Dosani, Josephine Etowa, and Cheryl van Daalen-Smith.

REVIEWERS

Jennifer Abbass Dick, University of Ontario Institute of Technology
Dianne Allen, Conestoga College
Sheila Blackstock, Thompson Rivers University
Marie Dietrich Leurer, University of Saskatchewan
Marilyn Evans, University of Western Ontario
Corinne Hart, Ryerson University
Ann MacLeod, Trent University
Sherry Poirier, Algonquin College
Billy Joel Reniva, Bow Valley College

This textbook is dedicated to my parents, Abdulrasul and Almas Mawji, who taught me nothing is impossible to achieve. To my husband, Naushad Dosani, who is always incredibly supportive. I hadn't realized until my nursing career that I had been thinking from a critical lens and advocating for social justice my entire life! Lastly, to our students, professors and instructors, and community health nurses across Canada—the energy and passion with which you learn and teach, and the exceptional work you do, ignites a flame in my soul that will never be extinguished!

—A.D.

This textbook is dedicated to my children: Ntami Enang (daughter) and Deval Enang (son), who have taught me so much about life in our community and the contexts of health care. To my brothers and friend, Christian Etowa, Egbe Etowa, and Francis Ukposidolo, for their unyielding support. And to all the students and community health nurses who continue to inspire me to engage in critical community health nursing.

—J.E.

What a whirlwind of humbling experiences this journey has provided! From the exhilarating experience of planning, shaping, and co-editing a critical text with two wise women, to meeting and standing beside numerous author teams as they took their respective chapters to a focus on power, upstream structural analyses, and community health nursing advocacy. The conversations have been a gift I'll be forever grateful for. We are indebted to Pearson Canada's editorial team and its commitment to ensuring our text begins to reflect our shared responsibility of reconciliation, permitting us the option to work toward its Indigenization. This textbook is dedicated to all the maverick CHNs across Canada who continue to speak up and act to reduce health inequities wherever their practice takes them.

—C.vDS.

Contributors

Sarah Alley, RN, BScN, MPH
Chapter 12—Communicable Diseases

Lisa Anne Ashley, RN, MEd, CCHN(C)
Program Lead, Professional Development, Canadian Nurses
Association
Chair, Chronic Disease Prevention Alliance of Canada
Chapter 2—Policy, Politics, and Power in Health Care

Megan Aston, RN, PhD
Professor, Dalhousie University School of Nursing
Chapter 18—Family Nursing

Annette Bailey, RN, BScN, MSN, PhD
Associate Professor and Associate Director, Collaborative
Degree Program, Daphne Cockwell School of Nursing,
Ryerson University
Chapter 28—Violence and Health

Louise Baptiste, RN, BN, MEd
Director of Indigenous Initiatives, Nursing Instructor, Faculty
of Nursing, University of Calgary
Chapter 8—Health Promotion

Heather D. Bensler
Director of Indigenous Initiatives (Faculty and Curriculum
Development), Faculty of Nursing, University of Calgary
Chapter 16—Maternal, Newborn, and Child Health

Claire Betker, RN, PhD, CCHN(C)
Executive Director, Active Living, Population and Public
Health Branch of Manitoba Health, Seniors and Active
Living
Chapter 7—Theoretical Foundations of Community Health
Nursing

Gwendyline Campbell McArthur
Indigenous Elder
Chapter 22—Indigenous Health

Kathleen Carlin, RN, MSc, PhD
Instructor, Department of Philosophy, Ryerson University
Chapter 6—Advocacy, Ethical, and Legal Considerations

Andrea Chircop
Assistant Professor, School of Nursing, Dalhousie University
Chapter 27—Ecological Determinants of Health and
Environmental Health Inequities

Karen Lauren Curry, RN, MN, CCHNc
Practice Educator, Victoria Order of Nurses Canada
Chapter 21—Older Adult Health

Alana Devereaux, RN, BN, PhD
Nursing Professor, Faculty of Health and Human Services,
Vancouver Island University
Chapter 32—Emergency Preparedness and Disaster Nursing

Katie Dilworth, RN, BSc, MHSc, CCHN(C)
President, Community Health Nurses of Canada (CHNC)
Chapter 1—The History of Community Health Nursing in
Canada

Aliyah Dosani, RN, BN, MPH, PhD
Associate Professor, School of Nursing and Midwifery, Faculty
of Health, Community and Education, Mount Royal
University; Adjunct Associate Professor, Department of
Community Health Sciences, Cumming School of Medicine,
University of Calgary
Chapter 4—Public Health Nursing
Chapter 11—Epidemiology
Chapter 16—Maternal, Newborn, and Child Health
Chapter 19—Gender and Community Health
Chapter 33—Global Health
Chapter 34—Critical Community Health Nursing: An Imperative

Nancy Christine Edwards, RN, PhD
Professor Emeritus and Distinguished Professor, School of
Nursing, University of Ottawa
Chapter 14—Community Health Planning, Monitoring, and
Evaluation

**Josephine Etowa, RM, RN, BScN, MN, PhD, FWACN,
FAAN**
Professor and Loyer DaSilva Chair in Public Health Nursing
School of Nursing, Faculty of Health Sciences, University of
Ottawa
Senior Investigator, Nursing Best Practice Research Centre,
University of Ottawa
Co-Chair, CHNC Standards of Practice Advisory Committee
Chapter 2—Policy, Politics, and Power in Health Care
Chapter 14—Community Health Planning, Monitoring, and
Evaluation
Chapter 16—Maternal, Newborn, and Child Health
Chapter 33—Global Health
Chapter 34—Critical Community Health Nursing: An
Imperative

Claire Farella, RN, BScN, MN
Manager of Infectious and Communicable Diseases,
Community Health Protection Department, Leeds Grenville
Lanark District Health Unit (Brockville, ON)
Chapter 32—Emergency Preparedness and Disaster Nursing

Linda Ferguson, RN, PhD
Professor, College of Nursing, University of Saskatchewan
Chapter 15—Digital Health

Rebecca Ganann, RN, PhD
Assistant Professor, School of Nursing, McMaster University
Chapter 10—Evidence-Informed Decision Making in
Community Health Nursing

Kathryn Hardill, RN(EC), MScN
Executive Director and Nurse Practitioner Lead, Peterborough
360 Degree Nurse Practitioner Led Clinic in Nogojiwanong
(Peterborough, Ontario)
Chapter 29—Poverty, Homelessness, and Food Insecurity

Mary Eleanor Hill, RN, PhD
Former Manager, Child, Youth, and Family Services,
Vancouver Island Health Authority
Chapter 7—Theoretical Foundations of Community Health
Nursing

Dave Holmes RN, PhD
Professor and Associate Dean Academic and Student Affairs,
Sue and Bill Gross School of Nursing, University of California-
Irvine.
Chapter 23—Community Mental Health

Lorraine Holtslander, RN, PhD, CHPCN(C)
Professor, College of Nursing, University of Saskatchewan
Chapter 25—Chronic Care, Long-Term Care, and Palliative
Care

Anne Judith Kearney, BN, MHSC, PhD, RN
Professor, School of Nursing, Memorial University
Chapter 4—Public Health Nursing

Kelley Kilpatrick, RN, PhD
Assistant Professor, Faculty of Nursing, Univerité de Montréal
Chapter 24—Rural and Remote Health

Megan Kirk, RN, MSc, BScN, PhD(c)
Nursing Doctoral Candidate, University of Victoria
Chapter 7—Theoretical Foundations of Community Health
Nursing

Mary Ellen Labrecque, RN(NP), PhD
Assistant Professor, College of Nursing, University of
Saskatchewan
Director, Nurse Practitioner Programs, University of
Saskatchewan
Chapter 24—Rural and Remote Health

Nancy Lefebre, RN, BScN, MScN, CHL, CCHL Fellow
Chief Clinical Executive and Vice President, Saint Elizabeth
Health Care
Chapter 5—Home Health Nursing in Canada

Debbie Sheppard LeMoine, RN, PhD
Assistant Director, Assistant Professor, Rankin School of
Nursing, St. Francis Xavier University
Chapter 18—Family Nursing

Candace Lind, RN, BN, MN, PhD
Associate Professor, Faculty of Nursing, University of Calgary
Chapter 8—Health Promotion

Wendi Lokanc-Diluzio, RN, BN, MN, PhD
Sexual and Reproductive Health Specialist, Alberta Health
Services
Instructor, University of Lethbridge
Instructor, University of Alberta
Co-Investigator, Faculty of Nursing, University of Calgary
Chapter 31—Sexually Transmitted and Blood-Borne
Infections

Sionnach Lukeman, RN, MScN
Assistant Professor, Rankin School of Nursing, St. Francis
Xavier University
Chapter 28—Violence and Health

Marjorie MacDonald, RN, PhD
Professor Emerita, School of Nursing, University of Victoria
Scientist, Canadian Institute for Substance Use Research
Chapter 7—Theoretical Foundations of Community Health
Nursing

Jo-Ann Macdonald, RN, BScN, MN, PhD
Associate Professor, Faculty of Nursing, University of Prince
Edward Island
Chapter 17—School Health

Joyce Mbugua, RN, MEd
Nurse Educator, Rankin School of Nursing, St. Francis Xavier
University
Chapter 9—Race, Culture, and Health

Elizabeth Ann McGibbon, RN, MN, PhD
Professor, St. Francis Xavier University
Chapter 9—Race, Culture, and Health
Chapter 28—Violence and Health

Christine McPherson, RN, PhD
Associate Professor, School of Nursing, University of Ottawa
Chapter 21—Older Adult Health

Esther Moghadam, RN, BScN, MEd
Director of Health Promotion, Chief Nursing Officer, Ottawa
Public Health
Chapter 2—Policy, Politics, and Power in Health Care

Jackie Muresan, RN, MSc
Advisor and Knowledge Broker, Region of Peel—Public Health
Chapter 10—Evidence-Informed Decision Making in Community Health Nursing

Abram Oudshoorn, RN, PhD
Assistant Professor, Arthur Labatt Family School of Nursing, Western University
Chapter 30—Substance Use and Community Health Nursing

Shelley C. Peacock, RN, BSc, PhD
Associate Professor, College of Nursing, University of Saskatchewan
Chapter 25—Chronic Care, Long-Term Care, and Palliative Care

Amélie Perron RN PhD
Associate Professor, School of Nursing, University of Ottawa
Co-founder, Nursing Observator
Chapter 23—Community Mental Health

Elizabeth Peter, RN, BScN, BA, MScN, PhD
Professor, Lawrence S. Bloomberg Faculty of Nursing, University of Toronto
Chair, Health Science Research Ethics Board, University of Toronto
Chapter 6—Advocacy, Ethical, and Legal Considerations

Cindy Peternelj-Taylor, RN, BScN, MSc
Professor, College of Nursing, University of Saskatchewan
Distinguished Fellow, International Association of Forensic Nurses
Editor-in-Chief, *Journal of Forensic Nursing*
Chapter 26—Correctional Health

Jeffrey Craig Phillips, RN, PhD, LLM, ARNP, ACRN, FAAN
Vice-Dean Governance and Secretary, Faculty of Health Sciences, University of Ottawa
Associate Professor, School of Nursing, University of Ottawa
Chapter 3—Nursing Roles, Functions, and Practice Settings

Caroline Porr, RN, BScN, MN, PhD, CHNC(C)
Associate Professor, School of Nursing, Memorial University
Chapter 4—Public Health Nursing

Shahirose Premji, RN, BSc, BScN, MScN, PhD, FAAN
Director and Professor, School of Nursing, Faculty of Health, York University
Chapter 33—Global Health

Karen L. Ray, RN, BScN, MSc
Former Manager of Knowledge Translation, Saint Elizabeth Health Care
Chapter 5—Home Health Nursing in Canada

Tracie Risling, RN, PhD
Associate Professor, College of Nursing, University of Saskatchewan
Communications Director, Canadian Nursing Informatics Association
Chapter 15—Digital Health

Elizabeth Saewyc, RN, PhD, PHN(Minn.), FSAHM, FCAHS, FAAN
Professor and Director, School of Nursing, University of British Columbia
Chapter 20—Lesbian, Gay, Bisexual, Transgender, Queer, and Two-Spirit Clients

Ruth Schofield, RN, BScN, MSc(T)
Assistant Professor, McMaster University
Clinical Instructor, Western University
Chapter 3—Nursing Roles, Functions, and Practice Settings

Tracy Scott, RN, MN
National Director of Education Services, Saint Elizabeth Health Care
Chapter 5—Home Health Nursing in Canada

Shirlee Sharkey, MHSc, BScN, BA, LLD (honoris causa)
President and CEO, Saint Elizabeth Health Care
Adjunct Professor, Lawrence S. Bloomberg Faculty of Nursing, University of Toronto
Chair, Excellence Canada
Chapter 5—Home Health Nursing in Canada

Victoria Smye, RN, PhD
Associate Professor and Director, Arthur Labatt Family School of Nursing, Western University
Chapter 30—Substance Use and Community Health Nursing

Lynette Leeseberg Stamler, RN, PhD, DLitt, FAAN
Professor, Associate Dean for Academic Programs, University of Nebraska Medical Center, College of Nursing
Chapter 11—Epidemiology

Louise Sweatman, RN, BScN, LLB, MSc
Director, Legal Services, Canadian Medical Association
Chapter 6—Advocacy, Ethical, and Legal Considerations

Dawn Tisdale, RN, BSN, MSN in progress
Chapter 22—Indigenous Health

Tammy Troute-Wood, RN, BScN, MN
Sexual and Reproductive Health Specialist, Alberta Health Services
Instructor, University of Lethbridge
Instructor, University of Alberta
Chapter 31—Sexually Transmitted and Blood-Borne Infections

Lisa Underhill, RN, MN, PHC, NP
Nurse Practitioner, Ottawa
Chapter 18—Family Nursing

Cheryl van Daalen-Smith, RN, BScN, PhD
Associate Professor, School of Nursing, York University
Chapter 17—School Health
Chapter 19—Gender and Community Health
Chapter 34—Critical Community Health Nursing: An
Imperative

Adele Ruth Vukic, RN, BN, MN, PhD
Faculty Member, School of Nursing, Faculty of Health,
Dalhousie University
Chapter 1—The History of Community Health Nursing in
Canada

Phil Woods, RPN, RMN, PhD
Professor and Associate Dean, College of Nursing, University
of Saskatchewan
Chapter 26—Correctional Health

Lucia Yiu, RN, BScN, BA, MScN
Associate Professor Emeritus, Faculty of Nursing, University of
Windsor
Chapter 13—Community Nursing Process

The History of Community Health Nursing in Canada

Adele Vukic and Katie Dilworth

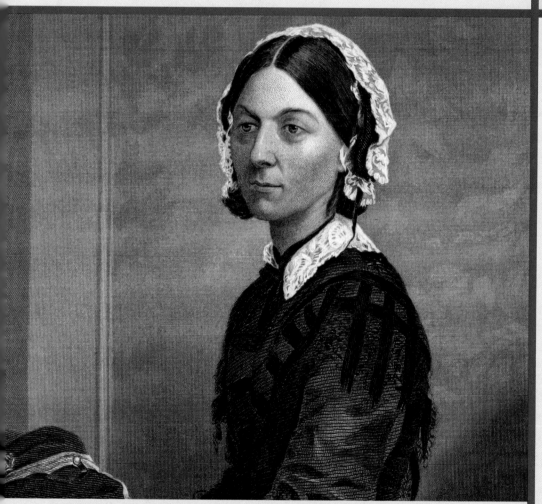

Source: Georgios Kollidas/Alamy Stock Photo

LEARNING OUTCOMES

After studying this chapter, you should be able to:

1. Analyze how the historical practices of community health nursing laid the foundation for current advocacy, health equity, and social justice work.

2. Describe the influence of the interplay of community health nursing and nursing education on the evolution of their practice, education, and research.

3. Identify the socioecological context of the development of community health nursing in Canada.

4. Identify the contributions and leadership of community health nurses, including Indigenous and racialized nurses in advancing primary health care, health equity, and Indigenous health.

5. Envision future community health nursing responsibilities toward enabling health for all, inclusive of the Truth and Reconciliation report and the complex needs of today's population.

INTRODUCTION

Community health nursing has evolved within dynamic sociopolitical, cultural, and economic contexts in Canada over the past five centuries. As a practice discipline and profession, nursing history inspires reflection on the questions and issues that persist through time. Nurse historian Patricia D'Antonio (2006) describes how research into nursing's past sheds light on challenges and opportunities in nursing's achievement of its social mission. Community health nurses (CHNs) advocate for the provision of **primary health care** and provide sociopolitical leadership for the development of the health system and global health in their practice

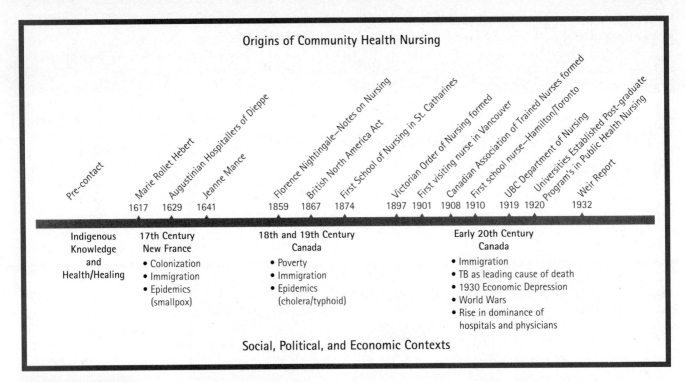

FIGURE **1.1** Origins of Community Health Nursing

(Armstrong-Reid, 2014; Falk-Rafael, 2005) yet community health nursing has been challenged to fulfill its mission of meeting the health needs of diverse communities over time.

The purpose of this chapter is to describe community health nursing practice in a historical context as a foundation for understanding subsequent chapters in this text. This chapter will examine the evolution and milestones of community health nursing in Canada (see Figure 1.1) and the challenges that confronted CHNs as they advanced their role in their profession. The chapter will also illustrate how CHNs develop relationships with individuals, families, and communities; provide leadership for health services; and promote the health of their clients. Their contributions to health, social justice, and public policy through political advocacy will be examined.

ORIGINS OF COMMUNITY HEALTH NURSING

The earliest forms of health care in Canada were the practices of First Peoples using traditional medicines and healing practices (Aboriginal Nurses Association of Canada, 2007; Bourque Bearskin, 2011). Later, Indigenous women provided essential health care, including curative midwifery services to European settlers in the western and northern regions of pre-Confederation Canada (Burnett, 2008). These practices have yet to be acknowledged within the history and modern practices of nursing and health care despite a growing awareness of their value (Bourque Bearskin, 2014). Epidemics of infectious diseases introduced by European settlers, wars, and the denigration of Indigenous culture and identity during the colonization of Canada by European immigrants led to social, health, and

economic disparities among Indigenous peoples that persist today. The history of the relationship between colonization and First Nation, Inuit and Métis peoples must be understood in the present-day context of Indigenous health. (See Chapter 22.) CHN practices were an integral part of this relationship and led to the evolution of health promotion and illness prevention.

Community health nursing is the earliest form of nursing practised in Canada and has a long and proud history of health promotion. Canadian nurse historian Margaret Allemang (2000) traces the introduction of community-oriented nursing to 17th-century New France and the Duchesse d'Aiguillon sisters, who established "essential health care and carried out work in homes, hospitals and communities" (p. 6). This early work of the sisters is emulated by the community health nursing practice of today with a focus on health inequities, the determinants of health, community outreach, and advocacy. The origins of community health nursing intersect with current trends in nursing, health care, and health equity.

Historians generally refer to the earliest forms of community health nursing as those practices in 17th century New France and the notable work and contributions of women and sisterhoods (Allemang, 2000). Gibbon and Mathewson (1947) chronicled the lasting and significant influence of the French in providing the earliest forms of organized community health nursing as practised by sisterhoods, including a small group of Augustinian Hospitallers of Dieppe, who worked to establish a hospital and provide care in villages and homes. Allemang (2000) further refers to "the Grey Nuns, established in 1738 by Marguerite d'Youville as Canada's first community nursing order" (p. 6). Also significant were the contributions of a laywoman, Marie Rollet Hebert, who worked alongside her surgeon husband in the early 17th century. Early accounts of

Hebert's work include relationships with First Nation people and how she learned about health and healing, including the "value of evergreen trees as a source of vitamin C during the long winter months" (Paul & Ross-Kerr, 2011, p. 20).

Although there is no complete agreement among historians, Canada's first nurse is most often identified as Jeanne Mance (1606–1673). After receiving practical training in nursing in France, Mance came to Canada and confronted political, social, and economic forces to establish a range of community health services that included the founding of the Hotel-Dieu Hospital of Montreal, and she is also described as the co-founder of Montreal (Allemang, 2000; Gibbon & Mathewson, 1947). This early nursing leader provided direct nursing care, advocated for social justice, and was the administrator of the hospital. Today, the Canadian Nurses Association (CNA) grants its highest and most prestigious award in her name.

The Grey Nuns were Canada's first community nursing order who understood health inequity and made significant contributions to providing access to health services, food, shelter, and education for the most vulnerable. Hardill (2006) refers to the order as the first form of "street outreach nursing" in the early 1700s when the Grey Nuns began public health visits to the "sick poor in what is now Quebec" (p. 91). Nurse historian Pauline Paul described contributions of the Grey Nuns and other religious nursing orders to the development of health services, nursing education, and hospital administration across the country:

> Nursing sisters were the first to provide health care in remote and frontier areas, and, when these areas became more settled, they were also among the first to establish and operate modern and urban hospitals . . . . Religious nursing orders have also been significant contributors to Canadian nursing education, operating schools of nursing within hospitals (such as the School of Nursing run by the hospital at the Edmonton General Hospital) and establishing university level nursing programs. (Paul, 2005, p. 137)

Early CHNs understood health inequity, focusing on the social determinants of health and concerns for vulnerable populations' access to housing, food, and the essentials of life. Health care delivery was not clearly demarcated as a separate entity of institutional and community-based care. Rather, the establishments of sick bays and hospitals were considered part of a continuum of health services that also included education, home visiting, clinics, and other avenues of access in the provision of services and advocacy for **social justice** and the essentials of life and health, including immunizations.

NATION BUILDING AND THE NIGHTINGALE ERA (MID- TO LATE 19TH CENTURY)

This period was marked by the political context of Canada's development as a nation, including immigration, challenges of providing basic health services to settlers, and Indigenous peoples experiencing a wave of epidemics introduced by immigrants. The 1867 British North America Act (BNA Act) made only limited provisions for the establishment and maintenance

of a health care system, specifying the federal government was responsible only for taxes, laws, quarantine, and the establishment of marine hospitals. First Nation legislative authority fell under the federal government with the signing of the BNA Act, and seven years later, in 1874, the Indian Act was proclaimed, which indicated health services be provided under the guise of the famous medicine chest and the pestilence clauses (Kue-Young, 1984). This legislation has significantly influenced community health nursing with Indigenous peoples. All other responsibilities for the organization of health care, including public health services, devolved to the provinces. Health care responsibilities were not specified within the Act, and the provinces, in the early years after Confederation, did not make much effort to undertake them. Organized health care was provided at the local (municipal) level through public welfare or, more frequently, charitable organizations. Many provinces passed legislation in the late 19th century to allow for the establishment of local and provincial departments of health. Challenging conditions, including social unrest created by industrial capitalism, immigration, urbanization, and harsh weather, were especially hard on vulnerable populations, creating vast health disparities. This helped shaped the provincial organization and financing of the public health system and nature of community health nursing.

The second half of the century was characterized by the development of the nursing profession, predominantly influenced by Florence Nightingale and women's groups. There was a rise in the dominance of medicine and hospitals as the centre of health care delivery. Nightingale was skilled in mathematics and one of the first community health nurses to understand the importance of health data (Winkelstein, 2009).

The Nightingale era in Canada saw the establishment of the first school of nursing in St. Catharines, Ontario, in 1874. The introduction of the Nightingale model of training nurses was a significant milestone in the development of the profession, offering formal training to nurses. During this period, nursing was confronted by the dominance of medicine and hospitals, as well as issues of class and gender, which remain today (Larsen & Baumgart, 1992; McPherson, 1996). Health promotion was present in the earliest forms of community health nursing practice. Florence Nightingale was a visionary epidemiologist who wisely collected and used statistics to identify population health concerns among soldiers during the Crimean War. An environmentalist, with a strong understanding of the social determinants of health, she identified "the five essential points in securing the health of houses as pure air, pure water, efficient drainage, cleanliness and light" (Nightingale, 1859/1946, p. 14). It is critical to note that Mary Seacole (1801–1881), a Jamaican born nurse, advanced the nursing care of the soldiers during the Crimean war; however, her expertise remains invisible during the era of Florence Nightingale's influence (Anionwu, 2006).

Women played a vital role in the development of community health services for the rural and poor communities in the late 19th and early 20th centuries. Lady Aberdeen, wife of the Governor General of Canada, led the development of the Victorian Order of Nurses (VON). Founded in 1897, the VON's goal was "to supply nurses, thoroughly trained in Hospital and District Nursing, and subject to one Central Authority, for the nursing of the sick who are otherwise unable to obtain trained nursing in their own homes, both in town and country districts" (Lady Aberdeen, cited in Gibbon, 1947, p. 8). The National Council of Women of Canada advocated for the development of the nursing profession through training and education as cited in Baker et al. (2012).

Significant points of conflict emerged between Lady Aberdeen's view of how to best meet the needs of prairie women and that of the National Council of Women. Her view that skilled, practical "home helpers" trained in midwifery and basic care could best reach rural women was opposed by physicians, nurses, and the National Council of Women. This opposition resulted in the creation of the VON, followed by the evolution of district and home nursing care in the country, resulting in the extinction of lay midwifery and the medicalization of obstetrics (Boutillier, 1994).

The VON's capacity to respond to local needs stemmed from its organizational structure, which included local branches with volunteers in various communities to sustain the organization. The VON encouraged local branches to extend their work and demonstrate their capacity to deliver a wide range of community health nursing services. Visiting nursing services became the backbone of these local branches and offered bedside nursing care to families who could not afford to hire private-duty nurses. The difference between the actual cost of the service and what was paid in fees by families was underwritten by charitable donations, fundraising, and, in some cases, grants from city or provincial governments. These local VON branches fulfilled a dual mandate: charitable work among the poor and provision of affordable nursing care to the working and middle classes.

The history of the VON has been documented in two monographs, one written on the occasion of its 50th anniversary (Gibbon, 1947) and one celebrating its 100th year of service in Canada (Penney, 1996). What started as a small group of nurses working to support people in their homes has since grown to 6000 staff and many volunteers. Although there have been significant changes in VON as a result of health care system reform and the rising population of older adults in Canada, the organization is partnering in new ways with new organizations while maintaining its initial vision from its first 120 years in service (Victoria Order of Nurses [VON], 2017).

EARLY 20TH CENTURY EVOLUTION OF COMMUNITY HEALTH NURSING

By the late 19th and early 20th centuries, the nursing profession was seen as having three distinct sectors: hospital nurses, private-duty nurses, and public health and home-visiting nurses (McPherson, 1996). Community health nursing emerged as a distinct specialty, and the majority of nurses were self-employed as private-duty nurses. CHNs such as public health and home-visiting nurses were considered among the profession's elite, and employment in this specialty practice required additional skills such as midwifery and, after World War I, post-diploma training from a university (Baldwin,

1997; McPherson, 1996; Penney, 1996). Public health and home-visiting nurses were different from nurses employed in other sectors of the health system. They tended to remain in their community practices longer than those employed in hospitals and private-duty nursing. They also enjoyed greater financial stability and higher salaries (McPherson, 1996). Their sense of adventure, independence, courage, and humanitarianism led pioneering Canadian CHNs to offer their services to people living in Canada's poorest urban districts and most isolated rural communities.

Pioneer CHNs worked to meet the immediate needs of communities for direct care and midwifery while also providing health and prevention education to individuals and families. The early practice of the CHN was characterized by considerable overlap between what we now identify as public health nursing roles and or home-visiting nursing roles. A growing distinction grew between direct care of individuals and families in the community and the focus on the health of the community as a whole as both home-visiting nursing and public nursing became specialized as forms of community health nursing that exist today (McKay, 2005). Significant other community health nursing roles have emerged, including occupational health nursing, outpost nursing, midwifery, culture- and community-based nursing, and, later in the century, community mental health nursing (Benoit & Carroll, 2005; Boschma, 2012; Dodd, Elliot, & Rousseau, 2005; Keddy & Dodd, 2005).

The role of women's volunteerism and leadership in communities continued to be an integral part in the development of community health nursing. At the local level, rural women's groups such as the Women's Institute and the United Farm Women made community development and the development of health care services a priority. These women lobbied local officials, served tea at child welfare clinics, sewed layettes for destitute families, provided transportation, made referrals, raised funds, and in untold other ways tried to enable CHNs to fulfill their professional obligations to the fullest extent possible (Riddell, 1991; Stuart, 1987).

Public Health Nursing as a Nursing Specialty

The term **public health nurse (PHN)** was first coined by American nurse Lillian Wald, who, with her colleague Mary Brewster, founded the Henry Street Visiting Nurse Service in the late 19th century. Their conception of practice was broad as they recognized the impact of the social determinants of health and attended to the issues of poverty, culture, and living conditions of the poor (Fee & Bu, 2010). Public health nursing emerged in Canada in the early 20th century when civic departments of health established health education and preventive programs to combat communicable diseases, infant mortality, and morbidity in school-age children. Nurses were perceived as the ideal professionals to deliver these programs because of their medical knowledge and their ability to interact with women and children in private homes and in the public school setting (Sears, 1995).

In the early 20th century, community health nursing evolved from the specialties of tuberculosis (TB) nursing and school nursing to programs focused on reducing infant mortality. Despite all efforts to improve urban sanitation and to regulate food and milk supplies, infant mortality rates in Canadian cities continued to climb until well into the second decade of the 20th century. Public health officials identified health education as a strategy to combat unnecessary disease and death. TB was the leading cause of death at the turn of the century, and it was at this point that nurses were first employed as civil servants in local health departments. Although the exact chronology varies from one city to another, the first PHNs were responsible for TB control, child hygiene programs, and school inspection programs.

Zilm and Warbinek (2002) refer to TB nursing and school nursing as the first two PHN specialties. The breadth and depth of these nursing specialties are revealed in the earliest issues of the *Canadian Nurse Journal* beginning in 1910, with the appointment of the first school nurses in Hamilton and Toronto. School PHNs participated in initiatives to preserve and promote the health of school-age children. As working-class children were removed from economic production and placed in the public school system, their significant health problems became fully visible (Peikoff & Brickey, 1991). Programs for the medical inspection of schoolchildren were established in major cities across Canada, and nurses were hired by boards of education. In many cities, such as Montreal, Toronto, Winnipeg, and Vancouver, school health programs were initially established by the boards of education. They were subsequently taken over by the health department as part of the process of consolidating all public health programs under one jurisdiction (City of Winnipeg Health Department, 1910; MacDougall, 1990).

Early accounts of school nursing had broad focus on the social determinants of health and their impact on health of children and families. Early school initiatives included medical inspections augmented by home visits to educate the parents and to ensure that all recommendations were followed (Sutherland, 1981). One school nurse described home visiting in connection with school nursing as an important part of holistic care:

> The child, having been examined by the School Medical Officer and being found to have any physical abnormality such as defective nasal breathing, defective vision or hearing, bad teeth or enlarged tonsils, etc., a notice is sent home to that effect and a visit is made to the parents of the child by the school nurse as soon as possible. She notes the home conditions and family circumstances, enquires as to the child's sleeping apartment, and often gives a few simple instructions in hygiene. When necessary she advises the mother to have treatment for the child, and although a great many of the parents are unable to afford even the simplest of treatments, we are able to a certain extent to overcome this difficulty through the kindness of the different specialists in the city . . . Often the nurse finds great poverty in the home, and sometimes the children have no boots or suitable clothing in which to come to school, or no sufficient food. (Ewart, 1916, p. 308)

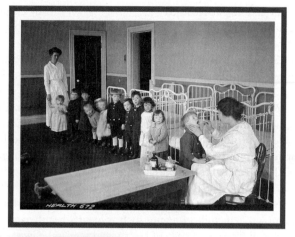

PHOTO 1.1 Inspecting children at daycare, 197 Euclid Avenue, February 13, 1923.

Source: Arthur S. Goss/City of Toronto Archives

The earliest maternal programs were the well-baby clinics established by the Red Cross Peace Program, which remain a signature program of public health nursing today. These early clinics were run by nurses who assessed the growth and development of children and provided mothers and caregivers with health teaching for the care and promotion of child health. Local physicians sometimes did not support public health programs because they feared that the PHNs would provide primary care and thus compete with them for both patients and income. It took considerable effort on the part of the nurses to lessen these concerns. Stuart (1987) found that PHNs often avoided giving advice to families about the prevention of communicable diseases, even when they knew more about immunization programs than did the local physicians. One of the strategies employed to silence the protests of local physicians was to refer all individuals found to have "abnormal" conditions to the attending physician for further follow-up, even in cases where the nurses could have provided this care themselves (Riddell, 1991). (See Photo 1.1.)

Public health officials and maternal feminists concluded that many parents, particularly the mothers, were "ignorant" and barely capable of providing a safe and healthy environment for the nation's future citizens (Meigs, 1916). Removing children from their parents was not a viable option; thus, educating mothers about infant feeding and hygiene became the intervention of choice (Peikoff & Brickey, 1991). Infant and child welfare and hygiene programs were carried out at milk depots, at well-baby clinics, and in private homes (Locke, 1918; MacNutt, 1913). Visiting nurses (VNs) staffed the clinics and visited the homes of newborn infants in the early postnatal period assessing the health of the infant and mother, the family's childcare practices, and the hygienic conditions in the home. A major focus was to promote breastfeeding of newborn infants.

Women volunteers played essential roles in developing the social, cultural, and health care services in smaller communities. As written by Yarmie (2013), the Red Cross established the first well-baby clinic with nurse Christina Thom in 1922, and "at the initial clinic over a dozen mothers had their babies' weight and height recorded . . . " (p. 114). Well-baby clinics developed across the country and contributed to the health and wellness of Canada's infants and children.

The establishment of public health nursing programs had limited success in rural and isolated areas. Many communities wanted the VNs to provide bedside nursing care, rather than the PHNs, who focused on health education and prevention of illness (Matthews, 1920; Stuart, 1987). By the beginning of World War II, the essential elements of community health nursing services were in place across the country. Provincial health departments had been organized, and local health departments operated in the majority of Canadian cities. The scope of work in health education and prevention of illness had grown to include programs such as mental health, control of venereal diseases, preschool health, and prenatal education. The VON continued to flourish by providing bedside nursing care in the home as a springboard to also providing public health programs in communities. Although the VON had been envisioned by its founders as a nursing service for individuals living in rural and isolated "country districts," it had attained its greatest success and stability in Canada's urban centres.

In the interwar years, the development of public health services was uneven and often unsuccessful. The time available for individual and family health education or preventive services was limited, and the nurses' ability to provide long-term follow-up in complex situations was significantly constrained. The need for home care and midwifery in rural and isolated areas also limited the successful establishment of public health nursing programs.

District and Visiting Nursing

Early programs of district or visiting nursing, the foundation of home health nursing as it exists today, were organized and operated by laywomen. Charitable organizations such as the Margaret Scott Nursing Mission in Winnipeg documented recognition of health inequities as they provided care to poor and destitute families (McKay, 2008). Working-class and lower-middle-class families also were recipients of visiting nursing services. These families could not afford to hire full-time private-duty nurses, and their homes were not large enough to provide accommodation for a nurse during the term of her employment. **District or visiting nursing** therefore provided a comprehensive array of services from bedside nursing to preventive health teaching. Pioneer nursing services such as Alberta's district nursing service provided essential emergency and obstetrical care and midwifery (Richardson, 1998). This was an early form of primary health care, as it encompassed access to essential curative, preventive, and health promotion services for people in their most immediate community setting—the home (World Health Organization [WHO], 1978).

Rural CHNs faced formidable challenges created by distance and climate. Although their urban counterparts, particularly in the early years, often walked many miles to visit homes at considerable distances from streetcar routes, urban nursing districts were measured in mere city blocks. Rural districts were enormous. One nurse stated, "I have a car for my school

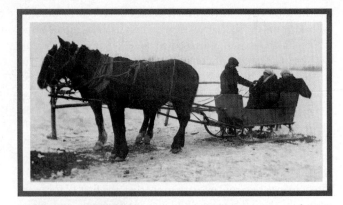

PHOTO **1.2** Travelling by sleigh, 1919

Source: Glenbow Archives NA-3956-1

inspection. It is the only way of covering 925 miles twice a year and paying home visits" (Matthews, 1920, p. 16). The first-hand accounts of early rural CHNs contain vivid descriptions of the various modes of transportation used and the dangerous road and weather conditions (Miller, 2000; Nevitt, 1978). (See Photo 1.2.)

Publicly funded health care programs changed the organization and work of visiting nursing associations in several ways (McKay, 2012). In the decade immediately following World War II, most programs were unable to sustain either their funding or the quality of their nursing programs (Richardson, 1997). Although the VON continued to grow during the postwar years, it was also forced to respond to the changing face of health care in Canada. Expanded local and provincial departments of health took over public health programs that previously had been provided by the VON (Penney, 1996). Hospital admission became the norm for Canadians requiring obstetrical, medical, or surgical care, shifting VON visiting nursing caseloads to the care of convalescent and chronically ill individuals. Further, the erosion of charitable donations, which had offset the cost of caring for the poor in the past, meant that VNs were more likely to be providing care to individuals who could afford to pay either directly or through third-party insurance arrangements.

Military Nursing

During the influenza epidemics, military nurses often were called upon to help care for the sick. Canadian nurse Elizabeth Smellie (1884–1968), who provided leadership for the war effort, was "the first woman, globally, to become a full colonel her career including leadership in public health, VON, and the CNA" (Toman, 2005, p. 171). Military nursing required the nurse to demonstrate the attributes and competencies of CHN: a broad vision; population health approaches; the ability to adapt practice in diverse settings across the spectra of primary, secondary, and tertiary prevention; and the ethical comportment to address complex conflicts that involve violence and human justice and rights. Today, emergency preparedness and disaster nursing are essential competencies for CHNs.

Indigenous Health Care

Considerable evidence demonstrates First Nation and Inuit peoples enjoyed good health at the time of first contact with Europeans. Shortly thereafter, epidemics of TB, diphtheria, smallpox, cholera, typhus, measles, and influenza were the greatest killer of many Indigenous populations (Royal Commission of Aboriginal Peoples [RCAP], 1996).

Since the Indian Act there have been numerous changes to the colonial health services for Indigenous peoples. (See Figure 1.2.) CHNs are an integral part of health services in the North. In 1922, mobile health services with PHNs delivering communicable disease control were initiated (Kue Young, 1984; RCAP, 1996). By the 1930s the first nursing station was established, and by the post-WWII era in the 1950s, there were numerous nursing stations throughout Canada. Outpost nursing refers to nurses providing services in the most remote geographic locations, serving settlers and Indigenous communities (Drees & McBain, 2001). Clinics were historically grounded in an infectious disease public health model dominated by the biomedical approach to treatment. Infant mortality rates and some morbidity rates had declined substantially, but the health disparities and poverty in these communities remained disproportionately high (RCAP, 1996). In situations where acute medical needs took precedence, the time and resources these nurses had to deliver preventive and health promotion services were more limited (Daigle, 2008).

NURSING EDUCATION

The first formal nurse training program was established at the General and Marine Hospital in St. Catharines, Ontario, in 1874. Early in the development of the nursing education program, hospital-based education had a limited breadth and a limited focus on public health nursing practice. The Red Cross played a pivotal role in advancing the education of PHNs by providing funding for certificate courses in public health at five Canadian universities as early as 1919. Nurses, including Ethel Johns, who was the first director of the Department of Nursing at the University of British Columbia (UBC), and other Canadian nurse leaders such as Edith Kathleen Russell, had a remarkable vision for the breadth and depth of education needed to prepare nurses and contributed to significant educational reforms needed to prepare CHNs (Carpenter, 1982; Kirkwood & Bouchard, 1992; Street, 1974; Zilm & Warbinek, 1994). In the same year, the first baccalaureate program in nursing was approved to begin at UBC; it was a five-year program in which, during the fifth and final year, students could elect a focus on public health nursing. The box that follows shows the original outline of the short course in public health nursing, as cited in the UBC calendar. This historical record of academic and field work, similar to some of the realities of community health nursing today, required PHNs to possess the knowledge and scope of practice with a focus on maternal child programs, communicable diseases, school health, and social welfare issues. Indigenous nurses have been a resource for expanding this discussion to include traditional medicines and processes (ANAC, 2007). They have been at the centre of

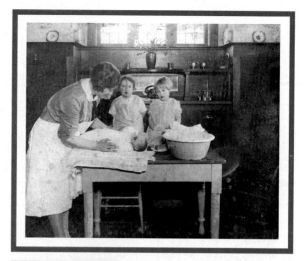

PHOTO 1.3 District nurse visits a home and demonstrates a baby bath.

Source: Image E-01177 courtesy of the Royal BC Museum and Archives

discussions educating nurses to improve health care access in Indigenous communities, including proposing a nursing specialization in Indigenous health nursing (ANAC, 2007).

As a specialist in education, Weir (1932) was commissioned to undertake a review of nursing education across the country and make recommendations. The Weir report describes the types of community nursing roles, activities, salaries, and numbers of nurses who were practising public health nursing at the time. Included in the classification were "visiting nurse, school nurse, industrial nurse, Red Cross, VON, director, staff nurse and supervisor" (Weir, 1932, p. 118). One of Weir's many recommendations was "in the immediate health interests of Canadians, as well as in their future economic interests, the number of PHNs in Canada should at least be doubled within

---

OUTLINE OF THE SHORT COURSE IN PUBLIC HEALTH NURSING, NOVEMBER 1920–MARCH 1921

Academic Work:

1. **Twelve lectures on each of the following:**
   a. Public Health Nursing
   b. School Hygiene
   c. Communicable Diseases
   d. Modern Social Problems

2. **Six lectures on each of the following:**
   e. Teaching Principles
   f. History of Nursing Education
   g. Social Service Problems
   h. Personal Hygiene
   i. Medical Aspects of Infant and Maternal Welfare
   j. Tuberculosis
   k. Mental Hygiene
   l. Sanitation

3. Occasional lectures on provincial legislation, municipal health departments, voluntary organizations, delinquent and deserted children, etc.

4. Excursions to special health features in and around Vancouver.

Field Work: For field work, the class was divided into sections of appropriate size, each of which received from one to two weeks' instruction and experience under trained workers in the actual operation of each of the following branches:

1. Urban School Nursing
2. Tuberculosis Problems
3. District Nursing
4. Health Centres and Rural School Nursing
5. Child Welfare
6. Medical, Social Service, and Relief Organizations

Source: UBC Calendar, 7th session, p. 36. Cited by G. Zilm & E. Warbinek (1994). *Legacy: History of nursing education at the University of British Columbia, 1919–1994* (p. 186). Vancouver, BC: UBC Press. Copyright © 1994 by University of British Columbia. Used by permission of University of British Columbia.

the next five or ten years" (p. 143). The report also contains recommendations for university standards of education and support of public health nursing as a nursing specialty (Duncan, Leipert, & Mill, 1999).

Diploma programs in public health nursing were also established in several Canadian universities to prepare nurses to meet the demands of this specialized practice. These programs prepared nurses without baccalaureate degrees to practise public health nursing. In the later part of the 20th century, the diploma programs in public health nursing were phased out, and the baccalaureate degree became an established requirement of entry-level public health nursing.

Questions about the unique nature of public health nursing practice and competencies remain a critical nursing education issue in the 21st century. The Community Health Nurses of Canada (CHNC) developed Standards of Practice in 2003 and continually revises them to ensure they reflect current practice. In 2014, the Canadian Association of Schools of Nursing (CASNb) convened an expert task force of educators and practitioners to identify the following entry-level competencies in public health nursing practice for undergraduate nursing students:

- public health sciences in nursing practice;
- population and community health assessment and analysis;
- population health planning, implementation, and evaluation;
- partnerships, collaboration, and advocacy; and
- communication in public health nursing. (Canadian Association of Schools of Nursing [CASN], 2014b)

Each competency domain encompasses the knowledge, skill, and attitudes essential for nursing practice (Tardif, 2006). Specific indicators contained within each domain further define the competency domains. These competencies emphasize the importance of developing and applying knowledge to address the determinants of health, building relationships with communities, and understanding the critical relationships among individual, family, and population health. It is significant to ponder how the competencies required of today's graduating students compare with those of early CHNs. Today's nursing education programs are challenged to balance opportunities for practice education in institutional settings and illness care with that of community health nursing and health promotion. Although these competencies relate specifically to the discipline of public health nursing, it is recognized that all nursing graduates have this preparation. The Community Health Nursing Education Interest Group affiliated with CASN established guidelines for best practices for clinical placements in community health nursing to insure the entry-level competencies for all undergraduate nursing students could be met (CASN, 2014c). In the face of these educational goals and challenges, one is reminded of the central role of community health nursing practice as the impetus for the ongoing evolution and advancement of baccalaureate nursing education.

MID-20TH CENTURY: EVOLUTION OF COMMUNITY HEALTH NURSING

Increased government responsibility for the health care of Canadians has had a significant impact on public health nursing. Between 1940 and 1970, health departments focused on the expansion of existing programs. This process included a general shift of emphasis from traditional programs such as child health, immunization, and communicable disease control to programs focusing on the reduction of morbidity and mortality from chronic illnesses and injuries. The early postpartum discharge home-visiting program placed significant demands on the time and resources of PHNs. In some instances, staffing patterns in health units and community health centres were modified to provide seven-day-a-week early postpartum services to mothers and neonates or to focus on just the very high-risk mothers. Staffing demand to improve maternal and newborn health outcomes continue to be an area of focus today, especially in Northern and Indigenous communities. According to Smylie et al. (2010), Indigenous infant mortality rates in Canada are higher than in the rest of the population.

In the early 1970s, rising hospital costs created both an opportunity and a crisis for the VON. Patients were discharged from the hospital earlier and required longer and more complex follow-up care in the community. However, these individuals were often unable to obtain bedside nursing care in their homes during their convalescence. No publicly insured programs for home care services existed until 1974, when the first such program was established in Manitoba (Shapiro, 1997). The VON realized that participation in publicly insured home care programs provided an opportunity to both consolidate and strengthen its organization. It commissioned a national report, which recommended that Canada's oldest and most experienced visiting nursing organization be given the mandate to deliver publicly insured home care programs (Pickering, 1976). Individual provincial governments have made a variety of decisions about the organization and funding of home care programs, not always including the VON. Today, as it did in the past, the VON continues to function by offering a mix of services shaped by local circumstances, with a particular focus on creating programs to respond to unmet needs among specific segments of the population (Penney, 1996).

Community mental health nursing emerged in the 1960s and 1970s in response to the deinstitutionalization of patients with mental illnesses. Community mental health nurses pioneered their new roles in the complex interface between psychiatry and nursing and between community and institutional care (Boschma, 2012).

Significant pressures on health care systems arising from the economic recession of the 1980s caused widespread loss of nursing positions in all sectors of health care, most evident in the hospitals. Particularly problematic was the trend to replace nurses who provided clinical leadership with managers who lacked this capacity, a trend that continues to impact nursing today. Governments replaced hospital-based care with community health services and home care, although this trend has yet to be fully realized. Publicly funded home care programs resulted in some growth in the number of nurses working in community settings. The role of home health nurses (HHNs), who provide nursing care and health education to the sick and convalescent in the home, is similar to that fulfilled by the VNs of the late 19th and early 20th centuries. The number of PHNs, however, has not increased. Their mandate has continued to emphasize health promotion, communicable disease control, healthy child development, and prevention of chronic illness. CHNs persistently respond to the social determinants of health and the needs of marginalized populations, advocating for equal access and social justice for all within the context of these programs.

The reduction in government spending during the 1980s and 1990s affected CHNs in all programs, both directly and indirectly reducing nursing staff numbers and levels of service for many programs. Infrastructure for communicable disease control was particularly hard hit. The loss of capacity to monitor, identify, and follow up on communicable diseases has been identified as one of the major reasons for the resurgence of TB and the recent emergence of new diseases such as acquired immune deficiency syndrome (AIDS), severe acute respiratory syndrome (SARS), and H1N1 influenza (Garrett, 1994, 2000). Deinstitutionalization of patients from acute care and psychiatric institutions has resulted in the need for innovative and comprehensive community-based health care programs and systems. Nursing leadership for the development of essential programs to meet client needs has become more important than ever. The CASN has created competencies for mental health nursing for all undergraduate nurses (CASN, 2014a).

CANADIAN RESEARCH 1.1

Swimming against the tide: A Canadian qualitative study examining the implementation of a province-wide public health initiative to address health equity. (McPerson, Ndumbe-Eyoh, Betker, Oickle, & Peroff-Johnston, 2016)

Effectively addressing the social determinants of health and health equity are critical yet still emerging areas of public health practice. This is significant for contemporary practice as the egregious impacts of health inequities on health outcomes continue to be revealed. More public health organizations seek to augment internal organizational capacity to address health equity, while the evidence base to inform such leadership is in its infancy. The purpose of this paper is to report on findings of a study examining key factors that influence the development and implementation of the social determinants of health public health nurse's (SDH-PHN) role in Ontario.

A descriptive qualitative case study approach examined the first Canadian province-wide initiative to add SDH-PHNs to each public health unit. Data sources were documents and staff from public health units (i.e., SDH-PHNs, managers, directors, chief nursing officers, medical officers of health), and external stakeholders. Data were collected through 42 individual interviews and 226 documents. Interview data were analyzed using framework analysis methods; Prior's approach guided document analysis.

Three themes related to the SDH-PHN role implementation were identified: (1) "swimming against the tide" to lead change as staff navigated ideological tensions, competency development, and novel collaborations; (2) shifting organizational practice environments impacted by initial role placement and action to structurally embed **health equity** priorities; and (3) bridging policy implementation gaps related to local provincial implementation and reporting expectations.

This study extends our understanding of the dynamic interplay among leadership, change management, ideological tensions, and local provincial public health policy impacting health equity agendas. Given that the social determinants of health lie outside public health, collaboration with communities, health partners, and non-health partners is essential to public health practice for health equity. The study findings have implications for increasing our knowledge and capacity for effective system-wide intervention toward health equity as a critical strategic priority for public health and for broader public policy and community engagement. Appropriate and effective public health leadership at multiple levels and by multiple actors is tantamount to adequately making inroads for health equity.

Discussion Questions

1. What are key factors influencing the development and implementation of the social determinants of health work in community health nursing?

2. What are some of the tensions in enabling nurses to address the social determinants of health?

3. What are some strategies CHNs can implement in practice for health equity?

LATE 20TH CENTURY: THE NEW PUBLIC HEALTH—PRIMARY HEALTH CARE AND HEALTH PROMOTION

The WHO adopted the Declaration of Alma-Ata at the 1978 International Conference on Primary Health Care and declared primary health care as the guiding vision for achieving health for all people. Since then, the WHO has consistently recognized nursing as the essential global workforce for achieving primary health care goals (WHO, 1978, 1989). Harnessing the skills and knowledge of CHNs is essential to achieving health equity, building on the historic foundation of how nurses have contributed to building essential services for people in their communities and advancing health systems.

CHNs have provided leadership for advancing the understanding and integration of primary health care principles in the Canadian health care system. (See Chapter 2.) The Canadian Nurses Association (CNA) (1980) submitted an influential brief titled "Putting Health into Health Care" to the federal government to review its health system. This was CNA's nationwide lobbying effort to endorse primary health care and health promotion.

Canada has provided strong international leadership in the evolution of health promotion. Its landmark documents, the Lalonde Report (1974) and the Ottawa Charter for Health Promotion (WHO, 1986), sparked a public health movement that focused the understanding of health and its determinants as value-based processes and identified broad health promotion strategies that remain foundational to community health nursing practice and to nursing education.

In 1987, the formation of the Community Health Nurses Association of Canada (CHNAC) marked a significant period of progress. Since that time, the CHNAC has evolved to become the CHNC, a specialty practice organization of the CNA. The CHNC serves as a centre of excellence for community health nursing and advances practice excellence. The CHNC represents the voices of, and advocates for, the role of CHNs, creates opportunities for partnerships across sectors and networks, and strengthens community health nursing leadership. The CHNC advocates for healthy public policy to address the social and environmental determinants of health and promotes a publicly funded, universal system for community health. Strategic organizational partnerships enable the CHNC to advance the practice of community health nursing through role definition, theory development, and research.

21ST CENTURY PROSPECTIVE: CONTINUITY WITH THEMES OF THE PAST

Events in the first decade of the 21st century continue to shape community health nursing. The Romanow Commission's report, titled "Building on Values: The Future of Health Care in Canada," continues to be recognized as a visionary document with recommendations for shifting resources and policy in the direction of primary health care, home health care, and health promotion, with nurses as the key players in the transformation of systems and services (Romanow, 2002). Many of these recommendations have been slow to take shape. Another pivotal event was the formation of the Public Health Agency of Canada (PHAC) in 2004 after the SARS crisis. It was created "in response to growing concerns about the capacity of Canada's public health system to anticipate and respond effectively to public health threats" (Public Health Agency of Canada [PHAC], 2018, para 1). In its first decade, the PHAC has drawn attention to the need to develop a sustainable public health workforce, including nursing, while emphasizing a vision of intersectoral policy development and interprofessional collaboration.

As in the past, CHNs of today must assume a strong policy advocacy role to ensure that essential nursing care and services are accessible to communities. From the earliest beginnings of Florence Nightingale using statistics to create a campaign of reform, advocacy has developed into a key mandate for nurses. With a health equity lens, PHNs increasingly focus their practice on the social determinants of health and examine the evidence pointing to the causes of poor health that are rooted in societal inequities and how marginalized populations experience homelessness, addiction, poverty, and injustice (Reutter & Kushner, 2010). This mandate is often difficult to achieve in hierarchical organizational structures, where there may be barriers to nurses voicing concerns and taking political action for change (Falk-Rafael & Betker, 2012).

In this context, Vukic and Keddy (2002) reinforced the need for outpost nurses to build a trusting working relationship to establish community development and health promotion strategies, as the majority of nurses and the services offered stemmed from a Eurocentric stance. The Aboriginal Nurses Association, now the Canadian Indigenous Nurses Association, has been instrumental in establishing culturally competent health care and cultural safety in the North (ANAC, 2007). Currently, the number of Indigenous nurses working in First Nation communities has increased, and most communities have established Indian health transfer of services (Waldrum, Herring, & Young, 1995). Vukic, Etowa, and Perley Dutcher (2014) demonstrate in the study on Aboriginal nurses' work-life that Indigenous nurses have the agency and talents necessary to create change in their communities and should play a leadership role in advocating for and addressing **Indigenous health care** needs (p. 98). Collectively, CHNs are responding to the health inequities found in Northern Indigenous communities, and nurse educators and nurse leaders are working with Indigenous communities and organizations to address the Truth and Reconciliation Commitment to Action (Truth and Reconciliation Commission, 2015). In light of all the changes, CHNs remain front and centre in promoting the principles of primary health care in Northern Indigenous communities.

Hardill (2006) pointed out that besides PHNs and the VON from the early days, CHNs can be inspired by the earliest forms of "street nursing" practised by the Grey Nuns, who cared for the "sick poor, in 18th century Quebec" (p. 91). The broad nature of community health nursing with its strong emphasis of evidence-informed practice, combined with their unique perspective from the eyes of their clients, provides CHNs an exceptional ability to understand the conditions that impact health.

Modern street nursing has been traced to Vancouver in 1946, when nurses began to provide antibiotic treatment and contact tracing for venereal diseases. Today, there is a strong legacy of CHNs' outreach, care, and advocacy to address the social and living conditions of the most vulnerable members of society. PHNs were actively involved in establishing the first needle exchange program in British Columbia after witnessing many of their clients dying from AIDS (www.nfb.ca). CHNs can be inspired by their roots of activism, advocacy, and outreach while finding ways to meet their standard of facilitating access and equity by recognizing the impacts of the social determinants of health and incorporating actions in their practice (Community Health Nurses of Canada [CHNC], 2019, revised).

In its earliest form, school nursing encompassed issues of the nurses' relationships with children, families, and the community as a whole. In fact, general public health nursing programs emerged from school nursing, whereas today PHNs are working to redefine their roles in schools, which became narrow and diminished in scope during the latter part of the 20th century. A renewed vision of comprehensive school health is revitalizing and extending the work of PHNs in schools; nurses can be proud of their legacy of contributions to school health over the past century.

It is significant that the early practice of community health nursing was generalist in nature, consisting of a comprehensive range of services, including home health care and health promotion. Nursing roles became differentiated and specialized over time in response to social, economic, and political forces, including the expanding knowledge of society.

Today, the competencies and role descriptions for CHNs include public health, home health, community mental health, and occupational health as distinct forms of community health nursing in Canada. Home health nursing is also undergoing specialization in the key areas of palliative care, chronic illness prevention and care, and long-term care. CHNs must also be equipped with knowledge about Indigenous health, emergency disaster preparedness, environmental health, and global health. In all areas, there is significant advancement in theory and research to support best practices and the development of the nursing profession into the 21st century. (See Figure 1.2.)

The CHNC has developed a professional practice model and standards for Canadian CHNs, specifying eight standards as benchmarks of excellence that define the practice of a registered nurse in the specialty area of community health nursing (CHNC, 2019, revised). (See Appendix A of this text.) Competencies have been developed to reflect to the practice of PHNs and HHNs with a minimum of two years' experience. (See Appendices B and C.) The standards reflect continuity with the early practice of nurses working in the community to promote health, prevent illness, advocate for services, partner with community organizations and women's groups, and provide courageous leadership for the establishment of essential services for vulnerable populations.

In 2006 the CNA developed a certification in community health nursing in recognition of this unique specialty of nursing practice. Canadian CHNs build on the legacy of the early nurses as they advance their practice to achieve the present-day goal of global health equity (Reutter & Kushner, 2010).

Many CHNs become strong advocates for healthy public policy, healthy environments, and conditions that enable health (Falk-Rafael & Betker, 2012; Reutter & Kushner, 2010). As indicated in the following Yes, But Why? box, childhood obesity is an area where the CHN's leadership and advocacy role can be maximized.

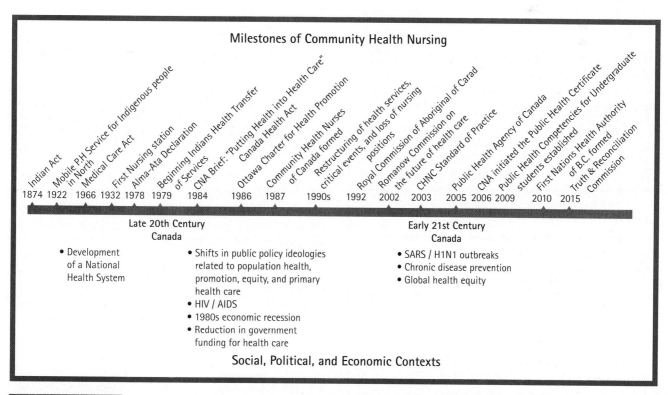

FIGURE 1.2 Critical Events Influencing the Milestones of Community Health Nursing, Mid-1960s to Present

YES, BUT WHY?

Childhood Obesity in Canada

What?

Despite the advances in community health nursing, the prevalence of obesity in children is increasing at alarming rates. Obesity rates among children and youth in Canada have nearly tripled in the last 30 years (Health Canada, 2017). The health impacts of this issue are tremendous. Children who are overweight or obese are more likely to grow up to be overweight or obese adults and struggle with their weight throughout their lives. As they age, they are more likely to experience type 2 diabetes, high blood pressure, heart disease, and arthritis (Morrison & Chanoine, 2007). Further, some overweight kids are bullied at school. They often have low self-esteem and suffer socially, and they are more likely to experience depression (Strauss, 2000). If nothing is done, the current generation of children will develop chronic illnesses much younger and will be more affected as they age (Katzmarzyk, 2011).

So What?

The social determinants of health and economic and political systems have an important influence on the conditions that influence people's health. Low-income children and adolescents are more likely to be obese than their higher-income counterparts (Odgen et al., 2010). Many factors contribute to this issue. The cost of organized sports or physical activities—and transportation to and from these activities—puts them out of the reach of low-income families. These activities, or facilities to host them, may not be available in their neighbourhoods.

Physical activity is a key issue in obesity prevention. Children are spending an increasing amount of time in front of computers and other screens that could be impacting their activity levels (Ontario Ministry of Health, 2013). In many families living in poverty, children without access to physical activities may be more likely to spend more time in front of screens than being physically active.

Low-income neighbourhoods often are not walkable or have poor access to fresh fruits and vegetables (Kakinami, 2015). When the only food available is in a convenience store or fast-food chain, the cost or availability of healthy food is limited. All of these can all increase the risk of being overweight.

Now What?

Canada needs a coordinated approach to create healthy communities and reduce or eliminate the broader social and health disparities that affect children's health and weight (Ontario Ministry of Health, 2013). PHNs can have tremendous influence in the area of obesity prevention at the individual, group, community, and system levels. Nurses promote a decrease in sedentary activities with emphasis on reducing the amount of time children spend watching TV and playing video games, and they can encourage physical activity. PHNs in schools can work to increase physical activity initiatives. Working with communities, PHNs can advocate for sports programs, green spaces, and playing fields.

At a population level, PHNs can influence the "built environment" by advocating for communities that encourage active transportation in the forms of walking, cycling, and using public transit, as well as recreational physical activity.

Standards of Practice Fulfilled

#1 Promoting Health
– Considers the determinants of health, the social and political context, and systemic structures in collaboration with the client to determine action.

#7 Health Equity
– Advocates for healthy public policy and social justice by participating in legislative and policy-making activities that influence determinants of health and access to services (CHNC, 2019, revised).

CASE STUDY

Early Childhood Development and Poverty

You are a CHN working in a public health organization in a diverse urban environment with many families coexisting within a wide variance of the social gradient. Your agency expects that you will provide best practices for early childhood development in your area. You are concerned that some families living in poverty, with minimal job opportunities and limited education, will not benefit from the programs as they are currently offered in your agency. Describe how you can advocate for health for all in your district by considering the following questions.

Discussion Questions

1. What are some lessons from past leaders in nursing that can influence your advocacy work to respond to the early childhood development in your district?

2. What current considerations does the PHN need to take into account when establishing priorities to respond to the inequities witnessed?

3. What are some opportunities the PHN can pursue to strive for health equity for the children in the community?

Advocacy can be challenging for CHNs, many whom work for government-funded organizations where advocacy is not supported. Professional organizations such as CHNC support the social justice framework of nurses in the community. In this time of fiscal constraint and system restructuring, it has never been so important for CHNs to continue to participate, with their interdisciplinary colleagues, in advocacy on behalf of their clients. It is particularly important for CHNs to be strong advocates for individuals who are rendered vulnerable by their social circumstances. See the Case Study on early childhood development and poverty, which illustrates the central role CHNs could play in diverse communities.

CONCLUSION

Community health nursing practice has evolved to address the impact that political, economic, and other macro systems

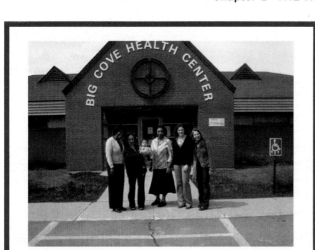

PHOTO 1.4 Increased representation of diversity of Community Health Nurses, in an Indigenous community, 2009

Left to right Dr J. Etowa, RN PhD Cheyenne Mary, RN MN, Cheyenne's infant, Dr E. Asuquo, RN PhD, M. Blacklows, B.S.W., Dr A. Vukic, RN, PhD

have on individual, family, aggregate, and population health. Knowledge development in health enables CHNs to shape their practices in ways that seek to engage both health care professionals and community members in finding new and innovative ways to achieve health for all.

Reflecting on the legacy of CHNs over the past three centuries, it is easy to recognize how the early practice of nurses was focused on promoting the health of individuals, families, populations, and communities, and included the prevention of infectious diseases. These nurses worked in partnership with women's groups and the communities they served to develop essential services, address what are now referred to as the social determinants of health, and advocate for marginalized and vulnerable people. Education for CHNs was developed by courageous leaders who had the vision for the difference these nurses can make. It is this legacy that positioned CHNs to meet the health goals for the 21st century.

Many factors influenced the early development of community health nursing as it exists today. CHNs continue to address health and social inequities in First Nation communities and in immigrant and refugee populations. Communicable and non-communicable disease prevention also remains a priority. A source of inspiration is found in the history of how nurses worked in partnership with, and gained strength from, dominant social movements and women's groups, and how they influenced policy in the development of health programs and organizations. Advocacy to increase the numbers of CHNs in all roles must remain a priority.

Finally, while the past inspires a vision for community health nursing in the 21st century, we must also acknowledge the vision and contributions of present-day leaders, including students who will move community health nursing forward to new achievements. In their final editorial after editing the journal *Public Health Nursing* for a decade, editors Abrams and Hays (2013) leave us with the vision that can apply to all forms of community health nursing today: "On the shoulders of younger giants, public health nursing moves forward" (p. 475).

KEY TERMS

district or visiting nursing (p. 6)
Indigenous health care (p. 10)
primary health care (p. 1)
public health nurse (PHN) (p. 4)
social justice (p. 3)
health equity (p. 9)

STUDY QUESTIONS

1. Summarize the early forms of community health nursing.

2. Which populations were the focus of early community nursing programs?

3. Briefly describe three of the earliest public health programs in which nurses were involved and the reasons for their implementation.

4. How did the British North America Act (1867) and 19th-century beliefs about the role of government influence the development of community health services?

5. Discuss how community health nursing contributed to the advancement of nursing education.

INDIVIDUAL CRITICAL-THINKING EXERCISES

The sources listed at the end of some of these questions are cited in full in the references section. Each source will provide additional insights into the controversies and debates surrounding the history of public health and visiting nursing.

1. Community health nursing has frequently been described as more autonomous than nursing practice in institutional settings. However, Eunice Dyke, Toronto's first supervisor of public health nursing, once stated that "public health nursing has in the medical profession its greatest friend and not infrequently its greatest stumbling block." How autonomous was the practice of early CHNs? (*Sources:* Comacchio, 1993; Stuart, 1992)

2. What role did middle-class ideas about class, ethnicity, and gender play in the development of public health programs to protect the health of infants and children? (*Sources:* Comacchio, 1993; Gleason, 2002; Chapter 3)

3. Reflecting on community health nursing education in your nursing program, what issues do you see that are continuous with the past as described in this chapter?

GROUP CRITICAL-THINKING EXERCISES

1. Social historians such as Alan Hunt (1999) argue that charity, philanthropy, and welfare programs are essentially efforts by the elite and middle classes to impose their behaviour, values, and culture upon others. Hunt describes these programs of moral or social regulation as being inspired by "the passionate conviction that there is something inherently wrong or immoral about the conduct of others" (p. ix). Locate

an issue of an early public health or nursing journal such as *The Public Health Journal* (now the *Canadian Journal of Public Health*) or *The Canadian Nurse* (particularly the section on public health). Conduct a brief content analysis of the issue, paying close attention to how the recipients of public health interventions are described. What conclusions can be drawn about the attitudes of health care professionals? What anxieties seem to underlie the interventions they describe and recommend to other health care practitioners?

2. Nurses were the intermediaries between the clients they served and the social and political elite who employed them to work in the community. However, their perspective on the objectives and effectiveness of community health programs is often absent from published histories of public health. To fill this gap in the historical record, do one of the following: (1) Locate a biographical account written by an early visiting or public health nurse, (2) locate an oral history of an early visiting or public health nurse in an archive, or (3) interview a retired visiting or public health nurse. How do their accounts resemble or differ from the history of community health nursing presented in this chapter? How would you account for any differences you identify?

3. Based on what you have learned about the history of community health nursing in Canada, what do you believe are the greatest challenges facing nurses in this practice setting today and in the future?

REFERENCES

Aboriginal Nurses Association of Canada [ANAC]. (2007). *Twice as good: A history of Aboriginal nurses*. Ottawa, ON: Author.

Abrams, S. E., & Hays, J. C. (2013). On the shoulders of younger giants public health nursing moves forward. *Public Health Nursing, 30*(6), 475–476. Published by John Wiley & Sons, Inc, © 2013.

Allemang, M. (2000). Development of community health nursing in Canada. In M. J. Stewart (Ed.), *Community nursing: Promoting Canada's health* (2nd ed., pp. 4–32). Toronto, ON: W. B. Saunders.

Anionwu E. (2006). About Mary Seacole. Thames Valley University, London: Mary Seacole Center for Nursing Practice.

Armstrong-Reid, S. (2014). *Lyle Creelman: The frontiers of global nursing*. Toronto, ON: University of Toronto Press.

Baker, C., Guest, E., Jorgenson, L., Crosby, K., & Boyd, J. (2012). *Ties that bind: The evolution of education for professional nursing in Canada from the 17th to the 21st Century*. A project report conducted by CASN National Office Staff to mark the occasion of the 70th Anniversary of the Canadian Association of Schools of Nursing.

Baldwin, D. O. (1997). *She answered every call: The life of public health nurse Mona Gordon Wilson (1894–1981)*. Charlottetown, PE: Indigo Press.

Benoit, C., & Carroll, D. (2005). Canadian midwifery: Blending traditional and modern practices. In C. Bates, D. Dodd, & N. Rousseau (Eds.), *On all frontiers: Four centuries of Canadian nursing* (pp. 27–41). Ottawa, ON: University of Ottawa Press.

Boschma, G. (2012). Community mental health nursing in Alberta, Canada: An oral history. *Nursing History Review, 20*, 103–135. doi:10.1891/1062-8061.20.103. Copyright © 2012 by University of British Columbia. Used by permission of University of British Columbia.

Bourque Bearskin, R. L. (2011). A critical lens on culture in nursing practice. *Nursing Ethics*, 1–12. doi:10.1177/0969733011480048

Bourque Bearskin, R. L. (2014). *Mâmawoh kamâtowin: Coming together to help each other: Honouring indigenous nursing knowledge*. (Unpublished doctoral dissertation.) University of Alberta Faculty of Nursing, Edmonton, Alberta.

Boutillier, B. (1994). Helpers or heroines? The National Council of Women, nursing and "women's work" in late Victorian Canada. In D. Dodd & D. Gorham (Eds.), *Caring and curing: Historical perspectives on women and healing in Canada* (pp. 17–48). Ottawa, ON: University of Ottawa Press.

Burnett, K. (2008). The healing work of Aboriginal women in Indigenous and newcomer communities. In J. Elliot, M. Stuart, & C. Toman (Eds.), *Place and practice in Canadian nursing history* (pp. 40–52). Vancouver, BC: UBC Press.

Canadian Association of Schools of Nursing (CASN). (2014a). *Entry-to-practice mental health and addiction competencies for undergraduate nursing education in Canada*. Ottawa, ON: Author. Retrieved from http://www.casn.ca/2015/11/entry-to-practice-mental-health-and-addiction-competencies-for-undergraduate-nursing-education-in-canada/

Canadian Association of Schools of Nursing (CASN). (2014b). *Entry-to-practice public health nursing competencies for undergraduate nursing education*. Ottawa, ON: Author.

Canadian Association of Schools of Nursing (CASN). (2014c). *Guidelines for quality community health nursing clinical guidelines*. Ottawa, ON: Author. Retrieved from http://casn.ca/wpcontent/uploads/2014/12/CPGuidelinesFinalMarch.pdf

Canadian Nurses Association (CNA). (1980). *Putting health into health care: Submission to the Health Services Review*. Ottawa, ON: Author.

Carpenter, H. (1982). *A divine discontent: Edith Kathleen Russell, reforming educator*. Toronto, ON: University of Toronto Faculty of Nursing.

City of Winnipeg Health Department. (1910). *Annual report for the year ending December 1909*. Winnipeg, MB: City of Winnipeg.

Comacchio, C. (1993). *Nations are built of babies: Saving Ontario's mothers and children 1900–1940*. Montreal, QC: McGill-Queen's University Press.

Community Health Nurses of Canada (CHNC). (2019, revised). *Canadian community health nursing professional practice model and standards of practice*. St. John's, NL: Author.

Daigle, J. (2008). The call of the North: Settlement nurses in the remote areas of Quebec. In J. Elliot, M. Stuart, & C. Toman (Eds.), *Place and practice in Canadian nursing history* (pp. 111–135). Vancouver, BC: UBC Press.

D'Antonio, P. (2006). History for a practice profession. *Nursing Inquiry, 13*(4), 242–248.

Dodd, D., Elliot, J., & Rousseau, N. (2005). Outpost nursing in Canada. In C. Bates, D. Dodd, & N. Rousseau (Eds.), *On all frontiers: Four centuries of Canadian nursing* (pp. 139–152). Ottawa, ON: University of Ottawa Press.

Drees, L. M., & McBain, L. (2001). Nursing and native peoples in northern Saskatchewan, 1930s–1950s. *Canadian Bulletin of Medical History, 18,* 43–65.

Duncan, S. M., Leipert, B. D., & Mill, J. E. (1999). Nurses as health evangelists? The evolution of public health nursing in Canada, 1918–1939. *Advances in Nursing Science, 22*(1), 40–51.

Ewart, M. (1916). Home visiting in connection with school nursing. *The Canadian Nurse, XII*(6), 307–309.

Falk-Rafael, A. (2005). Speaking truth to power: Nursing's legacy and moral imperative. *Advances in Nursing Science, 28*(2), 222.

Falk-Rafael, A., & Betker, C. (2012). The primacy of relationships: A study of public health nursing from a critical caring perspective. *Advances in Nursing Science, 35*(4), 315–332. doi:10.1097/ANS.ObO13e318271d127

Fee, E., & Bu, L. (2010). The origins of public health nursing: The Henry Street Visiting Service. *American Journal of Public Health, 100*(7), 1206–1207.

Garrett, L. (1994). *The coming plague: Newly emerging diseases in a world out of balance.* New York, NY: Penguin Books.

Garrett, L. (2000). *Betrayal of trust: The collapse of global public health.* New York, NY: Hyperion Press

Gibbon, J. M. (1947). *The Victorian Order of Nurses for Canada: 50th anniversary, 1897–1947.* Montreal, QC: Southam Press.

Gibbon, J. M., & Mathewson, M. (1947). *Three centuries of Canadian nursing.* Toronto, ON: Macmillan Co. of Canada.

Gleason, M. (2002). Race, class and health: School medical inspection and "healthy" children in British Columbia, 1890–1930. *Canadian Bulletin of Medical History/Bulletin Canadien d'histoire de la médicine, 19*(1), 85–112.

Government of Canada. (2017). *The chief public health officer's report on the state of public health in Canada 2017—Designing healthy living.* Retrieved from https://www.canada.ca/en/public-health/services/publications/chief-public-health-officer-reports-state-public-health-canada/2017-designing-healthy-living.html#a5_1

Hardill, K. (2006). From the Grey Nuns to the streets: A critical history of outreach nursing in Canada. *Public Health Nursing, 24*(1), 91–97.

Health Canada. (2017). *Childhood obesity.* Retrieved from https://www.canada.ca/en/public-health/services/childhood-obesity/childhood-obesity.html

Hunt, A. (1999). *Governing morals: A social history of moral regulation.* Cambridge, UK: Cambridge University Press.

Kakinami, K. (2015, June). Childhood obesity linked to poverty, parenting style. *Preventive Medicine, 75.*

Katzmarzyk, P. T. (2011). The economic costs associated with physical inactivity and obesity in Ontario. *The Health and Fitness Journal of Canada, 4*(4).

Keddy, B., & Dodd, D. (2005). The trained nurse: Private duty and VON home nursing (Late 1800s to 1940s). In C. Bates, D. Dodd, & N. Rousseau (Eds.), *On all frontiers: Four centuries of Canadian nursing* (pp. 43–56). Ottawa, ON: University of Ottawa Press.

Kirkwood, R., & Bouchard, J. (1992). *"Take counsel with one another": A beginning history of the Canadian Association of University Schools of Nursing 1942–1992.* Ottawa, ON: Canadian Association of University Schools of Nursing.

Kue Young, T. (1984). Indian health services in Canada: A sociohistorical perspective. *Social Science and Medicine, 18*(3), 257–264.

Lalonde, M. (1974). *A new perspective on the health of Canadians.* Ottawa, ON: Government of Canada.

Larsen, J., & Baumgart, A. J. (1992). Introduction to nursing in Canada. In A. Baumgart & J. Larsen (Eds.), *Canadian nursing faces the future* (pp. 3–22). St. Louis, MO: Mosby.

Locke, H. L. F. (1918). The problem of our infant population with special reference to the opportunity of the welfare nurse. *American Journal of Nursing, 18*(7), 523–526.

MacDougall, H. (1990). *Activists and advocates: Toronto's Health Department, 1883–1983.* Toronto, ON: Dundurn Press.

MacNutt, J. S. (1913). The Board of Health nurse: What she can do for the public welfare in a small city. *American Journal of Public Health, 3*(4), 344–350.

Matthews, O. (1920). Child welfare. *The Canadian Nurse, 16*(1), 15–16.

McKay, M. (2005). Public health nursing. In C. Bates, D. Dodd, & N. Rousseau (Eds.), *On all frontiers: Four centuries of Canadian nursing* (pp. 107–123). Ottawa, ON: University of Ottawa Press.

McKay, M. (2008). Region, faith and health: The development of Winnipeg's visiting nursing agencies. In J. Elliot, M. Stuart, & C. Toman (Eds.), *Place and practice in Canadian nursing history* (pp. 70–90). Vancouver, BC: UBC Press.

McKay, M. (2012). The history of community health nursing in Canada. In L. L. Stamler & L. Yiu (Eds.), *Community health nursing: A Canadian perspective* (3rd ed., pp. 1–20). Toronto, ON: Pearson Canada.

McPerson, N., Ndumbe-Eyoh, S., Betker, C., Oickle, D., & Peroff-Johnston, N. (2016). Swimming against the tide: A Canadian qualitative study examining the implementation of a province-wide public health initiative to address health equity. *International Journal for Equity in Health, 15,* 129.

McPherson, K. (1996). *Bedside matters: The transformation of Canadian nursing, 1900–1990.* Toronto, ON: Oxford University Press.

Meigs, G. L. (1916, August). Other factors in infant mortality than the milk supply and their control. *American Journal of Public Health, 6,* 847–853.

Miller, G. L. (2000). *Mustard plasters and handcars: Through the eyes of a Red Cross outpost nurse.* Toronto, ON: Natural Heritage/Natural History.

Morrison, K., & Chanoine, J. (2007). Clinical evaluation of obese children and adolescents. *Canadian Medical Association Journal, 176,* 8 suppl, 45–49.

Nevitt, J. (1978). *White caps and black bands: Nursing in Newfoundland to 1934.* St. John's, NL: Jefferson Press.

Nightingale, F. (1859/1946). *Notes on nursing.* London, UK: Harrison & Sons; Philadelphia, PA: Lippincott.

Ogden, C.L., Carroll, M.D., Curtin, L.R., Lamb, M.M., & Flegal, K.M. (2010). Prevalence of high body mass index in US children and adolescents, 2007–2008. *JAMA 303*(3):242–249.

Ontario Ministry of Health. (2013). *No time to wait: The Healthy Kids strategy.* ON: Author. Retrieved from http://www.health.gov.on.ca/en/common/ministry/publications/reports/healthy_kids/healthy_kids.pdf

Paul, P. (2005). Religious nursing orders of Canada: A presence on all western frontiers. In C. Bates, D. Dodd, & N. Rousseau (Eds.), *On all frontiers: Four centuries of Canadian nursing* (pp. 125–138). Ottawa, ON: University of Ottawa Press.

Paul, P., & Ross-Kerr, J. C. (2011). Nursing in Canada, 1600 to the present: A brief account. In J. C. Ross-Kerr & M. J. Wood (Eds.), *Canadian nursing issues and perspectives* (5th ed., pp. 18–41). Toronto, ON: Elsevier.

Peikoff, T., & Brickey, S. (1991). Creating precious children and glorified mothers: A theoretical assessment of the transformation of childhood. In R. Smandych, G. Dodds, & A. Esau (Eds.), *Dimensions of childhood: Essays on the history of children and youth in Canada* (pp. 29–61). Winnipeg, MB: Legal Research Institute of the University of Manitoba.

Penney, S. (1996). *A century of caring: The history of the Victorian Order of Nurses for Canada.* Ottawa, ON: Victorian Order of Nurses for Canada.

Pickering, E. A. (1976). *A case for the VON in home care.* Ottawa, ON: Victorian Order of Nurses for Canada.

Public Health Agency of Canada. (2018). © All rights reserved. About the Agency: Mandate. Public Health Agency of Canada, 2018. Adapted and reproduced with permission from the Minister of Health, 2018.

Report of the Royal Commission on Aboriginal Peoples. (1996). *Volume 3: Gathering strength.* Ottawa, ON: Ministry of Supply and Services.

Reutter, L., & Kushner, L. (2010). Health equity through action on the social determinants of health: Taking up the challenge in nursing. *Nursing Inquiry, 17,* 269–280.

Richardson, S. (1997). Women's enterprise: Establishing the Lethbridge Nursing Mission, 1909–1919. *Nursing History Review, 5,* 105–130.

Richardson, S. (1998). Political women, professional nurses, and the creation of Alberta's district nursing service, 1919–1925. *Nursing History Review, 6,* 25–50.

Riddell, S. E. (1991). *Curing society's ills: Public health nurses and public health nursing in rural British Columbia, 1916–1946.* Unpublished master's thesis, Simon Fraser University, Vancouver, BC.

Romanow, R. (2002). *Building on values: The future of health care in Canada.* Ottawa, ON: Government of Canada.

Sears, A. (1995). Before the welfare state: Public health and social policy. *Canadian Review of Sociology and Anthropology/Revue canadienne de sociologie et d'anthropologie, 32*(2), 169–188.

Shapiro, E. (1997). *The cost of privatization: A case study of home care in Manitoba.* Ottawa, ON: Canadian Centre for Policy Alternatives.

Smylie, J., Fell, D., Ohlsson, A., & the Joint Working Group on First Nations, Indian, Inuit, and Métis Infant Mortality of the Canadian Perinatal Surveillance System. (2010). A review of Aboriginal infant mortality rates in Canada: Striking and persistent Aboriginal/non-Aboriginal inequities. *Canadian Journal of Public Health, 101*(2):143–148.

Strauss R. S. (2000). Childhood obesity and self-esteem. *Pediatrics.* Jan; 105(1): e15.

Street, M. (1974). *Watch-fires on the mountain.* Toronto, ON: University of Toronto Press.

Stuart, M. E. (1987). *"Let not the people perish for lack of knowledge": Public health nursing and the Ontario rural child welfare project, 1916–1930.* (Unpublished doctoral dissertation.) University of Pennsylvania, Philadelphia.

Stuart, M. (1992). "Half a loaf is better than no bread": Public health nurses and physicians in Ontario, 1920–1925. *Nursing Research, 41*(1), 21–27.

Sutherland, N. (1981). "To create a strong and healthy race": School children in the public health movement, 1880–1914. In S. E. D. Short (Ed.), *Medicine in Canadian society: Historical perspectives* (pp. 361–393). Montreal, QC: McGill–Queen's University Press.

Tardif, J. (2006). *L'évaluation des compétences: Documenter le parcours de développement.* Montréal, QC: Chenelier Education.

Toman, C. (2005). "Ready, aye, ready": Canadian military nurses as an expandable and expendable workforce (1920–2000). In C. Bates, D. Dodd, & N. Rousseau (Eds.). *On all frontiers: Four centuries of Canadian nursing* (pp. 169–182). Ottawa, ON: University of Ottawa Press.

Truth and Reconciliation Commission of Canada. (2015). *Honouring the truth, reconciling for the future: Summary of the final report of the Truth and Reconciliation Commission of Canada.* Retrieved from http://www.trc.ca/websites/trcinstitution/File/2015/Honouring_the_Truth_Reconciling_for_the_Future_July_23_2015.pdf

Victorian Order of Nurses (VON). (2017). *Together in care annual report 2016–2017.* Ottawa, ON: Author. Retrieved from http://von.ca/sites/default/files/files/von_annualreport_2016-17_e04_web02.pdf

Vukic, A., & Keddy, B. (2002). Northern nursing practice in primary health care settings. *Journal of Advanced Nursing, 40*(5), 542–548.

Vukic, A., Etowa, J., & Perley-Dutcher, L. (2014). The sociopolitical impacts on health care that effect Aboriginal nurses working in Aboriginal communities. *International Journal of Nursing, 1*(2), 79–101. doi: 10.15640/ijn.v1n2a7.

Waldrum, J. B., Herring, D. A., & Young, T. K. (1995). *Aboriginal health in Canada: Historical, cultural and epidemiological perspectives.* Toronto, ON: University of Toronto Press.

Weir, G. M. (1932). *Survey of nursing education in Canada.* Toronto, ON: University of Toronto Press.

Winkelstein, W. (2009). Florence Nightingale founder of modern nursing and hospital epidemiology. *Epidemiology, 20*(2), 311.

World Health Organization (WHO). (1978, September). *Primary health care: Report on the international conference on primary health care, Alma Ata, USSR, 6–12 September.* Geneva, CH: Author.

World Health Organization (WHO). (1986, November). *The Ottawa charter for health promotion.* First International Conference on Health Promotion, Ottawa, ON. Retrieved from http://www.who.int/healthpromotion/conferences/previous/ottawa/en/index1.html

World Health Organization (WHO). (1989). *The role of nursing and mid-wifery personnel in the strategy of health for all.* Geneva, CH: Author.

Yarmie, A. (2013). *Women caring for Kamloops 1890–1975.* Kamloops, BC: Textual Studies in Canada and the Kamloops Museum and Archives.

Zilm, G., & Warbinek, E. (1994). *Legacy: History of nursing education at the University of British Columbia, 1919–1994.* Vancouver, BC: UBC Press.

Zilm, G., & Warbinek, E. (2002). Profile of a leader: Elizabeth Breeze. *Canadian Journal of Nursing Leadership, 15*(3), 28–29.

ABOUT THE AUTHORS

Adele Vukic, RN, BN, MN PhD, is currently a faculty member at the School of Nursing, Faculty of Health, Dalhousie University. She has practised Northern nursing for many years. Her teaching centres on population health, family nursing, and community health nursing. She is a strong advocate for social justice and reducing inequities in health and health care. Adele's main research is with Indigenous health, and she is also collaborating on research involving families with new babies. She has presented her work at conferences and published nationally and internationally.

Katie Dilworth, RN, BScN, MHSc, CCHN(C), has worked in community health nursing for over 30 years in both home health nursing and public health nursing. She holds a Bachelor's degree in nursing, a Master's degree in health science—health promotion, and a certification in community health nursing with the Canadian Nurses Association. Katie has volunteered with several community health associations, including the Community Health Nurses' Initiatives Group of the Registered Nurses Association of Ontario and the Canadian Public Health Association. Katie has volunteered extensively with Community Health Nurses of Canada, participating in several standing committees and serving as president.

ACKNOWLEDGEMENT

The authors acknowledge Dr. Susan Duncan and Dr. Marion McKay, authors of the previous versions of this chapter, whose work continues to provide a foundation for this presentation of the history of community health nursing in Canada.

CHAPTER 2

Policy, Politics, and Power in Health Care

Josephine Etowa, Lisa Ashley, and Esther Moghadam

LEARNING OUTCOMES

After studying this chapter, you will be able to:

1. Describe historical milestones in Canadian health care with a focus on community health.

2. Outline the paradigm shift to prevention, promotion, and the social determinants of health.

3. Describe organization of community health nursing care, including those that apply to Indigenous peoples and other populations that are vulnerable in Canada.

4. Examine how policy, politics, and power impact on health equity and community health nursing practice.

5. Discuss challenges in community health nursing.

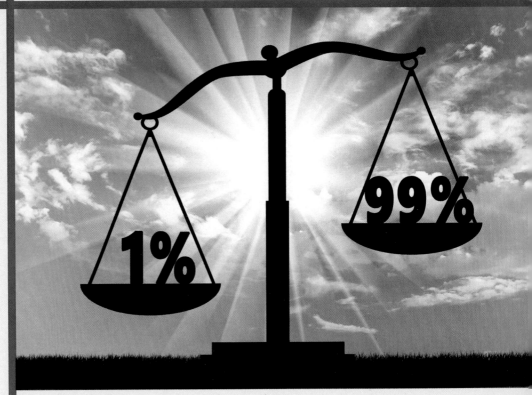

Source: Prazis/123RF

INTRODUCTION

A community health nurse's (CHN) professional practice can occur in a wide range of settings. CHNs are "accountable to a variety of authorities and stakeholders—the public, the regulatory body, and the employer—and are governed by legislative and policy mandates from multiple sources both internal and external to their employment situation" (Meagher-Stewart et al., 2004, p. 3). CHNs' practice is affected by the structure, processes, and leadership of the organizations they work in, enabled and constrained through funding, governance, values, policies, goals, and standards (Ganann et al., 2010; Meagher-Stewart et al., 2004; Molina-Mula & De Pedro-Gómez, 2012; Underwood et al., 2009).

Media reports assert that Canada is in crisis; spending is out of control and wait times are unreasonable. Substantive changes are needed to ensure sustainability of the health care system. There is also a chorus regarding the significance of health promotion and prevention and the critical role of community health nursing in addressing the social determinants of health and advancing health equity (Canadian Nurses Association [CNA], 2012a; Mahony & Jones, 2013; World Health Organization [WHO], 2008). CHNs need to understand how Canada's health care system has evolved and what factors influence how it is governed. This understanding will increase nursing leadership, visibility, and influence at decision-making tables in organizations and all levels of the health care system. The impact of this leadership has been identified as a particularly significant factor in the evolution of the health care system and in supporting community health nursing practice (Bekemeier, Grembowski, Yang, & Herting, 2012; Cummings et al., 2010).

This chapter begins with a description of historical milestones in Canadian health care, with the responsibilities of the federal, provincial or territorial, regional, and municipal governments for health care in Canada. Second, we outline the paradigm shift to prevention, promotion, and the social determinants of health. Third, we describe the organization of community health services, including delivery models and funding mechanisms in Canada. Fourth, we examine the impact of power, policy, and politics on health equity and community health nursing practice. Then we discuss some challenges facing community health nursing practice, including the invisibility of CHNs in health care leadership and the lack of CHN role clarity. The chapter concludes with key messages about these issues.

HISTORICAL MILESTONES IN CANADIAN HEALTH CARE

Between the 16th and 18th centuries, tens of thousands of people immigrated to Canada in search of a better future. They had significant social issues as well as communicable diseases such as cholera and typhus. In 1832, the first quarantine station, known as Grosse Isle, located in the St. Lawrence River near Quebec City, was established to assess all newcomers and isolate those arriving with communicable diseases. It remained in operation until 1932 and is now a national historic park. The realization that individuals and communities could do something to stop the spread of disease and benefit from early detection was known as the "sanitary" idea.

Following Confederation in Canada, additional community health strategies were introduced, such as public education; gathering and analyzing statistics; sewage and drinking water management; and maternal, infant, and child health care. In 1882, Ontario became the first provincial government to establish a full-time provincial board of health (with a $4000 budget). The Hudson's Bay Company took on the role and functions of the public health board in western Canada.

The 1867 Constitution Act (also known as the British North America Act) did not explicitly assign responsibility for health policy to either the federal government or the provincial governments; rather, government ensured the availability of and funding for health services. The Act did contain an equalization clause requiring provinces to provide "reasonably comparable levels of public service for reasonably comparable levels of taxation" (Sullivan & Baranek, 2002, p. 21).

Tommy Douglas, "father of medicare" and member of the Cooperative Commonwealth Federation party, introduced legislation to institute **medicare**, or publicly funded health care, with the first policy implemented at the provincial level in Saskatchewan in 1947. Ten years later, similar legislation, the Hospital Insurance and Diagnostic Services Act (HIDS), was passed by the Government of Canada (Rachlis & Kushner, 1994) whereby the federal government paid half the costs of insurance plans if key criteria were met.

Because provincial and territorial wealth varies considerably, the federal government's involvement has been necessary to equalize services across provinces and territories. It has done this by contributing funds (transferring money from wealthier to poorer provinces and territories) and by stipulating specific conditions the provinces and territories must meet to receive those funds. On December 12, 1983, Monique Bégin, Federal Minister of Health and Welfare, introduced Bill C-3, or the Canada Health Act, to Parliament. This legislation was in existence for 30 years (to April 16, 2014) and provided direction for cash contributions made by the federal government for essential medical and hospital services. The purpose of the Act was to "establish criteria and conditions in respect of insured health services and extended healthcare services provided under provincial law that must be met before a full cash contribution may be made" (Canada, House of Commons, 1984, p. 5). Bégin faced tough opposition to the Act from lobby groups, opposition parties, and members of the Liberal cabinet (Bégin, 2002). Intense lobbying and support by the Canadian Nurses Association (CNA) was instrumental in the bill being passed. In the words of Bégin, "Nursing became a big player during the Canada Health Act. They made the difference; it's as simple as that" (Rafael, 1997). The CNA is the national professional voice of registered nurses in Canada. The invaluable support provided by Canadian nurses was acknowledged by the Honourable Monique Bégin at the Canadian Public Health Association (CPHA) conference in Toronto in June 2010. She noted that not only were nurses instrumental in passing the Canada Health Act into law, but they were also successful in having it amended. As it was introduced to Parliament in 1983, Bill C-3 identified only physicians as providers of insurable services. The CNA amendment changed the language to include other health care workers as potential providers of insurable services (Mussallem, 1992).

Under the Canada Health Act, federal funding for essential medical services would continue so long as the provinces' health insurance plans met five criteria: (1) **publicly administered** (accountable to the public), (2) **comprehensive** (must cover necessary in-hospital, medical, and surgical–dental services), (3) **universal** (available to all), (4) **portable** (available after a maximum of three months of residency, and no extra charge for care out of province), and (5) **accessible** (no user fees, and health care providers must be reimbursed adequately). The **Canada Health Act** has ensured that Canadians have access to health care regardless of their ability to pay or where they live. It is held up as a symbol of the values that represent Canada. It articulates a social contract that defines health care as a basic right and reflects the values of social justice, equity, and community (Auditor General of Canada, 2002).

Health promotion, prevention of disease and injury, health protection, and home health were not emphasized in the Canada Health Act. Tommy Douglas had envisioned a second, more ambitious phase to medicare—one with a focus on keeping people well, as he understood that illness prevention and improved health were essential to controlling health care costs (Campbell & Marchildon, 2007). To realize this vision, a shift in the focus from individual conditions and behaviours to the social and economic determinants of health, such as education, poverty, hunger, and inadequate housing, is required (McBane, 2004).

In October 2006, the CNA again spoke up, with the then president, Dr. Marlene Smadu, presenting to the House of Commons Standing Committee on Finance. This CNA presentation outlined the position of nurses in Canada, stating that health promotion, funding to address the determinants of health, and support for control of drug costs were considerations as important as wait times and fears about financial sustainability (CNA, 2006).

In assessing the degree to which the Canada Health Act has been successful in ensuring that all Canadians have access to the health care they need, we need to look at the purpose of the Act and the extent to which other aspects of health care addressed by the Act have been implemented. The Canada Health Act implicitly and explicitly suggests a broader purpose. For example, Section 3 of the Act endorses **health promotion**, stating that the "primary objective of Canadian healthcare policy" is twofold: to facilitate reasonable access to health services and "to protect, promote, and restore the physical and mental well-being of the residents of Canada" (Canada, House of Commons, 1984, Section 3, p. 5). Despite this, the focus on adequate funding of community health services has been limited. Because the Canada Health Act establishes that only medically necessary physician services and hospital services are publicly funded, services such as home care fall outside the legislation. Provision of the funding for these services lies within the jurisdiction of each province and territory.

Because protective, preventive, and health promotion services were not required to meet the five criteria of medicare, they were not subject to the conditions of the Act. These services were left unprotected by federal legislation and were provided largely by provincial and territorial public health systems, although it is well recognized that these services add a critical balance to the treatment-focused insured service delivery addressed by the Canada Health Act. Each province, territory, and region determines what services are covered and to what extent. The result has been varied and fragmented community health service across the country (Tsasis, 2009). Today, public health systems in Canada continue to be confronted by ideologies that favour efficiency, effectiveness, and short-term outcomes, which tend to overshadow health promotion and prevention values, strategies, and activities (Kirk, Tomm-Bonde, & Schreiber, 2014). Effective chronic disease prevention and management will require broad policy options, including amending the Canada Health Act; promoting interdisciplinary teamwork; and supporting further integration of public health, home care, and other sectors of the health care system (Tsasis, 2009). Palliative care and community mental

health services are areas that need to be strengthened within the Canada Health Act (Marchildon, 2005). The review of the Act will require the involvement of professionals, citizens, and communities to provide insight and direction for the delivery and funding of health care.

A PARADIGM SHIFT TO PREVENTION, PROMOTION, AND THE SOCIAL DETERMINANTS OF HEALTH

When the legislative pillars of Canadian medicare were enacted in 1957, 1966, and 1984, the biomedical model dominated public and political thinking about health. The clinical definition of health was "the absence of disease," and the term "health promotion" was often used interchangeably with "disease prevention." Labelling the illness-oriented, treatment-focused physician and hospital services that were insured under the Act as "health care" contributed to this confusion. As challenges to the idea that health was related exclusively to the country's illness emerged, the federal government responded and provided leadership for the development of health promotion policies and resources.

An important acknowledgement of the limitations of the primacy of the funded medical/treatment system in Canada was the Lalonde Report of 1974 (Lalonde, 1974). This bold report presented a vision for health promotion services as a critical component of Canada's health care system. The forward-thinking framework identified four determinants of health: environment, lifestyle, human biology, and the health care system. This was the first acknowledgement that health was influenced by the social, economic, and environmental conditions in which people lived, worked, and played. The Lalonde Report was considered revolutionary by the global community and led to a reconceptualization of health promotion.

In 1978, Canada and other countries around the world met at the International Conference on Primary Health Care in Alma-Ata, USSR. Governments were urged to take action to "protect and promote the health" of the people of the world, and the Declaration of Alma-Ata (WHO, 1978) was issued. Canada was a signatory. The goal of **primary health care** is the attainment of better health services for all, which will be discussed in Chapter 7. The CNA continues to advocate for primary health care policy and practice that is consistent with the principles outlined in the World Health Organization (WHO) declaration (CNA, 2012b).

Afterward, federal leadership in forming a health promotion policy continued. In 1986, the federal Minister of Health, the Honourable Jake Epp, published "Achieving Health for All: A Framework for Health Promotion" (Epp, 1986), also known as the "Epp Framework." The Epp Framework expanded Lalonde's definition of health promotion, incorporated some of the tenets of primary health care, and emphasized the role of broad social, environmental, and political **determinants of health** (conditions that contribute to disease and disability). It concluded with a denouncement of strategies that focus on individual responsibility for health, or "blaming the victim," while ignoring the social and economic determinants.

The Epp Framework formed the basis for the Ottawa Charter for Health Promotion that emerged from the First International Conference on Health Promotion, hosted by the federal government in Ottawa in November 1986 (Epp, 1986). The Ottawa Charter (WHO, 1986), authored jointly by Health Canada, the CPHA, and the WHO, identified prerequisites for health, strategies for promoting health, and outcomes of those strategies (Kirk et al., 2014). The release of the Ottawa Charter marked a dramatic shift in health promotion. Peace, education, shelter, income, and food were among the determinants identified, and this broader view of health shifted the focus from providing illness care and identifying risk factors to an inclusive approach that also focused on socioenvironmental factors.

The Ottawa Charter acknowledged that caring for one's self and others is conducive to health, and it identified caring, holism, and ecology as essential concepts in health promotion (WHO, 1986). Federal government support for health promotion through policy making and development of resources has continued. Many of the resources that have been developed, such as the Population Health Template (Health Canada, 2001) and the Population Health Promotion Model (Hamilton & Bhatti, 1996), have been used to guide policy development and the practice and education of CHNs.

More than 30 years after the Declaration of Alma-Ata, the eighth Global Conference on Health Promotion was held in Helsinki in June 2013. At this international conference, participants affirmed that "Health for All is a major societal goal of governments and the cornerstone of sustainable development" (WHO, 2013, p. 1). (See Yes, But Why? box.) They called for a "Health in All Policies" approach and a commitment to equity in health. Health in All Policies is an approach to public policies across sectors that systematically takes into account the health implications of decisions, seeks synergies, and avoids harmful health impacts to improve population health and health equity. It improves accountability of policymakers for health impacts at all levels of policymaking. It includes an emphasis on the consequences of public policies on health systems and determinants of health and well-being (WHO, 2013).

health care systems. There is growing interest to address these structural determinants of health with strategies that include the implementation of Health in All Policies (HiAP) (Shankardass et al., 2018).

So What?

A 2008 report by Canada's chief public health officer noted that health inequalities and the social determinants of health can be addressed through public policy, individual action, and collective action (Butler-Jones, 2008). Studies have shown that these disparities are associated with structural differences, such as income, employment and working conditions, housing, education, food security, social inclusion, and the environment—the social determinants of health. Although targeted efforts to address the policy-level issues implicated in these determinants of health calls for a population health approach that includes both sociocultural values and government policies and processes, the complex nature of government institutions and their policy processes makes it difficult to tackle. HiAP is a tool to bolster health equity through inter-sectoral public policy efforts (Shankardass et al., 2018). It involves establishing governance structures and processes to enable effective evidence-based policy coordination and implementation. A HiAP approach is essential and helps avoid situations such as dropping compulsory physical education from schools or closing mental-health institutions without providing community services (CNA, 2013). HiAP can foster economic growth, productivity, and prosperity, while the health benefits are many: healthy children perform well in school, and citizens are more productive and more engaged in their communities (Keon & Pépin, 2009).

Now What?

CHNs need to advocate for the health of individuals living in Canada as core responsibility of government. Governments need to consider the consequences on population health of the policies, legislation, and programs they are developing. CHNs need to develop strategies to influence these government policies and processes at strategic points in their development and implementation. HiAP initiatives involve the use of diverse health equity interventions across multiple policy sectors. Therefore, CHNs need to use tools such as intersectionality lens to examine and influence the multiple stakeholders involved in HiAP initiatives and other policy processes.

CHNC Standards of Practice Fulfilled

#1 Promoting Health
- Considers the determinants of health, the social and political context, and systemic structures in collaboration with the client to determine action.

#7 Health Equity
- Advocates for healthy public policy and social justice by participating in legislative and policy-making activities that influence determinants of health and access to services (CHNC, 2019, revised).

YES, BUT WHY?

Health in All Policies (HiAP): A Tool for Population Health

What?

In Canada, broad sectors of public policy and legislation such as education policy; transportation, including highways and roads; environment; communication; natural resources; income security; and foreign trade are developed with little or no consideration for their population health implications. A policy with negative consequences for the health of the populations will put an extra burden on the economy and

ORGANIZATION OF COMMUNITY HEALTH CARE

"A strong community health system has the potential to effectively and efficiently address disease and injury issues upstream to prevent them from occurring, delay their onset, or care for those affected closer to home to restore health" (CHNC, 2011a, p. 17). Many factors influence how community health nursing is organized and delivered across Canada, including emerging diseases and health emergencies. Recommendations to address the central importance of public health in preventing the spread of diseases were highlighted in several reports. These include the Expert Panel on severe acute respiratory syndrome (SARS) and Infectious Disease Control (Walker, 2004), the National Advisory Committee on SARS and Public Health (Naylor, 2003) and two interim SARS Commission Reports (Campbell, 2004, 2005). As well, there was consensus that the water contamination in Walkerton, Ontario, in 2000 was a "wake-up call" for Canadian public health and occurred because "institutions vital to the infrastructure of public health were neglected" (Schabas, 2002, p. 1282). These reports posed questions about and made recommendations for funding, governance, and management of public health in Canada. The researchers monitored a series of communicable disease outbreaks, and their focus was on the health system's ability to respond adequately given the impact of the outbreaks on the communities, the health care system, and the economy.

Public Health Agency of Canada (PHAC)

The Public Health Agency of Canada (PHAC) was created in 2004 to deliver on the federal government's commitment to help protect the health and safety of all Canadians through activities that focus on preventing chronic diseases and injuries, responding to public health emergencies and infectious disease outbreaks, and strengthening the practice of public health in Canada. Confirmed as a legal entity in December 2006 through the Public Health Agency of Canada Act, it reports to the Parliament of Canada through the Minister of Health. National collaborating centres were created through the PHAC to strengthen the practice of public health across the country and integrate research into the delivery of services at the community level.

Each province and territory also examined the capacity of the public health component within their jurisdictional health care systems. Public health is not standardized across the provinces and territories, and each has a chief medical officer of health. There is a limited number of Indigenous-specific policies and frameworks. According to Lavoie (2013), "the federal policy framework informing issues of jurisdiction over Indigenous health is thin and loosely woven," and some provinces have no specific legislative framework for the responsibilities of health care in Indigenous communities. Ontario was the first province to develop an Indigenous Health and Wellness Strategy in 1990 and to develop the overarching Aboriginal Health Policy in 1994 (Ontario Ministry of Health and Long-Term Care, 2018). In Ontario, for example, the provincial government launched Operation Health Protection in 2003 (Ontario Ministry of Health and Long-Term Care, 2004), a three-year plan to rebuild public health. The intent was to address gaps in infectious disease control and broader concerns related to disease prevention and health promotion. Related activities included the establishment of two provincial committees to move public health renewal forward. The first committee, the Capacity Review Committee, was to assess and make recommendations as to the capacity and organizational framework for public health, and the second was to provide recommendations and a plan to establish a provincial arm's-length agency that would focus on research and practice excellence in public health (i.e., the application of research findings into the delivery of public health interventions).

Community Health Services

Most Canadian provinces and territories have moved to regional health authority structures for all health service delivery. This approach strives to integrate most or all health services (including CHN services) into a single organization. The timing, organization, and, in many cases, repeated reorganization of the regional health authorities and health regions have been unique to each province or territory. While community health services are organized and delivered differently across Canada, each province and territory provides primary health care, primary care, public health, and home care services. These are briefly discussed in the following sections.

1. Primary Health Care and Primary Care **Primary care** is a core component of primary health care but is focused on the services accessed at the first point of contact with the health system. The primary care system is the "first line" of clinical services that provides an entry point to the health care system. Primary care teams produce better health outcomes, improve access to services, ensure the most efficient use of resources, and lead to greater satisfaction for patients and providers. Primary care teams can achieve efficiencies by allowing each team member to function at the top of his or her skill set. Inter-professional teams are not only essential to providing comprehensive, continuous, and person-centred care to patients but are also critical in the mobilization of health care resources and assisting patients to navigate the health care system.

Primary care services across Canada have undergone major reforms in the past decade, responding to demographic changes, advances in health care and disease management strategies, and mounting evidence that strong systems are associated with better and more equitable health outcomes. Many of the reforms remain incomplete, and the potential improvement for patients, communities, and the health system has yet to occur.

A major obstacle to improving primary care through inter-professional teams is the lack of role clarity that has resulted from many professions joining together with little preparation or understanding of the other professions and of interprofessional practice. Reports and analysis of changes and improvements in the Canadian health systems suggest that these systems have achieved limited transformation and improvement in key areas where major care deficits persist, such as primary care, management of chronic diseases, home care, and mental health.

To be patient-centred and encourage complete care, primary care models are moving to incorporate different remuneration models. Many are characterized by blended payment arrangements, contractual requirements to provide a defined set of services, patient enrolment or rostering, and, in some cases, incentives and bonuses. Nurses working in primary care settings are almost exclusively salary-based. Investing in primary care would result in a health system that is more responsive to community needs by enabling screening, earlier diagnosis, and treatment; better management of chronic diseases; timely access to care by utilizing all available entry points to care; and a healthier population. Investment is still needed to support high-performing primary care models for a geographically and socioeconomically diverse population despite numerous initiatives across Canada introduced to strengthen infrastructure, improve access to after-hours care, and offer alternative funding models.

2. Public Health Whereas hospital and physicians' services have been governed by federal legislation for the last half of the 20th century, public health was decentralized at the outset. As a result, across Canada, the legal obligations and associated regulatory requirements for public health services are established under the provinces or territories. Therefore, funding for public health services generally involves a combination of regional, provincial, or territorial funds. The five main principles in the Canada Health Act have been hallmarks of Canadian public health services: comprehensiveness, universality, portability, public administration, and accessibility.

Health is greatly influenced by the environment, social factors, and access to health services (Bharmal, Pitkin, Felician, & Weden, 2015). Long before illness, health starts where we live, learn, work, and play. The social determinants of health, such as income, employment, housing, education, early child development, and social inclusion, affect people's lifestyle choices and their opportunities for optimal health (Robert Wood Johnson Foundation, 2010). Public health plays a critical role in the comprehensive system of care, including health and social services. The overarching goal of **public health** is to enhance and optimize the health status of communities and promote health equity. The core functions of public health are to assess population health status, protect and promote health, and prevent disease and injury. The discipline of public health is often cited as being at its best when invisible: doing its job well and preventing bad things like disease outbreaks that garner attention when they happen. Public health is now viewed as a sector that is embraced and increasingly called upon by the community. The changing societal recognition of the role of public health is resulting in a growing reliance on public health nursing in emergencies or situations that require an enhanced community response. SARS, listeriosis, and H1N1 are obvious examples. Public health nurses (PHNs) are being called upon to support situations that affect the physical, psychological, and social health and well-being of people, including flood

evacuations, food security during transit disruptions, resettlement of refugees, naloxone training of first-line responders, enforcement of immunization legislation, institutional flu, and gastrointestinal outbreak management. These examples illustrate the unique public health nursing contribution, including (a) conducting situational population health assessments to inform proactive and reactive response; (b) identifying populations affected by health threats or disproportionately experiencing negative health status or health impacts; and (c) leveraging their relationships with professionals, clients, and other stakeholders to drive collaboration and partnership to address the health needs.

PHNs have a rich history of providing service to some of the most vulnerable members in our communities. This is an excellent catalyst to propel practitioners into the next frontier of service to address specific barriers in disadvantaged neighbourhoods that make healthy behaviour choices challenging. PHNs can identify the social and economic factors, physical environment, and individual behaviours and conditions that affect health. They are in a unique position to be leaders of system change to foster excellent population health at all stages of life and in all neighbourhoods. See the Case Study that follows.

CASE STUDY

Alcohol is a widely used psychoactive substance in communities across Canada. Dependence on alcohol and its associated harms create public health and other societal problems. Vodina is an 18-year-old boy who lives with his mother in a two-bedroom public housing apartment in an Ottawa neighbourhood. His mother is unmarried and unemployed. They live on welfare assistance, which is barely adequate to cover food, rent, and transportation. They often visit the food bank to make ends meet. To supplement the family income, Vodina, who has not yet completed high school, has been doing odd jobs around their neighbourhood. However, his mother noticed he does not bring any money home. Instead, she found empty bottles of alcohol under his bed, and when she confronted him, he confessed to drinking alcohol regularly. His mother is worried and requested that he seek help from the local community health centre. During Vodina's first visit, the CHN noticed that he appeared anxious, flushed, and shabby. The CHN was concerned about his dry skin, brittle hair and fingernails, and the excessive smell of alcohol from his breath during his physical examination. Vodina told the CHN he drinks to help him deal with his mother's unpredictable temper.

Discussion Questions

1. How is health inequity implicated in this case?
2. What is the role of CHNs in addressing alcohol dependency?
3. What combination of policy and public health interventions could be used to reduce alcohol-related harms?

3. Cultural Competence Cultural competence is an important contribution to reducing health inequities and improving health outcomes. In Canada, it is absolutely critical for practitioners to understand the unique needs of individuals who experience marginalization such as First Nation, Inuit, and Métis peoples. Although the onus is on practitioners to provide culturally safe health services, the public health system can play a significant role to support health care organizations in the provision of culturally competent policies, structures, procedures, and practices (Antonello et al., 2016). Service barriers have been highlighted in Ontario's Urban Indigenous Action Plan Discussion Paper and the priorities of the Champlain Local Health Integrated Network's Indigenous Health Circle Forum. A growing body of research demonstrates the pervasive nature of racism against Indigenous peoples within the health care system, and scholars suggest that institutional racism has led to health disparities experienced by Indigenous peoples. According to the Health Council of Canada (2012), "this is one barrier to good health that lies squarely in the lap of the health care system itself. Many Aboriginal people don't trust—and therefore don't use—mainstream health care services because they don't feel safe from stereotyping and racism, and because the Western approach to health care can feel alienating and intimidating" (p. 1). Ensuring access to culturally safe health services has been identified as an essential part of any strategy to advance Indigenous health care equity. Although emerging evidence of the benefits of a culturally safe approach is promising, scientific evidence is currently scarce, largely qualitative, and anecdotal. From the perspective of Indigenous traditional knowledge, the evidence base for cultural safety is deeply rooted in traditional teachings, with relationships based on trust, acceptance, and safety seen as vital to the healing process.

Cultural safety training for health service providers is a critical next step. It is both an outcome defined by those who receive the service and a respectful process that pays explicit attention to understanding the historical, sociopolitical, and environmental context; the power imbalances inherent in health service delivery; and the need to fix these inequities through education and system change (Brascoupé & Waters, 2009). Multiple opportunities to reflect on one's own attitudes, beliefs, assumptions, and values, while addressing interpersonal and systemic racism toward Indigenous peoples, is required. Cultural safety training acknowledges history and responds to the Truth and Reconciliation Commission of Canada: Calls to Action (Truth and Reconciliation Commission of Canada, 2015) and other reconciliation-related priorities identified by the federal Department of Indigenous and Northern Affairs Canada as well as Ontario's Patients First approach and its commitment to Indigenous cultural competency and anti-racism training. As noted by Richmond and Cook (2016), the concept of reconciliation is a "fundamental precursor" for Indigenous health equity. In particular, the process of reconciliation fosters ongoing learning opportunities for health service providers, and addresses knowledge deficits related to the history, diversity, and contributions of Indigenous peoples. It also addresses the current impact of inter generational trauma and systemic racism on local Indigenous health outcomes.

CHNs can support the necessary system changes to improve access to culturally safe services for Indigenous peoples by promoting cultural safety training to each other and their respective health care organizations. CHNs can also use their skills in collaboration and partnership to work with local Elders, knowledge keepers, academic and education partners, curriculum developers, and community mobilizers and group facilitators to develop training that integrates relevant models of health and wellness for Indigenous peoples.

4. Home Care Health Canada defines **home care** as "a wide range of health services delivered at home and throughout the community to recovering, disabled, chronically, or terminally ill persons in need of medical, nursing, social, or therapeutic treatment and/or assistance with the essential activities of daily living" (Health Canada, 2010). The CHNC says, "Home health nurses are committed to the provision of accessible, responsive, and timely care which allows people to stay in their homes with safety and dignity" (CHNC, 2010c, p. 4).

Home care is not an insured health service under the Canada Health Act. Specifically, the Act does not require governments to provide or fund treatments given at home, although all governments offer basic coverage for home care, and some fund a broader range of services (Romanow, 2002a). This lack of legislative framework results in a wide variation in access to and availability of home care services across Canada (Canadian Institute for Health Information [CIHI], 2010). There is also wide variation in the availability of supportive services for individuals with long-term chronic conditions, which may include home support, homemaking, and options for assisted-living facilities. Provinces and territories differ in access to medical supplies, equipment, and drugs. In some jurisdictions these items must be paid for privately, either through a co-payment arrangement or entirely by the individual. While all home care services are provided based on assessed need, there is variation in the limits of home care services across Canada.

Several factors impact the need for a new approach to the provision of home health care:

- Canada is an aging nation with increasing rates of chronic disease.
- Across the country, there has been a reduction in numbers of family caregivers and support networks, and a decline in community support and volunteerism.
- Challenges exist in the recruitment and retention of health care workers.
- Increased use of technology for clients, providers, and the system allows for more home care.
- Governments recognize the need for a greater role for the home and community care sector and its critical function in terms of the efficiency and effectiveness of health systems given the rising costs of health care, greater strains on public health expenditures, and lower funding allocation for home- and community-based care (Canadian Healthcare Association, 2009).

The increase in use of and funding for home care has been attributed to several factors, most significantly the belief that services provided in the home are less costly and a more desirable means of delivering necessary care. These claims have yet to be proven. Another issue is that as the services shift to the home and community, they shift beyond the boundaries of public insurance (Deber, 2003). All of the provinces offer a package of basic services, but there are significant provincial variations in the degree to which services are publicly funded versus privately financed. This results in significant inequity in accessing publicly funded home care across different regions of the country. Although the actual figure is difficult to verify, the Canadian Alliance for Sustainable Heath Care (2012) calculated that private payment (a combination of out-of-pocket payment and private insurance coverage) for home care services in Canada was close to $2 million and represented approximately 23% of total home care expenditures in 2010. Savings associated with the provision of services in the home versus in an acute care setting may not reflect an actual decrease in cost so much as a transfer of costs to patients and their families (Shah, 2003).

POLICY, POLITICS, AND POWER IN HEALTH EQUITY AND CHN PRACTICE

Community health nursing practice occurs in a sociopolitical environment. CHNs work in a variety of settings, including community health centres, nursing homes, long-term care facilities, schools, government organizations, and other health care facilities outlined in Chapter 3. These are political environments where resources are finite, and CHNs must have the political savviness necessary to influence the allocation of resources for healthy workplaces and better client care (Mason, Gardner, Outlaw, & O'Grady, 2016). **Policy** guides the work of community health nursing, and policy making is carried out within a political context. **Politics** is "the use of relationship and power to gain ascendancy among stakeholders to influence policy and the allocation of scarce resources" (Mason et al., 2016, p. 10), and **power** is "the ability to act so as to achieve a goal" (p. 18). In the policy process, power is knowing the different players: who has power, who serves on key decision-making tables, and who are the thought leaders (Mason et al., 2016). These three concepts are analyzed within the context of **health equity** and **social justice** in community health nursing practice in this section.

Health Inequity

Community health nursing practice occurs in a milieu where multiple level policies, forces, and programs enable and support or interfere with and impede the ability of communities to address the conditions that lead to health inequity (Weinstein, Geller, Negussie, & Baciu, 2017). **Health inequity** refers to differences in health that are unnecessary, avoidable, unfair, and unjust or the absence of systematic disparities in health between social groups who have different levels of underlying social advantage or disadvantage (Braveman & Gruskin, 2003).

For example, on average, girl babies have a lower birth weight than boy babies; this is considered natural, biological variation and not associated with different health outcomes. Babies born to low-income mothers also have lower birth weight, but this is typically due to poorer nutrition, inadequate prenatal care, and other factors that are changeable. Thus, this is considered inequity.

Health equity means every person has an opportunity to achieve optimal health regardless of the colour of their skin, level of education, gender identity, sexual orientation, the job they have, the neighbourhood they live in, and whether or not they have a disability (Braveman, 2006). Health inequities within and between populations are produced and sustained through multiple, interconnected, and complex pathways. These pathways include complex interactions among biological, lifestyle, environmental, social, and economic circumstances—in other words, the social determinants of health and bad policies and politics. Health equity is undermined when these social conditions interact to prevent people from making decisions or taking actions that would promote health. Despite Canada's universal health care system, marginalized populations such as immigrants and refugees continue to experience barriers to accessing the health system (Ng, Pottie, & Spitzer, 2011; Pottie et al., 2011). Racialized people experience a disproportionately high burden of diseases and experience higher rates of mortality (Smylie, Fell, Ohlsson, & the Joint Working Group on First Nations, Indian, Inuit, and Métis Infant Mortality of the Canadian Perinatal Surveillance System, 2010). Smylie and colleagues (Smylie et al., 2010) found significant disparities persist in the infant mortality rates for First Nation, Inuit, and Métis babies when compared with the general Canadian population.

According to Marmot (2011), the unequal distribution of health that leads to health inequities is not "natural"; instead it is the result of toxic combinations of poor social policies and programs, unfair economic arrangements, and bad politics. To effectively navigate this complex policy environment, CHNs must acknowledge the sociopolitical processes that have implications for their practice at the micro (individual client) and macro (system) levels. As Mason, Gardner, Outlaw, and O'Grady (2016) assert, while the public needs to recognize nurses' important contribution to health care, nurses themselves must be prepared to fully engage in the important work and decisions of health and health care. It is not enough for nurses to influence service delivery at the point of care alone; they must be present at the tables where decisions are made. For example, although a CHN may practice in a culturally safe and competent manner with Indigenous and other racialized peoples, the values of Western health care models and systems may still undermine the health and well-being of these historically marginalized communities. The impetus is for CHNs to understand how policy and politics impact on the quality, safety, and accessibility of patient care and their working conditions.

Strategies to effectively address the challenges confronting community health nursing practice must target the many dimensions of causal pathways to inequities in health and health care. CHNs must unpack the many layers of the societal forces that create inequities in the system. Health equity work is deeply rooted in social justice. Community health nursing practice occurs "at that intersection where societal attitudes, government policies, and people's lives meet …[and] creates a moral imperative not only to attend to the health needs of the public but also, like Nightingale, to work to change the societal conditions contributing to poor health" (Falk-Rafael, 2005).

Social Justice

Social justice is "the view that everyone deserves equal rights and opportunities—this includes the right to good health." It suggests that "inequities in health are avoidable, unnecessary and unjust" (American Public Health Association [APHA], 2017). Fairness in the way we treat people or make decisions are core aspects of social justice. As CHNs, we must explicate the reasonableness of how common advantages and burdens are distributed. Racism and other forms of "isms" are forces that determine the distribution of the social determinants of health (APHA, 2017). A key part of ensuring good health for all is identifying and enhancing systemic disadvantage. Community organizations that have internal capacity anchored in social justice work in true partnership with communities to conduct equity-informed research, engage in policy change, and ensure programs and services meet the needs of diverse communities. Using a social justice lens involves collaborative partnership, intersectionality, and capacity building at all levels. A key focus of health equity work has been health and social policies (Mason et al., 2016). Politics shape institutional and public policy at every stage of its design and implementation. An understanding of politics and policy making would enhance CHNs' ability to intervene effectively during strategic points in the policy-making and implementation processes. Given that most health problems begin long before people seek health care, it is important for CHNs to be knowledgeable about the political aspects of the social determinants of health.

An understanding of the policy process is necessary for CHNs to advance healthier communities, strengthen the health care system, and advocate for an environment to effectively care for people with equity and skill. Mason and colleagues (2016, p. 4) assert that "Just as Florence Nightingale understood that health policy held the key to improving the health of poor Londoners and the British Military, so are today's nurses needed to create compelling cases and actively influence better health policies at every level of governance."

More recently, the Institute of Medicine (2011) reported on the future of nursing and called for CHNs to develop their internal capacity anchored in social justice, work in true partnership with communities to conduct equity-informed research, engage in policy change, and ensure programs and services meet the needs of diverse communities. One approach to addressing the needs of an increasingly diverse Canadian population is through effective integration of internationally educated nurses (IENs). (See Canadian Research 2.1.) CHNs' ability to shape this diverse work environment involves taking

an active role in evolving health care for positive impacts on the health of communities. Their action is often met with multiple challenges and barriers.

Power

The use of power requires "raising one's awareness about what is true and what is false. Being grounded in truth such as knowing the value of human caring and the role that nursing can have on individuals and populations" (Mason et al., 2016, p. 19). This is personal integrity and a form of power that is necessary for nursing to advance its policy agenda.

CANADIAN RESEARCH 2.1

Workforce diversity as a critical enabler for IENs' integration and health equity work (Ramji & Etowa, 2018)

Immigrants are a substantial part of the labour markets in most Western countries. In 2012, about 7% of the 365 422 nurses in Canada had graduated from an international nursing program (CIHI, 2012). In Ontario, Canada's largest province, IENs made up over 12% of the nursing workforce that year (CIHI, 2012). The growing number of Internationally Educated Nurses (IENs) is a reflection of the increasingly diverse Canadian population, and it has been a resource for increasing diversity in Canadian nursing. Organizational factors such as **workforce diversity**, leadership commitment to health equity, and community engagement serve as critical enablers for IENs' integration and effective cross-cultural care. Workforce diversity involves the recruitment and retention of diverse employees and organizational policies and practices that foster openness, acceptance, and camaraderie. Although the organizational priority of workforce diversity may be impressive, if policies and practices are left as neutral, they maintain the privilege of those who have traditionally held power and can have adverse impacts on historically marginalized people. Ramji and Etowa's (2018) instrumental qualitative case study approach informed by critical social theory revealed the dimensions of IENs' integration and the role of workforce diversity in workplace integration. They assert that workforce diversity is a key factor in "creating openness, acceptance, camaraderie and a sense of belonging for IENs" (p. 14). They found that integration of IENs is a two-way process requiring efforts on the part of the IENs and employer organizations alike. They highlight the significance of leadership commitment and organizational policies in managing workforce diversity and addressing equity.

Discussion Questions

1. Identify barriers to workplace integration of IENs.
2. What are the critical enablers of effective IEN integration?
3. What are the potential impacts of workplace diversity on health equity and community health nursing practice as whole?

Nursing as a profession has been historically marginalized, resulting in limited power in organized health care especially at the policy (macro) level. Nurses by the virtue of the body of knowledge they possess exert power over their clients, particularly at the micro-political level. Contemporary nurses are demonstrating power in a number of ways, including but not limited to the following:

- The authority that comes with the possession of knowledge ("knowledge is power")
- Legal power that is associated with the legitimatization of nursing roles (e.g., nurse practitioner)
- Changed self-perceptions to accept one's own ideas or the ideas of other nursing leaders instead of those imposed by others
- More involvement in the political process, labour unions, and organizational lobbying efforts

Power as an interpersonal construct involves the give and take or mutual exchange that occurs in interactions and is generally achieved through one party having a "base." This base can be information, reward, or coercion, which constitutes their power over others. Individual power is exercised within wider social structures and relationships (Hugman, 1991). CHNs' consistent contact and intimate knowledge of community health needs situate them in position of power that could be used to advocate for positive change (Buresh & Gordon, 2006). From this perspective, nurses do exert power, and it is usually exercised through the language they use in nurse–client interactions. Efforts to address health equity must also tackle power imbalance, the micro politics of social rituals, and the structural underpinnings that reinforce and perpetuate power relations. Also, more emphasis is placed on health policy. An upstream approach to health equity has a broader focus on the social determinants of health. **Policy and political competence** encompass the knowledge, skills, and behaviours that improve performance (Mason et al., 2016). This means CHNs should be sufficiently prepared to perform in the policy and political arenas. Traditionally nurses did not consider "playing politics" as critical for health care leadership; today they must advocate for others and influence policy (Ferris, Davidson, & Perrewe, 2005).

Community health nursing needs to address health equity using a social justice lens to unpack the many layers of societal forces that create health inequities, including analysis of the policy, political processes, and power dynamics surrounding policy making and implementation of effective programs. This includes building internal leadership capacity anchored in social justice and intersectionality, working in true partnership with stakeholders to conduct equity-informed research, engaging in policy change, and ensuring programs and services meet the needs of diverse communities. Nurses have traditionally shied away from politics. In today's health care arena, political awareness, political actions, and strategic use of the power of nursing to influence policy must become cornerstones of community nursing practice, education, and research.

CHALLENGES IN COMMUNITY HEALTH NURSING PRACTICE

Over the past decade, there has been significant growth in research and literature that describes the current situation for CHNs across Canada. The literature points to the strengths CHNs bring to positively influencing the health of individuals, families, communities, and society as a whole. It also paints a picture of numerous challenges, including health system challenges, lack of role clarity, need for strong leadership, and issues in interprofessional relationships.

Health System Challenges

Although nursing is the largest health care profession with great potential power, like many professions, it has struggled to increase its visibility and to collaborate with other stakeholders to influence health policy. CHNs' ability to shape this complex health care environment by playing an active role for positive impacts on the health of communities is often met with multiple challenges and barriers. For example, despite numerous calls for strengthening primary health care (Romanow, 2002b) and shifting toward community health and preventive care, an emphasis on illness care provided in institutions remains the current paradigm (Mahony & Jones, 2013). Inadequate funding and resources for disease prevention and health promotion remain an issue, and what exists is under constant and real threat. The lack of stable, long-term funding is cited as a major barrier to effective practice and service delivery (Dingley & Yoder, 2013; Underwood et al., 2009). CHNs themselves identify as priority in terms of the need for advocacy and collective action to shape system change (CHNC, 2010a; CHNC, 2011a; Schofield et al., 2011).

Role Clarity

Despite its long and rich history, community health nursing is in a vulnerable position today. The CHNC, the national voice to promote community health nursing in Canada, conducted a survey in 2008 to establish a vision for community health nursing in the year 2020 in Canada (CHNC, 2009a; Schofield et al., 2011). This visioning initiative included a national survey and several focus groups that included CHNs in different regions across Canada. The resulting "Community Health Nursing Vision 2020: Shaping the Future" (CHNC, 2009a) contains expressions of how community nurses experience their roles. For example, one CHN said, "I think public health nurses are undervalued by the community, by the consumer, by the nursing profession, by colleagues in different areas of nursing . . . people view it (community health nursing) as not really nursing, while it is really and truly the highest level of nursing that you're going to do (p. 9)."

This undervaluing mirrors the diminished funding and resources of previous decades. Others have identified the relative invisibility of CHNs. Two such examples can be found in post-SARS national and provincial reports. Campbell's report spoke generally of the public health system as "broken and need[ing] to be fixed . . . [T]he overall system is woefully inadequate . . . unprepared, fragmented, poorly led, uncoordinated, inadequately resourced, professionally impoverished and generally incapable of discharging its mandate" (Campbell, 2005, p. 24). Naylor (2003), in his report "Learning from SARS: Renewal of Public Health in Canada," stated that "the essential role of public health nurses throughout and following SARS received little attention" (p. 131).

Role clarity includes components such as shared common language to describe the role, working to the full scope of practice within the role, and an understanding of the role by others within the health system and the public. The ability to describe with confidence the CHN's role can contribute to a greater valuing of it by other professionals, the community, and the policy makers. The need for greater role clarity for CHNs is consistently noted in the literature (Brookes, Davidson, Daly, & Hancock, 2004; Kulbok, Thatcher, Park, & Meszaros, 2012), and this provides the basis for articulating the value of community health nursing.

Across Canada, there are differences in how CHNs are identified on official registration forms and in organizational structures, and therefore enumeration of CHNs is difficult. It remains unknown how many nurses actually work in the various sectors of community health and any associated demographics. A 2010 synthesis paper reviewed eight recent community health nursing reports, examining the common issues associated with community health nursing (CHNC, 2010b). Of the eight reports reviewed, seven specifically identified role clarity as an issue. As clear professional roles are foundational to a strong health care system and the ability to work effectively on interprofessional teams, CHNs, the organizations within which they work, and the professional associations that support them must continue to address this challenge. In response to this issue, the CPHA and CHNC released an updated role document for public health nursing in Canada (CPHA, 2010) to provide a common vision for the role and activities of CHN, including public health nursing in Canada.

Leadership

Leadership is a challenge contributing to the invisibility of CHNs. Leadership is about identifying a problem or new condition that requires a change, and then identifying the vision and skills to affect change and influencing and motivating others toward action. Although leadership is not limited to senior executives who occupy formal leadership positions, they are important decision makers and allies. Nurses are among the most trusted providers of information. CHNs are educators, seasoned collaborators, skilled communicators, and critical thinkers, and their intimate knowledge of health in communities equip them with the skills necessary to close health equity gaps through more visible leadership roles at decision-making tables. Although their client- and community-centric practice and advocacy work provide CHNs with a unique advantage in the leadership context, the perception of nursing profession as subservient jeopardizes its leadership role in community health and policy development platforms. Lack of public understanding of the nature of CHN work, lack of appreciation of CHN

expertise, and lack of value of their input marginalizes CHN voices in health leadership tables (Cusack, 2012). Recent studies reveal the marginal representation of CHNs in some health platforms. As Devereaux (2016) noted in her Knowledge-Power-Resistance Framework, the wealth of knowledge CHNs possess often remains untapped, including during public health crises such as the HINI pandemic. She further asserted that although PHNs played a key role in addressing the H1N1 crisis, operational decisions during the crisis were not based on these nurses' expertise, and there was limited acknowledgement in the pandemic documents of their central role in the success of the H1N1 immunization program. Similarly, MacNevin (2018) examined the role of PHNs in food insecurity work and found that while PHNs are ideally positioned to assume a leadership role in the monitoring efforts to address food insecurity, they often limited to frontline roles. As a PHN in MacNevin's study asserts, "if public health nurses are to assume a monitoring role in addressing health inequities at the [system redesign level], their role must expand beyond the realm of direct patient care" (p. 146).

This marginal CHN presence in health care leadership platforms calls for change. The accelerating pace of social change, including the evolving digital world, evolution of knowledge- and evidence-informed practices, and changing client preferences are a few of the more common drivers of change. Leaders recognize when these environmental changes create new future opportunities requiring organizations or teams to act and think in different ways. Leadership is proposed as a strategy that all CHNs can embrace and develop.

Leaders are acutely sensitive to the realities of navigating an organization or community with multiple legitimate but often competing priorities. Influencing others to take action is no small task. It requires a deliberate communication process that considers the strength of evidence and facts of the situation; the credibility, trust, and confidence that the leader holds; and the perception of risk and emotional investment of stakeholders (i.e., clients, funders, administrators, public, and employees). New ideas or actions constitute an opportunity to capitalize on stakeholders' attention and engagement. Despite the strongest evidence, it may still be very difficult for leaders to influence change. The process of influence allows a leader to build common ground that enables momentum to be created. Leaders are then required to continuously adapt their approach as they gain perspective from stakeholders, harnessing their enthusiasm and the enthusiasm and commitment of colleagues. One example of a tactic to begin the process of communicating to influence is the 4 Box Strategic Influencing Model (Harris, 2014). This model involves a series of steps to communicate change: (a) describing the rationale for change, (b) communicating benefits of the change, (c) addressing the disadvantage of the change, and (d) stating what is not changing and will remain the same.

Leaders know it is impossible to achieve change in isolation. It is critically important for leaders to foster relationships with community partners, decision makers, and funders. Leadership occurs within relationships, so understanding the impact of one's behaviour on others and being able to moderate and modify that behaviour or style are essential to effectively steering people and organizations toward a vision (Willcocks, 2012). Creating and articulating a clear purpose and vision is critical, and to do

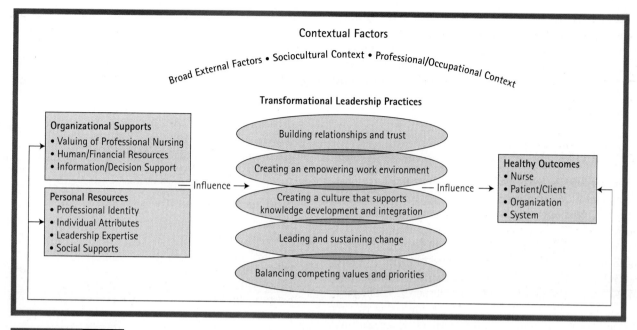

FIGURE 2.1 Conceptual Model for Developing and Sustaining Leadership

Source: RNAO (2013).

that effectively, CHNs must be able to see the long view, incorporating multiple aspects of the communities, the political environment, and the larger health and social systems. Conceptualizing oneself such that leadership is seen as a dimension of practice for all nurses is important to building leadership capacity in community health nursing (Scott & Miles, 2013). A lifetime commitment of self-reflecting on one's beliefs, strengths, weaknesses, and style of relating to others is required of effective leaders.

Leaders must remain flexible and dynamic on how to achieve overarching goals. A fundamental principle that enables this is humility. This includes the ability to listen to and embrace the wisdom of others. Effective leaders also bring energy, enthusiasm, and humour to the process and to the tasks at hand while remaining outcome-oriented (Brody, Barnes, Ruble, & Sakowski, 2012; Cummings et al., 2010). The literature does not identify people from any single discipline as having superior leadership skills; rather, each brings a unique set of perspectives, experiences, knowledge, skills, and attitudes that can be used to develop effective and collaborative leadership.

The outcomes of leadership have been described extensively. One such document is the Registered Nurses Association of Ontario's "Best Practice Guideline: Developing and Sustaining Nursing Leadership" (Registered Nurses Association of Ontario [RNAO], 2013), which discusses the significant impact of leadership in the workplace and community. For example, professionals working in health service organizations with strong leadership demonstrate increased organizational commitment, higher levels of organizational effectiveness, greater sense of affiliation with organizational goals, and increased ability to lead a diverse workforce.

Research completed through the development of the best practice guideline on nursing leadership (RNAO, 2013) found that the following attributes of nurse leaders contribute to effectiveness:

- communication and listening skills;
- resilience, persistence, and hardiness;
- comfort with ambiguity, uncertainty, and complexity;
- willingness to take risks;
- working from a foundational moral framework;
- confidence in own values and beliefs;
- self-confidence, self-awareness, social awareness;
- knowledge; and
- cultivation of professional and personal supports.

A conceptual model (see Figure 2.1) identifies contextual and personal factors that impact a nurse's approach to transformational leadership (Weberg, 2010). The model outlines individual and system components that contribute to effective nursing leadership (RNAO, 2013). For example, a nurse leader who strongly values professional nursing supports will approach relationship building in a way that is more likely to result in healthy and effective outcomes than a nurse leader who values individual successes and works alone in a chaotic environment where budgets are unstable. Leadership growth builds on organizational supports, personal resources, and past outcome experiences.

Organizational Supports

Within the context of community health nursing practice, important organizational supports that positively influence practice include a work culture that

- values the unique and combined contribution of staff;
- deliberately establishes leadership and mentoring plans;
- has a clear vision engendering commitment; and
- has stable funding and access to necessary resources to accomplish work.

Collaborative leadership at a national level will be strengthened by developing inter-sectoral relationships, promoting community health solutions across sectors, and addressing the wider determinants of health (Public Health Agency of Canada [PHAC], 2006). Mentoring is consistently identified as contributing to leadership development (Cooper & Wheeler, 2010).

CONCLUSION

To varying degrees, the federal, provincial, territorial, regional, and municipal levels of government are involved in Canadian health care. Medicare is one of the great achievements of Canada, and it is more than a public insurance program (Campbell & Marchildon, 2007). A universally accessible, publicly funded, not-for-profit health care system is steeped in Canadian values and embraced by the Canadian public. Efforts to enshrine those values in federal legislation began as early as 1919. The present legislation, the Canada Health Act, is limited in that its principles of public administration, portability, accessibility, universality, and public administration apply only to essential medical and hospital services. Nevertheless, the publicly funded and largely privately delivered health care system has served Canadians well with respect to health outcomes and cost-effectiveness (Starfield, 2010).

Pressures to reform medicare have come about not only because of its narrow focus on hospital and medical services but also because some favour augmenting the public system with services provided by the for-profit sector. Numerous reports at the provincial or territorial and federal levels have recommended reforms to the health care system. The most comprehensive of those, the Romanow Report, made 47 recommendations for the immediate future and the next 20 years (Romanow, 2002b).

The federal government has played a leadership role, not only in Canada but also in the world, in health promotion policy. A coordinated approach to implementing health promotion policy at the community and population levels has been hampered by the lack of a national public health plan. Prior to the SARS outbreak in 2004, there had been a steadily declining emphasis on the role of community health in the Canadian health system, in large part due to the exclusion of community health from the Canada Health Act. Restructuring of provincial health systems to regional models that include community health has played a role as community health issues compete with more pressing acute care concerns. There is a growing awareness of the need to address the upstream issues or root causes of illness if the current health care system is to be sustainable. Demands on limited home health and primary health care nursing services have challenged the community health system. Serious erosions to the public health system in Canada have led to the withdrawal and reduction of many public health nursing services and CHN presence in key settings such as schools, community places, and workplaces.

CHNs practise at the intersection of public policy and private lives and are in a position to include political advocacy and efforts to influence healthy public policy in their practice. The call for a revitalized public health and community health

system is being made. Strong leadership and action at all levels are required to answer this call. CHNs are well positioned and, in fact, morally obligated to act and provide leadership.

KEY TERMS

accessible   (p. 19)
Canada Health Act   (p. 19)
comprehensive   (p. 19)
determinants of health   (p. 20)
health equity   (p. 25)
health inequity   (p. 25)
health promotion   (p. 20)
home care   (p. 24)
leadership   (p. 28)
medicare   (p. 19)
policy   (p. 25)
policy and political competence   (p. 27)
politics   (p. 25)
portable   (p. 19)
power   (p. 25)
primary care   (p. 22)
primary health care   (p. 20)
public health   (p. 23)
publicly administered   (p. 19)
role clarity   (p. 28)
social justice   (p. 25)
universal   (p. 19)
workforce diversity   (p. 26)

STUDY QUESTIONS

1. Identify the origins of medicare in Canada, and summarize the laws that created the present Canadian health care system. What is considered to be phase two of the implementation of medicare?

2. Discuss the events that led to and necessitated passage of the Canada Health Act.

3. What role did organized nursing play in the passage of the Canada Health Act?

4. Discuss the federal and provincial responsibilities for health according to the Canada Health Act.

5. Contrast the funding mechanisms for public health and home health nursing services with the rest of the system.

6. To what degree was the Canada Health Act successful in achieving its intended goals. Are there issues with it?

7. Identify three key issues that intersect to contribute to health inequities.

INDIVIDUAL CRITICAL-THINKING EXERCISES

1. List your core values for health care in Canada. How do your values compare with the values reflected in the five key funding criteria described in the Canada Health Act?

2. How would your life be different if health care in this country was provided based on ability to pay rather than need?

3. This chapter has shown that health policy decisions leave a legacy for generations. Describe briefly one policy revision you would make in the areas of primary care, public health, and home care.

4. What examples can you describe of nurses' work to close the health equity gap?

5. What are some health problems in your community? How can you frame them as issues within a health policy context?

6. What opportunities have you encountered to promote the second phase of medicare development?

7. Leadership development is an ongoing process. What ideas do you have to develop your leadership skills and knowledge?

GROUP CRITICAL-THINKING EXERCISES

1. On what values was the health care system founded? How do your own values fit with the societal values that are reflected in the five funding criteria described in the Canada Health Act?

2. What are some of the solutions you and your group can generate to address issues in Canada's health care system? What role can CHNs play?

3. In an ideal world, create a health care system designed to provide the best care, to the most people, in the most cost-effective manner. Describe the mechanisms for financing, allocation, and delivery. Compare and contrast this system with the current Canadian system.

4. How can CHNs foster authentic relationships with community members to address health inequities?

REFERENCES

American Public Health Association (APHA). (2017). *Social justice and health.* Retrieved from https://www.apha.org/what-is-public-health/generation-public-health/our-work/social-justice

Antonello, D., Cohen, B., Janzen Le Ber, M., Kothari, A., Lemieux, S., Moran, K., . . . Wai, C. (2016). *Develop and test indicators of Ontario local public health agency work to address the social determinants of health to reduce health inequities Phase 2 Report: A case study approach to pilot test indicators.* Retrieved from http://www.publichealthontario.ca/en/ServicesAndTools/Documents

Auditor General of Canada. (2002). *1999 report of the Auditor General of Canada to the House of Commons* (Chapter 29). Retrieved from http://www.oag-bvg.gc.ca/internet/English/parl_oag_199911_29_e_10158.html

Bharmal, N., Pitkin Derose, K., Felician, M., & Weden, M. (2015, May). *Understanding the upstream social determinants of health.* RAND Corporation Working Paper, 1–18.

Braveman, P. (2006). Health disparities and health equity: concepts and measurement. *Annual Review of Public Health, 27,* 167–194.

Braveman, P., & Gruskin, S. (2003). Defining equity in health. *Journal of Epidemiology Community Health. 57*(4), 254–258.

Bégin, M. (2002). *Revisiting the Canada Health Act (1984): What are the impediments to change?* Address to the Institute for Research on Public Policy, 30th Anniversary Conference, Ottawa, ON. Retrieved from http://moniquebegin.telfer.uottawa.ca/files/032.pdf

Bekemeier, B., Grembowski, D., Yang, Y., & Herting, J. R. (2012). Leadership matters: Local health department clinician leaders and their relationship to decreasing health disparities. *Journal of Public Health Management and Practice, 18,* E1–E10.

Brascoupé, S., & Waters, C. (2009). Cultural safety: Exploring the applicability of the concept of cultural safety to Aboriginal health and community wellness. Retrieved from http://www.naho.ca/jah/english/jah05_02/V5_I2_Cultural_01.pdf

Brody, A. A., Barnes, K., Ruble, C., & Sakowski, J. (2012). Evidence-based practice council's potential path to staff nurse empowerment and leadership growth. *Journal of Nursing Administration, 42*(1), 28–33.

Brookes, K., Davidson, P., Daly, J., & Hancock, K. (2004). Community health nursing in Australia: A critical literature review and implications for professional nursing. *Contemporary Nursing, 16*(3), 195–207.

Buresh, B., & Gordon, S. (2006). *From silence to voice: What nurses know and must communicate to the public.* New York, NY: Cornell University Press.

Butler-Jones, D. (2008). The Chief Public Health Officer's Report on the State of Public Health in Canada: Addressing Health Inequalities. Accessed from https://www.canada.ca/content/dam/phac-aspc/migration/phac-aspc/cphorsphc-respcacsp/2008/fr-rc/pdf/CPHO-Report-e.pdf

Campbell, A. (2004). *SARS Commission interim report: SARS and public health in Ontario.* Toronto, ON: Ministry of Health and Long-Term Care. Retrieved from http://www.health.gov.on.ca/en/common/ministry/publications/reports/campbell04/campbell04_2.aspx

Campbell, A. (2005). *SARS Commission second interim report: SARS and public health legislation.* Toronto, ON: Ministry of Health and Long-Term Care. Retrieved from http://www.health.gov.on.ca/en/common/ministry/publications/reports/campbell05/campbell05.aspx

Campbell, B., & Marchildon, G. (2007). *Completing Tommy's vision.* Canadian Centre for Policy Alternatives. Retrieved from http://www.policyalternatives.ca/publications/commentary/completing-tommys-vision

Canada, House of Commons. (1984). *An act relating to cash contributions by Canada in respect of insured health services provided under provincial health care insurance plans and amounts payable by Canada in respect of extended health care services and to amend and repeal certain acts in consequence thereof (the Canada Health Act).* Ottawa, ON: Government of Canada. Retrieved from http://laws-lois.Justice.gc.ca/PDF/C-6.pdf

Canadian Alliance for Sustainable Health Care. (2012). *Home and community care in Canada: An economic footprint.* Ottawa, ON: Conference Board of Canada.

Canadian Healthcare Association. (2009). *Home Care in Canada: From the margins to the mainstream.* Ottawa, ON: Author.

Canadian Institute for Health Information (CIHI). (2012). *Regulated nurses: Canadian trends, 2007 to 2011.* Ottawa,

ON: CIHI. Retrieved from https://secure.cihi.ca/estore/productSeries.htm?pc=PCC449

Canadian Institute for Health Information (CIHI). (2010). *Home care, public sector expenditures and utilization of home care services in Canada: Exploring the data; and national health expenditure trends 1975 to 2010.* Retrieved from *https://secure.cihi.ca/free_products/NHEX%20Trends%20Report%202010_final_ENG_web.pdf*

Canadian Nurses Association (CNA). (2006). Report of Dr. Marlene Smadu (President, Canadian Nurses Association) at the Finance Committee. Retrieved from https://openparliament.ca/committees/finance/39-1/30/dr-marlene-smadu-1/only

Canadian Nurses Association (CNA). (2012a). Expert Commission (June, 2012). *A nursing call to action: The health of our nation, the future of our health system.* Retrieved from https://www.cna-aiic.ca/~/media/can/files/en/nec_report_e.pdf

Canadian Nurses Association (CNA). (2012b). *Primary health care: A position statement.* Retrieved from http://www.cna-aiic.ca/~/media/can/page-content/pdf-en/ps123_primary_health_care_2013_e.pdf?la=en

Canadian Nurses Association (CNA). (2013). *Optimizing the role of nursing in home health.* Retrieved from https://can-aiic.ca/~/media/can/page-content/pdf-en/optimizing_the_role_of_nursing_in_home_health_e.pdf?la=en

Canadian Public Health Association. (2010). *Public health, community health nursing practice in Canada: Roles and activities.* Ottawa: ON. Author. Retrieved from http://www.cpha.ca/uploads/pubs/3-1bk04214.pdf

Community Health Nurses of Canada. (2009a). *Vision statement and definition of community health nursing practice in Canada.* Toronto, ON: Author. Retrieved from http://www.chnig.org/documents/Definition_vision_Final.pdf

Community Health Nurses of Canada. (2010a). *Community health nurses speak out! Key findings from an environmental scan about the future of community health nursing in Canada.* Retrieved from http://www.chnc.ca/documents/Environmentalscan-CHNsspeakout.pdf

Community Health Nurses of Canada. (2010b). *A synthesis of Canadian community health nursing reports.* Retrieved from http://www.chnc.ca/documents/CommunityHealthNursing-keyreportssynthesis2010.doc

Community Health Nurses of Canada. (2010c). *Home health nursing competencies: Version 1.0.* Toronto, ON: Author. Retrieved from http://chnc.ca/documents/HomeHealthNursingCompetenciesVersion1.0March2010.pdf

Community Health Nurses of Canada (CHNC). (2011a). © Community Health Nurses of Canada. Reprinted with permission. Further reproduction prohibited.

Community Health Nurses of Canada (CHNC). (2019, revised). *Canadian community health nursing professional practice model and standards of practice.* St. John's, NL: Author.

Cooper, M., & Wheeler, M. M. (2010). *Building successful mentoring relationships. Canadian Nurse, 106*(7), 34–35.

Cummings, G., MacGregor, T., Davey, M., Lee, H., Wong, C., Lo, E., & Stafford, E. (2010). Leadership styles and outcome patterns for the nursing workforce and work environment: A systematic review. *International Journal of Nursing Studies, 4,* 363–385.

Cusack, C. (2012). Public health nurse service delivery: Development of a new model using Participatory Action Research. Unpublished doctoral thesis proposal. Winnipeg, MB.

Deber, R. (2003). Health care reform: Lessons from Canada. *American Journal of Public Health, 93*(1), 20–24.

Devereaux, A. (2016). Public health nurses' experiences during the H1N1/09 response. PhD in nursing dissertation completed at the University of Ottawa.

Dingley, J., & Yoder, L. (2013). The public health nursing work environment: Review of the research literature. *Journal of Public Health Management Practice, 19,* 308–321.

Epp, J. (1986). *Achieving health for all: A framework for health promotion.* Ottawa, ON: Health and Welfare Canada.

Falk-Rafael, A. (2005). Speaking truth to power: Nursing's legacy and moral imperative. *Advances in Nursing Science, 28*(3), 212–223.

Ferris, G., Davidson, S., & Perrewe, P. (2005). *Political skill at work: Impact on work effectiveness.* Mountain View: CA. Davies-Black Publishing.

Ganann, R., Underwood, J., Matthews, S., Goodyear, R., Stamler, L. L., Meagher-Stewart, D., & Munroe, V. (2010). Leadership attributes: A key to optimal utilization of the community health nursing workforce. *Canadian Journal of Nursing Leadership, 23*(2), 60–71.

Hamilton, N., & Bhatti, T. (1996). *Population health promotion.* Ottawa, ON: Health Canada, Health Promotion and Development Division. Retrieved from http://www.phac-aspc.gc.ca/ph-sp/php-psp/index-eng.php

Harris, R. (2014). *Getting buy-in for change.* Retrieved from http://www.fulcrumsearchscience.com/news/getting-buy-in-to-change-by-robert-harris

Health Canada. (2001). *The population health template: Key elements and actions that define a population health approach.* Retrieved from http://www.phac-aspc.gc.ca/ph-sp/pdf/discussion-eng.pdf

Health Canada. (2010). *Home and continuing care.* Retrieved from http://www.hc-sc.gc.ca/hcs-sss/home-domicile/index-eng.php

Health Council of Canada. (2012). *Empathy, dignity, and respect: Creating cultural safety for Aboriginal people in urban health care.* Retrieved from https://healthcouncilcanada.ca/files/Aboriginal_Report_EN_web_final.pdf

Hugman, R. (1991). *Power in caring professions.* London, UK: Macmillan.

Institute of Medicine. (2011). *The future of nursing: Leading change, advancing health.* Editors: Institute of Medicine (US) Committee on the Robert Wood Johnson Foundation Initiative on the Future of Nursing, at the Institute of Medicine. Washington (DC): National Academies Press (US).

Keon, W. J., & Pépin, L. (2009). *A healthy, productive Canada: A determinant of health approach.* The Standing Senate Committee on Social Affairs, Science and Technology Final Report of Senate Subcommittee on Population Health. Ottawa, ON: Senate Subcommittee on Population Health.

Kirk, M., Tomm-Bonde, L., & Schreiber, R. (2014). Public health reform and health promotion in Canada. *Global Health Promotion, 21*(2), 15–22.

Kulbok, P. A., Thatcher, E., Park, E., & Meszaros, P. (2012). Evolving public health nursing roles: Focus on community participatory health promotion and prevention. *Online Journal of Issues in Nursing, 17,* 1.

Lalonde, M. (1974). *A new perspective on the health of Canadians: A working paper.* Ottawa, ON: Health and Welfare Canada.

Lavoie, J. (2013). Policy silences: Why Canada needs a national First Nations, Inuit and Metis health policy. *International Journal of Circumpolar Health, 72*(22609), 1–7.

MacNevin, S. (2018). Understanding public health nurses' engagement in work to address food insecurity PhD in nursing. Dissertation completed at the University of Ottawa.

Mahony, D., & Jones, E. J. (2013). Social determinants of health in nursing education, research, and health policy. *Nursing Science Quarterly, 26,* 280–284.

Marchildon, G. (2005). *Health systems in transition: Canada.* Toronto, ON: University of Toronto Press.

Marmot, M. (2011). *Interim second report on social determinants of health and the health divide in the WHO European Region.* WHO.

Mason, D. J., Gardner, D. B., Outlaw, F. H., & O'Grady, E. T. (2016). *Policy and politics in nursing and health care* (7th ed.). St Louis, MO: Elsevier Inc.

McBane, M. (2004, December). *Medicare still on life-support.* Canadian Centre for Policy Alternatives. Retrieved from http://www.policyalternatives.ca

Meagher-Stewart, D., Aston, M., Edwards, N., Smith, D., Young, L., & Woodford, E. (2004). *Fostering citizen participation and collaborative practice: Tapping the wisdom and voices of public health nurses in Nova Scotia. The study of public health nurses' primary health care practice.* Dalhousie University, Halifax, NS: Author.

Molina-Mula, J., & De Pedro-Gómez, J. (2012). Impact of the politics of austerity in the quality of healthcare: Ethical advice. *Nursing Philosophy, 14*(1), 53–60.

Mussallem, H. K. (1992). Professional nurses' associations. In A. J. Baumgart & J. Larsen (Eds.), *Canadian nursing faces the future* (2nd ed., pp. 495–518). Toronto, ON: Mosby.

Naylor, D. (2003). *Learning from SARS: Renewal of public health in Canada: A report of the National Advisory Committee on SARS and Public Health.* Ottawa, ON: Health Canada.

Ng, E., Pottie, K., & Spitzer, D. (2011). Official language proficiency and self-reported health among immigrants to Canada. *Health Report, 22*(4), 15–23.

Ontario Ministry of Health and Long-Term Care. (2004). *Operation health protection: An action plan to prevent threats to our health and to promote a healthy Ontario.* Retrieved from http://health.gov.on.ca/en/common/ministry/publications/reports/consumer_04/oper_healthprotection.aspx

Ontario Ministry of Health and Long-Term Care. (2018). *Protecting and promoting the health of Ontarians. Ontario public health standard: Requirements for programs, services and accountability.* Queen's Printer for Ontario. Retrieved from http://www.health.gov.on.ca/en/pro/programs/publichealth/oph_standards/

Pottie, K., Greenaway, C., Feightner, J., Welch, V., Swinkels, H., Rashid, M., . . . coauthors of the Canadian Collaboration for Immigrant and Refugee Health. (2011). Evidence-based clinical guidelines for immigrants and refugees. *Canadian Medical Association Journal, 183*(12): E824–E925. doi: https://doi.org/10.1503/cmaj.090313

Public Health Agency of Canada (PHAC). (2006). *Health is everyone's business.* Retrieved from http://www.phac-aspc.gc.ca/ph-sp/collab/index-eng.php

Rachlis, M., & Kushner, C. (1994). *Strong medicine: How to save Canada's health care system.* Toronto, ON: Harper Perennial.

Rafael, A. (1997). Every day has different music: An oral history of public health nursing in Southern Ontario, 1980–1996. (Unpublished doctoral dissertation.) University of Colorado, Denver, CO.

Ramji, Z., & Etowa, J. (2018). Workplace Integration: Key Considerations for Internationally Educated Nurses and Employers. *Administrative Sciences, 8*(2): doi:10.3390/admsci8010002 www.mdpi.com/journal/admsci

Registered Nurses' Association of Ontario (RNAO). (2013). *Best practice guideline: Developing and sustaining nursing leadership* (2nd ed.). Toronto, ON: Author. Retrieved from http://rnao.ca/sites/rnao-ca/files/LeadershipBPG_Booklet_Web_1.pdf

Richmond, C., & Cook, C. (2016). *Creating conditions for Canadian Aboriginal health equity: The promise of healthy public policy.* Retrieved from https://publichealthreviews.biomedcentral.com/articles/10.1186/s40985-016-0016-5

Robert Wood Johnson Foundation. (2010). *A new way to talk about the social determinants of health.* Retrieved from http://www.rwjf.org/content/dam/farm/reports/reports/2010/rwjf63023

Romanow, R. (2002a). © All rights reserved. Discussion Paper: Homecare in Canada. Commission on the Future of Health Care in Canada. Health Canada, 2002 . Adapted and reproduced with permission from the Minister of Health, 2018.

Romanow, R. (2002b). *Shape the future of health care: Interim report.* Retrieved from http://dsp-psd.pwgsc.gc.ca/Collection/CP32-76-2002E.pdf

Schabas, R. (2002). Public health: What is to be done? *Canadian Medical Association Journal, 166*(10), 1282–1283.

Schofield, R., Ganann, R., Brooks, S., McGugan, J., Dalla Bona, K., Betker, C., . . . Watson, C. (2011). Community health nursing vision for 2020: Shaping the future. *Western Journal of Nursing Research, 33*(8), 1047–1068.

Scott, E. S., & Miles, J. (2013). Advancing leadership capacity in nursing. *Nursing Administration Quarterly, 37,* 77–82.

Shah, C. P. (2003). *Public health and preventive medicine in Canada* (5th ed.). Toronto, ON: Saunders Canada.

Shankardass, K., Muntaner, C., Kokkinen, L., Shahidi, F. V., Freiler, A., Oneka, G., . . . O'Campo, P. (2018). The implementation of health in all policies initiatives: A systems framework for government action. *Health Research Policy and Systems, 16*(1), 26.

Smylie, J., Fell, D., Ohlsson, A., & the Joint Working Group on First Nations, Indian, Inuit, and Métis Infant Mortality of the Canadian Perinatal Surveillance System. (2010). A review of Aboriginal infant mortality rates in Canada: Striking and persistent Aboriginal/non-Aboriginal inequities. *Canadian Journal of Public Health, 101*(2),143–148.

Starfield, B. (2010). Reinventing primary care: Lessons from Canada for the United States. *Health Affairs, 29*(5), 1030–1036.

Sullivan, T., & Baranek, P. (2002). *First do no harm: Making sense of Canadian health reform.* Toronto, ON: Malcolm Lester & Associates.

Truth and Reconciliation Commission of Canada. (2015). *Truth and Reconciliation Commission of Canada: Calls to Action.* Retrieved from http://www.trc.ca/websites/trcinstitution/File/2015/Findings/Calls_to_Action_English2.pdf

Tsasis, P. (2009). Chronic disease management and the home-care alternative in Ontario, Canada. *Health Services Management Research, 22,* 136–139.

Underwood, J. M., Mowat, D. L., Meagher-Stewart, D. M., Deber, R. B., Baumann, A. O., MacDonald, M. B., & Munroe, V. J. (2009). Building community and public health nursing capacity: A synthesis report of the National Community Health Nursing Study. *Canadian Journal of Public Health, 100*(5), I-1–I-13.

Walker, D. (2004). *For the public's health: A plan for action. Final report of the Ontario Expert Panel on SARS and Infectious Disease Control.* Toronto, ON: Ministry of Health and Long-Term Care. Retrieved from http://www.health.gov.on.ca/en/common/ministry/publications/reports/walker04/walker04_mn.aspx

Weberg, D. (2010). Transformational leadership and staff retention: An evidence review with implications for healthcare systems. *Nursing Administration Quarterly, 34*(3), 246–258.

Weinstein, J. N., Geller, A., Negussie, Y., & Baciu, A. (Eds.). (2017). *Communities in action: pathways to health equity.* A report of the National Academies of Sciences, Engineering, and Medicine. Washington, DC: National Academies Press.

Willcocks, S. G. (2012). Exploring leadership effectiveness: Nurses as clinical leaders in the NHS. *Leadership in Health Services, 25*(1), 8–19.

World Health Organization (WHO). (2013). Reprinted from Helsinki, Finland, *The Helsinki statement on health in all policies,* Copyright(2013).

World Health Organization, Health and Welfare Canada, & Canadian Public Health Association. (1986). *Ottawa charter for health promotion.* Ottawa: Canadian Public Health Association.

World Health Organization (WHO). (2008). *Closing the gap in a generation: Health equity through action on the social determinants of health.* Commission on the Social Determinants of Health, Geneva, CH: Author.

World Health Organization. (1978). *The declaration of Alma-Ata.* Geneva, Switzerland: Author.

ABOUT THE AUTHORS

Josephine Etowa, RM, RN, BscN, MN, PhD, FWACN, FAAN, is a Professor and Loyer-DaSilva Research Chair in Public Health Nursing at the University of Ottawa. She is a senior investigator with the Nursing Best Practice Research Centre at the University of Ottawa and a founding member and past president of the Health Association of African Canadians. Her program of research is grounded in over 25 years of clinical practice in maternal newborn and child health and community health nursing, with projects funded by local, national, and international organizations. She is currently the nominated principal investigator for a Canadian Institutes of Health Research–funded three-year, three-country study investigating infant feeding practices among Black women is living with HIV/AIDs in Ottawa, Port Harcourt (Nigeria), and Miami (United States). She serves on the boards of directors of the CPHA and the CHNC Research Committee, and she co-chairs CHNC's Standards of Practice Advisory Committee.

Lisa Ashley, RN, MEd, CCHN(C), is a senior nurse consultant with expertise in policy in the health care system. With a BScN in community health from Ryerson University and an MEd from the University of Ottawa, Lisa is certified in health management, multiple intervention programming, and community health nursing. She is dedicated to advancing nursing excellence and positive health outcomes by building strategic alliances to advance health care. She has conducted more than 70 presentations nationally and internationally, has contributed to more than 40 published articles, and has participated in more than 20 research projects. Lisa is an Academic Advisor to the School of Nursing, University of Ottawa and has guest lectured in faculties across Canada. As Chair of the Chronic Disease Prevention Alliance of Canada, Lisa led staff and volunteers to advance integrated population health advocacy and knowledge mobilization to prevent chronic disease. Lisa is currently working on her PhD Nursing at the University of Ottawa.

Esther Moghadam, RN, BScN, MEd, holds the dual role of Director of Health Promotion and Chief Nursing Officer at Ottawa Public Health. She has been a registered nurse for over 30 years working as a practitioner, researcher, educator, and manager in acute care and public and community health practice, including 10 years in executive roles. As chief nursing officer, she is responsible for promoting excellence in local public health nursing practice and collaborates on provincial public health nursing issues. In her role at Ottawa Public Health, Esther is responsible for public health functions of chronic disease, injury prevention, wellness, substance misuse, healthy growth and development, immunization, and school health. Her work as an academic advisor with the University of Ottawa School of Nursing has included teaching with the nursing program and advising for the Loyer-DaSilva Research Chair in Public Health Nursing. Esther holds a Bachelor of Science in Nursing, a Master of Education, and a post-graduate certificate in Population Health Risk Assessment and Management.

Nursing Roles, Functions, and Practice Settings

J. Craig Phillips and Ruth Schofield

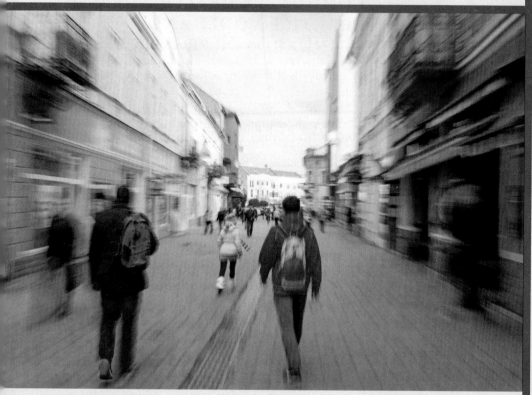

Source: Vbaleba/Fotolia

INTRODUCTION

Community health nursing practice describes the work of registered nurses, licensed/registered practical nurses, and nurse practitioners who work in a variety of settings within the community. The scopes of practice of the licensed/registered practical nurse and nurse practitioner are described under expansion and regulation of nursing practice in communities. (See page 49.) Unless noted otherwise, the registered nurse (RN) will be defined as the community health nurse. A **community health nurse (CHN)** works with people where they live, work, learn, worship, and play to promote health (Community Health Nurses of Canada [CHNC], 2009). The client means individuals, families, groups, communities, populations, and systems. CHNs work in various settings such as homes, schools, workplaces, streets, shelters, churches, field hospitals, community health centres, and outpost nursing stations. CHNs work with their clients to identify and address their barriers to health with them. These nurses view health as a dynamic process of physical, mental, spiritual, and social well-being and as a resource for everyday life that is influenced by circumstances, beliefs, and determinants of health (CHNC, 2011a). The title CHN most often refers to nurses working in Northern, rural, and remote areas of Canada and is a generalist role. Other CHNs in Canada may have titles such as public health nurse (PHN), home health nurse (HHN), occupational health nurse, primary care nurse, street nurse, parish nurse, forensic nurse, outpost/rural nurse, telehealth nurse, and community mental health nurse. The function of these various CHN roles are explained in this chapter. As indicated in Chapter 8, nurses work to promote health at various levels, sometimes implementing multiple interventions at different levels at the same time. This complex interplay of individual, group, community, and population-level interventions in promoting, protecting, or restoring health and preventing illness makes community health nursing unique, complex, and challenging. CHNs may undertake many roles and implement a range of interventions within the broad goal of promoting health.

In this chapter, we describe the community health nursing professional practice model, standards of practice, and the Blueprint for Action or national framework and action plan for CHNs. Examples of a broad range of community nursing roles, functions, and practice settings are presented. Trends affecting community health nursing practice are also included in this chapter.

BLUEPRINT FOR ACTION FOR COMMUNITY HEALTH NURSING IN CANADA

The **Blueprint for Action for Community Health Nursing in Canada** was released by the Community Health Nurses of Canada (CHNC) in 2011 (CHNC, 2011a). The Blueprint for Action provides a framework and a point of reference for ongoing dialogue on the development of community health nursing practice in Canada and was developed through an extensive consultation with many CHNs across the country and a scoping review of the literature. However, there is a need to collaborate with the Canadian Indigenous Nurses Association (CINA) to determine directions for future iterations of this Blueprint for Action. The intent of the framework is to inform the direction of CHNs in their practices and, ultimately, to promote and protect the health of Canadians. A continual call to action to advance community health nursing in Canada is realized at the CHNC annual national conference through the conference themes. For example, a current call to action is for CHNs to identify as Indigenous or non-Indigenous, know about Indigenous rights and history, recognize their own racist and stereotypical behaviours and attitudes, and complete cultural safety training to adapt their practice and education. Nurses need to understand traditional healing approaches and value this cultural health promotion work. The Blueprint for Action identifies six areas for action (CHNC, 2011a). CHNs need to:

■ Work across provinces and territories at full scope and with greater clarity for the role in all domains of practice, such as common scope of practice, practice roles, and nomenclature;

■ Support nursing leadership development and positions to advance community health nursing practice and to provide a voice for the profession;

■ Build on successful collaboration within nursing and strengthen partnerships with other professionals and sectors;

■ Transform the health care system into a system for (community) health;

■ Support strong educational preparation in community health nursing; and

■ Improve access to a range of professional development resources to advance community health nursing capacity.

COMMUNITY HEALTH NURSING PRACTICE MODEL AND STANDARDS OF PRACTICE

Community health nursing is one of 20 nursing practice specialties recognized in Canada (Canadian Nurses Association [CNA], 2015a, 2017a). Before World War II, about 60% of all nurses practised in private homes and community-based settings; but by 1989, with technological changes and medicare, about 85% of nurses were employed by hospitals (Bartfay, 2010). The trend toward hospital-based practice is slowly changing once again as a result of changes in primary health care in Canada. In 2014, 62% of nurses worked in the hospital setting (CNA, 2015b). The Canadian Nurses Association (CNA) recommends the solution to addressing the changing demographics and population health is the realignment of RNs between hospital and community settings (CNA, 2015b). In 2016, 15.8% of RNs were employed in the community health sector (Canadian Institute of Health Information [CIHI], 2016). This includes community health, public health, home health, occupational health, primary care, and telehealth nursing. CHNs embrace their nursing practice within a diversity of roles and practice settings. Combining their foundational nursing education with knowledge of community health nursing concepts, including a variety of service delivery models, nursing care encompasses the five key action areas for health promotion in the Ottawa Charter (build healthy public policy, create supportive environments for health, strengthen community action for health, develop personal skills, and re-orient health services; World Health Organization [WHO], 1986, 2015) and spans the complete prevention continuum from primordial prevention (prevents establishment of social, economic, environmental, and behavioural conditions through national policies supporting health) to primary prevention (prevention of illness or injury through health promotion activities and protective actions before the disease or injury) to secondary prevention (screening, early detection, and treatment) to tertiary prevention (maintaining and restoring health of clients with a chronic illness or condition) to quaternary prevention (a higher-level prevention that takes action to identify people at risk of over-medicalization; Betancourt et al., 2014; Pandve, 2014; Public Health Agency of Canada, 2013; Vollman, Anderson, & McFarlane, 2016).

The Community Health Nurses of Canada (CHNC) is an associate member of the CNA and a leader in community health nursing practice in Canada. The mission of the CHNC, as a national nursing organization for community health RNs, is to advance practice and to improve the health of Canadians. CHNC members view their values as ideals or beliefs that help to define and guide the organization. The values include health that is defined as a human right for all Canadians and a health care system that requires a balance of health promotion and illness care, leadership that is a requirement for system change and fundamental to supporting community health nursing practices, engagement of the voice of all populations so that they are full partners in determining approaches to health and wellness, and social justice and health equity that are foundational and central to community health nursing practices (CHNC, 2017a).

The CHNC represents the voices of CHNs. The members of the CHNC promote practice excellence and create opportunities for partnerships across sectors and networks through national conferences, webinars, local workshops, and online resources. These activities strengthen community health nursing leadership, and CHNC members advocate for healthy public policy to address social and environmental determinants of health and promote a publicly funded, not-for-profit system for (community) health (CHNC, 2012). Through substantial funding from the Public Health Agency of Canada, many structures and tools, including standards, competencies, and a Blueprint for Action, have been developed with the intent of strengthening the community health nursing workforce.

In 2011, the CHNC released the components of the Canadian community health nursing professional practice model. In 2013, a visual representation of the model was completed. (See Figure 3.1.) The CHNC (2019) outlines a professional practice model that includes a structure, process, and values supporting nurses' control over nursing care

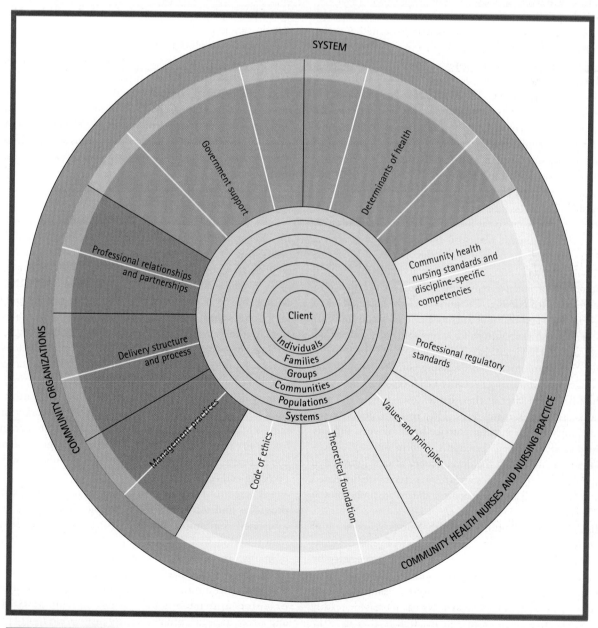

FIGURE 3.1 Canadian Community Health Nursing Professional Practice Model

delivery and the environment in which care is delivered. The community health nursing professional model of practice describes 13 components organized in four main categories: the client, CHNs and nursing practice, community organizations, and the system. The core of practice is the client, which includes individuals, families, groups, communities, systems, and populations. Informing the work of CHNs and nursing practice with clients is a code of ethics (CNA, 2017b), theoretical foundations, values and principles, professional regulatory standards, and community health nursing standards of practice and discipline-specific competencies. In the context of community organizations, community health nursing practice is influenced by management practices, delivery structures and process, and professional relationships and partnerships. The last category is the system that includes government support and determinants of health. During the development of the professional practice model, a national survey of 250 nurses reported that the model would provide them with a common framework for practice and would enable them to speak in a unified manner (Schofield, Currie, Filion, & Tao [2013]).

The original Canadian Community Health Nursing **standards of practice** were developed in 2003 and revised in 2011 and 2019 (CHNC, 2019, revised). The rationale for the revisions to the standards is noteworthy and reflects the growing practice of community health nursing. By changing the number of standards from five to seven, equal weighting and importance was given to health promotion, prevention and health protection, and health maintenance. The re-ordering of the original standards two and three reflects that professional relationships are an essential initial step in capacity building. A greater emphasis on social justice and the social and environmental determinants of health reflects current practice. The next version of the standards and the professional practice model will integrate Indigenous nursing and health.

Standards of practice represent a vision for excellence in community health nursing. The purpose of the standards is to define the scope and depth of nursing practice in the community and establish expectations for acceptable, safe, and ethical nursing care (CHNC, 2011a). The standards are the foundation for the community health nursing competencies in the community health nursing specialty CNA certification exam, which is described later in this chapter. (See Table 3.1.) The standards are used in many ways. They measure performance of community health nursing practice by employers, support professional development programs, inform nursing education curricula, and guide the development of new knowledge through research. The seven standards of practice are presented in Table 3.1. Details of each specific standard are found on the CHNC website.

In 2005, the Community Health Nurses Association of Canada (CHNAC), now the CHNC, received formal designation of community health nursing as a nursing specialty by the CNA national certification program. In 2006, the first CNA community health nursing certification examination was offered. The number of certified CHNs has increased steadily over the past five years, from 338 in 2008 to 874 in 2017 (CNA, 2017c). The certification is a voluntary national nursing

Table 3.1	Canadian Community Health Nurses Standards of Practice
1. Health promotion	
2. Prevention and health protection	
3. Health maintenance, restoration, and palliation	
4. Professional relationships	
5. Capacity building	
6. Health equity	
7. Evidence informed practice	
8. Professional responsibility and accountability	

Source: Community Health Nurses of Canada (2019, revised).

credential based on national standards released by CNA in 2003 and revised in 2012, but it is now often required or preferred by employers across Canada (CNA, 2017a). National certification is valid for five years.

In its standards of practice, the CHNC describes two sectors of CHNs: public health nurses and home health nurses (CHNC, 2011b). However, in the next version of the standards, the primary care nurses will be included, given their recent adoption of the Canadian Community Health Nursing standards of practice and inclusion in the CNA's CHN certification exam. In addition, modifications will be needed to the certification exam to integrate Indigenous nursing and health.

Key characteristics of CHNs are reflected in the standards and include a high level of independence, autonomy, resourcefulness, and collaboration with the client and his or her family and community. Strong community and individual health assessment skills, critical thinking and problem solving, and an understanding of the community and its resources as well as of the overall health care system are expected. All CHNs work within an array of provincial or territorial legislations and regulatory professional standards, but the concepts of health promotion are the foundation for their practices. Depending on the settings they work in, CHNs engage in the following activities: advocacy; building capacity; building coalitions and networks; care and counselling; case management; communication; community development; consultation; facilitation; health education; health threat response; leadership; social marketing and outreach; policy development and implementation; referral and follow-up; research; resource management; program planning, coordination, and evaluation; screening; surveillance; and team building and collaboration.

There are differences in the roles of CHNs across the provinces and territories. For example, in Quebec, there is a blended community health nursing model where a nurse may function within both hospital and community health domains. In Figure 3.2, the various roles of CHNs are identified and organized on the vertical axis as community-oriented or community-based approaches. A **community-oriented approach** is population- or community-focused and aimed at health promotion and disease and injury prevention in an entire population or community (WHO, 2010).

YES, BUT WHY?

Nursing Students' Perceptions of Community Health Nursing

What?

Community health nursing from a student's perspective in the last year of study reveals stereotypes such as "'pearls and pump' nurses, because they are the ones that can dress pretty, they are not the ones that are getting their hands dirty and doing all sorts of procedures" (Etowa, Duah, & Kohoun, 2017, p. 281). Similarly, first-year students perceive community care as a "low-status field" and associate it with a focus on senior care (van Iersel, Latour, de Vos, Kirschner, & Scholte op Reimer, 2018). Educators describe the devaluing of community health nursing education and the perception of being the "poor cousin" to acute care in baccalaureate programs (Schofield et al., 2011, p. 9; Valaitis et al., 2008).

So What?

Despite the Canadian Association of Schools of Nursing (CASN) accreditation requirements for the generalist preparation from the baccalaureate nursing curriculum, which includes community health nursing (Canadian Association of Schools of Nursing [CASN], 2014a), many factors play into the formation of these stereotypes in students. The disconnection between the theory-practice foundation to nursing education is present between expected and actual performance of new graduates in community health nursing practice (Pijl-Zieber, Barton, Awosoga, & Konkin, 2015). For example, this gap is exemplified in the commonly used non-traditional CHN placements where students identified the lack of RN mentorship that destabilized and confused their professional identity and perceived less experience in skill mastery and foundational nursing knowledge (Pijl-Zieber et al., 2015; Cohen & Gregory, 2009). Other underlying structural factors within the curriculum include the devaluing of community health nursing education illustrated by faculty's lack of knowledge and experience in community health, weak community health nursing leadership in the nursing program, the existence of a majority of faculty with an acute-care practice base, and inappropriate placements selected by individuals with minimal knowledge of community health nursing practice (Valaitis et al., 2008; Schofield et al., 2011). Moreover, an implicit message of less significance in nursing practice exists when fewer CHN placements are offered compared to multiple acute-care placements in the full program, thereby influencing students' preferred career choice (van Iersel et al., 2018). When entering nursing education, students come with preconceived ideas of nursing shaped by the media's portrayal of nursing in television shows such as *Grey's Anatomy* (Jubas & Knutson, 2012). The media image perpetuates the profile of the acute-care hospital nurse as the dominant area of nursing practice. This implies that students begin with a limited understanding and misconceptions of

community and the complexity of the field (van Iersel et al., 2018; Etowa et al., 2017). The invisible role of the CHN may negatively impact the attitudes of students.

Now What?

Community health nursing education can change these stereotypes in students. Strengthening community–academic partnerships, creating supportive curriculum structure and process, and identifying faculty champions can influence the content of the undergraduate curriculum (Valaitis et al., 2008; Betony, 2012). Re-examining CHN placements to expose students to a variety of community health nursing competencies, roles, and experiences will enable students to learn the extent and complexity of community health nursing practice (Pijl-Zieber et al., 2015). Integrating the CASN Guidelines for Quality Community Health Nursing Placements (CASN, 2010) can strengthen the selection of appropriate placements. Adopting exemplary CASN online public health teaching strategies to support practice development will expand the understanding and application of the CASN Entry-to-Practice Public Health Nursing competencies for undergraduate nursing education (CASN, 2014b, 2015) and the Canadian Community Health Nursing standards of practice (CHNC, 2019). Redesigning undergraduate programs can shift the focus from acute care to community (van Iersel et al., 2018). Introducing community health nursing earlier in the program can help change preferences not formed (van Iersel et al., 2018). Public knowledge of community health nursing will increase visibility and understanding of the impact it has on the health of individuals, families, communities, and populations (Etowa et al., 2017).

Standards of Practice Fulfilled

#6 Health Equity
- Evaluates and modifies efforts to increase accessibility to health and community services, and to advance health equity.

#8 Professional Responsibility and Accountability
- Participates in the advancement of community health nursing by mentoring students and new practitioners (CHNC, 2019, revised).

A **community-based approach** is the nursing care provided to individuals, families, and groups wherever they live, work, play, and learn; in other words, all nurses who practice outside the hospital (WHO, 2010). The Canadian Patient Safety Institute (Canadian Patient Safety Institute, 2016) defines community-based care as a coordinated and integrated approach to care provided in a range of community settings, such as people's homes, health care clinics, physicians' offices, public health units, hospices, and workplaces. On the horizontal axis, the roles of nurses are organized by their focus on a continuum of care from individuals, families, groups, communities, and populations.

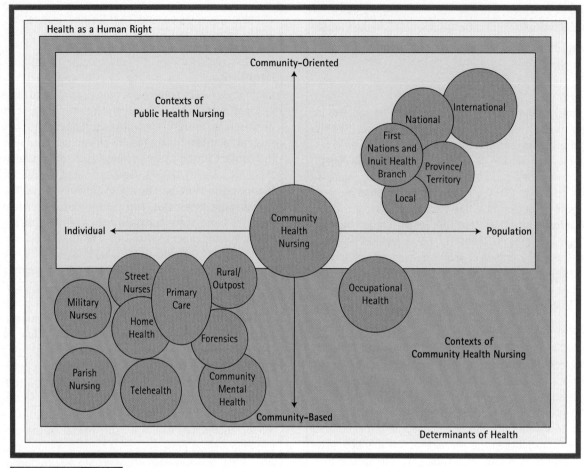

FIGURE   3.2   Community-Oriented and Community-Based Roles of CHNs

Source: Adapted from Phillips & Blais (2016).

Community Health Nursing with Indigenous Peoples and Minority Populations

In many community settings, CHNs are called upon to provide care to populations that experience health inequities and health disparities when compared to the Canadian population in general (Health Nexus, 2016a). These populations in Canada include, but are not limited to, First Nation, Métis, Inuit; LGBTQ2S or sexual orientation and gender identity minorities; and newcomers (immigrants and refugees) to Canada. The health disparities experienced by Indigenous peoples and their communities in Canada have been well documented (Anderson et al., 2016; Smylie, Fell, Ohlsson, & the Joint Working Group on First Nations, Indian, Inuit, and Métis Infant Mortality of the Canadian Perinatal Surveillance System, 2010), most recently in the Truth and Reconciliation Commission of Canada Report on the effects of the residential school system (Truth and Reconciliation Commission of Canada, 2015). Indigenous scholars advocate for the use of **wise practices**, which incorporate traditional knowledge, cosmology, and lifeways to guide health practices with Indigenous communities (Wesley-Esquimaux

& Snaowball, 2010). CHNs can address Indigenous health inequities by addressing prejudice among health workers, integrating trauma-informed care into their standards of practice, providing services for all Indigenous peoples not recognized by the Indian Act, and advocating for better supports for health workers in Indigenous communities, implementation of basic standards for supplies in nursing stations in remote communities, and inclusion of less addictive pharmaceutical options on formularies (Glauser, Tepper, & Konkin, 2016). Detailed information about Indigenous peoples is provided in Chapter 22.

LGBTQ2S persons experience worse physical and mental health outcomes than other Canadians as a result of barriers within the health care system, including health care providers who lack understanding of the needs of LGBTQ2S persons or outright stigma and discrimination perpetuated by health care providers. Further discussion about LGBTQ2S individuals is included in Chapter 20. Finally, newcomers to Canada, including immigrants and refugees, often encounter worse health outcomes as a result of not being able to find culturally appropriate services, language barriers, fear of deportation, and lack of access to familiar foods (Health Nexus, 2016b). More information about cross-cultural care is provided in Chapter 9.

NURSING ROLES IN COMMUNITY SETTINGS

Nursing with Indigenous Communities

Historical Perspective The history of on-reserve community health nursing services with First Nation peoples began in 1922 (Lavoie, Forget, & Browne, 2010). For further information about the history of nursing with Indigenous communities in Canada, read Chapter 1.

Practice Perspective Indigenous health nursing refers to "the way in which nursing care is provided to Aboriginal clients; and, also the way in which nursing interventions are targeted towards Aboriginal communities and populations (i.e., community empowerment, etc.)" (Nowgesic, 1999, p. 4). It is not about Indigenous nursing work in First Nation, Inuit, and Métis communities. CNA and the Aboriginal Nursing Association of Canada, now called the Canadian Indigenous Nurses Association, in charting a policy direction, described Indigenous nursing as nursing care and interventions informed by traditional knowledge, values, and beliefs (CNA, 2014). Indigenous nursing refers to clinical practice, education, research, administration, and policy that specifically involve First Nation, Inuit, and Métis nurses (CNA, 2014). Nursing in Indigenous communities is the focus of Chapter 22.

Public Health Nursing

Public health nursing utilizes knowledge from public health, nursing, social and environmental sciences, and research, integrating these with the concepts of primary health care, disease and injury prevention, community participation, community development, the social determinants of health, and health equity in order to promote, protect, and maintain the health of the population (CHNC, 2019, revised; Canadian Public Health Association [CPHA], 2010). The essential functions of public health are health promotion, disease and injury prevention, health protection, health surveillance, population health assessment, and emergency preparedness and response (CPHA, 2010). The definition of a PHN in Canada is a baccalaureate-prepared nurse and a member of good standing in an RN professional regulatory body (CPHA, 2010). Their population-based nursing practice is under the mandate of provincial and territorial public health legislation within official public health agencies (i.e., a health unit or health department of municipal, regional, or provincial or territorial government). PHNs' clients include individuals, families, groups, communities, populations, and systems. The conceptual frameworks familiar to public health nursing practice focus on the health promotion framework, where nurses enable the client to increase control over factors and conditions influencing their health, and the population health promotion framework, where nurses focus on improving the health status of the client population (Vollman et al., 2016). See Chapter 4 for an in-depth discussion of public health nursing.

CASE STUDY

You are a nursing student in your final year of study and will soon obtain your baccalaureate degree in nursing. You are determining your final focus for the nursing practicum. You have decided you would like to focus on the broader influences of health and work in the domain of social justice and overcoming health inequities. You are aware of the diversity in practice settings in the community, and the concept of working collaboratively, which seems to be a consistent feature among them, really appeals to you. You want to make your choice for the clinical practicum a good match for your clinical interests, skills, and the roles of the CHN within the specialty.

Discussion Questions

1. From reading all the descriptions of roles of CHNs in this chapter, assess which one appeals to you in terms of the kind of nursing roles and functions described.

2. What nursing knowledge, skills, and attitudes are required from you if you were working in the various specialties?

3. How would you prepare for practising in the community health nursing role you have chosen? What skill sets and theoretical knowledge would you review?

Home Health Nursing

Home health nursing is a specialized area of community health nursing practice in which the nurse, employed by a home health agency, provides clinical care in the client's home, school, or workplace. HHNs provide the resources to promote their clients' optimal level of well-being and functioning, and empower clients and their caregivers or families to take charge of their own care. **Home health nursing** activities include chronic disease management and curative practices, health promotion and health education, palliative care, rehabilitation, support and maintenance, social support, and support for the family so that the client can continue to live in the community (Canadian Home Care Association, 2014). More details on home health nursing are provided in Chapter 5. Table 3.2 describes the roles and functions of community health nurses (CHNs) in these practice settings.

Primary Care Nursing

Historical Perspectives Demand for primary care services has increased in developed countries such as Canada over the past two decades due to an aging population, rising client expectations, and a shift in focus from hospital to community care. Due to the high degree of specialization required for care of individuals, families, and communities, primary care nursing has also become specialized with regard to nursing knowledge, roles, and functions. Some of the titles for RNs in primary care settings in Canada are family practice nurse, primary care nurse, and **primary health care nurse**. In some jurisdictions, the

Table 3.2 Roles and Functions of CHNs in Varied Practice Settings

Roles	Work Setting	Aims	Roles/Function	Client Focus	Funding
Public health nurse	Client homes, schools, workplaces, shelters, streets, clinics, nursing stations, outpost nursing; First Nation, Inuit, and Métis communities	Promotes, protects, and preserves the health of populations Links the health and illness experiences of individuals, families, and communities to population health promotion (CPHA, 2010).	– Health promotion (e.g., supports healthy public policy to modify physical and social environments) – Disease and illness prevention (e.g., encourages healthy lifestyle choices) – Health protection (e.g., controls infectious diseases) – Health surveillance (e.g., collects and reports health data for tracking and forecasting health events) – Population health assessment (e.g., collects information about the population to initiate or evaluate services) – Emergency preparedness and response (e.g., plans for and evaluates public health's response to disasters)	Individual, family, group, community, population, and system	Municipal, provincial/territorial, federal governments
Home health nurse	Client homes, schools, workplaces, clinics, streets, nursing stations, outpost nursing; First Nation, Inuit, and Métis communities	Health promotion, prevention, health restoration and maintenance, or palliation and end-of-life care	– Manages chronic and terminal illness across the lifespan (e.g., management of intravenous infusion therapy, complex dialysis regimes) – Health teaching (e.g., new diabetics) – Rehabilitation (e.g., wound care in home and in clinics) – Palliation and end-of-life care – Support for individuals and caregivers	Individuals and families	Not-for-profit and for-profit agencies Provincial/territorial government
Rural nursing	Client homes, schools, clinics, streets, nursing stations, outpost nursing, health centres; First Nation, Inuit, and Métis communities	Focus on the roles of a PHN, HHN, and primary care in rural settings	See roles identified under PHNs, HHNs, and primary care	Individual, family, group, or population	Federal/provincial/territorial governments
Occupational health nurse	Workplace	Health promotion, maintenance and restoration, and injury and disease prevention in the workplace	– Needs assessments (e.g., health and safety risk assessments of workplace) – Injury prevention (e.g., establish policies and procedures) – Health promotion (e.g., healthy lifestyle programs) – Coordination (e.g., occupational health services)	Individual workers and worker populations	Employer

Table 3.2 Continued

Roles	Work Setting	Aims	Roles/Function	Client Focus	Funding
Community mental health nurse	Client homes, community health centres, nursing stations, outpost nursing, health centres; First Nation, Inuit, and Métis communities	Mental health care of people with serious mental illness living in the community, in collaboration with caregivers and the mental health care team	– Therapeutic relationship (e.g., long-term involvement) – Diagnosis and monitoring (e.g., risk assessment for alteration in mental health status) – Education (e.g., medication in partnership with health care team) – Teacher/coach (e.g., plans and supports choices to maximize mental health) – System navigation (e.g., advocates and supports access to community resources) – Treatment (e.g., administering medication)	Individual, family, group, or population	Provincial/ territorial government
Primary care nurse	Family health teams, nurse-practitioner-led clinics, public health units/departments, regional health authorities, post-secondary medical clinics, outposts, homeless services, nursing stations, health centres; First Nation, Inuit, and Métis communities	Episodic and chronic care across the lifespan in collaboration with physician and allied health team members	– Health promotion, injury and disease prevention, and management – Case management (e.g., helping clients navigate the health care system) – Health education – Triage and referral – Treatment (e.g., dressing changes, injections) – Counselling (works collaboratively with physician and health care team)	Individuals, families	Federal/ provincial/ territorial government
Forensic nurse	Prisons, hospital emergency rooms, police departments, coroner's office, lawyers	Nursing care and forensic sciences in the judicial system	– Conducts forensic investigations – Advocates for family/intimate partner violence prevention – Responds to and prevents family violence – Addresses online child abuse – Conducts sexual assault examinations	Individuals, families	Correctional facility or privately funded

(continued)

Table 3.2 Continued

Roles	Work Setting	Aims	Roles/Function	Client Focus	Funding
Military nurse	Military bases, operational units, outpatient or tertiary care facilities, overseas	Nursing officer is the title for a military nurse who is a commissioned member of the Canadian Forces Medical Service (CFMS)	– Focuses on sick and injured patients, not only in static facilities such as a garrison, base, or wing in a health care centre, but also in operational facilities such as a field hospital – Direct patient care – Policy development – Training and education	Military personnel and civilians	Federal government
Parish nurse	Faith communities	Called to minister and are affirmed by a faith to promote health, healing, and wholeness	– Health advocacy – Health education – Health counselling – Referrals to community resources	Individuals and families within a parish community	Private funding
Telehealth nurse	A variety of health care services delivered through computer-assisted and digital communication technologies; there is overlap with PHN and HHN roles	Support services across a spectrum of health care services, including health promotion, disease prevention, diagnosis, and treatment using computer-assisted and digital communication technologies; they facilitate increased access to health care services and enhance coordination of services across the continuum of care	– Health assessment – Triage – Health education – Monitors client status – Health counselling	The public and professionals	Federal/provincial government Private funding through physician offices
Outreach/street nurse	Streets, parks, homeless shelters, drop-in centres	Mostly secondary and tertiary health care services with people who are homeless	– Prevention (e.g., harm reduction through needle exchange) – Outreach – Counselling – System advocacy (facilitates access to services) – Legal support – Education	All ages of homeless population	Federal and provincial/territorial governments

title for advanced practice nurses can be **primary health care nurse practitioner**. Nurse practitioners in community settings will be described later in this chapter.

Practice Perspective Primary care nurses provide the first contact with the health care system in settings such as primary care networks; ambulatory care centres; long-term care facilities; physicians' offices; family health clinics; community health centres; correctional facilities; and community clinics in urban, rural, and remote communities (Primary Care Initiative, 2013). Primary care nurses might also focus on vulnerable groups such as the First Nations, Métis, Inuit, or immigrant and refugee communities, as well as individuals living with mental illness or experiencing homelessness, with specific evidence-based interventions designed for members of these groups (Health Canada, 2017). Primary care nursing focuses on health promotion, disease and injury prevention, cure, rehabilitation, and support. These CHNs work with other health care providers within a multidisciplinary and multi-sectoral clinic, or they might work independently for a community agency or within a vulnerable population.

Telehealth Nurses

Historical Perspectives **Telehealth** is the "remote delivery of health care services using technology and digital communications for assessment, information exchange, clinical decision making, interdisciplinary collaboration, and/or providing health care to individuals" (Nagel & Penner, 2016, p. 92). Nurses have used telephones to deliver nursing care for decades. More recent advances in computer-assisted and digital communication technologies allow nurses to provide nursing and other health care services through videoconferencing and other computer-mediated technologies such as email and text messaging (Nagel & Penner, 2016).

Practice Perspective Through telehealth, nurses are able to provide a range of services, including triage of health issues; consultations; provision of advice, counselling, support, and health education; and care coordination for chronic disease management (Barr, Vania, Randall, & Mulvale, 2017; Nagel & Penner, 2016). Telehealth nurses use strong communication, assessment, and critical-thinking skills to determine health care needs of individuals over the phone, computer, audio and video conferencing, and the internet (Nagel & Penner, 2016). A goal of **telehealth nursing** is self-care management and support for individuals and families living in the community and being monitored at home. The importance of relational practice and challenges within the dimensions of communication may influence effective client-provider relationships (Nagel & Penner, 2016). Nonverbal cues and touch are important aspects of communication that are diminished or lost in telehealth (Nagel & Penner, 2016). Despite these challenges, telehealth has been documented as a cost-effective approach to improving health access in Indigenous communities (Holyk, Pawlovich, Ross, & Hooper, 2017; Jones, Jacklin, & O'Connell, 2017; Liddy et al., 2017) to address child and

adolescent mental health delivery (Roberts, Hu, Axas, & Repetti, 2017), and to provide improved interprofessional collaboration for chronic disease management (Barr et al., 2017). Telehealth nursing opportunities in the future are promising because technologies continue to improve and facilitate access to health care for clients who want to remain in their homes or communities to receive care.

Outreach/Street Nurses

Outreach/street nursing is another area of nursing practice where nurses see their clients where they are. They provide primary care, home health care, mental health services, and public health services. They work in rural and urban areas across Canada with vulnerable individuals and populations such as people who are homeless in various settings, including shelters, First Nation people on or off reserve, and people in needle exchange sites, harm reduction clinics, community agencies, correctional facilities, medical clinics, and rehabilitation clinics.

Historical Perspectives Outreach/street nursing practice arose after World War II in an effort to meet the needs of marginalized individuals, and it grew in the 1970s and 1980s to address the high rates of sexually transmitted infections and the emerging HIV epidemic within inner city populations such as in Vancouver and Toronto (BC Centre for Disease Control, 2012). In 1988, the HIV/AIDS epidemic in Vancouver resulted in the development of the BC Centre for Disease Control's AIDS Prevention Street Nurse Program (Thumath, 2016). Thus, CHNs saw the need for and contributed to the development of the specific role of the street nurse (Hardill, 2007).

Practice Perspective Outreach/street nursing is often provided by PHNs, primary care nurses, and HHNs. It involves care focused on building relationships while maintaining the dignity of and respect for the clients, and creating an environment of cultural safety and empowerment. This relationship-building work often takes place between people who are homeless and community and government agencies. Street nurses rely on partnerships, community collaboration, and a client-centred approach in order to be successful and create change. Their work with government sectors and community services facilitates access to health services such as primary care or harm reduction strategies, job skills and retraining, and housing. They provide nursing services such as communicable disease support for those with HIV and tuberculosis, sexually transmitted infection follow-up and care, birth control, prenatal and postnatal supports, drug and alcohol rehabilitation, harm reduction, primary care, wound care, diabetic care, and mental health follow up.

Rural Nursing

Historical Perspective In Canada, nurses have been providing health care to remote and isolated communities such as the Northwest Territories and Newfoundland and Labrador as well as to Northern communities since the 1890s (Higgins, 2008). Visiting nurses often covered large geographic areas, travelling by horseback and eventually railway to provide health care to physically and socially isolated populations. In the early 1900s, programs became established in small towns or were set up temporarily on railway cars to handle disease outbreaks and teach families and communities about communicable diseases, proper nutrition, child development, school assessments, handling of drinking water, and proper disposal of sewage. Milk and food programs for vulnerable children were also set up (Abrams, 2008).

In order to legitimize the role of nurses working in isolated areas, provincial nursing programs across Canada developed specific nursing programs for providing health services in remote areas of Northern Canada and developed other programs that focused on expanding the role of nurses in primary care within community settings (Kaasalainen et al., 2010). In 1967, Dalhousie University in Nova Scotia established the first certification in midwifery and outpost nursing. Other universities followed suit in the early 1970s with nursing programs available in universities in Alberta, Manitoba, western Ontario, Toronto, Montreal, and Sherbrooke (Kaasalainen et al., 2010). In 2003, the Canadian Association of Rural and Remote Nurses (CARRN) became an emerging group and then gained affiliate group status of the CNA in 2004. CARRN is the voice of and represents rural and remote nurses in Canada (Canadian Association of Rural and Remote Nurses [CARRN], 2009). CARRN also developed and disseminated standards of practice regarding the roles and functions of the rural or remote nurse due to the complex and unique nature of this role and in order to increase awareness of it within community health nursing practice.

Practice Perspective In rural and Northern Canada, nurses in the community work in homes, schools, clinics, outpost nursing settings/stations health centres, and First Nation, Inuit, and Métis communities. Provision of nursing care in these parts of Canada is a challenge due to health disparities and subsequent health inequities that continue to the present day. The majority of Canada's land mass is rural and isolated. CHNs work within large geographic areas containing small numbers of inhabitants. A large portion of these populations are Indigenous with limited access to employment, transportation, health care services, clean water, and fresh food sources. Indigenous populations in the territories (Nunavut, Northwest Territories, and Yukon) as well as populations in Atlantic Canada are largely rural. Rural locations present challenges for the provision of adequate health care services, including midwifery and urgent care.

The multiple community roles of nurses in rural and remote areas include CHN, community nurse, PHN, HHN, and primary health care nurse. The functions of the PHN and HHN are similar to the urban descriptions with some exceptions. For example, in the Northwest Territories PHNs provide chronic care services along with public health programs, which are not part of public health nursing practice in urban settings (Government of Northwest Territories [GNWT], 2011a), and HHNs provide foot care and respite care in the home (GNWT, 2011b). CHNs usually provide primary care and often work in an expanded scope of practice

with other health care professionals (GNWT, 2011c; Yukon Health and Social Services, 2017). In Nunavut, the CHN provides broader community health roles, including health promotion, occupational health and safety, public health, community development, and curative treatment (Nunavut Department of Health, 2017). In the Yukon, nursing roles in the community are identified as home care nurses and community nurses where the work includes public health nursing and primary health care nursing (Yukon Health and Social Services, 2017). In addition to provincial and territorial funding of community health nursing services, Health Canada works with First Nation, Métis, and Inuit communities to provide nursing services. These rural nursing roles are complex and require strong clinical skills, critical-thinking skills, and the ability to work with established communities with community development initiatives. Health promotion and disease prevention are underdeveloped in rural and isolated locations due to other health care priorities in these communities. Access to physician care is scarce, and CHNs must work to their full scope of practice with the limited resources they have.

Occupational Health Nursing

Historical Perspective A significant milestone in the history of **occupational health nurses** was the formation of a national association in Canada that began over 30 years ago. Since then, there have been three national associations: the Canadian Council for Occupational Health Nurses (CCOHN), the National Association of Occupational Health Nurses, and the Canadian Occupational Health Nurses Association/Association Canadienne des Infirmières et Infirmiers en Santé du Travail. The CCOHN was responsible for certification until 1992. In 1994 the National Association of Occupational Health Nurses was renamed as the Canadian Occupational Health Nurses Association (Canadian Occupational Health Nurses Association [COHNA, 2014]). This association is a voice for influencing health and safety policy for Canadian workers and for advancing occupational health nursing practice excellence through conferences, national standards of practice, certification, and resources such as the *Disability Management Practice Standard Book*. Please refer to Chapter 27 for more details.

Practice Perspective Occupational health nurses base their practice on a nursing conceptual framework with four interrelated components: individual, health, occupational health nursing, and the environment (COHNA, 2014). The individual is viewed holistically, with rights to confidentiality and a healthy and safe workplace. Occupational health nursing is defined as a specialty area of nursing practice that focuses on the worker or worker group by promoting health, preventing illness or injury, protecting workers from risks, and recommending a safe and healthy work environment. Environment is described as a dynamic interaction between workers and their workplace, recognizing the interplay of social, physical, cultural, economic, and political factors. Health hazards are a particular focus (COHNA, 2014).

Parish Nursing

Historical Perspective **Parish nursing** arrived in Canada in 1992 (Canadian Association for Parish Nursing Ministry [CAPNM], 2014a). Reverend Granger Westberg, considered the founder of parish nursing, found that the professional knowledge and skills of RNs made a significant contribution to the health of people within faith communities (Solari-Twadell & McDermott, 1999). "Faith community" refers to a community of people who share similar history, values, and beliefs around their relationship with a higher power and others in the world. They often gather for purposes of worship and to support one another. "Ministry" refers to someone who represents the mission and purposes of a particular faith community, carries out his or her role in accordance with established standards, and is accountable to the public served rather than working in isolation or carrying out a personal agenda. Parish nurses in Canada began annual national conventions in 1998. In 2001, they incorporated as the Canadian Association for Parish Nursing Ministry (CAPNM). In 2004, parish nurses established core learning competencies and standards of practice (CAPNM, 2014b). In 2007, they became an associate member of CNA.

Practice Perspective A parish nurse is an RN with specialized knowledge to promote health, healing, and wholeness who is hired or recognized by a faith community and integrates faith and health into nursing practice (CAPNM, 2014b). Parish nurses often complete additional training, such as parish nursing courses. CAPNM (2014a) outlined 11 core competencies for basic parish nursing education programs and five standards of practice. Parish nurses core competencies include (a) baccalaureate of science in nursing (BScN), (b) orientation to parish nursing, (c) spiritual maturity and theological reflection, (d) personal and interpersonal skills, (e) teaching and facilitation, (f) worship, (g) faith community context, (h) collaboration, (i) management, (j) practicum, and (k) continuing education. Parish nurses standards of practice are similar to community health nursing standards of practice. In addition to health promotion and professional accountability, parish nurses are expected to facilitate spiritual care, collaboration, and advocacy.

Forensic Nursing

Historical Perspective **Forensic nursing** has its own distinct body of knowledge with a specific scope of practice and nursing standards, which have been developing since the 1970s (Zalon, Constantino, & Crane, 2013). To formalize this specialization in Canada, the Canadian Forensic Nurses Association (CFNA) (Canadian Forensic Nurses Association [CFNA, 2017]) was formed in 2006. CFNA facilitates networking and information exchange for forensic nurses across Canada and internationally to provide educational resources and collaborate on research topics related to forensic nursing practice. CFNA is an Associate Affiliate and Emerging (AAE) member of the CNA (CFNA, 2017). Forensic nurses are RNs who work in community psychiatry or are prepared as registered psychiatric nurses in BC, Alberta, Saskatchewan, and Manitoba. For further information on the role of forensic nurses and sexual assault nurse examiners, see Chapter 28.

Practice Perspective "Forensic" refers to the application of medical and nursing scientific knowledge to the care of clients and criminal offenders whose health issues have intersected with the law. The goals of forensic nurses are to provide for health care needs and to collect evidence for police and the legal system in a way that respects clients' dignity, right to choice, and self-determination. As well, within this nursing specialty, forensic nurses address the consequences of violence and trauma in society and work to prevent the reoccurrence of further liability incidents through advocacy and promotion of individuals' knowledge and coping skills. Forensic nurses also engage in the following activities: (a) community education regarding risk factors for violence, (b) social activism to prevent violence at the community and population levels, and (c) influencing healthy public policy to overcome challenges within social, economic, and cultural systems associated with violence (Speck & Faugno, 2013). Forensic nurses are part of a larger professional team and foster coalitions and networks with health care, law enforcement, social services, and community and government agencies. In addition, forensic nurses work with survivors of crime and with suspects and perpetrators of crimes and their families in settings such as the emergency room, intensive-care units, pediatrics, general medical and surgical care, long-term care, schools, prisons, coroner or medical examiner's offices, and outreach community settings (Zalon et al., 2013).

Within the specialty of forensic nursing are **sexual assault nurse examiners (SANE)**. SANEs respond specifically to calls relating to sexual assault or domestic violence in the emergency room and community settings. They provide comprehensive care to patients, collect evidence, and provide expert testimony during court cases that are brought forward in the legal system. Members of SANE teams are on call around the clock on a daily basis, and they respond quickly to calls from the emergency room and urgent care centres for survivors who are triaged as clinically stable but needing assessment, treatment, and possible referral for matters relating to sexual assault or domestic violence. SANEs aim to return control to survivors very early in the assessment phase of the interaction and strive to maintain a client-led approach throughout the intervention (Speck & Faugno, 2013; Zalon et al., 2013). SANEs possess knowledge of community resources and act as an initial liaison between survivors and community personnel and their agencies. SANEs must be non-judgmental and able to explain to the survivors the implications of reporting their violent event; this often is the concern of the survivors. Candid discussion of the possible consequences of reporting or not reporting incidents can assist the survivor in making informed decisions. SANEs must also possess confidence; knowledge; expert communication, assessment, and treatment skills; and knowledge of legal procedures. Care is taken to protect evidence, and documentation of assessment findings must be relevant, clear, objective, and, for the physical assessment, detailed (Speck & Faugno, 2013). SANEs may also provide care or counselling to perpetrators of sexual assaults or work with communities to develop sexual assault and domestic violence prevention programs.

Community Mental Health Nursing

Historical Perspective The history of community mental health nursing or psychiatric nursing in the community aligns with the deinstitutionalization of people with mental illness in Canada. The shift from hospital to a community focus for the care of people with mental illness began in the 1950s with the introduction of antipsychotic drugs (Forchuk et al., 2007). However, the shift in the focus of care did not happen until the late 1980s when community-based mental health programs were initiated across Canada (Sealy & Whitehead, 2004). An example of such a program found in many provinces is Assertive Community Treatment Teams that provide person-centred, recovery-oriented, and outreach mental health services (Fraser Health, 2017). Community mental health nurses (CMHN) are members of this multidisciplinary team. Similar to forensic nurses, a CMHN will often have psychiatric experience or, in the four western provinces and the Yukon, be a registered psychiatric nurse (Registered Psychiatric Nurse Regulators of Canada, 2017).

Practice Perspective The community mental health nursing role involves a blending of community nursing and mental health/psychiatric nursing. The CMHN collaborates with clients and other social and health care providers in the provision of client-centred services to individuals, families, groups, and communities. The settings where CMHNs provide services include primary care settings, home care, substance abuse/addiction programs, corrections institutions, community mental health programs, residential homes, and community outreach programs that visit homes, the street, and shelters (College of Registered Psychiatric Nurses of Manitoba, 2017).

Through a therapeutic relationship, the role of the CMHN involves service coordination, case management, symptom management and treatment, health promotion, crisis intervention, advocacy, support to achieve client goals of engagement in social and vocational activities, facilitation in accessing primary care, and other health services (Heslop, Wynaden, Tohotoa, & Heslop, 2016). Heslop et al. (2016) examined the roles of the CMHN and observed that coordination of care was the most significant aspect, demonstrating that well-developed networking and capacity-building skills in conjunction with advanced problem-solving and decision-making skills facilitated rapid responses to changing circumstances. Unfortunately, the role related to health promotion reported by CMHNs in the study was given less time; that part of the study, identified implications for individuals with mental illness who are significantly more likely than the general population to have a poor diet, experience poor sleep, and consume alcohol in excess (Heslop et al., 2016; Schofield et al., 2016).

Military Nursing

Historical Perspective **Military nursing** has been documented to occur as early as the 7th century, when Rufaida al-Asalmiya cared for wounded soldiers on battlefields outside her community of Medina, in what is now Saudi Arabia. In addition to her contributions to military nursing, Rufaida al-Asalmiya is credited with founding the first school of nursing for women, and she developed the first code of nursing conduct and ethics (Jan, 1996). Military nursing also has its formalized roots in one of the founders of modern nursing practice, Florence Nightingale, who practised during the Crimean War in the 1850s. The first recorded instance of military nursing in Canada was at the Northwest Rebellion in 1885 with the Métis uprising led by Louis Riel against the Canadian government, where nurses organized themselves to help the wounded. Nurses served as military nurses during World War I within the Royal Canadian Army. Nurses paid their own way to travel overseas when serving in organizations such as the Red Cross, Victorian Order of Nurses, and St. John's Ambulance (Canadian Military History Gateway, 2011). Canadian military nurses served on peacekeeping missions and responded to the 2014 Ebola outbreak in West Africa. Canada committed more than $110 million toward health, humanitarian, and security needs and to help fight the spread of Ebola and also donated the Canadian-developed Ebola vaccine (National Defence and the Canadian Armed Forces, 2015b).

Practice Perspective Military nurses are commissioned nursing officers of the Canadian Forces Medical Service. They possess leadership skills, and like civilian nurses, their primary duty is to care for sick and injured patients, and in this case, the population of Canadian Armed Forces members and insurgents either in Canada or on operations abroad. Nursing officers may work in military hospitals and outpatient health clinics or in moveable facilities such as field hospitals. Military nurses also provide disease prevention and outbreak response functions as part of international aid. The Ebola response in West Africa demonstrated how Canada, Canadian Forces, and Canadian Forces Nurses effectively collaborate with multinational organizations to avert further escalation of humanitarian disasters (National Defence and the Canadian Armed Forces, 2015b). Nursing officers work in several domains of nursing practice, including direct patient care within perioperative nursing, intensive care, mental health, air evacuation, and community health. Nursing officers are also involved in policy development, administrative duties, health education, and research. They provide preventive, occupational, and environmental health care services while working collaboratively with a larger health care team that includes physicians and medical technicians. Other career options for military nurses include humanitarian work and advocacy for the populations in which they serve. Military nursing goes beyond providing health care. A nurse working in the Canadian Forces needs to be physically fit, clinically adaptable to many different work environments with limited equipment and varied responsibilities, socially adaptable, and able to be deployed at short notice. Military nursing is challenging and provides nurses with the opportunity to use critical thinking and leadership skills in a variety of health care settings that nurses working with civilian populations are unlikely to experience (National Defence and the Canadian Armed Forces, 2015a).

EXPANSION AND REGULATION OF NURSING PRACTICE IN COMMUNITIES

In Canada there are four regulated nursing groups within the nursing profession (CNA, 2015a). These include: RNs, nurse practitioners, licensed/registered practical nurses, and registered psychiatric nurses. Licensed practical nurses have the designation of registered practical nurse in Ontario. Registered psychiatric nurses are educated and regulated only in the western provinces of British Columbia, Alberta, Saskatchewan, Manitoba, and the Yukon territory (CNA, 2015a). Members from each of these regulated nursing groups contribute to improving health outcomes for the Canadian population and practice in a variety of community settings across Canada. Current health care system transformation efforts have called for using each regulated nursing group to its full scope of practice. These efforts have resulted in new or expanded opportunities for members of the nursing profession that improve health care delivery and health outcomes, and contribute to achieving the human rights goal of health for all. This section focuses on the licensed/registered practical nurse and the nurse practitioner.

Licensed/Registered Practical Nurse

Between 2008 and 2012, the number of licensed/registered practical nurses (L/RPNs) increased by more than 18% in Canada compared to the RN workforce, which increased by less than 4% (Canadian Institute for Health Information, 2016). Consequently, this resulted in a shift in the composition of the regulated nurse workforce. L/RPNs now represent 24% of all regulated nurses (up from 22% in 2008), while RNs represent 74% (down from 77% in 2008) (CIHI, 2016). In 2015, the Registered Practical Nurses Association of Ontario reported that 19.3% of the RPNs, as they called in Ontario, were employed in the community sector (Registered Practical Nurses Association of Ontario, 2018).

Historical Perspective As early as 1914, the CNA identified the role of a practical nurse in the provision of care to clients at home (College of Licensed Practice Nurses in BC, 2017). Since 1996, the scope of practice of the L/RPN expanded as a result of a mandatory advanced education update and requirement of a two-year diploma (College of Licensed Practice Nurse of Alberta [CLPNA], 2017).

Practice Perspective The Canadian Council for Practical Nurse Regulators is a federation of the provinces' and territories' members and is responsible for the national regulation of L/RPNs. It establishes the national standards of practice outlining the expected practices for L/RPNs related to professional accountability and responsibility, knowledge-based practice, services to the public and self-regulations, and ethical practice (Canadian Council for Practical Nurse Regulators [CCPNR], 2013). A competency framework for entry to practice for L/RPNs was developed in 2013 (CCPNR, 2013). L/RPNs work in similar settings as RNs in the community (CNA, 2013). For

instance, beyond home care, they work in primary care, mental health, clinics, outreach/street nursing, nursing stations, occupational health, and public health (RPNAO, 2017). In public health their role focuses on immunization because legislation protects the title of PHN for baccalaureate-prepared RNs in some places such as Ontario (Health Promotion and Protection Act, 2017).

According to the College of Nurses of Ontario, there are guiding principles to distinguish RN and L/RPN practices. The RN has a greater foundational knowledge in clinical practice, decision making, critical thinking, leadership, research utilization, and resource management, resulting in more autonomous practice and capacity to respond to complex and unstable clinical situations (College of Nurses of Ontario [CNO], 2014). In more complex clinical situations in community health nursing, the L/RPN consults with or transfers care to the RN (CNO, 2014; CLPNA, 2017). The client for an L/RPN in community settings is the individual, family, or group (CCPNR, 2013).

Nurse Practitioners

Nurse practitioners (NPs) are advanced practice nurses. In community health settings, NPs may use titles such as primary health care nurse practitioner or family nurse practitioner. The titles used by NPs vary across practice settings and provinces and territories. They work within the community, often in remote areas. (See Photo 3.1.)

Historical Perspective The work of NPs evolved from decades of nurses working in isolated and remote areas in Canada, often as outpost nurses. In 1971, the Boudreau Report made the implementation of the expanded role of the RN a high priority in Canada's health care system. Many education programs began graduating NPs, but in the absence of supporting regulatory legislation, these nurses functioned as RNs working under medical directives (Nurse Practitioners' Association of Ontario [NPAO], 2011). The need for additional education

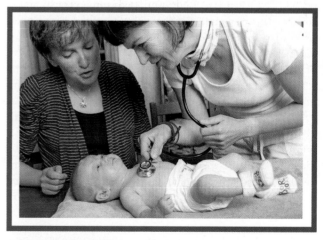

PHOTO 3.1 Primary health care nurse doing a well-baby check

Source: Edler von Rabenstein/Fotolia

for nurses working in specialty areas was recognized in the 1990s, and educational institutions began to offer certificate and graduate programs for NPs (CNA, 2011). In 2006, through federal funding, the CNA established the Canadian Nurse Practitioner Initiative (CNPI) to streamline practice expectations, optimize the contribution of NPs, and develop consistency in advanced nursing practice across the country (CNA, 2016b). The goal of the CNPI was to ensure sustained integration of the NP role in the health system through four action areas: legislation and regulation, education, communication, and health human resources (CNA, 2011). Major outcomes of the CNPI evolved around a legislative and regulatory framework that allows for a Canada-wide, consistent, principle-based approach for NP practice regulation. This approach gives provinces and territories flexibility in NP role implementation that facilitates mobility between jurisdictions and provides clarity for admitting internationally educated NPs (CNA, 2011).

The Canadian Nurse Practitioner Core Competency Framework (CNA, 2011) established core competencies for NP educational programs and a national NP exam, as well as a competency assessment framework for ongoing quality assurance of NP practices. It also recommends title protection for the NP so that only nurses with the defined qualifications are able to use the title NP. Therefore, Canadian NPs have a framework of consistent practice expectations and must demonstrate specific competencies in their expanded scope of practice. In 2014, the CASN published Nurse Practitioner Education in Canada: National Framework of Guiding Principles & Essential Components to insure consistency in NP training programs nationally (CASN, 2014).

Practice Perspective An NP is an RN with additional graduate-level education and strong clinical experience with the following competencies: autonomously diagnose, order, and interpret certain diagnostic tests; prescribe most pharmaceuticals but not controlled substances; and perform specific procedures within their legislated scope of practice (CNA, 2009). This RN category is known as "extended class" by regulatory bodies (CNO, 2017). All NPs work both autonomously and in collaboration to complement the roles of other health professionals as part of an interdisciplinary health care team to ensure optimal client care (CNA, 2011). The NP role includes health promotion, illness and injury prevention, and rehabilitation support to the individuals, families, communities, and systems in which they collaborate (NPAO, 2014).

In 2013, 32% of NPs worked in the community (CIHI, 2014) in areas such as community health centres, home care, public health, telehealth, ambulatory care, long-term care, mental health clinics, rural and outpost nursing stations, home visiting organizations, remote and Northern communities, and interprofessional family practice settings such as family health teams and primary care networks (CNA, 2012a). The focus of NP care in these settings varies considerably. Some NPs provide care to individuals of all ages and stages of life, whereas others work in settings with a specific health focus, such as sexual health, lactation support services, homeless services, primary health care in secondary schools, correctional facilities,

or palliative care. Opportunities for NPs in the community continue to expand.

NPs can diagnose a common disease, disorder, or condition; order and interpret prescribed diagnostic and screening tests, such as X-rays or ultrasounds; and prescribe specific medications. Authority to perform these advanced acts is subject to limits and conditions outlined by provincial and territorial regulatory bodies and the NPs' expertise. The NP will consult with a physician when the diagnosis or treatment plan is unclear or beyond the NP's scope of practice or competency level (CNA, 2012b).

TRENDS IN COMMUNITY HEALTH NURSING

Established and emerging trends in health care and nursing will continue to challenge CHNs to evolve their practices in order to continue to play a central role in the health system and provide effective and relevant care to their clients. These trends include an increasing focus on health equity and social justice, information communication technology, adapting to practice and system changes, and the changing profile of undergraduate nursing education.

Focus on Health Equity and Social Justice

CHNs historically have addressed health inequities, are aware of the need to change the living and working conditions for their clients and populations, and have advocated for community justice and social action (Abrams, 2008; Crowe, 2007; Fee & Bu, 2010; Jan, 1996). Trends in health care reorganization resulted in breaking down nurses' roles into a group of skills, tasks, or specialties such as postpartum care and immunization. This focus on social action has changed. However, standards of practice of community health nursing call for political and social advocacy to work with individuals, families, communities, systems, and populations to change underlying conditions that contribute to or perpetuate health disparities (CHNC, 2011a). Consequently, CHNs are not to just accept the conditions that contribute to marginalization and inequities but to take action to change them (CHNC, 2011a). Health equity, "attainment of the highest level of health for all people" (Healthy People 2020, 2017), implies that everyone, regardless of socially determined circumstances, has an equal opportunity to attain their full health potential. This requires an understanding of, and ability to analyze and advocate for, policies that increase access to health, as well as the ability to develop policies that address health disparities (Reutter & Kushner, 2010).

CHNs work with population groups such as Indigenous, homeless, LGBTQ2S, and new Canadians. In 2012, CNA's National Expert Commission was established to meet with Canadians and strategize how our health care system can better meet our needs (CNA, 2012a). As a result, an action plan was developed for all nurses and other interdisciplinary professionals to work collectively and collaboratively with other

Canadians to focus on health and the factors that influence it. It requires an application of health promotion approaches to address inequity and social injustices. Please see Chapter 8 for more details.

Information Communication Technology Advances

Information communication technology (ICT) innovation continues to expand in community health nursing practice. CHNs work with technology such as Bluetooth-enabled devices, handheld devices, smartphones, tablet computers, and computerized workstations. These devices are being used for electronic communication (e.g., email and voice mail), multimedia presentations (e.g., podcasts, blogs, and YouTube videos), and social networking (e.g., Twitter and Facebook). ICT assists CHNs in information and knowledge management and with communication in the delivery of community health nursing services (CASN, 2012). In some settings, CHNs update the client's health record by way of laptop or handheld electronic device. It is now possible to send test results electronically and receive a diagnosis and treatment order without having to transport a client to a medical centre. Telemonitoring applications are providing new opportunities for remote assessments of wound healing, cardiac and respiratory status monitoring, or assessing or monitoring other health indicators, thus making optimal use of scarce nursing and medical resources. Telephone nursing services are now available in many regions of Canada. CHNs are identifying and developing telehealth nursing competencies that support a therapeutic nurse–client relationship.

Social networking expands contacts and facilitates connections between individuals. Yet its full potential is just starting to be recognized. Knowledge of, comfort with, and use of this technology by CHNs is expected in order to identify, generate, manage, and process relevant data to support nursing practices (CHNC, 2011a). ICT challenges include keeping up with the trends, supporting appropriate use, and protecting staff and the public from a variety of services that can put the health of Canadians at risk. (See Canadian Research 3.1.) Chapter 15 provides an in-depth look at information technology.

Adapting to Practice and System Changes

The first significant practice change is that CHNs, and others in the health care system, need to adapt their practice to respond to the Calls to Action of the Truth and Reconciliation Commission of Canada (Truth and Reconciliation Commission of Canada, 2015). Recognizing and adopting cultural humility and cultural safety approaches are areas of professional development for all CHNs (Ward, Branch, & Fridkin, 2016). Traditional Indigenous Knowledge has been identified as the highest-ranked priority requiring action in nursing (CNA, 2014). Structural and policy changes are needed, such as greater representation of First Nation, Métis, and

---

CANADIAN RESEARCH 3.1

A content analysis of health and safety communications among internet-based sex work advertisements: Important information for public health (Kille, Bungay, Oliffe, & Atchison, 2017)

This study explored health and safety information included in the internet advertisements of sex workers in western Canada to describe how it may be used to develop e-health interventions for this population. Internet-based sex worker advertisements from 45 women, 24 men, and 6 transgender persons were examined using both content and thematic analysis. Four themes were identified: demographic characteristics, sexual services, health, and safety and security. Only 16% (12/75) of the advertisements included communications about sexually transmitted infections. The majority of advertisements that noted safety restrictions were women's advertisements. None of the men or transgender sex workers restricted alcohol or drug use. This study's findings offer health care providers and policy makers insights into how they might assist with promoting the health of internet-based sex workers and their clients.

Discussion Questions

1. What health and safety concerns can you identify for a person seeking sexual services through the internet and for a sex worker providing services through the internet?

2. Give an example from the Canadian community health nursing standards of practice indicating the relevance of this study to community health nursing practice.

3. Why is research that explores the sex and gender differences and internet use patterns important for community health nursing?

Inuit nurses in national leadership positions; public policy legitimizing the use of traditional medicine; and ceremony integration of these approaches with Western models of care. In 2017, CHNC passed a resolution at its annual general meeting titled "Integrating Action on Health Equity for Indigenous People" to integrate a culture-based focus into CHNC operations, offerings, and programs in partnership with the CINA (CHNC, 2017b). This will have implications for CHNs in practice, administration, policy, education, and research in the future.

The ever-evolving landscape of system transformation toward integration among the community services is another practice change faced by CHNs in various settings. The philosophy that home is better for recovery from illness and injury, for managing chronic conditions, and for end-of-life care is the key message in the new national home care action plan and is fast becoming a reality (CNA, 2016a). The population with the greatest demand for home care services is frail older adults over age 65, with one in six older adults receiving home care services. This demand for home care services will increase with the aging baby boomers. Integral to this shift to community care is the integration of community-based services. The CNA (2016) identified integration as a critical principle in harmonizing community-based health care services. Ploeg et al. (2016) found in their study on perspectives of older adults, family caregivers, and health care professionals on managing chronic conditions that funding structures in primary care and home care need modification with greater interprofessional collaborative practice. To strengthen the best approaches for primary care and public health to improve population and system outcomes, an Ecological Framework for Building Successful Collaboration Between Primary Care and Public Health (Valaitis et al., 2014) was developed with a user-friendly resource called Toolkit2Collaborate (www.toolkit2collaborate.ca). There exists a policy framework to integrate mental health and primary care for vulnerable populations, including people with serious mental illness who experience barriers to accessing primary care services for their physical and mental health care (Centre for Addiction and Mental Health, 2016).

The Changing Profile of Undergraduate Nursing Education

The preparation for community health nursing practice in undergraduate nursing programs is more important than ever with the shift to community-based and community-oriented roles in the Canadian health care system. (See Figure 3.2.) Several factors are influencing community health nursing education. In a scan of undergraduate nursing programs in Canada to determine the integration of community health nursing education, enablers and barriers were identified. Valaitis et al. (2008) found strong community–academic partnerships, supportive curriculum structures and processes, and faculty champions that were enablers; challenges identified were the devaluing of community health compared to acute care, lack of community health placements, lack of qualified faculty, and weak community health education leadership in academia. Further challenges were identified in a Canadian qualitative, descriptive national study of community health nursing leaders regarding practice, education, and research (Schofield et al., 2011). The findings of that study indicated a devaluing of community health nursing education in the curriculum, contributing to insufficient time in theoretical and clinical placements, something that is necessary to develop competencies in health promotion and disease prevention with individuals, families, and communities (Schofield et al., 2011). CHNs in this study boldly recommended a reorientation of basic baccalaureate content to strengthen community health nursing. In 2015, the introduction of the National Council Licensure Examination further challenged community health nursing educators and practitioners to speak out for the inclusion of content relevant to community health nursing practice in this national exam. Most recently the release of the Truth and Reconciliation Commission of Canada report urges modification to curriculum content to integrate Indigenous Traditional Knowledge, values, beliefs, and healing practices into nursing curricula. An enabler to support integration is the Cultural Competency and Cultural Safety in Nursing Education competency framework (Aboriginal Nurses Association of Canada [ANAC], 2009). This framework describes eight concepts, of which six are presented as core competencies. The foundational concepts include constructionist understanding of culture and cultural safety, and the core competencies are post-colonial understanding, communication, inclusivity, respect, traditional knowledge, mentoring, and supporting students for success (ANAC, 2009). This competency framework is intended for Indigenous and non-Indigenous undergraduate nurses upon graduation in Canada.

Other enablers to strengthen community health nursing in education are the Guidelines for Quality Community Health Nursing Clinical Placements to support undergraduate programs in the selection of quality placements (CASN, 2010). In 2014, CASN released Entry-to-Practice Public Health Nursing Competencies for Undergraduate Nursing Education. In 2015, the Public Health Nursing Teaching Strategies website was launched to support competency integration.

CONCLUSION

This chapter has described the diversity in roles and settings of community health nursing practice in Canada. With the shift in the health care system to community care and health promotion, and growing nursing research and use of information technology, the advancement of community health nursing education and practice is critical. National standards and the Blueprint for Action provide a framework to guide this change.

KEY TERMS

Blueprint for Action for Community Health Nursing in Canada (p. 36)
community health nurse (CHN) (p. 35)
community-based approach (p. 39)
community-oriented approach (p. 38)
forensic nursing (p. 47)
home health nursing (HHN) (p. 41)
information communication technology (ICT) (p. 51)
military nursing (p. 48)
occupational health nurses (p. 46)
outreach/street nursing (p. 45)
parish nursing (p. 47)
primary health care nurse practitioner (p. 45)
primary health care nurse (p. 41)
public health nursing (PHN) (p. 41)
sexual assault nurse examiners (SANEs) (p. 47)
standards of practice (p. 38)
telehealth (p. 45)
telehealth nursing (p. 45)
wise practices (p. 40)

STUDY QUESTIONS

1. Identify 10 types of practice settings for nurses working in community health nursing.

2. List five common roles that nurses working in community health nursing may perform in the various practice areas discussed in this chapter, and explain why each is important. Are these roles different when working with vulnerable populations? How? Why?

3. Describe the difference between community-oriented versus community-based nursing approaches.

4. Apply practice examples from any of the community health nursing practice areas discussed in this chapter to the seven community health nursing standards.

INDIVIDUAL CRITICAL-THINKING EXERCISES

1. Which area of community health nursing interests you most, and why?

2. Identify five key roles or functions of community health nursing that work toward achieving a healthier community.

3. What personal characteristics would draw nurses toward community health nursing rather than hospital-based nursing?

GROUP CRITICAL-THINKING EXERCISES

1. Create a concept map that interconnects the multiple roles and functions of nurses in a variety of community health settings in their work with individuals, families, groups, communities, and populations to promote health.

2. Identify strategies to promote an understanding of community health nursing roles among nurses in other sectors.

3. Debate the merits of legislation similar to the Canada Health Act that would provide standardized community health nursing services across Canada.

REFERENCES

Abrams, S. E. (2008). The best of public health nursing, circa 1941. *Public Health Nursing, 25*(3), 285–291.

Aboriginal Nurses Association of Canada (ANAC). (2009). *Cultural Competency and Cultural Safety in Nursing Education.* Retrieved from https://cna-aiic.ca/~/media/cna/page-content/pdf-en/first_nations_framework_e.pdf

Anderson, I., Robson, B., Connolly, M., Al-Yaman, F., Bjertness, E., King, A., . . . , Yap, L. (2016). Indigenous and tribal peoples' health (The Lancet–Lowitja Institute Global Collaboration): A population study. *The Lancet, 388*(10040), 131–157. doi:10.1016/S0140-6736(16)00345-7

Barr, N., Vania, D., Randall, G., & Mulvale, G. (2017). Impact of information and communication technology on interprofessional collaboration for chronic disease management: A systematic review. *Journal of Health Services Research & Policy, 22*(4), 250–257. doi:10.1077/1355819617714292

Bartfay, W. J. (2010). A brief history of community health nursing in Canada. In J. E. Hitchcock, P. E. Schubert, S. A. Thomas, & W. J. Bartfay (Eds.), *Community health nursing: Caring in action* (1st Canadian ed.). Toronto, ON: Nelson Education Ltd.

BC Centre for Disease Control. (2012). *Outreach street nurse program: History.* Vancouver, BC: Author. Retrieved from http://www.bccdc.ca/SexualHealth/Programs/StreetOutreachNurseProgram/SNHistory.htm

Betancourt, M. T., Roberts, K. C., Bennett, T. L., Driscoll, E. R., Jayaraman, G., & Pelletier, L., (2014). *Monitoring chronic diseases in Canada: the Chronic Disease Indicator Framework. 34*(1), 1–30.

Retrieved from https://www.canada.ca/en/public-health/services/reports-publications/health-promotion-chronic-disease-prevention-canada-research-policy-practice/vol-34-no-1-2014/supplement.html

Betony, K. (2012). Clinical practice placements in the community: A survey to determine if they reflect the shift in healthcare delivery from secondary to primary care settings. *Nurse Education Today, 32*(1), 21–26.

Canadian Association for Parish Nursing Ministry. (2014a). *Historical overview.* Retrieved from http://www.capnm.ca/historical_overview.htm

Canadian Association for Parish Nursing Ministry. (2014b). *Core competencies.* Retrieved from http://www.capnm.ca/core_competencies.htm

Canadian Association of Rural and Remote Nurses (CARRN). (2009). *Welcome to CARRN.* Retrieved from http://www.carrn.com/index.htm

Canadian Association of Schools of Nursing (CASN). (2010). *Guidelines for quality community health nursing clinical placements for baccalaureate nursing students.* Ottawa, ON: Author. Retrieved from http://casn.ca/wp-content/uploads/2014/12/CPGuidelinesFinalMarch.pdf

Canadian Association of Schools of Nursing (CASN). (2012). *Nursing informatics entry-to-practice competencies for registered nurses.* Ottawa, ON: Author. Retrieved from http://casn.ca/wp-content/uploads/2014/12/NursingInformaticsEntryToPracticeCompetenciesFINALENG.pdf

Canadian Association of Schools of Nursing (CASN). (2014a). *CASN accreditation program standards.* Retrieved from https://www.casn.ca/wp-content/uploads/2014/12/2014-FINAL-EN-Accred-standards-March-311.pdf

Canadian Association of Schools of Nursing (CASN). (2014b). *Entry-to-practice public health nursing competencies for undergraduate nursing education.* Ottawa, ON: Author. Retrieved from https://casn.ca/wp-content/uploads/2014/12/FINALpubli-chealthcompeENforweb.pdf

Canadian Association of Schools of Nursing (CASN). (2014c). *Nurse practitioner education in Canada: National framework of guiding principles & essential components.* Ottawa, ON: Author. Retrieved from http://casn.ca/wp-content/uploads/2014/12/FINALNPFrameworkEN20130131.pdf

Canadian Association of Schools of Nursing (CASN). (2015). *Public health teaching strategies website.* http://publichealth.casn.ca

Canadian Council for Practical Nurses Regulators (CCPNR). (2013). *Entry-to-practice competencies for licensed practice nurses.* Retrieved from http://www.ccpnr.ca/wp-content/uploads/2013/09/IJLPN-ETPC-Final.pdf

Canadian Forensic Nurses Association. (2017). *About.* Retrieved from http://forensicnurse.ca/about

Canadian Home Care Association. (2014). *Community home care association on the issues: Access to care.* Retrieved from http://www.cdnhomecare.ca/content.php?doc=180

Canadian Institute of Health Information. (2014). *RN workforce, by place of work and jurisdiction, Canada, 2009 to 2013.* Retrieved from https://secure.cihi.ca/estore/productFamily.htm?pf=PFC2646&lang=en&media=0

Canadian Institute for Health Information (CIHI). (2016). *Nursing workforce, by place of work and jurisdiction, Canada, 2007 to 2016.* Retrieved from https://www.cihi.ca/en/access-data-reports/results?query=nursing&Search+Submit

Canadian Military History Gateway. (2011). *Nurses: Canadian military*. Ottawa, ON: Author. Retrieved from http://www.cmhg.gc.ca/flash/gl-ga/index-eng.asp?letter=N&page=2

Canadian Nurses Association (CNA). (2009). *The nurse practitioner: A position statement*. Ottawa, ON: Author. Retrieved from http://cna-aiic.ca/~/media/cna/page-content/pdf-fr/ps_nurse_practitioner_e.pdf

Canadian Nurses Association (CNA). (2011). *Collaborative integration plan for the role of nurse practitioners in Canada*. Ottawa, ON: Author. Retrieved from http://www.npnow.ca/docs/Integration_Plan_for_the_Nurse_Practitioner_Role-En.pdf

Canadian Nurses Association (CNA). (2012a). *A nursing call to action*. Ottawa, ON: Author. Retrieved from www.cna-aiic.ca/~/media/cna/files/en/nec_report_e.pdf

Canadian Nurses Association (CNA). (2012b). *Workplace profile 2010 of nurse practitioners in Canada*. Ottawa, ON: Author. Retrieved from http://www.cna-aiic.ca/en/download-buy/nursing-statistics

Canadian Nurses Association (CNA). (2013). *Optimizing the role of nursing in home health*. Retrieved from http://cna-aiic.ca/~/media/cna/page-content/pdf-en/optimizing_the_role_of_nursing_in_home_health_e.pdf

Canadian Nurses Association (CNA). (2014). *Aboriginal health nursing and Aboriginal health: Charting policy direction for nursing in Canada*. Retrieved from https://www.cna-aiic.ca/~/media/cna/page-content/pdf-en/aboriginal-health-nursing-and-aboriginal-health_charting-policy-direction-for-nursing-in-canada.pdf?la=en

Canadian Nurses Association (CNA). (2015a). *Framework for the practice of registered nurses in Canada*. Retrieved from https://www.cna-aiic.ca/~/media/cna/page-content/pdf-en/framework-for-the-practice-of-registered-nurses-in-canada

Canadian Nurses Association (CNA). (2015b). *Latest nursing workforce report raises flags for population health*. Retrieved from https://www.cna-aiic.ca/news-room/news-releases/2015/latest-nursing-workforce-report-raises-flags-for-population-health

Canadian Nurses Association (CNA). (2016a). *Better home care in Canada: A national action plan*. Retrieved from https://www.cna-aiic.ca/~/media/cna/page-content/pdf-en/better-home-care-in-canada_a-national-action-plan%20copy.pdf?la=en

Canadian Nurses Association (CNA). (2016b). *The Canadian nurse practitioner initiative: A 10-year retrospective*. Retrieved from https://cna-aiic.ca/~/media/cna/page-content/pdf-en/canadian-nurse-practitioner-initiative-a-10-year-retrospective.pdf?la=en

Canadian Nurses Association (CNA). (2017a). *Certification and professional development*. Retrieved from https://cna-aiic.ca/~/media/nurseone/files/en/certification-statistics-2016-by-specialty-area-and-province-or-territory.pdf?la=en

Canadian Nurses Association (CNA). (2017b). *CNA certification program*. Ottawa, ON: Author. Retrieved from https://cna-aiic.ca/en/certification

Canadian Nurses Association (CNA). (2017c). *Code of ethics for registered nurses*. Retrieved from https://www.cna-aiic.ca/~/media/cna/page-content/pdf-en/code-of-ethics-2017-edition-secure-interactive.pdf?la=en

Canadian Occupational Health Nurses Association. (2014). *The scope*. Red Deer, AB: Author. Retrieved from http://www.cohna-aciist.ca/our-scope

Canadian Patient Safety Institute. (2016). *Community based care*. Retrieved from http://www.patientsafetyinstitute.ca/en/Topic/Pages/Community-Based-Care.aspx

Canadian Public Health Association (CPHA). (2010). *Public health-community health nursing practice in Canada: Roles and activities*. Retrieved from https://www.chnc.ca/upload/membership/document/2016-07/publichealth-communityhealthnursingincanadarolesandactivities2010.pdf

Centre for Addictions and Mental Health (CAMH). (2016). *Mental health and primary care policy framework*. Retrieved from https://www.camh.ca/en/hospital/about_camh/influencing_public_policy/Documents/PrimaryCarePolicyFramework_March2016.pdf

Cohen, B., & Gregory, D. (2009). Community health clinical education in Canada: Part 2—Developing competencies to address social justice, equity, and the social determinants of health. *International Journal of Nursing Education Scholarship*. 6(1), 1–17.

College of Licensed Practice Nurses of Alberta (CLPNA). (2017). *Accountability, competence, collaboration: Understanding LPN practice*. Retrieved from https://www.clpna.com/accountability-competence-collaboration-understanding-lpn-practice

College of Licensed Practice Nurses in BC (CLPNBC). (2017). *History of LPNs in BC and Canada*. Retrieved from https://clpnbc.org/What-is-an-LPN/History-of-LPNs-in-B-C-and-Canada

College of Nurses of Ontario (CNO). (2014). *Practice guideline: RN and RPN practice: The client, the nurse and the environment*. Retrieved from http://www.cno.org/globalassets/docs/prac/41062.pdf

College of Nurses of Ontario (CNO). (2017). *Extended class*. Toronto, ON: Author. Retrieved from http://www.cno.org/en/become-a-nurse/classes-of-registration/extended-class

College of Registered Psychiatric Nurses of Manitoba. (2017). *What RPNs do*. Retrieved from http://www.crpnm.mb.ca/psychiatric-nursing/what-rpns-do

Community Health Nurses of Canada (CHNC). (2009). *Vision and definition of community health nursing in Canada*. St John's, NL: Author. Retrieved from http://www.chnig.org/wp-content/uploads/2016/02/Vision.pdf

Community Health Nurses of Canada (CHNC). (2011a). *Blueprint for action for community health nursing in Canada*. St. John's, NL: Author. Retrieved from http://www.chnc.ca/documents/2011March03Blueprint_Final.pdf

Community Health Nurses of Canada (CHNC). (2011b). *Canadian community health nursing: Professional practice model and standards of practice*. St. John's, NL: Author. Retrieved from http://www.chnc.ca/documents/chnc-standardseng-book.pdf

Community Health Nurses of Canada (CHNC). (2019). © Community Health Nurses of Canada. Reprinted with permission. Further reproduction prohibited

Community Health Nurses of Canada (CHNC). (2012). *Community health nurses of Canada strategic plan 2012–2015*. St. John's, NL: Author. Retrieved from http://www.chnc.ca

Community Health Nurses of Canada (CHNC). (2017a). *About.* Retrieved from https://www.chnc.ca/en/vision-mission-statement-values

Community Health Nurses of Canada (CHNC). (2017b). *Integrating action on health equity for Indigenous people.* Retrieved from https://www.chnc.ca/upload/membership/document/2017-06/2017-resolution-integrating-action-on-health-equity-for-indigenous-people-486.pdf

Crowe, C. (2007). *Dying for a home: Homeless activists speak out.* Toronto, ON: Between the Lines.

Etowa, J., Duah, M. A., & Kohoun, B. (2017). The meaning of community health nursing: Voices of undergraduate nursing students. *Journal of Teaching and Education, 07*(01), 275–288. CD-ROM. ISSN: 2165-6266

Fee, E., & Bu, L. (2010). The origins of public health nursing: The Henry Street visiting nurse service. *The American Journal of Public Health, 100*(7), 1206–1207.

Forchuk, C., Turner, K., Joplin, L., Schofield, R., Csiernik, R., & Gorlick. C. (2007). Housing, income support and mental health: Points of disconnection. *Health Research Policy and Systems, 5*(14), 1–7.

Fraser Health. (2017). *Assertive community treatment teams.* Retrieved from http://www.fraserhealth.ca/health-info/mental-health-substance-use/mental-health-substance-use-community-services/assertive-community-treatment-team

Glauser, W., Tepper, J., & Konkin, J. (2016, January). 8 steps toward addressing Indigenous health inequities. *Healthy Debates.* Retrieved from http://healthydebate.ca/2016/01/topic/8-steps-toward-addressing-indigenous-health-inequities

Government of Northwest Territories (GNWT). (2011a). *Community health nurses.* Retrieved from http://www.practicenorth.ca/index.php?page=community-health-nurses

Government of Northwest Territories (GNWT). (2011b). *Home health nurses.* Retrieved from http://www.practicenorth.ca/index.php?page=home-care-nurses

Government of Northwest Territories (GNWT). (2011c). *Public health nurses.* Retrieved from http://www.practicenorth.ca/index.php?page=public-health-nurses

Hardill, K. (2007). From the Grey Nuns to the streets: A critical history of outreach nursing in Canada. *Public Health Nursing, 24*(1), 91–97.

Health Canada. (2017). *First Nations and Inuit Health.* Ottawa, ON: Author. Retrieved from http://www.hc-sc.gc.ca/fniah-spnia/index-eng.php

Health Nexus. (2016a). *Minority and vulnerable populations.* Toronto, ON: Author. Retrieved from http://en.healthnexus.ca/topics-tools/vulnerable-populations

Health Nexus. (2016b). *Newcomer populations.* Toronto, ON: Author. Retrieved from http://en.healthnexus.ca/topics-tools/vulnerable-populations/newcomer-populations

Healthy People 2020. (2017). *Health disparities and health equity.* Retrieved from https://www.healthypeople.gov/2020/about/foundation-health-measures/Disparities

Health Promotion and Protection Act. (2017). *Health Protection and Promotion Act,* R.S.O. 1990, c. H.7. Retrieved from https://www.ontario.ca/laws/statute/90h07

Heslop, B., Wynaden, D., Tohotoa, J., & Heslop, K. (2016). Mental health nurses' contributions to community mental health care: An Australian study. *International Journal of Mental Health Nursing, 25,* 426–433.

Higgins, J. (2008). *Grenfell Mission: Newfoundland and Labrador heritage.* Retrieved from http://www.heritage.nf.ca/society/grenfellmission.html

Holyk, T., Pawlovich, J., Ross, C., & Hooper, A. (2017). The role of Telehealth in improving continuity of care: The Carrier Sekani Family Services primary care model. *British Columbia Medical Journal, 59*(9), 459–464.

Jan, R. (1996). Rufaida al-Asalmiya, the first Muslim nurse. *Image: The Journal of Nursing Scholarship, 28*(3), 267–268.

Jones, L., Jacklin, K., & O'Connell, M. E. (2017). Development and use of health-related technologies in Indigenous Communities: Critical review. *Journal of Medical Internet Research, 19*(7), e256. doi:10.2196/jmir.7520

Jubas, K., & Knutson, P. (2012). Seeing and be(liev)ing: How nursing and medical students understand representations of their professions. *Studies in the Education of Adults, 44*(1), 85–100. doi: 10.1080/02660830.2012.11661625

Kaasalainen, S., Martin-Misener, R., Kilpatrick, K., Harbman, P., Bryant-Lukosius, D., Donald, F., . . . DiCenso, A. (2010). An historical overview of the development of advanced practice nursing roles in Canada. *Nursing Leadership, 23,* 25–60.

Kille, J., Bungay, V., Oliffe, J., & Atchison, C. (2017). A content analysis of health and safety communications among internet-based sex work advertisements: Important information for public health. *Journal of Medical Internet Research, 19*(4), e111. Retrieved from http://www.jmir.org/2017/4/e111

Lavoie, J. G., Forget, E. L., & Browne, A. J. (2010). Caught at the crossroad: First Nations, health care, and the legacy of the Indian Act. *Pimatisiwin: A Journal of Aboriginal and Indigenous Community Health, 8*(1), 83–100.

Liddy, C., McKellips, F., Armstrong, C., Afkham, A. Frase-Roberts, L. & Keely, E (2017). Improving access to specialists in remote communities: a cross-sectional study and cost analysis of the use of eConsult in Nunavut. *International Journal of Circumpolar Health, 76*(1), 1323493. doi: 10.1080/22423982.2017.1323493

Nagel, D. A., & Penner, J. L. (2016). Conceptualizing Telehealth in nursing practice: Advancing a conceptual model to fill a virtual gap. *Journal of Holistic Nursing, 34*(1), 91–104. doi:10.1177/0898010115580236

National Defence and the Canadian Armed Forces. (2015a). *Nursing officer.* Ottawa, ON: Author. Retrieved from http://www.forces.ca/en/job/nursingofficer-53?s=68&t=21#info-1

National Defence and the Canadian Armed Forces. (2015b). *Operation SIRONA.* Ottawa, ON: Author. Retrieved from http://www.forces.gc.ca/en/operations-abroad/op-sirona.page

Nowgesic, E. (1999). Aboriginal health nursing: A nursing specialty. *Aboriginal Nurse, 14*(2), 4.

Nunavut Department of Health. (2017). Community health nurse. Retrieved from https://www.gov.nu.ca/jobs/community-health-nurse-10-02-225-076la

Nurse Practitioners' Association of Ontario. (2011). *Nurse practitioner history in Ontario.* Toronto, ON: Author. Retrieved from http://npao.org/nurse-practitioners/history/#.VUvZJ2d0x9A

Pandve, H. T. (2014). Quaternary prevention: Need of the hour. *Journal of Family Medicine and Primary Care, 3*(4), 309–310. Retrieved from https://www.ncbi.nlm.nih.gov/pmc/articles/PMC4311333

Phillips, J. C., & Blais, K. K. (2016). Global health. In Blais, K. K., & Hayes, J. (Eds.), *Professional nursing practice: Concepts and perspectives, 7th ed.* Upper Saddle River, NJ: Pearson.

Pijl-Zieber, E. M., Barton, S., Awosoga, O., & Konkin, J. (2015). Disconnects in pedagogy and practice in community health nursing clinical experiences: Qualitative findings of a mixed method study. *Nursing Education Today, 35*(10), 43–48.

Ploeg, J., Fraser, K., Matthew-Maich, N., Dufour, S., Markle-Reid, M., McAiney, C., & Kaasalainen, S. (2017). *Research brief-managing multiple chronic conditions: A qualitative study of the perceptions of older adults, family caregivers and healthcare providers.* Retrieved from https://chru.mcmaster.ca/sites/default/files/research_briefs/Managing%20MCC.pdf

Primary Care Initiative. (2013). *What is a primary care initiative?* Retrieved from https://www.scpcn.ca/primary-care-initiative

Public Health Agency of Canada. (2013). *Implementing the population health approach.* Retrieved from http://www.phac-aspc.gc.ca/ph-sp/implement/index-eng.php

Registered Practical Nurses Association of Ontario. (2018). *What is a Registered Practical Nurse (RPN).* Retrieved from https://www.rpnao.org/rpncareers/what-rpn

Registered Psychiatric Nurse Regulators of Canada. (2017). *Home.* Retrieved from http://www.rpnc.ca

Ruetter, L., & Kushner, K. E. (2010). Health equity through action on the social determinants of health: Taking up the challenge in nursing. *Nursing Inquiry, 17*(3), 269–280.

Roberts, N., Hu, T., Axas, N., & Repetti, L. (2017). Child and adolescent emergency and urgent mental health delivery through telepsychiatry: 12-month prospective study. *Telemedicine and eHealth, 23*(10), 842–846. doi:10.1089/tmj.2016.0269

Schofield, R., Currie, G., Filion, F., & Tao, M. (2013). *Canadian community health nursing professional practice model graphic.* Paper presented at 7th Annual Community Health Nursing Conference, Kelowna, BC.

Schofield, R., Forchuk, C., Montgomery, P., Rudnick, A., Edwards, B., Meier, A., & Speechley, M. (2016). Comparing personal health practices: Individuals with mental illness and the general Canadian population. *Canadian Nurse. 112*(5), 23–27.

Schofield, R., Ganann, R., Brooks, S., McGugan, J., Dalla Bona, K., Betker, C., . . . , & Watson, C. (2011). Community health nursing vision 2020: Shaping the future. *Western Journal of Nursing Research, 33*(8), 1047–1068. doi: 0.1177/0193945910375819

Sealy, P., & Whitehead, P. (2004). Forty years of deinstitutionalization of psychiatric services in Canada: An empirical assessment. *The Canadian Journal of Psychiatry, 49*(4), 249–257.

Smylie, J., Fell, D., Ohlsson, A., & the Joint Working Group on First Nations, Indian, Inuit, and Métis Infant Mortality of the Canadian Perinatal Surveillance System. (2010). A review of Aboriginal infant mortality rates in Canada: Striking and persistent Aboriginal/non-Aboriginal inequities. *Canadian Journal of Public Health, 101*(2), 143–148. doi:10.17269/cjph.101.2370

Solari-Twadell, P. A., & McDermott, M. A. (1999). *Parish nursing: Promoting whole-person health within faith communities.* Thousand Oaks, CA: Sage.

Speck, P., & Faugno, D. (2013). Intimate partner, child, and elder violence and the three levels of prevention. In R. Constantino et al. (Eds.), *Forensic nursing: Evidence based principles and practice* (1st ed., pp. 117–139). Philadelphia: F. A. Davis.

Statistics Canada. (2007). *How Statistics Canada identifies Aboriginal peoples.* Ottawa, ON: Author. Retrieved from http://www.statcan.gc.ca/pub/12-592-x/12-592-x2007001-eng.pdf

Thumath, M. (2016). *The role of street nurses in increasing access to health care for marginalized populations.* Association of Registered Nurses of British Columbia. Retrieved from https://www.arnbc.ca/blog/the-role-of-street-nurses-in-increasing-access-to-health-care-for-marginalized-populations-by-meaghan-thumath-rn-bscn-msc-ph

Truth and Reconciliation Commission of Canada. (2015). *Honouring the truth, reconciling for the future: Summary of the final report of the Truth and Reconciliation Commission of Canada.* Retrieved from http://www.trc.ca/websites/trcinstitution/File/2015/Honouring_the_Truth_Reconciling_for_the_Future_July_23_2015.pdf

Valaitis, R., Rajsic, C. J., Cohen, B., Leeseberg Stamler, L., Meagher-Stewart, D., & Froude, S. A. (2008). Preparing the community health nursing workforce: Internal and external enablers and challenges influencing undergraduate nursing programs in Canada. *International Journal of Nursing Education Scholarship, 5*(1), 1–23.

Valaitis, R., MacDonald, M., Wong, S., Martin-Misener, R., O'Mara, L., & Meagher-Stewart, D. (2014). Development of an ecological framework for building successful collaboration between primary care and public health. *BMC Health Services Research, 14*(Suppl 2), P133. Retrieved from http://bmchealthservres.biomedcentral.com/articles/10.1186/1472-6963-14-S2-P133

van Iersel, M., Latour, C., de Vos, R., Kirschner, P., & Scholte op Reimera, W. (2018). Perceptions of community care and placement preferences in first-year nursing students: A multicentre, cross-sectional study. *Nurse Education Today, 60*, 92–97.

Vollman, A., Anderson, E., & McFarlane, J. (2016). *Canadian community as partner: Theory and multidisciplinary practice.* Philadelphia, PA: Wolters Kluwer Health.

Ward, C., Branch, C., & Fridkin, A. (2016). What is indigenous cultural safety and why should I care about it? *Visions, 11*(4). 29–32. Retrieved from http://www.heretohelp.bc.ca/sites/default/files/visions-indigenous-people-vol11.pdf

Wesley-Esquimaux, C. C., & Snowball, A. (2010). Viewing violence, Mental illness and addiction through a wise practices lens. *International Journal of Mental Health and Addiction, 8*(2), 390–407. doi:10.1007/s11469-009-9265-6

World Health Organization (WHO). (1986). *The Ottawa Charter for health promotion.* Geneva, CH: Author. Retrieved from http://www.who.int/healthpromotion/conferences/previous/ottawa/en/index4.html

World Health Organization (WHO). (2010). *A framework for community health nursing education.* Retrieved from http://apps.searo.who.int/PDS_DOCS/B4816.pdf

World Health Organization (WHO). (2015). *Primary health care.* Geneva, CH: Author. Retrieved from http://www.who .int/topics/primary_health_care/en

Yukon Health and Social Services. (2017). Community nursing. Retrieved from http://www.hss.gov.yk.ca/nurses.php

Zalon, M., Constantino, R., & Crane, P. (2013). Fundamentals of contemporary forensic nursing practice, education and research. In R. Constantino et al. (Eds.), *Forensic nursing: Evidence based principles and practice* (1st ed., pp. 2–26). Philadelphia, PA: F.A. Davis.

ABOUT THE AUTHORS

J. Craig Phillips, PhD, LLM, RN, ARNP, ACRN, FAAN, is Vice-Dean Governance and Secretary of the Faculty of Health Sciences and an associate professor in the School of Nursing at the University of Ottawa. He is an American-born Canadian whose ancestors are immigrant settlers from Sweden, Scotland, and Wales. He currently serves on the LGBT Expert Panel of the American Academy of Nursing, co-directs the International Nursing Network for HIV Research, is a senior scholar with the Nursing Best Practice Research Centre at the University of Ottawa, and is a member of the HIV Criminalization Working Group at the Center for Interdisciplinary Research on AIDS at Yale University. He has over 20 years in nursing practice as a nurse, clinical nurse specialist, nurse practitioner, educator, and higher education administrator. His program of research is titled "The Ecosocial Context of Health as a Human Right." His current research with Indigenous survivors of the child welfare system uses a two-eyed seeing approach to land-based healing interventions.

Ruth Schofield, RN, BScN, MSc(T), is an assistant professor at McMaster University and clinical instructor at Western University. For the past 14 years, she has developed, implemented, and evaluated innovative undergraduate curriculum in community health nursing education. She was president of the CHNC from 2011 to 2013 and has over 23 years of public health nursing practice experience in various programs and positions from front line to management. Her research focuses on community health nursing, mental health and housing, and nursing education.

Public Health Nursing

Caroline J. Porr, Anne J. Kearney, and Aliyah Dosani

LEARNING OUTCOMES

After studying this chapter, you should be able to:

1. Define public health.

2. Describe the roles of the public health nurse.

3. Describe the historical evolution of public health nursing in Canada.

4. Identify concepts, principles, and values fundamental to public health nursing practice.

5. List the discipline-specific competencies of public health nurses.

6. Appraise the roles of the public health nurse in relation to the core functions of public health.

7. Explain how social justice is significant to the role and responsibilities of the public health nurse.

8. Discuss public health nursing interventions as they relate to primordial, primary, secondary, tertiary, and quaternary levels of prevention.

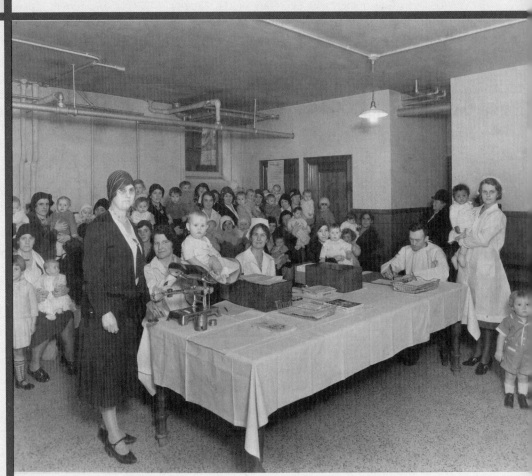

Source: Archives of Ontario. Reference code: RG 10-30-2, 1.14.5/Well Baby Clinic, Hamilton, Ontario, 1930.

INTRODUCTION

Public health is most commonly defined as the organized efforts of society to keep people healthy and prevent injury, illness, and premature death. It is a combination of programs, services, and policies that protect and promote the health of all Canadians (Last, 2001). In September 2004, the Public Health Agency of Canada (PHAC) was established with the mission to "promote and protect the health of Canadians through leadership, partnership, innovation, and action in public health" (Government of Canada, 2006; PHAC, 2015). In 2006, the Public Health Agency of Canada Act confirmed the agency as a legal entity and appointed a chief public health officer (CPHO). This legislation requires that the CPHO report annually on the state of public health in Canada. Under the leadership of the CPHO,

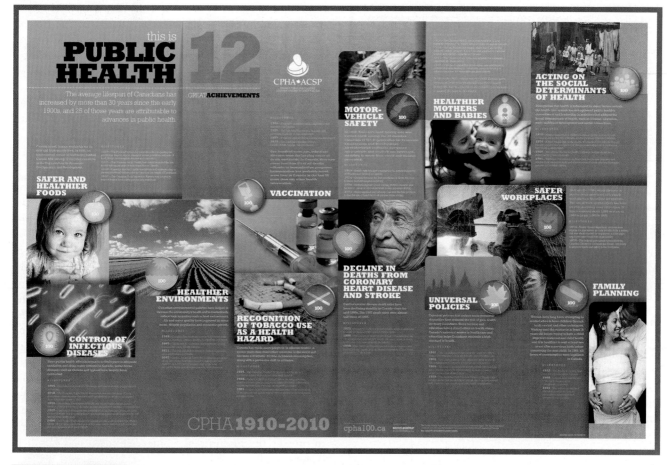

Source: Canadian Public Health Association. (n.d.). *This is public health: A Canadian history.* Ottawa, ON: Canadian Public Health Association. Retrieved from http://www.cpha.ca/uploads/history/cpha100-poster_e.pdf

various public health professionals focus on the health of the entire population in Canada to do the following:

- promote health;
- prevent and control chronic diseases and injuries;
- prevent and control infectious diseases;
- prepare for and respond to public health emergencies;
- serve as a central point for sharing Canada's expertise with the rest of the world;
- apply international research and development to Canada's public health programs; and
- strengthen intergovernmental collaboration on public health and facilitate national approaches to public health policy and planning (PHAC, 2018).

Canada has a remarkable record of public health achievements. The Canadian Public Health Association (CPHA) lists the 12 great achievements of public health in Canada (see Figure 4.1). It is significant to note that the average lifespan of Canadians has increased by more than 30 years since the early 1900s, and 25 of those years are attributable to advances in public health and the work of public health professionals (CPHA, n.d.). One type of public health professional is the **public health nurse (PHN)**. As discussed in Chapter 3, the PHN is one type of community health nurse. The PHN applies

public health science, the **principles of primary health care**, nursing science, and the social sciences to promote, protect, and preserve the health of populations (CPHA, 2010).

Having briefly introduced you to public health, we will now explore the roles and responsibilities of the PHN, beginning with the historical evolution of public health nursing in Canada. Concepts, principles, and values fundamental to public health nursing practice are interwoven throughout the chapter. At the end of the chapter are real-life exemplars from jurisdictions across Canada to illustrate the nature, diversity, and significant contributions of public health nursing practice. These exemplars will be discussed in terms of primordial, primary, secondary, tertiary, and quaternary prevention.

HISTORICAL EVOLUTION OF PUBLIC HEALTH NURSING

The earliest documented references to public health occurred before Canada became a nation. In 1831, the Colonial Office in England corresponded with the executive government in Quebec concerning the possible arrival of immigrants to Upper Canada with Asiatic sporadic cholera. In response, a sanitary commission and Canada's first board of health were

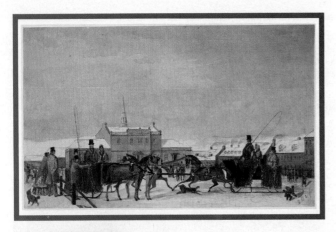

PHOTO **4.1** A Canadian scene in the 19th century

Source: Library and Archives Canada, Acc. No. R9266-45, Peter Winkworth Collection of Canadiana

immediately established, and directives were issued for the "preservation of health" (Bryce, 1910, p. 288). During this period there was little understanding of the nature, origin, and transmission of disease. Infectious diseases, particularly the cholera epidemic, accounted for the deaths of countless Indigenous peoples and early settlers. By the 1880s (see Photo 4.1), with scientific discoveries in the growing field of bacteriology, it became evident that personal hygiene and community sanitation were key to preventing malignant, contagious, and infectious diseases. Influenced by England's sanitary movement, Canadian sanitary reformers worked diligently to clean up water supplies and manage sewage removal and in so doing championed public health development in Canada. Public health initiatives that followed included legislation with detailed regulations for personal and environmental cleanliness (Allemang, 1995).

First Provincial Public Health Act

After Canadian Confederation in 1867, health and social welfare matters were the delegated responsibility of the provinces. In 1882, Dr. Peter Henderson Bryce was appointed the first secretary of the Provincial Board of Health of Ontario. He prepared the first Public Health Act, which was passed in Ontario in 1884 and became the model for legislation in other provinces across Canada (Bryce, 1910).

Other provinces in Canada soon established health acts and local boards of health. Local boards of health hired medical officers of health to protect Canadian citizens by responding to communicable disease outbreaks. Public health inspections and regulatory frameworks (e.g., environmental policies addressing contaminated water and sewage disposal systems) were soon added to the mandate of local boards of health. Local public health units oversaw such activities as proper pasteurization of milk, tuberculin testing of cows, tuberculosis isolation and quarantine practices, and the tracking of sexually transmitted infections. World War I made it necessary for preventive medicine to be integrated with clinical medicine to

control the spread of disease. A national Department of Health was founded by the Government of Canada at this time to enact legislation concerning disease surveillance and control measures as well as to safeguard public administration of food and drugs (Her Majesty the Queen in Right of Canada, represented by the Minister of Health, 2008).

The First Public Health Nurses in Canada

Lillian Wald coined the term "public health nurse." Wald was an American nurse and founder of the Henry Street Settlement in New York City. In 1893, Wald described nurses who worked with low-income communities as PHNs, setting them apart from nurses who cared for sick individuals in hospitals or in high-income homes (McKay, 2009). In Canada, public health nursing grew out of the religious persuasion and public conscience of the social gospel movement and maternal feminism. PHNs focused primarily on improving physical environmental conditions to reduce maternal and child morbidity and mortality. In the late 19th century, one out of every five infants died, and the rate of maternal deaths was high as well. In addition, at this time women were not recognized as people under the British North America Act (Ontario Ministry of Government Services, n.d.). Maternal feminists "were seeking sweeping social reform, particularly to protect the interests of women, children and families" (Harrison, 2011, p. 23).

Charitable Organizations Canada's first PHNs worked for charitable or religious organizations in several regions of the country. They were known as visiting nurses or district nurses. In 1885, a diet dispensary in Montreal employed a district nurse. The district nurses carried out nutrition counselling and assisted with volunteer distribution of nutritious meals to disadvantaged pregnant women and their families. Located in Toronto in 1889, the Nursing-at-Home Mission hired district nurses to visit disadvantaged families who lived close to the Children's Hospital. The Victorian Order of Nurses was founded in 1897 in Ottawa and served as a national district nursing association. It was not uncommon for PHNs to volunteer their expertise at Winnipeg's Margaret Scott Nursing Mission (constructed in 1905) or at the Lethbridge Nursing Mission (built in 1909), for example. Volunteer PHNs were also members of the St. Elizabeth Visiting Nurses' Association that was established in 1910 (McKay, 2009).

Civic Health Departments Increasingly, the delivery of public health programs to address complex issues of the more vulnerable populations (e.g., immigrants, urban poor, infants and children, and rural isolated families) was becoming too great a financial burden for charitable organizations. Many organizations sought government funding to maintain their programs. In 1910, Winnipeg's civic health department, through yearly grants, financed the local district nursing association and the milk depot to support their public health programs for children. The district nurse or PHN made visits to families armed

EUNICE HENRIETTA DYKE

Eunice Henrietta Dyke was born in Toronto and attended nursing school in the United States in 1905 (Johns Hopkins School for Nurses in Baltimore, Maryland). In 1911, Nurse Dyke began her employment with the Department of Public Health of the City of Toronto. She pioneered the idea of positioning child welfare services as the nucleus of the department's child health centres. The child's family became the focus of public health nursing services, and PHNs were responsible for families on a district basis. Decentralization of public health nursing services was truly innovative and was soon recognized around the world. Nurse Dyke also championed the coordination of public health and community welfare and social services. In 1937, she founded the Second Mile Club for seniors to combat elderly loneliness.

Source: Canadian Public Health Association. (n.d.). Profiles in public health. Retrieved from http://resources.cpha.ca/CPHA/ ThisIsPublicHealth/profiles/pages.php?l=E

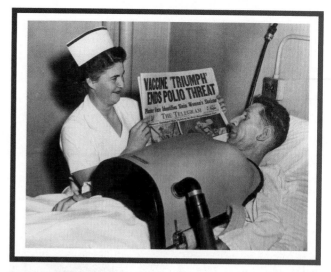

PHOTO 4.2 A patient in an iron lung: The "iron lung" was an artificial respirator used with patients suffering from paralytic polio. Patients with paralytic polio experienced paralysis of the diaphragm and intracostal muscles, which are essential for respiration.

Source: March of Dimes Canada

with milk supplies, health messages, and parenting instruction. The PHNs assisted mothers with childbirth, infant feeding, and childcare, including bathing children (Ontario Ministry of Government Services, n.d.). Universal public schooling in Canada began in the late 19th century. Local school boards began sponsoring school health programs and hired PHNs to conduct physical inspections of children and provide health education in the classroom. Children who were at risk were identified at schools, and PHNs often used this information to engage in home visits with vulnerable families. PHNs were instrumental in reducing high mortality rates among school-aged children by combatting tuberculosis and other communicable diseases. Civic health departments across Canada eventually took over voluntary public health programs, and before World War I, PHNs were hired to work in specific departments like Winnipeg's Child Hygiene Department. Nurse leader Eunice Henrietta Dyke spearheaded the opening of the Department of Public Health in the City of Toronto (McKay, 2009).

Families in rural regions of Canada received few public health nursing services because of a lack of municipal finances. Women's groups (e.g., Women's Institute or the United Farm Women) are cited as organizations that interceded and hired PHNs or physicians to hold child health clinics or to conduct school inspections. Eventually, public health programs and public health nursing services were solely the responsibility of the provinces. In 1916, Manitoba became the first province in Canada to establish a provincially funded public health nursing service. In 1919, Alberta provided its citizens with district nursing services, and British Columbia, in the same year, set up health centres for several communities that were staffed with PHNs (Allemang, 1995).

Vaccination Campaigns PHNs continued to battle diseases, including cholera, smallpox, typhoid fever, and several other communicable diseases. By the mid-1920s, following the discovery of diphtheria, pertussis, tetanus, and polio toxoids, PHNs were responsible for delivering substantial childhood immunization and vaccination programs. Polio, poliomyelitis, and infantile paralysis all refer to a disease that was terrifying for parents and children alike prior to the vaccine. This is because within a few hours of becoming ill a child could die or be permanently paralyzed (Harrison, 2011). In addition to delivering immunizations, PHNs were working in well-baby clinics, delivering prenatal classes, and conducting postnatal home visits where they discussed issues in parenting and the importance of childhood nutrition (PHAC, n.d.).

Public health nursing practice required advanced education, and the early PHNs were respected as "elite members of the nursing profession" (McKay, 2009, p. 250). Their work was both exciting and exhausting (see Photo 4.2; see Figure 4.2). It was not uncommon for PHNs to walk several miles in snowstorms or travel by dogsled or horseback to carry out their diverse roles and responsibilities. Gwen Thomas was a district nurse in Newfoundland after World War II. Her account is a captivating portrayal of a PHN:

> When I went to La Scie, it was 1949, and there was a lot of tuberculosis in Newfoundland. In quite a few families, one person or another was in bed with TB and eventually died. . . . The only way to get into La Scie was either by plane or in the winter by dog team, in the spring and summer by boat, or else across the woods road. I remember one time going to Shoe Cove, which was about four and a half miles, and we had to walk because there were no roads. When I arrived the patient was in labour. She had twins, which I delivered. (Marsh, Walsh, & Beaton, 2008, p. 183)

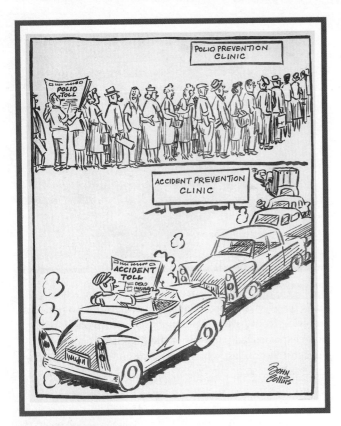

FIGURE **4.2** Polio Vaccination Campaign

Source: Collins, J. (circa 1959). *Too bad we can't have shots for this, too.* M965.199.6054 © McCord Museum, Montreal.

LYNN BLAIR

Lynn Blair grew up in Alexander, Manitoba. She received her nursing training from the Children's Hospital in Winnipeg, graduating in 1928. Nurse Blair obtained a diploma in public health nursing from the University of Minnesota 20 years later. Her nursing career included working at the San Haven State Sanatorium in North Dakota in 1928 and then at the new Department of Health and Welfare in Manitoba in 1929. As a PHN, she travelled extensively throughout Manitoba and assumed diverse responsibilities, including delivering veterinarian services, and she performed some services that were usually carried out by physicians at that time. She met the health needs of children with special needs and, as a nursing consultant in venereal disease, worked to prevent the spread of sexually transmitted infections. In 1940, Nurse Blair travelled 1000 miles a week seeking family placement for children evacuated from war-torn Britain. Nurse Blair was awarded the Canadian Public Health Association's Honorary Life Membership in 1975.

Source: Canadian Public Health Association. (n.d.). Profiles in public health. *Retrieved from http://resources.cpha.ca/CPHA/ ThisIsPublicHealth/profiles/pages.php?l=E*

ELEANORE LOUISE MINER

Eleanore Louise Miner of Regina, Saskatchewan, was a public health nursing leader. Her career spanned 35 years, and within that time she advanced primary prevention efforts and expanded the staff of public health professionals by including dental hygienists, nutritionists, speech therapists, psychologists, and physiotherapists. She focused on meeting the public health needs of vulnerable groups. From 1959 to 1961, she was president of provincial and national nursing associations. Nurse Miner published a series of articles on public financing of PHNs in the *Canadian Journal of Public Health*, documenting the important contributions of PHNs.

Source: Canadian Public Health Association. (n.d.). *Profiles in public health.* Retrieved from http://resources.cpha.ca/CPHA/ ThisIsPublicHealth/profiles/pages.php?l=E

PRIMARY HEALTH CARE AND PUBLIC HEALTH NURSING

The disturbing reality of health inequalities, worldwide, was the motivation behind the World Health Organization's (WHO) Health for All movement. In 1977, the World Assembly announced that the "main social target of governments and of the WHO should be attainment by all people of the world by the year 2000 a level of health that permits them to live socially and economically productive lives" (Little, 1992, p. 198). Assembly members, including Canada, endorsed the primary health care principles of public participation, intersectoral and interdisciplinary collaboration, health promotion, appropriate technology, and accessibility as key to achieving their goal. Former health minister Jake Epp's (1986) "Achieving Health for All" document and the release of the WHO, Health and Welfare Canada, and the Canadian Public Health Association (1986) document "Ottawa Charter for Health Promotion" were the impetus for Canadian health reform and the foundation of the "new" public health movement.

PHNs were to reduce and challenge health inequalities by enabling citizens to take action to improve their health. PHNs were called on to make a concerted effort to enact the principles of primary health care, to think upstream (i.e., to think about the many risk factors contributing to sickness and disease in an effort to prevent illness or injury) by addressing barriers to health (Butterfield, 2002; Raphael, 2011). Mahler (1985), then director general of the WHO, was confident PHNs could make a difference: "If millions of nurses in a thousand different places articulate the same ideas and convictions about Primary Health Care, and come together as one force, then they could act as a powerhouse for change" (p. 10). As Canadian provinces began preparing for major health care reform, nursing associations actively endorsed primary health care principles by submitting recommendations to provincial advisory committees, task forces, and commissions. "Health for all Canadians: A Call for Health Care Reform" by the

Canadian Nurses Association (CNA, 1988) led to position statements and projects pushing for nursing roles reflective of primary health care. Community nurses' resource centres, for example, were created in Manitoba. Alberta took steps to implement plans for the "Increased Direct Access to Nursing Services" project and reallocated $110 million from acute care to community health services. Between 1985 and 1995, the Canadian nursing profession lobbied for the shift from the medical model to a primary health care model.

Health care reform and health care restructuring in Canada since the mid-1990s have endeavoured to move health care services from institutions to communities and to place greater emphasis on health promotion, disease prevention, and public participation (Reutter & Ford, 1998). Public participation is a primary health care principle that is integral to PHNs achieving sustained change. Underwood (2010) asserted that the PHN's role is not just to educate, consult, or "do for" by providing services but to collaborate with individual citizens, families, and communities as active partners, addressing problems to promote, maintain, and restore health. This principle of public participation has been espoused by the Community Health Nurses of Canada (2011) in recognizing that citizens, collectively, have the knowledge and capacity to identify barriers to health and determine options to overcome those barriers. PHNs assume a strengths-based orientation by seeking information about capabilities of individual citizens, families, and communities, and by assisting them to mobilize resources. Capitalizing on strengths fosters a sense of optimism and hope, and citizens are apt to take charge and forge a healthier future for themselves (Gottlieb, 2013).

PUBLIC HEALTH NURSING DISCIPLINE-SPECIFIC COMPETENCIES

PHNs practise in various settings such as community health centres, homes, schools, workplaces, street clinics, youth centres, correctional facilities, outpost settings, and as part of community groups. Disease prevention, particularly infectious diseases, including preventing the introduction and spread of pandemic infections such as SARS and influenza A virus subtype H1N1, remains the responsibility of PHNs. Non-communicable chronic diseases (e.g., coronary heart disease and diabetes), injuries, and lifestyle risks to health due to tobacco, alcohol, and drug consumption require considerable time, effort, and expertise. PHNs continue to promote and advocate for the health and quality of life of mothers and children, in particular younger mothers and mothers of low socioeconomic status. The health of the environment is also a priority focus, especially with the threats brought on by global climate change, deterioration of the ecosystem, and land-use change. Such threats are interacting to create grave risks to community and population health, including exposure to infectious disease, water scarcity, food scarcity, natural disasters, and population displacement (Myers & Patz, 2009). In addition, food safety, sanitation, and occupational hazards remain part of the PHN's responsibilities.

Finally, PHNs focus on social justice as they work toward achieving equal rights and opportunities for individual citizens, families, communities, and populations (CNA, 2017), including the "right to good health" (American Public Health Association, 2018). By focusing on the basic prerequisites for health (i.e., peace, shelter, education, food, and income), PHNs are committed to reducing inequities in health (i.e., some citizens have a higher prevalence of disease and illness than others) that are unjust and avoidable. For example, poverty and homelessness are ongoing societal issues that PHNs have examined and addressed by lobbying for community-wide programs or systems-level policy change and through direct contact with individual citizens (Benbow, Gorlick, Forchuk, Ward-Griffin, & Berman, 2016).

Today, PHNs are the largest group of public health employees. PHNs function under the laws and regulations of various government bodies that oversee public health. Historically, public health programs have been delivered according to provincial mandates, and variance among programs and across jurisdictions continues. Sometimes PHNs must challenge current laws, regulations, or policies within their jurisdiction to better support the health of individual citizens, families, communities, and population groups, which we hope leads to reduced inequities. For this reason, the PHN needs to be knowledgeable about how federal, provincial, and territorial governments operate. Additionally, the PHN must have a working knowledge of the local operations of municipalities and Indigenous organizations (CPHA, 2010). Politics and public health administration are just some of the necessary elements of the PHN's knowledge base.

The PHN is expected to possess a comprehensive knowledge base to intervene effectively to contribute to the health of the population as a whole. For example, while the hospital nurse will require human pathophysiology to promote patient healing, the PHN requires the science of epidemiology to assess the magnitude of population-level health threats of specific diseases in society. Being population-oriented also means that the PHN is focused on the origins of health problems, such as those related to nutrition, income, employment, or the social and physical environments. PHNs look for risk factors that could be altered to prevent or delay illness or premature death. Similar to the systematic health assessment of a patient by the acute care nurse, the community is assessed systematically by the PHN. Using a population-oriented approach also equips PHNs for effective intersectoral collaboration, which means partnering with representatives from several sectors of society in addition to health (e.g., education, government, industry, recreation, nongovernmental agencies) to deal with, oftentimes, a vast array of factors (PHAC, n.d.).

The **public health nursing discipline-specific competencies** were established in 2009. This work was funded by the PHAC and led by members of the Community Health Nurses of Canada. The discipline-specific competencies include the following:

1. knowledge derived from public health and nursing science;

2. skills related to assessment and analysis;

3. conducting policy and program planning, implementation, and evaluation;

4. achieving partnerships, collaboration, and advocacy;

5. promoting diversity and inclusiveness;

6. effective communication exchange;

7. leadership capabilities; and

8. professional responsibility and accountability.

All of the eight discipline-specific competencies require that PHNs possess certain knowledge, skills, and attitudes, as outlined in Table 4.1. The PHN may have to rely on several competencies on a day-to-day basis to promote, protect, and preserve the health of the population. The attitudes are critical to the role, as are the broad knowledge base and diverse skills. A PHN would likely draw on all of the knowledge, skills, and attitudes presented in Table 4.1 while completing work that falls under one or more of the public health nursing discipline-specific competencies. Each PHN discerns which knowledge, skills, and attitudes are essential as he or she carries out responsibilities reflecting the competencies. Accordingly, a PHN may place more emphasis on certain knowledge, skills, and attitudes to inform his or her nursing practice.

Table 4.1	Public Health Nursing Discipline-Specific Competencies and Corresponding Knowledge, Skills, and Attitudes		
Competencies	**Knowledge**	**Skills**	**Attitudes**
1. Public health and nursing science	*The public health nurse has knowledge of*	*The public health nurse is equipped with skills to*	*The public health nurse considers*
2. Assessment and analysis	• behavioural and social sciences	• apply knowledge, critically appraise knowledge, and research new sources of knowledge	• health as multi-dimensional
3. Policy and program planning, implementation, and evaluation	• biostatistics • epidemiology • environmental public health	• collect, assess, analyze, and apply data, facts, concepts, and theories to determine individual, family, group, and community health concerns	• the influence of physical, sociocultural, political, and economic environments on health
4. Partnerships, collaboration, and advocacy	• demography • workplace health	• assess individual, family, group, and community levels of capacity to address health concerns	• support needs of individuals, families, groups, and communities to help them improve conditions conducive to health
5. Diversity and inclusiveness	• prevention of chronic diseases • infectious diseases	• identify and recommend appropriate interventions, including health promotion, health protection, and disease and injury prevention	• opportunities to address health inequities and promote social justice
6. Communication	• psychosocial problems and injuries • nursing theory	• lead policy and program planning, implementation, and evaluation	• accommodating diverse sociocultural, economic, and educational backgrounds
7. Leadership	• change theory • economics	• collaborate effectively with diverse individuals, families, groups, and communities	
8. Professional responsibility and accountability	• politics • public health administration	• promote positive team functioning	
	• community assessment • management theory	• initiate interdisciplinary and intersectoral partnerships and networks	
	• program planning and evaluation	• work to achieve interagency and intergovernmental co-operation	
	• population health principles	• act as spokesperson as needed on public health issues	
	• primary health care • determinants of health	• respond to public health emergencies	
	• community development theory		
	• social justice		
	• history of public health		

Source: Reproduction of Text: "Public Health Nursing Discipline-Specific Competencies and Corresponding Knowledge, Skills, and Attitudes", from The Public Health Nursing Discipline Specific Competencies (2009).

SIX ESSENTIAL FUNCTIONS OF PUBLIC HEALTH AND PUBLIC HEALTH NURSING ROLES

PHNs combine the knowledge, skills, and attitudes of the previously mentioned discipline-specific competencies to promote, protect, and preserve the health of all Canadians. PHNs perform the roles and responsibilities as outlined in the **six essential functions of public health** (CPHA, 2010):

1. **health protection**,
2. **health surveillance**,
3. **population health assessment**,
4. **disease and injury prevention**,
5. **health promotion**, and
6. **emergency preparation and response**.

PHNs concentrate their efforts on the population and the several prerequisites or determinants of health. Through ongoing surveillance and by examining vital statistics and other population data, the PHN decides when and where to intervene. PHNs carry out the essential public health functions previously listed by assuming various roles and employing an array of strategies, as illustrated in Table 4.2.

PUBLIC HEALTH NURSING AND LEADERSHIP

Leadership is one of the core competencies of public health nurses (Community Health Nurses of Canada, 2009). A leader in public health has the aptitude to influence, motivate, and enable others to achieve goals. As previously indicated, PHNs work at the "intersection where societal attitudes, government policies, and people's lives meet . . . [and this] creates a moral imperative to not only attend to the health needs of the public but also, like Nightingale, to work to change the societal conditions contributing to poor health" (Falk-Raphael, 2005, p. 219). Public health nursing leaders have "courage, vision, strategic agility, passion, and a moral core. They have substantial networks, keen understanding of issues and are solution focused while seeking root causes of problems" (Community Health Nurses of Canada, 2013, p. 23). Community Health Nurses of Canada (2015) recently released the Leadership Competencies for Public Health Practice in Canada. There are five domains of leadership competency:

1. transform systems,
2. achieve results,
3. lead self,
4. engage others, and
5. develop coalition.

More information regarding these leadership competencies can be found at https://www.chnc.ca. The following section is an overview of how PHNs function to create change in population health status through the six essential functions of public health systems in Canada.

LEVELS OF PREVENTION

It is important to note that PHNs intervene at five levels of prevention: primordial, primary, secondary, tertiary, and quaternary. **Primordial prevention** initiatives are those that prevent conditions that would enable the risk factors for disease from developing (Vollman, Anderson, & McFarlane, 2017). The initiatives are the establishment of conditions, actions, and measures that minimize hazards to health and that, hence, inhibit the emergence and establishment of processes and factors (environmental, economic, social, behavioural, cultural) known to increase the risk of disease (Porta, 2014). Primordial prevention is often accomplished through healthy public policy (Porta, 2014). Primordial prevention can also be viewed as the "focus on a more antecedent primary preventive strategy" (Starfield, 2001, p. 454). For example, iodized salt has been used for decades to prevent micronutrient deficiencies in populations around the world, including the Canadian population. There is emerging research indicating that we may be able to double fortify salt with iodine and folic acid (McGee, Sangakkara, & Diosady, 2017). PHNs will need to evaluate the value of double fortifying salt with iodine and folic acid and determine if advocacy is required at the national level to adopt such a policy. This action may help to improve the nutritional status of people who are living with a low socioeconomic status. In addition, legislation requiring an adequate minimum wage, or prohibiting hate crimes, or mandatory education for all children, are all examples of initiatives that can promote health for all and may be classified as primordial prevention. At the level of **primary prevention** the impact of specific risk factors is lessened, which leads to the reduction in the occurrence or incidence of disease (Vollman et al., 2017). Primary prevention initiatives are those that interrupt "the chain of causality at a point or points before a physiological or psychological abnormality is identifiable" (Starfield, 2001, p. 454). Primary prevention may entail both personal and communal efforts, such as decreasing environmental risks, enhancing nutritional status, immunizing against communicable diseases, or improving water supplies (Porta, 2014). Recently, researchers discovered that First Nations and Inuit communities in Quebec have an elevated risk of infant hospitalizations that could be related to poor rates of infant immunization (He et al., 2017). As an example of primary prevention, PHNs may enquire with various communities to determine how best to promote the uptake of infant immunization. This important work could be a start to decreasing the health status inequities we see between Indigenous and non-Indigenous populations in Canada (Smylie et al., 2016).

Secondary prevention initiatives are those that aim to identify disease processes as early as possible, usually at the preclinical stage, which may reduce the prevalence of disease by curbing its duration (Porta, 2014; Vollman et al., 2017).

Table 4.2	Public Health Nursing Roles		

Public Health Essential Functions	Description	Public Health Programming	Public Health Nursing Roles
Health protection	Health protection is a chief function of public health. Canada's water supply and food are protected from contamination. Regulatory frameworks protect the population from infectious diseases and from environmental threats.	• Water purification and monitoring • Air quality monitoring/ enforcement (Environmental Protection Act) • Restaurant inspections • Childcare facility inspections • Smoking cessation through public health policies, tobacco taxes, antismoking advertising campaigns, and product labelling	*Collaborator:* • Partners with health inspectors, government officials, and agency representatives to ensure all citizens have safe drinking water and food, and live, work, and play in safe environments • Establishes coalitions and networks as needed to enact or enforce public health legislation *Leader:* • Initiates action • Encourages citizens, the community, and those with power to initiate action *Policy Formulator:* • Identifies health protection issues in need of policy development • Participates in implementing and evaluating policy
Health surveillance	Public health professionals use health surveillance techniques to collect population data on an ongoing basis to detect early signs of illness and disease trends or outbreaks. Surveillance data provide the information needed to intervene in an effective manner to mitigate disease impact.	• Periodic health surveys • Cancer and other disease registries • Communicable disease reporting • Ongoing analysis of data to identify trends or emerging problems (e.g., recognition of increasing syphilis cases) • Reporting health threats to practitioners, what they need to look for, and intervention required	*Epidemiologist:* • Seeks health surveillance data • Coordinates systematic and routine collection and reporting of health data • Analyzes surveillance data for risk and forecasting of threatening events • Conducts surveillance of broad determinants of health • Disseminates surveillance findings and health implications to citizens, communities, and decision makers
Population health assessment	Public health professionals are well versed in what facilitates and what hinders the health of the Canadian population. Population health assessment is a tool to ensure public health programs, services, and policies are adequately meeting goals and objectives.	• Population or community health needs assessment • Health status report; system report card	*Epidemiologist:* • Applies health surveillance data to public health nursing practice • Conducts population health assessments and community health assessments • Justifies new initiatives or revisions to current programs or services with needs assessment

(continued)

Table 4.2	Continued		
Public Health Essential Functions	Description	Public Health Programming	Public Health Nursing Roles
			Outreach Worker: • Actively seeks information about the health of populations, communities, or aggregates • Uses health assessment findings to target issues (actual or potential) and to plan steps to address issues • Willing to reach out to high-risk communities (e.g., harm reduction strategies) if information indicates public health nursing interventions are warranted
Disease and injury prevention	Public health professionals contribute to the longevity and quality of life of Canadians through disease and injury prevention.	• Immunizations • Investigation and outbreak control • Screening for nutritional (e.g., scurvy), occupational (e.g., cancer of scrotum), and environmental (e.g., lead poisoning) diseases • Encouraging healthy behaviours (e.g., smoking cessation during pregnancy, healthy eating, breastfeeding, physical activity, bicycle helmet use)	**Service Provider:** • Manages and controls communicable diseases using prevention techniques, infection control, behaviour change counselling, outbreak management, and immunization • Conducts screening for disease • Informs individuals about screening procedures, rationale, and results • Monitors, documents, and evaluates screening activities • Uses effective strategies to reduce risk factors that may contribute to chronic disease, injury, and disability **Health Educator:** • Offers formal presentations, educational programs, and informal teaching sessions about healthy lifestyle behaviours • Applies teaching/learning principles to address health education needs and to ensure readiness of learner to change at-risk behaviours • Evaluates effectiveness of health education interventions • Uses marketing techniques to promote both community health programs and healthy living
Health promotion	Public health professionals improve the health of Canadians through healthy public policy, public participation, and community-based interventions.	• Intersectoral community partnerships (e.g., Heart & Stroke Foundation) to address factors affecting health • Advocacy for healthy public policies	**Capacity Builder:** • Involves communities, aggregates, and individual citizens in planning and priority setting of health promotion programs and services • Shares information about community resources • Fosters skill development of community members to mobilize resources, establish social networks, and navigate political processes

(continued)

Table 4.2	Continued		

Public Health Essential Functions	Description	Public Health Programming	Public Health Nursing Roles
		• Catalyzing the creation of physical and social environments to support health (e.g., bike paths, promoting access to social networks for institutionalized seniors)	***Community Developer:*** • Uses community development strategies to engage community members in identifying and addressing social, economic, cultural, and physical environment issues • Uses a strengths-based approach that supports community empowerment and decision making ***Facilitator:*** • Fosters interagency links and working relationships • Uses mediation skills to facilitate interagency and intergovernmental cooperation
Emergency preparedness and disaster response	Public health professionals are aware of the immediate and secondary threats to population health incited by natural disasters. Emergency preparedness and disaster response safeguard water supplies or food sources from contamination.	• Disaster planning to prepare communities to respond to floods, earthquakes, and fires • Leading institutions in emergency preparedness to respond to explosives or biological threats	***Consultant:*** • Uses knowledge and expertise in emergency preparedness and disaster response planning to inform individual citizens, nonprofit agencies, organizations, institutions, the public, and all levels of government of measures required to reduce the impact of public health emergencies • Acts as a resource person to communities, aggregates, and individual citizens • Plans for, is part of, and evaluates the response to both natural disasters (e.g., floods, earthquakes, fires, or infectious disease outbreaks) and human-made disasters (e.g., those involving explosives, chemicals, radioactive substances, or biological threats) to minimize serious illness, death, and social disruption • Uses effective risk-communication techniques to inform individual citizens and the public

Source: *Public Health—Community Health Nursing Practice in Canada: Roles and Activities* (4th ed.). Copyright © 2010 by Canadian Public Health Association. Used by permission of Canadian Public Health Association."

Secondary prevention disrupts "the chain of causality at a point where physiological or psychological abnormality is present but before there is manifestation as a symptom or sign noticed by the individual" (Starfield, 2001, p. 454). Usually secondary prevention initiatives target those individuals who are already accessing health services or patients who are already receiving care, thereby drawing their attention to an early disease process that may potentially exist (Vollman et al., 2017). These initiatives infrequently prevent disease occurrence but do so when early detection of a precursor lesion leads to complete removal of all such lesions (Porta, 2014; Vollman et al., 2017). PHNs may be involved in planning, implementing, and evaluating early clinical detection and population-based screening programs that usually aim at achieving secondary prevention (Porta, 2014; Vollman et al., 2017). For instance, women who are recent immigrants and those seeking asylum in Canada have been found to have a higher incidence of postpartum depression than women who are born in Canada (Dennis, Merry, & Gagnon, 2017). Therefore, PHNs will need to be creative in finding ways to reach vulnerable populations that require postpartum depression screening.

In **tertiary prevention**, measures aim at reducing the impact of long-term disease and disability by eliminating or reducing impairment or disability (Porta, 2014; Vollman et al., 2017). This type of intervention occurs "after sign or symptom is present, to reduce the likelihood of persistence or progression" (Starfield, 2001, p. 454). The focus is on rehabilitation that minimizes suffering and maximizes potential years of functional life (Porta, 2014; Vollman et al., 2017). Recent research evidence has demonstrated that marginalized women living with various vulnerabilities, including mental illness, active substance use, HIV, and unstable housing, show improved measures of HIV care (including viral load and medication adherence) when exposed to a weekly bidirectional text-messaging intervention (King et al., 2017). This evidence has significant implications for PHNs working with marginalized populations living with HIV because using innovative interventions, such as text-messaging, can be used as a form of tertiary prevention.

Quaternary prevention initiatives are those actions that identify individuals or populations at risk of over-medicalization (Tesser & Norman, 2016; Porta, 2014). Usually guidelines and policies that reflect operational knowledge are put into place that help to protect individuals from over-diagnosis or over-medicalization (Tesser, 2017; Tesser & Norman, 2016). Sometimes, this includes protecting populations from new medical procedures or interventions that are untested and proposing alternatives that are ethically appropriate for both populations and health care professionals alike (Tesser, 2017; Vollman et al., 2017). In a recent research study, patents who were diagnosed with a variant of uncertain significance (VUS) in a BRCA gene showed very high rates of bilateral prophylactic mastectomy, exceeding 38% (Welsh et al., 2017). Interestingly, over time, a significant proportion of BRCA VUS were reclassified as benign (Welsh et al., 2017). As an example of quaternary prevention, PHNs could engage this population group to participate in a support network to discuss the benefits and drawbacks of bilateral prophylactic mastectomy and whether it is considered to be a necessary form of intervention. Choosing Wisely is an international movement that began in the United States in 2012 to decrease unnecessary tests and procedures. It encourages dialogue between patients and clinicians to determine if a procedure is truly necessary. Choosing Wisely Canada was established in 2014 and works with various partners to create lists of tests and procedures that are not supported by evidence and may cause harm.

CANADIAN RESEARCH 4.1

Improving children's health and development in British Columbia through nurse home visiting: A randomized controlled trial protocol (Catherine et al., 2016)

Nurse-Family Partnership is a home visitation program designed for first-time lone-parent mothers experiencing socioeconomic disadvantage. During the program, PHNs visit mothers regularly during the prenatal period and for the first two years of the child's life. PHNs provide mothers with emotional and informational support, childcare guidance, and referral to other community services. The program began in the 1980s as the Perinatal/Early Infancy Project. It has been proven effective and has been replicated in 250 countries. Researchers have reported enhanced maternal outcomes such as better overall health, decreased substance use, and less depression, as well as safer home environments and diminished child abuse and neglect. The British Columbia Healthy Connections Project is conducting a randomized controlled trial to evaluate the effectiveness of the Nurse-Family Partnership in comparison to usual services in improving child development and mental health and mothers' life circumstances.

Discussion Questions

1. What levels of prevention exist within the Nurse-Family Partnership program?

2. Identify at least two essential functions of public health that the PHN may be carrying out when engaging in the Nurse-Family Partnership program.

3. Explain how the PHN may have to assume the public health nursing role of outreach worker while engaging in the Nurse-Family Partnership program.

YES, BUT WHY?

Inadequate Access to Food

What?

Did you know that many Canadians are having difficulty accessing food due to lack of money? Canadians are experiencing what has been termed "food insecurity," a persistent public health concern in every province and territory, especially among single-mother families and in Northern and remote regions of Canada (McIntyre & Anderson, 2016). Statistics Canada reported that in 2014, over 4 million Canadians could not access the food they needed to live a healthy life, and one in six Canadian children are living in food-insecure households (PROOF, n.d.). For example, 60% of Inuit children experience food insecurity (Findlay, Langlois, & Kohen, 2013). Most prevalent in Canada's North and the Maritimes are their experiences of not having enough to eat or, worse yet, going without eating for days at a time (Tarasuk, Mitchell, & Dachner, 2016).

So What?

Inadequate access to nutritious food places children at risk for physical and mental developmental delay and health problems (Council of Canadian Academies, 2014; Fram, Ritchie, Rosen, & Frongillo, 2015). Hunger, or severe food insecurity, experienced in childhood puts children at risk of developing respiratory complications, hyperactivity, and, depression and suicidal ideation as teenagers and young adults (McIntyre, Wu, Kwok, &

Patten, 2017). Access to nutritious food is not only a necessity but also a child's basic human right according to the Canadian Coalition for the Rights of Children (2012), which established the Convention on the Rights of the Child to better protect children's rights across Canada. Compared to other wealthy nations, Canada has done little to protect the basic rights of children and promote early child development (Raphael, 2016). Since the national income support policies (e.g., Universal Child Care Benefit and Child Tax Credit) were introduced in 2006 and 2007, child poverty has increased with greater decline in child well-being (Canadian Coalition for the Rights of Children, 2012; Raphael, 2016). We see inequities with less financial support offered for children in low-income households than for children in high-income households. Recently, the Liberal government announced an additional $200 in Canada Child Benefits for an average family with two children by July 2018 (MacGillivray, 2017).

Food insecurity continues to be a harsh reality for Inuit children such as those living in Nunavut, but in this Northern community the lack of sufficient income is not the only root cause. Other reasons include the decline of local, traditional foods from animal and plant sources, which for generations provided nutritious, cultural, and social benefits, and the imposition of store-bought foreign food that is transported at a high cost (Council of Canadian Academies, 2014). Although higher incomes will cover exorbitant food costs, are other measures warranted here to adequately address why food insecurity exists in Northern regions of Canada?

Now What?

PHNs can contribute to improving access to food by paying attention to research reports documenting the problem in their province or territory and by using the evidence to lobby for program and policy solutions at municipal, provincial, territorial, and federal levels of government (Tarasuk et al., 2016). PHNs can join global initiatives similar to the UN Special Rapporteur on the Right to Food, which has recommended a national food strategy to address the high rates of food insecurity in Canada's Inuit communities. At the community level, PHNs can advocate for higher social assistance benefits for single-parent families and can initiate or support school lunch programs (e.g., First Nations Nutrition Program).

Standards of Practice Fulfilled

#1 Health Promotion
- Seeks to identify and assess the root and historical causes of illness, disease and inequities in health, acknowledges diversity and the adverse effects of colonialism on Indigenous people, and when appropriate incorporates Indigenous ways of knowing including connectedness and reciprocity to the land and all life in health promotion.

 # 6 Health Equity
- Advocates for healthy public policy and social justice by participating in legislative and policy-making activities that influence determinants of health and access to services (CHNC, 2019, revised).

CASE STUDY

Matthew is a 42-year-old man who has been homeless for several years. A PHN, Heather, has been working with Matthew for the past three years. She is part of a team, including other nurses, an occupational therapist, a social worker, and a physician, which provides mobile outreach to the street-involved, including individuals who are using drugs and the homeless. The team's motto is, "We provide health care wherever you are." When Heather and other team members started working with Matthew, he told them he had epilepsy, which had caused trouble with the police, who once thought he was drunk when he fell while having a seizure. Since they started working with Matthew, he obtained a medical alert bracelet that will notify police and others of his epilepsy. Because Matthew is marginally literate, the team arranged for his medications to be dispensed in a blister pack with verbal explanation of how to use it so he more clearly understood when to take them. They helped him find affordable housing and taught him how to shop for affordable and nutritious food. Heather formed a committee consisting of the police and individuals working in homeless shelters, needle exchange programs, and crisis counselling centres to identify gaps in service and determine how best to address them. They have recruited volunteers from their target group to sit on their committee. A former homeless drug user is currently co-chairing the committee with Heather. The committee is developing a comprehensive strategy to provide employment training, supportive housing, and addiction treatment to enable individuals to achieve better health. She reported that one client said, "I feel valued as a human being again, the first time in a long time, because the nurse and others cared about me and helped me. I now take better care of myself and look forward to what the future may bring."

Discussion Questions

1. What core public health essential functions is the interprofessional team demonstrating in this situation?

2. Which public health nursing discipline-specific competencies does Heather demonstrate in this case study?

3. What public health nursing roles does Heather demonstrate in this case study?

CONCLUSION

PHNs have played and continue to play instrumental roles in the health and well-being of Canadians. Earliest documented accounts attest to the dedication, commitment, and visionary leadership of Canada's public health nursing pioneers. Today's PHNs face complex health-related issues locally, nationally, and globally. Safeguarding the health of the Canadian population entails assuming several roles, and PHNs must be equipped with diverse competencies. The career of the PHN will continue to be both challenging and exciting as PHNs work to fulfill the essential functions of health protection, health surveillance, population health assessment, disease and injury prevention, health promotion, and emergency preparation and response, for the betterment of all Canadians.

KEY TERMS

disease and injury prevention   (p. 65)

emergency preparation and response   (p. 65)

health promotion   (p. 65)

health protection   (p. 65)

health surveillance   (p. 65)

population health assessment   (p. 65)

primary prevention   (p. 65)

primordial prevention   (p. 65)

principles of primary health care   (p. 59)

public health   (p. 58)

public health nurse (PHN)   (p. 59)

public health nursing discipline-specific competencies   (p. 63)

quaternary prevention   (p. 69)

secondary prevention   (p. 65)

six essential functions of public health   (p. 65)

tertiary prevention   (p. 69)

STUDY QUESTIONS

1. What is the definition of public health?

2. When was the PHAC established, and why?

3. What is the role of the PHAC?

4. What are the six essential functions of public health in Canada?

5. What are the public health nursing disciplinary-specific competencies?

6. Discuss what you think are two of the most important contributions early PHNs have made and why.

INDIVIDUAL CRITICAL-THINKING EXERCISES

1. Consider the definition of public health presented in this chapter. Is there another component you think is critical to include in this definition?

2. Although the PHAC was established relatively recently, what other organizations in your province also contribute to public health?

3. How do you think PHNs may contribute to the work of the PHAC?

4. Why do you think it is important to have public health nursing disciplinary-specific competencies?

GROUP CRITICAL-THINKING EXERCISES

1. Discuss what course concepts you have learned in class that relate to the public health nursing discipline-specific competencies.

2. What public health activities are you able to identify in the communities in which you live?

3. What current events locally, nationally, or globally could benefit from critically examining the issues through a social justice lens? What role might PHNs play in addressing these issues?

REFERENCES

Allemang, M. (1995). Development of community health nursing in Canada. In M. J. Stewart (Ed.), *Community nursing: Promoting Canadians' health* (pp. 2–36). Toronto, ON: W. B. Saunders.

American Public Health Association. (2018). Our work. Retrieved from https://www.apha.org/what-is-public-health/generation-public-health/our-work

Benbow, S., Gorlick, C., Forchuk, C., Ward-Griffin, C., & Berman, H. (2016). Ontario's poverty reduction strategy: A critical discourse analysis. *Canadian Journal of Nursing Research, 48*(3–4), 100–109.

Bryce, P. (1910). History of public health in Canada. *The Canadian Therapeutist and Sanitary Engineer, 1,* 287–291. Retrieved from http://www.cpha.ca/uploads/history/book/History-book-print_chapter1_e.pdf

Butterfield, P. G. (2002). Upstream reflections on environmental health: An abbreviated history and framework for action. *Advances in Nursing Science, 25*(1), 32–49.

Canadian Coalition for Rights of Children. (2012). *Right in principle, right in practice: Implementation of the convention on the rights of the child in Canada*. Toronto, ON: Author. Retrieved from http://rightsofchildren.ca/wp-content/uploads/2016/01/CCRC-report-on-rights-of-children-in-Canada.pdf

Canadian Nurses Association (CNA). (1988). *Health for all Canadians: A call for health-care reform*. Ottawa, ON: Author.

Canadian Nurses Association (CNA). (2017). *Code of ethics for registered nurses* (2017 edition). Ottawa, ON: Author. Retrieved from https://www.cna-aiic.ca/~/media/cna/page-content/pdf-en/code-of-ethics-2017-edition-secure-interactive.pdf?la=en

Canadian Public Health Association (CPHA). (n.d.). 12 great achievements. Ottawa, ON: Author. Retrieved from http://www.cpha.ca/en/programs/history/achievements.aspp

Canadian Public Health Association (CPHA). (2010). *Public health/Community health nursing practice in Canada: Roles and activities* (4th ed.). Ottawa, ON: Author. Retrieved from http://www.cpha.ca/uploads/pubs/3-1bk04214.pdf

Catherine, N. L. A., Gonzalez, A., Boyle, M., Sheehan, D., Jack, S. M., Hougham, K. A., . . . Waddell, C. (2016). Improving children's health and development in British Columbia through nurse home visiting: A randomized controlled trial protocol. *BMC Health Services Research, 16,* 349. doi: 10.1186/s12913-016-1594-0

Community Health Nurses of Canada. (2009). *The public health nursing discipline specific competencies,* version 1.0. St. John's, NL: Author. Retrieved from http://www.chnc.ca/documents/competencies_june_2009_english.pdf

Community Health Nurses of Canada. (2019, revised). Canadian Community Health Nursing Professional Practice Model and Standards of Practice. St. John's, NL: Author.

Retrieved from https://www.chnc.ca/en/standards-of-practice?lang=switch1

Community Health Nurses of Canada. (2013). *Public health nursing leadership in Canada: Report to the National Collaborating Center on the Determinants of Health.* St. John's, NL: Author. Retrieved from https://www.chnc.ca/documents/PHNLeadershipDevelopmentinCanadaFinalReportwlogo-andacknowledgements2014Fub27.pdf

Community Health Nurses of Canada. (2015). *Leadership competencies for public health practice in Canada.* Version 1.0. St. John's, NL: Author. Retrieved from http://chnc.ca/documents/LCPHPC-EN

Council of Canadian Academies. (2014). *Aboriginal food security in northern Canada: Assessment of the state of knowledge.* Ottawa, ON: Expert Panel on the State of Knowledge of Food Security in Northern Canada. Retrieved from http://www.scienceadvice.ca/uploads/eng/assessments%20and%20publications%20and%20news%20releases/food%20security/foodsecurity_fullreporten.pdf

Dennis, C. L., Merry, L., & Gagnon, A. J. (2017). Postpartum depression risk factors among recent refugee, asylum-seeking, non-refugee immigrant, and Canadian-born women: Results from a prospective cohort study. *Social Psychiatry and Psychiatric Epidemiology, 52*(4), 411–422. doi:10.1007/s00127-017-1353-5

Epp, J. (1986). *Achieving health for all: A framework for health promotion in Canada.* Toronto, ON: Health and Welfare Canada.

Falk-Raphael, A. (2005). Speaking truth to power: Nursing's legacy and moral imperative. *Advances in Nursing Science, 28*(3), 212–223.

Findlay, L. C., Langlois, K. A., & Kohen, D. E. (2013). Hunger among Inuit children in Canada. *International Journal of Circumpolar Health, 72*(1), n.p. doi: 10.3402/ijch.v.72i0.20324

Fram, M. S., Ritchie, L. D., Rosen, N., & Frongillo, E. A. (2015). Child experience of food insecurity is association with child diet and physical activity. *The Journal of Nutrition, 145*(3), 499–504. doi: 10.3945/jn.114.194365

Gottlieb, L. (2013). *Strengths-based nursing care: Health and healing for person and family.* New York, NY: Springer.

Government of Canada: *Public Health Agency of Canada Act,* S.C., c. 5, 2006, c. Article 12. Retrieved from http://laws-lois.justice.gc.ca/eng/annualstatutes/2006_5/page-1.html

Harrison, C. (2011). *A passion for prevention: Public health nursing in Skeena health unit, 1937–1997.* Victoria, BC: First Choice Books.

He, H., Xiao, L., Torrie, J. E., Auger, N., McHugh, N. G. L., Zoungrana, H., & Luo, Z. C. (2017). Disparities in infant hospitalizations in Indigenous and non-Indigenous populations in Quebec, Canada. *Canadian Medical Association Journal, 189*(21), E739–E746. doi:10.1503/cmaj.160900

Her Majesty the Queen in Right of Canada, represented by the Minister of Health. (2008). *The chief public health officer's report on the state of public health in Canada 2008. Addressing health inequalities.* Ottawa, ON: Author. Retrieved from http://www.phac-aspc.gc.ca/cphorsphc-respcacsp/2008/fr-rc/index-eng.php

King, E., Kinvig, K., Steif, J., Qiu, A. Q., Maan, E. J., Albert, A. Y., . . . Murray, M. C. M. (2017). Mobile text messaging to improve medication adherence and viral load in a vulnerable Canadian population living with Human Immunodeficiency Virus: A repeated measures study. *Journal of Medical Internet Research, 19*(6), e190. doi:10.2196/jmir.6631

Last, J. M. (2001). *A Dictionary of epidemiology* (4th ed.). New York, NY: Oxford University Press.

Little, C. (1992). Health for all by the year 2000: Where is it now? *Nursing and Health Care, 13*(4), 198–201.

MacGillivray, S. (2017, October 23). Liberal government to boost Canada child benefit payments: Sources. *CBC News.* Retrieved from http://www.cbc.ca/news/politics/liberal-government-canada-child-benefit-boost-sources-1.4368019

Mahler, H. (1985). "Nurses lead the way." *New Zealand Nursing Journal, 78*(10), 10–11.

Marsh, M., Walsh, J., & Beaton, M. (2008). *A life of caring: Sixteen Newfoundland nurses tell their stories.* St. John's, NL: Breakwater Books.

McGee, E. J. T., Sangakkara, A. R., & Diosady, L. L. (2017). Double fortification of salt with folic acid and iodine. *Journal of Food Engineering, 198,* 72–80. http://dx.doi.org/10.1016/j.jfoodeng.2016.11.019

McIntyre, L., Wu, X., Kwok, C., & Patten, S. (2017). The pervasive effect of youth self-report of hunger on depression over 6 years of follow up. *Social Psychiatry and Psychiatric Epidemiology, 52*(5), 537–547.

McIntyre, L., & Anderson, L. (2016). Food insecurity. In D. Raphael (Ed.), *Social determinants of health: Canadian perspectives* (3rd ed., pp. 294–320). Toronto, ON: Canadian Scholars' Press.

McKay, M. (2009). Public health nursing in early 20th century in Canada. *Canadian Journal of Public Health, 100*(4), 249–250. Retrieved from http://journal.cpha.ca/index.php/cjph/issue/view/267

Myers, S. S., & Patz, J. A. (2009). Emerging threats to human health from global environmental change. *Annual Review of Environment and Resources, 34,* 223–252. doi:10.1146/annurev.environ.033108.102650

Ontario Ministry of Government Services. (n.d.). *Public health nurses: Bringing health home.* Retrieved from http://www.archives.gov.on.ca/en/explore/online/health_promotion/health_home.aspx

Porta, M. (Ed.). (2014). *A dictionary of epidemiology* (6th ed.). New York, NY: Oxford University Press.

PROOF. (n.d.). Children in food insecure households (brochure). Toronto: Research to Identify Policy Options to Reduce Food Insecurity (PROOF). Retrieved from http://proof.utoronto.ca/wp-content/uploads/2016/07/children-food-insecurity-factsheet.pdf

Public Health Agency of Canada. (n.d.). *Chapter 3: The role and organization of public health* [archived]. Ottawa, ON: Author. Retrieved from http://www.phac-aspc.gc.ca/publicat/sars-sras/naylor/3-eng.php#s3a

Public Health Agency of Canada (PHAC). (2018). © All rights reserved. *About the Agency: History.* Public Health Agency of Canada, 2018. Adapted and reproduced with permission from the Minister of Health, 2018.

Raphael, D. (2011). *Poverty in Canada: Implications for health and quality of life* (2nd ed.). Toronto, ON: Canadian Scholars' Press.

Raphael, D. (2016). Early child development and health. In D. Raphael (Ed.), *Social determinants of health: Canadian perspectives* (3rd ed., pp. 218–239). Toronto, ON: Canadian Scholars' Press.

Reutter, L., & Ford, J. S. (1998). Perceptions of changes in public health nursing practice: A Canadian perspective. *International Journal of Nursing Studies, 35*(1–2), 85–94. doi:10.1016/S0020-7489(97)00036-9

Smylie, J., Kirst, M., McShane, K., Firestone, M., Wolfe, S., & O'Campo, P. (2016). Understanding the role of Indigenous community participation in Indigenous prenatal and infant-toddler health promotion programs in Canada: A realist review. *Social Science & Medicine, 150,* 128–143. http://dx.doi.org/10.1016/j.socscimed.2015.12.019

Starfield, B. (2001). Basic concepts in population health and health care. *Journal of Epidemiology & Community Health, 55*(7), 452–454.

Tarasuk, V., Mitchell, A., & Dachner, N. (2016). *Household food insecurity in Canada, 2014.* Toronto, ON: Research to Identify Policy Options to Reduce Food Insecurity (PROOF). Retrieved from http://proof.utoronto.ca/wp-content/uploads/2016/04/Household-Food-Insecurity-in-Canada-2014.pdf

Tesser, C. D., & Norman, A. H. (2016). Differentiating clinical care from disease prevention: A prerequisite for practicing quaternary prevention. *Cadernos de Saude Publica, 32*(10), e00012316. http://dx.doi.org/10.1590/0102-311X00012316

Tesser, C. D. (2017). Why is quaternary prevention important in prevention? *Revista de Saude Publica, 51*(116), 9 pages. https://doi.org/10.11606/S1518-8787.2017051000041

Underwood, J. (2010). Maximizing community health nursing capacity in Canada: A research summary for decision makers. [Report of the national community health nursing study.] Ottawa, ON: Canadian Health Services Research Foundation. Retrieved from http://www.cfhi-fcass.ca/Migrated/PDF/ResearchReports/11510_Reiss_report_en_FINAL.pdf, http://site.ebrary.com/lib/memorial/Doc?id=10374331&ppg=10

Vollman, A. R., Anderson, E. T., & McFarlane, J. (2017). *Canadian community as partner: Theory and multidisciplinary practice* (4th ed.). Philadelphia, PA: Wolters Kluwer.

Welsh, J. L., Hoskin, T. L., Day, C. N., Thomas, A. S., Cogswell, J. A., Couch, F. J., & Boughey, J. C. (2017). Clinical decision-making in patients with variant of uncertain significance in BRCA1 or BRCA2 genes. *Annals of Surgical Oncology, 24*(10), 3067–3072. doi:10.1245/s10434-017-5959

World Health Organization, Health & Welfare Canada, & Canadian Public Health Association. (1986). *Ottawa charter for health promotion.* Ottawa, ON: Canadian Public Health Association.

ABOUT THE AUTHORS

Caroline J. Porr, BScN, MN, PhD, RN, CHNC(C), is Associate Professor in the School of Nursing at Memorial University in Newfoundland and Labrador. She is the recipient of Memorial's 2017 President's Award for Outstanding Teaching (Faculty). During her PhD research at the University of Alberta, she formulated a theoretical model of relationship building to inform public health nurses of how to establish therapeutic rapport when working with vulnerable and potentially stigmatized clients. One of her research pursuits has been to disseminate and test the model for its utility for front-line public health nursing practice. Dr. Porr has since facilitated several relational skills training workshops focused on helping public health nurses develop therapeutic relationships with lower-income lone-parent mothers.

Anne J. Kearney, BN, MHSC, PhD, RN, is Professor in the School of Nursing at Memorial University in Newfoundland and Labrador. All of her graduate work was in community health. Her PhD research explored women's practice of breast self-examination from a critical social perspective. She currently teaches community health nursing courses and has two programs of research. Her main program involves the critical appraisal of evidence related to the effectiveness of breast screening, particularly population-based mammography screening. She is also engaged in research to improve the conditions of nurses' worklife.

Aliyah Dosani, RN, BN, MPH, PhD, is Associate Professor in the School of Nursing and Midwifery, Faculty of Health, Community and Education at Mount Royal University in Calgary, Alberta. She is also an Adjunct Associate Professor in the Department of Community Health Sciences, Cumming School of Medicine, at University of Calgary in Calgary. She holds a PhD from the University of Calgary with a specialization in population/public health. Her nursing practice includes instructing students in the Bachelor of Nursing program, population/public health, community health nursing, and legal issues in nursing. Her work focuses on maternal, newborn, and child health. Her research interests include working on health equity and social justice issues through community-based programs and interventions. She also shares a passion for global health issues.

Home Health Nursing in Canada

Shirlee Sharkey, Nancy Lefebre, Karen L. Ray, Tracy Scott, and the Saint Elizabeth First Nations, Inuit and Métis Team

LEARNING OUTCOMES

After studying this chapter, you should be able to:

1. Summarize the evolution of home care and home health nursing in Canada.

2. Describe the role and unique characteristics of home health nursing.

3. Understand key areas of practice, key competencies, and desired outcomes of home health nurses.

4. Outline the organizational supports that are required for home health nurses to deliver high quality care.

5. Discuss current rewards and challenges in home health nursing.

6. Outline various issues related to health equity in home health nursing.

7. Articulate the opportunities and future for home health nursing.

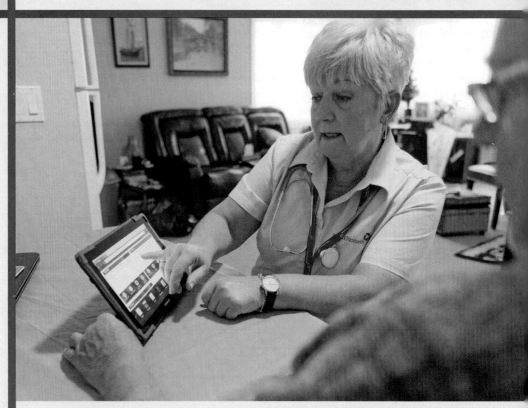

Source: Saint Elizabeth Health Care

INTRODUCTION

"People want to be at home and to direct their care, even when their health is compromised" (Canadian Nurses Association [CNA], 2013, p. iii). Keeping people at home is key to a sustainable health system, and **home health nurses (HHNs)** are the most utilized professional resource in home care. They are highly independent and autonomous and have the knowledge, interpersonal skills, and proven positive health outcomes to deliver care (CNA, 2013, p. iii). HHNs care for a diverse population of Canadians, with the goal of partnering with individuals and families to restore health, manage chronic health conditions, or gently transition to palliative care.

As described in Chapter 1, home health nursing was first evident in Canada in the early 17th century when nuns from religious orders arrived in Quebec to provide both direct nursing care and disease prevention (Community Health Nurses' Initiatives Group, 2000). To understand the role of HHNs in the Canadian health care system today, it is important to appreciate the foundations of home care and how it has evolved across the country.

Updating the Definition of Home Care

Canada's publicly funded health care system is based on values of fairness, equity, and support for individuals and their caregivers as established through the Canada Health Act (1984) (Government of Canada, 2017a). The Act sets the requirements that must be met by provinces and territories to ensure "reasonable access to medically necessary hospital and physician services." Through five core principles—portability, accessibility, universality, comprehensiveness, and public administration—the intent is to provide Canadians with health care "according to need and irrespective of their ability to pay" (Canadian Museum of Civilization, 1966). **Home care** is recognized as an "extended health service" and is not a publicly insured under the Canada Health Act.

Home care has evolved in response to providing health care services "closer to home" (see the Definition of Home Care and Home Health Nursing box that follows). By 1988, the federal government and all provinces and territories had launched home care programs, and in 1999, home care was extended to First Nation and Inuit communities (Canadian Home Care Association [CHCA], 2013) (see Figure 5.1). Several initiatives highlighted the need for further focus and investment in home care in Canada. For instance, the **Kirby Report** (Kirby, 2002) and the **Romanow Commission** (Romanow, 2002) described home care as an **essential service** of the health care system. These initiatives culminated with the creation of the **First Ministers Accord on Health Care Renewal**, which established a guarantee for first-dollar coverage for "a basket of services" in the home (Health Canada, 2003). However, despite this pledge, substantial variations are present in provincial home care funding, access, and services across Canada.

Home care consists of an array of services for people of all ages, provided in the home or community setting. Home care is designed to complement, not replace, the efforts of individuals to care for themselves with the assistance of family, friends, and community networks (CHCA, 2013). Although there is variation across the country, home care generally consists of the provision of nursing, personal care, physiotherapy, occupational therapy, social work, dietetics, speech language therapy, and medical equipment and supplies in the home. About 70% of home care is funded by the government through the public health care system, and the rest comes from private sources like supplemental insurance and out-of-pocket spending.

DEFINITION OF HOME CARE AND HOME HEALTH NURSING

Different types of home care services include acute, chronic, rehabilitative, and palliative care. With the aging Canadian population, home care is increasingly shifting toward a focus on chronic and rehabilitative health care needs in order to support people to live independently in their communities for as long as possible. When this is no longer viable, home care assists with coordinating and managing admission to long-term care (CHCA, 2013).

1970	Ontario
1972	Quebec
1974	Manitoba
1975	Newfoundland and Labrador
1978	British Columbia, Alberta, Saskatchewan, Northwest Territories
1979	New Brunswick
1981	Veterans Affairs Canada
1986	Prince Edward Island
1988	Nova Scotia, Yukon
1999	Nunavut, First Nations and Inuit Health Branch, Health Canada, Royal Canadian Mounted Police
2005	Canadian Forces

FIGURE 5.1 Year of Initiation of Publicly Funded Home Care Programs in Canada

Source: Canadian Home Care Association (CHCA), 2013.

Community Nurses

Home health nurses are just one of seven groups of nurses who work in the community. Although their job titles and workplaces may vary, studies show that nurses who work outside of institutions, in community settings such as ambulatory care, public health, occupational health, or home care, possess a common set of skills, knowledge, and attitudes (Underwood et al., 2009). Table 5.1 identifies the diverse roles of community health nurses, including those working in home health.

HOME HEALTH NURSING

As identified in Table 5.1, home health nursing is a specialized area of practice that is delivered in the client's home, school, or workplace, as well as in long-term care facilities, older adult residences, clinics, and other community settings. According to the Ontario Home Care Association (2011), the unique contribution of HHNs is their ability to combine knowledge from primary health care, such as the determinants of health (Chapter 1 and others), nursing science, and social science, to focus on prevention of illness or disease, health restoration, maintenance, or palliation. HHNs incorporate teaching and coaching into their care, and they initiate, manage, and evaluate the resources needed for each client. One of the unique aspects of home health nursing is the range of ages, diagnoses, and conditions among clients (Mildon & Underwood, 2010).

Who Are Home Health Nurses?

HHNs are registered nurses (RNs), licensed practical nurses (LPNs), and registered practical nurses (RPNs). For some clients, care may require the advanced assessment, critical decision-making skills, care planning, and supervision of unregulated workers consistent with RN practice. When the

Table 5.1		Clarifying Community Health Nursing Roles					
Title	Setting for Care	Primary Area of Focus	Defined Competencies	Funding	Target Population	RN/LPN
Public Health Nurse	Community venues such as schools, churches, community health centres, and homes	Disease and injury prevention, health promotion, and community development; program planning and policy development	Yes	Public health agency. In Ontario provincial and municipal funding. Rare federal funding for programs such as Canada Prenatal Nutrition Program (CPNP)	Individuals (babies, those with communicable diseases); population-based groups and the larger community	RN, some RPNs
Home Health Nurse	Home, school, clinic, and other residential settings, including shelters and on the street	Treatment of diseases or conditions that require surgical or clinical interventions; care coordination	Yes	Differs by province; some are employed by regional health authorities, whereas others are employed by not-for-profit and for-profit home care provider organizations	Individuals and their families or supports	RN LPN
Community Health Nurse	Community health centres (CHC)	Varies by CHC; could be disease prevention, treatment, health promotion, or community development; program planning	No	Provincial health budget	Individuals, families, and members of the local community, which quite often includes vulnerable groups	RN LPN

outcomes of care are more predictable, such as in chronic disease management or wound care, clients may benefit from the knowledge, skills, and expertise of LPN/RPNs. This delineation allows all categories of HHNs to work to their full scope of practice, provide high-quality care, and experience greater job satisfaction (CNA, 2013).

Currently, the number of nurses working in home care is difficult to determine due to the lack of delineation between community nursing job titles. We do know the number of nurses working in the community has increased since 2010 (see Table 5.2) and that 10 377 nurses in Canada state home care is their primary area of responsibility, representing 2.6% of the Canadian nursing workforce (Canadian Institute for Health Information [CHI], 2016).

Features of Home Health Nursing

HHNs utilize the **Community Health Nurses of Canada (CHNC)** model of care, which includes the application of general nursing Professional Regulatory Standards, Canadian Community Health Nursing (CCHN) Standards, Home Health Standards, and Home Health Nursing Competencies (Canadian Health Nurses of Canada [CHNC], 2019, revised). The **Competencies for Home Health Nursing** are discipline-specific competencies based on those previously devel-

oped by the Public Health Agency of Canada (2007) and place a strong emphasis on the highly independent and autonomous, flexible, and adaptive nature of the HHN, characterized best as being a "**guest in the home**" (CHNC, 2010).

The Competencies for Home Health Nursing consist of three overarching categories and 78 home health nursing discipline-specific competencies. The first competency category, **Elements of Home Health Nursing**, focuses on "the nursing activities, functions, goals and outcomes that are central to home health nursing practice" (CHNC, 2010, p. 9). The second competency category, **Foundations of Home Health Nursing**, focuses on "the core knowledge and primary health care philosophy that is central to home health nursing practice" (CHNC, 2010, p. 12) and includes health promotion, illness prevention, and health protection. The third competency category, **Quality and Professional Responsibilities**, focuses on "practice activities and/or strategies by which the HHN promotes quality of care and demonstrates professional responsibility" (CHNC, 2010, p. 13). (See Appendix C.)

HOME HEALTH NURSING CARE

In addition to the use of competencies and College of Nurses regulations, HHNs work according to local health authority policies and procedures, provincial legislation, nursing evidence,

Table 5.2	Regulated Nurses in Canada, 2016								

Registered Nurses (RNs) and Nurse Practitioners (NPs)

In 2016, a total of 44 609 RNs and NPs were employed in community care, 15.8% of all RNs across the provinces, with an increase of 7% since 2010.

Percentage of RNs in community health[1] in 2016

BC	AB	SK	MB	ON	QC	NB	NS	PE	NL
16.4%	17%	18.4%	16.1%	17.1%	13.1%	13.2%	11.3%	5%	14.4%

Licensed Practical Nurses (LPNs)/Registered Practical Nurses (RPNs)

In 2016, a total of 14 159 LPNs were employed in community care, 13.5% of LPNs/RPNs across the provinces, with an increase of 51% since 2010.

Percentage of LPN/RPNs in community health[1] in 2016

BC	AB	SK	MB	ON	QC	NB	NS	PE	NL
10.4%	26.5%	26.5%	15.2%	17.1%	1.9%	5.5%	17.1%	13.6%	4.3%

Note: 1. Community health includes data from community health centres, home care agencies, nursing stations (outposts or clinics), public health departments or units, and physicians' offices and family practice units.

Source: Canadian Institute for Health Information (2016).

and doctors' orders. On average, most HHNs have a caseload of 8–12 clients per day and generally travel from place to place to provide care. Workload depends on each client's condition and the nursing care required, which may be provided on either a visit or a shift basis. With the emergence of new care and funding models, some visits may be delivered virtually or augmented by technologies such remote patient monitoring. Type of care provided in the home is reflective of what other nurses see in the hospital, including management of chronic disease, and conditions affecting older adults such as dementia.

Generally, HHNs conduct a comprehensive assessment of the client in order to develop a care plan, monitor the condition, and make changes as needed (CHNC, 2010, p. 9). Client education is provided regarding their condition and treatment and includes such aspects as diet and mobilization to prevent complications. As well, the HHN plays a pivotal role in identifying and mitigating client risk at home, such as the potential for falls or medication errors (Canadian Patient Safety Institute, 2013; CHNC, 2010, p. 10).

HHNs also undertake care planning and care coordination, especially when working with clients with life-limiting illness (CHNC, 2010, p. 9). For clients who choose to remain at home for end-of-life care, the HHN works with the client, family, and health care team to provide pain and symptom management and psychosocial support. As part of this, the HHN assesses the family's ability to provide ongoing care or the need for additional services. It can be challenging for families to provide care, particularly if they are geographically dispersed or occupied with work and child rearing (Armstrong & Armstrong, 2008).

Facilitating Access and Equity

An important HHN core competency is to facilitate access to health care for all Canadians (CHNC, 2010, p. 11). Canada is a diverse nation with a multitude of cultures, identities, and approaches to health and living, and HHNs need to ensure their care is both respectful and culturally sensitive in order to avoid discrimination and ensure equitable care. As part of this,

it is vital that HHNs "optimize the allocation of human, financial and infrastructure resources" (CHNC, 2010, p. 11). This requires that they work collaboratively with other members of the interprofessional team or community resources designed to support people at home (Conference Board of Canada, 2012).

Building Relationships

Another aspect central to home health nursing is the ability to communicate and build a relationship with the client and their family during one or several visits. Being a guest in the home provides a unique opportunity for nurses to get to know the client in their everyday natural environment and support the family's role in promoting and maintaining health (CHNC, 2010, p. 11; Registered Nurses' Association of Ontario, 2002). To ensure care reflects the client and family needs and goals, HHNs practice **person- and family-centred care (PFCC)** (Institute for Patient and Family-Centred Care, 2017). PFCC acknowledges the expertise and experience that those receiving and providing care both bring to the relationship (Health Foundation, 2015; Saint Elizabeth, 2011). This represents a shift from a traditional "expert-driven" medical model where providers set the agenda and goals for care. PFCC is achieved by treating clients and their families with compassion, dignity, and respect and ensuring they have the information they need to make informed decisions about their care (CHNC, 2010, p. 11; Health Foundation, 2015).

Outcomes of Home Health Nursing

Monitoring HHN care outcomes through case review or chart audits helps ensure quality care and professional accountability (CHNC, 2010, p. 13). In Ontario, several home care organizations have collected nursing-sensitive outcomes over the last 10 years called **C-Health Outcomes for Better Information and Care (C-HOBIC)**. These indicators help assess the functional status of clients, their symptoms, therapeutic self-care, and risk of hospital readmissions or adverse events (Nagle & White, 2013; Nagle, White, & Pringle, 2010; Sun & Doran, 2014; Sun, Doran, Wodchis, & Peter, 2017; White, Nagle, & Hannah, 2017). Recently, some have suggested that in addition to clinical outcomes, patient-reported outcome measures and patient-reported experience measures should also be collected to provide a more comprehensive view of client health (Tourangeau, Kelly, Patterson, & Saari, 2016a; Tourangeau, Kelly, Patterson, & Saari, 2016b).

CANADIAN RESEARCH 5.1

Nurse-led health promotion interventions improve quality of life in frail older home care clients: Lessons learned from three randomized trials in Ontario, Canada.
(Markle-Reid, Browne, & Gafni, 2013)

Despite the general lack of data available to nurses on a regular basis, researchers have been able to painstakingly gather evidence to demonstrate that HHNs play a major role in home care by providing health assessment, support, access to resources, health promotion, and preventive care through regular home visits. This study helped to answer the question: Do home care interventions improve quality of life for clients?

A great focus is being placed on the frail older adult population due to their rising numbers and complex health needs. Not only is there a need to reduce the cost of hospitalization, but also home is where most people want to be. This study examined the lessons learned from three randomized controlled trials that included 498 community-living, frail older adults (65 years of age or more) using home health services in southern Ontario. Each study was designed to evaluate the effectiveness of different multicomponent, nurse-led health promotion and disease prevention interventions. The nurse-led interventions used evidence-based strategies to address known risk factors for functional decline and frailty. Across the three studies, a common approach was used to measure the change in health-related quality of life and the costs of health services.

The main lesson learned from the three studies is that nurse-led interventions for frail older home care clients provided greater improvements in quality of life and a foundation for "aging in place." The intervention included multiple home visits, multidimensional screening and assessment, evidence-based strategies, intensive case management, interprofessional collaboration, providers with geriatric training and experience, and referral to and coordination of community services.

Discussion Questions

1. What is the difference between a nurse-led and a medical model approach to care?
2. Since HHNs work in partnership with families, how do nurse-led home care programs benefit clients?
3. State why "aging in place" an important concept in today's Canadian society?

DEFINITION OF SERVICE PROVIDER ORGANIZATIONS

SPOs are usually incorporated entities and can be not-for-profit organizations; private corporations; municipal governments; or First Nation, Inuit, or Métis organizations. SPOs are responsible for providing nursing care, home support services, personal care, physiotherapy, occupational therapy, social work, dietetics, speech language therapy, and medical equipment and supplies in the home to individuals of all ages.

Source: healthcareathome.ca (2017).

Where Do Home Health Nurses Work?

In most provinces, home care is delivered through employees of **regional health authorities**, centre local de services communautaires or local community service centres (CLSCS; Quebec) or, in the case of Ontario, service provider organizations. Service provider organizations (SPOs) are agencies that have successfully completed a rigorous quality review and are contracted to provide publicly funded home care services to clients on behalf of Ontario's **Local Health Integration Networks (LHINs)** (see the Definition of Service Provider Organizations box that follows).

SPOs in Canada include not-for-profit organizations such as the Victorian Order of Nurses (VON) and Saint Elizabeth Health Care. Established in 1908, Saint Elizabeth is a national health care company that has been caring for Canadians and leading the development of community health for more than a century (see Photo 5.1). Leaders within these organizations strive to provide health care to the general population as well as to marginalized groups such as homeless or Indigenous communities who may face health inequities and barriers to such care.

Today, for-profit SPOs such as Paramed (www.paramed .com), the Visiting Homemakers Association (VHA) (www .vha.ca), and Bayshore Home Health (www.bayshore.ca) also deliver care in Canada. There has been much controversy regarding the role of not-for-profit and for-profit agencies in the health care system. Principles of the Canada Health Act of 1984 expect that health care is provided by not-for-profit organizations, is equitable regardless of region, and is accessible to all who are insured (Canadian Healthcare Organization [CHO], 2018).

ORGANIZATIONAL SUPPORTS FOR HOME HEALTH NURSING

Similar to other care settings, HHNs require supports and infrastructure to maintain high-quality clinical care and a positive work environment. These supports include the following:

Support for Evidence-Informed Decision Making and Evidence-Informed Practice

Evidence-informed decision making (EIDM) is an important part of the nursing care delivered in home health. EIDM making and practice has a long history in Canada, especially

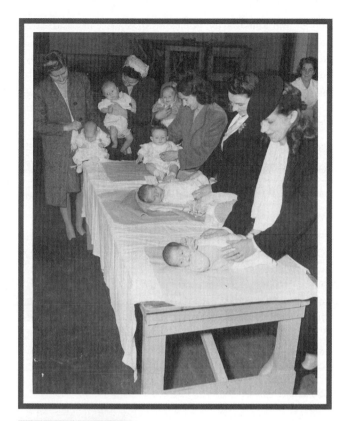

PHOTO 5.1 The historical roots of Saint Elizabeth Health Care are based on providing care through the Archdiocese of Toronto to mothers and young children in an effort to ensure their health and well-being (1947).

Source: Saint Elizabeth Health Care

in public health. Although there are a number of successful EIDM models for implementing evidence, one that has been successfully utilized in home care considers five aspects of clinical decision making—client preferences and actions; health care resources; clinical state, setting, and circumstances; clinical expertise; and research evidence to assist both clinicians and home care leaders (DiCenso, Callum, & Ciliska, 2008).

Leaders

As in all health care settings, leaders play a key role in shaping the workplace culture professional practice environment (Udod, 2012). Unlike an institution, HHNs often do not work in the same location as advanced practice or administrative leaders but rather in local client care teams that cover large geographical regions. Consequently, home care leaders have to work hard and adopt creative approaches to communicate effectively with HHNs, build relationships, advocate for staff, and support work–life balance. This requires a clear understanding of the HHN role, including its strengths and challenges, as well as ensuring access to orientation, safety training, ongoing education, and professional resources. It also requires the leader to work with the HHN to ensure quality outcomes. For example, facilitating chart audits and providing feedback to HHNs on clinical outcomes is an important role

for the leader in performance management and the quality-improvement process.

Professional Development

Self-regulation and the need for ongoing professional development is a high priority for nursing staff in all locales. Because HHNs are highly mobile and geographically dispersed, this requirement demands an innovative approach in home care. Digital and mobile technologies such as tablet computers and e-learning tools, webinars, and apps all play a key role in facilitating communication and ongoing knowledge and skill development for the HHN.

Clinical Networks and Organizational Structures

HHNs also need the support of clinical experts and other organizational infrastructures to provide care excellence (Chaillet et al., 2006; Flodgren et al., 2011; Ploeg et al., 2010). In some home care organizations, clinical program leaders are advanced practice nurses who directly manage the programs to ensure that they are based on home health standards, evidence-based guidelines, and nursing competencies. A clinical network of experts is typically available to provide timely clinical information, answer questions, and confirm policies and procedures. This is provided in person or through email, phone, e-learning products, or web-based knowledge repositories that make static information available anytime.

REWARDS AND CHALLENGES IN HHN

As with any profession, home health nursing has both rewards and challenges. Most HHNs love the autonomous nature of the role and when possible enjoy working to their full scope of practice. HHNs enjoy working as an important member of the interdisciplinary team and are often the lead for care coordination and access to additional resources and services to ensure that patient outcomes are achieved. The therapeutic relationship HHNs develop with the client and his or her family keeps the HHN working in the community. Most HHNs thrive on the variety of clients and clinical situations in their caseload, and following clients over time gives HHNs a sense of connection and accomplishment. HHNs also enjoy teaching and educating clients about their options for care and their ability to care independently for themselves. As part of this, HHNs coach people to change health behaviours, such as in the management of chronic diseases. Many HHNs also enjoy the advancement of technologies and the opportunity to care for clients in an entirely new way through virtual care, remote monitoring, and the exchange of information electronically.

However, a number of challenges are also present that impact the work of HHNs at the individual (client and nurse), organizational (employer, association, and academic institution), and systemic levels. These include the following:

Client and Nurse Issues

Changing Client Demographics In 2012, of the 2.2 million Canadians who received home care services, 45% were 85 years or older (Turcotte, 2014). As well, clients are now being discharged earlier, including those with mental health issues and those who wish to die at home (CHCA, 2013).

Difficult Working Conditions A study of Ontario HHNs found five recurrent occupational hazards: dangerous or aggressive pets, winter or night driving conditions, ergonomic issues, exposure to oxygen equipment or tanks, and environmental tobacco smoke exposure (Wong, Saari, Patterson, Puts, & Tourangeau, 2017).

Academic Institutions and Employers Issues

Lack of Education Regarding Home Care Nurses often lack exposure to home health in their education. When graduates seek employment in this sector, a more comprehensive orientation and preceptorship is required (Better Home Care in Canada Partners, 2016; Patterson, Hart, Bishop, & Purdy, 2013).

Challenges for Ongoing Professional Development As previously identified, the home care population is changing, which requires different knowledge and skills. Ongoing education can be more difficult because of the dispersed workforce.

Systemic Issues

In addition to the day-to-day challenges, some systemic issues also influence the way care is delivered (Coyte & McKeever, 2001).

Lack of a National Home Care Strategy Despite the desire for a comprehensive home care system, Canada does not have a **national home care strategy**. This has allowed provinces and territories to have variations in mandate, principles, and services due to jurisdictional priorities, available resources, and context (Better Home Care in Canada Parters, 2016; CHCA, 2013).

Inadequate Funding Current funding levels are not keeping pace with the growing demand for home care, leading to wait lists and in some regions restrictions on care through income testing, co-payments, caps on hours and type of professional services, and lack of coverage for drugs or supplies (CHCA, 2013).

Shift to Informal Caregivers Now more than ever, unpaid family caregivers are relied upon in order to keep clients at home. A 2012 Statistics Canada study found that 5.4 million people provide informal care to family or friends (Better Home Care in Canada Parters, 2016; Turcotte & Sawaya, 2015). Caregiving is often challenging and may result in out-of-pocket expenses, adverse employment implications, stress and mental health implications, strained relationships with other family members, and social isolation (Canadian Medical Association [CMA], 2016).

Lack of HHN Role Clarity A lack of role clarity has lead to the unfortunate underutilization of HHNs, with more emphasis on tasks and greater use of other providers (see Yes, But Why? box). Currently 70% of home care services are provided by unregulated workers, leading to gaps in care (Accreditation Canada & Canadian Home Care Association, 2015; Barken, Denton, Plenderleith, Zeytinoglu, & Brookman, 2015).

YES, BUT WHY?

The Move from Holistic Care to Task-Based Nursing

What?

Home care is growing in Canada. Approximately 2.2 million Canadians received home care visits in 2012, many of whom were much older and sicker than ever before (Turcotte, 2014). Although HHNs have advanced nursing education to deal with complex issues, they have recently seen their practice move from holistic care to a task-based approach (CNA, 2013). This change is primarily due to a lack of home care funding and a "fee for service" payment model that enables more client visits per day.

So What?

For the client, a task-based approach to care focuses on a procedure such as wound care, often missing many important client needs. However, if permitted to work to their full scope of practice, the HHN would use a person- and family-centred approach to conduct a detailed health assessment and develop a comprehensive plan for each unique client and family situation. Clients are assessed for underlying issues such as social isolation, risks that may predispose them to falls or medication errors, and their family's ability to cope with care requirements. The HHN is able to access other members of the health care team to address social issues and connect the client to supports in the community if needed. The HHN monitors the care plan and adapts it to ensure overall positive health outcomes. Task-based nursing does not allow for such fulsome practice.

Task-based nursing is also having a profound effect on HHNs, especially RNs. Today, although they learn from the same body of nursing knowledge as RPNs, RNs study for a longer period of time, allowing for greater foundational knowledge in clinical practice, decision making, critical thinking, leadership, research utilization, and resource management (College of Nurses of Ontario [CNO], 2014, p. 3). Specifically, they are also educated about issues that compromise health such as low income or poverty or the consequences of health inequity. Consequently, many nurses feel they are not working to their full scope or utilizing their knowledge and skills (CNA, 2013).

A task-based approach may also be having an impact on the health care system. Although it can enable more nursing visits, task-based care may cost the system more. For instance, issues that have not been adequately addressed in the home often cause rapid health decline and subsequent hospitalization. In fact, national statistics show that health care expenditures are at their highest when people are in their final days of life (Canadian Institute for Health Information

[CIHI], 2015). This may be due to the lack of care and planning as the client's condition changes.

Now What?

HHNs can help change the health inequities experienced by home care clients and their families across Canada. At a local level, HHNs can apply a strengths-based approach to interventions to promote health and well-being for people in their homes (Markle-Reid, Browne, & Gafni, 2013). They also can continue to work with the interprofessional health care team to help them understand and promote the HHN's scope of practice (di Costanzo, 2012). At the educational level, nurse educators can help make home health nursing more visible by advocating for curriculum and clinical placements in home and community care. HHNs can also participate in research to influence policy makers regarding the need for a full scope of practice, the consequences of the "fee for service" model, and new ways to fund and deliver holistic home care (Buurtzorg Neighborhood Nursing, 2017). At the government level, HHNs need to advocate for collection of health data to demonstrate the impact on client need (White, Nagle, & Hannah, 2017).

Standards of Practice Fulfilled

#3 *Health Maintenance, Restoration and Palliation*
- Uses a range of intervention strategies related to health maintenance, restoration and palliation to promote self-management of disease, maximize function, and enhance quality of life.

#6 *Health Equity*
- Health Equity: Advocates for healthy public policy and social justice by participating in legislative and policy-making activities that influence determinants of health and access to services (CHNC, 2019, revised).

HEALTH EQUITY IN HOME HEALTH NURSING

Given the systemic issues, it is not surprising that several vulnerable populations do not receive equitable home care in Canada. These include the following:

First Nation and Inuit Communities

Six hundred and eighty-six First Nation and Inuit (FNI) communities receive home care across Canada, many ranging in size and degree of isolation. The federal government funds services for FNI communities through the Department of Indigenous Services Canada. The governments of Nunavut and the Northwest Territories deliver their home care programs to all residents regardless of identity, and the Yukon Government has its own home care program accessible to all Yukon residents. The three First Nation bands in the Yukon without self-government agreements receive First Nation and Inuit Home and Community Care (FNIHCC) funds, which provide basic homemaking services to those in need, such as shopping, cleaning, and chopping wood (Health Canada, 2015).

To ensure that health care continues to meet FNI communities' needs, the FNIHCC developed a 10-year plan in collaboration with FNI partners and Health Canada's FNI Health Branch (see Figure 5.2). Its aim is to "provide a continuum of home and community care that is comprehensive, culturally safe, accessible, effective and equitable to that of other Canadians and which respond to the unique health and social needs of First Nations and Inuit" (Health Canada, 2015). Table 5.3 reflects the key priorities of the plan.

HHNs in FNI communities provide basic services that are comprehensive, culturally safe, accessible, and responsive to the unique health and social needs of the community. This often includes care for people with disproportionately high rates of disabilities and chronic or acute illnesses compared to the national average (Government of Canada, 2013). Many of these illnesses are the result of social determinants of health, such as compromised living conditions (e.g., food access or affordability, clean water, adequate housing, income, and resources) (Health Canada, 2015; National Collaborating Centre for Aboriginal Health, 2013).

Staff in FNI communities are employed directly by local communities, tribal councils, or provincial territorial organizations that determine the mix of providers required to meet the community's needs (CHCA, 2013). Frequently, individuals are sent outside of the community to receive care from physicians or allied professionals. This often results in fragmented care, communication breakdown, a lack of understanding regarding community care available, or conflict between federal and provincial funders regarding payment for services (Government of Canada, 2017b; Rahaman, Holmes, & Chartrand, 2017).

As the primary providers in many communities, most HHNs enjoy the benefits of working in a tight-knit community, but some feel overwhelmed with the working conditions, lack of clear role guidelines, and long work hours, resulting in poor job satisfaction, high turnover rates, and communities not receiving the care they need (Aboriginal Nurses Association of Canada, 2008). Nurses work according to HHN competencies and those relevant to cultural safety (National Collaborating Centre for Aboriginal Health, 2015). Ongoing education is delivered by eHealth to assist nurses to address complex health issues and to enable remote access to clinical experts and specialist care (Scott, Menzies, Chenard, & Spence, 2013).

Table 5.3	Principles of the FNIHCC (2013–2023) 10-Year Plan
Holistic Wellness: Respectful of both traditional and contemporary approaches to healing and wellness	
Community-centred: Delivered in consideration of community priorities	
Accessible: Available to those with assessed need	
Quality: Evidenced-informed, integrated quality	
Supportive: Supportive of individual, family, and community	
Sustainability: Sustainable funding and continuous care	

Source: Health Canada (2015).

First Nations and Inuit Home and Community Care (FNIHCC)
10-Year Plan (2013–2023)

Providing a path forward to assist staff, at all levels, anticipate and respond to the complex and changing health needs and challenges of First Nations and Inuit.

· OUR VISION ·

A continuum of home and community care services that are comprehensive, culturally safe, accessible, effective, and equitable to that of other Canadians and which respond to the unique health and social needs of First Nations and Inuit.

· OUR PRINCIPLES ·

Holistic Wellness
Respectful of both traditional and contemporary approaches to healing and wellness

Community-centered
Delivered in consideration of community priorities

Accessible
Available to those with assessed need

Quality
Evidenced-informed, integrated quality

Supportive
Supportive of individual, family and community

Sustainability
Sustainable funding and continuous care

· OUR GOALS ·

FNIHCC has committed to five goals which are intended to be achieved in accordance to the priorities of communities, regions, and the national office over the next 10 years.

Goal 1
A Home and Community Care Program that is based on a Holistic Wellness approach within a circle of care, offering high quality services and culturally safe care to clients through all phases of life.

Goal 2
New and innovative partnerships and planning that aligns with and enhances existing programs and services to improve health outcomes for Home and Community Care clients.

Goal 3
Promote sustainable and appropriate work environments in which Home and Community Care professionals and para professionals continue to be informed, competent, engaged and supported.

Goal 4
A sustainable Program that is supportive of the client, family and community, and is adaptable to changing needs, emerging trends, and is responsive to the Home Care needs of First Nation and Inuit.

Goal 5
A Program that is dedicated to quality improvement, based on high quality, consistent and standardized data collection and assessments.

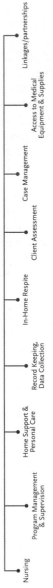

· WHAT WE DO ·

The FNIHCC Program provides basic essential services:

- Nursing
- Program Management & Supervision
- Home Support & Personal Care
- Record Keeping, Data Collection
- In-Home Respite
- Client Assessment
- Case Management
- Access to Medical Equipment & Supplies
- Linkages/partnerships

For more information about FNIHCC's 10-Year Plan go to **www.hc-sc.gc.ca/fniah-spnia/index-eng.php**

Pub : 140408

Canada

Health Canada   Santé Canada

FIGURE 5.2 FNIHCC 10-Year Plan Poster

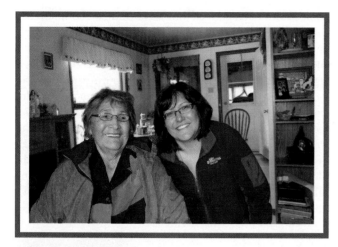

PHOTO **5.2** Home health nurse with client in FNI community

People Who Are Homeless or Vulnerably Housed

There are 235 000 people in Canada each year who are homeless or vulnerably housed (Gaetz, Dej, Richter, & Redman, 2016). People without a home face a higher risk of illness, have much shorter life expectancy, and may have mental health and addictions issues. Homeless individuals often experience significant gaps and barriers in accessing mainstream health services, including home care. Although care can be provided on the street, under bridges, or other places where people sleep, these environments have no running water or places to store medications or supplies. Consequently, when homeless people find it necessary to seek help, they often access it through hospital

---

CASE STUDY

A five-year old First Nation boy named Jordan River Anderson from Norway House Cree Nation suffered from Carey Fineman Ziter Syndrome, a rare muscular disorder that requires hospital medical treatment. After spending the first two years of his life in hospital, the doctors cleared him to live in a family home near the hospital in Winnipeg. However, the federal and provincial governments could not resolve who was financially responsible for the necessary home care. For over two years the governments argued over payment while the boy remained in hospital. The boy died in hospital, never having the opportunity to live in a family home and receive home care (Government of Canada, 2017b).

Discussion Questions

1. If you were an HHN in Winnipeg and knew of this case, what CHCN competencies might you have utilized in advocating for Jordan?

2. If Jordan had been allowed to be at home, what information from the health history would be important to consider when creating a nursing care plan?

3. What key principles of the FNIHCC 10-year plan were violated in this situation?

---

emergency departments or NP-led, street-based centres. In some urban areas, care for homeless persons is provided by HHNs in low-rent buildings, the shelter system, or a clinic setting. The key issues HHNs work with in these settings are sexual, physical, or emotional trauma; emergency medical issues such as stroke or traumatic injuries; respiratory and cardiovascular disease; and foot and wound care. HHNs also undertake health teaching related to disease prevention, management of chronic diseases, and linking individuals to medical and social resources.

One area where there is a profound gap is providing palliative care for the homeless. To address this need, in 2018 the Saint Elizabeth Foundation partnered with Hospice Toronto and Inner City Health Associates to open Journey Home Hospice, a specialized end-of-life facility for the homeless in downtown Toronto (Adams, 2017). The Journey Home Hospice is based on the Diane Morrison Hospice in Ottawa, which provides care to homeless people requiring palliation. In other areas of the country, similar supports have been tried, such as the Calgary Allied Mobile Palliative Program and the PORT project in Vancouver, but often funding becomes a problem to sustain services.

People Experiencing Mental Illness

In 2016, more than 7.5 million people in Canada, or one in five people, sustained some kind of mental health issue (Mental Health Commission of Canada, 2017). Care for people experiencing mental illness is lacking across all health care sectors, including home care. In the home, mental health services are provided for individuals who require immediate crisis interventions from assertive community treatment teams or monitoring for depression, delirium, and dementia. Care is provided through face-to-face visits, Telehealth communications, or new technology that facilitates communication and support with daily texting interactions with a counsellor who provides cognitive behavioural therapy (Mental Health Chatbot, 2018).

HHNs also provide care in community settings through mental health first-aid programs via the Mental Health Commission of Canada, harm reduction services for persons experiencing addictions and substance misuse, and the Canadian Mental Health Association (2017) in shelters, community clinics, or the school system. As well, some home care organizations provide supportive community programs for adults with mental health issues with a range of health, personal, social, and recreational activities and respite for family caregivers.

People Who Live in Rural and Remote Areas

A large portion of Canada is considered rural or remote, making accessibility one of the biggest obstacles to receiving high-quality home care. Travelling to urban areas can help to bridge this gap, but often transportation and costs may be prohibitive. In fact, many people do not want to leave their community and may avoid seeking outside help altogether. Individuals who do opt for care outside their community often experience lack of continuity, communication, and coordination of care (Kaasalainen et al., 2012).

Human resource shortages are also a challenge in rural and remote areas (CHCA, 2013). Recruiting and retaining an appropriate supply of qualified nurses and personal support workers is vital to ensuring high-quality and timely care. However, today Telehealth makes it possible for clients to connect with specialists or check in with HHNs through hand-held devices. For example, clients from across Nova Scotia can speak face-to-face with HHNs located anywhere on the Telehealth network without leaving their home communities (Nova Scotia, 2017).

As illustrated, one of the differences between nurses who work in the community and those employed in other sectors is the requirement for them to not only provide nursing services but also be an advocate for clients and families. This requires knowledge of health care and the social and political systems that enable outreach to vulnerable populations and equitable access to home care for all Canadians.

HOME HEALTH NURSES: THE FUTURE

Given our aging population, more care will be delivered at home in the future. This is a great opportunity for HHNs to bring their expertise to the forefront while advocating for equitable access to home care for all Canadians. Working in the natural home environment, HHNs are in a privileged position to observe, understand, and connect with clients and families, and to tailor care to their needs and lives. To fully realize the potential of this opportunity, Canada needs a national home care strategy as well as greater emphasis on home health nursing in education, clinical placements, and the development of new models of care and policy initiatives.

In today's health care context, access to information has transformed the role of the client to enable collaborative decision making with health care providers that reflects their individual knowledge, circumstances, and values. Clients and their caregivers expect to be engaged in decision making, to receive timely information and options for care, and to play an active role in healthy living and chronic disease management. This is wholly congruent with Canada's HHN competencies and our steadfast commitment to partner with clients and their families.

Tomorrow's HHN will need to focus not only on prevention and coordinating health care to address fragmentation but also on being technologically aware of the new health "ecosystem" that will wrap around the client and his or her family. Enabled by technology, HHNs will be required to manage multiple sources of data, synthesize information, and use it strategically to benefit client care. Yet undoubtedly the most essential role of the HHN will remain firmly rooted in the human side of health care—listening, guiding, informing, educating, advocating, and caring for clients (Sharkey & Lefebre, 2017).

CONCLUSION

Most Canadians have a desire to remain in their own homes, even when their health is less than optimum. This requires ongoing leadership to support the continued evolution of home health nursing, including research, new and innovative delivery models, better collection of health outcomes, role optimization within interprofessional teams, and integration and alignment across the health care system (CNA, 2012). It also requires that HHNs work with their organizations to provide holistic and responsive care, to develop innovative solutions, to advocate for access to home care for all, and to utilize technology to support community living. But health and wellness is truly anchored in the strengths of people and their networks and patterns of everyday life. It is the HHNs at the forefront of care who have the privilege of building strong relationships with clients and families to meet their own unique needs.

KEY TERMS

C-Health Outcomes for Better Information and Care (C-HOBIC) (p. 77)
Community Health Nurses of Canada (CHNC) (p. 76)
Competencies for Home Health Nursing (p. 76)
Elements of Home Health Nursing (p. 76)
essential service (p. 75)
First Ministers Accord on Health Care Renewal (p. 75)
Foundations of Home Health Nursing (p. 76)
guest in the home (p. 76)
home care (p. 75)
home health nurses (HHNs) (p. 74)
Kirby Report (p. 75)
Local Health Integration Networks (LHINs) (p. 78)
national home care strategy (p. 80)
person- and family-centred care (PFCC) (p. 77)
Quality and Professional Responsibilities (p. 76)
regional health authorities (p. 78)
Romanow Commission (p. 75)

STUDY QUESTIONS

1. How has the evolution of home care in Canada influenced nursing practice today?

2. What are the consequences to families of the expansion of home care within the health system?

3. How have social and societal expectations contributed to the evolution of home care in Canada?

4. Who qualifies to be an HHN?

5. List three roles of the HHN.

INDIVIDUAL CRITICAL-THINKING EXERCISES

1. What are the advantages or disadvantages of care delivered in the home?

2. What do you think the "lived experience" would be for clients and their families living at home with a chronic disease such as diabetes?

3. What mechanisms would you require for professional development in home health nursing?

GROUP CRITICAL-THINKING EXERCISES

1. It has been a "perfect world" for the last six months! What are some of the things that have changed in the work life of an HHN in home care? As a group, then choose the single most important change.

2. From the changes possible in question 1, what led your group to choose the one you did?

3. Based on your understanding of the significant factor you chose in question 2, how will the change affect the health outcomes of clients in the home? How does it impact the HHN's provision of care?

REFERENCES

Aboriginal Nurses Association of Canada. (2008). *Survey of nurses in isolated First Nations communities: Recruitment and retention issues.* Ottawa, ON: Aboriginal Nurses Association of Canada.

Accreditation Canada & Canadian Home Care Association. (2015). *Home care in Canada: Advancing quality improvement and integrating care.* Retrieved from http://www.cdnhomecare.ca/media.php?mid=4328

Adams, J. (March 16, 2017). Personal communication. Saint Elizabeth Health Care.

Armstrong, P., & Armstrong, H. (2008). Bring it home: Women's health work. *Women's Health and Urban Life: An International and Interdisciplinary Journal,* VII(2), 6–15.

Barken, R., Denton, M., Plenderleith, J., Zeytinoglu, I., & Brookman, C. (2015). Home care workers' skills in the context of task shifting: Complexities in care work. *Canadian Sociological Association,* 52(3), 289–309.

Better Home Care in Canada Partners. (2016). *Better home care in Canada: A national action plan.* Retrieved from http://www.thehomecareplan.ca

Buurtzorg Neighborhood Nursing. (2017). Retrieved from http://www.buurtzorgusa.org/aboutus

Canadian Healthcare Organization (CHO). (2018). *Canada health care.* Retrieved from http://www.canadian-healthcare.org/page2.html

Canadian Home Care Association (CHCA). (2013). *Portraits of home care in Canada, 2013.* Mississauga, ON: Author.

Canadian Institute for Health Information (CIHI). (2015). *National health expenditures: How has health spending on seniors changed?* Retrieved from https://www.cihi.ca/en/spending-and-health-workforce/spending/national-health-expenditure-trends/nhex2015-topic7

Canadian Institute for Health Information (CIHI). (2016). *Regulated nurses.* Retrieved from https://www.cihi.ca/en/regulated-nurses-2016

Canadian Medical Association (CMA). (2016). *The state of seniors health care in Canada.* https://www.cma.ca/En/Lists/Medias/the-state-of-seniors-health-care-in-canada-september-2016.pdf

Canadian Mental Health Association. (2017). Retrieved from https://cmha.ca

Canadian Museum of Civilization. (1966). *The Medical Care Act, 1966.* Retrieved from http://www.civilization.ca/cmc/exhibitions/hist/medicare/medic-5h23e.shtml

Canadian Nurses Association (CNA). (2012). *The health of our nation, the future of our health system: A nursing call to action.* Ottawa, ON: Author.

Canadian Nurses Association (CNA). (2013). *Optimizing the role of nursing in home health.* https://www.cna-aiic.ca/~/media/cna/page-content/pdf-en/optimizing_the_role_of_nursing_in_home_health_e.pdf?la=en

Canadian Patient Safety Institute. (2013). *Safety at home: A pan-Canadian home care safety study.* Edmonton, AB: Author.

Chaillet, N., Dubé, E., Dugas, M., Audibert, F., Trouigny, C., Fraser, W. D., & Dumont, A. (2006). Evidence-based strategies for implementing guidelines in obstetrics: A systematic review. *Obstetrics & Gynecology,* 108(5), 1234–1245. doi: 10.1097/01.AOG.0000236434.74160.8b

College of Nurses of Ontario (CNO). (2014). *RN and RPN practice: The client, the nurse and the environment.* Retrieved from http://www.cno.org/globalassets/docs/prac/41062.pdf

Community Health Nurses' Initiatives Group. (2000). *Home health nursing—A position paper.* Toronto, ON: Registered Nurses' Association of Ontario.

Community Health Nurses of Canada (CHNC). (2010). *Home health nursing competencies.* St. John's, NL: Author.

Community Health Nurses of Canada (CHNC). (2019, revised). *Canadian community health nursing professional practice model and standards of practice.* Retrieved from http://www.chnig.org/wp-content/uploads/2016/02/chnc-standards.pdf

Community Nursing Courses. (2017). Retrieved from http://www.yorku.ca/cvandaal/courses/community_as_partner.html

Conference Board of Canada. (2012). *Canadian Alliance for Sustainable Health Care (CASHC), annual report.* http://www.conferenceboard.ca/CASHC/aboutCASHC.aspx

Coyte, P., & McKeever, P. (2001). Home care in Canada: Passing the buck. *Canadian Journal of Nursing Research,* 33(2), 11–25.

DiCenso, A., Cullum, N., & Ciliska, D. (2008). Implementing evidence-based nursing: Some misconceptions. In N. Cullum, D. Ciliska, R. B. Haynes, & S. Marks (Eds.), *Evidence-based nursing: An introduction.* Oxford, UK: Blackwell.

di Costanzo, M. (2012). Full scope nursing. *Registered Nurse Journal,* November/December, 12–17.

Flodgren, G., Parmelli, E., Doumit, G., Gattellari, M., O'Brien, M. A., Grimshaw, J., & Eccles, M. P. (2011). Local opinion leaders: Effects on professional practice and health care outcomes. *Cochrane Database of Systematic Reviews,* 8(8).

Gaetz, S., Dej, E., Richter, T., & Redman, M. (2016). *The state of homelessness in Canada 2016.* Toronto, ON: Canadian Observatory on Homelessness Press.

Government of Canada. (2013). *Evaluation of First Nations and Inuit home care program. 2008–2009 to 2011–2012.* Retrieved from https://www.canada.ca/en/health-canada/corporate/about-health-canada/accountability-performance-financial-reporting/evaluation-reports/evaluation-first-nations-inuit-home-community-care-program-2008-2009-2011-2012.html#e2

Government of Canada. (2017a). *Canada Health Act.* Retrieved from https://www.canada.ca/en/health-canada/services/health-care-system/canada-health-care-system-medicare/canada-health-act.html

Government of Canada. (2017b). *Jordan's Principle*. Retrieved from https://www.canada.ca/en/health-canada/services/first-nations-inuit-health/jordans-principle.html

Health Canada. (2003). *First Ministers' accord on health care renewal*. Retrieved from http://www.hc-sc.gc.ca/hcs-sss/delivery-prestation/fptcollab/2003accord/index-eng.php

Health Canada. (2015). *First Nations and Inuit Home and Community Care (FNIHCC) 10-Year Plan (2013–2023)*. Retrieved from http://publications.gc.ca/collections/collection_2016/sc-hc/H34-282-2015-eng.pdf

Healthcareathome. (2017). Retrieved from http://healthcareathome.ca/serviceproviders/en/Home

Health Foundation. (2015). *Person-centred care resource centre. "What is person-centred care?"* Retrieved from http://personcentredcare.health.org.uk/area-of-care/what-is-person-centred-care

Institute for Patient and Family-Centred Care. (2017). *Patient and family-centred care?* Retrieved from http://www.ipfcc.org/about/pfcc.html

Kaasalainen, S., Brazil, K., Williams, A., Wilson, D., Willison, K., Marshall, D., & Taniguchi, A. (2012). Barriers and enablers to providing palliative care in rural communities: A nursing perspective. *The Journal of Rural and Community Development, 7*(4), 4–19.

Kirby, M. J. L. (2002). *The health of Canadians—The federal role. Final report, volume six: Recommendations for reform.* The Standing Senate Committee on Social Affairs, Science and Technology. Retrieved from http://www.parl.gc.ca/content/sen/committee/372/soci/rep/repoct02vol6-e.htm#CHAPTER%20ONE

Markle-Reid, M., Browne, G., & Gafni, A. (2013). Nurse-led health promotion interventions improve quality of life in frail older home care clients: Lessons learned from three randomized trials in Ontario, Canada. *Journal of Evaluation in Clinical Practice, 19*(1), 118–131.

Mental Health Chatbot. (2018). Retrieved from http://x2ai.com

Mental Health Commission of Canada. (2017). Retrieved from https://www.mentalhealthcommission.ca/English/focus-areas/mental-health-first-aid

Mildon, B., & Underwood, J. (2010). *Competencies for home health nursing: A literature review.* Toronto, ON: Community Health Nurses of Canada.

Nagle, L. M., & White, P. (2013). Evaluating nurses' use of HOBIC in home care. *Canadian Journal of Nursing Research, 45*(3), 92–114.

Nagle, L., White, P., & Pringle, D. (2010). Realizing the benefits of standardizing clinical outcomes. *Electronic Healthcare, 9*(2), e3–e9.

National Collaborating Centre for Aboriginal Health. (2013). Retrieved from https://www.ccnsa-nccah.ca/docs/context/FS-OverviewAbororiginalHealth-EN.pdf

National Collaborating Centre for Aboriginal Health. (2015). Retrieved from https://www.ccnsa-nccah.ca/495/Review_of_Core_Competencies_for_Public_Health__An_Aboriginal_Public_Health_Perspective.nccah?id=145

Nova Scotia Telehealth Network. (2017). Retrieved from https://novascotia.ca/dhw/ehealth/telehealth

Ontario Home Care Association. (2011). *Home care nursing in Ontario.* Retrieved from http://www.homecareontario.ca/

docs/default-source/HHR/hc-nsg-in-ontario—mar-2011—final-rev.pdf?sfvrsn=8

Patterson, E., Hart, C., Bishop, S., & Purdy, N. (2013). Deciding if home care is right for me: The experience of the new graduate nurse. *Home Health Care Management & Practice, 25*(4), 147–154. doi:10.1177/1084822312473828

Ploeg, J., Skelly, J., Rowan, M., Edwards, N., Davies, B., Grinspun, D., . . . Downey, A. (2010). The role of nursing best practice champions in diffusing practice guidelines: A mixed methods study. *Worldviews on Evidence-Based Nursing, 4*, 238–251. doi:10.1111/j.1741-6787.2010.00202.x

Public Health Agency of Canada. (2007). *Core competencies for public health in Canada: Release 1.0.* Ottawa, ON: Author.

Rahaman, Z., Holmes, D., & Chartrand, L. (2017). An opportunity for healing and holistic care: Exploring the roles of health care providers working within northern Canadian Aboriginal communities. *Journal of Holistic Nursing, American Holistic Nurses Association, 35*(2), 185–197.

Registered Nurses' Association of Ontario. (2002). *Supporting and strengthening families through expected and unexpected life events.* Toronto, ON: Author.

Romanow, R. J. (2002). *Building on values—The future of health care in Canada, final report. Commission on the future of health care in Canada.* Ottawa, ON: Government of Canada.

Saint Elizabeth. (2011). *Client-centred care in the Canadian home and community sector: A review of key concepts.* Retrieved from https://www.saintelizabeth.com/Services-and-Programs/Research-Centre/Person-and-Family-Centred-Care.aspx

Scott, T., Menzies, C., Chenard, G., & Spence, M. (2013). Bridging the gap: Innovative approaches to continuing education in rural, remote, and isolated First Nation communities. *Seminars in Dialysis, 26*(2), 164–168.

Sharkey, S., & Lefebre, N. (2017). Bringing nursing back to the future through people powered care. *Nursing Leadership, 30*(1), 11–22.

Sun, W., & Doran, D. (2014). Safety in the home: The association between therapeutic self-care ability and occurrence of adverse events for home care clients in Canada. *Journal of Nursing and Healthcare, 1*(2), 245–251.

Sun, W., Doran, D., Wodchis, D., & Peter, E. (2017). Examining the relationship between therapeutic self-care and adverse events for home care clients in Ontario, Canada: A retrospective cohort study. *BMC Health Services Research. 17*(206), 1–13.

Tourangeau, A., Kelly, S., Patterson, E., & Saari, M. (2016a). *Applied health research question 2.6a: Patient reported outcome measures in home-based care.* Toronto, ON: Ontario Ministry of Health and Long-Term Care. Retrieved from http://tourangeauresearch.com/wp-content/uploads/Tourangeau-Research-AHRQ-PROMs.pdf

Tourangeau, A., Kelly, S., Patterson, E., & Saari, M. (2016b). *Applied health research question 2.6b: Patient reported experience measures in home-based care.* Toronto, ON: Ontario Ministry of Health and Long-Term Care. Retrieved from http://tourangeauresearch.com/wp-content/uploads/Tourangeau-Research-AHRQ-PREMs-1.pdf

Turcotte, M. (2014). *Canadians with unmet home care needs. Insights on Canadian Society.* Cat. No. 75-006-X. Ottawa, ON: Statistics Canada. Retrieved from http://www.statcan.gc.ca/pub/75-006-x/2014001/article/14042-eng.pdf

Turcotte, M., & Sawaya, C. (2015). *Senior care: Differences by type of housing. Insights on Canadian Society.* Cat. No. 75-006-X. Ottawa, ON: Statistics Canada. Retrieved from http://www.statcan.gc.ca/pub/75-006-x/2015001/article/14142-eng.pdf

Udod, S. (2012). Process of seeking connectivity: Social relations of power between staff nurses and nurse managers. *Nursing Leadership, 25*(4), 29–47.

Underwood, J., Mowat, D., Meagher-Stewart, D., Deber, R., Baumann, A., MacDonald, M., . . . Munroe, V. J. (2009). Building community and public health nursing capacity: A synthesis report of the National Community Health Nursing Study. *Canadian Journal of Public Health, 100*(5), 1–11.

White, P., Nagle, L., & Hannah, K. (2017). *Adopting national nursing data standards in Canada.* Retrieved from https://canadian-nurse.com/en/articles/issues/2017/may-june-2017/adopting-national-nursing-data-standards-in-canada

Wong, M., Saari, M., Patterson, E., Puts, M., & Tourangeau, A. (2017). Occupational hazards for home care nurses across the rural-to-urban gradient in Ontario, Canada. *Health and Social Care in the Community, 25*(3), 1276–1286.

ABOUT THE AUTHORS

Shirlee M. Sharkey, CEO, CHE, MHSc, BScN, BA, LLD (honoris causa). Shirlee Sharkey is President and CEO of Saint Elizabeth, a national social enterprise providing home care, health solutions, and education to people where they are and when they need it. Under Shirlee's leadership, the not-for-profit charitable organization has enjoyed exponential growth and expansion, and facilitated transformative solutions in areas such as Indigenous health, end-of-life care, and caregiver wellness and support. Today, Saint Elizabeth delivers 20 000 care exchanges daily through its team of 9000 leaders and professionals. Passionate about giving back, Shirlee is the current Chair of Excellence Canada and a board member of the Canadian Centre for Aging and Brain Health Innovation. She is also member of the MaRS EXCITE International Advisory Council. Shirlee shares her knowledge and passion for social innovation as Adjunct Professor at the University of Toronto's Lawrence S. Bloomberg Faculty of Nursing and the Institute of Health Policy, Management and Evaluation.

Nancy Lefebre, BScN, MScN, CHL, CCHL Fellow. As Chief Clinical Executive and Senior Vice President, Nancy Lefebre is responsible for advancing Saint Elizabeth's shared value strategy, positioning the organization as a leader in social innovation and impact. Her special interests include end-of-life care, knowledge mobilization, and community partnerships. In her quest to ensure that a strong evidence base underpins health care practices, Nancy has established a collaborative research centre and a network of health career colleges. She is one of the first nursing leaders in Canada to complete the Executive Training for Research Application (EXTRA) Fellowship program. Nancy brings to Saint Elizabeth more than 25 years of experience in the North American health care sector. Nancy has a focus on community care from frontline practice to management, as well as the development of new business and clinical leadership.

Karen L. Ray, RN, BScN, MSc. Karen is the former Manager of Knowledge Translation at Saint Elizabeth. In her previous position, Karen provided leadership, direction, and support for the creation, management, dissemination, and exchange of knowledge through participation in evidence-to-practice initiatives and research. As a home health leader, Karen held a key role in enabling and operationalizing Saint Elizabeth's activities as a Registered Nurses' Association of Ontario "best practice spotlight" organization and also played an instrumental role in Saint Elizabeth's partnership with the Queen's University Joanna Briggs Collaboration to establish the first evidence translation group in North America focusing on home care.

Tracy Scott, RN, MN. Tracy Scott is National Director of Education Services for Saint Elizabeth Health Care and provides leadership to Saint Elizabeth Health Career Colleges as well as the Saint Elizabeth First Nations, Inuit and Métis Program (a national education program focused on supporting health care providers working in communities). Tracy has over 25 years of nursing experience, including primary care nursing, rural and remote community health nursing, and nursing administration. Tracy is supported in her work by members of the Saint Elizabeth First Nations, Inuit and Métis team. Team members contributing to this chapter are Melissa Spence and Charlene Frechette.

Advocacy, Ethical, and Legal Considerations

Elizabeth Peter, Louise Sweatman, and Kathleen Carlin

LEARNING OUTCOMES

After studying this chapter, you should be able to:

1. Describe the central ethical values of Canadian nursing and how they relate to community health nursing.

2. Examine the attributes of social justice as they relate to advocacy and to ethical and legal considerations for community health nursing.

3. Reflect critically on the central ethical issues in community health nursing.

4. Analyze the legal responsibilities of community health nurses.

5. Explain how capacity building is related to advocacy.

6. Analyze the political nature of ethical problems in the community.

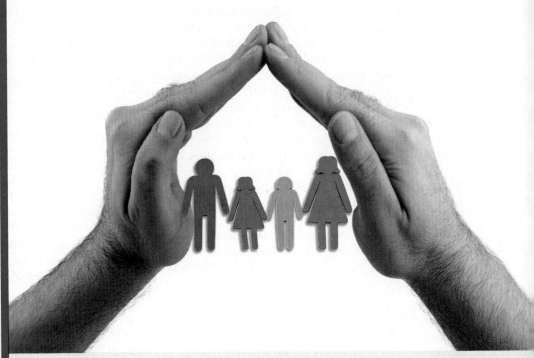

Source: Edu_oliveros/Fotolia

INTRODUCTION

Community health nurses (CHNs) encounter ethical issues in all facets of their everyday work. Ethical nursing practice requires CHNs to be able to reflect critically upon their practice, make sound ethical decisions, and take appropriate action.

Community nursing practice must reflect the central values of Canadian nursing expressed in the Canadian Nurses Association's (CNA, 2017a) "Code of Ethics for Registered Nurses." These values are listed in Table 6.1. The CNA code of ethics also recognizes ethical endeavours that address aspects of social justice related to broad societal issues in which nurses are asked to work toward eliminating social inequities.

The term "ethics" has been defined and used in numerous ways. For the purposes of this chapter, **ethics** refers to those values, norms, moral principles, virtues, and traditions that guide human conduct. Often, ideas that reflect what is good or right and what we ought and ought not to do are associated with ethics. Ethics is also a specialized area of philosophy. Moral philosophers study and reflect upon ethics and have developed formal ethical theories.

Table 6.1	Canadian Nurses Association Nursing Values and Ethical Responsibilities

A. Providing Safe, Compassionate, Competent, and Ethical Care

- Nurses provide safe, compassionate, competent, and ethical care.

B. Promoting Health and Well-Being

- Nurses work with persons who have health-care needs or are receiving care to enable them to attain their highest possible level of health and well-being.

C. Promoting and Respecting Informed Decision Making

- Nurses recognize, respect, and promote a person's right to be informed and make decisions.

D. Honouring Dignity

- Nurses recognize and respect the intrinsic worth of each person.

E. Maintaining Privacy and Confidentiality

- Nurses recognize the importance of privacy and confidentiality and safeguard personal, family, and community information obtained in the context of a professional relationship.

F. Promoting Justice

- Nurses uphold principles of justice by safeguarding human rights, equity, and fairness and by promoting the public good.

G. Being Accountable

- Nurses are accountable for their actions and answerable for their practice.

Source: From *Code of Ethics for Registered Nurses*. Copyright © 2008 by Canadian Nurses Association. Used by permission of Canadian Nurses Association.

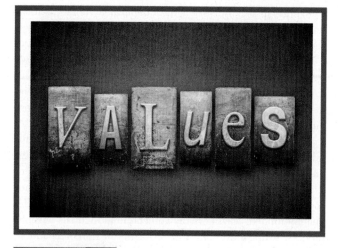

These theories can be helpful in identifying, articulating, and analyzing ethical issues. The term **bioethics**, also known as health care ethics, refers to the study of ethical issues that are related to health and health care. Nursing ethics examines ethical issues in health care "from the perspective of nursing theory and practice" (Johnstone, 2008, p. 16).

Bioethics and nursing ethics have made use of a range of ethical theories and approaches, including deontology, utilitarianism, casuistry, principlism, virtue ethics, and feminist ethics. It is beyond the scope of this chapter to describe all these in a meaningful and comprehensive fashion. Instead, the chapter will be framed using several Canadian nursing documents that articulate the central ethical values and concepts used in community health nursing, including the CNA's "Code of Ethics for Registered Nurses" (CNA, 2017a) and "Social Justice . . . a Means to an End, an End in Itself" (CNA, 2010) (see Photo 6.1). Occasionally, insights from other perspectives such as utilitarianism and feminist ethics will be drawn in to add depth to the understanding of the complex issues CHNs face. Ultimately, this chapter, with its emphasis on social justice and everyday ethical and legal concerns, will assist nurses and nursing students in gaining the capacity to reflect critically on the multiplicity of ethical and legal dimensions inherent in community health nursing.

SOCIAL JUSTICE

Social justice has been defined by the American Public Health Association (2017) as "the view that everyone deserves equal rights and opportunities—this includes the right to good health." Social justice also "focuses on the relative position of one social group in relationship to others in society, as well as on the root causes of disparities and what can be done to eliminate them" (CNA, 2017a, p. 26). It assumes that all societies experience broad, systematic oppression and inequities, such as racism, classism, sexism, and heterosexism, which affect some people more than others. Every individual contributes to oppression and inequity, even if unintentionally, and therefore is responsible also for contributing to the achievement of social, political, and economic parity. In this way, we are responsible not only for recognizing inequities and oppression but also for taking responsible action (CNA, 2010).

The descriptor "social" in social justice places emphasis on the application of justice to social groups, such as the need to address population health and unjust social institutions and relationships. From this perspective, the experiences of individuals are embedded within larger political, economic, cultural, and social contexts (Reimer, Kirkham, & Browne, 2006). For example, nurses must recognize the unique history of Indigenous people in Canada in order to promote justice (CNA, 2017a) because the Indian Act of 1876 has influenced the public's perception of Indigenous people as inferior, which has led to racist stereotypes (Richmond & Cook, 2016). Fundamental to community health nursing is an understanding of the socioenvironmental context of health, recognizing that basic resources and prerequisite conditions are necessary to achieve health (Community Health Nurses of Canada [CHNC], 2019, revised). Powers and Faden (2006) reinforce this notion by stressing that social justice is the foundational moral justification for public health as a social institution. A commitment is needed to address systematic disadvantage that severely limits the well-being of oppressed groups. Well-being involves multiple dimensions, including health, personal security, ability to reason, human attachment, and self-determination. Social justice strives to achieve sufficiently high levels in all these dimensions for everyone (Powers & Faden, 2006).

Social justice is also important when situating the ethical dimensions of health-care policy within a broad political understanding of the role of health care services in society. For example, Canadian home care services, because they are not covered by the Canada Health Act (1985), are often not adequately funded, leaving many vulnerable individuals without services. While most home care recipients are frail older adults, increasingly children with complex medical problems are cared for in the home. This cost-shifting to the home and family has led to excessive demands on unpaid caregivers, especially women (Peter, 2013).

Social justice is not just a means to an end or an approach to evaluate current circumstances. It has attributes that are desired results, or ends. Ten such attributes have been identified (see Table 6.2). They comprise equity (including health equity), human rights (including the right to health), democracy and civil rights, capacity building, just institutions, enabling environments, poverty reduction, ethical practice, advocacy, and partnerships (CNA, 2010). When recognizing and acting on problems of inequity in Canadian society, CHNs strive to achieve these attributes in their communities.

It is also important to note three features of social justice approaches that are useful to consider when using social justice as a framework for everyday community nursing practice. These features tend to distinguish this type of approach from principle-focused ones typically used in bioethics. First, social justice approaches tend to be concerned with the ethical use of power in health care. Broad political and structural dimensions of problems in health care and also the day-to-day use of power by health professionals are examined. Power, in itself, is ethically neutral. How power is used, however, is of ethical significance. Nurses and other health professionals can use their professional influence, which is a result of their knowledge and positions in health care systems, to improve the health and well-being of individuals, but they can also use this professional power to deny individuals the right to make choices regarding their health. This power can be exercised at the level of specific individuals and also used to address population-based inequities.

Second, a social justice approach, like feminist bioethics, tends to view persons relationally as unique, connected to others, and interdependent; that is, vulnerable and unequal in power. It is important to consider that persons' group membership, such as those defined by gender, class, race, age, and disability, must be taken into account (Sherwin & Stockdale, 2017). It focuses on how persons are situated or positioned in society; that is, the entire context of their lives, including culture, history, politics, and socioeconomic status. This relational definition of persons is appropriate for community health nursing because CHNs often work with vulnerable individuals and groups who are socially disadvantaged. Through their work, CHNs also emphasize the importance of their relationships with the clients they serve as a means of caring and empowerment.

Third, attending to social justice tends to elicit concern for issues of everyday life and not primarily with crisis issues. Not all ethical issues or problems are ethical or moral dilemmas. **Ethical dilemmas** "arise when there are equally compelling

Table 6.2	Social Justice: Ten Defining Attributes

Equity (including health equity)—Equity is based on the just treatment of all individuals, which includes equitable access and opportunity to meet health needs.

Human Rights (including the right to health)—These rights are defined by the United Nations Universal Declaration of Human Rights and the Canadian Charter of Rights and Freedoms.

Democracy and Civil Rights—These are outlined in the Canadian Bill of Rights. Democracy and civil rights exist when all have equal rights and power resides in the people and is not based on hereditary or arbitrary differences in privilege or rank.

Capacity Building—Capacity building refers to giving strength to individual and institutional skills, capabilities, knowledge, and experience through coaching, training, resource networking, and technical support.

Just Institutions—Just institutions engage in just practices and the fair treatment of all individuals in institutions.

Enabling Environments—Enabling environments support positive change, community empowerment, and policy development.

Poverty Reduction—The reduction of poverty through projects, programs, and structural reforms of an economic, social, or political nature increases the standard of living and the social and political participation of the poor.

Ethical Practice—The CNA code of ethics for registered nurses and ethics review boards defines ethical practice for nurses.

Advocacy—Advocacy involves the active support of individual rights and positive policy or system change.

Partnerships—Partnerships that foster social justice are based on the equitable sharing of roles and responsibilities among institutions and individuals across sectors.

Source: Based on Canadian Nurses Association. (2006). "Social justice . . . a means to an end, an end in itself." (February 2006). Further production prohibited.

reasons for and against two or more possible courses of action, and where choosing one course of action means that something else is relinquished or let go" (CNA, 2017a, p. 6). **Everyday ethics** in nursing refers to "how nurses pay attention to ethics in carrying out their common daily interactions, including how they approach their practice and reflect on their ethical commitment to persons receiving care or with health-care needs" (CNA, 2017a, p. 22). Everyday ethical concerns also can include those related to advocating for clients, working with limited resources, and relieving human suffering. Social justice expands the agenda of bioethics by examining broad health care issues that impact on everyday practice, such as the need to examine social inequities in Canada that prevent individuals from acquiring the determinants of health. It also recognizes that some perspectives, such as those of clients and nurses, have not been adequately brought into the dialogue and debate on ethical issues, nor have they been drawn upon fully in the development of bioethical theory.

ETHICAL AND LEGAL ISSUES ARISING IN COMMUNITY HEALTH NURSING PRACTICE

A number of specific ethical and legal issues can arise in community health nursing practice. These will be identified and addressed as they pertain to broad areas of community practice such as health promotion, prevention and health protection, and health maintenance, restoration, and palliation. Specific areas of ethical and legal concern as they relate to capacity building, access and equity, and professional responsibility and accountability will also be addressed. The content that follows is organized according to the seven standards of practice for community health nursing. Refer to Chapter 3 for a discussion on the seven standards of practice.

Health Promotion, Prevention, and Health Protection: Ethical Implications

Health promotion, prevention, and heath-protection policies and interventions have not always focused on the material and sociopolitical conditions necessary for health. Instead there has been an overemphasis on individual behaviour patterns (Wardrope, 2015). One way of addressing these ethical concerns has been to conceptualize prevention as consisting of five interlocking levels, primordial, primary, secondary, tertiary, and quaternary, to interrupt webs of causality that can lead to ill health (Starfield, 2001). For example, prevention interventions could be developed to reduce adolescent obesity to help prevent type 2 diabetes. Reducing the cost of wholesome food and increasing the minimum wage would be ways to reduce the incidence of obesity at the primordial level, particularly for families who are living in poverty. Poverty is a complex social problem with its roots in various disparities, including race. CHNs are also not always in a position to directly influence

sociopolitical factors that they have identified as moral concerns in their work. However, CHNs can influence change in many ways. There is a collective moral responsibility that goes beyond individual CHNs to bring about broad social and political change. Because we can be deeply connected as persons, it is possible to create social and professional groups that can better address social injustices. Organized professional groups can generally advocate for social change in ways that are more effective than individuals alone (Peter, 2011). For example, anti-poverty groups have brought greater public awareness of the problems facing many Canadians and the need to increase the minimum wage to a living wage.

Primary prevention interventions could include ensuring that schools have the facilities and equipment necessary for exercise and could eliminate unhealthy foods in cafeterias and vending machines. Schools could also provide education on healthy food choices and exercise. Nevertheless, there are potential moral harms in these activities that need to be discussed. CHNs can unwittingly become agents of social control. **Social control** refers "to the social processes by which the behaviour of individuals or group is regulated. Since all societies have norms and rules governing conduct, all equally have some mechanisms for ensuring conformity to those norms and for dealing with deviance" (Scott & Marshall, 2009). Obesity can mistakenly be viewed as a form of deviance. For example, given the current emphasis on obesity, a large body size in women has come to symbolize self-indulgence and moral failure, which in turn may lead women to question their sense of self and right to good health care (Wray & Deery, 2008). CHNs must strive to find the right balance of providing information to protect their clients without unduly undermining their self-esteem, alarming them, or restricting their autonomous choices because stigmatization can be the result of health promotion interventions (Wardrope, 2015). Nurses must respect the inherent **dignity** of the people they serve because it is a fundamental ethical responsibility (CNA, 2017a).

Secondary prevention could involve screening for diabetes; tertiary prevention could involve education for diabetes management, including programs in the community like cooking and exercise classes for people with diabetes. Tertiary prevention could include screening people for diabetes, and quaternary prevention could involve monitoring clients' progress as they continue with programs that reduce the need for insulin or medication for management. As much as possible, all approaches must resist over-medicalizing the prevention of type 2 diabetes because many of its causes are rooted in the social determinants of health. The concept of **medicalization** is "the process in which conditions and behaviours that were previously considered a normal part of life come to be understood as medical problems (e.g., the conceptualization of inattention and hyperactivity as Attention Deficit Hyperactivity Disorder)" (Gillett, Andrews, & Savelli, 2016, p. 275). Ultimately, health promotion, prevention, and health-protection activities are powerful tools that must be used with careful reflection as to their consequences for the health and well-being of individuals and communities. CHNs must be mindful of the social and professional power they possess as respected and trusted health professionals. There exists an ethical responsibility to reflect upon whose good and whose conception of health is being promoted and why.

Without a conscious awareness of the sociopolitical and economic factors that underlie health and illness, it is possible that CHNs could too easily blame clients who do not heed health information and acquire a disease. Alternatively, CHNs could view these clients as powerless victims of their circumstances, thereby absolving them from any responsibility for their health and absolving CHNs from any responsibility to provide information or other support to assist them in making health choices. Either extreme would not respect the dignity of these clients and would not promote social justice.

A more helpful perspective would put together these explanatory frameworks in a way that does not eliminate the possibility of choice but situates it. Feminist ethicists have developed the concept of relational autonomy that is helpful here (Sherwin, 1998; Sherwin & Stockdale, 2017). They describe how individuals are inherently social and relational beings who are significantly shaped by interpersonal and political relationships. Individuals exercise autonomy and choice within this web of interconnected and sometimes conflicting relationships. Options available to individuals are constrained by circumstances and the availability of resources. Pressure from significant others and social forces can also greatly influence decision making. For example, a young woman with limited financial means may engage in unprotected sexual intercourse with her male partner who refuses to wear a condom. She may understand the risk of unprotected sex but "choose" to have intercourse with him because she is financially dependent upon him and finds it difficult to say no to his requests for sex. Although she makes a choice, this choice is limited by her economic dependency and perhaps also by societal expectations upon women to sexually satisfy their male partners. Nevertheless, it is possible that future partners will be more receptive to her request, or her economic situation may improve. CHNs could become involved in primordial prevention activities such as challenging the roles of women in society and fighting for equal wages.

Interventions that Restrict Liberty It is important to recognize that efforts to prevent disease and injury restrict the liberty of individuals, thereby limiting their choice and autonomy. For example, seat-belt laws and speed limits restrict the liberty of individuals, but they are needed to protect health. Other strategies such as communicable disease surveillance and reporting can not only restrict liberty but also go against the ideals of confidentiality and privacy. Sound ethical reasons and legal authority must exist to impose these liberty-limiting strategies upon clients. In some instances, interventions are targeted to one group of people to protect another group's health, such as mandatory reporting of some communicable diseases (see Chapter 12). These interventions can be ethically justified if they fairly distribute benefits and burdens and limit burdens to the greatest extent possible.

Five justifications for public health programs and policies have been developed by Faden and Shebaya (2015) for ethical decision making about public health interventions that affect

Table 6.3	Five Justifications for Public Health Programs and Policies
1. Overall benefit	
2. Collective action and efficiency	
3. Fairness in the distribution of burdens	
4. The harm principle	
5. Paternalism	

liberty and privacy. These are overall benefit, collective action and efficiency, fairness in the distribution of burdens, the harm principle, and paternalism (see Table 6.3).

The first three justifications recognize that not everyone will benefit from a policy, or they may even object to it. The first justification for public health regulations, **overall benefit**, relies on statistics that indicate that regulations, in general, benefit society (Faden & Shebaya, 2015). For example, Health Canada (2017) controls what drugs and health products are made available to the public to project public safety. In doing so, they weigh the potential risks and benefits to the public.

The second justification, **collective action and efficiency**, recognizes that health as a public good requires that government institutions make decisions about health and safety given that all individuals cannot possess the expertise to make these decisions, nor would it be efficient for them to do so (Faden & Shebaya, 2015). For example, Health Canada employs experts who make decisions on behalf of Canadians given that it would be inefficient and often ill-informed if everyone made decisions independently about drugs and health products. Here again, individual liberties are restricted, but in the interests of the public good.

The third justification is **fairness in the distribution of burdens**, such as those associated with disease, disability, or public health interventions (Faden & Shebaya, 2015). For example, the rubella vaccination is given to children to protect pregnant women and their unborn children (Faden & Shebaya, 2015). Although children must bear the burden of the vaccination, the overall benefits to society are greater than the burden.

The fourth justification, the **harm principle**, developed by John Stuart Mill (1859, 1974), establishes the initial justification for restricting the liberty of people in a democratic society (Mill, 1974). He states, "The only purpose for which power can be rightfully exercised over any member of a civilized community, against his will, is to prevent harm to others. His own good, either physical or moral, is not a sufficient warrant" (p. 68). For example, a CHN would only be justified in quarantining individuals if they had a harmful communicable disease, such as severe acute respiratory syndrome (SARS).

The fifth justification, **paternalism**, can be defined as the interference of a person's liberty of action to promote his or her welfare, although normally this interference is only mild (Faden & Shebaya, 2015). For example, CHNs may persuade their communities through education to eat healthy meals even though their preference might be to eat high-fat snack foods.

Health Maintenance, Restoration, and Palliation: Ethical and Legal Implications

This section of the chapter will address the ethical dimensions of several aspects of this multifaceted CHN role, including community settings as sites of care, informed consent, family caregiving, and palliative care. Please see Chapter 3, Nursing Roles, Functions, and Practice Settings, for a more in-depth discussion.

Community Settings as Sites of Care Providing care in the community can be challenging because, unlike hospitals, many community settings were not designed primarily for the purposes of caregiving. Because of the variability of settings, CHNs must often adapt their approaches and procedures, and they must often travel significant distances or use technology to reach their clients. For example, CHNs working for the Saskatchewan Cancer Agency are able to provide mammography for Indigenous women, who are an under-screened population for breast cancer, by travelling hundreds of kilometres on gravel roads in a mobile mammography bus (Griffin & Layton, 2008). Another example includes a home care program in Ontario that serves clients with chronic obstructive pulmonary disease, congestive heart failure, and their associated comorbidities. Technology in the home permits monitoring and assessment along with health coaching, fostering the development of community-based care, and interprofessional collaboration among nurses and others (Canadian Home Care Association [CHCA], 2016a). The practices of these nurses and other providers are working toward social justice because their goals reveal a concern for health equity, the right to health and health services, the development of enabling environments, and advocacy.

Understanding the meaning and impact of various places or settings is central to community health nursing because CHNs deliver nursing services where clients live, work, learn, worship, and play (CHNC, 2011, revised), not in hospitals. Different places or settings accomplish different kinds of work; have different values, operational codes, and philosophies; and are influenced and structured by different kinds of knowledge and power. These factors combine to influence a person's moral agency within a particular place or environment (Peter & Liaschenko, 2018). The philosophy of Home is Best™ in the Fraser Health Authority in British Columbia asserts that home is the best place for illness and injury recovery, the management of long-term conditions, and end of life. It is an integrated approach to primary care, home care, and community care in which "surveillance nurses" maintain regular contact with clients to help support them to remain at home (CHCA, 2016b).

Thus, the experience of receiving and providing health care services cannot be overtly detached from the place in which it is received or provided (Andrews, 2016). Bioethics, including nursing ethics, has generally assumed that the hospital, not the community, is the setting of health care delivery, resulting in the neglect of many issues facing CHNs that are strongly shaped by the uniqueness of the settings or places in which they arise. Special ethical considerations arise when care is provided in the home because homes are highly significant and idealized places that are imbued with multiple meanings, including personal identity and autonomy, intimacy, normalcy, and security (Peter & Liaschenko, 2018). As nursing services are increasingly offered in homes rather than hospitals, it is necessary for nurses to become mindful of the social and ethical implications of this change.

Informed Consent To meet their ethical and legal responsibilities, CHNs must support and respect the informed choices of their clients. In order for CHNs to assist clients in making informed choices, at least two elements must be considered: the continuous exchange of information between the client and CHN, and respect for the client's autonomy by accepting his or her decisions. These two elements are part of the concept of **informed consent**. Consent is a basic principle underlying the provision of care, and without it a case for assault, negligence, or professional misconduct can be made against the nurse. The process of consent includes CHNs disclosing, unasked, whatever a reasonable person would want and need to know in the client's position. CHNs must provide information about the nature of the treatment and procedures they are offering, including benefits and risks, alternative treatments, and consequences if the treatment is not given. The presentation of this information must consider the client's education, language, age, values, culture, disease state, and mental capacity. When clients provide their consent, it must be done voluntarily—that is, without being coerced—and they must have the capacity, or mental competence, to do so. Exceptions exist in which consent for treatment is not needed, such as in emergency situations and as required by law.

Although clients have the right to make informed choices about their care, as their illnesses progress they often become unable to make decisions. When a client cannot understand and appreciate the consequences of his or her choices, a substitute decision maker, usually the next of kin, steps in to make decisions for the person. The CHN needs to be aware of the laws in his or her province or territory regarding the process for substitute decision makers. When the client and his or her family or substitute decision maker have discussed the client's preferences for treatment or withholding treatment, the substitute decision maker is able to make decisions based on what the client wishes. One of the ways that clients can communicate their wishes for care is by means of an **advance directive** (living will). An advance directive contains a person's wishes regarding future health care decisions. Advance directives are not only for people who are terminally ill. Anyone may stipulate what medical treatments he or she will accept or reject in certain situations, and an advance directive is used only if the person becomes incapable of making choices. The advantage of an advance directive is that it gives people an opportunity to express wishes about treatments such as cardiopulmonary resuscitation (CPR), artificial feeding, and pain control while they are capable of doing so. Advance directives, however, cannot substitute for communication between patients, their families, and their caregivers.

An advance directive contains two sections. The instructional directive sets out wishes for treatment. For example, people may state that if they become terminally ill, they do not want antibiotics for an infection. Others may stipulate that in a crisis they do not want to be transferred to hospital. The second section, the proxy directive, is a power of attorney for personal care, by which a person designates one or more substitute decision makers for health care. This could be a family member or a friend but should be someone who knows the person well and is comfortable carrying out his or her wishes. Each section of an advance directive may exist separately; wishes concerning treatment may be set down without naming a proxy, or a proxy may be named without making any stipulations about treatment.

Family Caregiving The family's role in caregiving, or informal care, has greatly expanded as responsibility for the provision of health care services has progressively shifted from the state to the family or individual. Like formal, or paid, caregiving in the home, women also provide a disproportionate amount of informal care in the home (Duxbury, Higgins, & Schroeder, 2009; Keefe, 2011). The level of care provision is extraordinary, encompassing both personal and high-tech care. It can include assistance with activities of daily living, such as bathing, eating, cooking, laundry, cleaning, and transportation, and also the provision and management of medications, injections, IVs, catheterizations, dialysis, tube feeding, and respiratory care. While most informal caregivers want to provide care (Keefe, 2011), there are inadequate public and workplace supports available (Canadian Cancer Network [CCN], Canadian Home Care Association, & Carers Canada, 2017). Increased rates of emotional and physical strain among informal caregivers have been reported (Duxbury et al., 2009), along with significant out-of-pocket costs and lifelong income losses (CCN et al., 2017; Keefe, 2011).

The transfer of caregiving responsibilities to family caregivers raises a number of ethical concerns. CHNs have a responsibility to promote and preserve the health and well-being of their clients, but because persons are relational, nurses also have a similar responsibility to a client's family. At times, it may be difficult to determine who is or should be the focus of care. The evidence previously cited illustrates that the health and well-being of clients may be threatened when caregivers are stressed and inadequately educated for their role. Moreover, when delegating responsibilities to family caregivers who do not have adequate support or resources, CHNs may be compromising safe, competent, and ethical care. Choice is also limited because clients may have no other option than to provide and receive care at home. Ultimately, however, the source of these ethical problems lies outside of the nurse–client relationship. It is important to recognize that the situations of both CHNs and their clients are the result of broader political forces and agendas that have limited the availability of resources in order to reduce costs. The CNA code of ethics (CNA, 2017a) addresses the importance of nurses upholding principles of justice and equity to ensure that people gain access to a fair share of health services and resources that are of their choosing. Advocacy for clients is one way for CHNs to promote justice. Advocating change for clients would also improve the health and well-being of CHNs because it would lessen the frequency of nurses practising in a way that compromises their ethical ideals.

Palliative Care A very special and increasingly frequent part of a CHN's practice is palliative care. Although most deaths occur in institutions, many people are now spending the last days of

their lives at home. Although the majority of Canadians would like to die at home, most die in hospitals and long-term care (Arnup, 2013). Advocacy groups like the Quality End-of-Life Care Coalition of Canada (QELCCC) strive for change, believing that "all Canadians have the right to die with dignity, free of pain, surrounded by their loved ones, in a setting of their choice" (QELCCC, 2017). The philosophy of palliative care is holistic and client-centred. The Canadian Hospice Palliative Care Nursing Standards of Practice (CHPC, 2014) guide nurses working in palliative care and complement the CNA (2017a) code. The CHPC standards emphasize the nurse's "respect for the personal meanings, specific needs, and hopes of the person throughout the illness trajectory and his/her family" (p. 14). Performing palliative care is extremely rewarding, but it can also be stressful for the CHN, the client, and the family. This intimate area of practice is one in which respecting a client's dignity and right to choice may be difficult for some CHNs (see Canadian Research 6.1). Each CHN may hold his or her own values regarding end-of-life care practices, such as withholding cardiopulmonary resuscitation and other treatments, artificial nutrition and hydration, pain control, and medical assistance in dying. When the CHN's values do not match the choices made by clients or their families, ethical dilemmas may arise. Clients often have cultural and religious practices or rituals that are important to them around the time of death. For example, a Catholic client may ask for a priest to administer the Sacrament of the Sick, and some religions have restrictions on who may care for the body after death. Respecting and facilitating these customs are part of the CHN's care.

CANADIAN RESEARCH 6.1

Navigating Conflicting Values in Palliative Home Care
(McClement, Edwards, Peter, & Roger, 2016)

This descriptive qualitative study drew on appreciative inquiry to examine the ethical dimensions of palliative home care from the perspective of nurses, physicians, administrators, and educators, along with clients and their families. Ethical practice was found to include the importance of accepting the clients' and families' lead, utilizing moral imagination, addressing conflicts in values, and reducing nurses' isolation. With respect to value conflicts, the authors described the need for clinicians to respect a client's wish to remain at home despite their perception that a client would be safer and better cared for elsewhere. The authors also reported the need to address conflicts that arise between clients and their families as an important dimension of ethical practice for clinicians.

Discussion Questions

1. What values can conflict when clinicians believe a client should no longer live at home?

2. What stereotypes might lead a CHN to believe that a client cannot remain at home?

3. What skills are required to address conflict?

Table 6.4	Criteria for MAID

1. Is at least 18 years old and capable,
2. Has voluntarily made the request,
3. Has provided informed consent,
4. Has a grievous and irremediable medical condition, which means:
   - Has a serious and incurable illness, disease, or disability;
   - Is in an advanced state of irreversible decline;
   - Has a condition that causes enduring physical or psychological suffering; and
   - Natural death is reasonably foreseeable.

Medical Assistance in Dying

In February 2015 the Supreme Court of Canada (SCC) rendered a decision (Carter v. Canada, 2015) that the Criminal Code infringed the rights of individuals to the extent that it prohibited medical assistance in dying (MAID)—within certain parameters. Within 16 months of the decision, the Canadian Parliament passed legislation (An Act to amend the Criminal Code and to make related amendments to other Acts [medical assistance in dying], 2016) supporting the right to die so long as the individual meets the criteria in Table 6.4.

Medical assistance in dying (MAID) is defined as (a) the administering by a medical practitioner or nurse practitioner of a substance, at a patient's request, that causes his or her death; or (b) the prescribing or providing by a medical practitioner or nurse practitioner of a substance, at a patient's request, so that he or she may self-administer the substance and in so doing cause his or her own death. Registered nurses or practical/licensed nurses may participate by providing care, but only medical practitioners and nurse practitioners may administer (or prescribe) the lethal substance if they have the knowledge, care, and skill.

In addition, numerous legal and regulatory safeguards are required of the medical practitioner and nurse practitioner, such as second opinions, documentation, independence of the practitioner providing the second opinion, and timing between the request and the administration. These are outlined in federal and provincial/territorial laws, rules, regulatory standards, and resources that practitioners involved in MAID should become familiar with.

The ethical debate that the practice of medical assistance in dying raises is the tension between the sanctity of life and quality of life. According to the sanctity of life view, life is inherently and equally valuable and inviolable. In this view, all lives, however they are lived, are worthy of respect, and ending a life under any circumstances is always a harm. According to the quality of life view, life should be measured on its extrinsic value; that is, on the basis of the person's quality of life or future quality of life. With this view, in some circumstances a continued life may be a fate worse than death; the prolongation of life itself is not worth the quality of life preserved. The ethical imperative to respect the duty to relieve unnecessary suffering by way of assistance with death, if that is what the person wants, finds justification in both promoting health and well-being and promoting and respecting informed decision-making (CNA, 2017a). In health care and in society today, there has been a gradual shift away from the notion of sanctity of life to quality of life and with that increased emphasis on autonomy. What ultimately grounds the SCC's decision and the federal legislation is an ethics of respect for persons or, as it translates into medical ethics, respect for patient autonomy.

In practice, the issue of the right of freedom of conscience gets raised. It protects and fosters a person's responsibility to maintain moral integrity by refusing, or choosing, to participate. One may choose to conscientiously object to or conscientiously participate in MAID. There are many reasons to accommodate or not to accommodate claims to conscientious objection, but ultimately it is a legitimate claim that participation in an act would go against a person's legitimately held beliefs and in doing so violate the person's moral integrity—and for a few, this includes refusing to refer to another health care professional.

The CNA (2017b) has developed a Framework on Medical Assistance in Dying based on its code of ethics, which details nurses' rights and responsibilities as well as more general information about the process. Nursing regulatory bodies have also developed guidelines with which nurses should become familiar.

The future is likely to bring changes in MAID legislation. For example, the Canadian Council of Academies will be releasing a report by the end of 2018 on MAID requests by mature minors, in advance directives, and where mental illness is the sole underlying condition. Legal challenges on the interpretation of "reasonably foreseeable" are also anticipated.

Professional Relationships: Ethical Implications

In building professional relationships, CHNs must recognize the uniqueness of their own attitudes, beliefs, and values regarding health as well as those of their clients. They must also maintain professional boundaries while involving and trusting clients as full partners in the caring relationship. Maintaining professional boundaries can become particularly challenging in the home environment where nurse and clients often spend sustained periods of time together in relative isolation. The **professional boundary** in a nurse–client relationship has been defined as "the point at which the relationship changes from professional and therapeutic to unprofessional and personal. Crossing a boundary means that the care provider is misusing the power in the relationship to meet his/her own personal needs, rather than the needs of the client, or behaving in an unprofessional manner with the client" (College of Nurses of Ontario, 2017a, p. 4). In other words, the CHN must be cautious that the focus of the relationship remains on meeting the needs of the client and not on his or her own needs. Nevertheless, relationships need not be distant and entirely clinical, given that they are often developed in familial settings within home and community.

Insite, a supervised injection facility in Vancouver, exemplifies the importance of building relationships that involve caring, trust, and advocacy in the work of CHNs. These nurses work in a harm-reduction setting to improve the health of individuals who use injection drugs. Relationship building is central to their activities, given that their clients experience barriers to accessing mainstream health services because often they face discrimination and lack financial resources and transportation. Without these nursing relationships, the role of these nurses in promoting health and reducing harm would not be possible. These roles involve a wide range of activities: needle exchange, primary nursing care, harm-reduction education, referrals to health and social services, and addiction treatment (Lightfoot et al., 2009).

Capacity Building: Ethical Implications

CHNs work collaboratively when building individual and community capacity. CHNs begin where individuals and communities are, helping them to identify relevant health issues and to assess their strengths and resources. CHNs use strategies that involve advocacy and empowerment (CHNC, 2011, revised). The World Health Organization (WHO, 2013, Track 1: Community Empowerment, para. 1) has described **empowerment** in the following way: "Community empowerment refers to the process of enabling communities to increase control over their lives . . . 'Empowerment' refers to the process by which people gain control over the factors and decisions that shape their lives. It is the process by which they increase their assets and attributes and build capacities to gain access, partners, networks and/or a voice, in order to gain control."

MacDonald (2013) argues that **advocacy** is the most common ethical orientation in public health nursing practice that embraces the character of the WHO's perspective on empowerment. It takes a stand for the practices, aims, and reforms that are in line with the moral goals of public health, which have a strong social justice orientation: "The moral aim is to promote the health of the population as a social good that allows people to pursue other valued ends" (MacDonald, 2013, p. 399). Public health ethics tends to be distinct from traditional bioethics in its focus on the health of populations as opposed to individuals, and in its concern for the social determinants of health as opposed to individual agency and responsibility (Upshur, 2012). Therefore, there is an emphasis placed on advocacy activities that involve collective interventions to promote and protect the health of populations and that are sensitive to health inequities and to marginalized and vulnerable populations (Dawson & Verweiji, 2007; MacDonald, 2013).

Actions based on empowerment and advocacy foster the everyday ethical practice of CHNs. Empowerment and advocacy enhance the choices and health and well-being of communities because they draw on a community's fundamental strengths and needs without the values of others being imposed upon them. CHNs can exercise their professional power ethically—that is,

in a manner that promotes, rather than restricts, the expression of community choices. For example, CHNs in a rural community near Edmonton, Alberta, initiated a project that through advocacy increased the number of community services accessed by pregnant women. These women were assessed by public health nurses who referred them to additional services as appropriate. Because prenatal anxiety, low self-esteem, and childcare stress are found to be predictors of postpartum depression, identifying and supporting women experiencing these issues are important during pregnancy (Strass & Billay, 2008). With this initiative, these nurses are demonstrating some of the core competencies for public health by building partnerships, collaborating, and advocating for potentially vulnerable pregnant women. These competencies are essential for achieving social justice (Edwards & Davison, 2008).

YES, BUT WHY?

Contaminated Water in Indigenous Communities on Reserves

What?

Most Canadians have sufficient access to safe and affordable drinking water, along with adequate sanitation. Yet for many First Nation communities, the water is contaminated, difficult to access, or at risk because of poor treatment systems (Human Rights Watch, 2016).

So What?

The Canadian government regulates the water for most communities but does not have binding regulations for water supplied on First Nation reserves. In addition, there has been a persistent lack of funding for the cost of water systems, a lack of capacity of water operators, and a declining quality of source water (Human Rights Watch, 2016). For example, the people of the Kashechewan First Nation in northern Ontario experienced *E. coli* in their drinking water supply and were subject to a boil-water advisory for over two years. In 2005 the situation worsened, which led to the evacuation and relocation of 800 people for an extended period, resulting in physical and psychosocial health effects (Bassil et al., 2017).

"**Environmental justice** refers to the inequitable exposures to environmental hazards or how environmental hazards disproportionately affect humans of lower socioeconomic status" (Bassil et al., 2017). Currently, disadvantaged communities, like Kashechewan First Nation, often experience increased exposure to pollutants as a result of a lack of adequate infrastructure while not benefitting from a higher standard of living (Bassil et al., 2017).

Now What?

Specifically, CHNs can take action by following some of the recommendations developed by Human Rights Watch (2016) that involve collaboration with First Nation communities and government, such as developing long-term plans to promulgate enforceable water and sanitation regulations, to create culturally acceptable water policies, to establish an independent water commission, and to foster water system knowledge-sharing. CHNs engaged in these actions need to recognize that from an Indigenous perspective, the quality of water is not merely environmental. Water is sacred, alive, and must be cared for with an ethic of thanksgiving, respect, and dignity (McGregor, 2012). More broadly, CHNs can address environmental injustices through voting, serving on a community board, or working on a local election campaign. Nurses can also move on to more involved political advocacy by running for local political office or becoming the spokesperson of an environmental justice group. At a deeper level, nurses can assume strategic positions in health care facilities, professional organizations, and government offices. Through these positions, nurses can become engaged with policy development with respect to the health impacts of environmental inequities on disadvantaged groups (Boswell, Cannon, & Miller, 2005).

Standards of Practice Fulfilled

#5 Capacity Building
- Uses a comprehensive mix of strategies such as coalition building, inter-sectoral collaboration, community engagement and mobilization, partnerships and networking to build community capacity to take action on priority issues.

#6 Health Equity
- Advocates for healthy public policy and social justice by participating in legislative and policy-making activities that influence determinants of health and access to services (CHNC, 2019, revised).

Health Equity: Ethical Implications

It is through facilitating access and equity that CHNs strive for social justice. CHNs must take into consideration that social factors such as age, sexual orientation, and socioeconomic status restrict equitable access and distribution of health services and determinants of health. Their activities can be at the local or global level and can involve promoting awareness and action regarding human rights, homelessness, poverty, unemployment, stigma, and so on.

Achieving social justice is extremely difficult. Although access to health care services is highly important, income security, housing, nutrition, education, and the environment are essential in improving the health of vulnerable populations (Lantz, Lichtenstein, & Pollack, 2007). Addressing these concerns requires policy changes and radical social change.

The story of Workman Arts Project, a partner program at the Centre for Addiction and Mental Health (CAMH) in Toronto, is an example of community health professionals facilitating access and equity. Lisa Brown, a mental health nurse, was the founder and executive artistic director of Workman Arts until June 2017. She was inspired and challenged by the talents of her clients and began to promote their creative expression through theatre. The Workman Arts Project

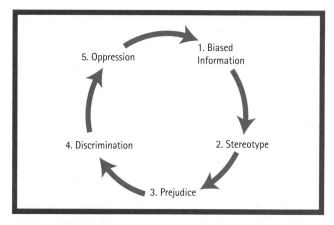

FIGURE   6.1   Cycle of Oppression

Source: McGibbon, E., Etowa, J., & McPherson, C. (2008). Healthcare access as a social determinant of health. *Canadian Nurse, 104*(7), 23–27.

employs both professional actors and people who receive mental health services. The mission of the Workman Arts Project is "to support aspiring, emerging and established artists with mental illness and addiction issues who are committed to developing and refining their art forms, and to promote a greater understanding of mental illness and addiction through film, theatre, visual arts, music, and literary arts" (CAMH, 2017). The activities of Workman Arts foster social justice because they promote health equity by helping and advocating for people with mental illnesses, an often marginalized group, to access some of the determinants of health, such as employment and income. In doing so, they reduce poverty and build the capacity of vulnerable people.

McGibbon, Etowa, and McPherson (2008) describe a cycle of oppression that in both practice and policy can result in inequities in access to care (see Figure 6.1). When biased information based on stereotypes is used to inform decision making, nurses and others can become highly prejudiced and discriminate against people. This discrimination can ultimately lead to barriers in accessing needed health care services, which is ultimately a form of oppression and social injustice that can lead to poor health. The authors provide the example of how people receiving social assistance are often falsely perceived as lazy when instead they may be unemployed because they lack childcare and transportation. This prejudice can result in disrespect and a failure to provide referrals that would facilitate access to employment and, ultimately, better health.

Professional Responsibility and Accountability: Ethical and Legal Implications

In demonstrating accountability, CHNs must adhere to regulatory standards, federal and provincial or territorial professional standards, laws, codes of ethics, and institutional policies. They have a responsibility to be knowledgeable and competent and must also help others around them, such as colleagues and students, to develop and maintain competence (CNA, 2017a).

Increasingly, attention has been given to the legal and ethical responsibility of nurses and other health care professionals to keep personal health information private and confidential. At both the federal and provincial or territorial levels, privacy legislation has been developed or is in the process of being developed. Because there are some variations across the country in terms of both the specifics of this legislation and its implementation within organizations, readers are urged to examine privacy regulations within their province or territory and employing organization.

The CNA (2017a), however, has described nurses' responsibilities for maintaining privacy and confidentiality, and this description can provide CHNs with some direction. It emphasizes people's right to control their personal information and the potential harm that could come to individuals, families, and communities if privacy and confidentiality are not maintained. Therefore, nurses are required to disclose health information only on a need-to-know basis, using only the amount of information needed. They also must abide by relevant privacy legislation.

Health information is considered confidential to the client. CHNs must normally get consent before disclosing personal or health information and in a practice setting may share this information with other team members within their organization on a need-to-know basis.

However, there are exceptions in which information can be disclosed without consent. These exceptions include a court order, subpoena, police investigation, or emergency situation to prevent serious harm or reduce significant risk to a person or a group of persons (CNO, 2017b). The most common exception for CHNs is the legal requirement to report child abuse and some infectious diseases. There are also less common situations in which CHNs encounter individuals who disclose information revealing that a client is a threat to others. The general principle is that when nurses are aware that a client represents serious and probable danger to the well-being of another, they owe a duty of care to take reasonable steps to protect the individual in danger. This principle is supported in law and by the CNA code of ethics (CNA, 2017a), which indicates that nurses may disclose information, after consulting with the heath care team, if there is substantial risk of serious harm to someone.

Negligence

When CHNs do not practise competently, allegations of negligence may be made against them. These situations are very stressful for nurses, and it is important to know what comprises negligence in Canadian law. There are four key elements that must be proven to make a finding of **negligence**: (a) that there was a relationship between the person bringing the claim (i.e., plaintiff; e.g., client, family) and the person being sued (i.e., defendant; e.g., nurse), (b) that the defendant

breached the standard of care, (c) that the plaintiff suffered a harm, and (d) that the harm suffered was caused by the defendant's breach of the standard of care.

A nurse–client relationship usually exists from the instant the nurse offers assistance and the client accepts it. A duty of care is established when a nurse owes a duty to another—the nature and extent will depend on the circumstances. The standard of care has been legally defined as bringing a reasonable degree of skill and knowledge and exercising a degree of care that could reasonably be expected of a normal prudent practitioner of the same experience and standing (Keatings & Smith, 2010). The standard of care determination is often based on professional standards, such as those set by regulatory bodies. Breaches of standard of care often stem from an action the nurse should have done (i.e., an omission) or an action the nurse did negligently (i.e., a commission). The mere breach of the standard of care, however, is insufficient to support a negligence claim. There must be harm suffered from the breach that was reasonably foreseeable, and there must be a causal connection between the harm suffered and the nurse's conduct.

CHNs, either individually or in partnership with others, also have the responsibility to take preventive and corrective action to protect clients from unsafe or unethical practice or circumstances. This action may entail reporting to appropriate authorities instances of unsafe or unethical care provided by family or others to children or vulnerable adults (CNA, 2017a). In every Canadian jurisdiction there is legislation that permits disclosure where there is a reasonable belief of real or suspected physical or sexual abuse of someone, in situations where a child's welfare is at risk, and when there is information related to communicable and sexually transmitted diseases. These circumstances are supported by a legislated duty to report, as the protection of the individual and community take priority over the confidentiality of the client.

CASE STUDY

Jane was recently hired by a visiting nurses agency. She is providing overnight nursing care for five-year-old Anthony, who is ventilator-dependent. Anthony lives with his mother, Susan, and two siblings, aged six months and three years. Susan asks Jane if she could care for all three children while she goes to buy groceries at a 24-hour grocery store. Although the children are all sleeping, Jane is reluctant to assume care for Anthony's siblings. She explains to Susan that she cannot. Susan then becomes upset, stating that she cannot afford to pay for a babysitter and that the other nurses have no problem looking after all of the children for short periods of time. Jane does not know what to do.

Discussion Questions

1. What ethical and legal issues are raised by this situation?

2. What sociopolitical factors situate these issues?

3. How could Jane help Susan in ways that do not violate professional and ethical standards?

CONCLUSION

In this chapter, common ethical and legal considerations in community health nursing were discussed. The CNA (2006) framework on social justice and the CNA (2017a) code of ethics were introduced as relevant ethical perspectives to articulate and address these considerations. The unique responsibilities of CHNs and the variable settings in which they work raise particular ethical concerns that must be understood sociopolitically. Health promotion and protection activities can enhance the well-being of clients, but they also can be means of social control that can compromise client choice and confidentiality. Legislation can often provide guidance to CHNs in these instances. In many cases, CHNs are in a position to advocate for social justice so that the health and well-being of their clients can be protected. Although Canada is a high income country, many Canadians do not have access to the determinants of health.

The health and well-being of CHNs and clients may be threatened when community settings are not suitable for providing care and when informal caregivers do not have the necessary resources for caregiving. CHNs providing palliative care to clients in their homes must possess an excellent knowledge of the ethical and legal considerations regarding end-of-life care, such as MAID, advance directives, and DNR ("do not resuscitate"). Like nurses in all settings, CHNs are required ethically to develop caring relationships with their clients that remain within the limits of professional boundaries. They must also be accountable for their work and must adhere to provincial or territorial and national ethical, legal, and professional standards.

KEY TERMS

advance directive   (p. 93)
advocacy   (p. 96)
bioethics   (p. 89)
collective action and efficiency   (p. 92)
dignity   (p. 91)
empowerment   (p. 96)
environmental justice   (p. 96)
ethical dilemmas   (p. 90)
ethics   (p. 88)
everyday ethics   (p. 91)
fairness in the distribution of burdens   (p. 92)
harm principle   (p. 92)
informed consent   (p. 93)
medical assistance in dying (MAID)   (p. 95)
medicalization   (p. 91)
negligence   (p. 98)
overall benefit   (p. 92)
paternalism   (p. 92)
professional boundary   (p. 95)
social control   (p. 91)
social justice   (p. 89)

STUDY QUESTIONS

1. Identify and define the seven central ethical values of Canadian nurses.
2. What are the 10 defining attributes of social justice?
3. List and define the five justifications for a public health intervention.
4. What does the process of informed consent involve? What information must CHNs provide, and what factors must they take into consideration?
5. What are the criteria for MAID in Canada?

INDIVIDUAL CRITICAL-THINKING EXERCISES

1. How are power and ethics related in community health nursing?
2. What aspects of community health nursing bring about social control? Can these be ethically justified? How?
3. What ethical responsibilities must community nurses consider when working with dying clients?

GROUP CRITICAL-THINKING EXERCISES

1. Identify a group in your community that experiences inequities that constrain their ability to meet their health needs. Discuss strategies that would promote social justice.
2. Ask each group member to write down his or her definition of health and then share it with the group. How are these definitions similar and different? How do they reflect different values?
3. Identify nursing leaders in your community who are promoting social justice. How are they accomplishing this?

REFERENCES

American Public Health Association (APHA). (2017). Social justice and health. Retrieved from https://www.apha.org/what-is-public-health/generation-public-health/our-work/social-justice

An Act to amend the Criminal Code and to make related amendments to other Acts (medical assistance in dying), SC 2016, c 3.

Andrews, G. J. (2016). Geographical thinking in nursing inquiry, part one: Locations, contents, meanings. *Nursing Philosophy, 17*, 262–281.

Arnup, K. (2013). *Death, dying and Canadian families*. Ottawa, ON: The Vanier Institute of Canada.

Bassil, K., Buzzelli, M., Lanphear, B., Peters, P., Moffatt, H., & Telfer, J. (2017). *Canadian environmental health atlas*. Retrieved from http://www.ehatlas.ca/environmental-justice/public-health/research-support-action

Boswell, C., Cannon, S., & Miller, J. (2005). Nurses' political involvement: Responsibility versus privilege. *Journal of Professional Nursing, 21*(1), 5–8.

Canada Health Act. 1985, C.6, s.1.

Canadian Cancer Network, Canadian Home Care Association, & Carers Canada (CCN, CHCA, & Carers Canada). (2017). *Advancing collective priorities: A Canadian carer strategy.* Retrieved from http://www.cdnhomecare.ca/media.php?mid=4918

Canadian Home Care Association (CHCA). (2016a). *High impact practices: Telehomecare in Ontario: Better health, at home.* Ottawa, ON: Author.

Canadian Home Care Association (CHCA). (2016b). *High impact practices: Home is Best*™. Ottawa, ON: Author.

Canadian Hospice Palliative Care Nursing Standards Committee (CHPC). (2014). Canadian hospice palliative care nursing standards of practice. Retrieved from http://www.chpca.net/interest_groups/nurses_ig.html

Canadian Nurses Association (CNA). (2006). *Social justice . . . a means to an end, an end in itself* (1st ed.). Ottawa, ON: Author.

Canadian Nurses Association (CNA). (2010). *Social justice . . . a means to an end, an end in itself* (2nd ed.). Ottawa, ON: Author.

Canadian Nurses Association (CNA). (2017a). *Code of ethics for registered nurses.* Ottawa, ON: Author.

Canadian Nurses Association (CNA). (2017b). National nursing framework on medical assistance in dying in Canada. Ottawa: ON, Author.

Carter v. Canada (Attorney General), [2015] 1 SCR 331, 2015 SCC 5.

Centre for Addiction and Mental Health (CAMH). (2017). *Workman Arts Project of Ontario.* Used by permission. Retrieved from http://www.camh.ca/en/hospital/about_camh/other_camh_websites/Pages/guide_asc_workman.aspx

College of Nurses of Ontario. (CNO). (2017a). *Therapeutic nurse–client relationship.* Toronto, ON: Author.

College of Nurses of Ontario (CNO). (2017b). *Confidentiality and privacy—Personal health information.* Toronto, ON: Author.

Community Health Nurses of Canada (CHNC). (2019, revised). *Canadian community health nursing standards of practice.* Retrieved from http://www.chnc.ca/nursing-standards-of-practice.cfm

Dawson, A., & Verwiji, M. (2007). *Ethics, prevention and public health.* New York, NY: Oxford University Press.

Duxbury, L., Higgins, C., & Schroeder, B. (2009). *Balancing paid work and caregiving responsibilities: A closer look at family caregivers in Canada.* Ottawa, ON: Canadian Policy Research Networks.

Edwards, N. C., & Davison, C. M. (2008). Social justice and core competencies for public health. *Canadian Journal of Public Health, 99*(2), 130–132.

Faden, R., & Shebaya, S. (2016). Public health ethics. In E. N. Zalta (ed.), *The Stanford encyclopedia of philosophy.* Retrieved from https://plato.stanford.edu/archives/win2016/entries/publichealth-ethics

Gillett, J., Andrews, G. J., & Savelli, M. (2016). *Health & society: Critical perspectives.* Don Mills, ON: Oxford University Press.

Griffin, S., & Layton, B. (2008). Bringing care closer to home. *The Canadian Nurse, 104*(6), 12–13.

Health Canada. (2017). Drugs and health products. Retrieved from https://www.canada.ca/en/health-canada/services/drugs-health-products.html

Human Rights Watch. (2016). Making it safe: Canada's obligation to end the First Nations water crisis. Retrieved from https://www.hrw.or/report/2016/06/07/make-it-safe/canadas-obligation-end-first-nations-water-crisis

Johnstone, M.-J. (2008). *Bioethics: A nursing perspective* (5th ed.). Sydney, AU: Harcourt Saunders.

Keatings, M., & Smith, O. (2010). *Ethical and legal issues in Canadian nursing* (3rd ed.). Toronto, ON: Elsevier.

Keefe, J. (2011). *Supporting caregivers and caregiving in Canada.* Montreal, QC: Institute for Research on Public Policy.

Lantz, P. M., Lichtenstein, R. L., & Pollack, H. A. (2007). Health policy approaches to population health: The limits of medicalization. *Health Affairs, 26*(5), 1253–1257.

Lightfoot, B., Panessa, C., Sargent, H., Thumath, M., Goldstone, I., & Pauly, B. (2009). Gaining Insite: Harm reduction in nursing practice. *Canadian Nurse, 105*(4), 16–22.

MacDonald, M. (2013). Ethics of public health. In J. Storch, P. Rodney, & R. Starzomski (Eds.), *Toward a moral horizon: Nursing ethics in leadership and practice* (2nd ed., pp. 398–429). Don Mills, ON: Pearson Education Canada.

McClement, S., Edwards, M., Peter, E., & Roger, K. (2016). Navigating conflicting values in palliative home care. *Journal of Pain and Symptom Management, 52*(6), e12.

McGibbon, E., Etowa, J., & McPherson, C. (2008). Health-care access as a social determinant of health. *Canadian Nurse, 104*(7), 23–27.

McGregor, D. (2012). Traditional knowledge: Considerations for protecting water in Ontario. *The International Indigenous Policy Journal, 3*(3), 1–21.

Mill, J. S. (1974). *On liberty.* London, UK: Penguin Books. (Original work published 1859).

Peter, E. (2011). Fostering social justice: The possibility of a socially connected model of moral agency. *Canadian Journal of Nursing Research, 43*(2), 11–17.

Peter, E. (2013). Home health care: Ethics, politics and policy. In J. Storch, P. Rodney, & R. Starzomski (Eds.), *Toward a moral horizon: Nursing ethics in leadership and practice.* (2nd ed., pp. 384–397). Don Mills, ON: Pearson Education Canada.

Peter, E., & Liaschenko, J. (2018). Nursing perspectives on health geography: Contributions and applications. In V. Crooks, G. Andrews, & J. Pearce (Eds.), *Routledge Handbook of Health Geography.* (In press.)

Powers, M., & Faden, R. (2006). *Social justice: The moral foundations of public health and health policy.* New York, NY: Oxford University Press.

Quality End-of-Life Care Coalition of Canada (QELCCC). (2017). Our mission. Used by permission of Canadian Hospice Palliative Care Association. Retrieved from http://www.qelccc.ca

Reimer Kirkham, S., & Browne, A. J. (2006). Toward a critical theoretical interpretation of social justice discourse in nursing. *Advances in Nursing Science, 29*(4), 324–339.

Richmond, C. A. M., & Cook, C. (2016). Creating conditions for Canadian Aboriginal health equity: The promise of healthy public policy. *Public Health Reviews, 37*(2), 1–16.

Scott, J., & Marshall, G. (2009). Social control. In *A dictionary of sociology.* Oxford University Press. Retrieved from http://www.oxfordreference.com.myaccess.library.utoronto.ca/views

Sherwin, S. (1998). A relational approach to autonomy in health care. In S. Sherwin (Ed.), *The politics of women's health: Exploring agency and autonomy* (pp. 19–47). Philadelphia, PA: Temple University Press.

Sherwin, S., & Stockdale, K. (2017). Whither bioethics now? The promise of relational theory. *IJFAB: International Journal of Feminist Approaches to Bioethics*, 10(1), 7–29.

Starfield, B. (2001). Basic concepts in population health and health care. *Journal of Epidemiology & Community Health,* 55(7), 452–454.

Strass, P., & Billay, E. (2008). A public health nursing initiative to promote antenatal health. *Canadian Nurse, 104*(2), 29–33.

Upshur, R. E. G. (2012). Setting the stage: Population and public health ethics. In Canadian Institutes of Health Research—Institute of Population and Public Health, *Population and public health ethics: Cases from research, policy, and practice.* Toronto, ON: University of Toronto Joint Centre for Bioethics.

Wardrope, A. (2015). Relational autonomy and the ethics of health promotion. *Public Health Ethics, 8*(1), 50–62.

World Health Organization (WHO). (2013). *7th global conference on health promotion.* Used by permission of World Health Organization. Retrieved from http://www.who.int/healthpromotion/conferences/7gchp/track1/en/index.html

Wray, S., & Deery, R. (2008). The medicalization of body size and women's healthcare. *Health Care for Women International, 29,* 227–243.

ABOUT THE AUTHORS

Elizabeth Peter, RN, BScN, BA, MScN, PhD, is Professor at the Lawrence S. Bloomberg Faculty of Nursing, University of Toronto. Dr. Peter's scholarship reflects her interdisciplinary background in nursing, philosophy, and bioethics. She has written extensively in nursing ethics, focusing her work on ethical concerns in community nursing, with a special emphasis on home care. Theoretically, she locates her work in feminist health care ethics and has explored the epistemology of nurses' moral knowledge, using the work of Margaret Urban Walker. Elizabeth is currently the chair of the Health Science Research Ethics Board at the University of Toronto, a member of the Joint Centre for Bioethics, and a faculty member on the Nurse Faculty Mentored Leadership Academy of Sigma Theta Tau International. During her studies, she worked for many years at the Centre for Addiction and Mental Health (Queen Street Site) in Toronto as both a staff nurse and a nursing coordinator.

Louise R. Sweatman, RN, BScN, LLB, MSc, is a lawyer and a registered nurse. She received her bachelor of nursing and master of science with a focus on ethics from the Faculty of Nursing, University of Toronto. She worked as a psychiatric nurse and then went back to school for a law degree from Osgoode Hall Law School, York University, in Toronto. She has worked in various provincial, national, and international organizations, including the Ontario Nurses Association, the Canadian Nurses Association, the International Council of Nurses, Assessment Strategies Inc., and the Canadian Medical Association. She is the founder and first chair of the Canadian Network of National Associations of Regulators. She co-managed the Canadian Gerontological Nursing Association and is currently Director of Legal Services at the Canadian Medical Association with special interest in health and public health law.

Kathleen Carlin, RN, MSc, PhD, specializes in health care ethics. She is currently an instructor in the Department of Philosophy at Ryerson University. She has been consultant to the ethics committee at St. Joseph's Healthcare, Centre for Mountain Health Services (formerly Hamilton Psychiatric Hospital) in Hamilton, Ontario, and has consulted in ethics for community agencies and long-term care institutions. With Louise Sweatman, she co-founded an annual community health ethics workshop day, which ran for several years at the University of Toronto's Victoria College. She was the lead author of the chapter on ethics in *A Guide to End-of-Life Care for Seniors* and has consulted on Ethics in Practice documents for the Canadian Nurses Association. She has given numerous presentations on ethics at conferences and to community and professional groups.

CHAPTER 7

Theoretical Foundations of Community Health Nursing

Claire Betker, Mary E. Hill, Megan Kirk, and Marjorie MacDonald

LEARNING OUTCOMES

After studying this chapter, you should be able to:

1. Explain what theory is and why an understanding of theory is essential to achieve the health equity and social justice aims of community health nursing.

2. Apply core public health concepts that contribute to community health nursing practice, including health equity, social justice, and the determinants of health.

3. Discuss the historical development of nursing theory relevant to community health nursing, and identify new directions for theory development, particularly with respect to integrating Indigenous perspectives.

4. Apply the theoretical and conceptual foundations of community health nursing, including levels of practice; community health nursing metaparadigm; philosophy, values, beliefs, and ethics; broad theoretical perspectives from other disciplines; nursing conceptual models and frameworks; and nursing theories.

5. Illustrate how theory-informed practice in community health nursing is important to clients, including Indigenous peoples and people experiencing social and health inequities, as well as to the health system, the profession, policy, and research.

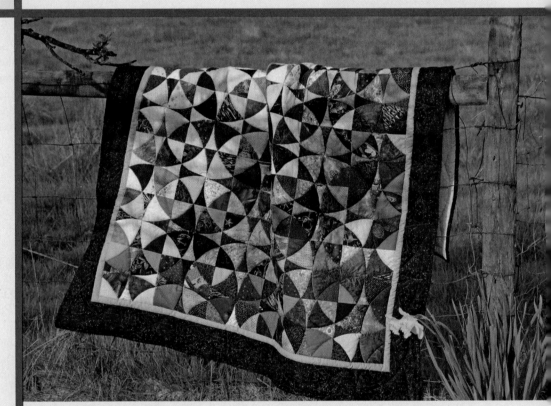

Source: Courtesy of Mary E. Hill

INTRODUCTION

There is no one theory that best describes community health nursing. Science is built on an array of theories, where advances often occur in areas of overlap and integration, much like the designs of a patchwork quilt (Risjord, 2010). Risjord (2010) argues that nursing knowledge is strengthened by joining together different views, making connections and bridging differences. This is no different for community health nursing theory.

Our focus in this chapter is on the theories, **conceptual models**, **conceptual frameworks**, and **theoretical foundations** and **philosophical foundations** of knowledge that guide community health nursing. The broad scope of practice, **values**, and principles underlying community health nursing require diverse and extensive **knowledge** that is grounded in and derived from theory, research, and practice, all of which are interconnected.

Theory provides roots that anchor both practice and research in the nursing discipline (Falk-Rafael, 2005b). Research, in turn, produces evidence to guide the practice of the community health nurse (CHN) in a variety of education, administration, policy, and practice roles. At the same time and in reciprocal fashion, the research and practice of nurses working in diverse community roles and settings contribute to community health nursing **theory development**. Thus, theory, research, and practice are integrated and interwoven.

As in the overlapping and integrated pieces of a patchwork quilt (Risjord, 2010), community health nursing is often described as synthesizing or integrating public health science and nursing theory to promote and protect the health of populations (Keller, Strohschein, & Schaffer, 2011). In fact, in the Community Health Nurses of Canada (CHNC) standards of practice (Community Health Nurses of Canada [CHNC], 2019, revised), the theoretical foundation of community health nursing practice is described as combining "**nursing theory** and knowledge (including social sciences and public health science) with home health and primary health care principles" (p. 6).

In addition to discussing the existing theoretical and philosophical foundations of community health nursing, we also discuss implications for community health nursing of new and emerging political and theoretical issues in Canada. A major issue that is important to take into consideration in the evolution of our theory and practice is the movement for decolonization and the recent release of the report of the Truth and Reconciliation Commission (2015b) with its associated Calls to Action (Truth and Reconciliation Commission, 2015a). We strongly support the Calls to Action and recognize the importance of Indigenous perspectives and ways of knowing as we discuss community health nursing theory and how it informs our practice, research, and education.

WHAT IS THEORY, AND WHY IS IT ESSENTIAL?

"A theory is an organized, coherent, and systematic articulation of a set of statements related to significant questions in a discipline and communicated as a meaningful whole" (Meleis, 2012, p. 29). Nurses have been heard to say that theory is not relevant in practice. Kurt Lewin (1951), the father of action research, said, "there is nothing more practical than a good theory" (p. 169). In fact, many theories used by CHNs are grounded in the practice experiences of nurses and the life experiences of clients, making these theories both relevant and practical. In this way theory supports understanding of why things are the way they are.

Nurses often have their own ideas about the cause of a particular issue or problem for a client or about the best way to work with individuals, families, and communities to address that issue. These ideas are actually "**informal theories**" or "theories in use" about the problem and the solution (Argyris & Schön, 1974). There are times when these informal theories may be inadequate or inappropriate. Nurses select and

integrate theory with past practice and experience to see and address issues in new ways. An intentional and systematic approach to using theories by CHNs contributes to meeting the standards of practice (CHNC, 2019, revised) and achieving better results for the people and communities with whom they work.

One way of understanding theory is to describe phenomena (objects, events, experiences), explain relationships among phenomena, predict consequences, and prescribe nursing care or actions (Meleis, 2012). As such, theory can assist practitioners, decision makers, educators, and researchers to explain what they see and experience, inform their actions and decisions, and articulate possible outcomes. Sometimes, particularly in community health nursing, there is no rigorous research-based evidence available to guide practice in specific situations. In the absence of evidence, theory can be very useful in informing practice in a way that provides a firmer foundation than that of just "doing what we have always done." Nurse scholars and researchers have developed many nursing theories that can guide community health nursing. In fact, nursing theories are integrated with theories developed in public health and the social sciences to guide the practice, research, and education of CHNs.

The story of Jason which is described in Chapter 8, page 149, is used throughout this chapter to demonstrate how theory and broader perspectives could be useful to understand and guide community health nursing practice. Jason is a young First Nation boy who came to the emergency department with a seriously infected cut on his leg. He lived in a neighbourhood where multiple issues such as unemployment, poverty, substandard housing, racism, discrimination, and classism contributed to circumstances that played a role in his injury and subsequent infection. The effects of intergenerational trauma resulting from colonization and the residential school experience have a bearing on the health and well-being of Indigenous communities, including Jason and his family. (See Chapter 22 for more information on the historical effects of colonization.) These broad factors, the social and structural determinants of health, need to be considered in providing care for Jason. In this chapter, we use Jason's situation as an example in order to explore the many elements that affected his health.

The core **concepts**, **patterns of knowing**, and different levels of theoretical knowledge in nursing are important foundations for understanding theory and how it can be used. We begin by describing these foundations. A short history of theory development in community health nursing is then presented, which will provide a context for understanding the current state and use of theory by CHNs. An organizing framework, adapted from the CHNC professional practice model (CHNC, 2013) introduced in Chapter 3 is used to provide a structure for discussing the diverse theoretical foundations of community health nursing, ranging from the very abstract to the more concrete. The chapter concludes with a discussion of the breadth and range of the theoretical foundations for community health nursing practice, education, and research, highlighting the need for further community health nursing theory application and development.

CORE CONCEPTS

Key public health concepts that contribute to the practice of public health nursing include "social justice, a population focus, reliance on epidemiology, health promotion and prevention, the greater good [or common good], and long-term commitment to community" (Keller et al., 2011, p. 251). Other concepts such as **health equity**, determinants of health, capacity building, a strengths-based approach, caring, cultural safety, and collaboration are important for community health nursing in Canada (CHNC, 2019, revised; Canadian Public Health Association [CPHA], 2010). Many of these concepts are addressed in more depth in other chapters throughout this text.

A key concept in public health is health inequity, which is defined as health differences among population groups—described in social, economic, demographic, or geographic terms—that are unfair and avoidable (National Collaborating Centre for Determinants of Health, 2013). Health equity, on the other hand, means that all people are able to reach their full health potential and are not disadvantaged because of circumstances such as age, race, ethnicity, gender, or social class (Whitehead & Dalgren, 2006). It "involves the fair distribution of resources needed for health, fair access to the opportunities available, and fairness in the support offered to people when ill" (p. 5). For further reading on these concepts, see the document "Public Health—Community Health Nursing Practice in Canada: Roles and Activities" (CPHA, 2010), where these and other core concepts are defined in the glossary.

PATTERNS OF KNOWING IN NURSING

Before considering theories, it is important to think about the various patterns or ways of knowing that CHNs use and integrate into their practice (CHNC, 2008). Carper (1978) identified four fundamental patterns of knowing in nursing, including aesthetic knowing, or the art of nursing that is actually feeling the experience with another; personal knowing, of oneself and the experiences that influence one's perspectives; ethical knowing, or a commitment of service with respect to human life and our moral obligations to society; and empirical knowing, which is using scientific processes and rigorous methodologies. White (1995) added sociopolitical knowing, which includes society's knowledge of nursing and nursing's knowledge of society and its politics. This pattern of knowing calls for nurses to find the "intersections between the health-related interests of the public and nursing and . . . become involved and active participants in these interests" (p. 85). The sociopolitical environment is multi-layered, and influences on health include the social context of the person and family as well as the sociopolitical context of the larger community. Building on White's work, Chinn and Kramer (2008) describe an emancipatory pattern of knowing that places the practice of nursing within the broader social, political, and economic context.

A CHN working in Jason's neighbourhood to address the health and safety of local children needs to consider the local First Nation perspectives as well as the sociopolitical environment. This is especially important when working with community members and organizations to facilitate community action. Emancipatory knowing is the capacity of the CHN "to recognize social and political problems of injustice or inequity, to realize that things could be different, and to piece together complex elements of experience and context to change a situation as it is to a situation that improves people's lives" (Chinn & Kramer, 2011, p. 64). Emancipatory knowing encourages CHNs to think beyond the simple treatment of Jason's wound to consider health equity by engaging the community, challenging locally held attitudes, questioning existing laws and regulations, developing and advocating for strategies to prevent further injuries, and promoting a healthier environment for children in that neighbourhood. Together these ways of knowing provide a basis for the development of knowledge to guide community health nursing practice, research, education, policy, and administration.

LEVELS OF THEORETICAL KNOWLEDGE IN COMMUNITY HEALTH NURSING

Theories are only one type of knowledge that provides direction for CHNs who seek ways to improve the health and quality of people's lives (Fawcett & DeSanto-Madeya, 2013). Other important types of nursing knowledge that inform community health nursing can be organized by level of abstraction (Fawcett & DeSanto-Madeya, 2013). The level of abstraction refers to the degree of complexity inherent in the knowledge component; the higher the level of abstraction, the less detail in the component. Starting with the most abstract, the types of knowledge are the community health nursing **metaparadigm**, philosophies, conceptual models and frameworks, and theories (Fawcett & DeSanto-Madeya, 2013). Later in this chapter, these are defined and elaborated on, and examples are provided. Briefly, a metaparadigm contains the global concepts essential to the practice of community health nursing. A philosophy is an abstract statement about what is believed to be true in terms of the development of knowledge and what is valued in terms of practice (Fawcett & DeSanto-Madeya, 2013). A conceptual model or framework contains abstract concepts and statements (or propositions) about their relationship and provides a way to organize and visualize them (Fawcett & DeSanto-Madeya, 2013). Theories are more concrete and can be derived from conceptual frameworks and from practice. Middle-range theories are concrete enough to be empirically tested (Fawcett & DeSanto-Madeya, 2013). See Table 7.1 for a list of many of the philosophies, theories, and conceptual models and frameworks that have been used to guide community health nursing practice. Our categorization of these levels of theoretical knowledge is derived from the academic literature; however, we are aware that various ways of knowing, worldviews, and perspectives from different cultures may not necessarily fit with this categorization.

Table 7.1	Examples of Philosophies, Theories, and Conceptual Frameworks used by CHNs

This table, adapted from Appendix E of the CCHN Standards of Practice document (CHNC, 2019, revised) and supplemented from other sources, includes over 80 examples of philosophies, theories, and conceptual frameworks that could be used by CHNs in different aspects of their work. The examples have been placed in a category that best aligns with the level of abstraction of the theory or model. As some theories and models were named before there was consistency in defining and labelling them, there is not always agreement about which is a theory and which is a model. As a result, some theories are listed as frameworks or models, some models and frameworks are called theories, and there are even several models listed as grand theories. In this chapter we discuss and define various types of theoretical foundations for nursing. Such a list will always be evolving, and we know there are many more theories and models that are not included in the table.

Category	Example
Nursing philosophies	– Florence Nightingale (1946) – Virginia Henderson (1966) – Watson's philosophy and science of caring (Watson, 1979, 2012)
Broad theoretical perspectives	– Complexity theory (Capra, 1996) (Cilliers, 1998) (Gambino, 2008) (Castellani & Hafferty, 2009) (Byrne & Callaghan, 2014) – Critical social theory (Held, 1980) (Stevens & Hall, 1992) – Feminist theory (various) – Intersectionality (Walby, Armstrong, & Strid, 2012) – Postcolonial theory (various) – Ecological systems theory (Bronfenbrenner, 1979) – Systems theory (Von Bertalanffy, 1972)
Conceptual models, frameworks, and practice models	– Albrecht nursing model for home health care (Albrecht, 1990) – Calgary family assessment model (Wright & Leahey, 2012) – Canadian community as partner (Vollman, Anderson, & McFarlane, 2012) – Canadian community health nursing professional practice model (CHNC, 2013) – Community health promotion model (Yiu, 2008, 2012) – Comprehensive multilevel nursing practice model (Ferketich, Phillips, & Verran, 1990) – Dimensions model of community health nursing (previously known as the epidemiologic prevention process model) (Clark, 1999) – Empowerment holosphere (Labonte, 1993) – Health literacy model (Koh, Brach, Harris, & Parchman, 2013) – Health promotion model (Pender, 1996) – Integrative model for holistic community health nursing (Laffrey & Kulbok, 1999) – Interactive and organizational model of community as client (Kuehnert, 1995) – Intervention wheel (Minnesota Department of Health) (Keller, Strohschein, Schaffer, & Lia-Hoagberg, 2004b) – McGill model (Gottlieb & Rowat, 1987) – Multiple interventions for community health framework (Edwards, Mill, & Kothari, 2004) – Neuman's systems model (Neuman, 1995) – Population health promotion model (Hamilton & Bhatti, 1996) – Prince Edward Island circle of health framework (Munro et al., 2000) – Public health nursing model (Kuss, Proulz-Girouard, Lovitt, Katz, & Kennelly, 1997) – Public health nursing practice model (Los Angeles County Health Department of Health Services) (Smith & Bazini-Barakat, 2003) – Transitional care model (University of Pennsylvania School of Nursing) (Lopez-Cantor, 2012) – Vulnerable populations conceptual model (Flaskerud & Winslow, 1998)

Table 7.1	Continued

Category	Example
Nursing theories	
• Grand nursing theories	– Interpersonal relations (Peplau, 1952) – Model of health (Newman, 1986) – Roy's adaptation model (Roy, 1987) – Science of unitary human beings (Rogers, 1983) – Self-care deficit model of nursing (Orem, 1985) – Theory of human becoming (Parse, 1992) – Transcultural/cultural care diversity and universality (Leininger, 1978) – Watson's human caring science (Watson, 1979, 2012)
• Middle-range nursing theories	– Theory of bureaucratic caring (Ray, 1989) – Critical caring (Falk-Rafael, 2005a) – Relational inquiry (Hartrick Doane, & Varcoe, 2005) – Strengths-based theory (Gotlieb & Gotlieb, 2013) – Translational environmental research in rural areas framework (TERRA) (Butterfield & Postma, 2009)
• Practice or substantive nursing theories	– Theory of collaborative decision making (Dalton, 2003) – Community energy theory (Helvie, 1981) – Construct for public health nursing (White, 1982) – Theory of hope (Duggleby et al., 2007) – Theory of maternal engagement (Jack, DiCenso, & Lohfeld, 2005) – Model of family caregiver relationships with home health providers (Funk & Stajduhar, 2011) – Neal theory of home health nursing practice (Neal, 1999) – Theory of peaceful end of life (Ruland & Moore, 1998) – Supportive care model (Davies & Oberle, 1990)
Other public health and social science theories, models, and frameworks	– Adult learning theory (Knowles, 1978) – Assets and strengths theory (Kretzman & McKnight, 1993) – Attachment theory (Bowlby, 1969) – Communications theory (various) – Community mobilization theory (Minkler, 2005) – Community organization theory (Lindeman, 1923) – Diffusion of innovation theory (Rogers, 2002, 2004) – Epidemiology theory (Krieger, 2001) – Health belief model (Strecher & Rosenstock, 1997) – Health literacy skills framework (Squires, Peinado, Berkman, Boudewyns, & McCormack, 2012) – Life course theory (Elder, 1996) – Leadership theory (various) (e.g., transformational leadership) – Management theory (various) – Organizational change (various) (e.g., Lewin's change management theory) (Lewin, 1951) – Theory of planned behaviour and reasoned action (Ajzen, 1991) – Reducing social inequities in health through settings-related interventions—a conceptual framework (Shareck, Frohlich, & Poland, 2013) – Social cognitive theory/self-efficacy theory (Bandura, 1977) – Social norms theory (Perkins, 2003) – Social ecological theory (Stokols, 1992, 1996) – Transtheoretical stages of change (Prochaska & DiClemente, 1985, 1992) – Ecosocial theory (Krieger, 1994)

HISTORY OF COMMUNITY HEALTH NURSING THEORY DEVELOPMENT AND USE

To gain an understanding of the current context of theory development and use in community health nursing, it is important to consider the history of theory in community health nursing. Over the past three decades, many nurses have written about the lack of theory development in community health nursing, particularly theories in which community is the explicit focus of practice (Bigbee & Issel, 2012; Clarke, 1998; Falk-Rafael, 2000; Hamilton & Bush, 1988; Kulig, 2000; Laffrey & Craig, 2000; McKnight & Van Dover, 1994; Sills & Goeppinger, 1985; Stewart, 2000). The problem is that nursing models and theories originally developed for practice with individuals and families within an illness context in clinical settings have been adapted for practice in the community, rather than being developed explicitly for the broad practice of community health nursing (Falk-Rafael, 2000). Thus, there can be a lack of fit between these theories and the demands of practice in and with the community.

This issue has not been raised in the home health care nursing literature, in part because nursing theories may be a better fit for home health care nursing practice than for public health nursing. For example, Orem's self-care deficit theory has been used to guide home health nursing practice (LaFerriere, 1995; Rice, 1994). Home health nursing focuses primarily on individuals and families dealing with illness, whereas public health nursing focuses on communities and populations from a health promotion perspective with a focus on primary and primordial prevention.

Theories with an illness focus directed at individual or family care can be relevant for CHNs who work primarily at that level (e.g., home health care nurses, primary care nurses, or even public health nurses [PHNs] in some aspects of their practice), but these theories provide limited guidance for the broad practice of community health nursing. This is particularly true for those aspects of practice aimed at promoting or maintaining the health of communities and populations. Furthermore, these adaptations have only been partially successful because they have not addressed social justice, social determinants of health, distribution and use of power, value systems, health equity, advocacy, and political processes essential to understanding and working with communities and populations (McKnight & Van Dover, 1994; Sheilds & Lindsey, 1998).

In 1987, Schultz argued that nursing theories often depict individuals' problems as isolated events rather than as representative of a pattern of responses in a community or population. This argument remains valid today. Most nursing theories do not acknowledge that communities and populations can exhibit a pattern of responses in health and illness; nor do they explain relationships among such patterns and the environment or social context. For this reason, they have not provided much guidance for CHNs in their efforts to take action on these larger patterns at the community or population level.

Fortunately, some theoretical development is occurring in which a community or population focus and an emphasis on health promotion and prevention are evident. Not only are general nursing theories being adapted for work in communities (e.g., Falk-Rafael, 2000; Green, 2013), but conceptual frameworks and models specific to community health nursing are being developed as well (e.g., Cohen & Reutter, 2007; Edwards et al., 2004; Keller, Strohschein, & Briske, 2012; Vollman et al., 2012). A few theories specific to community health nursing practice are beginning to emerge in the literature (Falk-Rafael, 2005a; Falk-Rafael & Betker, 2012a, 2012b). Some of these theories will be discussed in the next section of this chapter. Despite these developments, the Association of Community Health Nursing Educators (2010) in the United States identified theory development as a research priority for community health nursing, and it is a priority in Canada as well.

Indigenous Perspectives

What is not well represented in community health nursing theory and practice are First Nation, Métis, and Inuit (FNMI) perspectives. At the time the early theoretical development was going on in community health nursing, there was little acknowledgement of the colonial roots of all nursing theories, most of which were developed in the neo-liberal political environment of the United States (Browne, 2001, 2004). Despite the obvious congruence of many core principles of community health nursing with Indigenous perspectives (e.g., relational practice, social justice, solidarity, the common good, etc.) (Russell, 2000; Henry, Houston, & Mooney, 2004; Baylis, Kenny, & Sherwin, 2008; Shim, Benkert, Bell, Walker, & Danford, 2007), most nurse theorists assumed that community health nursing theories and models were relevant to practice with a range of populations and communities. They did not, however, explicitly draw on Indigenous perspectives in the development and application of theories to practice. In part, this may have been the result of very few FNMI nurses populating the ranks of community health nursing scholars, researchers, and leaders. However, recently "a significant shift is under way in which Indigenous knowledge and ways of knowing are being recognized as consisting of complex knowledge systems with integrity of their own" (Bourque Bearskin, 2011, p. 549/550). In the wake of the Truth and Reconciliation Commission of Canada and its Calls to Action (Truth and Reconciliation Commission of Canada, 2012), along with shifts in the governance of health services in Indigenous communities, development of community health nursing theory and practice that is more relevant to the needs of Indigenous populations is an imperative. This must be done in collaboration with FMNI scholars and community members.

Recognition of Indigenous perspectives reflects knowledge accumulated over thousands of years, and it reflects a view different from Western scientific approaches, which have often dismissed or undermined such knowledge (Martin, 2012). Two Indigenous perspectives that demonstrate an appreciation for both traditional Indigenous knowledge and Western scientific understanding are Two-Eyed Seeing and Two-Row Wampum. Two-Eyed Seeing, developed by Mi'kmaq Elders, describes learning to see with the strengths of traditional Indigenous ways of knowing with one eye while at the same time seeing with the strengths of Western knowledge with the other eye (Bartlett, Marshall, & Marshall, 2012). Two-Eyed seeing suggests that by recognizing and respecting a diversity of perspectives, we can come to better understand the health issues faced by Indigenous peoples (Martin, 2012).

Two-Row Wampum, based on a 1613 treaty between the Haudenosaunee and Dutch settlers, is a concept of coexistence originating in the ways that various First Nation groups had hoped to work with European settlers (Keefer, 2014; McGregor, 2002). The wampum belt, with two rows of purple beads on a white background depicting two boats travelling down a river, reflects each side maintaining its own worldview while at the same time sharing information and working together on shared concerns (McGregor, 2002). The Equity Lens in Public Health research group at the University of Victoria, which includes Indigenous scholars, developed an Indigenous framework to guide analysis in that project with the Two-Row Wampum as a model (Kent, Loppie, Carriere, MacDonald, & Pauly, 2017). These two approaches are examples of the diverse perspectives held by First Nation communities in different parts of the country and can be used to guide collaborative work between Indigenous and Western researchers, CHNs, and other practitioners.

CHNs working with different populations do not need to shed their own perspectives but need to build awareness and respect for other views they encounter, including Indigenous perspectives. A nurse might consider reaching out to the local First Nation to learn more about local beliefs and traditions, which may differ among First Nation communities. These efforts could help to inform how the nurse would interact and work with Jason and his family.

THEORETICAL FOUNDATIONS OF COMMUNITY HEALTH NURSING

As already discussed, despite significant theory development in nursing, there has actually been very little theory developed in, of, and for community health nursing that takes into account the specific focus and concerns of community health nursing practice, including a focus on those populations disadvantaged by the social determinants of health. As a result of such limited specific community health nursing theory, it is important to consider a wider range of theoretical knowledge, such as broad theoretical perspectives, conceptual models, frameworks, and Indigenous perspectives. Not only can these types of knowledge provide the theoretical foundation for new community health nursing theory development, but in the absence of relevant theory, they can also provide a solid grounding for practice, research, and education.

The ideas that make up the theoretical basis of community health nursing are difficult to represent visually in a way that illustrates their interconnectedness. The CHNC professional practice model graphic (CHNC, 2013) is used to organize the discussion of CHNs' foundations. (See Figure 7.1.) The section of the CHNC model called "theoretical foundations" is described in more depth here. Using a fan graphic (Figure 7.2), the most important types of

theoretical knowledge in community health nursing are presented as individual blades. These include the community health nursing metaparadigm; philosophies that encompass values, beliefs, and ethics central to the unique focus of community health nursing; broad theoretical perspectives used in community health nursing; conceptual models and frameworks; and nursing grand, middle-range, and practice theories, as well as public health and other social science theories relevant to community health nursing. The theoretical concepts inherent in various theories, models, and frameworks are listed around the theoretical foundations model, and as mentioned earlier, some of the core concepts are described in detail in this chapter. Of course, not all elements in this framework are always used to guide community health nursing practice or develop theory, but they represent important components of theory and theory development. In the next sections, each blade of the organizing framework shown in Figure 7.2 is described, highlighting how each relates to other elements in the framework and is illustrated in Jason's story.

LEVELS OF PRACTICE

As reflected in the centre of the CHNC professional practice model (Figure 7.1), community health nursing theory, practice, and research, informed by all of the elements listed, is directed at multiple **levels of practice**, either separately or in concert. Practising in diverse settings, including homes, clinics, schools, organizations, community spaces, and the street, CHNs support the health and well-being of individuals, families, groups, communities, systems, and populations (CHNC, 2019, revised). Individual-level practice involves working with people to change knowledge, attitudes, practices, and behaviours. When working with individuals, CHNs consider families as both context and influence on individual-level health. They also consider families as the unit of care and use interventions that promote the health of the whole family. Families, of course, make up a healthy neighbourhood and community. Although Jason and his family are one small unit in their neighbourhood, other families would likely share similar concerns for safe play areas for their children. Community-level practice looks to change community norms, attitudes, behaviours, and practices to promote the health of its members. Interventions are directed toward entire populations, or to sub-populations "under threat" (McGibbon, 2012) and require partnership, inter-sectoral collaboration, and community engagement.

CHNs might work with Jason's family to educate them about safe play while at the same time connecting with the local First Nation to work together to support families in Jason's neighbourhood, while also working in conjunction with the local regional government to advocate for improvements. Systems-level practice is aimed at society-wide change and works to change laws, organizations, policies, or power structures, including the historical effects of colonization, that influence health. Advocacy is an important strategy for CHNs at the broader societal level. The Canadian Nurses

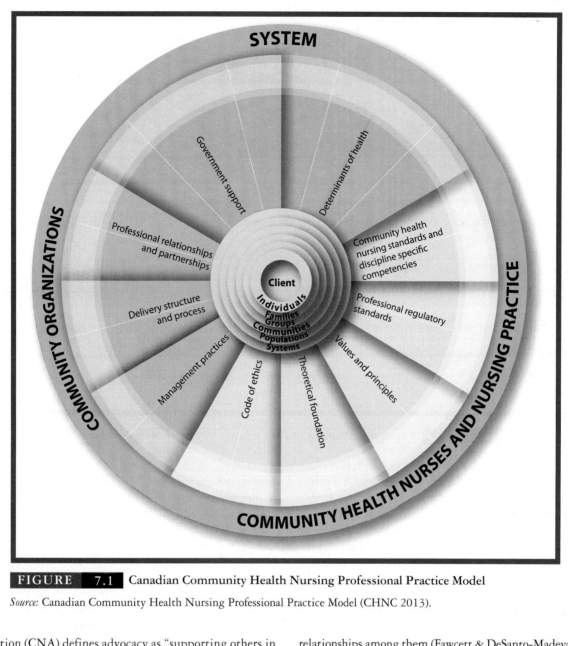

FIGURE 7.1 Canadian Community Health Nursing Professional Practice Model

Source: Canadian Community Health Nursing Professional Practice Model (CHNC 2013).

Association (CNA) defines advocacy as "supporting others in speaking for themselves or speaking on behalf of those who cannot speak for themselves" (Canadian Nurses Association [CNA], 2017, p. 20). We need to consider all levels of community health nursing practice as we explore in more detail the theoretical foundations in the next sections.

THE COMMUNITY HEALTH NURSING METAPARADIGM

Over the years, there has been dialogue about the domains and boundaries of knowledge in nursing, which has implications for the definition of community health nursing as a synthesis of nursing, public health, and social science. Early theoretical work in nursing focused on identifying and describing the concepts that defined nursing and that could provide the basis for theory development in nursing science. A metaparadigm, the most abstract level of knowledge, identifies the phenomena of central concern to a discipline and describes the concepts and the relationships among them (Fawcett & DeSanto-Madeya, 2013). There is general agreement that the central concepts in nursing include person or client, environment, health, and nursing. Although a nursing theorist may conceptualize each term somewhat differently, when these concepts are considered together, they provide the broad parameters of nursing and help to articulate what the work is about (Fawcett & DeSanto-Madeya, 2013).

It is difficult to see the focus of community health nursing practice reflected in the early writing on the metaparadigm and in the descriptions of the defining concepts. However, conceptual work that took place in the 1980s and 1990s extended these foundational concepts to encompass the focus of community health nursing. For example, Schultz (1987) discussed the client as being "more than one." Most nursing theorists tended to focus on client, or person, as an individual, not taking into account a focus on a "community as client." Chopoorian (1986), Stevens (1989), and Kleffel (1991) extended the foundational concept of environment and challenged nursing's narrow conceptualization of it as "the immediate surroundings or circumstances of the individual or family or as an interactional field

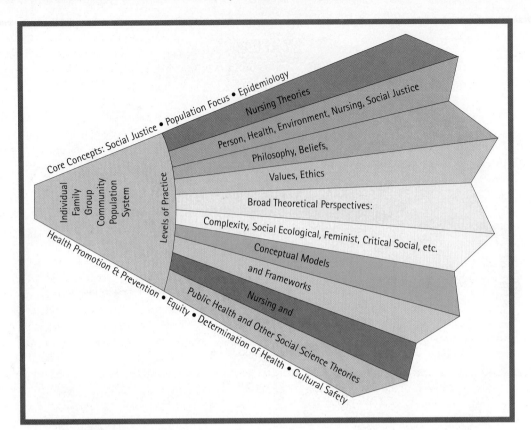

FIGURE 7.2 Theoretical Foundations of Community Health Nursing Model

to which individuals adapt, adjust, or conform" (p. 42). Finally, many theories do not include in their definition of nursing those actions taken by nurses to influence change in the larger social, political, and economic environment. Thus, a reconceptualizion of the scope and definition of nursing was required to take into account community, population, and societal levels of practice, and sociopolitical or emancipatory knowing.

Given these challenges to the relevance of the nursing metaparadigm for community health nursing, Shim and colleagues (2007) reconceptualized these concepts from a community health nursing perspective and added social justice as a new metaparadigm concept. (See Figure 7.3.) They argued that because health inequities can only be addressed by consistently pursuing change at the system and population levels using political and economic solutions, social justice must be the central concept and philosophy that guides community health nursing. Just as we faced challenges in integrating ideas relevant to community health nursing into our metaparadigm and our theories, we now face the challenge of ensuring relevance of our basic paradigm and theories to practice with Indigenous populations and communities. Much work remains to be done, but in the remainder of this chapter, we discuss various theories, models, and frameworks that help to guide community health nursing practice, using Jason's story to illustrate possible approaches. The first major blade in our model of the theoretical foundations of community health nursing (Figure 7.3) is the metaparadigm.

The CHNC (2019, revised) and the Canadian Public Health Association (CPHA, 2010) draw on Shim et al.'s (2007) work in defining the theoretical basis for community health

nursing in Canada. Social justice is explicitly named as a value of community health nursing and is incorporated into each of the seven standards (CHNC, 2019, revised). Social justice is defined and discussed throughout this text (e.g., Chapters 3 and 8) in the context of ethics, and it draws on work of the CNA (2006). Social justice is a central concept in the CNA code of ethics for registered nurses (CNA, 2008, 2017). CNA (2006) identified 10 defining attributes of social justice and included equity, human rights, enabling environments, and poverty reduction among them. These attributes of social justice are integrally related to other important theoretical

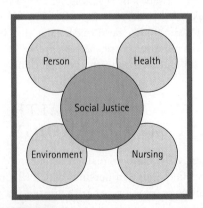

FIGURE 7.3 Key Aspects of Nursing Knowledge (Metaparadigm)

Source: Based on Canadian Public Health Association. (2010). Public health—Community health nursing practice in Canada: Roles and activities.

concepts in community health nursing (e.g., the social determinants of health). Social justice "focuses on the relative position of one social group in relation to others in society as well as on the root causes of disparities and what can be done to eliminate them" (CNA, 2017, p. 26).

Equity and inequity are discussed earlier in this chapter, and the social determinants of health are defined in Chapters 3 and 8. However, these are central concepts to consider in a discussion of community health nursing theory and theory development. There is strong evidence that the conditions of our lives influence our health, and the term "the social determinants of health" refers to the social conditions that "interact to influence our health and well-being and affect how vulnerable we are to disease and injury" (National Collaborating Centre for Public Health, 2012, p. 1). The World Health Organization (WHO) (2013) defined the social determinants of health as "the circumstances in which people are born, grow up, live, work and age, and the systems put in place to deal with illness" (p. 1). These circumstances influence health at global and national levels but also at the local level where Jason and his family live and play.

How can these broader notions of social justice, equity, and social determinants of health be applied by CHNs? In Jason's story, the concept of social justice took centre stage. With no safe place for children to play, the likelihood of further injuries was significant. Taking an upstream (i.e., a prevention or health promotion) approach, and viewing the situation from the perspective of critical social justice, the CHNs in Jason's area might engage with local band council members, Elders, politicians, businesses, and religious leaders among others to initiate a community development process to work toward safer and more stimulating environments for children who have limited resources. Social justice is informed by theories about the equitable or fair distribution of resources, including power, wealth, assets, privileges, and advantages, and includes a vision of a community that is equitable and in which all members are safe and secure. Using this perspective, a CHN in Jason's neighbourhood would consider the information about injuries and play space, engage with members of the community to consider solutions, together to take action at multiple levels to build capacity, propose policy changes, and ensure safety (Browne et al., 2012; Levy & Sidel, 2006).

NURSING PHILOSOPHY, VALUES, BELIEFS, AND ETHICS

The second major blade in our model of the theoretical foundations of community health nursing is nursing philosophy. This encompasses values, **beliefs**, and **ethics** and is central to the unique focus of community health nursing. Philosophy is about the nature of reality, knowledge, and knowing (Chinn & Kramer, 2011). Philosophies "communicate what the members of a discipline believe to be true in relation to the phenomena of interest to that discipline" (Fawcett & DeSanto-Madeya, 2013, p. 8). Philosophy provides an outline of basic beliefs about a subject and offers guiding principles. It challenges us to consider or to engage in inquiry and reflection about questions

we face in daily practice: questions about issues such as power, equity, social justice, oppression, and racism. It is philosophy that stands behind the CHN's decision to walk away from Jason and his injury or to stay and consider how to make a difference within the neighbourhood and for a larger population of children.

Critical inquiry and the examination of beliefs and meaning are the processes of philosophy. Philosophies make significant contributions to nursing knowledge in that they provide broad understanding of nursing and bases for theory development. Philosophy is more than a statement of beliefs; it is also the application of those beliefs to situations that are both known and unknown (Poliferoni, 2011). Florence Nightingale, the founder of modern nursing, developed a very early and enduring philosophy of nursing when she wrote Notes on Nursing: What It Is and What It Is Not in 1859 (Nightingale, 1946). In this small book, Nightingale sought to describe nursing and the general rules for nursing practice (Masters, 2011). What Nightingale described in the mid-1800s reflects community health nursing today and our emphasis on illness and injury prevention, health promotion, and social justice (Pfettscher, 2010). Nightingale identified a key strategy for promoting health, which is to make health issues visible to the public and to politicians. Nightingale's perspective on nursing, social justice, and our role in advocacy and addressing the broader determinants of health informed "critical caring," a **middle-range theory** developed by Canadian scholar Dr. Adeline Falk-Rafael (Falk-Rafael, 2005a) and described later in this chapter.

The fact that critical inquiry and the examination of beliefs and values are the very processes of philosophy suggests that there is a place within the basic foundations of community health nursing for us to reflect deeply on and explore how our values and beliefs have led us to participate unknowingly in practices that reinforce the colonization of Indigenous peoples. This framework of nursing foundations provides a critical space for us, as CHNs, to dig deeply within ourselves as individuals and collectives to surface our unacknowledged racism, ethnocentrism, heterosexism, and the other "isms" (McGibbon & McPherson, 2011) that might cause harm in our practice. In the sections that follow, we attempt to point out opportunities for integrating consideration of Indigenous perspectives into our theories, frameworks, and models, recognizing that many of us are new to this and will need the support and patience of our colleagues and allies to do this well.

An important philosophical value in community health nursing is to promote the common good (Keller et al., 2011). Canadian feminist ethicists, in their relational perspective on public health ethics, state that the common good refers to the pursuit of shared human interests in survival, safety, and security for the good of all (Baylis et al., 2008). There are problems in the application of general nursing theory to community health nursing because most nursing theories reflect the value of individualism (Browne, 2001, 2004; Williams, 1989). Implicit in this is the notion that the interests of the individual should take precedence or be valued over the interests of the community or population. This is not necessarily a value shared by community health nursing (MacDonald, 2013). Not only

Reorienting public health nurses' practice with a professional practice model (Cusack, Cohen, Mignone, Chartier, & Lutfiyya, 2017)

This recent study used a participatory action research approach to develop a professional practice model to support PHNs to work to the full scope of equity-focused practice. The model refocused PHN roles to population health and equity.

The population of a large urban health authority reflected many varied and increasing health inequities. PHNs working in that health authority had requested clarity in their role, priorities, and focus of their activities. They identified the lack of a service-delivery model to guide their practice and decision making as contributing to their lack of role clarity. The issue was bought to the Regional Practice Council for resolution. In response, the first author initiated an innovative participatory action research project and invited the PHNs in the region to participate. The researcher and nurses worked as a team to focus on the issue and developed a professional practice model to address differing population needs.

The professional practice model is being used for collaborative planning as well as delivery and evaluation of public health nursing services. Developing and using the model assisted PHNs to prioritize activities and to practice to full scope. They reported a shift in practice to be more "population based and equity focused" and that their interactions with families were informed through the use of an equity lens. An important finding of this study was the need for clarification of the concept of equity and its application in practice. Because action on the social determinants of health and advancing health equity are foundational concepts for community health nursing practice in Canada, there was an assumption that PHNs would all hold these beliefs. However, these values were not universal, and the development of the practice model provided an opportunity to clarify and reinforce these concepts and how they are applied in practice.

Discussion Questions

1. What are some of the challenges facing a CHN to practising from an equity perspective?

2. What would support a CHN in using a population health approach to address the social determinants of health reflected in Jason's story?

3. How could a practice model such as the one developed through this research be used to encourage reflection and dialogue on values and concepts important to community health nursing practice and research?

that the value of individualism is inherent in most nursing theories (Browne, 2001, 2004). An individualist ethic or value has been less apparent in Canada, at least until recently, where people are more likely to support government programs and regulation (e.g., health care and the Canada Health Act) in the public interest. Canada's health care system is based on principles of universality, accessibility, and public administration (Government of Canada, 1985) and reflects Canadians' greater support of a collectivist ethic. This is evident in the widely shared belief among Canadians (Romanow, 2002) that all of us are entitled to health care that is available to all regardless of ability to pay, accessible wherever one lives in the country, and administered without profit by a public institution. These principles oppose an individualist ethic. Nonetheless, individualism is still a value held by many Canadians that goes counter to the basic philosophy of community health nursing practice, which reflects collectivist values and the notion of the common good (MacDonald, 2013).

An example of individualism is to prioritize the right of individual nurses to refuse flu vaccination over the rights of an entire group of patients and the larger community to avoid risk imposed by others, nurses in particular. A collectivist value is reflected in policies that require vaccination or some other mechanism to prevent viral transmission. Another example of collectivist values would be legislation requiring the use of seat belts or bicycle helmets. In this case, the common good is prioritized over an individual's right to choose to engage in risky behaviour.

These conflicting values in nursing make population-focused practice a real challenge for some nurses who have been educated and socialized to focus on individuals. As Laffrey and Craig (1995) pointed out, "There is constant tension between nursing's concern for human beings as individuals and their concern with the larger community and the aggregates of which it is composed" (p. 126). Theories to guide practice with individuals and families in communities are necessary, and the lack of theory to guide community health nursing practice at the other levels—community, population, systems, and society—is problematic.

BROAD THEORETICAL PERSPECTIVES

The third blade of the theoretical foundations model (Figure 7.2) identifies some broad theoretical perspectives that have been used to inform community health nursing theory, research, and practice. A theoretical perspective encompasses a variety of theories that differ in significant ways from one another but share some core concepts. These perspectives originate outside of nursing but contribute to a CHN's knowledge synthesis. They are also interconnected in part by including many of the same concepts that are discussed throughout this chapter (e.g., social justice, health equity, a population focus). Each perspective can provide a framework for incorporating more concrete and specific theories. This will become clear where an overview of six perspectives is provided in this section. Others are described in Table 7.2.

is individualism an implicit value in most areas of nursing, but also it is a predominant value in Western society at large (MacDonald, 2001; Minkler, 1989). This is particularly true in the United States, where, historically, much of our nursing literature and theory originates. It should be no surprise then

Table 7.2	Broad Theoretical Perspectives Relevant to Community Health Nursing		
Theory	**Unique Features**	**Similarities and Differences to Other Theories**	**Relationship to Community Health Nursing Standards of Practice and Examples from Community Health Nursing Practice**
Complexity science theory	The view that in any given situation there are numerous and diverse parts interacting with the potential to evolve to a new situation. There is no single complexity theory or approach to complexity. Some of the core concepts include interconnectedness, non-linearity, self-organization, and co-evolution.	Complexity moves away from linear cause-and-effect dynamics. It encourages CHNs to think differently about complex public health problems. Complexity theory is similar to intersectionality in that there may be overlapping influences; however, intersectionality does not consider the characteristics of the changing relationships.	All of the CHNC standards of practice reflect issues ranging from very simple to very complex and occasionally to chaotic. Complexity theory can be useful at any of the practice levels, from an individual perspective to a systems perspective.
Social ecological theory	The health of individuals, communities, and populations is influenced by the interplay between people and their environment.	Like complexity and intersectionality, social ecological theory recognizes the impact of many different influences and the overlap among them.	CHNs engage in health promotion activities and consider the array of factors affecting the health of the client and family (e.g., well-child clinics). CHNs consider broad determinants of health, such as income, education, employment opportunities, physical environment, and support systems. An ecological perspective is reflected in the CHNC standards related to capacity building, professional relationships, and health equity (CHNC, 2019, revised).
Critical social theory	Considers the multiple social and economic forces resulting in power differentials within society.	Places equity issues in the foreground. From this perspective, a CHN challenges the status quo and engages with the problems of society.	Whether implementing strategies at the individual level or a broad population level, CHNs need to appreciate the multiple intersecting forces at play shaping the lives and well-being of those cared for.
Feminist theory	Focuses on the role of sexism and oppression in creating inequities.	Feminism is a component part of intersectionality.	This may come into play at multiple levels of practice. Feminist theory is a consideration for all of the eight CHNC standards of practice.
Intersectionality theory	Considers the multiple oppressive forces at play.	Similar to complexity, critical social, and social ecological theories with multiple influences; however, intersectionality has more of a focus on feminism as well as other isms, such as racism and classism, and the compounding effect of the overlap among them.	As with feminism, intersectionality affects all levels of community health nursing practice and all of the eight CHNC standards of practice.
Postcolonial theory	Considers the role of race and history in creating inequities.	Similar to feminist theory with the focus of oppression in causing inequities in health.	Working with many different groups in the community, CHNs need to be aware of the influence and expectations of the dominant culture, what impact that could have on the local community, and their place within it.

Complexity Science Theory

Complexity science is a relatively recent addition to nursing's theoretical toolbox. It has a diverse range of interconnected disciplinary and theoretical roots, but an elaboration of these is beyond the scope of this chapter. Complexity science is sometimes equated with and referred to as "complexity theory" or "complex adaptive systems theory," but these are only a small component of the broad map of complexity science. The evolution of complexity science has proceeded along several parallel yet interconnected paths. Much of the health care application of complexity science, including nursing applications (e.g., Anderson, Crabtree, Steele, McDaniel, & Reuben, 2005; Davidson, Ray, & Turkel, 2011) has been originally derived from systems theory. Examples include King's (1981) theory of goal attainment and Neuman's (1972) systems model, which are based on the notion that human beings are open systems that interact constantly with their environments.

In general, the environments and structures within which CHNs practice can be considered complex adaptive systems (CAS), which are "a collection of individual agents with freedom to act in ways that are not always totally predictable and whose actions are interconnected" (Plsek & Greenhalgh, 2001, p. 625). Although there is no single complexity theory or approach to complexity, there are concepts central to any complexity science approach. These include interconnectedness or interdependency, non-linearity, self-organization, emergence, and co-evolution, which have been well described in the nursing literature (e.g., Anderson et al., 2005).

Interconnectedness occurs as agents in the system interact locally and exchange information to create new connections that allow information to spread through the system. Interactions at the local level give rise to global patterns. Relationships in the system are non-linear in that there is a disproportionate relationship between cause and effect; a small change might result in a very large effect, and vice versa. In self-organization, people mutually adjust their actions to cope and adapt to changing environmental or contextual circumstances. This self-organization arises through the interrelationships and interdependencies of the agents in the system. Emergence occurs through the processes of self-organization and non-linear interactions, whereby there is an emergence of system-level properties that are distinct from the properties of the interacting agents. Herd immunity is an excellent example of a system-level property that arises from immunization of only some members of the system (MacDonald, 2004). Finally, co-evolution means that because a CAS is open, agents within the system interact with others beyond the system so that both the CAS and the world beyond evolve and change in relation to each other.

Complexity theory helps nurses to understand their relationship to the systems within which they work, and the theoretical principles have implications for their practice (Ray, Turkel, & Cohn, 2011). For example, from a complexity science perspective, rigid rules and protocols have limited application or may even be counterproductive. In an era of standardization and protocols in nursing, complexity requires consideration of whether a one-size-fits-all approach to policy and practice is appropriate. Each situation and community is unique and may require a unique solution. In a complex system, the success of a given action or practice is dependent on the context, so success on one occasion does not mean there will be success the next time. Understanding phenomena requires us to see the whole in the part and the part in the whole (MacDonald, 2004), which is, of course, very congruent with notions of holism and ecocentric approaches in nursing (Kleffel, 1996). In complexity science, the essence of a phenomenon exists in the interrelationships and interdependencies among people, events, actions, and experiences (Westley, Zimmerman, & Patton, 2007). It is the interconnectedness of people and their environments that is a primary focus in complexity science. It is these notions of relationship and connection that are consistent with nursing values and all the theoretical perspectives discussed in this chapter.

Looking at Jason's story through a complexity lens enables the CHN to see the many influences on his current situation. With this in mind, the nurse can work on an individual basis with Jason as well as with his family and at a community level. Complexity theory pushes us to consider the web-like influences at play in any situation and the interrelationships among the multiple agents in the system. Focusing on these relationships and how they are connected to one another will assist the CHN in ensuring that he or she is engaging appropriate actors in the process. The notion of emergence helps the CHN recognize that multiple smaller actions by many actors in concert across the various levels can result in a significant positive outcome. The concept of co-evolution guides the CHN to note unintended consequences in a related system as a result of actions in one system. As in Jason's story, what appears as a simple problem (a cut on the leg) is now seen as a much more complex problem involving poverty, racism, and intergenerational trauma. A complexity approach helps CHNs to peel back the layers and consider the various interconnected influences and actions, which are important in helping us to consider appropriate solutions.

Social Ecological Theory

The fundamental theoretical assumption in social ecological theory is that health is influenced by the interplay among individuals or communities and their surroundings—family, community, culture, and physical and social environment (Stokols, 1992). Social ecology "pays explicit attention to the social, institutional, and culture contexts of people–environment relations, and draws on both large-scale preventive strategies of public health and individual-level strategies of behavioural sciences" (McLaren & Hawe, 2005, p. 12). Social ecology draws on systems concepts of adaptation (what people do to adapt to the demands of context), succession (interventions are influenced by the history of the setting with its norms, values, policies, and social structures), cycling of resources (interventions must build on existing strengths of individuals, groups, communities, and institutions), and interdependence (settings are systems, and changes in one aspect of the setting influence other aspects) (Stokols, 1996). The socioenvironmental approach to health promotion described in Chapter 8 of this text is a social ecological perspective.

The social ecological perspective is also reflected in the field of social epidemiology, one of the important sciences that informs the synthesis in community health nursing (Keller et al., 2011), and it has been referred to as an "ecosocial" perspective or a "social ecological systems" perspective (Krieger, 2001). Social epidemiology seeks to uncover and explain social inequalities in health and how these are distributed in the population. As in all ecological perspectives, the influences on health are multilevel and interconnected. Indigenous theoretical perspectives have drawn on social ecological theories in a variety of ways, particularly in the areas of environmental health and natural resource management (Dudgeon & Berkes, 2003; Bohensky, Butler, & Davis, 2013), so the use of social ecological theory and our attempts to draw on Indigenous perspectives seem to be a good fit for community health nursing and public health.

In relation to Jason's story, a CHN working in this community from a social ecological perspective would need to consider the various determinants of health at multiple levels to address systematic barriers to health equity. For instance, a CHN in collaboration with concerned community members could advocate at the political level for legislation around adequate funding to ensure proper disposal of unsafe materials on neighbourhood streets. The CHN could work with community members and other community organizations to create a safe environment for local children. At the highest ecological level, the political structure, CHNs can be involved in activities that are far upstream from the immediate determinants of injury but that address the societal conditions (e.g., poverty or racism) that create inequity that results in injuries among particular segments of the population, such as children like Jason.

Critical Social Theory

The need to address the underlying power differentials and social inequities that affect health leads us to consider another broad theoretical perspective. Critical social theory is one perspective that has been used by CHNs for many years to inform their work with population groups that have been disadvantaged by social circumstances (Allen, 1985; Butterfield, 1990; Cohen & Reutter, 2007; Kleffel, 1991; Stevens & Hall, 1992). CHNs are committed to promoting the health of marginalized groups and populations "under threat" (McGibbon, 2012). This requires nurses to work with not only individual clients and families but also collaboratively with other sectors to influence public policy and address the structural and systemic determinants of health. Although others often use the term "vulnerable" to describe groups experiencing social disadvantage, McGibbon has moved away from the notion of vulnerability and instead uses the term "under threat" to indicate that the source of oppression and marginalization is not within the individuals themselves but in the social and political structures that create systematic disadvantage.

Critical social theory provides a vantage from which to examine issues of community health practice and policy to see what is possible within the current situation. This perspective challenges the status quo and assumes a deliberate engagement with the problems of society and the processes of social transformation. In Jason's situation one can see that the simple act of attending to his leg wound alone misses the underlying factors that led to his injury in the first place. Asking "why" illuminates various social and community issues. This provides

an opportunity for CHNs to engage with local policies and services to work toward improvements benefitting the larger community. Critical social theory allows the CHN to take the historically situated sociopolitical perspective, analyze it, and then challenge the social inequities and injustices that resulted from it (Chinn & Kramer, 2011). A critical social theorist "takes the stance that some values are better than others and makes an explicit commitment to social justice" (Strega, 2005, p. 207).

Feminist Theory

Feminism encompasses the perspectives and methods committed to political and social changes that improve the lives of women and, in turn, the lives of all people (Chinn & Kramer, 2011). Feminism is defined by hooks (2000) as "a movement to end sexism, sexist exploitation, and oppression" (p. viii). Although there are multiple perspectives, debates, and disagreements within feminist theory, there are some commonalities among them. In general, feminism is focused on equity, oppression, and justice, which are central concerns in public health (Rogers, 2006) and community health nursing. A feminist theorist sees inequality as based on social oppression rather than individual misfortune (McGibbon & Etowa, 2009). Lack of power, diminished opportunities, discrimination, and oppression are some of the less-noticeable aspects of inequality (Rogers, 2006). While equity is considered key to public health, a feminist perspective on equity suggests that simply being female is also a risk factor for increased inequity (Rogers, 2006).

Because much of the work of CHNs is directed toward reducing the effects of poverty, their activities have the potential to make a difference in the lives of women and children who are over-represented in the population of the disadvantaged (Rogers, 2006). As well, women as family care providers are traditionally the ones most often mediating the preventive aspects of diet, exercise, and other aspects of health within the household (Rogers, 2006). Very often it is these women whom CHNs work with individually, in families, and in groups. CHNs advocate for their clients in ways that promote health, empowerment, justice, and equality (Leipert, 2001).

Reading between the lines in Jason's story, it is possible to see that issues of injustice and oppression are likely present. A CHN working in this community would want to consider how plans for improving health could be informed by a feminist perspective. This would start by considering the perspectives of the local population, building on their strengths, offering a range of options, and supporting efforts for change (Leipert, 2001). In working with Jason's neighbourhood, the CHN would develop closer connections and cooperation with community members and recognize needs identified by this group while taking into consideration cultural and economic diversity as well as the perceived power of his or her own position as a CHN and health expert (James, 1996, as cited in Leipert, 2001). Feminist theory assists CHNs in taking a stand with groups that experience conditions creating vulnerability, questioning oppressive situations, facilitating strategies developed by the group, and dealing with the broader social, political, and economic roots of poor health (Leipert, 2001).

Intersectionality Theory

Another broad theoretical perspective, intersectionality, provides a way to understand how multiple social identities such as gender, race, disability, socioeconomic status, and other inequalities intersect at the level of the individual and reflect social constructions of oppression and privilege (Bowleg, 2012). Intersectionality examines difference and the influence of power on an individual or group who have their own histories within the context of their current surroundings (Corbin & Tomm Bonde, 2012). Like roads that meet at an intersection, the interweaving of multiple social determinants and mechanisms offers a more inclusive look at the factors of sexism, racism, and other isms that come together as oppression, which negatively impacts the health of individuals and populations.

Intersectionality has been described as a framework that accounts for the synergistic or amplifying influence of multiple forms of oppression (McGibbon, 2008). Yet it has been noted that intersectionality has been defined and represented in a number of ways (McGibbon & Etowa, 2009). For instance, within nursing, intersectionality has been discussed as a useful paradigm for approaching research (e.g., Van Herk, Smith, & Andrew, 2011). It has also been used to better understand social justice for nursing action, education, practice, research, and policy (e.g., Pauly, MacKinnon, & Varcoe, 2009). For another example of intersectionality in nursing, turn to Chapter 28.

In Jason's case, the combination of his First Nation heritage, his poor economic situation, and the impoverished neighbourhood in which his family lives culminate in the lack of a safe environment for children to live and play. CHNs need to be aware of how these factors may intersect to deepen the disadvantage experienced by Jason and his family as they struggle to ensure a safe environment in the context of racism, discrimination, and poverty. Nurses need to keep these in mind as they work with Jason, his family, other First Nation members and local community partners to improve safety, prevent injuries, and ultimately improve the health of the community.

Postcolonial Theory

Postcolonial theory, as a broad theoretical perspective, challenges us to consider oppressive structures that assume a view reflecting dominant discourse and culture, and to give "voice to subjugated and Indigenous knowledge, especially non-Western voices" (Reimer-Kirkham et al., 2009, p. 155). A postcolonial theoretical perspective can contribute to "understanding how continuities from the past shape the present context of health and health care" (Browne, Smye, & Varcoe, 2005, p. 19). A better understanding of historical influences on the current experiences of individuals receiving care allows an appreciation of the lasting consequences of colonization on identity, race, and health. Postcolonial theory is an important theoretical perspective to draw on in community health nursing practice; it challenges our assumptions through encouraging self-reflection and exploration of the forms of oppression at play within any given nurse–client or nurse–community interaction.

Postcolonial theory is also beneficial for nurse researchers in guiding the research process. For instance, it informs research question development, study design, and data analysis. Canadian nurse researchers have used postcolonial theory extensively in working with Indigenous families, and communities (e.g., Smith, Edwards, Martens, & Varcoe, 2007; Smith, Varcoe, & Edwards, 2005; Van Herk, Smith, & Tedford Gold, 2012). As well, nurse researchers' interest in gender analysis in postcolonial theory has led to the use of postcolonial feminist theory to get at the root causes of racialized and gendered inequities (Reimer-Kirkham, Baumbusch, Schultz, & Anderson, 2009).

Postcolonial theory is important and useful within community health nursing research and practice to challenge the privileging of knowledge within Canada, but it is also useful within a global health context. For instance, in Chapter 33, postcolonial theory may explain the differences among international health, global health, and public health, and lead to questions regarding the dominance and authority of Western knowledge in nursing practice throughout the world.

Thus, no matter a nurse's location, it is important to become aware of and question our ways of thinking and being. For instance, a CHN coming from a white middle-class background needs to be aware of the importance of cultural safety when working with Jason and his family, by providing care with an understanding that the impoverished state of this family (which led to Jason's need for health care) is related to the loss of cultural values and norms. Assumptions about ways to address health issues may not always fit with the standardized view of the dominant culture. Care needs to be given in a way that respects both cultural differences and acceptable solutions.

CONCEPTUAL MODELS AND FRAMEWORKS

As the fourth blade in the theoretical foundations of community health nursing model (Figure 7.2), conceptual models and frameworks are the "scaffolding" for theories. Much of the development of theory in community health nursing has been in conceptual models and frameworks. A conceptual model or framework is defined as a set of relatively abstract and general concepts, the propositions that describe those concepts, and the general relations between the concepts. As discussed earlier in the section on broad theoretical perspectives, a model or framework can integrate theories. This was illustrated with the social ecological perspective already discussed. Similarly, the community health nursing models and frameworks discussed in this section incorporate specific middle-range and practice or substantive theories.

Although the terms "framework" and "model" are often used interchangeably, some theorists suggest that a framework is less formal than a conceptual model and does not usually contain propositions (Fawcett & DeSanto-Madeya, 2013). In this chapter, conceptual frameworks and models are categorized together. For a list of several conceptual models and frameworks that are particularly relevant to community health nursing, refer to Table 7.3. The next section describes some conceptual models or frameworks that have been developed and used widely to guide community health nursing practice.

Table 7.3	Conceptual Models and Frameworks	
Conceptual Model or Framework	**Key Points**	**Relationship to Community Health Nursing Standards of Practice and Examples from Community Health Nursing Practice**
Canadian community as partner (Vollman et al., 2003, 2008, 2012)	This conceptual model depicts the community as a dynamic system that interacts with its environment and moves iteratively through the phases of community assessment, analysis, diagnosis, planning, intervention, and evaluation. It sees interventions as primary, secondary, or tertiary preventive levels, and is consistent with the broad determinants of health.	CHNC standards 1 and 2, health promotion and prevention, and health protection, are incorporated in this model, as are standards 3, 5, 6, and 7. An example from practice is a local community demand for birth control services for teens and the subsequent involvement of CHNs with teens and community partners to establish accessible and welcoming clinic services.
Population health promotion: An integrated model of population health and health promotion (Hamilton & Bhatti, 1996)	This widely used Canadian model demonstrates the link between population health and health promotion at various levels of action. The model is used to identify specific actions as well as demonstrate how to combine various actions to create a comprehensive action strategy. Attention is directed to individual, family, and community levels.	An example of a specific health concern might be the development of community support groups for young parents. This model fits well with public health nursing discipline-specific competencies 3, 4, and 5 (CHNC, 2009) as well as CHNC standards 1, 2, 4, 5, 6, and 7.
Multiple interventions for community health framework (Edwards et al., 2004)	This Canadian model is based on the assumption that interrelated social, cultural, political, and economic factors influence the health of individuals. Multiple intervention programs are based in a socioecological framework where a combination of interventions are used to target individual, community, and political levels as well as different sectors such as education, transportation, housing, health, and others. It considers nested determinants of health and recognizes that effects may change over time with changing players and leadership, both locally and politically.	In Duncan, BC, CHNs improved breastfeeding rates within their community by promoting the WHO's "10 Steps" with colleagues in acute care. CHNs were involved in the development of health authority and school board policies to support breastfeeding. CHNs worked with local grocery stores and food banks to reduce formula promotions. They initiated photo contests, breastfeeding calendars, World Breastfeeding Day events, and parent support groups to change the local culture related to breastfeeding. CHNC standards 1, 2, 4, 5, and 7 are closely linked to this framework.
Health promotion model (Pender, 1996)	This American nursing conceptual model focuses on health promoting behaviour directed toward positive health outcomes at an individual level. It identifies how a range of individual experiences and characteristics affect the health promoting behaviour of individuals. It is particularly useful in changing personal health especially in home health care, but less so for changing social determinants as it does not address the broader population.	CHNs develop a smoking cessation clinic after community assessments indicated higher-than-average smoking rates in the perinatal population. CHNs use motivational interviewing to assist clients in resolving health issues and refer to other community resources as needed. Although it has some connections with all of the CHNC standards, this model relates particularly well with standards 1, 3, 5, and 7.

Table 7.3	Continued	
Conceptual Model or Framework	**Key Points**	**Relationship to Community Health Nursing Standards of Practice and Examples from Community Health Nursing Practice**
Calgary family assessment model (Wright & Leahey, 2012)	The Calgary family assessment model is an integrated, multidimensional framework based on systems, cybernetics, communication, and change theory. This is a model that can be used to assess a family or as an organizing framework for clinical work with individual families. It focuses on the interaction among all individuals within a family and is inclusive of past, present, and future family members.	A home health nurse can use this model, for example, with a family experiencing a major illness or facing death to assess the relationships within the family support network. This model relates especially well to CHNC standards 3, 5, and 7.
An integrative model for holistic community health nursing (Laffrey & Kulbok, 1999)	This American model outlines nursing care for the individual, family, and community. CHNs practising in different settings will have different areas of practice and require different kinds of expertise. Multilevel practice is described within a population-centred perspective. An integrated approach supports the broad scope of practice in the community and provides a basis for collaboration and partnership.	CHNC standards related to this model include 1, 2, 3, 5, and 7 in particular, although the remaining standards are also relevant. A practice example is the home health nurse who may be initially involved with a client recovering from an injury. The nurse soon recognizes the challenges inherent within the family and the community and connects with the PHN to follow up with the broader issues, planning together what could be done with the community to prevent similar injuries.
Intervention wheel (Keller & Strohschein, 2012)	Also known as the Minnesota intervention wheel, this model demonstrates the relationships between interventions and outcomes for different levels of practice. It depicts how PHNs improve population health through interventions with individuals, families, and communities, as well as the systems that impact on the health of communities. It considers the determinants of health and emphasizes health promotion and prevention interventions to improve population health.	A PHN might focus on ways to improve breastfeeding and immunization rates while working with a population of perinatal women. This may be accomplished through individual contact with moms as well as by engaging with local partners to shift the prevailing community culture. CHNC standards 1, 2, 4, 5, 6, and 7 fit particularly well with this model.
First Nations Perspective on Health and Wellness model (First Nations Health Authority of British Columbia (2018))	Developed in conjunction with First Nations in British Columbia to depict shared understanding of wellness, this model extends from individual responsibility for health and wellness to the broader determinants of health. It consists of concentric circles that emphasize the balance among the mental, emotional, spiritual, and physical aspects of health. The overarching values of this model demonstrate respect and honouring First Nation languages, cultures, and traditions.	This model reflects all of the CHNC standards of practice.

Canadian Community as Partner

Consistent with Neuman's (1995) theory, the emphasis is on understanding the community as a dynamic system that interacts with its environment (Vollman et al., 2008). The model assists users in moving iteratively through the phases of community health nursing: assessment, analysis, diagnosis, planning, intervention, and evaluation. The Canadianization of community as partner grounded it more explicitly in health promotion, drawing on the Ottawa Charter (Vollman et al., 2012). Assessment is guided by the assessment wheel with the people of the community whose health is affected by and affects various subsystems at its core. The authors explain that the subsystems are consistent with the broad determinants of health (see Chapter 8), an important aspect of community health nursing practice. For example, the education subsystem in the wheel parallels the education determinant of health.

Keep in mind Jason's neighbourhood as the phases of the community health nursing process are considered. Through analysis of the data collected in the assessment phase (in partnership with the community), a community diagnosis is made about the priority issues to address. The CHN engages local partners in planning interventions to reduce the community stressors and build community resilience. Using the model, interventions are conceptualized as primary (to prevent disease from occurring), secondary (early detection of disease), or tertiary (to slow or reduce disease processes). CHNs can intervene with activities directed at one or more levels of prevention, which progress from health promotion before disease processes have begun to reduce the symptoms or progress of a disease. Thus, theories of health promotion are relevant within this model. In fact, the Canadian community as partner (Vollman et al., 2012) discussion in this text is built around intervention strategies from the five action areas of the Ottawa Charter. (See Chapter 8.) Each action area points to the need for specific theories to guide practice. For example, in the action area "strengthening community action," theories and principles of community development would be relevant. Once implemented, these interventions are evaluated. This process of assessment, analysis, planning, intervention, and evaluation is reflected in each of the eight standards of practice (CHNC, 2019, revised).

Using this model, a CHN would begin by collecting information about the number and nature of childhood injuries in Jason's neighbourhood. The CHN might also gather local information and stories about individual events to illustrate the effects on families and the community, all the while working with community members to raise awareness of the issues. Through this process, the CHN demonstrates caring, communication, and a commitment to the community through the development of relationships that facilitate the achievement of collaboratively identified health goals.

The Intervention Wheel

The intervention wheel (Figure 7.4) is an evidence-based, widely tested, and validated public health nursing conceptual model (Keller, Strohschein, Lia-Hoagberg, & Schaffer, 1998). The intervention wheel depicts how public health nursing improves population health through interventions with individuals, families, and communities, as well as with the systems that affect community health. It incorporates evidence that demonstrates the relationships between interventions and outcomes for different levels of practice.

The model was inductively derived from the practice of PHNs and some home care nurses. The authors used grounded theory research method to identify 17 core public health nursing interventions that were common to the work of PHNs. Later, these interventions were subjected to an extensive systematic review of evidence to support their effectiveness. Each intervention is accompanied by a set of steps and recommended best practices that are grouped together in coloured wedges of the wheel. Each colour represents a different class of public health nursing intervention.

The model is population-based in that—at all levels of practice, even the individual level—interventions are carried out in the service of improving population health. Using this model, it is possible to imagine how a CHN in Jason's neighbourhood can work at various levels to make a difference in his community. Drawing on the interventions in the orange wedge of the wheel (collaboration, coalition building, and community organizing), the CHN can raise awareness of the issue of safety and injury prevention with community organizations and begin to collaborate with them, building a coalition to advocate (yellow wedge) for improvements in safety. By advocating with local municipal government officials and other sectors like education and housing on the issue of safe environments, CHNs in collaboration with others can initiate a conversation and set in motion the wheels of action for change.

Although this model is focused on the practice of PHNs, there are situations in which other CHNs will engage in public health functions and carry out interventions. For example, a home health nurse might follow Jason after his visit to the hospital to assist with his wound care and may engage in one or more of the interventions at the individual or family level (Keller et al., 2004a, 2004b). A home health nurse might enact interventions in the blue wedge of the wheel: health teaching, counselling, and consultation. The nurse might also use advocacy strategies (yellow wedge), screen for diseases (purple wedge), or engage in collaboration (orange wedge) with others in the community. Because the wheel includes individual and family levels of practice within a population focus, which may include health promotion and disease prevention, these interventions would be quite appropriate for a home health nurse.

An Integrative Model for Holistic Community Health Nursing

This model provides an integrated and holistic approach to community health nursing across settings and goes beyond the traditional nursing focus on the individual and family levels to include group and community levels (Laffrey & Kulbok, 1999). The model is conceptualized within a holistic and ecocentric perspective (Kleffel, 1996) in which the "human and non-human are one within the same organic system" (p. 4). Practice

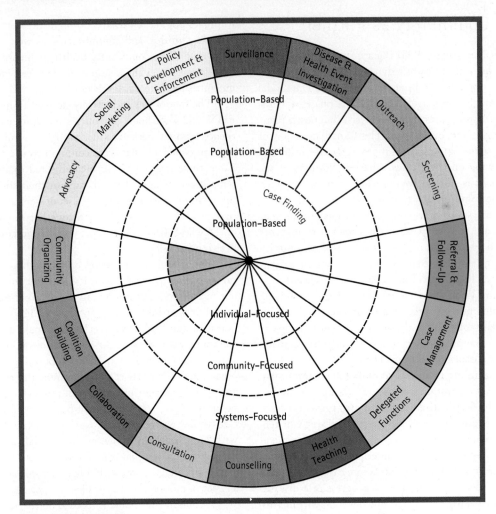

FIGURE 7.4 The Intervention Wheel

Source: Public Health Interventions Applications for Public Health Nursing Practice, March 2001. Copyright © 2001 by Minnesota Department of Health. Used by permission of Minnesota Department of Health.

is conceptualized within a primary health care framework (Laffrey & Craig, 2000), and multilevel practice is described within a population-centred perspective (Kulbok, Laffrey, & Chitthathairattm, 2008). Primary health care is described in detail in Chapter 8.

This model (Figure 7.5) contains two dimensions: (1) the "client system" (individual, family, group, and community) and (2) the "focus of care," which encompasses health promotion at the core, including prevention of illness, disease, injury, and disability, as well as illness care. The fact that care is directed at different levels of clients and different foci of practice means that the model can be used to conceptualize the broad and diverse practice of CHNs. For example, home health nurses who primarily provide care for individuals and families might emphasize illness care but could also incorporate a focus on prevention. There are various levels of prevention considered in the delivery of community health nursing services. Primordial prevention aims to impede the development of environmental conditions, such as economic, social, and cultural factors that increase the risk of disease (Porta, 2008) and that may contribute to health inequities. Primary

prevention addresses more immediate ways to prevent disease or injury from actually occurring. This is sometimes referred to as "upstream" prevention. Secondary prevention relates to early detection of disease, while tertiary prevention aims to slow or reduce disease processes. Quaternary prevention endeavours to prevent inappropriate or unnecessary medical interventions to minimize the suffering of a chronically ill client; for instance, the promotion of a healthy death (Last, 2007). CHNs use interventions directed at one or more levels of prevention, progressing from health promotion before disease processes have begun to reducing the symptoms and progress of a disease. Levels of prevention are also discussed throughout this text.

In Jason's situation, the home health nurse may have been initially involved in his wound care, but recognizing the challenges inherent within the family and the community, that nurse might have connected with the PHN to follow up with the broader issues, planning together about what could be done with the community to prevent further such injuries. The authors emphasize that no single practitioner can do everything, so collaboration and coordination across teams of nurses and other providers is essential in maintaining the integrity of the model.

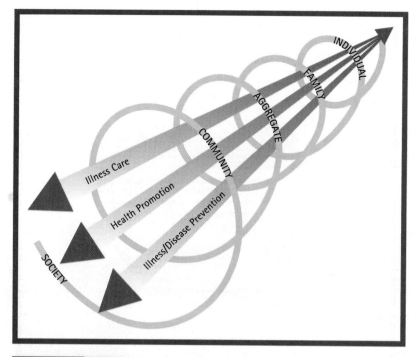

FIGURE **7.5** An Integrative Model for Holistic Community Health Nursing

Source: Based on Laffrey, S. C., & Kulbok, P. A. (1999). An integrative model for holistic community health nursing. *Journal of Holistic Nursing, 17*(1), 88–103.

This model is one of the few available in the literature that can be used by nurses working across diverse community health nursing–client systems and foci of practice. The model fully encompasses the holistic and integrative vision of the CHNC (2019, revised) that CHNs collectively share a common history, values, skills, traditions, and beliefs, and that their distinctive practices are complementary within a shared philosophical base.

First Nations Health Authority Perspective on Health and Wellness

In 2013, the BC First Nations Health Authority assumed responsibility for the health services and programs previously operated by the federal government to improve health care for First Nations in the province. Its First Nations Perspective on Health and Wellness model (First Nations Health Authority of British Columbia, 2018) (see Figure 7.6) visually represents a holistic understanding of health and wellness, drawing on feedback and teachings from BC First Nations. The First Nations Perspective on Health and Wellness denotes the alignment and continuous interaction of the physical, emotional, mental and spiritual realities, and how these aspects of wellness connect and intersect with the social determinants of health. (See Chapter 22 for further elaboration.)

The First Nations Perspective on Health and Wellness model is used to guide care and create shared understanding. It communicates a conceptual framework that acts as an anchor to decolonize and redesign health programs and services for First Nations in BC (First Nations Health Authority of British

Columbia, 2018). Community health nursing services in First Nations communities across BC are central in this model of delivery, which is under the control of the communities.

NURSING THEORIES

The last blade of the theoretical foundations of community health nursing model (Figure 7.2) considers nursing theories as well as theories from public health and the social sciences. Nurses in all areas of practice know about and have used a range of theories, models, and frameworks to guide their practice both from within and outside of nursing. Theories contain relatively concrete and specific concepts (e.g., caring, self-care, adaptation) and propositions that define those concepts and their relationships. Nursing theories, like the broad range of knowledge components in this chapter, can be categorized by the degree of abstraction, ranging from fairly concrete and situation-specific **practice theories**, through middle-range theories, to more abstract **grand theories**. Exemplar theories in each of these categories that have either been developed for community health nursing or adapted for use in community health nursing practice, education, and research are highlighted and briefly described in the following sections.

Grand Nursing Theories

Grand theories are broad in their scope, and the concepts are described in abstract terms. As such, they can be used in a broad range of practice situations and provide high-level

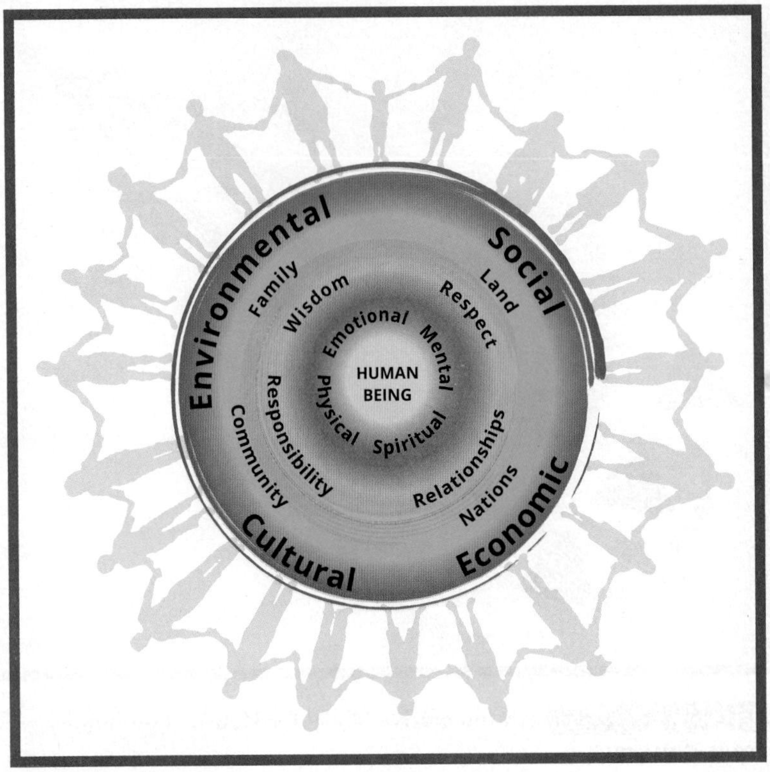

FIGURE   7.6   First Nations Perspective on Health and Wellness Model

Source: First Nations Health Authority of British Columbia (2018).

guidance to practice and research. A brief summary of several grand nursing theories is presented in Table 7.4. Two theories that relate particularly well to community health nursing are examined more closely.

Human Caring Science   In the development of this grand nursing theory, Jean Watson focused on the concept of caring (Watson, 2012). Her work reflects the influences of some non-nursing theories, such as physics, psychology, and education (Falk-Rafael, 2000). Although initially aimed at the relationship between a nurse and an individual, Watson also considers the determinants of health (Watson, 1979), health promotion, and the health of communities (Falk-Rafael, 2000). This theory reflects the socioenvironmental context of community health nursing and recognizes the interdependence of the health of individuals and the health of a community. Watson (2012) describes caring as "a truly life-giving presence of being open and giving from the heart, receptive with respect, compassion, and dignity, creating a trusting relationship that is human-to-human" (p. 45). She describes 10 carative processes reflected by nurses in a caring relationship with clients, including, for example, practising loving kindness, being authentically present, seeking creative solutions, and creating a healing environment (Watson, 2012).

Watson (2012) emphasizes the role of nurses helping individuals to gain more self-caring, self-knowledge,

self-control, and inner healing regardless of their health condition. CHNs working with individuals, families, and communities recognize the importance of such a relationship in the development of prevention and health promotion activities. Without a caring relationship, CHNs would not be invited back into homes to continue working with families; nor would they be identified as valuable and trusted resources in the community.

In the example of Jason, when a CHN follows up with Jason and his family after their encounter in the emergency department, being authentically present and working together with the family to seek mutually agreed-upon and culturally relevant solutions to prevent further injuries could make a difference in the way the family accepts nursing support. Developing a trusting relationship with Jason's family facilitates next steps to begin working with friends and neighbours in the local community to find solutions for safe play areas for children.

Self-Care Deficit Nursing Theory   Another relevant grand theory used in community health nursing practice is Dorothea Orem's (1985) "self-care deficit nursing" theory. Comprising three interrelated theories—theory of self-care, theory of self-care deficit, and theory of nursing systems—the central focus of Orem's work is the self-care needs of individuals and the nurse–client interaction aimed at preserving or improving client self-care. Orem (1985) outlined the need for nursing care

Table 7.4	Grand Nursing Theories Relevant to Community Health Nursing	
Grand Theory	**Key Points**	**Relationship to CHNC (2019, revised) Standards of Practice and Examples from Community Health Nursing Practice**
Roy's adaptation model (Roy, 1987)	This grand nursing theory focuses on the interaction between individuals and their environment. Roy identified four modes of adaptation to achieve health, including physiological, self-concept, role function, and interdependence. The purpose of this theory is to explain how nurses can facilitate the change process toward an individual's intended goals.	In practice, a CHN might work with an older adult person recovering from a hip fracture who wishes to achieve mobility and independent living. The CHN works collaboratively with clients and their families to identify resources and provide support in adapting to a new level of ability. This connects with all of the CHNC standards of practice.
Watson's human caring science (Watson, 1979)	Human caring science is based on 10 carative processes that reflect a deep respect for life and the power of human caring. It recognizes that human-to-human environmental and ecological associations are important, and it values the subjective experiences of both the individual and the nurse and the relationship between them.	This theory reflects the socioenvironmental context of community health nursing and recognizes the interdependence of the health of individuals and the health of a community. CHNs working with families in the perinatal period recognize the importance of their relationship with those families and their connections with the community. Whether working with individuals or families, communities or co-workers, the importance of developing a relationship is an important part of all of the CHNC standards.
Self-care deficit theory of nursing (Orem, 1985)	The self-care model aims to facilitate the client–nurse interaction to preserve the integrity of human beings through self-care by offering 10 self-care actions. The agency and capacity of the client are enhanced by strategies directed at controlling, maintaining, and motivating actions toward self-care. Orem explains the need for nursing as the inability to provide self-care due to situations of personal health.	The importance of the client–nurse interaction is an essential component of each of the eight CHNC standards of practice.
Theory of human becoming (Parse, 2003)	Three principles comprise this theory. The first is that people structure and knowingly choose the meaning of their reality. The second is that people create patterns in their life, which convey meaning and value. The third principle is that people continuously change in life as they engage with and choose from an infinite range of possibilities. Parse's theory of human becoming fits well with the work of CHNs. The ebb and flow of relationships, altered by changing environmental or personal circumstances, make up the fabric of the work CHNs engage in. Understanding and using Parse's approach helps in moving toward desired outcomes from the client's perspective and guides nurses to practise in a wholly respectful way.	Parse's approach is apparent when CHNs use motivational interviewing as an aspect of client-centred care or by engaging in self-reflection after caring for a palliative patient, assessing their own awareness and assumptions that influence the care of the client. Whether working with individuals, families, or communities, an important aspect of community health nursing work is the development of relationships, and this is clearly reflected in each of the eight CCHN standards of practice.

when an individual is unable "to maintain continuously that amount and quality of self-care which is therapeutic in sustaining life and health" (p. 55).

Even though nursing practice guided by Orem's principles is most often directed at individual self-care abilities and deficits, Orem (1985) also considers how nurses provide care for individuals who are part of larger units, such as families, groups, and communities. Consequently, Orem's work has been used to guide community health nursing practice in family nursing (Reutter, 1984; Taylor, 2001) and hospice care (LaFerriere, 1995), and as the basis in developing a community nursing model (Taylor & McLaughlin, 1991).

Reutter (1984) uses Orem's theory of self-care to develop a family assessment guide that is useful for CHNs and explains how "the presuppositions underlying the self-care philosophy have been embraced by community health nursing for years, and indeed are necessary when working with individuals in the area of health promotion (p. 3)." Within this theory, clients are conceptualized as active participants in maintaining health and reaching health goals that are congruent with aims of community health nursing practice. Similarly, within a palliative care home setting, CHNs can find guidance in Orem's theory of self-care deficit, assisting clients and their families to manage care deficits in hopes of enhancing quality of life of those involved (LaFerriere, 1995).

Using this grand theory, a CHN could assist Jason's family to identify their needs and desires in relation to the unsafe debris left on neighbourhood streets. In addition to assisting Jason's family to identify their self-care needs, a CHN could help this family connect with other concerned community members to build capacity and could partner with local agencies to address adequate clean-up of their neighbourhood streets and proper disposal of harmful debris. In this way, the CHN is helping to surface and address the needs of Jason, his family, and the broader community to protect neighbourhood children from unsafe debris on local streets. This theory provides little guidance to intervene at the level of the broader social and political context of Jason and his family.

Middle-Range Theories

Middle-range theories contain a limited number of variables or concepts, are fairly narrow in their scope, and have a lower level of abstraction than either grand theories or conceptual models. These characteristics increase their usability for theory-based practice and research (Peterson, 2009). Middle-range theories not only provide direction for practice, but they are also used to generate testable hypotheses for research. Knowledge generated through middle-range theory development and validation has contributed to the maturation of the larger nursing discipline (Smith, 2003), which, in turn, contributes to more effective practice, enhanced impact, and improved health outcomes for individuals, families, and communities. The generation of more middle-range theories in community health nursing would be helpful in developing the specialty of community health nursing. An outline of several middle-range theories is presented in Table 7.5. Critical caring theory, as one that was developed

specifically for community health nursing in Canada, will be examined more closely.

Critical Caring Theory Critical caring, a middle-range theory, "integrates critical feminist theories into nursing science and builds on previous work that linked caring science and empowered caring to public health nursing practice" (Falk-Rafael, 2005a, p. 47). It transforms the caritas processes, or caring practices described in Jean Watson's (1979) caring science (Falk-Rafael, 2000), a grand nursing theory, into seven carative health promoting processes that "form the 'core' of public health nursing practice and reflect the legacy and reality of public health nursing practice" (Falk-Rafael, 2005a, p. 38). Further, critical caring is proposed as a way of being (ontology), knowing (epistemology), choosing (ethics), and doing (praxis) (Falk-Rafael, 2005a). It is a nursing theory informed by the ethics of caring and social justice and, as such, is considered an appropriate framework to guide nursing actions directed toward taking up the challenge by the Commission on the Social Determinants of Health to "close the gap" in health equity.

Critical caring "root(s) public health nursing practice in an expanded nursing caring science that reincorporates the social justice agenda" (Falk-Rafael, 2005a, p. 38). Falk-Rafael used the metaphor of a tree (practice) anchored by its roots (theory) to describe the reciprocal relationship between theory and practice, where "theory that is nourished by practice is a living and growing entity that provides support for practice while dynamically defining the characteristics and parameters of practice" (p. 39).

The theory illustrates the PHN's caring and social justice moral centre, and how PHNs' practice is informed and guided by it. Practising this way, CHNs are ideally suited to take up the challenge to reduce health inequities through working with others to effect change in the social, cultural, economic, political structures, systems, and policies that create social injustice (Falk-Rafael & Betker, 2012b). Critical caring theory has the potential to be a tool of resistance to counter the forces that limit CHNs from working to their full scope of practice and fulfilling their potential in the challenge to close the health equity gap (Falk-Rafael & Betker, 2012a).

Critical caring was used as a theoretical framework in a doctoral dissertation by Hill (2017) to explore organizational influences on the practice of PHNs with priority perinatal families. The themes identified by PHNs validated the carative health-promoting processes and identified an additional process, that of navigating organizational complexity. This process describes how PHNs manage to continue providing service at individual, community, and systems levels within the ongoing and ever-changing influences of a complex health care organization. Although not always based on resistance to change or moral distress, as described by Falk-Rafael and Betker (2012b), PHNs spoke about the many ways in which they would go the extra mile for their clients and communities in order to achieve better outcomes (Hill, 2017).

The seven carative health promoting processes described by Falk-Rafael help CHNs to consider the knowledge they bring to the situation, the importance of a helping-trusting relationship, and the value of reflexive practice. This theory

Table 7.5	Middle-Range Theories	
Middle Range Theory	**Key Points**	**Relationship to CHNC (2019, revised) Standards of Practice and Examples from Community Health Nursing Practice**
Critical caring theory (Falk-Rafael, 2005a)	Canadian nurse scholar Falk-Rafael identifies seven carative health-promoting processes that reflect the core of public health nursing. This middle-range theory uses a broad definition of client to encompass communities and populations. The carative health-promoting processes include the process of teaching and learning, the creation of supportive and sustainable environments, social justice, building capacity, and honouring local belief systems.	This theory connects with all of the CHNC standards of practice. An example of this is found in the approach taken by PHNs in the Nurse-Family Partnership/Healthy Connections program implemented in BC in 2012, with the goal of developing and maintaining helping and trusting relationships with families at increased need.
Strengths-based theory (Gottlieb & Gottlieb, 2013)	This Canadian approach incorporates thinking about the positives, the things that work well, and what holds potential. It is about finding the balance between focusing on client strengths while at the same time dealing with problems. It is oriented to the individual, family, and community levels of intervention.	This approach is highlighted by CHNC standard 5, capacity building. An example would be CHNs who offer a chronic disease management clinic by providing support and strategies to manage and improve health for adults in low-income housing who have experienced a recent cardiac event.
Relational inquiry (Hartrick Doane & Varcoe, 2005, 2007, 2008)	These Canadian nurse scholars explain how relational practice focuses on the way that personal, interpersonal, and contextual elements shape people's experiences and life situations. This approach considers how capacities and socioenvironmental limitations influence people's health and illness experiences, decision making, and the various ways of managing health and illness. It recognizes that health, illness, and experiences are shaped by social, economic, cultural, family, historical, and geographical contexts as well as by biology, gender, age, and ability.	This theory particularly addresses CHNC standards 4 and 5: professional relationships and capacity building. An example from practice is work that CHNs do with families living in poverty and the importance of developing a trusting and respectful relationship with individuals and families as well as the larger community.

also considers the processes of teaching and learning, the creation of supportive and sustainable environments, building capacity, and honouring local belief systems. Falk-Rafael (2005a) notes that these processes have been identified as the core of community health nursing practice. It is a caring relationship based on these elements that a CHN brings when engaging with members of Jason's community to begin to work together toward positive change. Falk-Rafael (2005b) describes community health nursing practice as being "at that intersection where societal attitudes, government policies, and people's lives meet. Such privilege creates a moral imperative not only to attend to the health needs of the public but also, like Nightingale, to work to change the societal conditions contributing to poor health" (p. 219)—that is, to engage in social justice.

The carative health promoting processes of the critical caring theory identify the importance of developing and maintaining helping-trusting relationships as well as a reflexive approach to caring and at the same time "being open and attending to spiritual-mysterious and existential dimensions" (Falk-Rafael, 2005a, p. 46). These underlying values align with the perspectives of Two-Eyed Seeing and Two-Row Wampum, as well as with the First Nations Health Authority of British Columbia's (2018) Health and Wellness model, which depicts the environmental, social, economic, and cultural values that shape health. Even the first health promoting process of "preparation of self" (Falk-Rafael, 2005a, p. 41) links to the Truth and Reconciliation Commission of Canada's (2012) Call to Action # 26.

CHNs are "leaders of changes to systems in society that support health, and they play key roles in disease, disability and injury prevention, as well as in health promotion" (CPHA, 2010, p. 6). Reducing health inequities and ensuring access to health and health care is clearly within nursing's mandate. Reutter and Kushner (2010) called upon CHNs to take up the challenge to "close the gap" posed by the WHO's Commission on Social Determinants of Health, which demonstrated that "social injustice is killing people on a grand scale" (WHO Commission on Social Determinants of Health, 2008, p. 26). Reutter and Kushner further advocated for PHNs to use a "critical caring approach" to guide their work of promoting health equity. Using this nursing theory as a guide, CHNs will be better able to understand the social, political, economic, and historical context of health inequities; provide sensitive empowering care through informed action; and work to change the underlying social conditions that result in and perpetuate health inequities (Reutter & Kushner, 2010).

Practice or Substantive Theories in Nursing

Practice or substantive theories in nursing are the least complex, contain fewer concepts, and refer to specific, well-defined phenomena. Practice theories tend to be prescriptive and thus provide direction for practice (McEwen, 2011). For example, Funk, Stajduhar, and Purkis (2011) developed a practice theory that considers the relationship between home health nurses and families when providing end-of-life care. A number of Canadian substantive theories that provide guidance and direction for some specific areas of community health nursing are presented in Table 7.6. This table provides information about the nature of these substantive theories, some practice examples to illustrate them, and their links to the CHNC (2019, revised) standards of practice. One substantive theory is highlighted.

Table 7.6 Practice or Substantive Theories

Practice Theory	Key Points	Relationship to CHNC (2019, revised) Standards of Practice and Examples from Community Health Nursing Practice
Theory of maternal engagement with PHNs and family visitors (Jack et al., 2005)	This grounded theory, developed by Canadian nurses and epidemiology researchers, describes the process by which mothers identified as being at risk of poor parenting practices engage with PHNs. This theory helps PHNs to identify client anxieties and perceptions related to the provision of home visits. It highlights the importance of the development of a trusting relationship between mothers and the PHNs.	CHNC standards 4 and 5 are particularly relevant to this theory. Home visits are a key strategy for PHNs in providing support for parents of young children. To increase the effectiveness of home visiting and to establish a relationship, it is essential for nurses to engage in a process of building trust, seeking mutuality, and understanding the perspectives of mothers.
Supportive care model (Davies & Oberle, 1990)	This Canadian model of support in palliative nursing considers six dimensions of nursing care: valuing, maintaining integrity, connecting, empowering, doing for, and finding meaning. This model focuses on community health nursing practice at the individual and family levels.	This model aligns well with CHNC standard 3, health maintenance, restoration, and palliation; with standard 4, professional relationships; and with standard 5, building capacity. The palliative care work that home health nurses do involves individuals as well as their families.
Theory of hope (Duggleby & Wright, 2005)	This Canadian theory describes the process through which palliative patients live with hope and acknowledge life as it is. This theory discusses how health status can be assessed and mutual plans developed among nurse, client, and family in order to maximize the abilities of the individual and family within the context of the community.	Home health nurses working with patients requiring palliative care consider how individuals and families endure and cope with suffering. This model aligns with CHNC standard 3, health maintenance, restoration, and palliation; standard 4, professional relationships; and standard 5, building capacity.
Model of family caregiver relationships with home health providers (Funk , Stajduhar, & Purkis, 2011, 2013)	This Canadian model considers the relationship between home health nurses and families, particularly during end-of-life experiences, and looks at ways to enhance those relationships and the satisfaction with those services.	This model is particularly relevant to home health nurses in their work with palliative patients, and it connects directly to CHNC standard 3, health maintenance, restoration, and palliation.

A Theory of Maternal Engagement with Public Health Nurses and Family Visitors This grounded theory was developed by a group of Canadian nurses and epidemiology researchers (Jack, DiCenso, & Lohfield, 2005). They describe the process by which mothers identified as being at risk of poor parenting practices engage with PHNs. This theory helps PHNs identify client perceptions about the provision of home visits and highlights the importance of developing a trusting relationship between mothers and PHNs. Mothers often cope with feelings of vulnerability and powerlessness during the initial phase of engagement with an unfamiliar nurse working to protect their families and limit their vulnerability. This involves moving through the phases of *overcoming fear*, *building trust*, and *seeking mutuality*. To increase the effectiveness of home visiting and to establish a connected relationship, this theory guides the CHN to understand and assimilate the perspectives of mothers as they move through the previous three phases in establishing a relationship.

Limitations of Current Nursing Theories While acknowledging the importance of these theories to the development of nursing, we can point out certain limitations for community health nursing from critical, feminist, intersectional, and Indigenous perspectives. For example, there is a lack of social justice and equity focus in many of the main grand nursing theories, which makes them limited for use in community health nursing. In addition, some grand theories focus more on individuals and not on the broader community or systems levels of practice. Orem's (1985) theory, for instance, is about self-care and is very individual focused, as is Parse's (2003) theory of human becoming. Although most nursing theories have not explicitly included Indigenous perspectives or focused on Indigenous peoples, there are some parallels between several nursing theories and Indigenous perspectives. For example, Watson's (1979) human caring science and Falk-Rafael's (2005a) critical caring theories stress the importance of relationships, the connections with community, and upstream thinking by recognizing the value of sustainable environments. Falk-Rafael's (2005a) critical caring theory reflects the importance of honouring local belief systems; however, many nursing theories do not take into consideration history, culture, or past experience to a sufficient degree. By overlooking these differences, we assume shared understanding where this may not be the case.

Public Health and Other Social Science Theories There is a wide range of public health and other social science theories that have relevance for community health nursing, such as epidemiology, communications, leadership, management, and learning. One public health theory that is an important foundation for understanding population health is the ecosocial theory. In an attempt to move beyond the limitations of the web of causation, Nancy Krieger (1994) developed the ecosocial theory, which goes beyond an individualistic focus to better understand the social influences of health and disease. Based on the question of "who and what drives current and changing patterns of social inequalities in health" (p. 672), the ecosocial theory helps us to think critically and systematically

CASE STUDY
A Story about Care

This is a palliative and end-of-life care story illustrative of home health nursing. Please watch the video entitled *A Story about Care* on YouTube. In this vignette Jim Mulcahy shares his experience with end-stage lymphoma and that of his wife, Sarah, who is living with Huntington's disease. He talks about how meaningful a simple and genuine touch is. Jim's story demonstrates the power of a caring relationship with health care providers who can see the person and not merely the disease. After viewing this video, consider how a CHN working with home health could relate to the individuals and families with whom she or he works and see people holistically as complex individuals who have a life outside and apart from their medical history.

Canadian nurse scholars Betty Davies and Kathy Oberle developed the supportive care model for palliative nursing that consists of six central dimensions of nursing care (Davies & Oberle, 1990). The first of these dimensions is valuing or the attitude that a nurse brings toward the person she or he is caring for. The second dimension is maintaining integrity of the nurse in terms of psychological, moral, and emotional well-being. Following that is connecting, which relates to establishing a relationship. Empowering involves helping people to identify and develop their inner strength to do what they need or would like to do. "Doing for" comprises the physical care provided to individuals. And finally, finding meaning involves making personal sense of what is happening or has happened. This enables CHNs to feel that they are doing the best they can to contribute to the healing of a patient.

In the same vein, Duggleby and Wright (2005) offer a theory of hope related to older adult palliative patients—how they endure and cope with suffering. This theory describes the process through which these patients live with hope and acknowledge life as it is. Both models align with CHNC standard 3, health maintenance, restoration, and palliation, and with standard 4 regarding professional relationships (CHNC, 2011, revised). These theories reflect the way in which health status can be assessed and mutual plans developed among nurse, client, and family that maximize the abilities of the individual and family within the context of the community. Core community health nursing concepts that are significant in this case study and in the supportive care model include caring, a strengths-based approach, hope, well-being, relationships, and empowerment.

A broad theoretical perspective that is reflected in this example is social ecological theory, in that the nurse needs to consider the multiple influences at play that have an impact on the health and well-being of patients and their families.

As health care has changed, greater focus has been placed on tasks, doing of procedures, and "doing for" clients even in the home setting. However, this model urges nurses to maintain a focus of care on people as whole persons and not solely on procedures and administrative aspects of care. With that being said, there are challenges that could confront a home health nurse, including a heavy caseload, time constraints, or other unexpected events. However, a key aspect of promoting health is the development of a therapeutic relationship throughout the course of care.

Discussion Questions

1. How would you ensure you are prepared to develop a relationship with a palliative patient?

2. In addition to providing direct care to Jim, how would you support the family?

3. How will you support Jim to live with hope, recognizing that you have limited time to spend given your heavy caseload?

about multiple connections between the social and biological production of disease and health inequities (Krieger, 2001).

As discussed previously, CHNs often use theories from other disciplines to inform their practice; for example, the stages of change (Prochaska, DiClemente, & Norcross, 1992). This theory considers the various stages of change that individuals progress through, such as precontemplation, contemplation, determination, action, and maintenance, in dealing with addictive or other problem behaviours (Prochaska et al., 1992). For example, in Jason's situation, if his parents smoked cigarettes and recognized that their addiction to smoking not only affects the health of their family but also places an additional economic strain on the household. They may have tried unsuccessfully to quit in the past, but using this approach, the CHN may help them to anticipate and work through the challenges of quitting.

The theory of diffusion of innovation by Rogers (2002) has also been used by CHNs in assisting community members to take up new approaches. This theory is described as "the process through which an innovation, defined as an idea perceived as new, spreads via certain communication channels over time among the members of a social system" (Rogers, 2004, p. 13). In an effort to improve the availability of fresh fruits and vegetables in Jason's impoverished neighbourhood, a CHN might facilitate the establishment of a "good food box" system in the hope that it would benefit not only Jason's family but many other families in the area as well. CHNC standards (CHNC, 2019, revised) relating to health promotion and health maintenance reflect both of these social science theories.

These are a few examples of the many different theories from the public health and social sciences that may be useful for CHNs to consider in their day-to-day practice. See the last section of Table 7.1 for a long but not exhaustive list of theories from other disciplines.

YES, BUT WHY?

Social Determinants of Breastfeeding

What?

There are many health benefits for both mother and infant with exclusive breastfeeding for the first six months of life (WHO, 2018). Compared to formula, breastfeeding is the least expensive option (Leon-Cava, Lutter, Ross, & Martine, 2002), saving an estimated $1500 annually for families as well as indirect savings from fewer days of lost work with sick children (Association of Women's Health, Obstetric, & Neonatal Nurses, 2015). However, although most mothers can breastfeed successfully with accurate information and support from family, health care providers, and the larger community, breastfeeding is not without its challenges (WHO, n.d.). Research by Renfrew et al. found that "infant feeding is strongly related to inequalities in health, and far from being an individual decision made by each woman, is influenced most strongly by structural determinants of health" (Renfrew, McCormick, Wade, Quinn, & Dowswell, 2012, p. 3), such as social acceptance, lay and professional support, and public policy. Social and economic conditions are known to affect the health of families and children, increasing the risk of poor mental and physical health outcomes for families living in disadvantaged conditions. Inequalities lead to health disparities between neighbourhoods and populations. When these differences are avoidable, unfair, and systematic (National Collaborating Centre for Determinants of Health, 2013), they are considered inequities and require intervention at multiple levels.

So What?

The WHO has identified breastfeeding as the best way to provide infants with the nutrients they require for healthy growth and development (WHO, n.d.). For as long as humans have existed, they have depended on breast milk to survive. However, by the 1940s global breastfeeding rates declined when the use of breastmilk substitutes became popular, aided by aggressive marketing by formula companies (Stevens, Patrick, & Pickler, 2009). Although rates of breastfeeding have improved over the past few decades, challenges continue to negatively impact the practice of breastfeeding (Stevens et al., 2009), some of which stem from policy decisions. For example, consider the recent U.S. official opposition to a breastfeeding resolution at the May 2018 United Nations–affiliated World Health Assembly (Jacobs, 2018). They opposed the use of a language requiring governments to "protect, promote, and support breast-feeding."

Now What?

CHNs play an important role in supporting breastfeeding at different levels. Using critical caring theory (Falk-Rafael, 2005a; Falk-Rafael & Betker, 2012b, 2012a), CHNs recognize the sociopolitical context that influences the infant feeding decisions individuals, families, and communities make.

Effectively addressing these issues upstream requires CHNs to be politically savvy. CHNs also need to understand that a trusting relationship with individual women, families, and communities is foundational to effective practice. Clinical expertise about breastfeeding, knowledge of community supports and resources, a transpersonal teaching approach, development of supportive environments within the community and the health care organization, building community capacity, and respecting local belief systems all reflect the roles CHNs play to support breastfeeding (Falk-Rafael & Betker, 2012b). For CHNs this means understanding the science behind breastfeeding, assisting individual women, collaborating with local partners, and helping to shift community and organizational attitudes to support breastfeeding.

Standards of Practice Fulfilled:

#1 Health Promotion
- Considers the determinants of health, the social and political context, and systemic structures in collaboration with the client to determine action.

#6 Health Equity
- Advocates for healthy public policy and social justice by participating in legislative and policy-making activities that influence determinants of health and access to services (CHNC, 2019, revised).

CONCLUSION

In this chapter the importance of theory in guiding community health nursing practice and research is emphasized. There has been limited development of theories, however, that are specific to the phenomena that concern CHNs. Clearly, more theory development is needed so that the work of CHNs at the community and population levels is informed by theories that explicitly reflect our concerns and do not have to be adapted from theories developed in an illness context for the care of individuals. At the same time, while there are few community health nursing theories per se, there has been a considerable amount of theoretical development in community health nursing that reflects a broad synthesis of knowledge from the public health sciences, social sciences, and nursing. This development was illustrated in an organizing framework that drew on the CHNC professional practice model graphic (theoretical foundations).

Drawing on nursing's metaparadigm, CHNs have developed a unique metaparadigm that defines the concepts in ways that reflect their phenomena of concern, explains the levels of practice, and places social justice at the core. CHNs' work has been informed for many years by theoretical perspectives such as social ecological theory, feminism, and critical social theory, and more recently by emerging perspectives such as complexity science, postcolonial theory, and intersectionality. CHNs have also developed a range of models and frameworks to guide research and practice that (a) draw from the core theoretical concepts of community health nursing, (b) reflect CHNs' values base, (c) direct action at the multiple levels of intervention for CHNs, ranging from the individual to society, and (d) encompass the full range of community health nursing competencies across the continuum of care, including health promotion, disease prevention, health maintenance and restoration, and palliation.

Through Jason's story, it is evident that the core concepts of community health nursing and the kinds of actions that might be taken to address community health issues are related and interconnected as well as common to all the theoretical perspectives, models, frameworks, and theories discussed in this chapter. Jason's story demonstrates how the living conditions in which people are born, live, and play influence their health and increase the chances of preventable injury. These unfair and avoidable circumstances are commonly referred to as the social determinants of health, where an imbalance of money, resources, opportunity, and power result in health inequities between people in society. Actions to address these conditions that ensure access to health (versus access to health care) take place at multiple levels, and CHNs work at all of these levels. CHNs do not work solely with individuals to help them address the problems they encounter after they occur, but they work upstream to prevent them from occurring—not only for the individuals concerned but also for the communities of which they are members. CHNs collaborate and work with families, communities, and populations as well as at the political level to build capacity for people to take action on improving their own health, advocating for the determinants of health in order to promote equity and social justice.

Finally, community health nursing has a very broad scope of practice, and the values and principles underlying community health nursing practice require a diverse and extensive knowledge base grounded in theory, research, and practical experience, all of which are intimately interconnected. Theory informs the conduct of community health nursing research, which produces the evidence used to guide the practice of CHNs in educational, administrative, and practitioner roles. At the same time, in an iterative fashion, research and the practical experience of nurses working in diverse community roles and settings contribute to the development of community health nursing.

KEY TERMS

beliefs   (p. 111)
concepts   (p. 103)
conceptual frameworks   (p. 102)
conceptual models   (p. 102)
ethics   (p. 111)
grand theories   (p. 121)
health equity   (p. 104)
informal theories   (p. 103)
knowledge   (p. 102)
levels of practice   (p. 108)
metaparadigm   (p. 104)
middle-range theory   (p. 111)
nursing theory   (p. 103)
patterns of knowing   (p. 103)

STUDY QUESTIONS

1. Which of the following elements make up the community health nursing metaparadigm?

   a. Health, healing, person, environment, and nursing

   b. Person, environment, nursing, health, and social justice

   c. Person, health, nursing, and environment

   d. Communities, nursing, prevention, equity, and environment

2. Which of the following components contribute to the theoretical foundations of community health nursing?

   a. Determinants of health, prevention, health inequities

   b. Practical experience, research

   c. Grand nursing theories

   d. Social ecological theory, feminist theory, complexity theory

   e. Values, beliefs, and ethics

   f. All of the above

3. How are theory, research, and practice integrated?

4. What key concepts in community health nursing practice are drawn from public health?

5. Why is the individual-based approach to community health nursing so widespread? How is the individual-based approach to health promoted in current theories?

INDIVIDUAL CRITICAL-THINKING EXERCISES

1. The Canadian Public Health Association (CPHA, 2010) states that "the public/CHN combines knowledge from public health science, primary health care (including the determinants of health), nursing science, and the social sciences" (p. 8). Given this statement, what aspects of nursing science do nurses bring to the practice of community or public health nursing?

2. In order to enhance cultural safety, it is important for health care providers to reflect on and consider their own values, beliefs, and biases. Reflect on the influences in your life that might shape your approach to client care.

3. Some nurses believe that theory is not relevant to nursing practice. What do you think about this statement, and why? What factors contribute to this belief about the relevance of theory to practice?

4. What kind of theory might you use as a CHN working with a family with multiple health problems? What would support you in the use of that theory?

5. When a PHN provides immunizations to an individual, how does this contribute to population health? What is one conceptual model that helps to explain this?

GROUP CRITICAL-THINKING EXERCISES

1. Some portions of the population tend to experience greater health inequities than others; for example, First Nation populations or families living in poverty. Discuss with your group how a postcolonial perspective might help you to view this situation differently.

2. Discuss how a social ecological view might influence health promotion activities related to improving childhood immunization rates in a small community.

3. Using critical social theory, brainstorm and then discuss strategies you would use to address Jason's situation. How would you go about advocating for policies that would help to address preventable injuries in Jason's community (i.e., what would be your first steps)?

REFERENCES

Ajzen, I. (1991). The theory of planned behavior. *Organizational Behavior and Human Decision Processes, 50*, 179–211.

Albrecht, M. N. (1990). The Albrecht model for home health care: Implications for research, practice, and education. *Public Health Nursing, 7*(2), 118–126.

Allen, D. G. (1985). Nursing research and social control: Alternative models of science that emphasize understanding and emancipation. *Image: The Journal of Nursing Scholarship, 17*(2), 58–64.

Anderson, R. A., Crabtree, B. E., Steele, D. J., McDaniel, J., & Reuben, R. (2005). Case study research: The view from complexity science. *Qualitative Health Research, 15*(5), 669–685.

Argyris, C., & Schön, D. (1974). *Theory in practice: Increasing professional effectiveness.* San Francisco, CA: Jossey-Bass.

Association of Community Health Nursing Educators. (2010). Research priorities for public health nursing. *Public Health Nursing, 27*(1), 94–100.

Association of Women's Health, Obstetric, & Neonatal Nurses. (2015). Breastfeeding: AWHONN position statement. *Journal of Obstetric Gynecologic and Neonatal Nursing, 44*(1), 83–88.

Bandura, A. (1977). Self-efficacy: Toward a unifying theory of behavioral change. *Psychological Review, 84*(2), 191–215.

Bartlett, C., Marshall, M., & Marshall, A. (2012). Two-eyed seeing and other lessons learned within a co-learning journey of bringing together indigenous and mainstream knowledges and ways of knowing. *Journal of Environmental Studies and Sciences, 2*(4), 331–340.

Baylis, F., Kenny, N., & Sherwin, S. (2008). A relational account of public health ethics. *Public Health Ethics, 1*(3), 196–209.

Bigbee, J. L., & Issel, M. (2012). Conceptual models for population focused public health nursing interventions and outcomes: State of the art. *Public Health Nursing, 29*(4), 370–379.

Bohensky, E. L., Butler, J. R. A., & Davies, J. (2013). Integrating Indigenous ecological knowledge and science in natural resource management: Perspectives from Australia. *Ecology & Society, 18*(3), 20. http://dx.doi.org/10.5751/ES-05846-180320

Bourque Bearskin, R. L. (2011). A critical lens on culture in nursing practice. *Nursing Ethics, 18*(4), 548–559.

Bowlby, J. (1969). *Attachment and loss: Vol. 1 Attachment.* New York, NY: Basic Books.

Bowleg, L. (2012). The problem with the phrase "women and minorities": Intersectionality—an important theoretical framework for public health. *American Journal of Public Health, 102*(7), 1267–1273.

Bronfenbrenner, U. (1979). *The ecology of human development: Experiments by nature and design.* Cambridge, MA: Harvard University Press.

Browne, A. J., Varcoe, C. M., Wong, S. T., Smye, V. L., Lavoie, J., Littlejohn, D., . . . Lennox, S. (2012). Closing the health equity gap: Evidence-based strategies for primary health care organizations. *International Journal for Equity in Health, 11*(59), 1–15.

Browne, A. J. (2001). The influence of liberal political ideology on nursing science. *Nursing Inquiry, 8*(2), 118–129.

Browne, A. J. (2004). Response to critique of "The influence of liberal political ideology on nursing science." *Nursing Inquiry, 11*(2), 122–123.

Browne, A. J., Smye, V. L., & Varcoe, C. (2005). The relevance of postcolonial theoretical perspectives to research in Aboriginal health. *Canadian Journal of Nursing Research, 27*(4), 16–37.

Butterfield, P. G. (1990). Thinking upstream: Nursing a conceptual understanding of the societal context of health behavior. *Advances in Nursing Science, 12*(2), 1–8.

Butterfield, P., & Postma, J. (2009). The TERRA framework: Conceptualizing rural environmental health inequities through an environmental justice lens. *Advances in Nursing Science, 32*(2), 107–117.

Byrne, D., & Callaghan, G. (2014). *Complexity theory and the social sciences: The state of the art.* New York, NY: Routledge.

Canadian Nurses Association (CNA). (2006). *Social justice . . . a means to an end, an end in itself.* Ottawa, ON: Author.

Canadian Nurses Association (CNA). (2008). *Code of ethics for registered nurses.* Ottawa, ON: Author.

Canadian Nurses Association (CNA). (2017). *Code of ethics for registered nurses.* Ottawa, ON: Author.

Canadian Public Health Association. (2010). *Public health—Community health nursing practice in Canada: Roles and activities.* Ottawa, ON: Author. Retrieved from http://www.cpha.ca/uploads/pubs/3-1bk04214.pdf

Capra, F. (1996). *The web of life: A new synthesis of mind and matter.* London, UK: HarperCollins.

Castellani, B., & Hafferty, F. W. (2009). *Sociology and complexity science: A new field of inquiry.* Berlin, Germany: Springer.

Carper, B. (1978). Fundamental patterns of knowing in nursing, *Advances in Nursing Science, 1*(1), 13–23.

Chinn, P. L., & Kramer, M. K. (2008). *Integrated theory and knowledge development in nursing* (7th ed.). St. Louis, MO: Elsevier, Mosby.

Chinn, P. L., & Kramer, M. K. (2011). *Integrated theory and knowledge development in nursing.* (8th ed.). St. Louis, MO: Elsevier, Mosby.

Chopoorian, T. J. (1986). Reconceptualizing the environment. In P. Moccia (Ed.), *New approaches to theory development.* New York, NY: National League for Nursing.

Cilliers, P. (1998). *Complexity and postmodernism: Understanding complex systems.* London, UK: Routledge.

Clark, M. J. (1999). *Nursing in the community: Dimensions of community health nursing.* Stamford, CT: Appleton & Lange.

Clarke, P. N. (1998). Nursing theory as a guide for inquiry in family and community nursing. *Nursing Science Quarterly, 11*(12), 47–48.

Cohen, B., & Reutter, L. (2007). Development of the role of public health nurses in addressing child and family poverty: A framework for action. *Journal of Advanced Nursing, 60*(1), 96–107.

Community Health Nurses of Canada (CHNC). (2008). *Canadian community health nursing standards of practice.* Toronto, ON: Author.

Community Health Nurses of Canada (CHNC). (Ed.). (2009). *Public health nursing discipline specific competencies.* Toronto, ON: Author.

Community Health Nurses of Canada (CHNC). (2019, revised). *Canadian community health nursing: Professional practice model & standards of practice.* St. John's, NL: Author. Retrieved from https://www.chnc.ca/documents/CHNC-ProfessionalPracticeModel-EN/index.html

Community Health Nurses of Canada (CHNC). (2013). *Canadian community health nursing professional practice model.* Toronto, ON: Author.

Corbin, J., & Tomm Bonde, L. (2012). Intersections of context and HIV/AIDS in sub-Saharan Africa: What can we learn from feminist theory? *Perspectives in Public Health, 132*(8), 8–9.

Cusack, C., Cohen, B., Mignone, J., Chartier, M. J., & Lutfiyya, Z. (2017). Reorienting public health nurses' practice with a professional practice model. *Canadian Journal of Nursing Research, 49*(1), 16–27.

Dalton, J. M. (2003). Development and testing of the theory of collaborative decision-making in nursing practice for triads. *Journal of Advanced Nursing, 41*(1), 22–33.

Davidson, A. W., Ray, M. A., & Turkel, M. C. (Eds.). (2011). *Nursing, caring, and complexity science: For human-environment well-being.* New York, NY: Springer Publishing Co.

Davies, B., & Oberle, K. (1990). Dimensions of the supportive role of the nurse in palliative care. *Oncology Nursing Forum, 17*(1), 87–94.

Dudgeon, R. C., & Berkes, F. (2003). Local understandings of the land: Traditional ecological knowledge and indigenous knowledge. In H. Selin (Ed.), *Nature across cultures: Views of nature and the environment in non-western cultures* (pp. 75–96). Great Britain: Khllver Academic Publishers.

Duggleby, W., & Wright, K. (2005). Transforming hope: How elderly palliative patients live with hope. *Canadian Journal of Nursing Research, 37*(2), 70–84.

Duggleby, W., Wright, K., Williams, A., Degner, L., Cammer, A., & Holtslander, L. (2007). Developing a living with hope program for caregivers of family members with advanced cancer. *Journal of Palliative Care, 23*(1), 24–31.

Edwards, N., Mill, J., & Kothari, A. (2004). Multiple intervention research program in community health. *Canadian Journal of Nursing Research, 36*(1), 40–55.

Elder, G. H. (1996). Human lives in changing societies. In R. B. Cairns, G. H. Elder, & E. J. Costello (Eds.), *Developmental science* (pp. 31–62). Melbourne, Australia: Cambridge University Press.

Falk-Rafael, A. R. (2000). Watson's philosophy, science, and theory of human caring as a conceptual framework for guiding community health nursing practice. *Advances in Nursing Science, 23*(2), 34–49.

Falk-Rafael, A. R. (2005a). Advancing nursing theory through theory-guided practice: The emergence of a critical caring perspective. *Advances in Nursing Science, 28*(1), 38–49.

Falk-Rafael, A. R. (2005b). Speaking truth to power: Nursing's legacy and moral imperative. *Advances in Nursing Science, 28*(3), 212–223.

Falk-Rafael, A. R., & Betker, C. (2012a). The primacy of relationships: A study of public health nursing practice from a critical caring perspective. *Advances in Nursing Science, 35*(4), 315–332.

Falk-Rafael, A. R., & Betker, C. (2012b). Witnessing social injustice downstream and advocating for health equity upstream: "The trombone slide" of nursing. *Advances in Nursing Science, 35*(2), 98–112.

Fawcett, J., & DeSanto-Madeya, S. (2013). *Contemporary nursing knowledge: Analysis and evaluation of nursing models and theories* (3rd ed.). Philadelphia, PA: F. A. Davis Co.

Ferketich, A. L., Phillips, L. R., & Verran, J. A. (1990). *Comprehensive multi-level nursing model for rural Hispanics.* (Agency for Health Care Policy and Research Grant HSO 6801-01). Bethesda, MD: Agency for Health Care Policy and Research.

First Nations Health Authority of British Columbia. (2018). *First Nations perspective on health and wellness.* Retrieved from http://www.fnha.ca

Flaskerud, J., & Winslow, B. (1998). Conceptualizing vulnerable populations health related research. *Nursing Research, 47*(2), 69–78.

Funk, L.M, Stajduhar K.I, & Purkis, M.E. (2011). An exploration of empowerment discourse within home-care nurses' accounts of practice. *Nursing Inquiry, 18*(1):66-76. doi: 10.1111/j.1440-1800.2010.00502.x.

Funk, L. & Stajduhar, K. (2013). Analysis and proposed model of family caregivers' relationships with home health providers and perceptions of the quality of formal services. *Journal of Applied Gerontology, 32*(2):188-206. doi: 10.1177/0733464811408699.

Gambino, M. (2008). Complexity and nursing theory: A seismic shift. In C. Lindberg, S. Nash, & C. Lindberg (Eds.), *On the edge: Nursing in the age of complexity* (pp. 49–72). Bordentown, NJ: PlexusPress.

Gottlieb, L. N., & Gottlieb, B. (2013). *Strengths-based nursing care: Health and healing for person and family.* New York, NY: Springer Publishing Company.

Gottlieb, L., & Rowat, K. (1987). The McGill model of nursing. *Advances in Nursing Science, 9*(4), 51–61.

Government of Canada. (1985). *Canada Health Act.* Retrieved from http://laws-lois.justice.gc.ca/eng/acts/C-6

Green, R. (2013). Application of the self-care deficit nursing theory: The community context. *Self-Care, Dependent-Care and Nursing, 20*(1), 5–15.

Hamilton, N., & Bhatti, T. (1996). *Population health promotion: An integrated model of population health and health promotion.* Ottawa, ON: Public Health Agency of Canada.

Hamilton, P. A., & Bush, H. A. (1988). Theory development in community health nursing: Issues and recommendations. *Scholarly Inquiry for Nursing Practice, 2*(2), 145–160.

Hartrick Doane, G., & Varcoe, C. (2005). *Family nursing as relational inquiry: Developing health-promoting practice.* Philadelphia, PA: Lippincott Williams & Wilkins.

Hartrick Doane, G., & Varcoe, C. (2007). Relational practice and nursing obligations. *Advances in Nursing Science, 30*(3), 192–205.

Hartrick Doane, G., & Varcoe, C. (2008). Knowledge translation in everyday nursing: From evidence-based to inquiry-based practice. *Advances in Nursing Science, 31*(4), 283–295.

Held, D. (1980). *Introduction to critical theory: Horkheimer to Habermas.* Berkeley, CA: University of California Press.

Helvie, C. O. (1981). *Community health nursing: Theory and practice.* New York, NY: Harper & Row.

Henderson, V. (1966). *The nature of nursing: A definition and its implications for practice, research, and education.* New York, NY: McMillan.

Henry, B. R., Houston, S., & Mooney, G. (2004). Institutional racism in Australia. *Medical Journal of Australia, 180*(10), 517–520.

Hill, M. E. (2017). Public health nursing: What difference does it make for priority perinatal women? (Doctoral dissertation, University of Victoria, 2017). *Dissertation Abstracts.* Retrieved from https://dspace.library.uvic.ca/handle/1828/8475

hooks, b. (2000). *Feminist theory: From margin to center* (2nd ed.). London, UK: Pluto Press.

Jacobs, A. (2018, July 8). Opposition to breast-feeding resolution by U.S. stuns World Health officials. *The New York Times.* Retrieved from https://www.nytimes.com/2018/07/08/health/world-health-breastfeeding-ecuador-trump.html

Jack, S. K., DiCenso, A., & Lohfeld, L. (2005). A theory of maternal engagement with public health nurses and family visitors. *Journal of Advanced Nursing, 49*(2), 182–190.

Keefer, T. (2014). A short introduction to the two-row wampum. *Briarpatch,* 14–15.

Keller, L. O., & Strohschein, S. (2012). Population-based public health nursing practice: The intervention wheel. In M. Stanhope & J. Lancaster (Eds.), *Public health nursing: Population-centered health care in the community* (8th ed., pp. 186–215). Maryland Heights, MO: Elsevier.

Keller, L. O., Strohschein, S., & Schaffer, M. A. (2011). Cornerstones of public health nursing. *Public Health Nursing, 28*(3), 249–260.

Keller, L. O., Strohschein, S., Lia-Hoagberg, B., & Schaffer, M. (1998). Population-based public health nursing interventions: A model from practice. *Public Health Nursing, 15*(3), 207–215.

Keller, L. O., Strohschein, S., Lia-Hoagberg, B., & Schaffer, M. (2004a). Population-based public health interventions:

Practice-based and evidence supported. Part 1. *Public Health Nursing, 21*(5), 453–468.

Keller, L. O., Strohschein, S., Schaffer, M., & Lia-Hoagberg, B. (2004b). Population-based public health interventions: Innovation in practice, teaching and management. Part II. *Public Health Nursing, 21*(5), 469–487.

Keller, L. O., Strohschein, S., & Briske, L. (2012). Population-based public health nursing practice: The intervention wheel. In M. Stanhope & J. Lancaster (Eds.), *Public health nursing—Revised reprint: Population-centered health care in the community* (8th ed.). Maryland Heights, MO: Elsevier.

Kent, A., Loppie, C., Carriere, J., MacDonald, M., & Pauly, B. (2017). Xpey' relational environments: An analytic framework for conceptualizing Indigenous health equity. *Health Promotion and Chronic Disease in Canada, 37*(12), 273–280.

King, I. M. (1981). *A theory for nursing: Systems, concepts, process.* New York, NY: Wiley & Sons.

Kleffel, D. (1991). Rethinking the environment as a domain of nursing knowledge. *Advances in Nursing Science, 14*(1), 40–51.

Kleffel, D. (1996). Environmental paradigms: Moving toward an ecocentric perspective. *Advances in Nursing Science, 18*(4), 1–10.

Knowles, M. S. (1978). Andragology: Adult learning theory in perspective. *Community College Review, 5*(3), 9–20.

Koh, H. K., Brach, C., Harris, L. M., & Parchman, M. L. (2013). A proposed "health literate care model" would constitute a systems approach to improving patients' engagement in care. *Health Affairs, 32*(2), 357–367.

Kretzmann, J. P., & McKnight, J. L. (1993). *Building communities from the inside out: A path toward finding and mobilizing a community's assets.* Chicago, IL: ACTA Publications.

Krieger, N. (1994). Epidemiology and the web of causation: Has anyone seen the spider. *Social Science & Medicine, 39*(7), 887–903.

Krieger, N. (2001). Theories for social epidemiology in the 21st century: An ecosocial perspective. *International Journal of Epidemiology, 30*(4), 668–677.

Kuehnert, P. L. (1995). The interactive and organizational model of community as client: A model for public health nursing practice. *Public Health Nursing, 12*(1), 9–17.

Kulbok, P. A., Laffrey, S. C., & Chitthathairatt, S. (2008). Integrating muiltilevel approaches to promote community health. In M. Stanhope & J. Lancaster (Eds.), *Public health nursing: Population-centered health care in the community* (7th ed.). St. Louis, MO: Mosby Elsevier.

Kulig, J. (2000). Community resiliency: The potential for the development of community health nursing theory. *Public Health Nursing, 17*(5), 374–385.

Kuss, T., Proulz-Girouard, L., Lovitt, S., Katz, C. B., & Kennelly, P. (1997). A public health nursing model. *Public Health Nursing, 14*(2), 81–91.

Labonte, R. (1993). Health promotion and empowerment: Practice frameworks. *Centre for Health Promotion, HP-10-0102.*

Laferriere, R. H. (1995). Orem's theory in practice: Hospice nursing care. *Home Healthcare Nurse, 13*(5), 50–54.

Laffrey, S. C., & Craig, D. M. (1995). Health promotion for communities and aggregates: An integrated model. In M. Stewart (Ed.), *Community nursing: Promoting Canadians' health* (pp. 125–145). Toronto, ON: W. B. Saunders.

Laffrey, S. C., & Craig, D. M. (2000). Health promotion for communities and aggregates: An integrative model. In M. Stewart (Ed.), *Community nursing: Promoting Canadians' health* (pp. 105–125). Toronto, ON: W. B. Saunders.

Laffrey, S. C., & Kulbok, P. A. (1999). An integrative model for holistic community health nursing. *Journal of Holistic Nursing, 17*(1), 88–103.

Last, J. M. (Ed.). (2007). *A dictionary of public health.* New York, NY: Oxford University Press.

Leininger, M. (Ed.). (1978). *Transcultural nursing: Concepts, theories, and practice.* New York, NY: John Wiley & Sons.

Leipert, B. D. (2001). Feminism and public health nursing: Partners for health. *Scholarly Inquiry for Nursing Practice, 15*(1), 49–62.

Leon-Cava, N., Lutter, S., Ross, J., & Martin, L. (2002). *Quantifying the benefits of breastfeeding: A summary of the evidence.* Washington, D.C: Pan American Health Organization.

Levy, B. S., & Sidel, V. W. (2006). The nature of social injustice and its impact on public health. In B. S. Levy & V. W. Sidel (Eds.), *Social injustice and public health* (pp. 5–24). New York, NY: Oxford University Press.

Lewin, K. (1951). *Field theory in social science: Selected theoretical papers by Kurt Lewin.* D. Cartwright (Ed.). Oxford, UK: Harpers.

Lindeman, E. C. (1923). Aspects of community organization in relation to public policy. *Annals of the American Academy of Political and Social Science, 105*, 83–87.

Lopez-Cantor, M. T. (2012). Transitional care. In F. Chiappelli, X. M. C. Brant, & C. B. Cajulis (Eds.), *Comparative effectiveness and efficacy research and analysis for practice (CEERAP)* (pp. 165–180). New York, NY: Springer.

MacDonald, M. (2001). Health promotion: Historical, philosophical and theoretical perspectives. In L. E. Young & V. E. Hayes (Eds.), *Transforming health promotion practice: Concepts, issues, and applications* (pp. 22–45). Philadelphia, PA: F. A. Davis Co.

MacDonald, M. (2004). From miasma to fractals: The epidemiology revolution and public health nursing. *Public Health Nursing, 21*(4), 380–391.

MacDonald, M. (2013). Public health ethics. In J. Storch, P. Rodney, & R. Starzomski (Eds.), *Toward a moral horizon: Nursing ethics for leadership and practice* (pp. 398–429). Toronto, ON: Pearson.

Martin, D. H. (2012). Two-eyed seeing: A framework for understanding Indigenous and non-Indigenous approaches to Indigenous health research. *Canadian Journal of Nursing Research, 44*(2), 20–42.

Masters, K. (2011). Models and theories focused on nursing goals and functions. J. B. Butts & K. L. Rich (Eds.), *Philosophies and theories for advanced nursing practice* (pp. 383–412). Sudbury, MA: Jones & Bartlett Learning.

McEwen, M. (2011). Overview of theory in nursing. In M. McEwen & E. M. Wills (Eds.), *Theoretical basis for nursing* (3rd ed.). Philadelphia, PA: Lippincott, Williams & Wilkins.

McGibbon, E. A. (2008). Health and health care: A human rights perspective. In D. Raphael (Ed.), *Social determinants of health: A Canadian perspective.* Toronto, ON: Canadian Scholars' Press.

McGibbon, E. A. (2012). People under threat. In E. A. McGibbon (Ed.), *Oppression: A social determinant of health.* Halifax, NS: Fernwood Publishers.

McGibbon, E. A., & Etowa, J. (2009). *Anti-racist health care practice.* Toronto, ON: Canadian Scholars' Press.

McGibbon, E., & McPherson, C. (2011). Applying intersectionality and complexity theory to address the social determinants of women's health. *Women's Health and Urban Life, 10*(1), 59–86.

McGregor, D. (2002). Traditional ecological knowledge and the two-row wampum. *Biodiversity, 3*(3), 8–9.

McKnight, J., & Van Dover, L. (1994). Community as client: A challenge for nursing education. *Public Health Nursing, 11*(1), 12–16.

McLaren, L., & Hawe, P. (2005). Ecological perspectives in health research. *Journal of Epidemiology and Community Health, 59,* 6–14.

Meleis, A. I. (2012). *Theoretical nursing: Development and progress* (5th ed.). Philadelphia, PA: Lippincott Williams & Wilkins.

Minkler, M. (1989). Health education, health promotion, and the open society. *Health Education and Behavior, 16*(1), 17–30.

Minkler, M. (Ed.). (2005). *Community organizing and community building for health.* New Brunswick, NJ: Rutgers University Press.

Munro, M., Gallant, M., MacKinnon, M., Dell, G., Herbert, R., MacNutt, G., . . . Roberston, K. (2000). The Prince Edward Island conceptual model for nursing: A nursing perspective of primary health care. *Canadian Journal of Nursing Research, 32*(1), 39–55.

National Collaborating Centre for Determinants of Health. (2013). *Let's talk: Health equity.* Antigonish, NS: NCCDH, St. Francis Xavier University.

National Collaborating Centre for Public Health. (2012). *What are the social determinants of health?* Retrieved from http://www.nccph.ca/docs/NCCPHSDOHFactsheet_EN_May2012.pdf

Neal, L. J. (1999). The Neal theory: Implications for practice and administration. *Home Healthcare Nurse, 17*(3), 181–187.

Neuman, B. N. (1972). A model for teaching total person approach to patient populations. *Nursing Research, 21*(3), 264–269.

Neuman, B. (1995). *The Neuman systems model* (3rd ed.). Norwalk, CT: Appleton & Lange.

Newman, M. A. (1986). *Health as expanding consciousness.* St. Louis, MO: Mosby.

Nightingale, F. (1946). *Notes on nursing.* Philadelphia, PA: Edward Stern & Company. (Original work published 1859.)

Orem, D. E. (1985). *Nursing: Concepts of practice* (3rd ed.). New York, NY: McGraw Hill.

Parse, R. R. (1992). Human becoming: Parse's theory of nursing. *Nursing Science Quarterly, 5,* 35–42.

Parse, R. R. (2003). *Community: A human becoming perspective.* Sudbury, MA: Jones & Bartlett Learning.

Pauly, B. M., MacKinnon, K., & Varcoe, C. (2009). Revisiting "Who gets care?" Health equity as an arena for nursing action. *Advances in Nursing Science, 32*(2), 118–127.

Pender, N. J. (1996). *Health promotion in nursing practice* (3rd ed.). Stamford, CT: Appleton & Lange.

Peplau, H. E. (1952). *Interpersonal relations in nursing.* New York, NY: G. P. Putnam's Sons.

Perkins, H. W. (Ed.). (2003). *The social norms approach to preventing school and college age substance abuse: A handbook for educators, counselors, and clinicians.* San Francisco, CA: Jossey-Bass.

Peterson, S. J. (2009). Introduction to the nature of nursing knowledge. In S. J. Peterson & T. S. Bredow (Eds.), *Middle range theories: Application to nursing research* (2nd ed., pp. 3–45). Philadelphia, PA: Lippincott Williams & Wilkins.

Pfettscher, S. (2010). Florence Nightingale 1820–1910: Modern nursing. In M. R. Alligood & A. M. Tomey (Eds.), *Nursing theorists and their work* (7th ed., pp. 71–90). St. Louis, MI: Mosby Elsevier.

Plsek, P., & Greenhalgh, T. (2001). The challenge of complexity in health care. *British Medical Journal, 323*(7313), 625–628.

Poliferoni, E. C. (2011). Philosophy of science: An introduction. In J. B. Butts & K. L. Rich (Eds.), *Philosophies and theories for advanced nursing practice* (pp. 3–18). Sudbury, MA: Jones & Bartlett Learning.

Porta, M. (2008). *Dictionary of epidemiology.* New York, NY: Oxford University Press.

Prochaska, J. O., & DiClemente, C. C. (1985). Common processes of change in smoking, weight control, and psychological distress. In S. Shiffman & T. Wills (Eds.), *Coping and substance abuse* (pp. 345–363). San Diego, CA: Academic Press.

Prochaska, J. O., DiClemente, C. C., & Norcross, J. C. (1992). In search of how people change: Applications to addictive behaviors. *American Psychologist, 47*(9), 1102–1114.

Ray, M. (1989). The theory of bureaucratic caring for nursing practice in the organizational culture. *Nursing Administration Quarterly, 13*(2), 31–42.

Ray, M. A., Turkel, M. C., & Cohn, J. (2011). Relational caring complexity: The study of caring and complexity in health care hospital organizations. In A. W. Davidson, M. A. Ray, & M. C. Turkel (Eds.), *Nursing, caring, and complexity science: For human-environment well-being* (pp. 95–117). New York, NY: Springer Publishing.

Reimer-Kirkham, S., Varcoe, C., Browne, A. J., Lynam, M. J., Khan, K. B., & McDonald, H. (2009). Critical inquiry and knowledge translation: Exploring compatibilities and tensions. *Nursing Philosophy, 10,* 152–166.

Reimer-Kirkham, S., Baumbusch, J. L., Schultz, A. S. H., & Anderson, J. (2009). Knowledge development and evidence-based practice: Insights and opportunities from a postcolonial feminist perspective for transformative nursing practice. In P. G. Reed & N. B. Crawford Shearer (Eds.), *Perspectives on nursing theory* (5th ed., pp. 349–364). Philadelphia, PA: Wolters Kluwer Health; Lippincott Williams & Wilkins.

Renfrew, M. J., McCormick, F. M., Wade, A., Quinn, B., & Dowswell, T. (2012). Support for healthy breastfeeding mothers with healthy term babies. *Cochrane Database of Systematic Reviews, 5.*

Reutter, L. (1984). Family health assessment—An integrated approach. *Journal of Advanced Nursing, 9,* 391–399.

Reutter, L., & Kushner, K. (2010). Health equity through action of the social determinants of health: Taking up the challenge in nursing. *Nursing Inquiry, 17*(3), 269–280.

Rice, R. (1994). Conceptual framework for nursing practice in the home: The Rice model of dynamic self-determination. *Home Healthcare Nurse, 12*(2), 51–53.

Risjord, M. (2010). *Nursing knowledge: science, practice, and philosophy.* Chichester, UK: John Wiley & Sons Ltd.

Rogers, E. M. (2002). Diffusion of preventive innovations. *Addictive Behaviors, 27,* 989–993.

Rogers, E. M. (2004). A prospective and retrospective look at the diffusion model. *Journal of Health Communication, 9,* 13–19.

Rogers, M. E. (1983). Science of unitary human beings: A paradigm for nursing. In I. W. Clements & F. B. Roberts (Eds.), *Family health: A theoretical approach to nursing care* (pp. 219–227). New York, NY: John Wiley & Sons.

Rogers, W. A. (2006). Feminism and public health ethics. *Journal of Medical Ethics, 32,* 351–354. doi:10.1136/jme.2005.013466

Romanow, R. (2002). *Building on values: The future of health care in Canada, final report.* Commission on the Future of Health Care in Canada: National Library of Canada.

Roy, C. (1987). Roy's adaptation model. In R. R. Parse (Ed.), *Nursing science: Major paradigms theories and critiques* (pp. 35–45). Philadelphia, PA: W. B. Saunders.

Ruland, C. M., & Moore, S. M. (1998). Theory construction based on standards of care: A proposed theory of the peaceful end of life. *Nursing Outlook, 46*(4), 169–175.

Russell, D. (2000). *A people's dream: Aboriginal self-government in Canada.* Vancouver, BC: UBC Press.

Shareck, M., Frohlich, K. L., & Poland, B. (2013). Reducing social inequities in health through settings related interventions—a conceptual framework. *Global Health Promotion, 20*(2), 39–52.

Schultz, P. R. (1987). When client means more than one: Extending the foundational concept of person. *Advances in Nursing Science, 10*(1), 71–86.

Sheilds, L. E., & Lindsey, A. E. (1998). Community health promotion nursing practice. *Advances in Nursing Science, 20*(4), 23–36.

Shim, S., Benkert, R., Bell, S., Walker, D., & Danford, C. (2007). Social justice: Added metaparadigm concept for urban health nursing. *Public Health Nursing, 24*(1), 73–80.

Sills, G., & Goeppinger, J. (1985). The community as a field of inquiry in nursing. *Annual Review of Nursing Research, 3,* 1–57.

Smith, D. A., Edwards, N. C., Martens, P. J., & Varcoe, C. (2007). Making a difference: A new care paradigm for pregnant and parenting Aboriginal people. *Canadian Journal of Public Health, 98*(4), 321–325.

Smith, D., Varcoe, C., & Edwards, N. (2005). Turning around the intergenerational impact of residential schools on Aboriginal people: Implications for health policy and practice. *Canadian Journal of Nursing Research, 37*(4), 38–60.

Smith, K., & Bazini-Barakat, N. (2003). A public health nursing practice model: Melding public health nursing principles with the nursing process. *Public Health Nursing, 20*(1), 42–48.

Smith, M. J. (2003). Evaluation of middle range theories for the discipline of nursing. In M. J. Smith & P. R. Liehr (Eds.), *Middle range theory for nursing* (pp. 189–211). New York, NY: Springer Publishing.

Squires, L., Peinado, S., Berkman, N., Boudewyns, V., & McCormack, L. (2012). The health literacy skills framework. *Journal of Health Communication: International Perspectives.* doi:10.1080/10810730.2012.713442

Stevens, P. E. (1989). A critical social reconceptualization of environment in nursing: Implications for methodology. *Advances in Nursing Science, 11*(4), 56–68.

Stevens, P. E., & Hall, J. M. (1992). Applying critical theories to nursing in communities. *Public Health Nursing, 9*(1), 2–9.

Stevens, E. E., Patrick, T. E., & Pickler, R. (2009). A history of infant feeding. *Journal of Perinatal Education, 18*(2).

Stewart, M. (2000). Framework based on primary health care principles. In M. Stewart (Ed.), *Community nursing: Promoting Canadians' health* (pp. 58–82). Toronto, ON: W. B. Saunders.

Stokols, D. (1992). Establishing and maintaining healthy environments: Toward a social ecology of health promotion. *American Psychologist, 47*(1), 6–22.

Stokols, D. (1996). Translating social ecological theory into guidelines for community health promotion. *American Journal of Health Promotion, 10,* 282–298.

Strecher, V. J., & Rosenstock, I. M. (1997). The health belief model. In A. Baum, S. Newman, J. Weinman, R. West, & C. McManus (Eds.), *Cambridge handbook of psychology, health and medicine* (pp. 113–116). New York, NY: Cambridge University Press.

Strega, S. (2005). The view from the poststructural margins: Epistemology and methodology reconsidered. In L. Brown & S. Strega (Eds.), *Research as resistance: Critical, indigenous and anti-oppressive approaches* (pp. 199–236). Toronto, ON: Canadian Scholars' Press.

Taylor, S. G., & McLaughlin, K. (1991). Orem's general theory of nursing and community nursing. *Nursing Science Quarterly, 4*(153), 153–160.

Taylor, S. G. (2001). Orem's general theory of nursing and families. *Nursing Science Quarterly, 14*(7), 7–9.

Truth and Reconciliation Commission of Canada. (2012). *Truth and reconciliation commission of Canada: Calls to action.* Retrieved from http://www.trc.ca

Truth and Reconciliation Commission of Canada (2015a). *Calls to action.* Author: Winnipeg, MB. Retrieved from http://www.trc.ca

Truth and Reconciliation Commission of Canada. (2015b). *Honouring the truth, reconciling for the future: Summary of the final report of the Truth and Reconciliation Commission of Canada.* Winnipeg, MB. Retrieved from http://www.trc.ca

Van Herk, K. A., Smith, D., & Andrew, C. (2011). Examining our privileges and oppressions: Incorporating an intersectionality paradigm into nursing. *Nursing Inquiry, 18*(1), 29–39.

Van Herk, K. A., Smith, D., & Tedford Gold, S. (2012). Safe care spaces and places: Exploring urban Aboriginal families' access to preventive care. *Health and Place, 18,* 649–656.

Vollman, A. R., Anderson, E. T., & McFarlane, J. (2003). *Canadian community as partner.* Philadelphia, PA: Lippincott Williams & Wilkins.

Vollman, A. R., Anderson, E. T., & McFarlane, J. M. (2008). *Canadian community as partner: Theory and practice in nursing.* Philadelphia, PA: Lippincott Williams & Wilkins.

Vollman, A. R., Anderson, E. T., & McFarlane, J. (2012). *Canadian community as partner: Theory and multidisciplinary practice* (3rd ed.). Philadelphia, PA: Wolters Kluwer; Lippincott Williams & Wilkins.

Von Bertalanffy, L. (1972). The history and status of general systems theory. *Academy of Management Journal, 15*(4), 407–426.

Walby, S., Armstrong, J., & Strid, S. (2012). Intersectionality: Multiple inequalities in social theory. *Sociology, 46*(2), 224–240.

Watson, J. (1979). *Nursing: The philosophy and science of caring.* Boston, MA: Little, Brown & Co.

Watson, J. (2012). *Human caring science.* Sudbury, MA: Jones & Bartlett.

Westley, F., Zimmerman, B., & Patton, M.Q. (2007). *Getting to maybe: How the world is changed.* Toronto, ON: Vintage Canada.

White, J. (1995). Patterns of knowing: Review, critique and update. *Advances in Nursing Science, 17*(4), 73–86.

White, M. S. (1982). Construct for public health. *Nursing Outlook, 30*, 527–530.

Whitehead, M., & Dahlgren, G. (2006). *Concepts and principles for tackling social inequities in health: Levelling up* (Part 1). Geneva, CH: World Health Organization.

Williams, D. M. (1989). Political theory and individualistic health promotion. *Advances in Nursing Science, 12*(1), 14–25.

World Health Organization (WHO). (2010). *Backgrounder 3: Key concepts.* Used by permission of World Health Organization. Retrieved from http://www.who.int/social_determinants/final_report/key_concepts_en.pdf

World Health Organization Commission on Social Determinants of Health. (2008). *Closing the gap in a generation: Health equity through action on the social determinants of health.* Geneva, CH: Author.

World Health Organization (WHO). (Ed.). (n.d.). *Health topics: Breastfeeding.* Retrieved from http://www.who.int/topics/breastfeeding/en

World Health Organization (WHO). (Ed.). (2018, February 16). *Infant and young child feeding.* Retrieved from http://www.who.int/news-room/fact-sheets/detail/infant-and-young-child-feeding

Wright, L. M., & Leahey, M. (2012). *Nurses and families: A guide to family assessment and intervention* (6th ed.). Philadelphia, PA: F. A. Davis Co.

Yiu, L. (2008). Community care. In L. L. Stamler & L. Yiu (Eds.), *Community health nursing: A Canadian perspective* (2nd ed., pp. 176–195). Toronto, ON: Pearson Canada Inc.

Yiu, L. (2012). Community care. In L. L. Stamler & L. Yiu (Eds.), *Community health nursing: A Canadian perspective* (3rd ed., pp. 213–235). Toronto, ON: Pearson Canada Inc.

ABOUT THE AUTHORS

Claire Betker, RN, PhD, CCHN(C), is Executive Director, Active Living, Population and Public Health Branch of Manitoba Health, Seniors and Active Living. Claire has worked as a registered nurse in community health for more than 40 years at local, regional, provincial, and national levels in mental health, home health, primary health care, and public health. Claire is a certified Community Health Nurse and has been very involved with the Community Health Nurses of Canada in Manitoba and nationally, participating in several standing committees and serving as president and past president. Claire is the president of the Canadian Nurses Association. Completed in 2016, her PhD dissertation examined public health leadership to advance health equity.

Mary E. Hill, RN, PhD, was formerly a manager of Child, Youth, and Family Services with the Vancouver Island Health Authority. She has over 35 years of experience in public health nursing and community health services management. She has maintained a particular interest in perinatal services, breastfeeding supports, and tobacco prevention activities. Her doctoral dissertation explored how the routine, day-to-day practice of PHNs affected breastfeeding, immunizations, and tobacco outcomes among priority perinatal women, as well as the effect of organizational factors on the ability of PHNs to provide that service.

Megan Kirk, RN, PhD(c), MSc, BScN, is currently a nursing doctoral candidate at the University of Victoria. She has been interested in the area of prevention in both of her graduate degrees. In her master's thesis, she explored the influence of work hours on the cardiovascular health of female hospital employees. Now, in her doctorate, she is focusing on the work of public health nurses and elucidating the impact of their efforts on the health and well-being of individuals, families, communities, and populations. She hopes to highlight the difference that public health nurses make in the communities they serve.

Marjorie MacDonald, RN, PhD, is Professor Emerita with the School of Nursing at the University of Victoria Faculty of Human and Social Development, and a Scientist with the Canadian Institute for Substance Use Research. Marjorie's research interests include public health nursing, public health policy and practice, health services research related to public health services and systems renewal, primary health care, adolescent health promotion, smoking and drug use prevention, adolescent health literacy, and advanced practice nursing, particularly in a public health context.

Health Promotion

Candace Lind and Louise Baptiste

CHAPTER 8

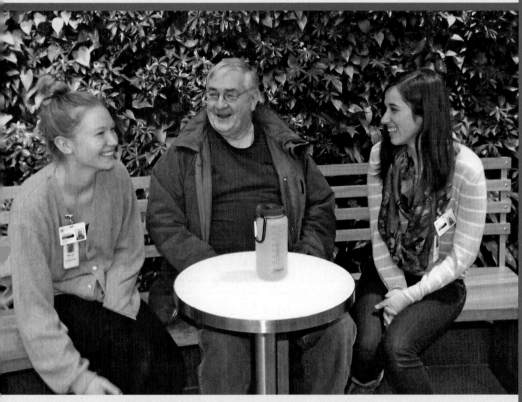

Source: Courtesy of Nikita Baker

INTRODUCTION

Canada is credited with being a birthplace of the worldwide **health promotion** movement. Health promotion is a complex social and political process that has been the focus of much international discussion over the last few decades; however, many of the large-scale potential benefits of health promotion have yet to be realized. Numerous complex factors have affected the advancement of health promotion, which are discussed in this chapter. The chapter starts with an overview of health, including definitions of health, health promotion, Indigenous health and health promotion, and upstream and downstream approaches to promoting health. The history of primary health care (PHC) (including description of values, principles, and elements), the Ottawa Charter and subsequent international or global charters for health promotion, and social determinants of health are presented. Population health promotion and the population health promotion model are introduced and discussed. The sections that follow include social marketing, population health indicators, "at risk" populations, risk communication, levels of prevention used in health promotion, harm reduction, and safe injection sites. The chapter closes with a discussion of research, advocacy, and activism in health promotion practice.

DEFINITIONS OF HEALTH AND HEALTH PROMOTION

Health is a difficult concept to define. The Oxford etymological dictionary (Hoad, 1996) describes health as a state of sound body, mind, and spirit; a state of wholeness. The traditional Euro-Canadian understanding of health and health care rests within the biomedical model where health has been understood as the absence of disease and illness, rather than a state of wholeness. From a biomedical perspective, to achieve health one needs only attend to physical pathology (Kaplan, 2000). However, health is more than a static biomedical concept. Health is a dynamic process with multiple assumptions and understandings that evolve over time and evolve with varying professional perspectives and purpose. Although the practice of medicine views health mainly through the biomedical model, nursing has defined the concept of health as an evolving, holistic human experience, informed by multiple professions, recognizing the medical definition is just one aspect of health (Payne, 1983).

Promoting health is the foundation of nursing practice (Canadian Nurses Association [CNA], 2009). Nurses work alongside multiple professions (in interprofessional and multisectoral teams) to promote, support, maintain, and restore health in individuals, families, communities, and populations. The international concept of health had been disease focused until 1946, when the World Health Organization (WHO) broadened the definition from just the absence of disease to "a state of complete physical, mental and social well-being and not merely the absence of disease or infirmity" (World Health Organization [WHO], 1948, para. 1). This change in the conceptualization of health shifted the understanding of health away from disease control to include more comprehensive aspects of being human. This broad definition of health has been adopted as a foundational understanding to inform many professions concerned with the health of humans and societies. With a need to expand on the notion of health as a state of complete well-being, health-related professions have adapted the WHO's definition to create definitions tailored to inform and guide their unique practices. Nursing, anthropology, sociology, and social work are some professions that have adopted the WHO's definition, adding their own unique views of health to meet the needs of their professional focus. For example, anthropology (the study of human societies and cultures) defines the concept of health as being bound within the political, economic, and religious domains of a society (Kleinman & Petryna, 2001). Within the practice of sociology, person-centred care is a movement to expand health care's definition of health to include human capabilities, such as the ability to use imagination and senses to enjoy everyday experiences (Frank, 2013). This movement identifies the value of social factors, capabilities, and strengths of a person, as well as the quality of the health care provider–client relationship, as important considerations of a person's overall health (Frank, 2013; Venkatapura, 2013). The profession of social work considers health within the broad context of integrating services to improve function, longevity, and access to quality care (Fisher & Elnitsky, 2012).

These broad concepts of health have been adopted to guide nurses to help people achieve their full potential mentally, physically, spiritually, and socially, so they can experience a life worth living. Community health nurses (CHNs) define health as "a resource for everyday life that is influenced by circumstances, beliefs, and the determinants of health" (Community Health Nurses Association of Canada [CHNAC], 2008, p. 10). Founded on the principles of social justice, CHNs strive to promote and protect the health of individuals, families, and communities regardless of where they live, work, or play (CHNAC, 2008). Nursing's holistic view of health acknowledges that it can be a unique experience for individuals, families, and communities. Individuals or families may view health through a lens aligned with their immediate needs: being able to socialize with friends during rapidly declining health, having a supportive family in the face of crisis or life-altering illness, having a warm meal and place to sleep on a cold night, or having the right to happiness as well as the freedom and autonomy to live life one's own way. Community members hold values and preferences that differ from mainstream society, where being healthy may mean living without fear of persecution. Within the broad and inclusive lens of social justice, health may mean living in a just and fair society where equitable distribution of resources can support universal education, access to equitable health care, and the freedom to contribute as a full member of society with equal rights, privileges, and rewards (CNA, 2010). Health might be described as having support to live to one's full potential within a family, community, or society that can love, support, and care for its members.

Health promotion has a long history in Euro-Canada and globally; however, its full implementation continues to be challenging. Health promotion is still sometimes narrowly used or conceptualized as the equivalent of health education. Health education is a common information-sharing health promotion strategy used to increase people's knowledge and oftentimes used to assist with individual behavioural change or to help produce more healthful environments. However, health education is only one of several key components and action areas of health promotion, as illustrated in the Ottawa Charter and the population health promotion model (PHPM) below. What is health promotion? According to the WHO (2009a),

> Health promotion is the process of enabling people to increase control over, and to improve, their health. To reach a state of complete physical, mental and social well-being, an individual or group must be able to identify and to realize aspirations, to satisfy needs, and to change or cope with the environment. Health is, therefore, seen as a resource for everyday life, not the objective of living. Health is a positive concept emphasizing social and personal resources, as well as physical capacities. Therefore, health promotion is not just the responsibility of the health sector, but goes beyond healthy lifestyles to well-being. (p. 1)

This definition is the most widespread in use and remains unchanged since the landmark **Ottawa Charter for**

Health Promotion (WHO, 1986) was written, as an outcome from the First International Conference on Health Promotion. The WHO's health promotion glossary of terms adds that health promotion represents a comprehensive social and political process. Therefore, health promotion actions must go beyond simply strengthening people's skills and abilities to manage their own health and instead move toward action to change social, environmental, and economic conditions to alleviate their impact on public and individuals' health (WHO, 1998). People are helped to increase control over the determinants of their health as the means of improving their health. Health promotion should be an integral part of nursing practice in any setting. Nurses must work together with people to understand their needs from their perspectives and work within those perspectives to set up the conditions to facilitate healthy change—and help people feel empowered to create the changes that will help themselves. In recent years, the increased need for political advocacy, investment in strategies that address the determinants of health, building health promotion capacity, and partnership development have been deemed critical for dealing with the challenges of living in an increasingly global world (Smith, Tang, & Nutbeam, 2006). Health promotion is often viewed as a process or a framework in which people work together to create conditions that sustain health and address broader social and economic conditions that affect a population's health (Fawcett et al., 2010) by applying a wide range of activities and approaches to achieve outcomes (Raphael, 2010a). In essence, health promotion seeks to enhance people's ability to exercise control over the environmental, social, and behavioural conditions that affect their quality of life. Health promotion strategies encourage citizen engagement in improving the determinants of health and well-being, which improves quality of life (Raphael, 2010a). Health promotion therefore goes well beyond simply addressing healthy lifestyles, to improve overall well-being. Health promotion is an amalgamation of values and practices that promote health. Health promotion has also been described as a combination of educational, political, regulatory, or organizational activities or conditions of living that are conducive to the health of individuals or communities (McKenzie, Neiger, & Thackeray, 2013). Partnerships and community involvement have been described as the main contributing factors that achieve long-term impacts (Franco-Paredes, Zeuli, Hernandez-Ramos, & Santos-Preciado, 2010).

Raeburn and Rootman (2007) stated that health promotion has a positive and action-oriented nature, whereby it builds healthiness rather than just focuses on prevention or treatment of illness and other conditions. Ultimately, "health promotion aims to reduce differences in health status and vulnerability, and to ensure equal opportunities and resources to enable all people to achieve their fullest health potential and quality of life" (Frankish, Moulton, Rootman, Cole, & Gray, 2006, p. 176). Therefore, "health promotion represents a comprehensive social and political process, it not only embraces actions directed at strengthening the skills and capabilities of individuals, but also action directed toward changing social, environmental and economic conditions so as to alleviate their

impact on public and individual health" (Hills, Carroll, & Vollman, 2007, p. 330).

Nurses act upon many levels and across many sectors of society to promote the health of people. The **social determinants of health** are just as important and often can be even more important than the biological or physical determinants of a person's health. Therefore, although caring for people when they are sick or injured is an important component of nursing work, nursing practice is not just focused on looking after people in hospitals or in their homes when they are ill or focused on teaching them about health. Nursing must also be involved in activism, advocacy, and other ways of creating social change to improve people's health. Cathy Crowe's multifaceted work to raise awareness and address the issues of homelessness and Cheryl Forchuk's work advocating for discharged mental health patients' safe integration into communities are Canadian examples of nursing activism efforts to raise awareness and create change to improve people's health.

Indigenous Health and Health Promotion

A Euro-Canadian understanding of health and health promotion has been conventionally framed from an individualistic and biomedical lens. An Indigenous understanding of health, however, arises from a broader, more holistic, community-focused lens where " . . . wellness is achieved through a balance of the body, mind, emotion and spirit, and holistic health requires the family and community to work together . . . Each part enhances, supports, and affects the other. Individual wellness is the result of how each of these factors is addressed" (Cameron, del Pilar Carmargo Plazas, Salas, Bourque Bearskin, & Hungler, 2014, p. E10). Good health is therefore connected to having a sense of community, personal identity, and the practice of cultural and spiritual traditions (Cameron et al., 2014). The land plays a critically important role in forming and maintaining cultural identities, social relationships, and health and well-being (Richmond, 2015). Living in harmony with nature has traditionally been an integral component of the health of Indigenous peoples around the world (Bourque Bearskin et al., 2016; Cameron et al., 2014).

The WHO definition of health promotion may be particularly germane to Indigenous populations in Canada in the recovery from cultural genocide, attributable at least in part to the residential school system (see Chapter 22). The colonization of Indigenous populations in Canada has led to the loss of traditional systems of health and wellness, and which now " . . . being told from the outside how to be healthy and well, no longer sits well with us." (Dion Stout, 2015, p. 145). Health promotion as the process involved in regaining control and power in reclaiming culture is important. However, as McPhail-Bell, Bond, Brough, and Frederick (2015) caution, ethical **Indigenous health promotion** requires health practitioners to relinquish control over the health promotion process, not an easy task in a Euro-Canadian health care system. It is critically important that **empowerment** is viewed as a key component of health promotion processes health care practitioners use, not just as a way to engage with people to effect behavioural change (McPhail-Bell et al., 2015). This shift is starting, for example, in the changes that have been occurring in the way research with Indigenous populations is conceptualized and carried out, employing Indigenous methodologies, ways of knowing, and control over the research. The Truth and Reconciliation Commission of Canada's Calls to Action to redress the legacy of the residential schools (2012) and the United Nations Declaration of the Rights of Indigenous Peoples (United Nations, 2008) provide starting points in raising awareness and creating action for health-promoting change that calls upon every Canadian's involvement in the healing process.

UPSTREAM AND DOWNSTREAM APPROACHES TO PROMOTING HEALTH

McKinlay (1994) offers a story as an example of health promotion offering upstream and **downstream approaches** to improving the health of populations. What follows is an adaptation of that story.

Imagine a town situated in a valley where the river provides most of the drinking water. Despite its idyllic appearance, every year many people experience episodes of diarrhea, vomiting, and dehydration, with the most severely impacted including young children, the vulnerable, and older adults. The town health department has implemented many strategies to help people stay well, such as boiled water advisories advertised on television, radio, billboards, and posters. There are a few wells that have clean drinking water, but these have low flow rates with only enough clean water for the few families who can afford it. The town health department has enough funds to provide antibacterial pills to the people most impacted and pay for medications such as antibiotics for the people who get sick. However, despite all these yearly efforts, the morbidity and mortality rates in this town due to gastrointestinal infections remain 10 times the national average. What is not well known is that upstream is a factory that dumps unfiltered sewage into the river (Photo 8.1). The factory owner obtained approval to dump years ago because the products being discarded into the river are organic and biodegradable. However, in recent years the number and size of factory operations have increased dramatically. One day a group of public health nurses received permission to do a community assessment and environmental scan to investigate the problem. They tested the river water and learned the bacterial count was much higher than recommended. From municipal and district reports, they learned it had been 15 years since the policies regarding sewage dumping into the river had been addressed. Driving upstream, they observed the factory sewage pipes steadily dumping large quantities of waste products into the river. Coming back to their town they encouraged the town health department to take action upstream to ensure that the water the townspeople were drinking downstream was cleaner. However, town council

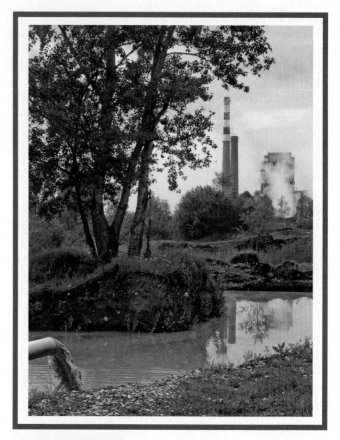

PHOTO 8.1 Dirty water stems from pipe polluting the river.

Source: Ngaga/Shutterstock

replied that due to the high costs of treating the ill townspeople, providing antibacterial products to clean the water, and providing boiled water advisories, there was no money left over to address the upstream issues.

The upstream story may sound bizarre, but there are many similar situations in Canada where there is less-than-adequate health care funding available for prevention and promotion strategies due to the high cost of providing acute-care services. Acute-care services are usually tertiary prevention measures, are focused on individual treatment and cure, and are considered downstream interventions. **Upstream approaches** are oftentimes prevention and promotion strategies focused on policy interventions that benefit the whole population, or primary health care interventions that focus on people's well-being by addressing and taking action on the root causes of preventable diseases and injuries. Examples of upstream approaches could include nursing actions that advocate for safer environments—those that encourage safe and affordable exercise, such as walking, running, inline skating, and biking—or lobbying for higher tobacco taxes that encourage people to quit or reduce tobacco use (Canadian Public Health Association [CPHA], 2011; Public Health Agency of Canada [PHAC], 2013a). Upstream approaches usually extend beyond addressing individual behaviours and identify programs, policies, and environmental changes that will impact the health of a population. The earlier examples of creating environments that encourage exercise and increase the cost of tobacco make it easier for people to make healthy lifestyle choices. Policies such as adding fluoride to municipal water supplies (to prevent dental caries), adding iodine to salt, or adding vitamin D to milk are upstream interventions made by elected officials to improve the health of the populations they represent.

PRIMARY HEALTH CARE

History of Primary Health Care

Canada is considered an international leader in the **health promotion movement**, **population health**, and **primary health care (PHC)** (CPHA, 2010). Almost immediately after Canada became a country in 1867, Canadians began lobbying for improvements to the determinants of health, such as safe water and sewage disposal systems, and for the government to take action on overcrowded and slum housing, poverty, malnutrition, and unsafe food and milk supplies (CPHA, 2010). An early example of the principles of PHC arose in the 1940s in Canada. Members of the Co-operative Commonwealth Federation political party in Saskatchewan (under Tommy Douglas's leadership) were concerned that the poorest people in the province could not afford hospital services. They implemented a provincial hospital insurance program in 1947. Eliminating exclusion from health care services based on inability to pay for services was also the rationale for introducing a national hospital insurance program in 1957, a program that paid hospitalization fees for all Canadians. Despite this program, the inability to pay a doctor's fees remained common. Therefore, in 1966 Canada instituted a national medicare program that would pay for costs incurred for treating people in hospital, clinics, and doctors' offices (Canadian Health Coalition, 2009). Health care service is one component of PHC. Addressing the needs of the poor ensured that they could receive health care services, and this became a precursor to future PHC initiatives.

From 1974 to 1994 the Canadian federal government played a large part in establishing Canada as a leader in health promotion. This began with the release of "A New Perspective on the Health of Canadians" in 1974 written by Marc Lalonde, then Minister of National Health and Welfare, Canada, currently called Health Canada. Four elements of the health field concept were presented: human biology, environment, lifestyle, and health care organization. The purpose of this working document was to unfold a new perspective on the health of Canadians and stimulate interest in future health programs for Canada. However, it achieved much more. It shifted national thinking toward health promotion, albeit mainly focused on lifestyles, and led to the establishment of Canada as an initiator and world leader in health promotion. ParticipACTION, a well-known program encouraging individual exercise and healthy living, was launched in the 1970s as one initiative resulting from the Lalonde Report (ParticipACTION Archive Project, n.d.).

In Canada, the health promotion programs that arose from the Lalonde Report were under-resourced, and the public face of health promotion became focused on lifestyle programs such as tobacco, alcohol, drugs, and nutrition. What was not taken forward well from the report was the call for a focus on environment as one of the causes of ill health. Lalonde had identified environmental risks as those that include the physical and social environments. He stated, "One of the most important but least understood environmental problems is the effect of rapid social change on the mental and physical health of Canadians . . . [and] the number of economically deprived Canadians is still high, resulting in a lack of adequate housing and insufficient or inadequate clothing. All the foregoing environmental conditions create risks which are a far greater threat to health than any present inadequacy of the health care system" (Lalonde, 1974, p. 18). In 1974, Lalonde stated that the health care system was mainly oriented to treating illness, which, unfortunately, remains the case today. Most health care dollars are still allocated for acute care or hospital treatment.

The Lalonde Report received international attention, helping stimulate the WHO to convene a meeting of member countries to address the disparities in health status between developed and undeveloped countries. In 1978, an international conference on PHC resulted in the Declaration of Alma-Ata (WHO, 1978). An important component of the declaration was the statement that health "is a fundamental human right and that the attainment of the highest possible level of health is a most important worldwide social goal whose realization requires the action of many other social and economic sectors in addition to the health sector" (WHO, 1978, p. 1). This declaration drew attention to the inequalities in health care status between high-income and low-income countries and stated that interventions should be practical, scientifically sound, socially acceptable, and universally accessible to individuals and families in the community, at a cost the people and country could afford. In the Canadian context, community participation at all levels of intervention should, as much as possible, use local resources, including educating and hiring Indigenous health care professionals.

In 1984 the WHO wrote a small discussion document on the concept and principles of health promotion, introducing the principles of involving the population as a whole and directing action to the determinants of health. This was taken up in a 1985 Canadian federal policy review initiated by federal bureaucrats and supported by Honourable Jake Epp, the Federal Minister of Health at the time. In 1986 the minister released a report titled "Achieving Health for All: A Framework for Health Promotion," more commonly called the Epp Report. This report defined the three mechanisms of health promotion as (a) self-care, (b) actions people take to help each other cope, and (c) healthy environments (Epp, 1986). As a part of setting a new direction, Minister Epp agreed to host the First International Conference on Health Promotion in Ottawa in collaboration with the WHO and the Canadian Public Health Association (CPHA). The conference representatives built on the Epp Report, creating the Ottawa Charter for Health Promotion, which contributed to establishing Canada as a leader in PHC—in addition to leadership in health promotion.

Programs aimed at changing individual behaviour have limited effectiveness; therefore, health strategies must be broadened to include political, economic, social, and cultural interventions, with the empowerment of people to engage in public policy changes as one of their main objectives (Navarro, 2009). Even Lalonde (1974) had identified the important role of governments in improving the health of Canadians, along with individual citizens, health care professionals, and institutions. He acknowledged, however, that "this fragmentation of responsibility has sometimes led to imbalanced approaches, with each participant in the health field pursuing solutions only within his [sic] area of interest" (Lalonde, 1974, p. 33). In 1985, Taylor and Rieger stated, "the social origins of illness are no longer disputed, yet 130 years after the publication of the Virchow's Report, governments are still unwilling to accept the corollary; that is, that socioeconomic improvements are more necessary than medical ones" (Taylor & Rieger, 1985, p. 557). What are our governments' priorities today? What are their areas of interest, if they follow a neo-liberal agenda (a political agenda that includes reduced government involvement in and funding for social and other services, and favours privatization and a market economy)? How does that affect their view of health, and whose responsibility it is to create the conditions for a healthy society?

Reflecting the continuing global issues in health promotion, challenges in implementing health promotion in Canada continue. In partnership with the Canadian Health Services Research Foundation, the Canadian Nurses Association (CNA) commissioned a research report to analyze public policy and programming focused on the determinants of health and health outcomes in Canada (Muntaner, Ng, & Chung, 2012). The issue is that all levels of governments (federal to municipal) have taken minimal action to narrow health inequalities by focusing on social determinants of health and public policy, even though income, housing, food insecurity, and social exclusion form the major modifiable social determinants of health over the life course (Muntaner et al., 2012). A scoping review of the literature indicated a clear central finding of a large, negative, and statistically significant association between the social determinants of health and health inequalities in Canada (Muntaner et al., 2012). Although the social determinants of health have been recognized as important to nursing practice for many years, this review suggests specific action nurses can take to address this pressing issue. Action includes nursing collaboration with government, civil, and health sectors, with roles in advocacy, policy analysis, and political activities—that is, to become active social change agents. A call for nurses to refocus practice on social justice (characteristic of early public health nursing) has led to CHNs in Canada calling for practice focused on reducing health and social inequalities to become a standard and core competency of nursing practice (Muntaner et al., 2012). Nurses must focus on the root causes of health inequalities, identify which determinants of health require action, implement the principles of social justice, and engage in advocacy for the most disadvantaged groups in society (Muntaner et al., 2012). Policy recommendations include initiatives to reduce child and adult poverty (through financial assistance and social wages), increases in minimum wages to a "living wage" necessary for supporting housing and food needs, campaigns and social movements for the rights of socially excluded groups, advocacy for intersectoral action on health inequalities across levels of government to coordinate social determinant of health policies, support for political candidates who are receptive to taking action on social determinants of health, and encouragement for greater workplace democracy to protect and increase worker bargaining power (Muntaner et al., 2012).

Primary Health Care Values, Principles, and Elements

PHC is defined as:

> essential health care based on practical, scientifically sound and socially acceptable methods and technology made universally accessible to individuals and families in the community through their full participation and at a cost that the community and country can afford to maintain at every stage of their development in the spirit of self-reliance and self-determination. It forms an integral part both of the country's health system, of which it is the central function and main focus, and of the overall social and economic development of the community. It is the first level of contact of individuals, the family and community with the national health system bringing health care as close as possible to where people live and work, and constitutes the first element of a continuing health care process. (WHO, 1978, p. 2–3)

Primary care is sometimes confused with PHC; however, primary care is a narrower concept that refers to a person-centred comprehensive approach (often biomedical) to care delivery at the point of entry into the health care system (WHO, 2008). For example, nurse practitioners working in the community provide primary care services to clients, and their practices may also be informed by the values and principles of PHC.

The WHO describes PHC as the route to better health for all, with five key components required to achieve that goal:

- reducing exclusion and social disparities in health (universal coverage reforms);
- organizing health services around people's needs and expectations (service delivery reforms);
- integrating health into all sectors (public policy reforms);
- pursuing collaborative models of policy dialogue (leadership reforms); and
- increasing stakeholder participation. (WHO, 2013a, p. 1)

The underlying values of PHC are social justice and equity. As explained in Chapter 6, social justice refers to the fair distribution of society's benefits and responsibilities, and focuses on eliminating the root causes of inequities (CNA, 2010), leading to equality of opportunities for health. Equity refers to the fair distribution of resources for health. Philosophically, PHC permeates all of society and social justice, and equity directs nursing's focus toward improving the health of the most disadvantaged, thereby giving all people the same opportunities for health and quality of life. Strategically, PHC strategies may focus on developing strengths or assets; offering opportunities for change to address deficits or needs; maximizing the involvement of the community; including all sectors that impact the determinants of health (but avoiding duplication of services); and using only health methods and technologies that are accessible, acceptable, affordable, and appropriate for each situation (University of Saskatchewan, 2011).

There are five principles of PHC: accessibility, public participation, health promotion, appropriate technology, and intersectoral collaboration or cooperation. *Accessibility* means that health care is universally available to all people regardless of geographic community and is delivered in a timely manner. This means the distribution of health care providers must include rural, remote, and urban communities. However, barriers to accessibility go well beyond geographic barriers—they can also refer to barriers created by health care providers' assumptions about, or biases against, certain groups of people. For example, if a health care provider refuses to provide sexually transmitted infection screening to a lesbian couple because of a belief that sexually transmitted infections occur primarily through heterosexual transmission, this is an accessibility barrier. Additionally, health care providers who actively stigmatize vulnerable populations (such as people living with homelessness, people with addictions, or people involved in sex work) by the way they treat them in emergency departments are also creating barriers to accessible health care service. People who feel discriminated against may avoid seeking health care when needed because of fear of stigmatization.

The second principle of PHC is *public participation*. This means people are actively encouraged to participate in making decisions about their own health and in identifying the health needs of their communities. The design and delivery of health care must be flexible, responsive, and ensure respect for diversity. The third principle of PHC is *health promotion*. Through health promotion, people build understandings about the social determinants of health and develop skills to improve and maintain their own health and well-being.

Appropriate technology means that the appropriate modes of care are available based on a society's social, economic, and cultural development. Equity is an important component of appropriate technology. Appropriate technology does not mean an MRI in every village; rather, it means that alternatives to high-cost or high-technology services must be developed in many environments. Appropriate models of health care must be developed and tested before implementation.

Intersectoral collaboration or cooperation means that because health and well-being are linked to economic and social policy, intersectoral collaboration is needed to establish national and local health goals, healthy public policies, and planning and evaluation of health services. Providers from different health professions and sectors of society must collaborate and function interdependently to meet the needs of the public. They must all also participate in government policy formation that impacts the health and well-being of people in their society.

Optimal PHC approaches involve full participation of the community of people they will impact. Community involvement includes development, coordination, delivery, and evaluation of initiatives and should include laypeople, community leaders, and practitioners with PHC implementation experience and expertise. The WHO has outlined eight essential elements of PHC, and these are used as guiding principles to set direction and measure success:

1. *Education about health problems and prevention techniques.* Education serves the purpose of identifying and preventing (or controlling) dominant health challenges for a target population. A solid understanding of PHC and the health challenges for the target population is necessary before the first steps are taken to create healthier populations. Research and application of knowledge occur throughout the process.

2. *Promotion of food supply and proper nutrition.* This element includes the provision of an appropriate, nutritious food supply. In resource-poor nations the focus is on providing an adequate food supply for the population, whereas in resource-rich countries such as Canada, strategies focus more on obesity and nutrition (Canadian Obesity Network, 2013).

3. *Adequate supply of safe water and basic sanitation.* Basic sanitation includes removal of garbage and safe disposal of bodily waste products.

4. *Maternal and child health care, including family planning.* Evidence shows that adequate and quality health services are associated with improvements in maternal, perinatal, neonatal, and child mortality rates and health outcomes. Worldwide, yearly approximately 303 000 women die during pregnancy and childbirth, and many of these can be avoided if pregnant women have access to quality skilled care before, during, and after childbirth (WHO, 2016).

5. *Immunization against major infectious diseases.* Globally, 2 to 3 million deaths per year are averted because of immunization, but an additional 1.5 million deaths could be prevented with an improvement in vaccination coverage (WHO, 2018).

6. *Prevention and control of locally endemic diseases.* Endemic diseases are those that are prevalent in people in a particular group, community, or region, but in relatively low numbers. A Canadian example of an endemic disease is tuberculosis in populations that reside in Northern Canada. A multifaceted PHC approach is required to eradicate this endemic disease (Health Canada, 2012).

7. *Appropriate treatment of common diseases and injuries using the PHC principle of appropriate technology.* Appropriate technology means using the right intervention or initiative, at the right time, so that the needs of the entire population are met. It is based on the best scientific evidence demonstrating effectiveness. It also includes using the right resources and the right health care providers, based on the local economy, using the PHC value of equity.

8. *Provision of essential drugs* (WHO, 2013b). Drugs sustain and can improve life in the case of many acute and chronic illnesses, providing an otherwise unattainable higher quality of life for many people.

Implementation of the PHC elements may be hampered by numerous factors, such as political will, cultural values (including race, age, or gender biases), lack of resources, or inadequate infrastructure. Poor outcomes of PHC initiatives may also result from misguided but well-intended decisions that reflect the values and norms of the dominant culture rather than those that involve the target population in all levels and aspects of decision making, from resource allocation to the parameters of projects or initiatives. In recognition of this type of bias, the Canadian Institutes of Health Research (2013) developed the Institute of Aboriginal Peoples' Health to better understand why Aboriginal/Indigenous morbidity and mortality rates are significantly worse than non-Indigenous Canadians' rates and to promote innovative research that will serve to improve the health of Indigenous people in Canada. Before receiving research funding, researchers must have demonstrated a good relationship with the Indigenous community they seek to work with, including consultation, information sharing, partnering with Indigenous community members, and demonstrating respect for the community.

THE OTTAWA CHARTER FOR HEALTH PROMOTION

The first international conference on health promotion was held in Ottawa in November 1986 with 212 participants from 38 countries (WHO et al., 1986). This conference resulted in the production of the Ottawa Charter for Health Promotion. The document was intended to be a worldwide charter for action, presenting strategies and approaches for health promotion that were considered vital for major progress toward individual and collective commitment to an earlier set, ambitious goal of "Health for All by the Year 2000" in a movement toward a "new public health."

A logo that represented this call for action was developed to include the following key components in a schematic representation (see Figure 8.1). The main graphic elements of the health promotion logo are one outer circle, one inner circle, and three wings that originate from this inner circle, one of which is breaking the outside circle. The logo incorporates five key action areas for health promotion:

a. Build healthy public policy. This means health must be on the agenda of policy makers across all sectors and levels of society—not just the health sector.

b. Create supportive environments for health. The way that society is organized (e.g., living and working conditions) must be addressed, as health cannot be separated from other goals.

c. Strengthen community action. At the heart of this action strategy is community empowerment—for communities to have a greater sense of ownership and control over their own endeavours and destinies. Community development is an important component of this strategy.

d. Develop personal skills. Enhancing people's life skills enables them to exercise more control over their own health. Education and institutional action are required.

e. Reorient health services toward preventing diseases and promoting health. The responsibility for health promotion in health services is one that is shared by all citizens; we must work together toward creating a health-care system that contributes to the pursuit of health (WHO et al., 1986).

The outside circle represents the goal of building healthy public policies, symbolizing the need for policies to "hold things together." The three wings inside the circle symbolize the need to address all key action areas of health promotion identified in the Ottawa Charter in an integrated and complementary manner. The upper wing that is breaking the outer circle suggests that society and communities, as well as individuals, are constantly changing, and therefore the policy sphere has to constantly react and develop to reflect these changes to enable building healthy public policies. The inner circle of the logo represents the three basic strategies for health promotion: enabling (strategies that ensure equal opportunity for people to achieve health), mediating (strategies that mediate among different sectors of society), and advocating (strategies that aim to make social and other conditions favourable for health), which are needed and applied to all health promotion action areas. Overall, the logo (Figure 8.1) is a visual representation of a comprehensive, multi-strategy approach to health promotion. Health promotion applies diverse strategies and methods in an integrated manner for effective action. Since 1986, the WHO has kept this symbol as the health promotion logo. It has undergone some visual modifications for subsequent health promotion conferences, but its essence has remained the same. The Ottawa Charter remains the key policy document of the international health promotion movement (Lindstrom & Eriksson, 2009), and its continuing value has been reaffirmed repeatedly during a further eight international conferences on health promotion.

Other Charters for Health Promotion

To date, there have been nine global conferences on health promotion. The second international conference on health promotion was held in Adelaide, South Australia, in 1988. Health

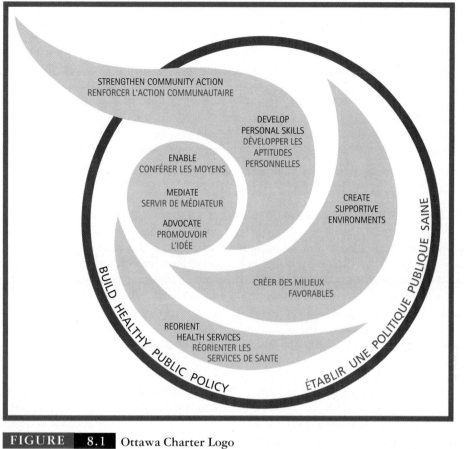

was asserted as a human right and a sound social investment; therefore, health is a fundamental social goal (WHO, 2009a). Recommendations arose for people's involvement in health policy creation and cooperation between sectors of society (WHO, 2009a). In 1991 the third international conference on health promotion was held in Sweden. At the time of this conference, public concern about global environmental threats had grown, and the need for a focus on sustainable development was highlighted (WHO, 2009a). The call for action that arose from this conference included addressing inequities and social justice, with millions of people living in extreme poverty and deprivation in increasingly degraded environments. Women were particularly highlighted as a population that remains oppressed in much of the world, with sexual exploitation and discrimination hampering their meaningful contributory capacity in creating supportive environments for health (WHO, 2009a). Education was declared a basic human right and a key catalyst to causing the political, economic, and social change required to ensure health. Military expenditure was identified as causing much more than deaths and disability to populations; it was also recognized as the cause of new forms of "ecological vandalism" (WHO, 2009a).

The fourth international conference on health promotion was held in Jakarta, Indonesia, in 1997. Health promotion action was declared to have a marked impact on the social

determinants of health and was the path to improving human rights and reducing inequities in health status. Poverty was identified as the greatest threat to health (WHO, 2009a). New partnerships for health must arise between and across different sectors at all levels of a society's government. For example, additional resources for education and housing, not just for the health sector, are needed. New investments for health should reflect the needs of vulnerable or marginalized groups, such as older people, children, women, Indigenous peoples, and populations living in poverty (WHO, 2009a). Empowering principles were woven throughout the declaration, and it was noted, particularly, in the declaration that "health promotion is carried out by and with people, not on or to people" (WHO, 2009a, p. 20).

The fifth global conference on health promotion in Mexico in 2000 led to the Mexico Ministerial Statement for the Promotion of Health and strategies to move ideas to action (WHO, 2009a). The ministerial statement acknowledged promotion of health and social development as a central duty and responsibility of governments (WHO, 2009a). It appeared that the main issue was no longer a lack of evidence of the effectiveness of health promotion, but rather that the problems lie elsewhere; for example, in political will to change.

The sixth global conference on health promotion, held in Thailand in 2005, led to the **Bangkok Charter for Health**

Promotion in a Globalized World (WHO, 2009a). This charter affirmed that policies and partnerships to empower communities and improve health and equity should be at the centre of global and national development (WHO, 2009a). Health promotion is based on the critical human right to have the highest attainable standard of health, without discrimination. The charter recognized that, worldwide, the vulnerability of children and exclusion of marginalized populations has increased, with increasing inequities within and between countries (WHO, 2009a). Although progress had been made in placing health at the centre of development, progress in the areas of political action, broad participation, and sustained advocacy had not occurred, and many proven-effective health promotion strategies had not been fully implemented (WHO, 2009a).

The seventh global conference on health promotion was held in the Republic of Kenya in 2009, and its findings were published in a document entitled "**The Nairobi Call to Action**" (WHO, 2009b). In this document, health promotion was affirmed as remaining the core and most cost-effective strategy to improve health and quality of life and reduce health inequities and poverty worldwide. The Ottawa Charter was also affirmed as remaining as relevant then for leading health promotion efforts as it had been in 1986. The eighth global conference on health promotion took place in Helsinki, Finland, in 2013. Leaders in health promotion came together to discuss how political decisions related to health are implemented in the form of practical actions. The **Helsinki Statement on Health in All Policies** that resulted from conference deliberations affirmed the importance of considering the health implications of decisions across sectors of government (WHO, 2013b).

Implementation gaps still exist in policy, practice, governance, and political will, resulting in the continuation of avoidable illness and suffering for individuals, as well as various social and economic implications for populations (WHO, 2009b). The issue is not lack of evidence of the effectiveness of health promotion interventions, but it is multi-factorial, stemming from deeper issues and mandates that drive policies and practices. Issues and barriers may be related to the difficulties inherent in situating health promotion responsibilities beyond just those of the health sector and in understanding that health promotion goes far beyond just promoting healthy lifestyles. Putting health on the agendas of policy makers, governments, social and economic sectors, industry, the media, and voluntary organizations, as outlined in the Ottawa Charter, is a daunting task.

Navarro (2009) reflected on the root cause of this continuing lack of progress in health promotion, which he attributes to the continuation of neo-liberal government policies that accentuate and promote class dominance and class alliances based on power. The result is a continuation of poverty as the major determinant of health of people in most countries (both low income and high income), so the "urgent public health project is to recover the representativeness of political institutions and make them accountable to the large sections of the population that have been disenfranchised . . . [as] disease is a social and political category imposed on people within an enormously

repressive social and economic capitalist system" (p. 15). This statement was not new. Rudolf Virchow (a pathologist) had been contracted by the Polish government to survey the 1848 typhus epidemic and submit a report for recommendations. He concluded in a now-famous statement: "Medicine is a social science, and politics nothing but medicine on a grand scale" (Taylor & Rieger, 1985, p. 548). Virchow's recommendations included improving income, employment, housing, and nutrition for the citizens, calling for political reforms in the areas of democracy, universal education, disestablishment of the church, taxation reform, and others. His recommendations were unacceptable to the government, and he was suspended in 1849 (Taylor & Rieger, 1985).

The ninth global conference on health promotion occurred in 2016 in Shanghai, China, and focused on creating a new vision for health promotion based on the United Nations 2030 Sustainable Development Goals (SDGs). For the first time, health promotion was positioned as the key means to achieve global sustainable development. Investments in health promotion can lead to a wide range of societal transformations offering benefit to the most disadvantaged members of society while improving the health, well-being, and quality of life for everyone (WHO, 2017). The conference was called a "political watershed" for health promotion, as "Over 1260 high-level political stakeholders were engaged in the conference, emphasizing the need for bold political action across sectors to promote health. The message is clear: health is a political issue and, therefore, political choices and commitments are crucial" (WHO, 2017, p. 1). The thematic areas of the conference focused on three pillars of health promotion: good governance, healthy cities, and health literacy (WHO, 2017). Over 100 mayors attended the conference to exchange ideas for creating healthy cities within the context of the SDGs.

SOCIAL DETERMINANTS OF HEALTH

Social Determinants of Health: Variations in the Literature

The concept of the social determinants of health has origins attributed to the discussion of the impact of physical and social environments in the Lalonde Report and expanded upon in 1996 by Tarlov to include housing, education, social acceptance, employment, and income (Raphael, 2009). These determinants of health were developed out of attempts to understand why members of different socioeconomic groups experience different health outcomes (Raphael, 2009). The CNA has understood for some time that it is critical for nurses to assess the multitude of factors that affect their clients' health. For example, ask an individual where their position is in their workplace hierarchy; "those lower in the [job] hierarchy experienced three times the risk of death from heart disease, stroke, cancer, gastrointestinal disease, accident, and suicide compared with those at the top of the hierarchy. These differences could not be explained by differences in medical care" (CNA, 2005, p. 1).

It is paramount that nurses understand that serious illness and early death related to poverty are connected to low social standing. Poor health and early death then are linked to social determinants of health, not just to accessibility to health care.

Poverty can have a hugely negative effect on people's health, extending across and highlighting the interconnectedness of many of the social determinants of health, such as social environments, social support networks, educational attainment, gender, employment status, and income and social status. Stewart et al. (2009) compared experiences of social isolation and perceptions of belonging among low-income and higher-income people in two Canadian jurisdictions. They found that low-income people experienced greater isolation and a lower sense of belonging than did higher-income people. Poverty was also closely connected to a sense of feeling prejudged, stigmatized, avoided, and isolated, preventing some lower-income people from becoming involved in community activities, thereby leading to further distancing and self-isolating behaviours (Stewart et al., 2009). This internalized marginalizing process can further magnify a person's feelings of disempowerment and worthlessness and lead to other detrimental effects on emotional, mental, and physical health. Stewart et al. (2009) suggest that programs and policies to reduce income inequalities by tackling the root causes of poverty may help increase a sense of belonging and decrease the social isolation of vulnerable populations. Children's health is particularly hard-hit by poverty; as Raphael (2010b) indicated, not only do children's living circumstances have an immediate effect on their health, but they also contribute to their health status as adults.

Various authors have added to or modified the social determinants of health. The Public Health Agency of Canada has retained the 12 determinants described in the PHPM (see Figure 8.2) but expanded on some: education and literacy, employment or working conditions, personal health practices and coping skills, and biology and genetic endowment (PHAC, 2011). In a Chief Public Health Officer's report on the State of Public Health in Canada, Butler-Jones (2012) stated that the determinants of health factors include income and social status, social support networks, education and literacy, employment and working conditions, social environments, physical environments, personal health practices and coping skills, healthy child development, biology and genetic endowment, health services, gender, and culture, all of which affect Canadians throughout their life course. These are very similar to the original 12 listed in Figure 8.2.

Newer additions to the social determinants of health have included more specific or narrowed areas, such as housing and Indigenous background. War or conflict and hope have been put forward and are being considered as determinants of health in the future. Raphael (2016) most recently suggested there are 16 social determinants of health: disability, early life, education, employment and working conditions, Indigenous ancestry, food security, gender, geography, housing, health care services, immigrant status, income and its distribution, race, social safety net, social exclusion, and unemployment and employment security. Raphael shared Indigenous ancestry is not often explored in most conceptualizations of the determinants of health but should be because "It represents the interaction of culture,

WHICH TIPS FOR BETTER HEALTH ARE CONSISTENT WITH RESEARCH EVIDENCE?

The messages given to the public by governments, health associations, and health workers are heavily influenced by the ways in which health issues are understood. Contrast the two sets of messages provided below. The first set is individually oriented and assumes individuals can control the factors that determine their health. The second set is societally oriented and assumes the most important determinants of health are beyond the control of most individuals. Which set of tips is most consistent with the available evidence on the determinants of health?

The Traditional Ten Tips for Better Health

1. Don't smoke. If you can, stop. If you can't, cut down.
2. Follow a balanced diet with plenty of fruit and vegetables.
3. Keep physically active.
4. Manage stress by, for example, talking things through and making time to relax.
5. If you drink alcohol, do so in moderation.
6. Cover up in the sun, and protect children from sunburn.
7. Practise safer sex.
8. Take up cancer screening opportunities.
9. Be safe on the roads: follow the Highway Code.
10. Learn the First Aid ABCs: airways, breathing, circulation. (Donaldson, 1999)

The Social Determinants Ten Tips for Better Health

1. Don't be poor. If you can, stop. If you can't, try not to be poor for long.
2. Don't have poor parents.
3. Own a car.
4. Don't work in a stressful, low-paid manual job.
5. Don't live in damp, low-quality housing.
6. Be able to afford to go on a foreign holiday and sunbathe.
7. Practise not losing your job and don't become unemployed.
8. Take up all benefits you are entitled to, if you are unemployed, retired, or sick or disabled.
9. Don't live next to a busy major road or near a polluting factory.
10. Learn how to fill in the complex housing benefit/asylum application forms before you become homeless and destitute. (Gordon, 1999; personal communication)

Source: Raphael (2009). Used by permission of Canadian Scholars' Press.

public policy, and the mechanisms by which the history of colonialism and systematic exclusion from participation in Canadian life profoundly affects health" (Raphael, 2016, p. 10). Statistics Canada (2016) published a report from a study of the relationship between social determinants of health and health outcomes for off-reserve Indigenous populations aged 15 and older, using data from the 2012 Aboriginal Peoples Survey. Outcomes were analyzed from the perspective of proximal (health behaviours, physical and social environments), intermediate (community infrastructure, systems, and resources), and distal (historic, political, social, and economic) factors. Key intermediate and distal factors predictive of poor health outcomes included living in a home needing major repairs, having less than high school education, being unemployed, having household income in the lowest tercile, experiencing food insecurity, and having no one to turn to for support (Statistics Canada, 2016).

Toronto Charter on the Social Determinants of Health A national conference called "Social Determinants of Health across the Lifespan: A Current Accounting and Policy Implications" was held at York University in Toronto in 2002. The conference focused on a discussion and analysis of the state of the social determinants of health in Canada. Policy implications to strengthen the social determinants of health were discussed, and a **Toronto Charter on the Social Determinants of Health** was written (Raphael, 2009). These determinants closely parallel the PHPM determinants of health, with specific differences, including identification of Aboriginal status as a separate determinant of health in Canada (as it is related to poor health outcomes), and the issues of food security and housing meriting their own stand-alone determinant status as well.

The Toronto Charter recognized that Canadian women, Canadians of colour, and new Canadians were significantly more at risk than others when there is deterioration in the quality of any of the determinants of health (Raphael, Bryant, & Curry-Stevens, 2004; "Strengthening the Social Determinants of Health," 2003). At the conference, the 12 proposed social determinants of health of the Toronto Charter (see Table 8.1) were examined as focal points for efforts to promote health and social justice for all Canadians by improving the quality of the determinants of health. The Community Health Nurses of Canada (CHNC) expanded the list to include 27 determinants of health, which are offered for comparison in Table 8.1 (CHNC, 2019, revised).

Other determinants of health could include mental health and obesity (International Association for the Study of Obesity, Canadian Obesity Network, & Centre for Addiction and

Table 8.1	Social Determinants of Health: Comparison of Terminology
Social Determinants of Health: Toronto Charter	**Social Determinants of Health: Community Health Nurses of Canada**
Aboriginal status	Aboriginal/Indigenous status
Early life	Early childhood development (early life)/Childhood experiences/ Healthy child development
Education	Education/Literacy/Education systems
Employment and working conditions	Employment and working conditions
Food security	Food insecurity
Gender	Gender
Health care services	Access to health services/Health service systems
Housing	Housing
Income and its distribution	Income and income distribution/Poverty
Social safety net	Social safety (support) networks/Social capital
Social exclusion	Social exclusion
Unemployment and employment security	Unemployment and job security/Precarious employment
	Physical environment Environment
	Biology and genetic endowment
	Social environment
	Social status
	Personal health practices and coping skills/Healthy behaviours
	Culture
	Race/Racism
	Having different abilities
	Migration/Dislocation
	Immigration
	Cultural continuity
	Relationships with territory/land
	Colonization
	Politics/War/Conflict
	Self-reliance and self-determination

Mental Health, 2012). Action strategies have been developed. The "Toronto Charter for Physical Activity" (Global Advocacy Council for Physical Activity & International Society for Physical Activity and Health [GACPA & ISPAH], 2010) advocates for governments, organizations, and communities to create environments to support physical activity for whole populations, as it "promotes well-being and mental health, prevents disease, improves social connectedness and quality of life, provides economic benefits and contributes to environmental sustainability" (GACPA & ISPAH, 2010, p. 1). Physical activity is identified as a powerful way to decrease non-communicable diseases and improve the health of Canadians and people worldwide. Policies and practices throughout societies influence whether or not physical activity becomes socially acceptable, is physically achievable, or remains unattainable. Urban design, school policies, accessibility to public transportation, and the media profoundly influence whether or not individuals have the opportunity to engage in healthy daily physical activity. Non-communicable diseases such as heart disease, stroke, diabetes, and many cancers are directly linked to physical inactivity, making it the fourth leading cause of death worldwide. Since the factors that influence physical inactivity are complex and multi-sectoral, multiple sectors of society should be included in the search for feasible solutions to the issue of inactivity. For governments and policy makers ready to motivate, inspire, and support communities and individuals to become participants in physical activity, a complementary document was developed with seven recommended "best investments" to increase population levels of physical activity:

1. "Whole-of-school" programs. This investment advocates for highly active activities for children, as well as opportunities for staff and families to participate in physical activities.

2. Transportation policies and systems that prioritize walking, cycling, and public transportation. This investment helps to improve air quality and ease traffic congestion.

3. Urban design regulations and infrastructure that provide for equitable and safe access to recreational physical activity, and opportunities for transport-related walking and cycling, targeted for people across the life course.

4. Physical activity and non-communicable disease prevention integrated into PHC systems. Health care workers, including nurses and physicians, have the opportunity to screen for potential issues and educate a large portion of the population on the importance of incorporating physical activity into daily life.

5. Public education, including using mass media to reach people to raise awareness and change social norms on physical activity.

6. Community-wide programs involving multiple settings and sectors, and that mobilize and integrate community engagement and resources. To successfully implement this investment in population health, whole-community

approaches are more successful at encouraging physical activity than are single-program delivery approaches.

7. Sports systems and programs that promote "sport for all" and encourage participation across the lifespan. This investment promotes adapting sports programs to reduce financial and social barriers; to appeal to women, men, girls, and boys of all ages; and to be accessible and inclusive for people with mental and physical disabilities (GACPA & ISPAH, 2010).

Jason's Story

The following story is offered as an example that shows the complex interplay of factors that determine the health of Canadians:

Why is Jason in the hospital?

Because he has a bad infection in his leg.

But why does he have an infection?

Because he has a cut on his leg and it got infected.

But why does he have a cut on his leg?

Because he was playing in the junk yard next to his apartment building and there was some sharp, jagged steel there that he fell on.

But why was he playing in the junk yard?

Because his neighbourhood is kind of run down. A lot of kids play there and there is no one to supervise them.

But why does he live in that neighbourhood?

Because his parents can't afford a nicer place to live.

But why can't his parents afford a nicer place to live?

Because his dad is unemployed and his mom is sick.

But why is his dad unemployed?

Because he doesn't have much education and he can't find a job.

But why . . . ?

(Federal, Provincial, and Territorial Advisory Committee on Population Health, 1999, p. vii)

Jason's story shows the cascade of societal inequities that contributed to a young boy's injury and hospitalization. As this story indicates, the health of Canadians may be determined more by societal values than by individual lifestyle and behaviour. The most appropriate question to ask should not be "Why doesn't Jason play somewhere other than a junk yard?" but rather, "Why is there a junkyard and not a safe playground in Jason's neighbourhood?" (Photo 8.2). The condition of the places where we live, work, and play directly affects the psychological and physical health of all the Jasons of the world, and also of their families, friends, neighbours, and the broader community (Mikkonen & Raphael, 2010). Without some form of post-secondary education, people like Jason's father are not likely to work for much more than minimum wage, thereby restricting the options of where a family can afford to live. Low-cost housing often exists in high-density population

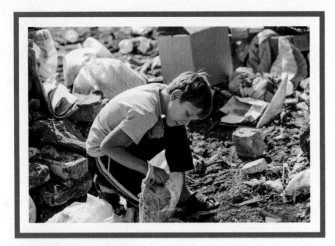

neighbourhoods, which may not have safe green spaces and parks for children and families to relax and play in.

The health of Canadians is largely determined by the social conditions people live within, and many of these social conditions are out of their reach or control as they are related to the distribution of income and societal wealth, affordable post-secondary education, employment status and working conditions, high-quality affordable housing, safe neighbourhoods, the availability and accessibility of health care, affordable medications, and the availability of social services during times of need (Mikkonen & Raphael, 2010). Nursing actions that would help promote Jason's health include addressing the root causes of poverty and an unjust society (Lind, Loewen, & Mawji, 2012). It does very little to change Jason's outcome to simply tell him to play somewhere else when the environment he lives in provides no other options for him and society does little to support the necessary social changes to make his living environment healthy (Frankish et al., 2006). Because they work closely with individuals, families, and communities, CHNs see opportunities to address health promotion issues as well as advocate for and support vulnerable communities to move toward self-empowerment and to work to create change through social action.

The CNA encourages all nurses to support the health of society by promoting public policies that address the social determinants of health. Nurses are in an opportune position to act as advocates, as nurses have more contact time with the population than any other health care professional (Mildon, 2013a). Because of this contact time and their educational preparation, nurses have a collective wealth of experience and knowledge. By participating in health research, nurses can also add to what is known about the relationship between the determinants of health and the state of health of Canadians (CNA, 2009) and use that knowledge to inform their work as agents of social change. Perhaps by changing the unhealthy environments and social conditions that a large number of Canadians have little choice but to live within, stories like Jason's would become less common.

Canadian Nurses Association Role in the Social Determinants of Health

In 2011, CNA president Judith Shamian and several CNA staff members attended a commemorative event in Ottawa to celebrate a quarter century of the Ottawa Charter and met the charter's Canadian (Irving Rootman), American (David McQueen), and European (Ilona Kickbusch) pioneers. These leaders described how the charter changed our definition of health care so that it focused on social justice and "offered three challenges to health professionals globally: to continue to focus on the social determinants of health to build the capacity for health promotion within individuals, communities, and society as a whole; to reaffirm our commitment for a more equitable world; and to encourage investment in public health through public support and working beyond the health sector with education and private industry" (Ashley, 2011, p. 20).

Nurses have the opportunity to reduce social inequalities and inequities and positively influence the health of Canadians through engaging in politics and policy analysis and acting as advocates. By upholding the principles of social justice, nurses can ensure the most marginalized and disadvantaged groups in society have access to services that address multiple determinants of health, which, once accessed, have positive benefits for the quality of health and living for all Canadians (Muntaner et al., 2012). Examples of opportunities to have a positive influence on the health outcomes of Canadians include the following nursing actions:

- supporting initiatives that reduce child and adulthood poverty levels by increasing financial assistance and social wages (social determinants of health provided through public funds);
- supporting initiatives that increase minimum wages to "living wages," to ensure that economic security, stable housing, and food needs are met;
- supporting campaigns and social movements that advocate for progressive taxation (where tax rate is based on income), the right to food security and affordable housing, and the enforcement of laws that protect the rights of socially excluded groups;
- advocating for intersectoral action on health at municipal, provincial or territorial, and federal levels of government to coordinate action undertaken by sectors outside the health sector;
- supporting political parties at provincial or territorial and federal levels of government that are receptive to taking action on the social determinants of health (such as those that are pro-labour or pro-redistribution of wealth); and
- encouraging greater workplace democracy to increase the number of unionized workplaces since labour unions are important determinants of generous welfare states, narrower social inequalities and better population health (Muntaner et al., 2012, p. 3).

To address health inequalities and the social determinants of health for all Canadians, the CNA (2012) recognizes the need for nurses to advocate for improvements in the social determinants of health approaches to address the disparities in physical and mental health outcomes for Canadians across the lifespan. The profession of nursing has a vast body of knowledge and experience and holds the potential to offer a strong and powerful voice for change, augmented by large numbers of nurses across the country. Collectively, nurses are the largest group of health care professionals in Canada. Nurses have a professional and social responsibility to become a significant part of re-shaping Canada's health care system into one that addresses the social determinants of health for all Canadians, rather than simply standing by and watching a re-shaping of health care focused on meeting the requirements of institutions (CNA, 2012).

POPULATION HEALTH PROMOTION

Health promotion involves a comprehensive, multi-strategy approach, applying diverse strategies and methods in an integrated manner. This characteristic is one of the preconditions for health promotion to be effective. Health promotion addresses the key action areas identified in the Ottawa Charter in an integrated and coherent manner.

Population health promotion is a process of taking action on the interrelated conditions (i.e., social determinants of health) that affect a population's health to create healthy change. Population health promotion focuses on maintaining or improving the health of populations and reducing disparities in health status between people, evident in the health issues that those with inadequate income face. In population health promotion, population health concepts are integrated with the principles that guide action on health promotion. The PHPM (Flynn, 1999) explains the relationship between population health and health promotion. It shows how a population health approach can be implemented through action on the full range of health determinants by using the multiple health promotion strategies outlined in the Ottawa Charter for Health Promotion.

There remains debate about the use of evidence in health promotion practice. However, an evidence base for health promotion practice does exist (Juneau, Jones, McQueen, & Potvin, 2011). If a narrow view of evidence prevails among practitioners, such as a belief that it consists solely of rigid empirical research, then the evidence base may appear to be slim. However, if an expansion into multiple styles of research is valued, then there is much research evidence that practitioners can (and do) use. There is a current trend away from individual-centred health promotion interventions toward those that target groups or entire populations, which reflects a long-awaited evolution of the field of health promotion from lifestyle-based health education to environmental and social justice–oriented health promotion (Juneau et al., 2011). Local relevance is now understood to be paramount in planning health promotion, and examples of participatory research projects are now emerging in the health promotion literature (Potvin, Junea, Jones, & McQueen, 2011) as some of the best examples of improving

local interventions. This approach to health promotion holds promise, whereas decades of attempts to change individuals' behaviour have met with little or no long-term health-promoting results.

Health promotion, not public health, has been described as our best link to social justice, social change, and social reform, because of its focus on the reduction of disparities that have an impact on health. This was espoused originally in the Ottawa Charter and this focus has remained since then (Dupere et al., 2007). As Marie-Claude Lamarre (2011) of the International Union for Health Promotion and Education put it, health promotion is a multi-dimensional cross-sectoral concept. Key values and principles provide a common basis for health promotion practice, which include "… a socioecological model of health that takes into account the cultural, economic, and social determinants of health; a commitment to equity, and social justice; a respect for cultural diversity and sensitivity; a dedication to sustainable development; and a participatory approach to engaging the population in identifying needs …" (Lamarre, 2011, p. 3).

The Population Health Promotion Model

The **population health promotion model (PHPM)** is a Canadian-developed model (visually represented in the form of a cube) for understanding the who, what, how, and why of intervention or action on multiple levels across a society to create healthy change. Nancy Hamilton and Tariq Bhatti from the Health Promotion Development Division of Health Canada developed this model in 1996, and Larry Flynn from Health Canada revised (streamlined) the model in 1999. To promote the health of populations, we need to understand what the determinants of health are, which goes well beyond an understanding based on genetics or biology. We also need to understand what people's needs are, develop action strategies for promoting health, look at where action should be targeted (i.e., at one level or across multiple levels), and understand the foundation and evidence base for helping guide nurses in choosing what interventions to implement. What are our decisions based on? Evidence includes research, evaluation, experiential learning, values, and assumptions, which are at the base of this cube because they are the foundations of professional decision making that create the frame of possibilities a nurse will view—what she or he may be limited by or opened up toward considering for interventions. All of the components of the cube, and the decisions that have to be made, arise from this foundation for evidence-based decision making (Figure 8.2).

The PHPM incorporates a number of values and assumptions: comprehensive action needs to be taken on all the determinants of health; multiple entry points for planning and implementing are essential; health problems may affect some groups more than others; solutions to problems involve changing social values and structures; one's health is a result of a combination of one's own health practices plus the impact of social and physical environments in which we live, work,

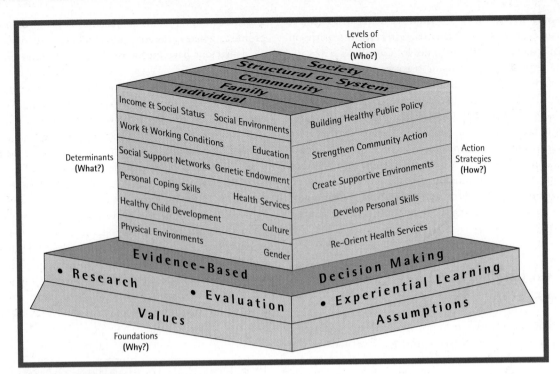

FIGURE 8.2 The Population Health Promotion Model

Source: © All rights reserved. Population Health Promotion: An Integrated Model of Population Health and Health Promotion. Public Health Agency of Canada, modified: 2001. Adapted and reproduced with permission from the Minister of Health, 2018.

learn, pray, and play; health-promoting opportunities arise in environments with social justice and equity and where relationships are built on mutual respect and caring (rather than on power and status); and meaningful participation of community members is needed. Understanding your own values and assumptions is important as this may create openings to listening to and valuing other perspectives, realizing that you do not hold the one "truth" and there may be multiple perspectives on a situation. Self-understanding creates the opportunities for working in true partnerships with others, especially if they feel you are willing to listen and include them in an authentic, non-token manner. The PHPM addresses the root causes of problems people face, and therefore suggests areas where the most powerful interventions to create healthy change should occur.

The social determinants of health include economic and social conditions that shape the health of individuals, communities, and societies (Raphael, 2010a). Health problems may affect certain groups more than others. If it is the responsibility of society as a whole to take care of its members, then solutions to problems might necessitate changing social values and structures.

Explanation of the Four Sides of the Cube The PHPM is a four-sided cube. The sides of the cube include social determinants of health, levels of action, action strategies, and the foundations of the cube become the fourth side. The intent of this model is to help guide actions to improve health, asking the following: On what should we take action, how should we take action, and with whom should we act? (PHAC, 2001). The social

determinants of health on the PHPM cube consist of income and social status, social environments, work and working conditions, education, social support networks, genetic endowment, personal coping skills, health services, healthy child development, culture, physical environments, and gender.

The side of the cube called "levels of action" draws attention to the fact that action must be taken at various levels within society, including at the individual, family, and community levels, including people linked by a common interest or by geographic setting; at the structural or system level (e.g., housing or education sectors); and within society as a whole (PHAC, 2001).

A comprehensive set of action strategies derived from the Ottawa Charter comprises the side of the cube called "action strategies." The base of the model provides a foundation giving direction for action on population health that is grounded in evidence-based decision making, research, evaluation, experiential learning, values, and assumptions.

Population Health and Population Health Indicators

Population health is an approach used to understand and improve the health of an entire population or subpopulations, such as children, older adults, or newcomers to Canada. Linked to health promotion that is not focused on individual people, a **population health approach** identifies and takes action to improve the root causes of health issues that impact the health of the overall population (PHAC, 2013a). Health inequities are addressed through research to determine the primary factors that influence health at the population level and strategies are subsequently developed, implemented, and evaluated to address influential and modifiable risk factors (Vollman, Anderson, & McFarlane, 2017). The factors that influence a population's health are usually interrelated conditions that occur over the life course. Applications of knowledge from past interventions can make a measurable difference to the health of populations.

Population health indicators are used to measure the health of populations as well as the progress made toward creating healthier citizens. Health indicators are closely related to the determinants of health, and examples of indicators include self-rated well-being surveys, life expectancy, number of people with a specific diagnosis or type of injury (e.g., lung cancer, hip fractures), number of hospitalization days per injury or diagnosis, death rate, potential years of life lost, and number and reason for emergency room visits, to name a few. Many of these measurement indicators are collected and collated annually to allow health care professionals to compare data, track changes, and identify areas of success and areas for improvement. Health status indicators can be found in Statistics Canada publications, community health profiles, census data, and health indicator reports (Health Canada, 2017) as well as in other reports and publications from government and large organizations.

As components of a population health assessment, it is necessary to have additional information on the protective factors and risk factors specific to a population (Kindig & Stoddart, 2003; Vollman, Anderson, & McFarlane, 2017). Assessments could include a community's levels of physical activity, breastfeeding practices, diet, tobacco use, alcohol and illegal drug usage, living and working conditions, number of crosswalks and safe places to cross busy streets, schools and their entrance requirements, number and condition of playgrounds and green spaces, presence of recreational centres, and pollution levels. Environmental scans are reports that summarize changes or noteworthy data in health status indicators and include current and emerging issues to support health care decision making, and these are discussed further in Chapter 13.

Population health interventions include policy and program development to address social, economic, and physical environment factors that influence people's decision making (Hawe & Potvin, 2009). Developing a population health intervention may begin by obtaining information from other health providers regarding past successful and unsuccessful strategies. Information gathered from online searches, literature reviews, and key informant interviews will help prevent duplication of unsuccessful interventions and may encourage health professionals to build on interventions that have been successful elsewhere. The population health approach coupled with the PHPM (Flynn, 1999) provides a framework to plan how to target the health of a population and develop interventions. An identified population could be either geographically located or an aggregate of people with commonalities such as age, interests, diagnosis, culture, or religious affiliation. Population health interventions may be implemented at community,

sector, or societal levels. Strategies developed to change the health of a population are generally different from those used to work with individuals. Development of personal skills at a population level is facilitated by social marketing interventions, which may include use of websites; bus, billboard, or television advertisements; and radio interviews or newspaper columns. Many people do not change their behaviour based solely on knowledge of what is best for their health. For example, smokers may believe smoking is bad for their health but because it is an addiction they continue to smoke. As a result, multiple action strategies to improve population health frequently include building healthy public policies that legislate healthy behaviour (e.g., tobacco bylaws, seat-belt laws, speed limits) or create supportive environments (e.g., tobacco cessation programs, soft playground surfaces, safe bike paths) for health.

Developing and implementing successful population health strategies that will make a positive and measurable difference in a population's health is challenging even when health care professionals have information identifying the social, economic, and physical forces impacting the health concern. Achieving health promotion goals can take years, oftentimes requiring multiple health promotion strategies implemented at various levels (ranging from individual to society) while simultaneously addressing multiple determinants of health. For example, one group may be lobbying government to pass healthy public policies while another is working with community members to develop personal skills at an individual level. Tobacco cessation initiatives are an example of a successful multifaceted population health intervention strategy. Over 60 years ago tobacco was identified as a cause of lung cancer, and in 1959 the CPHA began an anti-tobacco educational campaign targeting smokers. Over the following decades multiple strategies were implemented to move toward creating a tobacco-free society. Approaches used to build healthy public policy included (a) increasing taxes on tobacco to make it less affordable (especially for children and teens), (b) leveraging substantial penalties for selling tobacco products to those under 18 years of age, (c) lobbying efforts that resulted in bylaws that decreased secondhand smoke exposure, and (d) banning tobacco advertising. Efforts implemented simultaneously focused on developing personal skills through campaigns to raise the awareness of the dangers of tobacco use and provided strategies smokers could use to assist them to quit smoking. Targeted strategies for disadvantaged and high-risk groups with significantly higher smoking rates included reorienting health services to offer increased numbers and types of cessation services for individuals and included strengthening community groups to take action in creating environments where smoking behaviour was less convenient, along with social marketing campaigns that de-normalized smoking (Cancer Council Australia, 2013; CPHA, 2011; Gilmore, Tavakoly, Taylor, & Reed, 2013). In Canada smoking rates have decreased substantially; in 2011 22.3% of males and 17.5% of females smoked (Janz, 2015). Nevertheless, more population interventions are required as for example, in 2008 there were 19 000 lung cancer deaths in Canada, accounting for approximately 27% of all cancer deaths (Janz, 2015).

SOCIAL MARKETING: AN EXAMPLE OF A POPULATION HEALTH INTERVENTION

Social marketing is a term that was introduced in 1971 to describe the use of marketing principles and techniques to advance a social cause, idea, or behaviour (Kotler & Roberto, 1989). Social marketing is a strategy that uses proven concepts and techniques from the commercial sector to promote changes in social behaviours. The goal of social marketing is to encourage health-promoting behaviours, or to eliminate or significantly reduce behaviours that negatively impact a population's health. It has been described as a health intervention approach (Gordon, McDermott, Stead, & Angus, 2006). Used appropriately, social marketing holds enormous potential to create healthy change and influence social issues (Andreasen, 1995). Examples of successful long-running social marketing campaigns include ParticipACTION, with exercise promotion strategies. Other examples include promotions to increase breastfeeding or to decrease unprotected sex. Social marketing is most effective for populations that are considering change or have been unsuccessful when they try to change. Social marketing is also used when health promoters have a goal of improving the health of communities or populations that are not easy to reach via other methods. For example, it could be fairly easy to intervene with children who attend school as they are a "captive audience," but to reach other audiences, such as working adults, social marketing is one of the few successful strategies. Even though similar approaches may be used, social marketing campaigns are not education campaigns where the objective is just to create awareness of an issue. The objective of social media campaigns is to promote "socially beneficial behaviour change" (Grier & Bryant, 2005, p. 319). Although social marketing can be highly effective, one caution is that it is not always appropriate to use. Social marketing would be ineffective for people who actively resist change or who are entrenched in a particular behaviour with no interest in change. Alternate strategies may be required. For example, legislative intervention (passing a law that required everyone to comply) was required to achieve high percentages of seat-belt use in Canadian populations.

Six essential benchmarks of a successful social marketing intervention (see Table 8.2) have been described as (a) voluntary behaviour change with measurable objectives; (b) consumer research, whereby the intervention is derived from knowledge of consumers' values and needs; (c) segmentation and targeting, where different variables are considered for a more focused selection of target groups; (d) a marketing mix that uses the "four Ps" described in Table 8.2; (e) exchange, meaning the target group feels it receives a reward (tangible or intangible); and (f) competition, whereby competing behaviours are identified and strategies are developed to minimize competing forces to the targeted behaviour change (Gordon et al., 2006).

Before initiating a social marketing strategy, nurses must have a clear understanding of their target audience and what specific behaviour they want that group to change or adopt, and there must be a clear and concise statement of the desired

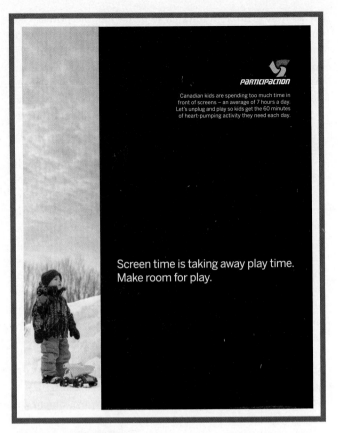

Screen time is taking away play time. Make room for play.

FIGURE 8.3 ParticipACTION Social Marketing Poster

Source: Courtesy of ParticipACTION

change. Most health promotion practitioners have many important messages they want delivered to a target audience. It is usually challenging to determine which one is the highest priority, and which is most likely to achieve measurable change. An important question to ask is therefore, "If the target population follows the suggested action, will I achieve my program goal?"

Social marketing is based on the four Ps of commercial marketing, which include offering the right product, at the right price, presented in the right time and right place, and promoted in the right way. The product being "sold" is an idea or behaviour related to better health—a social practice or a tangible object, with service or support offered to assist the target audience to adopt the desired behaviour. Examples of products could be weight loss or tobacco cessation programs. An important concept in social marketing is having a clear call to action. A call to action is not suggesting that a smoker quits or a sedentary person exercises but, rather, is giving them the next step toward attaining that goal, such as a phone number to call for help.

"AT RISK" POPULATIONS

"**At risk**" is a term often used to describe a group or population that has a higher risk of a particular illness (morbidity) or negative life outcome (such as mortality) than might be experienced by other populations (Kozier et al., 2014;

Table 8.2	Andreasen's Benchmarks of a Successful Social Marketing Intervention

Benchmark	Explanation
1. Behaviour Change	Intervention seeks to change behaviour and has specific measurable behavioural objectives.
2. Consumer Research	Intervention is based on an understanding of consumer experiences, values, and needs. Formative research is conducted to identify these. Intervention elements are pre-tested with the target group.
3. Segmentation and Targeting	Different segmentation variables are considered when selecting the intervention target group. Intervention strategy is tailored for the selected segment(s).
4. Marketing Mix	Intervention considers the best strategic application of the "marketing mix." This consists of the four Ps of "product," "price," "place," and "promotion." Other Ps might include "policy change" or "people" (e.g., training is provided to intervention delivery agents). Interventions that only use the promotion P are social advertising, not social marketing.
5. Exchange	Intervention considers what will motivate people to engage voluntarily with the intervention and offers them something beneficial in return. The offered benefit may be intangible (such as personal satisfaction) or tangible (such as rewards for participating in the program and making behavioural changes).
6. Competition	Competing forces to the behaviour change are analyzed. Intervention considers the appeal of the current behaviour to the alternative healthier behaviour and uses strategies that seek to remove or minimize this competition.

Source: Adapted from McDermott, Stead, & Hastings, 2005.

Roach, 2000). Although offering useful awareness of issues for prevention to focus upon, this approach can also devolve into creating or perpetuating stigmas such as racism, sexism, ageism, and other prejudices that affect health care professionals' assumptions about particular groups and their behaviours toward those groups, potentially leading to oppressive behaviours directed toward people considered to be at risk. For example, a common assumption made about social assistance recipients is that they are lazy and choose to be unemployed. If health care practitioners hold this stereotyped view of recipients, they may discriminate against them while developing care plans, and minimize their full access to competent and compassionate health care and resources. Similarly, another population at risk of further stigma by this labelling is Indigenous peoples. Although many morbidity (e.g., rates of diabetes) and mortality (e.g., deaths related to disease and suicide) statistics are higher for Métis and First Nations populations, and even higher among the Inuit, a deficit-driven approach situates the problems as lying within individuals rather than serving as a reflection of the wider social and historical contexts and inequities (Adelson, 2005). Discriminatory practices based on racism make the health care system unsafe for many Indigenous people (Health Council of Canada, 2012). See Chapter 22 on Indigenous health for more in-depth discussion.

As described by Roach (2000), dangerous assumptions could occur "if the basis for the excess mortality among certain racial groups is an intrinsic characteristic of the group, some might consider this a sign of 'racial inferiority'" (p. 261), and act accordingly. However, to believe the causes are solely external to that particular group may not be welcomed by politicians or other decision makers because "if the excess mortality rate is entirely due to various types of social injustices (such as racism and discrimination, resulting in a lack of education, underemployment, and poor access to care, resulting in a fatalistic self-destructive lifestyle), the moral and financial implications would be staggering" (Roach, 2000, p. 261).

Labelling a group of people "at risk" may be a double-edge sword, with either or both good and bad implications or outcomes. For example, this labelling can bring attention to and address the causes of health inequities, consider longer-term risk exposure, provide easier access to resources to address issues, and bring public and political attention and support to an issue. The downside of labelling a group at risk is that this practice may further marginalize and stigmatize a group, expanding societal assumptions of their incapacity or incompetence and providing a continuing justification of oppressive practices. This may lead to nurses making paternalistic assumptions that drive actions directed toward a group, as nurses may be rendered blind and deaf to that group's decision-making capabilities and voice.

Many traditional research approaches or programs for a population that has been labelled at risk have included interventions to prevent disease or promote health that focus exclusively on requiring those people to learn the facts and then change their own high-risk behaviour. These interventions have been less successful than those that have targeted government regulation or action (i.e., clean water, adequate sewage, housing standards, highway safety, or occupational safety) (Syme, 2000). The multiple risk factor intervention trial (MRFIT) has been described as one such classic failure by its own lead researcher (Syme, 2000). This was a multimillion-dollar randomized control trial conducted across 20 cities in the United States. The research focused on reducing the death rate from heart disease in men by lowering men's risk through behavioural change. Interventions with 6428 men targeted tobacco reduction, diet change, and control over hypertension. The men were closely followed by clinic staff and counsellors over a six- to eight-year period. They found that the men in the intervention group did not have better results than the men in the control (non-intervention) group (Syme, 2000). In addition to postulating why this and other trials had failed, Syme realized that the focus of health promotion interventions must shift. "In trials like MRFIT, nothing is done to change the distribution of disease in the population because such programs do not address the forces in society that caused the problem in the first place" (p. 80). He concluded, "it is . . . social, economic, organization, or political situations that are at the root of most problems" (p. 92). However, multiple levels for interventions are also important, and the most important of these may be the necessity of empowering individuals as a first step in the movement toward societal change (Syme, 2000).

Risk Communication

Risk communication refers to the transmission of information about an existing or imminent health or environmental risk, the anticipated severity of the risk, and the percentage of people it will impact. Communication of risk is vital because in our current social environment, risks change rapidly with the introduction of new and varied technologies. Providing people with timely information is the single most influential way to shape their decision making and subsequent behaviour. Communication must be strategic, appropriate for the target audience, and grounded in evidence from both social and physical science (Health Canada, 2006). Contact tracing is a form of risk communication that is discussed further in Chapter 12.

Risk management refers to the broad collection of activities involved in addressing health or safety risks. Risk management within health promotion identifies subpopulations or target populations that have a unique health concern or similar risk factors that can lead to several different health concerns. The subpopulation may have social, cultural, economic, or geographic commonalities. Risk factors can then be targeted in a way that is most effective for that population, where a generalized approach may have been too diluted and not specific enough to create a measurable change. Additionally, this approach is often more amenable to implementing several different concurrent strategies to address multiple determinants of health. It is easier to identify and involve community leaders, and the evaluation process is simpler (PHAC, 2013b). One example would be smoking cessation strategies that specifically target pregnant women rather than targeting the population in general.

LEVELS OF PREVENTION USED IN HEALTH PROMOTION

When nurses look at health promotion and the levels of prevention, they widen their lenses beyond disease prevention to include injury prevention, thereby capturing a broad area to promote the health of individuals, families, and communities.

Prevention interventions can occur at primordial, primary, secondary, tertiary, or quaternary levels (Starfield, 2001; Vollman et al., 2017). Primordial prevention (at a distal level) and primary prevention (at a more proximal level) promote health through an upstream approach using the identification of potential risk factors and the mobilization of policy and public awareness to avoid injury or illness. Primordial prevention refers to preventing risk factors from existing, whereas in primary prevention risk factors may occur; but for both, disease or injury has not yet occurred in the population (McPherson, Belton, & Watson-Creed, 2017). The focus is on the avoidance of illness or injury, addressing issues at a distal level (primordial prevention) before they become risk factors, or by identifying specific risk factors, or targeting particular populations (primary prevention) and then intervening to prevent or reduce the risk through health promotion activities and protective actions. Strategies can be aimed at preventing or reducing the risk of disease or injury from occurring at multiple levels; for example, by including health considerations across all sector policies, by improving or maintaining health, boosting the immune system, or preventing injury. An example of primordial prevention would be the more distal initiative of completely removing access to tobacco products and tobacco smoke from public venues (McPherson et al., 2017). Nursing interventions at the level of primary prevention could include (a) promoting properly installed CSA-approved car seats to transport newborn infants home, (b) offering smoking cessation programs, and (c) public education to help stop the spread of sexually transmitted infections (STIs) in all age groups. Safe housing, sanitation, and nutrition are other initiatives. Included at this level are immunizations against childhood diseases as well as nurse-managed mass immunization clinics against the influenza virus (CHNC, 2012).

The value of primary prevention is visible in Canada's history with the influenza virus. At the end of World War I, in 1918, Canadian soldiers returned home unwittingly transporting the Spanish influenza with them. From 1918 to 1919 the influenza virus spread quickly, becoming a worldwide epidemic that took the lives of an estimated 2 million people. The Canadian death toll from the four-year war was 60,000, but in sharp contrast, the Canadian death toll from the one-year Spanish influenza epidemic was 50,000 people. Many who succumbed were young, healthy people who died within a day of contracting the virus. In an attempt to control this epidemic, many non-essential services throughout the country were shut down, quarantines were imposed by each province, and face masks were required to be worn in all public spaces. As a direct result of this epidemic, in 1919 a department of health was created in Canada (Canadian War Museum, n.d.). Primary prevention interventions such as yearly mass immunizations against influenza have helped to prevent a repeat epidemic of such magnitude and devastation. Primary prevention actions have also minimized the spread of preventable childhood diseases, minimized the risk of injuries from car crashes, and helped to slow the spread of many communicable diseases, thereby helping to preserve the health of all Canadians.

YES, BUT WHY?

Hugh Papik's story of health inequity and social injustice

What?

On August 3, 2016, Maggie Papik received a phone call from staff at her uncle Hugh's Elders' home, telling her she needed to come and deal with him because he was drunk. Staff had found him lying on the ground covered in his own urine (Bird, 2016). Hugh was a 68-year-old Inuvialuit man who had had several strokes in the past and no history of drinking. Maggie transported her uncle to the local health centre, but the nurses there also insisted he was drunk; and he did not receive a physical assessment (Weber, 2016a). Six hours later a medevac was ordered to transport him to the nearest hospital, 120 km away in Inuvik (Bird, 2016). Subsequently, a CT scan of his brain showed he had a stroke, which had remained undiagnosed and untreated until it was too late. He was pronounced brain dead and later died (Bird, 2016).

So What?

Unfortunately, health care examples like this abound—to the point where they have been declared endemic in the Canadian health care system (Boyer, 2017). Hugh's experience therefore cannot be explained as a health care provider assessment and diagnosis error. Why did home care staff and clinic staff assume Hugh Papik was drunk and forego investigating the cause of his symptoms? On a surface level, one symptom of a stroke can be slurred speech, so that could be mistaken for the slurred speech of drunkenness. However, in a person who had a history of strokes, why wouldn't the first assumption from a care provider be that he may have had another stroke, and then a thorough assessment be undertaken? His medical history would support this as the logical first possibility to be ruled out, but that is not what occurred. The question cannot be answered without digging into the root causes underlying mistreatment or lack of treatment for Indigenous peoples. Racism is the root cause. A systematic review of empirical literature measuring direct and indirect health care provider racism suggested over two-thirds of providers show evidence of racist beliefs, emotions, and behaviours toward patients (Paradies, Truong, & Priest, 2014). There is a plethora of research confirming that " . . . Indigenous peoples frequently experience individual and systemic racism when interfacing with the health care system." (Browne, 2017, p. 24). Therefore, the extent of the issue is deep and pervasive, and a "Lack of provider awareness of institutional racism and the resultant structural barriers that patients . . . face are areas that need examination" (Nelson, 2016).

Now What?

In addition to examining personal nursing practices that contribute to disparities in health (Hall & Fields, 2013), solutions lie upstream. The systemic problems are poorly understood, or worse—not even perceived to exist by many health care professionals (Boyer, 2017). The structural and historical forces that influence racial disparities in health care must first be understood (Goodman et al., 2017; Hall & Fields, 2013). In this case, Northwest Territories health minister Glen Abernethy committed to addressing recommendations arising from an investigation into Hugh Papik's death, sharing that his death was a symptom of widespread systemic racism in health care delivery (Weber, 2016b). From the 16 recommendations, there are key areas CHNs could contribute to: (a) Recommendation 14 is to develop and initiate policies for cultural safety training for all health care workers (Government of Northwest Territories [GNWT], 2017). CHNs have expertise in partnering with communities; this expertise can be used to partner with an Indigenous community to develop cultural safety training that is grounded in an anti-oppression framework and a community's collective wisdom and strengths. Community strengths- and capacity-building health promotion is a hallmark of CHN practice (CHNC, 2011; Lind & Smith, 2008). (b) Recommendation 16 is to affect change within the health care system to incorporate Indigenous healing practices (GNWT, 2017). CHNs build relationships and trust in the communities they work with and could act as advocates and bridges to honour and support Indigenous healers in having their voices heard in a collective planning process for infusing Indigenous healing strategies into institutional health care practices.

Standards of Practice Fulfilled

#1 Health Promotion
- Considers the determinants of health, the social and political context, and systemic structures in collaboration with the client to determine action.

#5 Capacity Building
- Recognizes the unique history of Indigenous people, and incorporates Indigenous ways of knowing and culturally safe engagement strategies in capacity building efforts.

#6 Health Equity
- Participates with community members and advocates for health in intersectoral policy development and implementation to reduce health equity gaps between populations.
- Understands historical injustices, inequitable power relations, institutionalized and interpersonal racism and their impacts on health and health care and provides culturally safe care.

#4 Professional Relationships
- Recognizes own personal beliefs, attitudes, assumptions, feelings and values including racism and stereotypes and their potential impact on nursing practice.

#8 Professional Responsibility and Accountability
- Provides leadership in collaboration with the community to advocate for healthy public policy based on the foundations of health equity and social justice (CHNC, 2019, revised).

At the level of secondary prevention, the focus is to halt an illness if possible and perhaps effect a cure, or at least slow the progression of a disease through therapeutic treatments and medications. Examples of secondary prevention include (a) screening measures such as examining skin for signs of melanoma, (b) blood tests for diabetes, (c) testicular self-exam, (d) yearly cholesterol tests, and (e) colonoscopies. A remarkable example of successful secondary prevention was the advent of the Papanicolaou (Pap) smear. Used to screen for early detection of cervical cancer, the routine use of Pap smears has had a significant impact on women's deaths from this cancer. Since the 1950s the use of Pap smears has decreased the number of deaths by over 70% (Daley et al., 2013). The availability of and easy access to blood pressure machines throughout communities (i.e., in local grocery or drug stores) is an example of self-monitored secondary prevention. Individuals can become active participants in monitoring their cardiovascular health in part by checking their own blood pressure. When an unusual blood pressure reading arises, individuals can arrange to have their blood pressure assessed more thoroughly by a health care provider, potentially preventing damage from undetected and untreated hypertension.

In tertiary prevention, the goal is to limit disability and to rehabilitate or restore the affected person to the maximum possible capability, maximize their quality of life, and meet their self-identified goals. Examples of tertiary prevention include rehabilitation for people who have experienced a stroke or counselling for a rape victim. Nurses identify potential complications and implement strategies to help a person adapt, considering their vulnerabilities, strengths, and preferences. Nurses may provide education, monitor treatment effectiveness, or address adverse side effects. An example of nursing interventions using tertiary prevention is described in Chapter 32. In cases of a disaster such as the 2013 floods in Calgary and southern Alberta that left thousands of people homeless, CHNs may intervene at multiple different levels. These can include providing a range of services such as door-to-door first aid in the disaster zone, emotional support, safety and sanitation education, assessing individual and family needs, and connecting people with basic necessities such as housing, food, and medications. Community-level tertiary interventions include consultation and collaboration with community partners to focus on helping restore a community to its prior level of function. Quaternary prevention draws attention to identifying people who may be at risk for medical mishaps such as untested treatments or over-medicalization to address issues such as patient safety (McPherson et al., 2017) and the necessity of evidence-informed decision making to guide practice. In quaternary prevention the focus shifts to ethical practices that examine unnecessary investigations or treatment that may lack benefit or create harm and the inclusion of the affected people and even society in examining these issues (Alber, Kuehlein, Schedlbauer, & Schaffer, 2017). An example of quaternary prevention at a population level could include the recognition of the trauma incurred in a population affected by a natural disaster, consulting with them and minimizing their over-exposure to population health assessments or research on their experience.

HARM REDUCTION

Harm reduction is a philosophy and approach to health care delivery, programs, or policies, implemented with a goal to protect the health of, and reduce secondary harm for, individuals who engage in high-risk activities that are associated with poor health outcomes. The goal is not cessation of the high-risk behaviour, but rather it is to reduce the more immediate and related harms arising from engaging in that behaviour. A harm reduction approach ensures access to evidence-based information for individuals to make informed decisions about their lives and health and equal access to promotive health care services. Harm reduction requires a nonjudgmental stance that focuses on reducing potential harm from high-risk activities while treating individuals with respect and dignity. It is a health-promoting strategy whereby individuals who engage in high-risk lifestyles and behaviours can receive specialized health care services to address their concerns and minimize potential negative health outcomes and harms (International Harm Reduction Association, 2010; Pauly, 2007). These individuals may have difficulty accessing health care for a wide variety of reasons, including negative past experiences or fear of being judged.

Harm reduction strategies seek to address health inequities and bring meaningful health care to individuals who might otherwise be marginalized by some health care providers. Nurses working within this philosophy understand that the goal of care is to protect health by reducing harm but also recognize that complex social issues form the root causes of many high-risk behaviours (Pauly, 2007). Harm reduction seeks to ensure there is equitable access to promotive health care, medical care, counselling, and social services for marginalized persons. Harm reduction is not concerned with fixing problems or offering solutions; it is about meeting people "where they are at," providing nonjudgmental, compassionate care with the goal of reducing the secondary harm people might experience from engaging in particular high-risk behaviours (International Harm Reduction Association, 2010; Pauly, 2007; Taylor & Caine, 2013). Abuse of illegal and prescription drugs or alcohol; engaging in unsafe, unprotected sexual activities; and limiting exposure to secondhand tobacco smoke are examples of behaviours that harm reduction safety nets address. Providing at-risk individuals with products and health care services while they are actively engaging in harmful behaviours not only promotes health and reduces overall negative health outcomes, but it also ensures that the universal right to health care is accessible to some of the most marginalized, vulnerable Canadians (Taylor & Cain, 2013). As a philosophy, harm reduction recognizes the deeply complex relationship between root causes, social determinants of health, social justice, and health inequities that exist among different socioeconomic groups (Pauly, 2007).

Harm reduction programs benefit the health of the public as well as the individual by helping to control the spread of communicable diseases like human immune deficiency virus (HIV), hepatitis C, STIs, and preventable lung diseases. For example, tobacco smoke causes physical harm to smokers, but secondhand smoke also harms bystanders who are exposed to it in locations where tobacco use is not regulated (e.g., personal cars and homes). One harm-reduction alternative to smoking is the use of electronic cigarettes. For individuals who are unable or unwilling to abstain from smoking, electronic cigarettes provide the means to continue the habit under a model of tobacco harm reduction (THR) (Phillips & Rodu, 2013). Electronic cigarettes and other alternatives for THR, such as smokeless tobacco (oral snuff) and nicotine patches, do not create smoke that harms others (although further research is required on the effects of e-cigarettes). These are examples of harm reduction that benefits a community as the risk is reduced to only the user.

Examples of other harm reduction programs that nurses participate in include promoting the use of helmets with bicycles, distributing condoms to help control the spread of STIs, and promoting clean needle exchange programs to reduce the incidence of needle sharing and subsequent spread of blood-borne illnesses with people who use intravenous drugs (IVD). At the individual level, harm reduction models provide a safety net that mitigates the potential harm individuals may be exposed to. Nurses practise harm reduction in part by ensuring individuals have access to clean IVD supplies, access to safe disposal for used syringes, and supportive services to promote physical and mental safety for both the individual and the public. With mounting concern arising from the fentanyl overdose death crisis in Canada, there has been a call for extending harm reduction initiates to include promoting safe consumption for opioid users by providing medically safe alternatives to the drugs sold on the streets (Webster, 2017). Harm reduction in the context of STIs is discussed further in Chapter 31.

Safe Injection Sites

Vancouver's "Insite" is North America's first safe injection facility, operated by nurses. Operating from a harm reduction model, Insite opened in 2003 in Vancouver's Eastside. IVD use in the area was high, as were mortality rates among that community. Prior to the opening of Insite's 12-booth safe injection sites, users self-injected in alleys where they were at a high risk of experiencing theft, violence, arrest, or accidental overdose. After the opening of Insite, the fatal overdose rate decreased by 35% in and around the area, compared to a fatal overdose rate decrease of only 9.3% in the rest of the city (Marshall, Millroy, Wood Montaner, & Kerr, 2011). In this nurse-run clinic (employing nurses, counsellors, and support staff), clients who were traditionally hard to reach now had a safe place to inject, in addition to access to health care, addiction treatment, mental health counselling, social support, and a way to connect with outside services (Bard, 2011). At Insite, clients are given clean needles and supplies, can exchange dirty needles, are monitored for potential overdose while they inject, and are provided with emergency care if an overdose happens. There they can have their health concerns addressed and learn about the importance of using only clean supplies to protect themselves and others against the spread of blood-borne diseases (Jozaghi & Andresen, 2013). Expanded well beyond offering a needle exchange program, Insite addresses the need for health services and a way to connect people with other support services, mental, and physical care.

Insite's harm reduction IVD program has demonstrated its value by saving taxpayers $1.9 million a year in HIV and accidental overdose-related health care costs (Pinkerton, 2011). Nurses are instrumental in providing harm reduction services to Insite as well as to many other harm reduction programs and have been at the forefront of the movement to protect Insite from closure. In 2011, the Supreme Court of Canada ruled against the Conservative federal government's attempts to have the safe injection site permanently closed. Nursing organizations across Canada supported the program and its nurses during the long court battle (Keepnews, 2011). Nurses argued that "people at risk of addiction or people dealing with an addiction have a constitutional right not to be denied access to health services that reduce the risk of morbidity and mortality related to addiction" (Lynkowski, 2011, para. 4). The nurses' legal argument advocating for the constitutional rights of this marginalized group of citizens influenced the outcome of the Supreme Court's decision to keep North America's only supervised injection facility open at that time (Lynkowski, 2011). At the heart of the court battle was the drive to ensure the health and safety of a marginalized, vulnerable group of Canadian citizens. It became the responsibility of nurses to speak out against the closure of Insite and protect these vulnerable people by addressing immediate issues as well as confronting the social forces that create an environment of health inequity. The CNA tirelessly advocated for supervised injection sites, as shared by the president of CNA: "We presented to the provincial/territorial health ministers on harm reduction; called on the federal government to replace Bill C-65 with a new bill based on the principles of harm reduction, established best practices and sound research; and appeared before the media to further drive home the message" (Mildon, 2013b, p. 4).

Following the election of a Liberal federal government in 2015, the political landscape changed to one supportive of harm reduction initiatives, with the subsequent removal of many of the barriers to approving and opening safe injection facilities across Canada (Kerr, Mitra, Kennedy, & McNeil, 2017). Although multiple municipalities across Canada (e.g., Montreal, Toronto, Ottawa, and Victoria) have opened facilities or have plans to develop facilities, there are challenges with implementing these services. Issues still exist, arising from bureaucratic requirements and inconsistent levels of support locally, from municipal, provincial, or federal politicians (Kerr et al., 2017), and from NIMBYism (not-in-my-backyard) attitudes in non-supportive communities (Bardwell, Scheim, Mitra, & Kerr, 2017). Employing multiple strategies for gaining support from a diversity of community stakeholders has been suggested, as public and stakeholder opinions impact policy decisions (Bardwell et al., 2017).

More broadly, nursing's roles in harm reduction include developing, managing, operating, and promoting harm reduction programs; advocacy work to educate governments and society about the foundational principles and positive benefits of harm reduction programs; and reducing barriers to accessing health care that exist for people who are homeless, people who abuse substances, people who engage in sex work, or others whose lifestyles place them at risk for increased morbidity and mortality (Pauly, 2007). At a political level, nurses address harm reduction by confronting and addressing the underlying root causes of harmful behaviours: (a) poverty, (b) inequity,

CASE STUDY

(adapted from Benita Cohen)

One of the key roles of the CHN working in a public health setting is to support the family in the first year of the life of a new child. This includes assisting parents in their new role(s), promoting optimal child development, and connecting the family with appropriate community resources.

Imagine that you are a CHN who has been given a postpartum referral from the local hospital. The referral contains the following information: first-time mother, 17 years old; newborn male born at 36 weeks' gestation, weighing six pounds; unclear if infant's father is involved; very little contact with the health care system prior to giving birth; receiving social assistance; has no phone. You arrive at the address, which is located in a low-income neighbourhood, and find the mother alone with her infant in a tiny one-bedroom apartment on the third floor of a poorly maintained building without an elevator. You observe that the apartment has very few furnishings, dirty dishes piled in the sink, and empty junk food wrappers and containers everywhere. The mother quickly becomes tearful, stating that she doesn't have enough money to pay the rent, is estranged from her family and culture, and has few friends in the community. Her family immigrated to Canada from Saudi Arabia when she was 10 years old, but she dropped out of school when she was 16 because she was continuously bullied, hearing repeated messages that "her kind" were not welcome here.

Using the PHPM as a guide, answer the discussion questions.

Discussion Questions

1. What information do you already know, and what additional information do you need to obtain about the determinants of health affecting this family?

2. Give specific examples of one or more health promotion strategies that you as the CHN could use at the individual, family, or community level to address each of the following determinants of health affecting this family:

   a. Income and social status

   b. Social support networks

   c. Personal health practices and coping

   d. Healthy child development

   e. Access to health services

   f. Culture

   g. Race

3. What knowledge, skills, or attitudes does a CHN require in order to effectively promote the health of this family?

and (c) social injustice. Nurses act as advocates and are activists for social change to address the root causes that determine the health of Canadians. Nurses lobby governments and sectors across society to provide safe neighbourhoods, affordable housing, food security, fair working conditions and remuneration, safe and affordable educational childcare programs for working parents, timely psychological support for survivors of trauma or abuse, and the rights of women and children to be full members of society.

RESEARCH, ADVOCACY, AND ACTIVISM IN HEALTH PROMOTION PRACTICE

Nurses provide care for people from conception to death and in a variety of settings ranging from acute-care institutions to community-based settings and people's homes with the goal of helping people achieve and maintain their maximum level of health and wellness. Many of the people nurses care for have health conditions, illnesses, or injuries that could have been prevented with early intervention or prevention strategies, so nurses are well aware that an "ounce of prevention is worth a pound of cure." Nurses work closely with individuals, which results in an appreciation of the challenges that illness and injury cause, not only for the individual but also for their families, communities, and the larger society. They repeatedly hear about the chain of events that lead to life-threatening or life-altering outcomes for individuals and families. Nursing passion for health promotion and prevention activities results from knowledge of the effects of real-life situations on real people. The following Canadian Research 8.1 is an example of nursing research and action that seeks to partner with and promote the health of individuals and communities.

CANADIAN RESEARCH 8.1

Women-centred and culturally responsive heart health promotion among Indigenous women in Canada.
(Ziabakhsh, Pederson, Prodan-Bhalla, Middagh, & Jinkerson-Brass, 2016)

The goal of this research was to investigate the outcomes of a pilot project co-led by nurse practitioners and First Nation community-based women, using a balance of women-centred practices and Indigenous processes for heart health promotion that is situated in and responsive to a community's needs. Learning was shared from this Seven Sisters pilot project intervention and outcomes. "The Seven Sisters project was piloted as a gender- and culturally responsive model to promote heart-healthy activities among indigenous women" (Ziabakhsh et al., 2016, p. 816). Western biomedical approaches to health promotion may contradict (and even be harmful to) Indigenous approaches to health and healing and, in particular, neglect the mental and spiritual aspects of well-being. Traditional Indigenous processes (e.g., Talking Circles) were used to integrate Indigenous knowledge with Western knowledge to promote a holistic approach to heart health among women. Seven Sisters ran as a two-hour weekly women's group for eight weeks. Eight women (from different First Nations) with at least one cardiac risk factor participated regularly in the sessions, which each started with a Sacred Blanket ceremony and Talking Circle facilitated by a Cultural Lead, then an educational component and discussion led by two nurse practitioners, addressing a number of heart health topics. The nurse practitioners modified their teaching approach to be less didactic as they became more familiar with Indigenous teaching perspectives. Goals unfolded in the Talking Circles, which although initially envisioned as an ice-breaker to open conversations, they quickly evolved to become the main process used in all group sessions. Program outcomes included women eating more healthfully, and changes in the women's emotional health. Program participants shared the most meaningful outcomes for them were the integration of Indigenous cultural elements into the program format, the importance of fostering relationships among all the participants (nurse practitioners and the community women), and honouring one another's knowledge. The Talking Circles had fostered these connections, relationship development, spirituality, and traditional learning. The women valued being the recipients of teachings but also valued that they were able to pass along their own wisdom to others. Particularly important feedback on the nurse practitioners' role was an appreciation for their openness and willingness to modify the process and to partner with the women, becoming their sisters sharing power with them rather than exerting power over them.

Discussion Questions

1. What were key components of the heart health promotion intervention that were successful, and why were they successful?

2. How can Indigenous ways of knowing inform Western practise to provide a culturally safe model to promote heart-healthy activities among Indigenous women?

3. Using the PHPM as a guide, with a group of fellow students discuss potential interventions to support this population of women beyond the pilot project intervention.

The profession of nursing has a history of **social action** and **activism**. This includes leaders such as Florence Nightingale, who shaped the profession of nursing as a social movement intent on reform, and Lillian Wald. Early in the 20th century, Lillian Wald used activism as a public health intervention to effect change for the people living in poverty in the College Settlement on Henry Street in New York City. Her lobbying work led to changes for child labour and the development of a federal Children's Bureau (De Leeuw & De Leeuw, 1961). Lavinia Dock was at the forefront of the fight for women's right to vote, and Margaret Sanger, credited with creating the term "birth control," was indicted and jailed for her efforts to distribute birth control information to women.

Although social activism is a component of nursing's past, nurses have not used the route of social expression on a major scale since the days of Lillian Wald. In recent history, because more nurses practise in an environment that gives preference to the individual, they are not perceived as social activists but more as patient advocates. It is the attention to society, as a whole, that makes advocacy a social justice issue and a mandatory component of public health and community nursing practice. Nursing practice settings are already starting to shift from hospitals to work based more in community settings in Canada (Bartfay, 2010), which will create more opportunities for nursing practice focused on health promotion and different forms of advocacy and activism.

Ignoring the political realities of health, particularly health inequities, is one way of habituating them and rendering them invisible. We do not see what we have become used to, and worse, we make assumptions that normalize certain situations. Health professionals have an important and necessary role to play in countering this process through objective debate. To remain silent over injustices is an unacceptable—and political—act. According to the CNA (2000), the primary determinants of health and illness are social, political, and economic in nature. "To be concerned with health is to be concerned with the social context, and that nursing is, indeed a political act" (CNA, 2000, p. 1). Nurses have the ability to see the bigger picture, and this is where the roots of political activism lie. To be advocates for clients, patients, or communities may require becoming political activists. A rhetorical question can help nurses reflect personally on this issue: Should I focus on helping people adapt to poverty or focus on helping people learn how to influence the environment that has contributed to their situation of poverty? Which is most likely to lead to lasting change?

If nurses use upstream approaches to engage in health promoting practice with communities, it means they must move away from patching societal wounds with ineffective programs and instead look for the structural and foundational changes required to effect change on the social determinants of health. Structural changes arise from policy changes that direct the focus of interventions. Nursing action could include support for political action to modify the environment and strengthen resources for healthy living, reinforce social networks and social support within a community, and develop the material resources and economic base available to the community. In Jason's story, using community development principles (see Chapter 7), one example of an effective nursing intervention could include a focus on mobilizing support by creating awareness of unsafe play spaces and lobbying for the resources for building a safe playground for Jason and other neighbourhood children.

CONCLUSION

Health promotion planning and programming will always include multiple levels in which nurses can and must take action. Individual-level interventions will likely always include key components such as nutrition and lifestyle teaching; however, they will remain simply not enough if we wish to create better health for whole populations. This means that the social determinants of health must play a key part in all interventions if we wish to have any lasting changes occur. It is not enough to teach people about the hazards of smoking and implement stop-smoking programs; for every adult who quits smoking, there is a child somewhere who starts smoking. What stops us from addressing the root causes and engaging in primary prevention efforts? Often we implement band-aid solutions in a downstream approach when what is really needed are large-scale structural, systemic, and societal changes. These changes are urgently required to improve the health of Indigenous populations and address entrenched systemic and societal racism. These are the types of changes that require political will and political intervention, as expressed over and over again throughout the international health promotion charters. Nursing's scope of practice includes advocacy, which can be translated as the need for social action and activism on a larger scale, similar to the earlier pioneer nursing work of Lillian Wald and Margaret Sanger. Nurses must practise from a position of cultural safety, employing the principle of social justice, and must speak out. To remain silent, refuse to act, or refuse to even acknowledge that nursing practice addresses root causes of the health issues faced by people is to remain part of the problem and to condone the status quo. Do we want to continue to contribute to marginalizing practices that harm individuals and populations? Do we want to continue to provide ineffectual band-aids for all the Jasons who become entrapped in a revolving door of health risks they may not be able to change?

KEY TERMS

activism   (p. 161)
at risk   (p. 154)
Bangkok Charter for Health Promotion in a Globalized World   (p. 145)
downstream approaches   (p. 140)
empowerment   (p. 139)
harm reduction   (p. 158)
health   (p. 138)
health promotion   (p. 137)
health promotion movement   (p. 141)
Helsinki Statement on Health in All Policies   (p. 146)
Indigenous health promotion   (p. 139)
The Nairobi Call to Action   (p. 146)
Ottawa Charter for Health Promotion   (p. 138)
population health   (p. 141)
population health approach   (p. 152)
population health indicators   (p. 153)
population health interventions   (p. 153)
population health promotion   (p. 151)
population health promotion model (PHPM)   (p. 151)
prevention interventions   (p. 156)
primary care   (p. 142)
primary health care (PHC)   (p. 141)
risk communication   (p. 156)
risk management   (p. 156)
social action   (p. 161)

social determinants of health   (p. 139)
social marketing   (p. 154)
Toronto Charter on the Social Determinants of Health   (p. 148)
upstream approaches   (p. 140)

STUDY QUESTIONS

1. Describe Indigenous understandings of health and the role that ethical health promotion practices can play in empowering the First Nation, Inuit, and Métis populations.

2. Describe the differences and similarities among PHC, population health, and health promotion.

3. Define PHC, and describe its two values, five principles, and eight elements.

4. Identify the role that social justice plays in addressing the root causes of inequity within Canada's marginalized populations.

5. What is the limitation of using an approach to health promotion that focuses exclusively on behaviour change?

INDIVIDUAL CRITICAL-THINKING EXERCISES

1. Prior to reading this chapter, what did the term "health promotion" mean to you? Has your initial interpretation changed, and if so, how?

2. You are a CHN in an Indigenous community where there appears to be an increasing number of children with non-insulin dependent diabetes mellitus. Describe an upstream approach to community health promotion in this situation.

3. Visit the website of your provincial/territorial nursing association. Search for policy or position statements on PHC. Look for descriptions of activities that influence health care reform for Indigenous communities. Identify opportunities for CHNs to participate in the initiative. Reflect on how you can become involved.

GROUP CRITICAL-THINKING EXERCISES

1. Discuss your answers to Individual Critical-Thinking Exercise 1 with one or more partners. How do your responses compare? What factors influenced your original understanding of health promotion? How are these different from those of your partners?

2. What is the definition of health promotion that the WHO uses, and why is this the definition that CHNs use?

3. With a partner, interview a CHN in your community. Ask the following questions: What does the term "health promotion" mean to you? What are the main health issues in your area? Describe some of the health promotion activities in your practice. What are the barriers to engaging in health promotion activities? Analyze the responses with your partner. How would you summarize this CHN's approach to health promotion?

REFERENCES

Adelson, N. (2005). The embodiment of inequity: Health disparities in Aboriginal Canada. *Canadian Journal of Public Health, 96*(2), S45–S61.

Alber, K., Kuehlein, T., Schedlbauer, A., & Schaffer, S. (2017). Medical overuse and quaternary prevention in primary care – A qualitative study with general practitioners. *BMC Family Practice, 18*(99), 1–13. doi: 10.1186/s12875-017-0667-4

Andreasen, A. (1995). *Marketing social change*. San Francisco, CA: Jossey-Bass.

Ashley, L. (2011). Health promotion charter rings true after 25 years. *Canadian Nurse, 107*(7), 20. Copyright © 2011 by Canadian Nurses Association. Used by permission of Canadian Nurses Association.

Bard, R. (2011). Let's not lose Insite. *Canadian Nurse, 107*(4), 3.

Bardwell, G., Scheim, A., Mitra, S., & Kerr, T. (2017). Assessing support for supervised injection services among community stakeholders in London, Canada. *International Journal of Drug Policy, 48,* 27–33.

Bartfay, W. J. (2010). A brief history of community health nursing in Canada. In J. E. Hitchcock, P. E. Schubert, S. A. Thomas, & W. J. Bartfay (Eds.), *Community health nursing: Caring in action* (1st Canadian ed., pp. 11–22). Toronto, ON: Nelson Education.

Bird, H. (2016, August 15). Inuvialuit woman says uncle's stroke mistaken for drunkenness. *CBC News.* Retrieved from http://www.cbc.ca/news/canada/north/hugh-papik-stroke-racism-1.3719372

Bourque Bearskin, R. L., Cameron, B. L., King, M., Weber-Pillwax, C., Dion Stout, M., Voyageur, E., . . . Martial, R. (2016). Mamowoh Kamatowin, "Coming together to help each other in wellness": Honouring Indigenous nursing knowledge. *International Journal of Indigenous Health, 11*(1), 18–33.

Boyer, Y. (2017). Healing racism in Canadian health care. *Canadian Medical Association Journal, 189*(46), E1408–E1409.

Browne, A. (2017). Moving beyond description: Closing the health equity gap by redressing racism impacting Indigenous populations. *Social Science & Medicine, 184,* 23–26. https://doi.org/10.1016/j.socscimed.2017.04.045

Butler-Jones, D. (2012). *The Chief Public Health Officer's report on the state of public health in Canada, 2012: Influencing health—The importance of sex and gender.* Retrieved from http://publichealth.gc.ca/CPHOreport

Cameron, B. L., del Pilar Carmargo Plazas, M., Salas, A. S., Bourque Bearskin, R. L., & Hungler, K. (2014). Understanding inequalities in access to health care services for Aboriginal people: A call for nursing action. *Advances in Nursing Science, 37*(3), E1–E16.

Canadian Health Coalition. (2009). The history of health care. Retrieved from http://medicare.ca/main/the-facts/the-history-of-medicare

Canadian Institutes of Health Research. (2013). About Institute of Aboriginal Peoples' Health. Retrieved from http://www.cihr-irsc.gc.ca/e/8172.html

Canadian Nurses Association (CNA). (2000). Nursing is a political act—The bigger picture. *Nursing Now: Issues and Trends in Canadian nursing, 5*(8), 1–4.

Canadian Nurses Association (CNA). (2005). Social determinants of health and nursing: A summary of the issues. Retrieved from http://www.cna-aiic.ca/~/media/cna/page%20content/pdf%20en/2013/07/26/10/38/bg8_social_determinants_e.pdf

Canadian Nurses Association (CNA). (2009). *Determinants of health.* Ottawa, ON: Author.

Canadian Nurses Association (CNA). (2010). Social justice . . . a means to an end, an end in itself (2nd ed.). Retrieved from http://www2.cna-aiic.ca/CNA/documents/pdf/publications/Social_Justice_2010_e.pdf

Canadian Nurses Association (CNA). (2012). A nursing call to action: The health of our nation, the future of our health system. Retrieved from http://www2.cna-aiic.ca/CNA/documents/pdf/publications/nec/NEC_Report_e.pdf

Canadian Obesity Network. (2013). Creating a credible community for change. Retrieved from http://www.obesitynetwork.ca/about

Canadian Public Health Association (CPHA). (2010). Canada's leadership in addressing the social determinants of health. Retrieved from http://www.cpha.ca/en/programs/history/achievements/01-sdh/leadership.aspx

Canadian Public Health Association (CPHA). (2011). The winnable battle: Ending tobacco use in Canada. Retrieved from http://www.cpha.ca/uploads/positions/position-paper-tobacco_e.pdf

Canadian War Museum. (n.d.). Retrieved from http://www.warmuseum.ca/cwm/exhibitions/guerre/influenza-e.aspx

Cancer Council Australia. (2013). National cancer prevention policy: Tobacco control. Retrieved from http://wiki.cancer.org.au/prevention/Tobacco_control/Effective_interventions

Community Health Nurses Association of Canada (CHNC). (2008). *Canadian community health nursing standards of practice.* Retrieved from http://www.chnc.ca/documents/chn_standards_of_practice_mar08_english.pdf

Community Health Nurses of Canada (CHNC). (2019, revised). *Canadian community health nursing: Professional practice model & standards of practice.* St. John's, NL: Author. Retrieved from https://www.chnc.ca/documents/CHNC-ProfessionalPracticeModel-EN/index.html

Community Health Nurses of Canada (CHNC). (2012). *Public health nursing: Primary prevention of chronic diseases.* Retrieved from http://www.chnc.ca/documents/2012maychnccdpreport.pdf

Daley, E., Perrin, K., Vamos, C., Hernandez, N., Anstey, E., Baker, E., . . . Ebbert, J. (2013). Confusion about Pap smears: Lack of knowledge among high risk women. *Journal of Women's Health, 22*(1), 67–74. doi:10.1089/jwh.2012.3667

De Leeuw, A., & De Leeuw, C. (1961). *Nurses who led the way.* Racine, WI: Whitman.

Dion Stout, M. (2015). Atikowisi miyw-ayawin, ascribed health and wellness, to kaskitamasowin miyw-ayawin, achieved health and wellness: Shifting the paradigm. In M. Greenwood, S. De Leeuw, N. M. Lindsay, & C. Reading (Eds.). *Determinants of Indigenous peoples' health in Canada: Beyond the social* (pp. 143–151). Toronto, ON: Canadian Scholars' Press.

Dupere, S., Ridde, V., Carroll, S., O'Neill, M., Rootman, I., & Pederson, A. (2007). Conclusion: The rhizome and the tree. In M. O'Neill, A. Pederson, S. Dupere, & I. Rootman (Eds.),

Health Promotion in Canada: Critical perspectives (2nd ed., pp. 371–388). Toronto, ON: Canadian Scholars' Press.

Epp, J. (1986). *Achieving health for all: A framework for health promotion.* Ottawa, ON: Minister of Supply and Services Canada.

Fawcett, S., Abeykoon, P., Arora, M., Dobe, M., Galloway-Gilliam, L., Liburd, L., & Munodawafa, D. (2010). Constructing an action agenda for community empowerment at the 7th Global Conference on Health Promotion in Nairobi. *Global Health Promotion, 17*(4), 52–56.

Federal, Provincial, and Territorial Advisory Committee on Population Health. (1999). *Towards a healthy future: Second report on the health of Canadians.* Charlottetown, PEI: Author.

Fisher, M. P., & Elnitsky, C. (2012). Health and social services integration: A review of concepts and models. *Social Work in Public Health, 27*(5), 441–468. doi:10.1080/19371918.201 0.525149

Flynn, L. (1999). *Population health promotion model.* Revised from original model developed by N. Hamilton and T. Bhatti, Health Promotion Development Division, Health Canada, 1996. Winnipeg, MB: Health Canada, Manitoba/ Saskatchewan Region.

Frank, L. (2013). Person centered care, autonomy, and the definition of health. *The American Journal of Bioethics, 13*(8), 59. doi:10.1080/19371918.2010.525149

Frankish, C. J., Moulton, G., Rootman, I., Cole, C., & Gray, D. (2006). Setting a foundation: Underlying values and structures of health promotion in primary health care settings. *Primary Health Care Research and Development, 7*(2), 172–182.

Franco-Paredes, C., Zeuli, J., Hernandez-Ramos, I., & Santos-Preciado, J. I. (2010). Preserving idealism in global health promotion. *Global Health Promotion, 17*(4), 57–60.

Gilmore, A. B., Tavakoly, B., Taylor, G., & Reed, H. (2013). Understanding tobacco industry pricing strategy and whether it undermines tobacco tax policy: The example of the UK cigarette market. *Addiction, 108*(7), 1317–1326.

Global Advocacy Council for Physical Activity & International Society for Physical Activity and Health (GACPA & ISPAH). (2010). *The Toronto charter for physical activity: A global call to action.* Used by permission of Global Advocacy Council for Physical Activity, International Society for Physical Activity and Health. Retrieved from http://www.activecanada2020.ca/background-documents/toronto-charter

Goodman, A., Fleming, K., Markwick, N., Morrison, T., Lagimodiere, L., Kerr, T., & Western Aboriginal Harm Reduction Society. (2017). "They treated me like crap and I know it was because I was Native": The healthcare experiences of Aboriginal peoples living in Vancouver's inner city. *Social Science & Medicine, 178,* 87–94.

Gordon, R., McDermott, L., Stead, M., & Angus, K. (2006). The effectiveness of social marketing interventions for health improvement: What's the evidence? *Public Health, 120*(12), 1133–1139.

Government of Northwest Territories (GWT). (2017). Recommendations from the external investigation. Retrieved from www.cbc.ca/news/canada/north/hugh-papik-aklavik-stroke-death-review-recommendations-1.4001297

Grier, S., & Bryant, C. A. (2005). Social marketing in public health. *Annual Review of Public Health, 26,* 319–330. doi: 10.1146/annurev.publhealth.26.021304.144610

Hall, J. M., & Fields, B. (2013). Continuing the conversation in nursing on race and racism. *Nursing Outlook, 61,* 164–173.

Hawe, P., & Potvin, L. (2009). What is population health intervention research? *Canadian Journal of Public Health, 100*(1), I8–I14.

Health Canada. (2006). Strategic risk communications framework. Retrieved from http://www.phac-aspc.gc.ca/publicat/2007/risk-com/pdf/ris-comm_e.pdf

Health Canada. (2012). First Nation & Inuit health: Tuberculosis. Retrieved from http://www.hc-sc.gc.ca/fniah-spnia/diseases-maladies/tuberculos/index-eng.php

Health Canada. (2017). *Health indicators.* Retrieved from https://www.canada.ca/en/health-canada/services/health-care-system/health-indicators.html

Health Council of Canada. (2012). *Empathy, dignity, and respect: Creating cultural safety for Aboriginal people in urban health care.* Toronto, ON: Author.

Hills, M., Carroll, S., & Vollman, A. (2007). Health promotion and health professions in Canada: Toward a shared vision. In M. O'Neill, A. Pederson, S. Dupere, & I. Rootman (Eds.), *Health promotion in Canada: Critical perspectives* (2nd ed., pp. 330–346). Toronto, ON: Canadian Scholars' Press.

Hoad, T. F. (Ed.). (1996). *The concise Oxford dictionary of English etymology.* Oxford, UK: Oxford University.

International Association for the Study of Obesity, Canadian Obesity Network, & Centre for Addiction and Mental Health. (2012). *Toronto charter on obesity & mental health.* Retrieved from http://www.worldobesity.org/site_media/uploads/Toronto_Charter_on_Obesity_Mental_Health.pdf

International Harm Reduction Association. (2010). What is harm reduction? Retrieved from http://www.ihra.net/files/2010/08/10/Briefing_What_is_HR_English.pdf

Janz, T. (2015). *Current smoking trends.* (Statistics Canada Catalogue no. 82-624-X). Retrieved from https://www.statcan.gc.ca/pub/82-624-x/2012001/article/11676-eng.htm

Jozaghi, E., & Andresen, M. A. (2013). Should North America's first and only supervised injection facility (In Site) be expanded in British Columbia, Canada? *Harm Reduction Journal, 10*(1), 1–9. doi:10.1186/1477-7517-10-1

Juneau, C.-E., Jones, C. M., McQueen, D. V., & Potvin, L. (2011). Evidence-based health promotion: An emerging field. *Global Health Promotion, 18*(1), 79–89.

Kaplan, R. M. (2000). Promoting wellness: Biomedical versus outcomes models. In M. S. Jamner, & D. Stokols (Eds.), *Promoting human wellness: New frontiers for research, practice, and policy* (pp. 44–77). Berkeley, CA: University of California.

Keepnews, D. M. (2011). Canada's Insite decision: A victory for public health. *Policy, Politics, & Nursing Practice, 12*(3), 131–132. doi:10.1177/1527154411431154

Kerr, T., Mitra, S., Kennedy, M. C., & McNeil, R. (2017). Supervised injection facilities in Canada: past, present and future. *Harm Reduction Journal, 14*(28), 1–9. doi: 10.1186/s12954-017-0154-1

Kindig, D., & Stoddart, G. (2003). What is population health? *American Journal of Public Health, 93*(3), 380–383.

Kleinman, A., & Petryna, A. (2001). Health, anthropological aspects. In *International encyclopedia of the social & behavioral sciences*. New York, NY: Elsevier.

Kotler, P., & Roberto, E. L. (1989). *Social marketing: Strategies for changing public behavior*. New York, NY: The Free Press.

Kozier, B., Erb, G., Berman, A., Snyder, S. J., Buck, M., Yiu, L., & Stamler, L. L. (2014). *Fundamentals of Canadian nursing: Concepts, process, and practice* (3rd Canadian ed.). Toronto, ON: Pearson.

Lalonde, M. (1974). *A new perspective on the health of Canadians: A working document*. Ottawa, ON: Government of Canada.

Lamarre, M.-C. (2011). 2011 . . . a year of celebrations. *Global Health Promotion, 18*(4), 3–4. Copyright © 2011 by Sage Publications Ltd. (UK). Used by permission of Sage Publications Ltd. (UK).

Lind, C., & Smith, D. (2008). Analyzing the state of community health nursing: Advancing from deficit to strengths-based practice using appreciative inquiry. *Advances in Nursing Science, 31*(1), 28–41.

Lind, C., Loewen, S., & Mawji, A. (2012). Health promotion. In D. D'Amico, C. Barbarito, C. Twomey, & N. Harder (Eds.), *Health & Physical Assessment in Nursing* (Canadian ed., pp. 22–36). Toronto, ON: Pearson Canada.

Lindstrom, B., & Eriksson, M. (2009). The salutogenic approach to the making of HiAP/healthy public policy: Illustrated by a case study. *Global Health Promotion, 16*(1), 17–28.

Lynkowski, D. (2011). CPHA applauds Supreme Court decision on Vancouver's supervised injection facility. *CPHA Health Digest, 35*(3). Copyright © 2011 by Canadian Public Health Association. Used by permission of Canadian Public Health Association. Retrieved from http://www.cpha.ca/en/about/digest/xxxv-3/xxxv-3-02.aspx

Marshall, B. D. L., Millroy, M.-J., Wood, E., Montaner, J. S. G., & Kerr, T. (2011). Reduction in overdose mortality after the opening of North America's first medically supervised safer injecting facility: A retrospective population based study. *Lancet, 377*, 1429–1437. doi:10:1016/S01406736(10)62353-7

McDermott, L., Stead, M., & Hastings, G. (2005). What is and what is not social marketing: the challenge of reviewing the evidence. *Journal of Marketing Management, 21*(5–6), 545–553.

McKenzie, J. F., Neiger, B. L., & Thackeray, R. (2013). *Planning, implementing & evaluating health promotion programs: A primer* (6th ed.). Boston, MA: Pearson.

McKinlay, J. (1994). *An annotated bibliography of works held in the library of Australasia*. Adelaide, Australia: Royal Geographical Society of Australasia, South Australian Branch.

McPhail-Bell, K., Bond, C., Brough, M., & Fredericks, B. (2015). 'We don't tell people what to do': Ethical practice and Indigenous health promotion. *Health Promotion Journal of Australia, 26*, 195–199.

McPherson, N. C., Belton, K. L., & Watson-Creed, G. (2017). Population health action: Prevention and harm reduction. In A. R. Vollman, E. T. Anderson, & J. McFarlane (Eds.), *Canadian community as partner: Theory & multidisciplinary practice* (4th ed., pp. 157–170). Philadelphia, PA: Wolters Kluwer.

Mikkonen, J., & Raphael, D. (2010). *Social determinants of health: The Canadian facts*. Toronto, ON: York University School of Health Policy and Management.

Mildon, B. (2013a). Turning awareness into advocacy. *Canadian Nurse, 109*(8), 4.

Mildon, B. (2013b). A force for social good. *Canadian Nurse, 109*(9), p. 4.

Muntaner, C., Ng, E., & Chung, H. (2012). *Better health: An analysis of public policy and programming focusing on the determinants of health and health outcomes that are effective in achieving the healthiest populations*. Ottawa, ON: Canadian Health Services Research Foundation.

Navarro, V. (2009). What we mean by social determinants of health. *Global Health Promotion, 16*(1), 5–16.

Nelson, S. (2016). Race, racism, and health disparities: What can I do about it? *Creative Nursing, 22*(3), 161–165.

Paradies, Y., Truong, M., & Priest, N. (2014). A systematic review of the extent and measurement of healthcare provider racism. *Journal of General Internal Medicine, 29*(2), 364–387.

ParticipACTION Archive Project (n.d.). *Historic timeline*. Retrieved from http://scaa.sk.ca/gallery/participaction/english/structure/timeline.html

Pauly, B. (2007). Harm reduction through a social justice lens. *International Journal of Drug Policy, 19*, 4–10. doi:10.1016/j.drugpo.2007.11.005

Payne, L. (1983). Health: A basic concept in nursing theory. *Journal of Advanced Nursing, 8*, 393–395.

Phillips, C. V., & Rodu, B. (2013). Tobacco harm reduction: opportunity and opposition. *Drugs and Alcohol Today, 13*(2), 73–78. doi:10.1108/DAT-032013-0015

Pinkerton, S. D. (2011). How many HIV infections are prevented by Vancouver Canada's supervised injection facility? *International Journal of Drug Policy, 22*(3), 179–183. doi: 10:1016/j.drugpo.2011.03.003

Potvin, L., Juneau, C.-E., Jones, C. M., & McQueen, D. V. (2011). How is evidence used for planning, implementation and evaluation of health promotion? A global collection of case studies, *Global Health Promotion, 18*(1), 7–8.

Public Health Agency of Canada (PHAC). (2001). © All rights reserved. Population Health Promotion: An Integrated Model of Population Health and Health Promotion. Public Health Agency of Canada, modified: 2001. Adapted and reproduced with permission from the Minister of Health, 2018.

Public Health Agency of Canada (PHAC). (2011). What determines health? Retrieved from http://www.phac-aspc.gc.ca/ph-sp/determinants/index-eng.php

Public Health Agency of Canada (PHAC). (2013a). What is the population health approach? Retrieved from http://www.phac-aspc.gc.ca/ph-sp/approach-approche/appr-eng.php

Public Health Agency of Canada (PHAC). (2013b). Health promotion. Retrieved from http://www.phac-aspc.gc.ca/hp-ps/index-eng.php

Raeburn, J., & Rootman, I. (2007). A new appraisal of the concept of health. In M. O'Neill, A. Pederson, S. Dupere, & I. Rootman (Eds.), *Health promotion in Canada: Critical perspectives* (2nd ed., pp. 19–31). Toronto, ON: Canadian Scholars' Press.

Raphael, D. (2009). *Social determinants of health* (2nd ed.). Toronto, ON: Canadian Scholars' Press.

Raphael, D. (2010a). Setting the stage: Why quality of life? Why health promotion? In D. Raphael (Ed.), *Health promotion and quality of life in Canada: Essential readings* (pp. 1–13). Toronto, ON: Canadian Scholars' Press.

Raphael, D. (2010b). The health of Canada's children. Part III: Public policy and the social determinants of children's health. *Paediatrics & Child Health, 15*(3), 143–149.

Raphael, D. (2016). *Social determinants of health: Canadian perspectives* (3rd ed.). Toronto, ON: Canadian Scholar' Press.

Raphael, D., Bryant, T., & Curry-Stevens, A. (2004). Toronto Charter outlines future health policy directions for Canada and elsewhere. *Health Promotion International, 19*(2), 269–273.

Richmond, C. (2015). The relatedness of people, land, and health. In M. Greenwood, S. De Leeuw, N. M. Lindsay, & C. Reading (Eds.), *Determinants of Indigenous peoples' health in Canada: Beyond the social* (pp. 47–63). Toronto, ON: Canadian Scholars' Press.

Roach, M. (2000). Race and health: Implications for health care delivery and wellness promotion. In M. S. Jamner & D. Stokols (Eds.), *Promoting human wellness: New frontiers for research, practice, and policy* (pp. 258–293). Berkeley, CA: University of California Press.

Smith, B. J., Tang, K. C., & Nutbeam, D. (2006). WHO health promotion glossary: New terms. *Health Promotion International Advance Access*, 1–6. doi:10.1093/heapro/dal033

Starfield, B. (2001). Basic concepts in population health and health care. *Journal of Epidemiology & Community Health, 55*(7), 452–454.

Statistics Canada. (2016). *Aboriginal peoples survey, 2012. Social determinants of health for the off-reserve First Nations population, 15 years of age and older, 2012*. Retrieved from https://www.statcan.gc.ca/pub/89-653-x/89-653-x2016010-eng.htm

Stewart, M. J., Makwarimba, E., Reutter, L. I., Veenstra, G., Raphael, D., & Love, R. (2009). Poverty, sense of belonging and experiences of social isolation. *Journal of Poverty, 13*(2), 173–195. doi:10.1080/10875540902841762

Strengthening the Social Determinants of Health: The Toronto Charter for a Healthy Canada. (2003). Retrieved from http://depts.washington.edu/ccph/pdf_files/Toronto%20Charter%20Final.pdf

Syme, S. L. (2000). Community participation, empowerment, and health: Development of a wellness guide for California. In M. S. Jamner & D. Stokols (Eds.), *Promoting human wellness: New frontiers for research, practice, and policy* (pp. 78–98). Berkeley, CA: University of California Press.

Taylor, M., & Caine, V. (2013). Exploring practices of harm reduction. *Alberta RN, 68*(4), 17–19.

Taylor, R., & Rieger, A. (1985). Medicine as social science: Rudolf Virchow on the typhus epidemic in upper Silesia. *International Journal of Health Services, 15,* 547–559.

Truth and Reconciliation Commission of Canada. (2012). *Truth and Reconciliation Commission of Canada: Calls to action.* Retrieved from http://www.trc.ca

United Nations. (2008). *United Nations declaration on the rights of Indigenous peoples.* Retrieved from http://www.un.org/esa/socdev/unpfii/documents/DRIPS_en.pdf

University of Saskatchewan. (2011). Definition of primary health care. College of Medicine, Primary Health Care Group. Retrieved from http://www.medicine.usask.ca/research/health-research-groups/primary-health-care-research-group-1/definition-of-primary-health-care

Venkatapuram, S. (2013). Health, vital goals, and central human capabilities. *Bioethics, 27*(5), 271–279. doi: 10.1111/j.1467-8519.2011.01953.x

Vollman, A. R., Anderson, E. T., & McFarlane, J. (2017). *Canadian community as partner: Theory & multidisciplinary practice* (4th ed.). Philadelphia, PA: Wolters Kluwer.

Weber, B. (2016a, August 17). Hugh Papik, Aboriginal elder, dies after stroke misdiagnosed as drunkenness. *The Canadian Press.* Retrieved from http://www.huffingtonpost.ca/2016/08/17/n-w-t-to-probe-stroke-death-of-elder-who-was-misdiagnosed-as-drunk_n_11569178.html

Weber, B. (2016b, March 1). N.W.T. report into elder's death will help address 'systemic racism' in health care: Minister. *The Canadian Press.* Retrieved from https://www.thestar.com/news/canada/2017/03/01/nwt-report-into-elders-death-will-help-address-systemic-racism-in-health-care-minister.html

Webster, P. C. (2017). Calls for medically safe heroin mount in Canada. *The Lancet, 389,* 239.

World Health Organization (WHO). (1948). Preamble to the Constitution of the World Health Organization as adopted by the International Health Conference, New York, 19–22 June, 1946; signed on 22 July 1946 by the representatives of 61 States (Official Records of the World Health Organization, no. 2, p. 100) and entered into force on 7 April 1948.

World Health Organization (WHO). (1978). Reprinted from *Declaration of Alma-Ata*, pp. 2–3. World Health Organization. Copyright © 1978.

World Health Organization (WHO). (1986). Reprinted from *The Ottawa charter for health promotion.*

World Health Organization (WHO). (1998). *Health promotion glossary.* Geneva, CH: Author.

World Health Organization (WHO). (2008). *Primary health care: Now more than ever.* Geneva, CH: Author. Retrieved from http://www.who.int/entity/whr/2008/en

World Health Organization (WHO). (2009a). *Milestones in health promotion: Statements from global conferences.* Geneva, CH: Author.

World Health Organization (WHO). (2009b). *The Nairobi call to action for closing the implementation gap in health promotion.* Geneva, CH: Author.

World Health Organization (WHO). (2013a). *Primary health care.* Retrieved from http://www.who.int/topics/primary_health_care/en

World Health Organization (WHO). (2013b). *The Helsinki statement on health in all policies.* Retrieved from http://www.who.int/healthpromotion/conferences/8gchp/8gchp_helsinki_statement.pdf

World Health Organization (WHO). (2016). *True magnitude of stillbirths and maternal and neonatal deaths underreported.* Retrieved from http://www.who.int/mediacentre/news/releases/2016/stillbirths-neonatal-deaths/en/

World Health Organization (WHO). (2017). *Promoting health in the SDGs. Report on the 9th global conference for health promotion: All for health, health for all, 21-24 November 2016.* Retrieved from http://apps.who.int/iris/bitstream/10665/259183/1/WHO-NMH-PND-17.5-eng.pdf?ua=1

World Health Organization (WHO). (2018). *Immunization coverage: Fact sheet.* Retrieved from http://www.who.int/mediacentre/factsheets/fs378/en

World Health Organization, Health and Welfare Canada, & Canadian Public Health Association. (1986). *Ottawa charter for health promotion.* Ottawa, ON: Author.

Ziabakhsh, S., Pederson, A., Prodan-Bhalla, N., Middagh, D., & Jinkerson-Brass, S. (2016). Women-centered and culturally responsive heart health promotion among Indigenous women in Canada. *Health Promotion Practice, 17*(6), 814–826.

ABOUT THE AUTHORS

Candace Lind is an RN with a BN, MN, and PhD in Nursing from the University of Calgary and a completed post-doctoral fellowship in Community Health Nursing from the University of Ottawa. She is Associate Professor in the Faculty of Nursing at the University of Calgary, where her program of research focuses on child and youth health promotion and encompasses research that is relationship-based, informs interprofessional practice and policy development, and addresses the ways in which youth and other marginalized populations are conceptualized in society. Her research and community health undergraduate teaching are informed by the attributes of social justice and the social determinants of health, and she is particularly interested in strengths-building, health-promoting approaches to practice and research.

Louise Baptiste is an RN with a BN from Athabasca University and a Master of Education degree from the University of Calgary. She is Director of Indigenous Initiatives with a focus on student supports and community outreach, as well as a nursing instructor, for the Faculty of Nursing, University of Calgary. She is a proud member of Samson Cree Nation and has worked with Indigenous and non-Indigenous populations in Treaty 7 and Métis Nation Region 3 territory. Her career focus has been on emergency nursing and health promotion, and nursing education. She is particularly interested in social justice, cultural safety, and health promotion for Indigenous populations.

Race, Culture, and Health

Elizabeth McGibbon and Joyce Mbugua

LEARNING OUTCOMES

After studying this chapter, you should be able to:

1. Discuss important assumptions and characteristics of culture.

2. Discuss cultural diversity in Canada.

3. Describe the relationships among culture, race, and racism.

4. Analyze the four areas of the cycle of oppression to show how these areas are related, how they apply in community health nursing practice, and how oppression creates barriers in access to care.

5. Compare and contrast cultural competence, cultural safety, and cultural humility in community health nursing practice.

6. Describe examples of racism in nursing, with specific attention to the history of the profession of nursing, white privilege, and settler privilege.

7. Identify and discuss the components of an anti-racist, anti-oppressive lens for community health nursing practice.

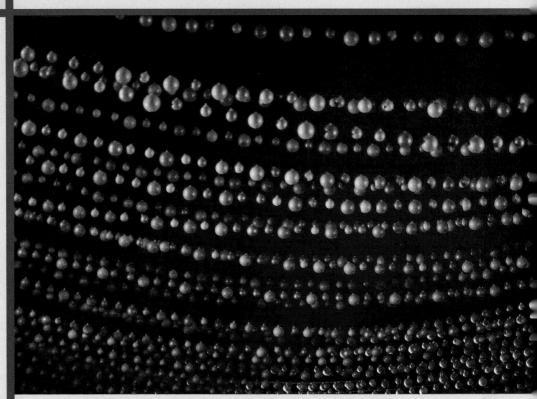

Source: © *Riley Smith Photography*

INTRODUCTION

Culture is a central concept for community health nursing. In this chapter, we explore different meanings of culture, and ethnic and racial diversity. We also analyze how these meanings influence our own understandings of communities and how they intimately influence community health nursing practice. We begin with assumptions about culture and definitions of associated concepts, and continue with an overview of diversity in Canada, including immigrant and migrant health. The chapter emphasizes how community health nurses (CHNs) can deepen their understandings of societal power and privilege to move forward with anti-racist, anti-oppressive practice.

ASSUMPTIONS AND CHARACTERISTICS OF CULTURE

Culture includes language, gestures, tools, customs, and traditions that define a group's values and organize social interactions. According to the Aboriginal Nurses Association of Canada (ANAC) (Aboriginal Nurses Association of Canada [ANAC], 2009), culture is more than beliefs, practices, and values. In other words, it is important that nurses move beyond simplistic and essentialist lists of what we think might constitute the "culture" of our clients, families, and communities. Instead, it is crucial that we focus on the ways culture is defined and redefined, along with the power and privilege that comes with being able to define the cultures of "others." Our values and assumptions unfold in social, historical, and political contexts, and they impact our perceptions and nursing actions. According to Allender, Rector, and Warner (2014), characteristics shared by cultures include the following:

- *Culture is a* **social construction.** Cultural norms, behaviours, and values are learned through socialization within the family and community. However, culture is interpreted and shaped individually as well as being situated, negotiated, and transformed within complex social and power relations and the broader structural forces that affect us (e.g., mass media, social media). "Socially constructed means that it is an idea that has been constructed, built, made-up, over time, by society, and by dominant social and cultural systems such as government, education, and health care" (McGibbon & Mbugua, 2017, p. 135).
- *Culture is an integrated system embedded in everyday life.* Beliefs and health care practices are usually consistent with the overall paradigms that are used to make sense out of the world.
- *Culture is shared.* Beliefs that have meanings and are shared by a group are called cultural values. These values are transmitted within a group and imparted over time. Values shared by people form cultural stability and security. They guide members about what to believe and how to act. Notably, individuals may not share, or may even find constraining, the values of their cultural groups or their communities.
- *Culture is largely implicit and tacit.* Culture shapes us at an unconscious level. Most of the time, we do not stop to consider assumptions and expectations that ground our behaviours and decisions.
- *Culture is fluid and dynamic.* Culture is always adapting and changing, especially with increased global migration and access to technology. For example, racialized cultures have been influenced by the dominant Canadian Eurocentric culture. Growing diversity and global interconnectedness have influenced the Canadian culture in return.
- *Culture is expressed and intersects* with other social constructs such as **race**, gender, **ethnicity**, class, language, and disability. For example, people with both visible and invisible disabilities may consider themselves to be sharing common cultural identities and experiences rather than having

a "pathological" disorder (Marks, 2007). The historical and current importance of French language rights in Quebec is an outward expression of cultural identity.

One of the main barriers to nurses' understandings of culture is the biomedical Eurocentric foundation of nursing practice. **Eurocentrism** refers to the dominance of white, European ways of thinking and knowing. An almost exclusive focus on the individual has implications for CHNs, providing "little or no guidance for addressing how we act as a community, the duties and obligations, and the mutual and disparate moral interests of individuals, families, and communities" (Shirley, 2007, p. 14). The Community Health Nurses of Canada (CHNC) (2011) standards and competencies, as well as the Canadian Public Health Association's (2010) guidelines for public health and community health nursing practice, emphasize a greater and more explicit emphasis on assumptions regarding cultural contexts of the broader **societal structures** that underpin society. These are the political, economic, and social structures of society and the culture that informs them (e.g., law, religion, health care, government) (Navarro, 2002).

CULTURAL DIVERSITY IN CANADA

Statistics Canada (2016) estimates that in the next two decades, First Nation, Métis, and Inuit (FNMI) populations are likely to exceed 2.5 million persons. First Nation populations—including both registered and treaty Indians under the Indian Act as well as those who are non-status, grew by 39.3% in 2006 to 977 230 people in 2016. The Métis population (587 545) had the largest increase over the 10-year span, rising 51.2% between 2006 and 2016. The Inuit population (65 025) grew by 29.1% from 2006 to 2016. The median age of FNMI peoples is 10 years younger, on average, when compared to the general population in Canada. The Canadian Census profile (Statistics Canada, 2016) reported that there were 1 198 540 people who identified as Black Canadians (the term used in the census). Just as FNMI peoples are not a homogenous group, Black Canadians also identify in many different ways, including African Canadian, Caribbean Canadian, and Black Canadian. High rates of successful immigration from Africa continue to increase Black populations in Canada.

According to the 2016 Canadian Census, there were 7 540 830 foreign-born individuals who came to Canada through the immigration process, representing over one-fifth (21.9%) of Canada's total population during the period of 2011–2016 (Statistics Canada, 2017). For the first time, Africa ranked second, ahead of Europe, as a source continent of recent immigrants to Canada, with a share of 13.4% in 2016. Asia (including the Middle East) remains the top source continent of recent immigrants. In 2016, the majority (61.8%) of newcomers were born in Asia. People from more than 200 different ethnic groups, speaking 150 different languages, live in Canada. Each year more than 250 000 new immigrants enter the country, making it one of the most ethnically diverse in the world (Statistics Canada, 2013).

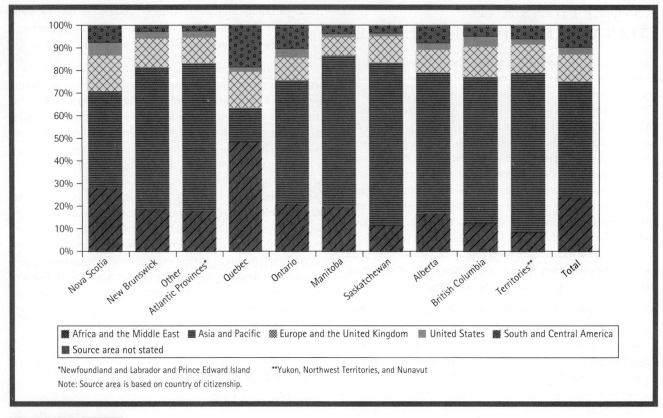

Source: Citizenship and Immigration Canada (2015). *Canada facts and figures: Immigrant Overview, Permanent Residents.* Ottawa: Citizenship and Immigration Canada.

The term *immigrant* refers to individuals who are eligible for permanent residency, including people accepted in the categories of economic immigrants (people selected for their skills and ability to contribute to Canada's economy), family class immigrants (people sponsored by a Canadian citizen or permanent resident), and government-assisted and privately sponsored refugees (Citizenship and Immigration Canada [CIC], 2015). Currently, the top source countries for immigrants are the Philippines, China, and India. The vast majority of newcomers live in large urban areas, and 95% settle in Ontario, British Columbia, Quebec, and Alberta. Canada's largest cities, such as Toronto, Vancouver, and Montreal, became home to 63.4% of recent immigrants in 2011. Provincial and territorial settlement diversity is reflected in Figure 9.1. Quebec controls its own immigration policy and requires commitment to living in a francophone society for acceptance. A higher proportion of people from Africa and the Middle East, which include French-speaking countries, immigrate to Quebec compared to Canada as a whole (48.3% versus 23.9%) (CIC, 2015).

In the midst of rapidly increasing immigration and the resulting enrichment of Canada, there are significant barriers. Although successful results in a full medical examination are required before immigrants are deemed eligible to enter Canada, perceptions of immigrants as "disease breeders" and "health fraudsters" still exist. Canadian Research 9.1 provides current research about attitudes toward immigrants in Canada. Media coverage, an important source of information, can potentially influence and shape public opinion and policy agendas regarding the health and medical issues of immigrants.

CANADIAN RESEARCH 9.1

"Immigrants Can Be Deadly": Critical Discourse Analysis of Racialization of Immigrant Health in the Canadian Press and Public Health Policies. (Reitmanova, Gustafson, & Ahmed, 2015)

There is current and historical evidence of stereotyping, **discrimination**, and **oppression** of immigrants in Canada. The authors examined 273 articles from 10 major Canadian daily newspapers over the period of one decade. They analyzed the articles in terms of how immigrants were described and characterized. The researchers used critical discourse analysis of newspaper articles to highlight issues of power and social injustice through which immigrant health was constructed and handled by Canada's health policies. By examining the role of the Canadian press in framing health and social issues of immigrants, the researchers showed pre-existing racializing discourses that treated the immigrant body as a disease breeder, promoting immigrants as health fraudsters who abuse health benefits and forge their health records. Immigrants were found to be variously described as "imposters" or "scroungers" and often associated with "specific forms of 'ethnic' crime, such as aggression, mugging, rioting, theft, prostitution, and especially drugs" (Henry & Tator, 2009).

The researchers concluded that the contemporary Canadian press continues to reproduce long-standing ways of racializing immigrants through how they are described in

Newcomer Health

Immigrants bring significant strengths, such as determination, resilience, and diversity, yet they can also experience significant challenges, some of which arise from differing migration pathways. New immigrants to Canada rate their health more highly than Canadian-born people. Reasons for this difference include medical screening before their acceptance and entry into Canada and evidence that non-refugees often have healthier pre-migration lifestyles. However, health status declines quickly after arrival, though in variable ways (Kim et al., 2013). Foreign-born visible minority women have reported the greatest health decline after 10 years in Canada (Spitzer, 2012).

Language acquisition is challenging and underlies many recent immigrants' lives. Although limitations in English or French fluency affect job attainment, there are other factors that influence obtaining secure employment, including **racism** in employment processes (Galabuzi, 2012). All of these factors, in turn, impact the social determinants of immigrant health, including limited social support, especially for individuals without extended families. Social isolation, experiences of refugee camps and multiple translocations related to war, and awareness of hardships experienced by family members remaining in the country of origin result in the potential for post-traumatic stress. There may also be waiting periods of three months in order to be eligible for provincial health coverage. New Canadians often have difficulty finding a nurse practitioner or a physician; thus, the health services they receive are often limited to episodic treatment rather than comprehensive care. In 2012, changes were made to Canadian health care eligibility for refugees through the Interim Federal Health (IFH) program. Instead of receiving comprehensive health care, most refugee claimants, who are considered to be temporary residents, receive limited health care services, often only when their disease is considered a danger to public health. National public protest and public policy advocacy from health and social service providers, including a successful Federal Court challenge, led to

the media. In response to this coverage, the press ran stories calling for tightening of borders and immigration policies, and improving medical screening and surveillance of immigrants to protect the health of Canadian-born citizens (Reitmanova et al., 2015). A more balanced and fair media coverage of immigrant health will require de-racialization of immigrant health issues as well as the transformation of the Canadian press toward greater inclusivity.

Discussion Questions

1. Where do nurses get the majority of their information about immigrants in Canada?
2. Why do you think negative stereotypes of immigrants persist in Canada, despite evidence to the contrary?
3. How do you think these negative views of immigrants may impact their health status and their success in accessing health care?

Figure 9.2 describes common attitudes toward levels of immigration in Canada and toward immigrants who are members of visible minorities. Canada is not an outlier; the same hardening of attitudes can be observed in other countries (Drinkwater, Eade, & Garapich, 2009; Hugo, 2002). Governments and media play mutually reinforcing roles in stigmatizing refugees, using illness and uncleanliness as both literal and symbolic threats (Reitmanova et al., 2015). Discrediting refugees sells newspapers and can be an effective tool to justify politically motivated decisions, but the tactic is likely jeopardizing the mental health of many already traumatized people. It is well documented that immigrants bring significant strength, determination, resilience, and diversity, and they are usually in good health. However, once they enter Canada, their health status starts to decline, and this process has been associated with low income, unemployment, experiences of discrimination, and barriers to assessing health and social care services (Kim, Carrasco, Muntaner, McKenzie, & Noh, 2013).

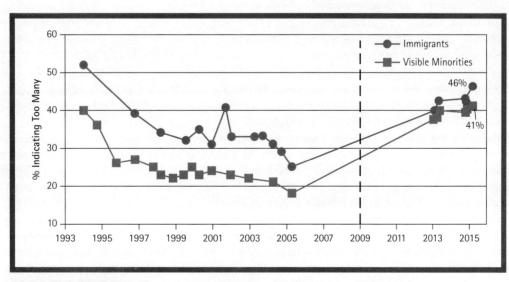

FIGURE 9.2 Attitudes about Immigration and Visible Minorities

Source: Graves (2015).

reversal of some reductions in IFH services. Changes to IFH coverage highlight the role of government policy and ideology in determining who is deserving of what types of immigration classification and which services of publicly funded health care.

Issues such as immigration status, precarious employment, insecure housing, and lack of knowledge about Canadian health care systems are made more complex by language barriers and differing cultural meanings regarding health, illness, and care practices. Building trust is an essential first step in building relationships, and often interpreters are necessary. Family members, especially spouses or children, should not be asked to interpret. It is important for CHNs and student nurses to know policies related to working with interpreters and the services available in their institutions and clinical placements. The CHN working with migrant and refugee families and communities must be knowledgeable about public policy related to immigration and settlement.

CULTURE, RACE, AND RACISM

Canada has a complex history when it comes to culture, race, racism, and **racialization**. Few of us have been systematically educated about Canada's history regarding racialized peoples. Or, more accurately, we have often been systematically educated in a way that reinforces racism. One of the most successful ways to perpetuate racism is to ensure the erasure of historical facts and stories. Chapters 1 and 22 provide a comprehensive discussion of important historical contexts. Critical perspectives help us understand

the root causes of discriminatory practices such as racism and identify some of their unjust structural public-policy-created origins.

When we think about race, one of the first things that comes to mind is that race only applies to people who are not white or who are not historically descendant from Europeans. However, race refers to any group of people who share the same physical characteristics, such as skin tone, hair texture, and facial features (McGibbon & Mbugua, 2017). Although people can be grouped by any number of physical differences (height, foot size, resistance to certain diseases), race is an artificial, socially constructed way to categorize people (Etowa & McGibbon, 2012). Although there is only 0.1% variation in the human genome (Shampo & Kyle, 2011), race continues to be a foundational way to categorize people in the health fields, including nursing. Race and ethnicity are used interchangeably. Table 9.1 describes important terms for understanding culture, race, and racism in community health nursing.

Since race is a social construction, a primary function of continuing to use race as a category is to perpetuate racism. Williams (1999) defines racism as "an ideology of inferiority that is used to justify unequal treatment (discrimination) of members of groups defined as inferior, by both individuals and societal institutions" (p. 176). Racism is the systematic practice of denying people access to rights, representation, or resources based on racial differences. It is neither natural nor inevitable. As we explore in this chapter, racism involves more than personal actions of individuals. Racism is also a comprehensive system of discrimination that involves social institutions, and it impacts

Table 9.1	Important Terms for Understanding Culture in Context
Culture	Culture is a very broad term that encompasses areas such as language, ways of communicating and developing a sense of community, relationships with the land and with food, as well as rituals, art, customs, beliefs and attitudes. These areas help to define a group's values and influence their social interactions and ways of formal and informal governance. It is important to note that culture intersects with religion and faith. Cultural groups are not homogenous. People with a European heritage have many different cultural traditions (e.g., Irish, Roma, Italian). There are many different African Canadian cultures, immigrant cultures, First Nations, Métis cultures, LGBTQ2S cultures, youth cultures, deaf cultures, to name a few.
Ethnicity	When people describe their ethnicity, they refer to a common language, culture, country of origin, and ancestry. Ethnicity is often self-defined and it also intersects with identities such as culture and religion. People of the same race may describe themselves as having different ethnicities. For example, people in the African diaspora may describe themselves as Ghanaian, South African, or Caribbean. People with a Celtic heritage may describe themselves as Scottish or Irish.
Nationality	Nationality refers to how people describe where they live or where they are a citizen. Sometimes, people refer to their nationality in terms of their country of origin. So, a family who has immigrated to Canada from Syria may describe their nationality as Canadian, Syrian, or both.
Race	Although race is universally used as a way to stratify or categorize people, race has absolutely no scientific meaning. Race is a social construction that serves the purpose of justifying racist notions of the supremacy of whiteness. Racism has a long history in the medical sciences, where everything from "scientific" measurement of human head shape to gait have been used to "prove" the inferiority of people who are not defined as "white". It is important to note that whiteness is also a social construction.
Religion	Religion has historically referred to a system of faith-based practices, rituals and beliefs, often based in superhuman agency, such as Gods. Spirituality and faith are often central when people describe their religion, and these foundations often provide life-long guidance for religious individuals, families, and communities. Religion and ethnicity are often conflated, which often deepens discrimination and oppression. An example is the persistent blurring of the religion of Islam with terrorist groups such as Al Qaeda and the Islamic State.

Sources: Peoples, J. & Bailey, G. (2014). *Humanity: An introduction to cultural anthropology.* Toronto: Nelson Education; McGibbon, E. (2018). *Social justice and health.* Course Materials. St. Francis Xavier University; Etowa, J. & McGibbon, E. (2012). Race and racism as determinants of health. In E. McGibbon (Ed.) *Oppression: A social determinant of health* (pp. 73–88). Halifax: Fernwood Publishing.

virtually every aspect of society (McGibbon & Etowa, 2009). It is important to note that although racism is a systematic process that is created and sustained across Canada, Canadians, including nurses, can take action to dismantle it.

The perpetuation of racism becomes especially evident when we consider that the term *race* is exclusively used to describe people of colour, as if they are the only people who have a race. This process is referred to as racialization. According to Ahmad (1993), "Racialization assumes that race is the primary, natural, and neutral means of categorization, and that the groups are also distinct in behavioral characteristics, which result from their race" (p. 18). Another way to think about racialization in health care is racial profiling, where health care providers tend to generalize about certain groups, creating an inaccurate profile about members of these groups (Tang & Browne, 2008). Minority registered nurses also report that they experience racial profiling and marginalization in their nursing practice (J. Mbugua, personal communication, April 12, 2017), describing situations where they entered a patient's room and family members would automatically tell them to take the breakfast or dinner tray away. When nurses, individuals, families, communities, and nations are racialized or racially profiled, it means they are negatively categorized in a particular way, based on their skin colour and other physical attributes. Most significantly, this inaccurate categorization is largely negative, derogatory, demeaning, and often dangerous to health and well-being.

YES, BUT WHY?

Health and the Racialization of Poverty in Canadian Communities

What?

Even though we live in a country with seemingly equal opportunity for families to obtain employment that will sustain the health and well-being of communities, racialized people are persistently less likely to gain employment, regardless of their educational attainment (Block & Galabuzi, 2011). Racialized communities face high levels of poverty. The 2006 Canadian Census (the last census to collect this information) showed that the overall poverty rate in Canada was 11% in 2006. However, for racialized persons it was 22%, compared to 9% for non-racialized persons (Statistics Canada, 2011). Racialized women have even higher levels of poverty. Women form the majority (about 53%) of people living in poverty in Canada, a process called the feminization of poverty (Women's Legal Education and Action Fund, 2011). Forty-four percent of First Nation women living off reserve and 47% of First Nation women living on reserve live in poverty. Poverty, in turn, creates significant compromises in all of the social determinants of health, leading to intergenerational health impacts across the life course.

So What?

This process is referred to as the racialization of poverty in Canada, a process where poverty becomes disproportionately concentrated and reproduced among racialized

group members, in some cases inter-generationally (Block & Galabuzi, 2011). The impact of these forces accentuates historical forms of racial discrimination in the Canadian labour market and creates a process of social and economic marginalization (Galabuzi, 2012). According to Block and Galabuzi (2011), the racialization of poverty is also linked to the entrenchment of privileged access to the economic resources in Canadian society by a powerful minority. The results are large inequities in the social determinants of health, such as income and wealth in Canada as a whole (McGibbon, 2017; Raphael, 2016). Consequently, health outcomes are severely impacted. These inequities are disproportionately experienced by racialized Canadians, especially new Canadians, African Canadians, and FNMI peoples.

Now What?

The CCHN Standards of Practice provide clear direction about how you can act for change. CHNs have professional responsibility and accountability to educate themselves about how racism operates to decrease chances for adequate family income to sustain a quality of life that promotes family and community health and well-being. An excellent way to begin or enhance this process is to explore the facts and stories on key Canadian websites such as the Center for Social Justice (www.socialjustice.org), The Canadian Council for Refugees (http://ccrweb.ca), Black Lives Matter (http://art.blacklives-matter.com), and Idle No More (www.idlenomore.ca). These websites demonstrate first-voice calls for action, including action from allies in the fight against the racism and ongoing colonization that seriously impacts chances of meaningful employment, health, and well-being for individuals and families across the life course. In order to honor CCHN standards, it is essential to begin or continue a lifelong professional nursing process of educating ourselves and others about racism and access to sustained and meaningful family employment.

Standards of Practice Fulfilled

#1 Health Promotion
– Seeks to identify and assess the root and historical causes of illness, disease and inequities in health, acknowledges diversity and the adverse effects of colonialism on Indigenous people, and when appropriate incorporates Indigenous ways of knowing including connectedness and reciprocity to the land and all life in health promotion.

#3 Health Maintenance, Restoration, and Palliation
– Includes cultural safety and cultural humility approaches in all aspects of health maintenance, restoration, and palliation interventions.

#4 Professional Relationships
– Recognizes own personal beliefs, attitudes, assumptions, feelings, and values including racism and stereotypes and their potential impact on nursing practice.

#6 Health Equity
– Understands historical injustices, inequitable power relations, institutionalized and interpersonal racism and their impacts on health and health care and provides culturally safe care (Community Health Nurses of Canada [CHNC], 2019, revised).

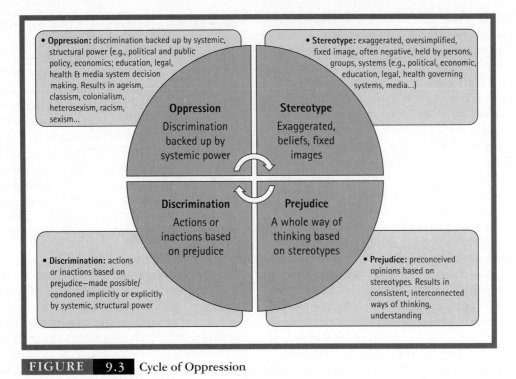

FIGURE 9.3 Cycle of Oppression

Source: Adapted from McGibbon and Mbugua (2017)

THE CYCLE OF OPPRESSION

There are many ways to think about culture, race, and racialization in societal systems and in community health nursing practice. CHNs are often very familiar with the ways that unfairness, such as **prejudice** and discrimination, creates barriers across the life course. The cycle of oppression is a way to help us understand how stereotyping and prejudice lead to societal or systemic oppressions, including ableism, ageism, classism, genderism, heterosexism, racism, and sexism. (See Figure 9.3.)

The cycle begins when we create and maintain stereotypes about individuals, families, and communities. A **stereotype** is an exaggerated, oversimplified, often negative fixed image held by persons, groups, and political and economic decision makers. We all hold numerous stereotypes that we have absorbed over time, through our gender and social class socialization, the media, and our education at the primary and secondary levels, to mention a few. For example, since we have all grown up in a racist, sexist society, we have all absorbed some of these stereotypes (e.g., girls are not very good at math, FNMI students all get free tuition, African Canadian women have a higher pain tolerance than white Euro-Canadian women). We are not often aware of the basket of stereotypes we carry with us in our everyday lives and into our nursing practice.

Prejudice is a preconceived opinion and whole way of thinking based on stereotypes. Stereotypes deeply impact the way we think about individuals, families, and communities. These prejudices usually operate without our direct knowledge—they are embedded in our thinking, and in order to "see" them, we need to make a specific effort. Discrimination is action or inaction based on prejudice. When we engage in discriminatory practices as nurses, we are usually not aware of our discrimination. Oppression is discrimination backed up by

systemic power, for example, in public policies and in education, legal, and health systems (e.g., ageism, classism, racism, sexism, and **colonialism**). In all the areas in the cycle, the one that is most difficult to understand is oppression because it involves thinking about the very underpinnings of society and how they influence nursing practice. The Case Study on page 175 illustrates how the cycle of oppression can be applied to help us understand how we may be practising discrimination and therefore how we can educate ourselves for culturally safe care.

Oppression and Barriers in Access to Care for Racialized Peoples

The cycle of oppression illustrates the ways that nursing practice can, and does, produce culturally unsafe actions and inactions. Discrimination produces significant barriers in access to health and nursing care—underscoring the urgent need for CHNs to understand and apply the cycle. In a systematic review of Canadian literature (1990–2010) on the impact of race and racism on health, researchers found that health care providers unconsciously racialized patients' explanations by applying cultural or overly simplified characteristics (Nestel, 2012). Racism has been measured in many access-to-care areas and includes inadequate or under treatment of disease, less systematic or vigorous basic care, and less access to quality care. For example, FNMI peoples are diagnosed at later stages of various kinds of cancer, thus contributing to higher mortality rates (Morrisseau, 2009). These rates have been attributed to limited access to screening and treatment services, and provider lack of cultural knowledge and cultural competency (National Collaborating Center for Aboriginal Health, 2011).

CASE STUDY

Mr. Brian Sinclair and the Cycle of Oppression in Health Care

Mr. Sinclair was a vulnerable First Nation man who was also a double amputee. He went to the Health Sciences Centre in Winnipeg in 2008 complaining of abdominal pain and a catheter problem. "He was told to go and wait in the waiting room. He was never called back. Ever. He was ignored to death. He had a bladder infection. He just needed antibiotics and a catheter change. [At the inquest] the chief medical examiner said: 'If the treatment had been given . . . he would not have died on that day'" (Zbogar, 2014, p. A9). Hospital staff walked past Mr. Sinclair many times and did not intervene. He vomited as he went into shock, and someone gave him a basin. This was the sum total of medical intervention. The inquest revealed that some of the staff assumed that he was drunk and "sleeping it off." Mr. Sinclair was left in distress and without the emergency care he needed for the duration of 34 hours. He died in the emergency department and was ignored for several more hours until rigor mortis set in.

At the inquest, the Sinclair family and their lawyer, Mr. Victor Zbogar, rejected the euphemisms that were used to identify causation of the death: "access block" and "patient flow" problems. Rather, we see the cycle of oppression operating here: *stereotyping* about Mr. Sinclair as a drunk and homeless Indigenous man led clinicians to a *prejudice* that he did not need emergency care; stereotyping led to *discrimination*, in this case lack of action, until he died. *Oppression* happens when discrimination is backed up by institutional power. In the nursing and medical care, or lack thereof, of Mr. Brian Sinclair, discrimination was backed up and justified by institutional power, in this case, a health care system with embedded allowances for clinical incompetence related to the social determinants of health and a legal system that hid racist clinical practice under the guise of patient-flow problems.

Discussion Questions

1. How do nurses develop stereotypes of FNMI peoples in Canada?

2. How do nurses learn (or not learn) about the historical contexts of FNMI peoples in Canada?

3. How can you, as community health nursing students, act to embed cultural safety in your classroom and clinical learning?

In caring for racialized individuals, families, and communities, provider bias dovetails with an overarching lack of fit with Eurocentric, Western service delivery models in the care of FNMI peoples, Black Canadians, and immigrant populations, to name a few.

In a 2012 report about racism and stereotyping of urban Indigenous peoples in Canada, some patients were refused painkillers, in spite of severe pain, due to a belief they were at a higher risk of becoming addicted or were already abusing prescription drugs (Health Council of Canada, 2012). "Significant disparities exist between access to health care services for First Nation, Inuit, and Métis peoples and other Canadians . . . If the system responds poorly to Indigenous people, they do not come for health care or do not respond well to health care" (p. 24). A 2015 Canadian study (Park, Tjepkema, Goedhuis, & Pennock, 2015) reported avoidable mortality for First Nation people in Canada—a measure of deaths that potentially could have been averted through effective prevention practices, public health policies, and provision of timely and adequate health care. The researchers' longitudinal analysis compared avoidable mortality among First Nation and non-Indigenous adults. First Nation women had almost 2.5 times the rate of avoidable mortality rates when compared to non-First Nation women (Park et al., 2015).

Barriers in access to care are significant for many racialized groups. There is a growing awareness of the role played by discrimination in the provision of health care services to immigrants and refugees across Canada (Pollock, Newbold, Lafrenière, & Edge, 2012). Numerous authors and groups have also identified systemic racism and anti-Black racism within the health care system (Sinai Health System Human Rights & Health Equity Office, 2017).

When we think of complex patients, we picture an aging population with multiple chronic diseases. It's important we all understand that inequity and racism are disease equivalents in terms of their impact. They contribute to complexity and poor outcomes in the same way diabetes and hypertension do (Newton, 2017, p. 2).

CULTURAL COMPETENCE, CULTURAL SAFETY, AND CULTURAL HUMILITY

According to ANAC (2009), **cultural safety** happens along a continuum from cultural awareness, cultural sensitivity, and **cultural competence** to cultural safety. ANAC (2009) emphasizes that cultural awareness approaches could be a starting point in the development of cultural safety. However, these approaches all have similar and distinct limitations, including their assumptions that "others" are seen as bearers of culture, or culturally exotic. Another limitation is that cultural awareness approaches are based in the social locations of the dominant culture. There is no responsibility to change the health care system or to engage in related social action. Finally, they do not involve practitioners reflecting on their own perspectives regarding their actions (ANAC, 2009).

First described by Leininger (2006), cultural competence was seen as a way to address culturally specific health needs. The concept of cultural competence integrates the knowledge, attitudes, and skills that nurses would use in order to plan effective and appropriate interventions. Dudas (2012) identified three dimensions of cultural competence: *awareness*, which means having some knowledge of cultural similarities and differences combined with self-reflection; *attitudes*, which include sensitivity, openness, being nonjudgmental, and respecting differences; and *behaviours*, which require creativity while providing care through a "cultural lens." Camphina-Bacote (2002) described five constructs that inform the *process of cultural competence*: cultural awareness (self-examination), cultural knowledge, cultural skill (collecting and assessing data), cultural encounters (the process of relationships), and cultural desire (motivation of the health care provider).

A key strength of cultural competence is that it suggests action (ANAC, 2009). However, in addition to a lack of attention to responsibility for changing the health care system or to engaging in related social action, culture is sometimes reduced to technical skills for which clinicians can develop expertise, and cultural lifescapes are homogenized as a way to simplify the learning of "cultural others" (ANAC, 2009). Leininger's (2006) transcultural nursing model was similarly critiqued because it rests on a broadly defined concept of culture that is narrowly applied. The focus is on individual identity within an understanding of culture that "essentializes" or emphasizes the similarities of experiences and simplifies differences (Gustavson, 2005). The culture of origin is accentuated and often perceived to be static, rather than recognizing the multiple identities and the relational processes involved in all our encounters as well as changes that occur through migration (Gray & Thomas, 2006; Williamson & Harrison, 2010).

Cultural safety involves understanding and naming power and privileges in the therapeutic relationship. The concept is grounded in a critical social science perspective where structural, systemic processes such as oppression and colonialism are explicitly discussed in the context of nursing practice, education, research, policy making, and leadership. Strengths of a cultural safety approach include drawing our attention more explicitly to addressing inequities, supporting CHNs in the following:

- "improving healthcare access for patients, aggregates, and populations;
- acknowledging that we are all bearers of culture;
- exposing the social, political, and historical contexts of healthcare;
- enabling practitioners to consider difficult concepts, such as racism, discrimination, and prejudice;
- acknowledging that cultural safety is determined by those to whom nurses provide care;
- understanding the limitations of 'culture' in terms of having people access and safely move through healthcare systems and encounters with care providers; and
- challenging unequal power relations" (ANAC, 2009, p. 2).

Cultural humility is a relatively recent term that enhances and extends culturally safe care. It is a process of self-reflection where health care providers make a commitment to understand their personal and systemic biases through education and reflection, and to maintain respectful processes and relationships based on mutual trust (First Nations Health Authority, 2015). In their #itstartswithme movement, the First Nations Health Authority states that system-wide change begins with every individual who works in health. Cultural humility and cultural competence are very much consistent with CHNC (2011) standards and competencies, and can provide CHNs with a clear road map for personal and systems change in their communities, organizations, and governance structures.

RACISM AND WHITE SETTLER PRIVILEGE IN NURSING

Racism in nursing historically has been theorized by numerous scholars, including nurses. Areas of discussion include racism as a barrier to health equity and social justice (Anderson, Reimer-Kirkham, Browne, Khan, & Lynam, 2009); culture, values, and racism and their application to nursing (Cortis, 2003); teaching about race, racism, and health in nursing (Drevdahl, 2002); systemic racism toward nurses of colour and racialist discourses in nursing (Das Gupta, 2009); white privilege in the nursing profession (Puzan, 2003); and nurse education through a white lens, including racism in the mentor–student relationship (McGibbon, Mulaudzi, Didham, Barton, & Sochan, 2013; Scammell & Olumide, 2011).

Nursing education, practice, research, leadership, and policy making are immersed in historical injustices that create and sustain racism. According to Georges (2003), "the events and multiple discourses that have brought us to this present moment in nursing recede endlessly backward into a Eurocentric cultural context with sexism, racism, and classism at its heart, and we carry this context within us" (p. 45). The profession itself has been colonized over time and across global boundaries. Theoretical and overall intellectual development is based in mainstream white Euro-Canadian and class privilege. Historical accounts of the evolution of nursing as a profession render invisible the leadership of Black and FNMI nurses (McGibbon et al., 2013). For example, Jamaican-born Mary Seacole, who served not only as a nurse but also as a financial benefactor in the Crimean War (1853–1856), is invisible in nursing history. Public attention to Florence Nightingale, who was white and from an upper-class English family, overshadowed Seacole's significant contributions to the profession (Anionwu, 2006; McGibbon et al., 2013).

Nursing's grand theories, still a cornerstone of nursing education, demonstrate the near erasure of the complex economic, social, and political history of racism, including colonialism. Some would argue that nursing theories such as those of Henderson, Newman, Orem, Parse, Peplau, and Rogers do indeed integrate sociopolitical ideas (McGibbon et al., 2013). However, finding the language of power, privilege, oppression, and the isms will be akin to looking for a "needle in a haystack" (McGibbon & Etowa, 2009). A focus on cultural diversity, diet, dancing, and dress of "others" persists without an examination of power, privilege, and oppression. Embracing multiculturalism and diversity without an anti-racist lens serves to reinforce the privilege of dominant groups (Berman & Paradies, 2010) and a Eurocentric focus on nursing knowledge development.

White privilege is the other side of the coin, the hidden side of the racism equation in nursing. As discussed in this chapter, race is a socially constructed designation, where white people, as Puzan (2003) states, are seen neutrally—they have no race.

White privilege is a core pillar of racism in nursing, whether it is individual acts of racism, such as treating racialized individuals and families unethically in the emergency department, or deeply entrenched and less identifiable systemic racism, such as lack of university administrative support for increasing FNMI, African Canadian, and new Canadian student nurse enrolment. Understanding white privilege is complex because it involves "nice" nurses, be they practitioners, administrators, or policy makers, being complicit with racism, even if their lack of awareness renders their racism "invisible" (McGibbon et al., 2013). **White Euro-Canadian privilege** in Canada is increasingly being linked to what is called **settler privilege**. Here, settler generally refers to people whose ancestors came to Canada from Europe over the last few centuries. The European colonization of FNMI lands and the dispossession of resources made room for settlement and settler resource "development" (McGibbon, 2018). Therefore, although settlers today may not link these original dispossessions to the disenfranchisement of FNMI peoples today, settlers nonetheless stand on the economic, environmental, political, and sociocultural

benefits of the dispossessions created by their ancestral fore-mothers and forefathers. Settler privilege involves unearned, current, and historical advantages that settler Canadians rely on by virtue of the historical relationship to the original settlers of Canada. White privilege and settler privilege offer invisible advantages across the lifespan. Table 9.2, based in MacIntosh's (1998) analysis of white privilege, provide specific examples of how white and settler privilege operate in the health fields.

The unearned gains that privilege bestows on white Euro-Canadian persons carries a logic of disadvantaging others, thus creating a duality of dominance/subordination, freedom/restriction, access to correct means/lacking access to correct means, and order/disorder (Hagey & McKay, 2000). Settler privilege happens in tandem with white privilege—they operate in synergy. Settler privilege confers both explicit and tacit advantages that are just as invisible to settlers as white privilege. All health care in what is now known as Canada takes

Table 9.2	Examples of How White Settler Privilege Operates in Health Care

- When I require pain medication after knee surgery, I can be pretty sure that I will not be refused pain relief because: "Black women have a high pain tolerance."

- When I ask my community health practitioner for pain medication to treat a serious workplace back injury, I can be pretty sure that I won't be accused of "drug seeking, because Natives are usually addicts and alcoholics."

- When one of my family members is hospitalized and critically ill, I can be pretty sure that I can access on-call spiritual caregivers that match my faith.

- When I leave my community to be admitted to a hospital maternity unit to give birth to my fourth baby, I won't hear one of the nurses say: "Oh, Native women are used to having lots of babies. She won't need much attention from us."

- After I give birth to my baby, and my parents, grandparents, and children arrive with a celebration meal, I can be pretty sure that one of the health care staff will not say: "There's always so many of them. They always travel in packs and there's no room for them here."

If I Am a White Settler Health Care Student

- If I decide to further my education at the baccalaureate, master's, or doctoral level, I can be pretty sure that most of my professors will be persons of my race.

- When I study for my exams, my textbooks will mostly depict persons of my race.

- When I study health care theories and perspectives, I can be sure that the theorists are of my race.

- In my class about historical health influences, when I speak up about the Irish potato famine, I can be pretty sure that I won't be accused of being stuck in the past or taking things too seriously.

- When I learn about family and community health, I can be pretty sure that my textbooks, assignments, and class discussions largely reflect my own white settler perspective.

If I Am a White Settler Health Care Provider, Teacher, or Researcher

- When I am employed in my first clinical practice position, I can be pretty sure that most of my colleagues will be of my white settler race.

- If I ask to speak to the "person in charge" when I am advocating for ethical patient/family/community care, I can be pretty sure that I will be facing a person of my own white settler race.

- In my community nursing placement, when I assess newborns with the Apgar score, I can be sure that the instrument is designed to assess white settler newborns.

- If I lobby my municipal, provincial/territorial, or national political representatives about increasing community health care, I will most likely be talking to a person of my white settler race.

- When I attend conferences and professional meetings, and when I search health literature, I can be nearly certain that the worldview underpinning the thinking will be aligned with my worldview—Eurocentric and biomedical.

Source: Adapted from McGibbon (2018).

place on ancestral and many unceded territories of FNMI peoples. Unceded refers to the traditional lands of First Nations that were not negotiated by treaty with European settler officials. The peoples whose territories were negotiated by treaty process have been largely subjected to the illegal disregard of those historic agreements by the Canadian government.

One of the key ways for CHNs to enact change is to decolonize nursing. As described in Chapter 22, decolonizing involves actively seeking knowledge about postcolonial power imperatives. Donald (2009) further explains that although the outcomes were vastly different, the process of colonization happened synergistically among the colonized and the colonizers, and hence, decolonization should integrate this shared history (McGibbon et al., 2013).

If colonialism is indeed a shared condition, then **decolonization** needs to be a shared endeavour. Decolonization in the Canadian context can only occur when Indigenous peoples and Canadians face one another across historic divides, deconstruct their shared past, and critically engage with the realization that both the present and future are similarly tied together (Donald, 2009, p. 5).

TOWARD ANTI-OPPRESSION, ANTI-RACISM COMMUNITY HEALTH NURSING PRACTICE

It is very difficult for white Euro-Canadian settlers in the health care system (providers, researchers, government policy makers, and so on) to come to grips with their ongoing participation in

racialization and colonization, including their everyday microaggressions and their health-damaging and sometimes deadly neglect at point of care (McGibbon, 2018). According to Dei (1996), an anti-racism framework:

> explicitly names the issues of race and social difference as issues of power and equity, rather than as matters of cultural and ethnic variety . . . while the notion of culture(s) and cultural differences are relevant to anti-racism discourse, it stresses that a romanticized notion of culture, which fails to critically interrogate power, is severely limited in the understanding of social reality." (pp. 25–27)

Understanding privilege, understanding how the cycle of oppression operates, and acting for social change are key components of anti-oppression practice, including anti-racism. Figure 9.4 illustrates an anti-oppressive, anti-racist theoretical framework for practice. The beginning of this overall process is for CHNs to learn how to actively "see" stereotyping, prejudice, and discrimination—to see how the cycle of oppression unfolds in our everyday practice, education, research, policy making, and social action leadership. The discussions and activities associated with this chapter are designed to promote the development of skills and tools for *seeing* this cycle. Along with seeing oppression comes seeing our own privileges, such as white Euro-Canadian and settler privilege, and how these privileges support the disadvantaging of our clients, our colleagues in nursing practice, and racialized peoples across Canada and globally.

When we identify, or "see" specific ways that oppression and privilege operate in our everyday practice, education,

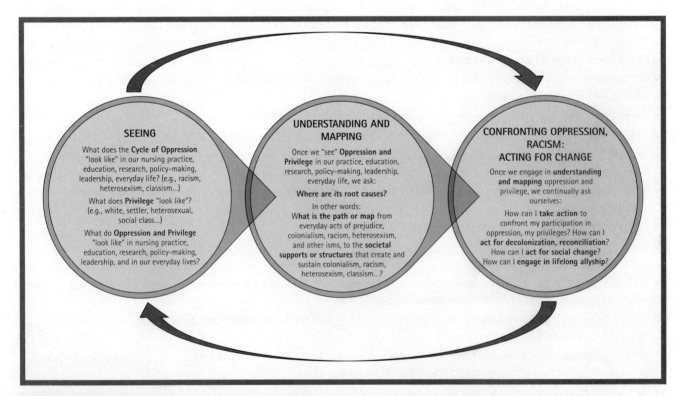

FIGURE 9.4 Toward Anti-Oppression, Anti-Racism Community Health Nursing Practice

Source: McGibbon (2017).

Table 9.3	Looking through a Critical Lens Using Multiple Filters

Part 1: Inquire at the Contextual Level:

Pick a specific community to whose members you will be providing care. Try to select a community with which you are not very familiar . . . Use literature, media, the internet, and other resources to answer the following questions:

- What key historical, economic, and political forces predominantly influence this community? (Think about migration in and out of the community, wars, settlement, and economic recessions.)
- Which groups tend to be privileged over others in this community?
- What are the most common race, social class, and gender dynamics within this community?
- What key, taken-for-granted beliefs, labels, and stereotypes might be operating in relation to this community?
- What changes in the status quo (think structures, inequities, and taken-for-granted thinking) can you see that might improve health and health care for this community?

Part 2: Inquire at the contextual and interpersonal levels:

Pick a specific person or family from that community.

- What structural conditions and inequities are advantaging and/or disadvantaging the health and health care experiences of *this* person or family?
- What power dynamics are most advantaging and/or disadvantaging the health and health care experiences of *this* person or family?
- What stereotyping and labelling practices might be affecting this person or family?
- What changes in the status quo can you see that would benefit this person or family?

Part 3: Inquire at the intrapersonal level.

Think about your own inquiry process.

- What differences and similarities do you see between yourself and this community and person or family?
- Which of your values, beliefs, assumptions, and practices are confirmed or challenged as you inquire?
- How might you relate differently at the intrapersonal, interpersonal, and contextual levels?

Source: Based on Doane, G. H. & Varcoe, C. (2014). *How to Nurse: Relational Inquiry with Individuals and Families in Shifting Contexts.* New York: Wolters Kluwer.

research, policy making, and leadership, we then engage in understanding and mapping this process: Where are its root causes? As discussed earlier in the chapter, root or structural causes are the systemic, societal supports for oppression (e.g., the isms held in public policy and in related legal, health, education, and community services systems). In other words, we commit to a sustained practice of asking ourselves: What is the path or map from everyday acts of prejudice, colonialism, classism, racism, heterosexism, and other isms in nursing practice to the societal supports or structures that create and support these isms? Once we engage in understanding and mapping oppressions, including racism, and the privileges that support and sustain oppressions, CHNs can continually ask: How can I take action to recognize my own privilege and my participation in oppressive practices? How can I act for decolonization and reconciliation? How can I engage in social change and lifelong allyship in my nursing practice and in my everyday life? It is important to note that the processes of seeing, understanding and mapping, and acting for change often overlap in a circular way, as depicted in the diagram. For example, when we take action, we may see new forms of oppression and privilege that inspire us take further action.

Anti-oppressive, anti-racist practice involves constant engagement in examining our own values, assumptions, and ways of thinking. Doane and Varcoe (2014, p. 80) refer to nurses becoming involved in an ongoing process of inquiry that focuses on looking through a critical lens using multiple filters in our nursing care with communities. (See Table 9.3.) These authors help us analyze the isms and their historical and current contexts in our practice with individuals, families, and communities.

CONCLUSION

Race and culture are foundational influences on CHNs and on the individuals, families, communities, and nations with whom they practise. As this chapter explores, these socially constructed ideas have a profound impact on the ways that racialized peoples are perceived and treated in economic, governance, education, health, and media systems, to name a few. These social constructions and stereotyping heavily influence CHNs' practice, as well as the practice of our colleagues, policy makers, and individuals in a position to take leadership roles. It is now well known that the cycle of oppression is embedded in health systems and in society as a whole—the very structures and systems that CHNs seek to change. However, privileges such as white Euro-Canadian and settler privilege can make it difficult to even see these structures and systems. CHNs may also be positioned very differently, where some have intersecting privileges, and some struggle with the day-to-day impacts of oppressions, including racism, on "the other side of the coin." Although educating ourselves is a foundation for social change, it is not enough. When we commit to taking action, we enhance our own learning by working with as many people, groups, communities, and institutions as is necessary to make meaningful and sustained change in communities and ultimately in public policy and the structural systems that underpin policy at all levels.

KEY TERMS

colonialism (p. 174)
cultural competence (p. 175)
cultural humility (p. 176)
cultural safety (p. 175)
culture (p. 168)
decolonization (p. 178)
discrimination (p. 170)
ethnicity (p. 169)
Eurocentrism (p. 169)
oppression (p. 170)
prejudice (p. 174)
race (p. 169)
racialization (p. 172)
racism (p. 171)
settler privilege (p. 177)
social construction (p. 169)
societal structures (p. 169)
stereotype (p. 174)
white Euro-Canadian privilege (p. 177)

STUDY QUESTIONS

1. Describe the characteristics of culture.

2. Describe the similarities and differences between cultural competence and cultural safety. What are the implications of these similarities and differences for CHNs' practice?

3. Describe how cultural beliefs and values shape the interactions between nurses and clients.

INDIVIDUAL CRITICAL-THINKING EXERCISES

1. What implications does the Canadian Charter of Rights and Freedoms (Government of Canada, 1982) have on nursing practice when working with culturally diverse families?

2. In your work as a public health nurse, you meet a family new to Canada at a community health fair. Communicating using very limited English, the parents tell you that money is very scarce, the mother is pregnant with her fifth child, the family does not have permanent residence status in Canada, and they are uncertain whether they will be allowed to stay. They are worried they will be deported to their country of origin. What community supports and services would you assist this family to access in order of priority, and why?

3. How does culture influence health and illness within diverse communities? What roles do the social determinants of health and public policies play?

GROUP CRITICAL-THINKING EXERCISES

1. How would you go about gaining and demonstrating the skills and behaviours for culturally safe practice?

2. Are the members of your nursing class representative of your community's population? Why or why not?

3. Discuss as a group the similarities and differences between your understandings of diversity and multiculturalism.

REFERENCES

Aboriginal Nurses Association of Canada. (2009). *Cultural competence and cultural safety in nursing education: A framework for First Nations, Inuit and Métis nursing*. Ottawa, ON: Author. Used by permission of Aboriginal Nurses Association of Canada. Retrieved from http://www.anac.on.ca/Documents/Making%20It%20Happen%20Curriculum%20Project/FINALFRAMEWORK.pdf

Ahmad, W. I. U. (1993). *"Race" and health in contemporary Britain*. Buckingham, UK: Open University Press.

Allender, J. A., Rector, C., & Warner, K. (2014). *Community health nursing: Promoting and protecting the public's health* (7th ed.). Philadelphia, PA: Lippincott, Williams & Wilkins.

Anderson, J., Reimer-Kirkham, S., Browne, A., Khan, K. B., & Lynam, M. (2009). Inequities in health and healthcare viewed through the ethical lens of critical social justice: Contextual knowledge for the global priorities ahead. *ANS. Advances in Nursing Science, 32*(4), 282.

Anionwu, E. (2006). *About Mary Seacole*. Thames Valley University, London: Mary Seacole Center for Nursing Practice.

Berman, G., & Paradies, Y. (2010). Racism, disadvantage and multiculturalism: Towards effective anti-racist praxis. *Ethnic and Racial Studies, 33*(2), 214–232.

Block, S., & Galabuzi, G.-E. (2011). *Canada's color-coded labour market: The gap for racialized workers*. Ottawa, ON: Canadian Center for Policy Alternatives.

Camphina-Bacote, J. (2002). The process of cultural competence in the delivery of healthcare services: A model of care. *Journal of Transcultural Nursing, 13*(3), 181–184.

Canadian Public Health Association. (2010). *Public health—community health nursing practice in Canada: Roles and activities* (4th ed.). Ottawa, ON: Author.

Citizenship and Immigration Canada. (2015). *Canada facts and figures 2014: Immigration overview—permanent residents*. Retrieved from http://www.cic.gc.ca/english/pdf/2014-Facts-Permanent.pdf

Community Health Nurses of Canada. (2011, 2019, revised). *Canadian community health nursing: Professional practice model and standards of practice*. St. John's, NL: Author.

Cortis, J. D. (2003). Culture, values and racism: Application to nursing. *International Nursing Review, 50*, 55–64.

Das Gupta, T. (2009). *Real nurses and others: Racism in nursing*. Halifax, NS: Fernwood Publishing.

Dei, G. S. (1996). *Anti-racism theory and practice*. Halifax, NS: Fernwood Publishing.

Doane, G. H., & Varcoe, C. (2014). *How to nurse: Relational inquiry with individuals and families in shifting contexts*. New York, NY: Wolters Kluwer.

Donald, D. (2009). Forts, curriculum, and Indigenous métis-sage: Imagining decolonization of Aboriginal-Canadian relations in educational contexts. *First Nations Perspectives, 2*, 1–24.

Drevdahl, D. (2002). Teaching about race, racism, and health. *Journal of Nursing Education, 40*, 285–289.

Drinkwater, S., Eade, J., & Garapich, M. (2009). Poles apart? EU enlargement and the labour market outcomes of immigrants in the United Kingdom. *International Migration, 47*, 161–190.

Dudas, K. I. (2012). Cultural competence: An evolutionary concept analysis. *Nursing Education Perspectives, 33*(5), 317–321.

Etowa, J. & McGibbon, E. (2012). Race and racism as determinants of health. In E. McGibbon (Ed.) *Oppression: A social determinant of health* (pp. 73–88). Halifax: Fernwood Publishing.

First Nations Health Authority. (2015). *#itstartswithme, Creating a climate for change: Cultural safety and humility in health services delivery for First Nations and Aboriginal peoples in British Columbia*. Vancouver, BC: FNHA. Retrieved from http://www.fnha.ca/wellness/cultural-humility

Galabuzi, G.-E. (2012). Social exclusion as a determinant of health. In E. A. McGibbon (Ed.), *Oppression: A social determinant of health* (pp. 97–112). Halifax, NS: Fernwood Books.

Georges, J. M. (2003). An emerging discourse: Toward epistemic diversity in nursing. *Advances in Nursing Science, 26*(1), 44.

Government of Canada. (1982). *Canadian charter of rights and freedoms*. Ottawa, ON: Government of Canada.

Gray, D. P., & Thomas, D. J. (2006). Critical reflections on culture in nursing. *Journal of Cultural Diversity, 13*(2), 76–82.

Graves, F. (2015). *Tolerance under pressure*. Ottawa, ON: EKOS. Retrieved from http://www.ekospolitics.com/index.php/2015/03/tolerance-under-pressure

Gustafson, D. L. (2005). Transcultural nursing theory from a critical cultural perspective. *Advances in Nursing Science, 28*(1), 2–16.

Hagey, R., & MacKay, R. W. (2000). Qualitative research to identify racialist discourse: Towards equity in nursing curricula. *International Journal of Nursing Studies, 37*, 45–56.

Health Council of Canada. (2012). *Empathy, dignity, and respect: Creating cultural safety for Aboriginal people in urban health care*. Ottawa, ON: Health Council of Canada.

Henry, F., & Tator, C. (2009). *The color of democracy: Racism in Canadian society* (4th ed.). Toronto, ON: Nelson College Indigenous.

Hugo, G. (2002). From compassion to compliance? Trends in refugee and humanitarian migration in Australia. *GeoJournal, 56*(1), 27–37.

Kim, I., Carrasco, C., Muntaner, C., McKenzie, K., & Noh, S. (2013). Ethnicity and postmigration health trajectory in new immigrants to Canada. *American Journal of Public Health, 103*(4), e104.

Leininger, M. (2006). Culture care diversity and universality theory and evolution of the ethnonursing method. In M. Leininger & M. R. McFarland (Eds.), *Culture care diversity and universality: A worldwide nursing theory* (2nd ed., pp. 1–41). Boston, MA: Jones and Bartlett.

Marks, B. (2007). Cultural competence revisited: Nursing students with disabilities. *The Journal of Nursing Education, 46*(2), 70.

McGibbon, E. (2017). Embodied oppression: The social determinants of health. In W. Antony, J. Antony, & L. Samuelson (Eds.). *Power and resistance: Canadian thinking about Canadian social issues* (pp. 165–194). Halifax, NS: Fernwood Publishing.

McGibbon, E. (2018). Decolonizing health care: Reconciliation roles for white settlers. *Women's Health and Urban Life, 13*(2). Retrieved from https://ojs.scholarsportal.info/uoit/index.php/whul/article/view/65

McGibbon, E. (2018). *Social justice and health*. Course Materials. St. Francis Xavier University.

McGibbon, E., & Etowa, J. (2009). *Anti-racist health care practice*. Toronto, ON: Canadian Scholars Press.

McGibbon, E., & Mbugua, J. (2017). Race and racialization in health, health care, and nursing education. In M. McIntyre & C. McDonald (Eds.), *Realities of Canadian nursing* (5th ed.). New York, NY: Wolters Kluwer Health.

McGibbon, E., Mulaudzi, F. M., Didham, P., Barton, S., & Sochan, A. (2013). Toward decolonizing nursing: The colonization of nursing and strategies for increasing the counter-narrative. *Nursing Inquiry, 21*(3), 179–191.

McIntosh, P. (1998). White privilege: Unpacking the invisible knapsack. *Best of Pact Press: A Collection of the Best Articles on Racial Identity*. North Carolina: Pact Press.

Morrisseau, K. (2009). *Aboriginal cancer control progress report*. Winnipeg, MB: Aboriginal Services. Retrieved from http://www.cancercare.mb.ca/resource/File/AboriginalCancerControlProgressReport_07-08.pdf

Navarro, V. (2002). *The political economy of social inequalities*. Amityville, NY: Baywood.

Nestel, S. (2012). *Color-coded health care: The impact of racism on Canadians' health*. Toronto, ON: Wellesley Institute.

National Collaborating Center for Aboriginal Health. (2011). *Access to health services as a social determinant of First Nations, Métis, and Inuit health*. Prince George, BC NCCAH.

Newton, G. (2017). Keynote address. *Black experiences in health care (BEHC) symposium*. Toronto, ON: Sinai Health System.

Park, J., Tjepkema, M., Goedhuis, N., & Pennock, J. (2015). Avoidable mortality among First Nations adults in Canada: A cohort analysis. *Health Reports, 26*(8), 10.

Peoples, J. & Bailey, G. (2014). *Humanity: An introduction to cultural anthropology*. Toronto: Nelson Education.

Pollock, G., Newbold, K., Lafrenière, G., & Edge, S. (2012). Discrimination in the doctor's office: Immigrants and refugee Experiences. *Critical Social Work, 13*(2), 60–79.

Puzan, E. (2003). The unbearable whiteness of being (in nursing). *Nursing Inquiry, 10*(3), 193–200.

Raphael, D. (2016). *The social determinants of health*. Toronto, ON: Canadian Scholars Press.

Scammell, J. M. E., & Olumide, G. (2011). Racism and the mentor–student relationship: Nurse education through a white lens. *Nurse Education Today, 32*, 545–50.

Shampo, M. A., & Kyle, R. A. (2011). J. Craig Venter: The human genome project. *Mayo Clinic Proceedings, 86*(4), e27.

Shirley, J. (2007). Limits of autonomy in nursing's moral discourse. *Advances in Nursing Science, 30*(1), 14–25.

Spitzer, D. (2012). Oppression and immigrant health in Canada. In E. A. McGibbon (Ed.), *Oppression: A social determinant of health* (pp. 113–122). Halifax, NS: Fernwood.

Statistics Canada (2011). Census profile: 2011 Census. Ottawa, ON: Statistics Canada. Retrieved from http://www12 .statcan.gc.ca/census-recensement/2011/dp-pd/prof/index .cfm?Lang=E

Statistics Canada. (2013). *Immigration and ethnocultural diversity in Canada: National household survey 2011.* (Government No. 99-010-X2011001). Ottawa, ON: Author. Retrieved from http://www12.statcan.gc.ca/nhs-enm/2011/as-sa/99-010-x/99-010-x2011001-eng.pdf

Statistics Canada. (2016). Census profile: *2016 Census.* Ottawa, ON: Statistics Canada. Retrieved from: https:// www12.statcan.gc.ca/census-recensement/2016/dp-pd/prof/index.cfm?Lang=E

Statistics Canada. (2017, October 25). Immigration and ethnocultural diversity: Key results from the 2016 Census. *The Daily.*

Reitmanova, S., Gustafson, D. L., & Ahmed, R. (2015). "Immigrants can be deadly": Critical discourse analysis of racialization of immigrant health in the Canadian press and public health policies. *Canadian Journal of Communication, 40*(3), 471.

Sinai Health System Human Rights & Health Equity Office. (2017). *Black experiences in health care (BEHC) Symposium.* Toronto, ON: Sinai Health System.

Tang, S. Y., & Browne, A. J. (2008). "Race" matters: Racialization and egalitarian discourses involving Aboriginal people in the Canadian health care context. *Ethnicity & Health, 13*(2), 109–127.

Women's Legal Education and Action Fund. (2011). *Women and poverty.* Toronto, ON: LEAF.

Williams, D. R. (1999). Race, socioeconomic status, and health the added effects of racism and discrimination. *Annals of the New York Academy of Sciences, 896*(1), 173–188.

Williamson, M., & Harrison, L. (2010). Providing culturally appropriate care: A literature review. *International Journal of Nursing Studies, 47*(6), 761–769.

Zbogar, V. (2014, June 16). Brian Sinclair's death was a homicide: But call it whatever you want, just address the discrimination. *Winnipeg Free Press Print Edition*, A9.

ABOUT THE AUTHORS

Elizabeth McGibbon, RN, MN, PhD, is a professor at St. Francis Xavier University, Nova Scotia. Her teaching, research, and publications focus on embodied oppression, access to health care, health equity and public policy, and the political economy of health. She leads a Social Sciences and Humanities Research Council-funded project, Mapping Health Equity in Canadian Public Policy, and is a co-researcher with Debwewin: The Truth of our Hearts, a study aiming to diversify our dialogue and understanding of heart health in Manitoban First Nations people (Canadian Institutes of Health Research). Her books include *Anti-racist Health Care Practice* (with Dr. Josephine Etowa) and *Oppression: A Social Determinant of Health* (edited volume). She is an invited chapter author in four multiple-edition Canadian books about critical perspectives on health and society. She was one of three leads in establishment of the National Collaborating Center, Determinants of Health. Along with social justice colleagues, her awards include recognition from the Nova Scotia Human Rights Commission (anti-racism community action) and the Canadian Armed Forces (refugee humanitarian work).

Joyce Mbugua, RN, MEd, a Black woman and a Black nurse, started her nursing career in Kenya, where she graduated as an enrolled nurse-midwife and worked for eight years before moving to Canada with her family in 2000. She graduated with Bachelor of Science in Nursing in 2004. Her 2017 Master of Education focused on curriculum, with concentration in nursing/health sciences. She worked full-time as a registered nurse in Antigonish (St. Martha's Hospital, the R.K. MacDonald Nursing Home) for 10 years before joining St. Francis Xavier University Rankin School of Nursing as a nurse educator in 2014. She teaches clinical and simulation components in medical-surgical and pediatric nursing, as well healthy aging. She has worked with students at all levels from first year to fourth year. Her graduate research was focused on how to retain and graduate minority nursing students in order to diversify the nursing profession. Her teaching and research is informed by her years of clinical experiences and her experience as a mature international nursing student.

Evidence-Informed Decision Making in Community Health Nursing

Jackie Muresan and Rebecca Ganann

CHAPTER 10

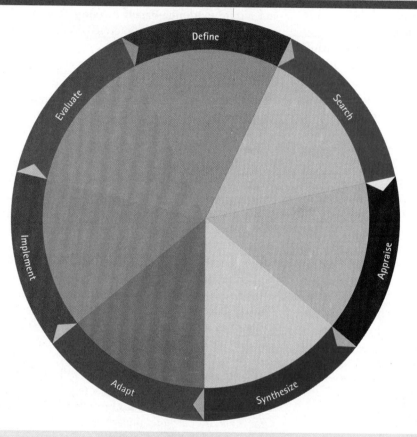

Source: Adapted from National Collaborating Centre for Methods and Tools {NCCMT}. (2018). "Model for evidence-informed decision making in public health." Adapted with permission.

INTRODUCTION

Through critical thinking and reflection, community health nurses (CHNs) can ask important questions about nursing practice and how it may be improved. CHNs participate in research and have opportunities to use research evidence to inform their practice. CHNs can be critical consumers of information and influence decision making by using high-quality research evidence to improve client outcomes. The professional practice model (introduced in Chapter 3) indicates that CHNs are active participants in integrating knowledge into their practice; they engage in **evidence-informed decision making** (Community Health Nurses of Canada [CHNC], 2019, revised). CHNs may pose the following practice questions:

- As the Canadian population ages, falls among older adults living in the community are an issue relevant to CHNs working in home care, primary care, and public health. A CHN may ask how falls among community-dwelling older adults can be prevented. (Tricco et al., 2017)

- School-aged children are a population group that CHNs may work with. A key period to teach healthy lifestyle habit development is during the formative school years. The local school board is concerned that there is too little time to teach the required curriculum, so members of the board are considering reducing the time children spend in physical activity. At the same time, the region is concerned about the increasing numbers of overweight children. Are school-based physical activity programs effective in improving activity duration in children? (Dobbins, Husson, DeCorby, & LaRocca, 2013)
- There are many opportunities for CHNs to promote health during the perinatal period. For example, a CHN could be interested in what prenatal interventions promote nutritional outcomes such as breastfeeding or infant birthweight among Indigenous women and their infants. (Ashman, Brown, Collins, Rollo, & Rae, 2017)
- CHNs may also be interested in population-based approaches to support healthy weights before, during, and after pregnancy (see Photo 10.1). A woman's weight before and during pregnancy can impact the health of both the woman and her infant. Women of childbearing age in Canada are significantly heavier than they were in the past (Health Canada, 2010). Approximately one-third of Canadian women (35%) are overweight or obese as they enter pregnancy (Public Health Agency of Canada [PHAC], 2009). During pregnancy, 35% of women gain more weight than is recommended (PHAC, 2009). In the postpartum period, weight retained from pregnancy can put a woman at risk of entering her next pregnancy at a higher body mass index. A CHN could be interested

in whether technological interventions could be used to (1) support women to experience appropriate gestational weight gain and (2) achieve and maintain a healthy weight in the postpartum or interpregnancy period. You find a recent systematic review that addresses these questions (Sherifali et al., 2017) (see Canadian Research 10.1).

CHNs are faced with questions like these every day. After graduation, how can nurses continue to be educated critical thinkers whose practice is based on high-quality research evidence? How can busy nurses keep current with the research findings? How can nurses meet provincial nursing standards for using evidence in practice, the national public health core competencies (PHAC, 2008), or the national Community Health Nursing Standards of Practice (CHNC, 2019, revised)? This chapter highlights strategies CHNs can use to develop and sustain **evidence-based nursing (EBN)** practice and enable them to be evidence-informed decision makers.

PHOTO 10.1 A woman's weight before and during pregnancy can impact the health of both the woman and her infant.

Source: Tanis Saucier/Shutterstock

CANADIAN RESEARCH 10.1

The effectiveness of e-health technologies on weight management in pregnant and postpartum women (Sherifali et al., 2017)

The purpose of this systematic review was to summarize the evidence on whether e-health technologies targeting physical activity, nutrition, or both are effective for weight management during and/or after pregnancy. Of the 1837 titles identified and screened and 176 articles retrieved, 10 studies were relevant and included in the review. The authors concluded that e-health technologies are not effective for managing weight gain during pregnancy (mean difference −1.62 kg, 95% CI: −3.57 to 0.33 kg). However, in the postpartum period, there is evidence from four studies (of mixed quality) that e-health technologies using the Web or texts to target nutrition and physical activity are effective in reducing weight (mean difference −2.55 kg, 95% CI: −3.81 to −1.28 kg). Only 10 studies were identified for this review with relatively small samples, so the results must be interpreted with caution. This is a relatively new area of research, and several clinical trials are currently under way to further explore the use of e-health technologies during and after pregnancy.

Discussion Questions

1. Some people naively look at systematic reviews and see that many titles were discarded; in this example, they found 10 studies of the initial 1837 titles. They then claimed that not all studies were used; large numbers were thrown out, making a systematic review not really a look at all the available research. How would you respond?

2. Is this conclusion convincing—that e-health technology can reduce postpartum weight? It is a clinically important change? Is it worth putting resources into e-health lifestyle interventions for postpartum women? Why or why not?

3. What would need to be considered before providing this type of intervention in the community?

WHAT IS EVIDENCE-INFORMED DECISION MAKING?

Evidence-informed decision making (EIDM) involves considering valuable evidence from a variety of sources, including client or community health issues and local context; client, community, and political preferences and actions; resources; and the best available research evidence (National Collaborating Centre for Methods and Tools [NCCMT], 2012). CHNs must use their clinical expertise to integrate all these factors into a decision or recommendations (NCCMT, 2012).

In Figure 10.1, the elements of EIDM are presented. Each element in the model appears to have equal weight; however, the process of EIDM may be more complicated. For example, CHNs have the knowledge and skills to provide effective web-based and text message support to pre- and postnatal women to promote healthy lifestyles in pregnancy. We know from the research evidence that the e-health interventions to support healthy maternal postpartum weights are effective (Sherifali et al., 2017). However, weight management is a potentially sensitive issue, and some new mothers may see this support as intrusive and not be open to receiving e-health interventions focused on this topic. Further, important contextual barriers, such as socioeconomic factors, levels of overall and technological literacy, and language barriers among the local population of postpartum women, would need to be considered prior to deciding to implement this strategy, along with the resources available to offer this type of intervention.

Evidence-informed decision making has evolved from the initial work done in evidence-based medicine and later evidence-based nursing (EBN). EBN is defined as the conscientious, explicit, and judicious use of current best evidence in making decisions about the care of individual patients (DiCenso, Guyatt, & Ciliska, 2005). Evidence-based practice is not discipline specific and means integrating individual clinical expertise with the best available external clinical evidence from systematic research (Sackett, Rosenberg, Gray, & Haynes, 1996). In evidence-based practice, research is integrated with other information that might influence the management of health issues and problems, such as clinical expertise, preference for alternative forms of care, and available resources.

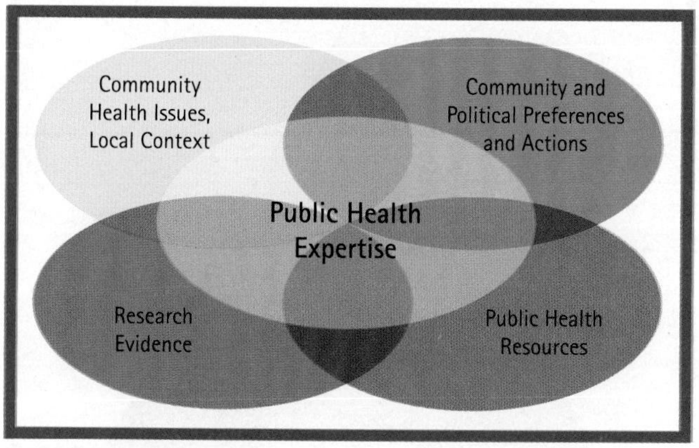

Evidence-based practice may have been misunderstood in the past to mean the application of research findings to a decision, regardless of the context or patient preferences. To overcome this type of confusion, some authors have removed the word "based." They now call the process "**evidence-informed practice**" to reflect the variety of factors that shape decisions particularly in relation to the use of evidence in policy making (Canadian Health Services Research Foundation, 2004).

Evidence-informed practice is broader than research utilization. For individuals who work in public health, the steps of the evidence-informed public health process (see figure on first page of this chapter) have been developed; the process is the same for CHNs working in any setting. This process is circular in nature, beginning with *defining* the question and moving through various phases. This is an iterative process. When the evaluation phase is complete, you may have new questions to define and can move through the cycle again. Engaging in this iterative process assists CHNs to inform their practice with the best available evidence. What difference does the use of research make? Heater, Becker, and Olson (1988) conducted a meta-analysis to determine the contribution of research-based practice to client **outcomes**. They found 84 nurse-conducted studies involving 4146 patients and reported that clients who received research-based nursing care made "sizable gains" in behavioural knowledge and in physiological and psychosocial outcomes compared with those receiving routine nursing care. The same review would be a massive undertaking today, as there are so many more studies that would need to be included.

Why Don't All Nurses Use Research Evidence in Decision Making?

Even though awareness has improved over the last few decades, nurses lack the knowledge and skills to be able to find, access, and interpret the best available research evidence and then apply, implement, and evaluate its impact (Alspach, 2006; Melnyk et al., 2004). In addition, organizational barriers, such as lack of time and support for research use and system barriers may contribute to some inability to use research evidence (Squires, Moralejo, & LeFort, 2007). More current research has switched focus from measuring use of research to understanding the factors that determine research utilization, such as the characteristics of the health professional, the organization, and the change to be implemented (Dobbins, Davies, Danseco, Edwards, & Virani, 2005; Farmer et al., 2008; Graham et al., 2006).

The sheer volume of research available is more than any nurse can manage. Nurses working individually could only hope to find and read a small proportion of the research that is published each year. This is compounded by the fact that research relevant to community health nursing may be published in non-nursing journals. In addition to barriers faced

FIGURE 10.1 A Model for Evidence-Informed Decision Making

Source: Adapted from NCCMT (2018). "Model for evidenceinformed decision making in public health." Adapted with permission.

by individual nurses, there are political, cultural, economic, and other environmental barriers that must be overcome to practice in an evidence-informed way. Furthermore, there is a substantial time lag of 8 to 17 years between the time technical information is generated and the time it is used in actual practice (Lomas, 1991; Morris, Wooding, & Grant, 2011). The following section describes the process of evidence-informed practice.

THE PROCESS OF EVIDENCE-INFORMED PRACTICE

1. Define

Nurses need to ask critical questions to evaluate interventions and consider alternative options. To find relevant research, practice questions need to be structured, usually consisting of the P—population, I—intervention, C—comparison, and O—outcomes. It may also be framed as the P—population and S—situation for qualitative questions about how and why. The population refers to the patient, client, group, community, or population; the intervention is the action that is under consideration for some health promotion, disease prevention, or treatment effect; and the outcome is the result of interest from the client or clinical perspective. To return to some of the questions at the start of this chapter, a CHN may ask the following answerable questions:

- For new mothers (population), can e-health technology (intervention) be used to achieve a healthy weight in the postpartum period (outcome)?
- What is the effect of school-based physical activity programs (intervention) on duration of physical activity (outcome) among school-aged children and youth (population)?
- What do community-dwelling older adults and their caregivers (population) perceive as the facilitators and barriers to falls prevention and maintaining independence (situation)?

2. Search

There is a considerable amount of research in many topic areas of community health. In practice, CHNs need skills to be able to find high-quality relevant information quickly. An internet search engine may overwhelm you with the number of "hits." It is important to note that literature from search results on the internet appear in order of the frequency of other people choosing them as opposed to any quality criteria. However, there are several free- (or open-) access databases that either contain articles that have already been critically appraised or will allow you to use quality filters, such as limiting by study design. When you conduct a literature search, you can consider synonymous terms for the populations, situations, interventions, and outcomes. For example, for the population, new mothers might be found using other search terms such as postpartum, maternal,

primipara, or multipara. The same process is followed for the interventions and outcomes. This will allow you to find all the possible search terms, leading to a more efficient search. The most effective search may be done with the assistance of a health sciences librarian. Taking the original question, the list of synonyms for each component of the question, and any articles already found on the subject will allow the librarian to see how this type of article is indexed in databases.

It is also important to be clear about the purpose of finding this literature. Is the goal to find a guideline about a topic that would give direction on policy and procedure decisions? For example, should sexually active teens be screened for cervical cancer? The answer to this question is likely to be a policy decision at the provincial or regional level. What are the Canadian recommendations? You can go to the Canadian Task Force on Preventive Health Care and find the answer (https://canadiantaskforce.ca). Or is the goal to find a systematic review that will provide a synthesis of the individual studies on a topic? (See the section "What Is a Systematic Review?" later in this chapter.) Or has a policy decision been made, and what you are looking for are the detailed interventions that nurses need to put into action? You are likely to find the answers to this question in more detail in the individual intervention studies rather than the systematic review. However, keep in mind that the systematic review would identify those individual studies for you. Not everyone has access to a librarian. The following will discuss how to access reputable information quickly.

One tool that can help you to find the best available evidence most efficiently and effectively is the hierarchy of pre-processed research evidence also known as the 6S pyramid (DiCenso, Bayley, & Haynes, 2009). The bottom of the pyramid is made of single studies. Each level of the pyramid (see Figure 10.2) draws on research evidence from the layers below it. Starting at the top of the pyramid to do your search can help you find the most synthesized evidence first, for instance guidelines at the summaries level and then systematic reviews at the

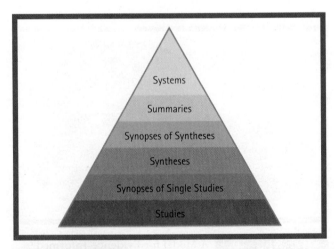

FIGURE 10.2 The 6S Search Pyramid

Source: Adapted from NCCMT (2018). Resources for Evidence-Based Practice: The 6S Pyramid. Retrieved from https://hslmcmaster.libguides.com/ebm. Adapted with permission.

syntheses level. If you are lucky, you may even find a source of evidence that has been pre-appraised (continue reading for more information about pre-appraised research).

Guidelines are the highest level of evidence found on the 6S pyramid available for community health. These systematically developed statements or recommendations provide guidance for decision making about a health issue (Woolf, Grol, Hutchinson, Eccles, & Grimshaw, 1999). Guidelines could cover the treatment or management of a disease as well as other topics such as health promotion, prevention, screening, or diagnosis. A high-quality guideline is informed by a systematic review, and thus the evidence from lower levels in the 6S pyramid is incorporated. In addition to the Canadian Task Force on Preventive Health Care guidelines mentioned earlier, other places to search for guidelines include, the National Institute for Health and Clinical Excellence (NICE) (www.nice.org.uk), and the Registered Nurses Association of Ontario (http://rnao.ca/bpg/guidelines). Guidelines are an important source of evidence for CHNs, but their quality should still be assessed before using them to make a decision. This chapter will not provide detailed information about critical appraisal of guidelines, but you can find out more on the AGREE Enterprise website (www.agreetrust.org).

The most time-efficient sources of good information are the websites that give you "pre-appraised" research. They have selected the best articles through critically appraising, rating, and summarizing the research, thus giving you the "gold nuggets" of good-quality research. For CHNs in Canada, one "go-to" place for pre-appraised research is Health Evidence™ (www.healthevidence.org). This service searches databases broadly (e.g., Medline, Embase, Cochrane Library, Campbell Collaboration Library, and others) on a regular basis for systematic reviews that are relevant to community health in Canada. Any relevant reviews are entered into the Health Evidence™ database and rated for quality on a scale of one to ten, independently, by two different qualified raters. You can search by free text or by the narrowed categories or strategies offered for different populations, different intervention types, and different intervention locations. Some of the high-quality reviews have a three- to four-page synopsis that provides a brief description of the background of the issue, results of the review, level of evidence for different outcomes, and implications for practice and policy. Levels of evidence is a categorization of quantitative study designs that go in descending order or strength (increasing potential for bias), from systematic reviews (with or without statistical summary, which is called meta-analysis), followed by randomized controlled trials, then **observational studies**. Using Health Evidence™ is of additional benefit, since reviews (particularly Cochrane reviews) may be 60 pages or more in length. By reading a summary statement (synopsis), you will be able to assess whether the respective research is useful for your purposes. You may then decide if you would like to continue reading the entire document or move on. Another source of pre-processed information is Clinical Evidence (http://clinicalevidence.bmj.com). It is an evidence-based tool organized around common primary care and hospital-based problems. It provides concise accounts of the current state of knowledge, ignorance, and uncertainty about the prevention and treatment of a wide range of clinical conditions based on thorough searches of the literature. Clinical Evidence uses information from the Cochrane Library (see the following paragraph) and the abstraction journals. However, it starts not with the journals but with **clinical questions** such as prevention and treatment of pressure sores or management of acute stroke or acute myocardial infarction. This source may be more useful to those CHNs who work in home care (Chapters 3 and 5) or primary care (Chapters 3 and 8). The McMaster Optimal Aging Portal (www.mcmasteroptimalaging.org) is another useful source of pre-processed research evidence for CHNs working with older adults through public health, home care, primary care, and policy roles.

The Cochrane Collaboration is an international organization that aims to help people make informed decisions about health by preparing, maintaining, and ensuring the accessibility of rigorous, systematic, and up-to-date reviews (including meta-analyses where appropriate) of the benefits and risks of specific health care interventions (Jadad & Haynes, 1998). Examples of the Cochrane Collaboration's relevance to community health include smoking cessation in the workplace, parent training for improving maternal psychosocial health, and prevention of falls in older adults. The Cochrane Library is the product of the Collaboration's work and includes reports and protocols over 7000 systematic reviews produced within the Collaboration, and abstracts of more than 20 000 reviews summarized and critically appraised by the Centre for Reviews and Dissemination at the University of York, UK. You can search the Cochrane Library online (www.thecochranelibrary.com) without charge for abstracts of reviews and through subscription for full access to their resources.

Like the Cochrane Collaboration, the Campbell Collaboration generates high-quality synthesized evidence using rigorous methods, but it is specifically focused on providing evidence to inform policy and decision making about social justice issues (https://campbellcollaboration.org).

If you are specifically looking for evidence about health equity, the Campbell Collaboration is one place to look. However, research on health equity could be indexed in any of the traditional electronic databases. Your search could include terms such as "equity" or "health disparities" or "social determinants of health" or "social equality" along with the terms for the population, intervention, or situation in your answerable question. For example, in a search on the effectiveness of school-based interventions for physical activity, you will find a scoping review about the equity effects of interventions to promote children's physical activity. This type of evidence could help you to understand whether there are different effects of school-based interventions for physical activity among different sub-groups in the population and whether these interventions could contribute to inequalities in health. It is important to note that some populations considered "at risk" may not be represented (or may be underrepresented) in the research literature. It then becomes very important to consider if the existing research can be applied to your population (or not) and whether you can anticipate the same results.

If you can't find pre-appraised literature to answer your question, it is necessary to go to other databases. Free online access is available for PubMed (www.ncbi.nlm.nih.gov), which can be searched with key words, setting limits for type of publication, year of publication, language, a nursing subset of journals, and so on. Another useful place to search is the Cumulative Index of Nursing and Allied Health Literature (CINAHL). Similar to PubMed, CINAHL allows for limits to be set and to search by author or key word. In all cases, there is a mixture of free access and pay-per-view access to full-text articles, unless you have access through an established library consortium.

3. Appraise

Once the articles are found and retrieved, you must decide if their quality is sufficient so that you can be confident in using them. Some health care research is too poor in quality to be used in decision-making. As previously stated, this is less critical with some of the pre-appraised sources of research. Several checklists for quality (validity) have been developed (Ciliska, Thomas, & Buffett, 2012) to help people acquire and hone their **critical appraisal skills**; that is, the ability to decide if an article is of sufficient methodological quality that it warrants attention for decision making. With a little practice, these skills become easier and quicker to apply.

Outcomes or intervention research answers questions about effectiveness or harm and has a **quantitative research** design. As stated in Chapter 11, Epidemiology, different research designs are best for answering particular types of questions. For example, questions about effectiveness or harms of certain interventions and prevention are best answered by **randomized controlled trials** in which the investigators have no control over who is placed in the intervention group versus the control group. The most efficient way to access evidence of this type that may inform your practice is a systematic review of randomized controlled trials. However, randomized controlled trials may be unethical, such as randomizing mothers to breastfeed or not to see if breastfeeding is associated with eczema, or randomizing preteens to smoke to see if it causes lung cancer. Also, trials are very expensive. If a trial cannot be done due to ethical or financial reasons, the next best design to answer the question is a **cohort design**, where at least two groups are compared before and after one group receives an intervention. Questions exploring perceptions, feelings, and experiences are best answered through a **qualitative research** design such as phenomenology or grounded theory. Questions and interventions that evolve through partnerships between researchers and participants are best dealt with through **participatory action research (PAR)**. PAR is action-oriented research in which the researchers and participants are partners in developing the question, intervention, and evaluation. PAR helps to ensure that the group under study gets the questions that are most important to them asked and answered and that the information is immediately useable for them. Participatory approaches are critical to ensuring ethical conduct of research when working with Indigenous populations. See the Yes, But Why? box for an example of a PAR study with Indigenous women and health care providers in their communities. Participatory client-oriented research approaches are becoming increasingly common through the support of policies such as the Ontario

Patients First bill and research funding such as the Canadian Institutes of Health Research Strategy for Patient-Oriented Research (http://www.cihr-irsc.gc.ca/e/41204.html).

YES, BUT WHY?

Cervical Cancer among Indigenous Women in Canada

What?

Cervical cancer rates have dropped significantly over time in Canada due to regular Papanicolaou (Pap) screening. The media has reported that cervical cancer is becoming rare in Canada. However, for specific populations such as Indigenous women, there is an increased risk of morbidity and mortality from cervical cancer (Wakewich, Wood, Davey, Laframboise, & Zehbe, 2016). For example, two recent analyses, from Ontario and British Columbia respectively, indicate that incidence rates for cervical cancer are significantly higher for Indigenous women when compared to other women (Chiefs of Ontario, Cancer Care Ontario, & Institute for Clinical Evaluative Sciences, 2016; McGahan et al., 2017). These findings are similar in other provinces and territories (Maar et al., 2016).

So What?

The increased risk of cervical cancer among Indigenous women in Canada is likely due to a lack of access to and low participation in screening and follow-up (Maar et al., 2016). To understand the factors that influence this issue and explore strategies to address it, researchers have partnered with First Nation communities in rural Ontario (Maar et al., 2013). Using a PAR method, in-depth interviews and focus groups were conducted with health and social-service providers as well as Indigenous women to explore community attitudes about cancer, cervical screening, barriers and facilitators to screening, and strategies to promote it. The findings from this program of research suggest that inequities in cervical cancer screening among Indigenous women are the result of broader societal- and community-level influences rather than individual health behaviours (Maar et al., 2013). Participants identified numerous barriers to cervical cancer screening, including a shortage of appropriately trained health care providers; no recall system for regular Pap testing; lack of transportation; socioeconomic, health literacy, and educational inequalities; and generational effects (Maar et al., 2013). Negative experiences with government health services among Indigenous people have also created distrust of health authorities. Distrust is the result of past government policies and a lack of control over how health care is provided for Indigenous people. In addition, the colonial legacy has affected body perceptions among Indigenous women and led to stigma about body and sexual health (Wakewich et al., 2016).

Now What?

Strategies to increase cervical cancer screening rates in Indigenous communities need to go beyond individual-level educational and behavioural approaches to remove structural obstacles to participation (Maar et al., 2013). In addition, this research suggests that promotion of cervical cancer screening among Indigenous women should include explaining the value of screening, using educational strategies to raise awareness among women and health professionals, embedding screening into community events, creating a trusting rapport with women, integrating screening recruitment into existing services, creating a regular dialogue about screening, and incorporating an Indigenous perspective on body into screening techniques (Maar et al., 2016). CHNs can incorporate these findings into their practice and advocate for evidence-informed approaches to cervical screening for Indigenous women.

Standards of Practice Fulfilled

#1 Health Promotion

- Collaborates with client to do a comprehensive, evidence informed, and strength-based holistic health assessment using multiple sources and methods to identify needs, assets, inequities, and resources.
- Uses a collaborative relationship with the client and other partners to facilitate and advocate for structural system change and healthy public policy using multiple health promotion strategies.

#4 Professional Relationships

- "Acknowledges that the current state of Aboriginal health in Canada is a direct result of previous Canadian government policies" in working with Indigenous people as stated in the Truth and Reconciliation Commission of Canada: Calls to Action.

#5 Capacity Building

- Recognizes the unique history of Indigenous people, and incorporates Indigenous ways of knowing and culturally safe engagement strategies in capacity building efforts.

#6 Access and Equity

- Understands historical injustices, inequitable power relations, institutionalized and interpersonal racism and their impacts on health and health care and provides culturally safe care.

#7 Evidence Informed Practice

- Uses professional expertise in considering best available research evidence, and other factors such as client context and preferences, and available resources to determine nursing actions.

#8 Professional Responsibility and Accountability

- Provides leadership in collaboration with the community to advocate for healthy public policy based on the foundations of health equity and social justice (CHNC, 2019, revised).

One principle when critically appraising articles is to ensure that the appropriate design was used to answer the question. More recently, researchers are realizing that health care topics are very complex and that **mixed methods research** may be most appropriate. Mixed methods include both quantitative and qualitative methods, either concurrently or sequentially. For example, the research described in the Yes, But Why? box was part of a larger mixed methods study. In addition to using qualitative methods to explore the factors influencing cervical cancer screening and strategies to improve it, the team conducted a randomized controlled trial to compare the effectiveness of two different cervical cancer screening modalities for Indigenous women (Wood et al., 2014; Zehbe et al., 2016).

The Additional Research Boxes in MyNursingLab discuss criteria for critical appraisal of systematic reviews, single intervention studies, and qualitative research and demonstrate the application of the criteria to actual research studies.

CRITICAL APPRAISAL OF INTERVENTION STUDIES (TREATMENT OR PREVENTION)

It is likely that you will find several studies that relate to your question. If your search did not identify a relevant systematic review that summarizes these studies, you may need consider using a single study. The decision to use an **intervention study** (treatment or prevention) to inform decisions depends on the quality of the study design and your confidence in the findings. These are the major questions used to evaluate primary studies of interventions or prevention:

- Are the results valid?
- What were the results?
- Will the results help me in improving the health of clients? (Ciliska, Cullum, & Marks, 2001; Sackett, Strauss, Richardson, Rosenberg, & Haynes, 2000)

The following section discusses more specific critical appraisal criteria that help to answer these questions.

Are the Results Valid?

This question considers whether the reported results are likely to reflect the true size and direction of the treatment effect. Was the research designed to minimize bias and lead to accurate findings? (See the box "Questions Used to Critically Appraise Intervention Studies [Treatment or Prevention]".)

Was the assignment of participants to treatment groups randomized, and was the randomization concealed? The purpose of randomization is to remove any control over who is assigned to an intervention or control group. As well, groups should be similar in all respects, except for exposure to the intervention. Known and unknown factors (age, gender, socioeconomic status, disease severity) that could influence the outcome of the study are evenly distributed among the groups. Different methods, such as a table of random numbers or computer-generated random numbers, ensure that all participants have an equal chance of being in each of the study groups. The methods section of the article should tell if and how participants were randomized.

The person recruiting the participants into the study should not know to which group each person is allocated. This is called *allocation concealment*. Concealment could happen through a process of calling a central office to get the allocation of the participant or using numbered, opaque, sealed envelopes.

In this way, the recruiter does not know until after participants are registered to which group they will be assigned, and the participant does not know at all. This prevents the recruiter from exercising bias in recruitment.

Was follow-up sufficiently long and complete? The first of these two criteria must be judged by the reader. The definition of appropriate length of follow-up varies with different practice questions. For example, success in weight loss measured at six months after a year-long intervention does not give a true picture of how many people are able to maintain the weight loss over time. A minimum expectation would be a one-year follow-up. Similarly, with early childhood interventions, follow-up for only two years may mean that important child or family outcomes that occur later in life are missed.

The second part of these criteria relates to completeness of follow-up. Seldom are studies able to retain all participants until the end of the follow-up. If large numbers are lost, it reduces confidence in the results. To continue with the example of e-health interventions to support weight loss in postpartum women, large dropouts are usual during treatment and follow-up. If the author reports on only those who remained in the study, those participants are more likely to be doing well in terms of their weight loss. Participants who were unsuccessful with the intervention are more likely to drop out, thereby making the intervention look far more effective than it really is. A retention rate of 80% is considered good; however, this is somewhat topic dependent, as one would expect the dropout rates of a transient population (e.g., homeless individuals) to be much higher.

Were participants analyzed in groups to which they were assigned? Participants should be analyzed in the group to which they were randomized, regardless of whether they received the treatment or not, or completed treatment as assigned. This is also used in relation to **intention-to-treat analysis**. If the participants who discontinued treatment—for example, due to unpleasant side effects—were omitted from analysis, we would be left only with participants who had better outcomes, making the treatment look more effective than it was. Intention-to-treat analysis includes data (often baseline) for all dropouts so the effect is no change in dropouts. This gives a more conservative estimate of the effect of the intervention, compared to the analysis that leaves them out and only includes those who completed the intervention.

Were participants, clinicians, outcome assessors, and data analysts unaware of (blinded to or masked from) participant allocation? Several of the groups involved in a trial have the potential to bias outcomes if they know whether a participant is in the intervention or control group. **Bias** means any systematic tendency to produce an outcome that differs from the truth. It includes the tendency to look more carefully for particular outcomes or to probe more deeply for outcomes in one group and not the other. Participants are also more likely to recall an event or exposure if they have an adverse outcome than if they do not, which could bias results. Studies can be labelled single, double, or triple blinded depending on how many of the groups were unaware of the allocation of the participants. Authors should clearly state which groups were blinded or masked. For example, if participants know they are in the intervention group, they may have increased sensitivity to the good or bad effects of the treatment. Participant blinding is easier to do in drug trials where placebos can be made to look identical to the active drug. However, in community nursing it is difficult to blind participants to a nurse coming into their home or to a psychosocial intervention. Potential bias can be minimized by ensuring that the participant does not know the specific outcome(s) being examined. Similarly, clinicians who care for the participants and know the allocation may unconsciously alter care and may have a heightened awareness of positive outcomes or adverse outcomes in a way that biases the evaluation.

The most important group to be blinded is the one that measures the outcomes. Ideally, clinicians providing care are not assessing outcomes. The measurement of key outcomes can be unconsciously distorted by the clinicians' beliefs about the intervention and its side effects. Objective outcome measures, such as antibody titres for measles, are less subject to outcome assessor bias than self-report of full measles immunization. Similarly, data analyses should be done with coded data that do not allow for identification of treatment groups. Consequently, readers of randomized trials should look for reports of which groups were and were not blinded to the participant allocation. If blinding is not possible, the authors should report on steps taken to minimize possible biases.

QUESTIONS USED TO CRITICALLY APPRAISE INTERVENTION STUDIES (TREATMENT OR PREVENTION)

1. **Are the results of this study valid?**
   a. Was the assignment of participants to treatment groups randomized, and was the randomization concealed?
   b. Was follow-up sufficiently long and complete?
   c. Were participants analyzed in the groups to which they were assigned?
   d. Were participants, clinicians, outcome assessors, and data analysts unaware of (blinded to or masked from) participant allocation?
   e. Were participants in each group treated equally except for the intervention being evaluated?
   f. Were the groups similar at the start of the trial?

2. **What were the results?**
   a. How large is the effect? Is it clinically important?
   b. How precise is the treatment effect?

3. **Will the results help me in working with my clients?**
   a. Are my clients so different from those in the study that the results do not apply?
   b. Is the treatment feasible in our setting?
   c. Were all the clinically important outcomes (harms as well as benefits) considered?
   d. What are my clients' or community's values and preferences for both the outcomes we are trying to prevent and the unintended consequences that may arise?

Source: Adapted from Cullum, N. (2001). Evaluation of studies of treatment or prevention interventions, part 2: Applying the results of studies to your patients. *Evidence-Based Nursing, 4*(1), 7–8. Reproduced with permission of the BMJ Publishing Group Ltd.

Were participants in each group treated equally except for the intervention being evaluated? Randomization should ensure that the only difference between study groups is the treatment being evaluated. An important principle is that additional treatments, or extra care, should not be given. Readers of randomized trials should look carefully at the descriptions of interventions received by all groups, especially if the practitioners are not blinded to allocation.

Were the groups similar at the start of the trial? Randomization should ensure that the groups of study participants were similar at the beginning. Usually, a table of baseline characteristics is prepared, and some analysis is done to check that randomization actually "worked." If the groups show statistically significant differences at the beginning, the impact of the intervention may be altered, which can affect the validity of the result. If imbalances do exist at baseline, adjustment in the analysis can be done with statistical techniques such as using baseline values as a covariate.

What Were the Results?

Once you have determined that the results are valid, it important to understand what the results really mean. The questions discussed and explained below will guide you through this process.

How large is the effect? Is it clinically important? How precise is the treatment effect?

The effects of treatment are measured using one or more outcome measures. They can be **dichotomous** (yes/no; alive/dead; pregnant/not pregnant) or **continuous** (weight, blood pressure, self-esteem rating). Different statistical tests are used for different types of data. Often statistical test results are reported as p value. The convention is that any p value less than 0.05 is considered statistically significant and means that the intervention has an effect on the outcome. More information may be gained about the extent of that difference using other statistical tests, such as **relative risk reduction (RRR)** and **absolute risk reduction (ARR)**.

The RRR is the proportional reduction in rates of poor outcomes (e.g., death or readmission) between the experimental (better outcomes) and control (greater poor outcomes) participants. For example, an RRR of 50% means that there were 50% fewer deaths in the experimental group compared with the control group.

$$RRR = \frac{\text{Event rate in control group} - \text{Event rate in experimental group}}{\text{Event rate in the control group}}$$

Relative risk (RR) is the proportion of participants experiencing an outcome in the intervention group divided by the proportion experiencing the outcome in the control group. However, RR does not account for the number of people in the study who would have died anyway without the intervention. This is called the absolute risk reduction (ARR). For example, an ARR of 2% means that there were 2% fewer deaths in the experimental group than the control group.

$$ARR =$$
Event rate in control group – Event rate in experimental group

Yet another approach is to report the **number needed to treat (NNT)**. This describes the number of people who must be treated with the intervention to prevent one additional negative outcome (e.g., death) or promote one additional positive outcome (e.g., smoking cessation).

$$NNT = \frac{1}{ARR}$$

When researchers report statistical significance, it is imperative to ask if this is **clinically important** or whether it has a meaningful impact on client outcomes. It is quite possible that results are statistically significant but clinically unimportant. In a hypothetical example studying weight-loss interventions for obese women, the group with a more intensive intervention lost a mean of five kilograms more than the group in the less intensive intervention. Though the researchers found this statistically significant ($p = 0.03$), it was not personally meaningful to morbidly obese women. Researchers had predetermined that weight loss would not be clinically meaningful unless the participants reached 10% weight loss. Therefore, this five-kilogram weight loss was not a clinically meaningful result.

Precision of the results can never be absolute but is estimated by calculating **confidence intervals (CIs)** around the RRR or ARR. CIs are a range of values with a specified probability (usually 95%) of including the true effect, which can never be known absolutely. Wide CIs indicate less precision in the estimated effect of the intervention. There is no magic number of what constitutes wide or narrow CIs; that judgment takes exposure to many studies. Also, it involves being able to make the same practice decision at the end of the confidence interval closest to no difference, as you would make from the overall results. Precision increases with larger sample sizes.

Will the Results Help Me in Working with My Clients?

- Are my clients (individuals, families, communities, systems, or populations) so different from those in the study that the results do not apply?
- Is the treatment feasible in our setting?
- Were all the clinically important outcomes (harms as well as benefits) considered?
- What are my clients' values and preferences for both the outcome we are trying to prevent and the unintended consequences that may arise?
- Are there implications of this study applicable at the broader policy level?

This set of questions is context dependent. That is, you need to understand your client's needs and values, and consider the benefits against the risks and costs to the client, population, and your organization or agency. This is rarely a decision of an individual practitioner, and in community health it is more often an agency, government policy, or population-level decision.

To use the findings of a study, you need to consider these questions and make judgments in relation to your own client population. Consider how similar the characteristics of the study participants are to your own clients. Think about any reasons why you should *not* apply the study results to your population, rather than looking for evidence that the study participants are exactly the same as your clients. Feasibility in your setting depends on factors such as cost, organizational resources, nursing skills, availability of special equipment, and acceptability to clients. For example, if we are considering e-health interventions to support weight loss in postpartum women it will be important to consider how applicable the results are for women who may face socio-economic, language, or literacy barriers to technology-based interventions. Harms and benefits should be included in the research by including various obvious outcomes such as health impacts but also other outcomes like quality of life and economics. Negative effects should also be included.

CRITICAL APPRAISAL OF SYSTEMATIC REVIEWS

A **systematic review** is a summary of research evidence that relates to a specific question. It could involve causation, diagnosis, or prognosis but more frequently involves effectiveness of an intervention. The terms "systematic review" and "overview" are often used interchangeably. Basing a practice decision on a single study may be a mistake, as the study may have an inadequate sample size to detect clinically important differences between treatments, leading to false conclusions. Discrepant findings across studies of the same question may occur due to chance or subtle differences in study design or participants. Therefore, it is useful to look at a summary of all the research related to a focused question.

In a narrative literature review, authors may selectively pick articles that support their viewpoint and ignore those that do not, so that the conclusion is set before the articles are selected. Systematic reviews differ from an unsystematic narrative literature review in that they attempt to overcome possible biases by following a rigorous methodology of search, retrieval, relevance and validity (quality) rating, data extraction, synthesis, and report writing. Explicit pre-set criteria are used for relevance and validity. Two people conduct each stage independently and then compare results and discuss discrepancies before moving on to the next stage. Details of the methods used at every stage are recorded.

A **meta-analysis** is a type of systematic review in which the quantitative results of several studies are combined to get an overall summary statistic that represents the combined effect of the intervention across different study populations. The reviewers must decide whether the statistical combination (meta-analysis) is appropriate by using both clinical judgment and a statistical test for heterogeneity. The clinical judgment requires the reviewers to examine the methodologies and statistical tests completed in the studies under review and ascertain if it is reasonable to combine them in a meta-analysis. The statistical tests determine whether the differences among results of individual studies are greater than one would expect if all studies were measuring the same underlying effect and the observed differences were due only to chance. The more significant the test of heterogeneity, the less likely that the observed differences are from chance alone and that some other factor, such as design, participants, intervention, or outcome, is responsible for the differences in the treatment effect across studies (Sackett et al., 2000). Readers must use their expertise to decide whether the statistical combination is reasonable. Systematic reviews help to answer questions without having to access large numbers of research reports; they overcome the obstacles of lack of time and, sometimes, lack of skills necessary to conduct the critical appraisal. But can one be confident in using all reviews? A search may easily yield more than 200 reviews—are they all of equal value? What does one do if they give conflicting results?

Common misconceptions of systematic reviews are that they include *only* randomized trials, they must adopt a biomedical model, and they must have some statistical synthesis (Petticrew, 2001). If these were true, there would be few reviews of interest in community health, as many community health questions have not been or cannot be addressed by randomized trials. Fortunately, review methods are improving to include non-randomized studies, such as cohort studies; to use a population health model; and to synthesize without necessarily including meta-analysis. The Cochrane Public Health Group (http://ph.cochrane.org) has been a leader in promoting the methods, conduct, and use of systematic reviews and meta-analyses in community healthcare. Many websites contain high-quality systematic reviews relevant to community health and resources for skill building in critical appraisal of reviews. (See MyNursingLab for additional resources.)

In this section, we look at how to critically appraise systematic reviews to decide if the methods are strong enough that the results may be applied to decisions. The same major questions used for evaluation of intervention studies can be used to evaluate systematic reviews (see the box "Questions Used to Critically Appraise Systematic Review Articles"). You will have a chance to practice appraising a systematic review article in the case study found at the end of the chapter.

Are the Results Valid?

Is this a systematic review of randomized trials? Questions about the effectiveness of treatment or prevention are best answered by randomized controlled trials if it is ethically possible to do so, whereas questions about harm or prognosis are best answered by cohort studies (Roberts & DiCenso, 1999). You should look to see if the authors used randomized trials (if ethically possible) or the next most rigorous design that included a comparison group (quasi-experimental or cohort analytic designs).

Does the systematic review include a description of the strategies used to find all relevant studies? Every systematic review grows from a focused question, through the development of the search strategies and terms for each database, to retrieval of studies. Explicit inclusion or exclusion criteria are predetermined, and the review should state that two people independently reviewed each article for inclusion. A thorough search for both published and unpublished studies should be done. The publication of research in a journal is more likely to occur in studies that have statistically significant results. Studies in which a new intervention is not found to be effective are frequently not published, a phenomenon known as publication bias. Systematic reviews that do not include unpublished studies may overestimate the effect of an intervention; that is, it will appear that the intervention is more effective than it really is. Therefore, in addition to searching through relevant databases such as CINAHL, MEDLINE, Embase, PsycINFO, ERIC, or Cochrane Library, researchers should hand-search relevant journals; review reference lists from retrieved articles; contact experts, authors, and relevant manufacturing companies; and review abstracts presented at relevant scientific meetings. For policy-related reviews, it may be important that the authors have searched for unpublished studies, also known as "grey literature," such as an evaluation of local implementation of a policy conducted by a health region or authority. Unless the authors of the reviews tell us what they did to locate relevant studies, it is difficult to know if any were missed.

Does the systematic review include a description of how the validity of individual studies was assessed? A narrative review often reports on study findings without considering the methodological strengths of the studies. Differences in study quality often explain differences in results across studies, with those of poorer quality tending to overestimate the effectiveness of the interventions (Kunz & Oxman, 1998). Quality ratings are sometimes used in the analysis to compare outcomes across

studies by study strength. Or, if there are many studies to consider, the authors may choose to apply a quality rating threshold for inclusion (i.e., include only high-quality studies) or give greater attention and weight to the stronger studies. This predefined quality checklist minimizes reviewer bias by helping to ensure that reviewers appraise each study consistently and thoroughly. Having two or more raters helps to reduce mistakes and bias and increases the reader's confidence in the systematic review. The quality rating tools usually include criteria such as those presented for evaluating interventions.

Were the results consistent from study to study? The reader would be most confident using the results of a review if the results were similar in all included studies; that is, showing the same direction of effect—all being positive, all negative, or all showing no effect. But what if the direction of effect differs across studies? Differences may be due to types of clients included; the timing, duration, and intensity of the intervention; the outcomes measured; or the ways in which the outcomes were measured. If there are differences in results, the reader may also consider if there are differences in the quality of the primary studies that could influence the effect estimates (as discussed earlier).

What Were the Results?

How large was the treatment effect? How precise was the estimate of treatment effect? Comparing a simple count of studies that helped, harmed, or showed no difference in treatments would assume that all studies had equal validity, power of the sample size to detect a difference, duration and intensity of interventions, and follow-up. Meta-analysis, when appropriate, can assign different weights to individual studies so that those with greater precision or higher quality make a greater contribution to the summary statistic. Summary statistics often used include **odds ratio (OR)**, relative risk (RR, defined earlier), and **weighted mean difference**. The OR describes the likelihood of a participant in the experimental group having an event (e.g., pregnancy) divided by the likelihood of a participant in the control group having the event. In a study such as prevention of pregnancy, one would consider that an RR or OR of less than 1 represents a beneficial treatment. Weighted mean difference is the mean of the difference found between control and intervention groups across studies entered into a meta-analysis. Both OR and RR are used for dichotomous data (dead/alive, pregnant/not pregnant, smoking/not smoking), whereas weighted mean difference is used for continuous data (weight, blood pressure, blood glucose). For more information on OR and RR, see Chapter 11.

The precision of the results is estimated by calculating confidence intervals (CI, defined earlier) around the summary statistic. The CI is useful for decision making because we can look at both extremes of the effect. For a dichotomous outcome, if the lower extreme is 1 or close to it, the effect of the intervention is quite small and probably not worthwhile. A hypothetical display is shown in Figure 10.3 to demonstrate how **forest plots** from a meta-analysis are read. The summary odds ratio of the three studies in Figure 10.3 is 0.69 (95% CI: 0.51–0.90), which indicates that the treatment was effective in producing the desired outcome.

QUESTIONS USED TO CRITICALLY APPRAISE SYSTEMATIC REVIEW ARTICLES

1. **Are the results of this systematic review valid?**
   a. Is this a systematic review of randomized trials?
   b. Does the systematic review include a description of the strategies used to find all the relevant articles?
   c. Does the systematic review include a description of how the validity of individual studies was assessed?
   d. Were the results consistent from study to study?

2. **What were the results?**
   a. How large was the treatment effect?
   b. How precise was the estimate of treatment effect?

3. **Will the results help me in working with my clients?**
   a. Are my clients so different from those in the study that the results do not apply?
   b. Is the treatment feasible in our setting?
   c. Were all the clinically important outcomes (harms as well as benefits) considered?
   d. What are my clients' values and preferences for both the outcomes we are trying to prevent and the unintended consequences that may arise?

Sources: Adapted from Ciliska, D., Cullum, N., & Marks, S. (2001). Evaluation of systematic reviews of treatment or prevention interventions. *Evidence-Based Nursing, 4*(4), 100–104; Sackett, D. L., Strauss, S. E., Richardson, W. S., Rosenberg, W., & Haynes, R. B. (2000). *Evidence-Based Medicine: How to Practice and Teach EBM.* London, UK: Churchill Livingstone.

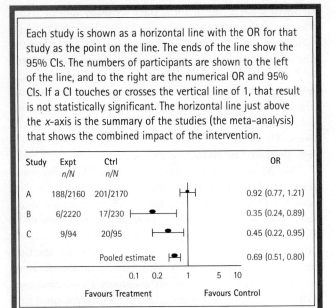

Each study is shown as a horizontal line with the OR for that study as the point on the line. The ends of the line show the 95% CIs. The numbers of participants are shown to the left of the line, and to the right are the numerical OR and 95% CIs. If a CI touches or crosses the vertical line of 1, that result is not statistically significant. The horizontal line just above the x-axis is the summary of the studies (the meta-analysis) that shows the combined impact of the intervention.

Study	Expt n/N	Ctrl n/N		OR
A	188/2160	201/2170		0.92 (0.77, 1.21)
B	6/2220	17/230		0.35 (0.24, 0.89)
C	9/94	20/95		0.45 (0.22, 0.95)
		Pooled estimate		0.69 (0.51, 0.80)

0.1 0.2 1 5 10

Favours Treatment   Favours Control

FIGURE   10.3   Example of Meta-Analysis Display

Will the Results Help Me in Working with My Clients?

- Are my clients so different from those in the study that the study results do not apply?
- Is the treatment feasible in our setting?
- Were all the clinically important outcomes (harms as well as benefits) considered?
- What are my clients' values and preferences for both the outcome we are trying to prevent and the unintended consequences that may arise?

These questions are context dependent; that is, you need to understand your client's preferences, know the resources in your setting, and consider the benefits against the risks and costs. For example, feasibility in a school-based multifaceted sexual health program intervention would relate not only to the skills of the nurses and resources of the health department to deliver the intervention, but also to the ability of the school board to withstand the parental pressures for abstinence programs. In addition, researchers look for all outcomes, both positive and negative, that might affect the participants and the health care system. Outcomes might include mortality, morbidity, costs, quality of life, and participant satisfaction. Participant and family values must be considered. If, in the example above, families are unwilling to have their children exposed to multifaceted sexual health education programs, the students must be given an alternative during that school time.

Where possible, decisions should not be made based on a single study. Systematic reviews allow for much more confidence in the research evidence. This is particularly important for policy decisions.

CRITICAL APPRAISAL OF QUALITATIVE RESEARCH

Qualitative research is important for the development of nursing knowledge. Qualitative research describes, explores, and explains phenomena and is concerned with the process or experience rather than outcomes. To obtain rich data, sampling is purposive as opposed to the random or probability sampling used in quantitative research. Data collection is done in many ways, but the most common are observation and group or individual interviews. Data analysis is completed using codes, themes, and patterns, not by statistical techniques, and it produces rich, deep descriptions rather than numbers. Qualitative research does not allow inference to a population as a whole but allows the researcher to generalize to a theoretical understanding of the phenomena being studied (Grove, Burns, & Gray, 2012).

Major types of qualitative research used in nursing include (a) phenomenology, (b) grounded theory, (c) ethnography, (d) case study, (e) qualitative description, and (f) PAR. The first three are the most common. **Phenomenology** seeks to describe the lived experiences of people (Creswell, 2012), such as the experience of people returning home after a stroke. **Grounded theory** generates theories or models of the phenomena being studied (Creswell, 2012), such as the development of a model of coping used by family caregivers of people who have HIV. **Ethnography** describes a culture (Creswell, 2012) and answers questions such as what it is like to be a pregnant teen trying to continue with school. Reading qualitative research deepens our understanding of the perceptions and experiences of people we work with and has the potential to enrich our interactions and care through a more complete understanding of a situations. When researchers want to explore a program, activity, or event in detail, they use case study design. This method involves multiple modes of in-depth data collection over a sustained period (Creswell, 2012). The purpose of qualitative descriptive studies is to provide a comprehensive summary of events in everyday terms. The methods of sampling, data collection, and analysis can vary, but researchers stay close to the data (Sandelowski, 2000). As stated earlier, action-oriented research questions and interventions that evolve through partnerships between researchers and participants are best dealt with through PAR (Grove et al., 2012).

The questions used to evaluate primary treatment studies or systematic reviews can be used to evaluate qualitative research (see the box titled "Questions Used to Critically Appraise Qualitative Research Reports"). For application of these criteria to Canadian studies, see Case Study B about a grounded theory study and Case Study C about participatory action study in MyNursingLab.

Are the Findings Valid?

Is the research question clear and adequately substantiated? This question will determine whether the qualitative study will be read. The article should clearly establish the question and what is already known about the topic.

Is the design appropriate for the research question? Overall, it is important to determine if the authors used the appropriate method for their question (e.g., phenomenology is used to explore experience and meaning for clients following colostomy, rather than using an ethnographic approach). A more sophisticated appraisal considers whether the specific design and its theoretical or philosophical roots (the types of questions the methodology is designed to address) fit with the purpose of the study.

Was the method of sampling appropriate for the research question? The study should report on how participants were selected. Many different types of sampling are used in qualitative research, including theoretical sampling or purposeful sampling for maximum variation, typical cases, extreme cases, or critical cases.

Were data collected and managed systematically? The study should try to define the breadth (variation, multiple perspectives) and depth (numbers and types of data collected). Also, has each investigator kept track of the process—data collection, exploring hunches, decision making, and data analysis procedures—using journaling and memos?

Were the data analyzed appropriately? The researcher should report on how the data were organized and reduced to identify patterns. Are there clear links between the data (e.g., the narrative and quotes) and the themes that were developed out of the data? Often the analysis identifies further areas for data collection and analysis. Usually, the researcher uses other team members to assist in the analysis, providing various interpretations of the data. Member checking (taking the results back to the participants or people associated with the issue under study) is often done to validate the findings, assess for resonance of findings with participant experience, and gather alternative interpretations of the analysis.

QUESTIONS USED TO CRITICALLY APPRAISE QUALITATIVE RESEARCH REPORTS

1. **Are the findings valid?**
   a. Is the research question clear and adequately substantiated?
   b. Is the design appropriate for the research question?
   c. Was the method of sampling appropriate for the research question?
   d. Were data collected and managed systematically?
   e. Were the data analyzed appropriately?

2. **What were the findings?**
   a. Is the description of findings thorough?

3. **Will the results help me in working with my clients?**
   a. What meaning and relevance does the study have for my practice?
   b. Does the study help me understand the context of my practice?
   c. Does the study enhance my knowledge about my practice?

Source: Adapted from Russell, C. K., & Gregory, D. M. (2003). Evaluation of qualitative research studies. *Evidence-Based Nursing, 6*(2), 36–40. Reproduced with permission of the BMJ Publishing Group.

What Were the Findings?

Is the description of findings thorough? Qualitative research is difficult to write within the word limit of standard journals. It is difficult to fit the rich description of results and analysis into one publication. It is expected that authors have used direct quotations from participants to illustrate the descriptions and conceptualizations.

Will the Results Help Me in Working with My Clients?

- What meaning and relevance does the study have for my practice?
- Does the study help me understand the context of my practice?
- Does the study enhance my knowledge about my practice?

As with the other critical appraisal tools, this final section is focused on contextualizing the research. The authors should establish the need for and relevance of the research and discuss the results in the context of other existing knowledge. Readers must use their critique of the study as well as the information presented in the report to decide if any parts of the research findings are potentially transferable to their own practice and policy decisions at the local, provincial, or national level.

4. Synthesize

The synthesis stage requires that you (a) consider the evidence found, (b) determine how to deal with conflicting results in different studies, and (c) identify which evidence you will use for decision making. To decide which evidence to use, consider which source is the most highly synthesized evidence (e.g., guideline, systematic review) according to the 6S pyramid. Next, select the article(s) you appraised to be of highest quality. Third, you should examine the date of publication, particularly guidelines or systematic reviews, published within the past two years (otherwise the studies are old). Alternatively, for an older review, you can replicate the search and find studies that have come out since the search in that review ended. If there are conflicting results from reviews or individual studies of equal quality, then fourth consider relevance to your population, and lastly, the resources required to implement the intervention.

In community health nursing, many decisions to implement a change in practice or policy are beyond the individual; they are decided by a team. In every case, the decision involves all five aspects of Figure 10.1: research evidence, community health issues and local context, community and political preferences and actions, public health resources, and public health expertise. Furthermore, if the decision goes beyond individual clients or small groups, political and organizational elements become involved. This is particularly evident in the final decision of the example of an intervention around school-based sexual health education. The students, parents, and high school would all have to be involved in the decision if there is any chance for a school-based intervention for sexual health to be successful.

What should you do if no research evidence is found during the database search? Or if the research that comes up is of consistently poor quality? In those cases, expert opinion or usual practice is the standard for decision making. You may be able to find practice guidelines on the topic. These depend on a thorough literature review and then consensus meetings with expert panels to make practice decisions, particularly where research evidence does not exist (Registered Nurses Association of Ontario, 2010; U.S. Department of Health and Human Services, Agency for Healthcare Research and Quality, 2010). Similarly, "best practice" documents describe programs or interventions that seem to be effective but may not yet have been rigorously evaluated.

Caution must be exercised when implementing interventions for which there is no good evaluation. Rationale for decisions needs to be documented. CHNs must be particularly vigilant in observing for effects, both positive and negative, then ensuring that they are documented. Unfortunately, many effects are not evident until years after the intervention when no one is observing any longer! Areas of interest where evaluation does not exist are prime research questions that should receive priority attention from funding agencies.

5. Adapt

Once your team decides which research evidence to use, you must consider all the population and political factors involved in making a program or policy decision. A tool was developed, based on a literature review, that helps you to consider a multitude of factors in addition to the research results. It is called the Applicability and Transferability Tool by Buffett, Ciliska, and Thomas (2011) and may be found at www.nccmt.ca/pubs/A&Trevised-startEN.pdf. In the decision-making process, the tool prompts team members to think about how the intervention needs to be adapted to the local population. Factors that need to be considered include the magnitude of the issue in your population, the social acceptability of the program or policy you are considering implementing, the political acceptability of your intervention, and the ability to garner resources for the program or policy you have chosen to implement.

6. Implement

After you've found the best available evidence to answer your question and adapted it to your client or community, you and your team will need to decide about whether to change practice. Once a decision has been made and organizational support is achieved, a comprehensive plan must address how everyone within the organization will be informed of the proposed change. Regardless of whether you are changing key messages you share with clients for health teaching, starting a new program or revising a policy, change within your organization or agency is usually required. Changing the practice of health care professionals has been studied extensively with mixed and unclear results. The "Effective Practice and Organization of Care" review group (www.epoc.cochrane.org/en/index.html) within the Cochrane Collaboration conducts systematic reviews of educational,

behavioural, organizational, financial, and regulatory interventions related to changing the practice of health care professionals or the organization of health care. One large systematic review studied strategies for guideline dissemination and implementation (Grimshaw et al., 2004). They found that the median absolute improvements in performance across interventions was 14.1% in comparisons of reminders, 8.1% in comparisons of dissemination of educational materials, 7.0% in comparisons of audit and feedback, and 6.0% in comparisons of multifaceted interventions involving educational outreach. This is somewhat surprising, as you might expect that there would be enhanced performance improvements with multiple interventions.

The implementation plan should include a diagnostic analysis (environmental scan) to identify barriers and supports to the characteristics of the innovation (the change being introduced), the client (individual, families, communities, systems, or populations), the practitioners, the organization, and the environment so that barriers can be reduced and supports strengthened. It is important to consider characteristics of the innovation, such as the resources it will require (will it cost more or be time/resource saving?) and how different it is from current practice. Relevant characteristics of individual practitioners include level of education, years of experience, and general acceptance or resistance to change. Organizational characteristics include affiliation with an academic setting, size, level of care, funding sources, organizational structure, research participation, research orientation, and usual valuing of research findings. The environment includes factors such as rural or urban setting, economic status of the community, and health issues valued by the community (Dobbins, Ciliska, Cockerill, Barnsley, & DiCenso, 2002).

Important stakeholders must be identified. They may include the nurses, medical staff, clients, and accounting staff. A champion may be needed with the enthusiasm and energy to push for practice change. Identifying opinion leaders and influencing their understanding and attitudes about the proposed practice change is another strategy worth pursuing, despite the inconclusive evidence that this strategy is effective. Interventions to promote dissemination, uptake, and utilization of research results is an area that requires further focused research to complete the cycle of evidence-informed practice, from question identification to implementation and evaluation.

7. Evaluate

After implementing a practice or policy change, an evaluation period is needed to see if it is working. This does not mean replicating the original study that was used as a basis for the practice change. It does, however, mean a period of data collection from baseline to ensure that the rates of the desired outcomes are like those in the original study. Additionally, participation rates could be used to understand client (individual, family, community, system, or population) acceptability. It is also significant to note if any potential negative outcomes are like those listed in the study. Finally, it is important to let others who work with similar populations know about what you did and how it worked. This dissemination can be done through formal mechanisms (e.g., conference presentations and papers, educational meetings) or informally through dialogue within networks and online forums.

USING RESEARCH IN PRACTICE

Although CHNs often work within an organization or agency, they have a professional responsibility as individual nurses to reflect on areas of uncertainty in their practice. CHNs can use their critical thinking skills to ask questions and use the best available evidence to make decisions. As part of CHNs' professional responsibility and accountability (standard seven), CHNs are expected to "provide leadership by creating change in communities and systems," "use current evidence and informatics to identify, generate, manage and process relevant data to support nursing practice," "participate in research," and "advocate for effective and efficient use of health care resources" (CHNC, 2011 revised, pp. 22–23). To fulfill this standard, CHNs can use the process of evidence-informed practice described in this chapter.

Using Research for Management Decisions and Policy Development

While research evidence is useful for practitioners working with individual clients, it is also important that management decisions be evidence informed. Decisions regarding the implementation of a new intervention in a community are usually made where there is no additional funding. Therefore, if the organization wishes to begin a new program, it must be done with existing resources. This may mean taking staff away from other programs or activities to dedicate their time to the new initiative. Reviewing the research evidence for both the proposed activity and any existing programs helps managers to make those decisions.

The actual conduct (as opposed to the search and discovery) of systematic reviews has contributed to their use by clinicians and policy-level decision makers. Potential review questions are sought from the policy, management, and front-line clinician perspectives. Groups that conduct the reviews typically include the methodological experts along with the community practitioners and policy decision makers chosen for their content expertise and their understanding of the context and relevance to community health. These expert partners can assist in identifying and refining the priority questions, rating articles for relevance to the question, reviewing drafts, and helping to write clinical, management, and policy implications. People working at institutional or government policy levels are increasingly aware of and value the need for research evidence, yet they face other competing factors (e.g., public opinion and pressures, fiscal restraints) when making policy decisions.

CASE STUDY

Critical Appraisal of a Systematic Review
(Durepos et al., 2017)

Scenario: The prevalence of dementia in Canada is increasing. Dementia is a progressive neurodegenerative disease that causes physical, psychological, and behavioural symptoms. As a CHN, you are seeing an increasing number of community-dwelling older adults with dementia. Care for this disease is challenging for the patient themselves as well as their family members and other caregivers. The home and community care agencies, local hospital, and long-term care homes in your area have established a committee to collaboratively identify best practice recommendations for consistent dementia care. Given that this disease is chronic and life-limiting, the committee needs to identify a dementia care guideline that provides comprehensive recommendations, including palliative care. As a CHN, you were invited to be a committee member and are tasked with looking for the best available evidence.

You try the search skills you learned through a free online learning module about searching (www.nccmt.ca). The approach to searching should allow you to find high-quality pre-processed research evidence in a short time. You decide to look for published evidence first and go to PubMed (www.pubmed.gov) and click "Clinical Queries" in the centre of the page, under "PubMed Tools." You enter the search terms *dementia* AND *palliative* AND *guideline*. Based what you learned about the 6S pyramid,

you hope to identify a guideline or systematic review first, rather than looking at single studies. You get a short list of results under the heading "systematic reviews." The second result by Durepos and colleagues (2017) is recent and looks relevant. You quickly scan the rest of the results for systematic reviews and don't see anything else recent and relevant. You retrieve the article, which is open access.

The purpose of the review by Durepos et al. was to assess palliative care content in current guidelines for dementia. The review has a clearly focused question that is relevant to your situation. The review includes international guidelines focused on comprehensive care for people with dementia and/or Alzheimer's disease. You decide to read on.

You think back to the questions used to critically appraise systematic review articles described earlier in this chapter. This is not a review of randomized controlled trials, but the authors have looked for the right type of research evidence (clinical practice guidelines) to answer their question.

The review involved a comprehensive search of health and psychological databases, including CINAHL, MEDLINE, Embase, and PsycINFO. The review team also used other techniques to locate published and unpublished literature such as searching the websites of organizations focused on neurology or cognitive impairment and contacting them for more information, as well as checking reference lists of relevant documents. Two reviewers used predetermined inclusion criteria to independently assess each reference identified in the search for relevance.

The quality of included guidelines was appraised using the Appraisal of Guidelines for Research and Evaluation II (Agree II) tool, a standardized international tool for assessing guideline quality (Brouwers et al., 2010). A cut-off score of 60% or greater on the rigour of development domain and an overall quality score of four or more out of seven was used to ensure the highest quality evidenced was synthesized. Quality assessment and data extraction were completed by two independent reviewers to minimize bias. After completing the appraisal of this review, you have confidence in the findings.

The review team used the Square of Care Model to Guide Palliative Care (Canadian Hospice Palliative Care Association, 2015) to organize the data extraction from each guideline and summarized findings in a table. Since this review is not about the effectiveness of an intervention, the findings do not include numerical results or an overall estimate of a treatment effect. However, you can view the consistency of findings across the included guidelines presented in the table in the article.

Reading the article in more detail you see 11 guidelines are included in the analysis. The National Institute for Health and Clinical Excellence (NICE) (2006, updated 2016) guideline on dementia includes content on all domains of the square of care model except for loss and grief. It also received the highest quality rating of the guidelines reviewed. You retrieve this comprehensive guideline from the United Kingdom, which provides recommendations on disease management, physical and cognitive function, as well as psychological, social, practical, spiritual, and end-of-life care. You think it would be relevant to adults with dementia living in your community. This review you located has quickly helped you to identify a high-quality guideline that will be of interest to your committee.

Discussion Questions

1. Will you present this systematic review and the relevant guideline identified from it at your next committee meeting? How could this research evidence inform your next steps?

2. How did finding and using a systematic review in this scenario help to overcome some of the barriers to research use among nurses?

3. Let's say you hadn't identified a systematic review or a guideline in your initial search of PubMed. What are three other sources you could search to identify guidelines?

PARTICIPATING IN COMMUNITY HEALTH RESEARCH

CHNs are involved in many different types of research, the most common being program evaluation using process outcomes such as numbers of clients, numbers of groups, hours spent, and reasons for home visits. These types of data are important for tracking uses of services and how resources are spent within the agency. Client outcome measurement is the next most likely information collected; for example, client mortality, morbidity, immunization status or coverage, communicable disease outbreak, goals met, or breastfeeding rates. CHNs are usually asked to capture these data, at least in formal records. They also may be required to report it in other formats, or the agency may conduct periodic chart reviews or database summaries. These local data often feed into provincial and national databases and registries of statistics. Some of these databases are available to regions within a province so that local rates can be followed.

CHNs could also be involved in recruiting, collecting data, and analyzing qualitative or quantitative information for a research study. For example, a CHN may facilitate focus groups with new immigrant women to understand their experience as a first-time parent living in a new country. CHNs could also be involved in gathering survey data for a study about the health of the homeless to better understand the health issues impacting this vulnerable population.

CONCLUSION

In this chapter, we reviewed evidence-informed decision making as it relates to community health nursing. Although evidence can be observations made by the nurse, expert "gut hunches," or advice of colleagues, we too often ignore the evidence from research (Estabrooks, Chong, Brigidear, & Profetto-McGrath, 2005). Therefore, this chapter focused on research evidence—finding, critiquing, and using it through the process of evidence-informed decision making. Particular detail was presented in relation to critical appraisal of research articles on effectiveness questions (primary studies or systematic reviews) and qualitative research to judge whether it should be used in practice, management, or policy decisions. The process of using quality research evidence does not end with critical appraisal and individual client decisions. In community health nursing, evidence-informed practice more often involves getting organizational "buy-in" and changing policies and procedures or interventions. We presented information about understanding the barriers to using research to change community health nursing practice, management decisions, and policies.

Research, in the form of process evaluation, currently takes place daily in every community organization in Canada. Therefore, CHNs have many opportunities to become involved in research. Further, as the valuing of research evidence increases in community health nursing, the critical attitude necessary for evidence-informed decision making will increase so that health care professionals will more frequently ask questions about their practice. Since there is not a research-based answer for every practice question within community health, the need to conduct research in community health will continue. CHNs will find they are asked to participate in research by collecting data, providing interventions, or developing research proposals.

KEY TERMS

absolute risk reduction (ARR)   (p. 191)

bias   (p. 190)

clinical questions   (p. 187)

clinically important   (p. 191)

cohort design   (p. 188)

confidence intervals (CIs)   (p. 191)

continuous   (p. 191)

critical appraisal skills   (p. 188)

dichotomous   (p. 191)

ethnography   (p. 194)

evidence-informed decision making (EIDM)   (p. 183)

evidence-based nursing (EBN)   (p. 184)

evidence-informed practice   (p. 185)

forest plot   (p. 193)

grounded theory   (p. 194)

guidelines   (p. 187)

intention-to-treat analysis   (p. 190)

intervention study   (p. 189)

meta-analysis   (p. 192)

mixed methods research   (p. 189)

number needed to treat (NNT)   (p. 191)

observational studies   (p. 187)

odds ratio (OR)   (p. 193)

outcomes   (p. 185)

participatory action research (PAR)   (p. 188)

phenomenology   (p. 194)

qualitative research   (p. 188)

quantitative research   (p. 188)

randomized controlled trials   (p. 188)

relative risk (RR)   (p. 191)

relative risk reduction (RRR)   (p. 191)

systematic review   (p. 192)

weighted mean difference   (p. 193)

STUDY QUESTIONS

1. Identify four factors to consider for evidence-informed decision making.

2. What attitude provides the basis for the EIDM to begin?

3. In what ways might you conduct research as part of your daily role in community health nursing?

4. Name the four major categories of factors to consider when planning to implement a clinical practice or policy change. Give a few examples under each category.

5. Give examples of client-related questions that would most appropriately be answered by phenomenology, grounded theory, and ethnography.

INDIVIDUAL CRITICAL-THINKING EXERCISES

1. Pick an intervention that has been shown to be effective, and discuss how you would plan to implement that practice change in an agency or organization. (You could search www.healthevidence.org to find an effective intervention relevant to community health.) What factors would you assess? What processes would you use?

2. Answer the following using Figure 10.3.

   a. How many studies were involved in this meta-analysis?

   b. Which of those studies had statistically significant findings?

   c. How would you interpret the result? Is the intervention effective? Is it statistically significant? Is it precise?

   If you need help with interpreting the results of a meta-analysis to answer this question, review the brief video on understanding research evidence from the NCCMT called *Forest Plots* at www.nccmt.ca.

3. In a study of an intervention to increase school students' use of helmets when in-line skating, the intervention consisted of an in-school educational video plus free helmets, versus the video alone. The odds ratio for observed helmet use was 3.85 in favour of the video plus free helmets (CI 3.05 to 4.11). Was this a statistically significant result? Put the results into words using the odds ratio.

   If you need help with interpreting an odds ratio, review the brief video on understanding research evidence from the NCCMT called *How to Calculate an Odds Ratio* at www.nccmt.ca.

GROUP CRITICAL-THINKING EXERCISES

1. Select an article that evaluates an intervention relevant to community health nursing. Use the criteria in the box titled "Questions Used to Critically Appraise Intervention Studies (Treatment or Prevention)" to critically appraise the article and come to a decision about using the intervention in your own practice.

2. As in question 1, critically appraise a systematic review article using the criteria in the box titled "Questions Used to Critically Appraise Systematic Review Articles."

3. As in question 1, critically appraise an article on qualitative research using the criteria in the box titled "Questions Used to Critically Appraise Qualitative Research Reports." If it is a valid study, discuss what the study findings contribute to your understanding of the issue that was explored.

REFERENCES

Alspach, G. (2006). Nurses' use and understanding of evidence-based practice: Some preliminary evidence. *Critical Care Nurse, 26*(6), 11–12.

Ashman, A., Brown, L., Collins, C., Rollo, M., & Rae, K. (2017). Factors associated with effective nutrition interventions for pregnant Indigenous women: A systematic review. *Journal of the Academy of Nutrition & Dietetics, 117*(8), 1222–1253.

Buffet, C., Ciliska, D., & Thomas, H. (2011). *It worked there. Will it work here? Tool for assessing applicability and transferability of evidence (A: When considering starting a new program)*. Hamilton, ON: National Collaborating Centre for Methods and Tools. Retrieved from http://www.nccmt.ca/uploads/media/media/0001/01/bfb0cda5aaa62c5b-5d9894e5c98804b85b41cf36.pdf

Brouwers, M., Kho, M., Browman, G. P., Burgers, J. S., Cluzeau, F., Feder, G., . . . Zitzelsberger, L. (2010). AGREE II: Advancing guideline development, reporting and evaluation in health care. *Canadian Medical Association Journal, 182*(18), E839–E842. doi: 10.1503/cmaj.090449

Canadian Health Services Research Foundation. (2004). *What counts? Interpreting evidence-based decision-making for management and policy*. Report of the 6th CHSRF Annual Invitational Workshop. Ottawa, ON: Author. Retrieved from http://www.cfhi-fcass.ca/migrated/pdf/event_reports/2004_workshop_report_e.pdf

Canadian Hospice Palliative Care Association (CHPCA). (2013). A model to guide hospice palliative care. Ottawa, ON. Available from www.chpca.net/media/319547/norms-of-practice-eng-web.pdf

Chiefs of Ontario, Cancer Care Ontario, & Institute for Clinical Evaluative Sciences. (2016). *Cancer in First Nations people in Ontario: Mortality, survival and prevalence*. Toronto, ON: Author. Retrieved from: https://www.cancercareontario.ca/en/statistical-reports/cancer-first-nations-people-ontario-incidence-mortality-survival-and-prevalence

Ciliska, D., Cullum, N., & Marks, S. (2001). Evaluation of systematic reviews of treatment or prevention interventions. *Evidence-Based Nursing, 4*(4), 100–104.

Ciliska, D., Thomas, H., & Buffett, C. (2012). *A compendium of critical appraisal tools for public health practice*. Hamilton, ON: National Collaborating Centre for Methods and Tools. Retrieved from http://www.nccmt.ca/pubs/Compendium-ToolENG.pdf

Community Health Nurses of Canada (CHNC). (2019, revised). *Canadian community health nursing: Professional practice model & standards of practice*. St. John's, NL: Author. Retrieved from https://www.chnc.ca/documents/CHNC-ProfessionalPracticeModel-EN/index.html

Creswell, J. W. (2012). *Qualitative inquiry and research design: Choosing among five approaches*. Thousand Oaks, CA: Sage Publications.

DiCenso, A., Guyatt, G., & Ciliska, D. (2005). *Evidence-based nursing: A guide to clinical practice*. St. Louis, MO: Mosby.

DiCenso, A., Bayley, L., & Haynes, B. (2009). Accessing pre-appraised evidence: Fine tuning the 5S model into a 6S model. *Evidence-Based Nursing, 12*(4), 99–101.

Dobbins, M., Ciliska, D., Cockerill, R., Barnsley, J., & DiCenso, A. (2002). A framework for the dissemination and utilization of research for health care policy and practice. *Online Journal of Knowledge Synthesis in Nursing, 9*(7), 149–160. doi:10.1111/j.1524- 475X.2002.00149.x

Dobbins, M., Davies, B., Danseco, E., Edwards, N., & Virani, T. (2005). Changing nursing practice: Evaluating the usefulness of a best- practice guideline implementation toolkit. *Nursing Leadership, 18*(1), 34–45.

Dobbins, M., Husson, H., DeCorby, K., & LaRocca, R. L. (2013). School-based physical activity programs for promoting physical activity and fitness in children and adolescents aged 6 to 18. *Cochrane Database of Systematic Reviews, 2*. Art. No.: CD007651. doi:10.1002/14651858.CD007651.pub2

Durepos, P., Wickson-Griffiths, A., Hazzan, A. A., Kaasalainen, S., Vastis, V., Battisella, L., & Papaioannou, A. (2017). Assessing palliative care content in dementia care guidelines: A systematic review. *Journal of Pain and Symptom Management, 53*(4), pp. 804–813. doi: 10.1016/j.jpainsymman.2016.10.368

Estabrooks, C. A., Chong, H., Brigidear, K., & Profetto-McGrath, J. (2005). Profiling Canadian nurses' preferred knowledge sources for clinical practice. *Canadian Journal of Nursing Research*, 37(2), 118–40.

Farmer, A. P., Légaré, F., Turcot, L., Grimshaw, J., Harvey, E., McGowan, J. L., & Wolf, F. (2008). Printed educational materials: Effect on professional practice and health care outcomes. *Cochrane Database Systematic Reviews, 16*(3), Art. No.: CD004398.

Graham, I. D., Logan, J., Harrison, M. B., Straus, S. E., Tetroe, J., Caswell, W., & Robinson, N. (2006). Lost in knowledge translation: Time for a map? *Journal of Continuing Education in the Health Professions, 26*(1), 13–24.

Grimshaw, J. M., Thomas, R. E., MacLennan, G., Fraser, C., Ramsay, C. R., Vale, L., . . . Donaldson, C. (2004). Effectiveness and efficiency of guideline dissemination and implementation strategies. *Health Technology Assessment, 8*(6), 1–72. doi:10.3310/hta8060

Grove, S. K., Burns, N., & Gray, J. (2012). *The practice of nursing research: Appraisal, synthesis and generation of evidence*. St. Louis, MO: Elsevier.

Heater, B. S., Becker, A. M., & Olson, R. (1988). Nursing interventions and patient outcomes. A meta-analysis of studies. *Nursing Research, 37*(5), 303–307.

Health Canada. (2010). Prenatal nutrition guidelines for health professionals: Gestational weight gain [Internet]. Ottawa, ON: Health Canada. Retrieved from http://www.hcsc.gc.ca/fn-an/alt_formats/pdf/nutrition/prenatal/ewba-mbsa-eng.pdf

Jadad, A. R., & Haynes, R. B. (1998). The Cochrane collaboration: Advances and challenges in improving evidence-based decision making. *Medical Decision Making, 18*(1), 2–9.

Kunz, R., & Oxman, A. (1998). The unpredictability paradox: Review of empirical comparisons of randomized and non-randomized clinical trials. *British Medical Journal, 317*(7167), 1185–1190.

Lomas, J. (1991). Words without action? The production, dissemination, and impact of consensus recommendations. *Annual Review of Public Health, 12*(1), 41–65.

Maar, M., Burchell, A., Little, J., Ogilvie, G., Severini, A., Yang, J. M., & Zehbe, I. (2013). A qualitative study of provider perspectives of structural barriers to cervical cancer screening among First Nations women. *Women's Health Issues, 23*(5), e319–e325. doi:10.1016/j.whi.2013.06.005

Maar, M., Wakewich, P., Wood, B., Severini, A., Little, J., Buchell, A. N., . . . Zehbe, I. (2016). Strategies for increasing cervical cancer screening amongst First Nations communities in Northwest Ontario, Canada. *Health Care for Women International, 37*(4), 478–495. doi:10.1080/07399332.2014.959168

McGahan, C. E., Linn, K., Guno, P., Johnson, H., Colman, A. J., Spinelli, J. J., & Caron, N. R. (2017). Cancer in First Nations people living in British Columbia, Canada: An analysis of incidence and survival from 1993 to 2010.

Cancer Causes Control, 28(10), 1105–1116. doi: 10.1007/s10552-017-0950-7

Melnyk, B., Fineout-Overholt, E., Feinstein, N. F., Li, H., Small, L., Wilcox, L., & Kraus, R. (2004). Nurses perceived knowledge, beliefs, skills, and needs regarding evidence-based practice: Implications for accelerating the paradigm shift. *Worldviews on Evidence-Based Nursing, 1*(3), 185–193.

Morris, Z. S., Wooding, S., & Grant, J. (2011). The answer is 17 years, what is the question: Understanding time lags in translational research. *Journal of the Royal Society of Medicine, 104*(12), 510–520.

National Collaborating Centre for Methods and Tools (NCCMT). (2012). A model for evidence-informed decision making in public health. [fact sheet]. Retrieved from http://www.nccmt.ca/uploads/media/media/0001/01/4504c27e14836059b8fd3ce3b3eaac2ed2ce6ed6.pdf

National Institute for Health and Clinical Excellence. (2006, updated 2016). Dementia: supporting people with dementia and their carers in health and social care. Retrieved from https://www.nice.org.uk/guidance/cg42

Oxman, A., Guyatt, G., Cook, D., & Montori, V. (2002). Summarizing the evidence. In G. Guyatt & D. Rennie (Eds.), *Users' guides to the medical literature: A manual for evidence-based clinical practice* (pp. 155–173). Chicago, IL: AMA Press.

Petticrew, M. (2001). Systematic reviews from astronomy to zoology: Myths and misconceptions. *British Medical Journal, 322*(7278), 98–101.

Public Health Agency of Canada (PHAC). (2008). *Core Competencies for Public Health. 1.0.* Ottawa, ON: Author. Retrieved from http://www.phac-aspc.gc.ca/ccph-cesp/index-eng.php

Public Health Agency of Canada (PHAC). (2009). What mothers say: The Canadian maternity experiences survey. Ottawa. Retrieved from http://www.phac-aspc.gc.ca/rhs-ssg/pdf/survey-eng.pdf

Registered Nurses Association of Ontario. (2010). *Best practice guidelines*. Toronto: ON: Author. Retrieved from http://www.rnao.org

Roberts, J., & DiCenso, A. (1999). Identifying the best research design to fit the question, part 1: Quantitative designs. *Evidence-Based Nursing, 2*(1), 4–6.

Sackett, D. L., Rosenberg, W., Gray, J. A. M., & Haynes, R. B. (1996). Evidence-based medicine: What it is and what it isn't. *British Medical Journal, 312*(7050), 71–72.

Sackett, D. L., Strauss, S. E., Richardson, W. S., Rosenberg, W., & Haynes, R. B. (2000). *Evidence based medicine: How to practice and teach EBM.* London, UK: Churchill Livingstone.

Sandelowski, M. (2000). Whatever happened to qualitative description? *Research in Nursing & Health, 23*(4), 334–340.

Sherifali, D., Nerenberg, K. A., Wilson, S., Ali, M. U., Redman, L. M., & Adamo, K. B. (2017). The effectiveness of eHealth technologies on weight management in pregnant and postpartum women: Systematic review and meta-analysis. *Journal of Medical Internet Research, 19*(10), 1–14.

Squires, J. E., Moralejo, D., & LeFort, S. M. (2007). Exploring the role of organizational policies and procedures in promoting research utilization in registered nurses. *Implementation Science, 2*(1), 17.

Tricco, A. C., Thomas, S. M., Veroniki, A. A., Hamid, J. S., Cogo, E., Strifler, L., . . . Straus, S. E. (2017). Comparisons of interventions for preventing falls in older adults: A systematic review and meta-analysis. *Journal of the American Medical Association, 318*(17), 1687–1699.

U.S. Department of Health and Human Services, Agency for Healthcare Research and Quality. (2010). National guideline clearinghouse. Retrieved from http://www.ahrq.gov

Wakewich, P., Wood, B., Davey, C., Laframboise, A., & Zehbe, I. (2016). Colonial legacy and the experience of First Nations women in cervical cancer screening: A Canadian multi-community study. *Critical Public Health, 26*(4), 368–380. doi:10.1080/09581596.2015.1067671

Woolf, S. H., Grol, R., Hutchinson, A., Eccles, M., & Grimshaw, J. (1999). Clinical guidelines: Potential benefits, limitations, and harms of clinical guidelines. *British Medical Journal, 318*(7182): 527–530.

Wood, B., Burchell, A. N., Escott, N., Little, J., Maar, M., Ogilvie, G., & Zehbe, I. (2014). Using community engagement to inform and implement a community-randomized controlled trial in the Anishinaabek cervical cancer screening study. *Frontiers in Oncology, 4*(27). doi:10.3389/fonc.2014.00027

Zehbe, I., Jackson, R., Wood, B., Weaver, B., Escott, N., Severini, A., . . . Little, J. (2016). Community-randomised controlled trial embedded in the Anishinaabek Cervical Cancer Screening Study: Human papillomavirus self-sampling versus Pananicolaou cytology. *British Medical Journal Open, 6*(10): e011754. doi:10.1136/bmjopen-2016-011754

ABOUT THE AUTHORS

Jackie Muresan, RN, MSc, is an Advisor and Knowledge Broker at Region of Peel—Public Health. She has worked in the community as a public health nurse and prenatal educator. Her areas of expertise are evidence-informed decision making and knowledge translation in public health.

Rebecca Ganann, RN, PhD, is an Assistant Professor in the School of Nursing, McMaster University. Her research interests include community health, knowledge translation, primary health care, patient engagement, health equity, aging, implementation science, health services, and policy research.

CHAPTER 11

Epidemiology

Lynnette Leeseberg Stamler & Aliyah Dosani

LEARNING OUTCOMES

After studying this chapter, you should be able to:

1. Describe the theoretical underpinnings of the epidemiologic process and its historical and present value to community health nurses (CHNs).

2. Differentiate between association and causality, and explain some of the criteria that suggest a causal relationship.

3. Differentiate between screening and surveillance, and give examples of each.

4. Discuss the various measurements used in epidemiologic research and reports and their meaning for CHNs.

5. Describe the research study designs commonly used in epidemiologic research, and link the research question with the appropriate design.

6. Discuss how epidemiology has expanded to the study of disease and health promotion.

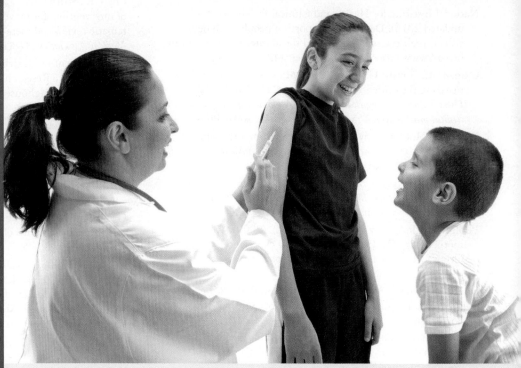

Source: Levent Konuk/Shutterstock

INTRODUCTION

Throughout history, humans have ascribed different causes for disease. It was not until the 1870s that specific bacteria were recognized as causing disease. During the past century, health professionals have come to understand that there are multiple factors or influences on many diseases and health challenges. In addition to learning the many causes of disease, health researchers are working to discover the factors that promote health. In this chapter you will learn the basics of the science of epidemiology, understand the types of data used in community health nursing, and begin to acquire the skills to identify and ask questions, using epidemiologic data to find some of the answers.

WHAT IS EPIDEMIOLOGY?

Epidemiology is defined as "the study of the occurrence and distribution of health-related states or events in specified populations, including the study of the determinants influencing such states and the application of this knowledge to control the health problem" (Porta, 2008, p. 81). The most well-known of these is public health epidemiology (or infectious disease epidemiology). Some authors stratify the concept with sub-definitions, such as exposure-oriented (e.g., nutritional, environmental) and disease-oriented (e.g., cancer, injury).

Friis and Sellers (2014) note that the purpose of epidemiology is to describe, explain, predict, and control challenges to population health. Epidemiologists first seek to describe health-related events by answering the questions who, what, when, and where, and by following trends in the population. Further explorations expand descriptions by answering the questions how and why, and by examining causality and modes of transmission. From this information come predictions that guide interventions and the use of health care resources. Finally, controls are implemented to prevent new illness; cure, if possible, individuals who are ill; and rehabilitate or prevent complications for those with a chronic disease.

Historical Background of Epidemiology

Though large-scale, focused epidemiologic studies are a relatively new phenomenon, the basis of understanding for such studies has been noted throughout history. Hippocrates is credited with being the first to notice and record a possible relationship between the environment and the health or disease of people. He suggested that physicians study "the mode in which the inhabitants live and what are their pursuits, whether they are fond of eating and drinking to excess, and given to indolence, or are fond of exercise and labor, and not given to excess in eating and drinking" (Hippocrates, 400 BCE).

Though history has recorded the existence and duration of epidemics such as the plague or the Black Death, few large-scale efforts were made to accurately record data that would increase the understanding of these epidemics. By the 1600s, statistics such as numbers of births and deaths were being recorded in London, England, and a haberdasher, John Graunt, was the first to study these statistics. He noted, for instance, gender differences in births (more males than females), seasonal variations in deaths, and high levels of infant deaths.

It was not until 1839 that Dr. William Farr initiated a more complete gathering of statistical data in England. During a cholera epidemic in the mid-1850s, Dr. John Snow noticed an apparent relationship between the number of cholera deaths in various neighbourhoods and the source of the drinking water. He clearly demonstrated that people who lived in areas or homes served by particular water companies had much higher death rates from cholera than those in neighbourhoods served by other water companies.

Florence Nightingale, a contemporary of Snow and Farr, was also convinced of the effect of the environment on disease and death. When she arrived at Scutari during the Crimean War, she discovered horrendous conditions and a lax method of recording deaths and their causes. She stressed accurate recording of these statistics and used them to explain and publicize the reality of the situation. Her polar diagrams, for instance, clearly demonstrated that in January 1855, 2761 soldiers died from contagious diseases, 83 from wounds, and 324 from other causes. It became clear that without ongoing recruitment, the entire army could have been wiped out from disease alone (Cohen, 1984). It was through her influence and her record-keeping that she was able to persuade authorities to allow her to implement sanitation practices that significantly decreased the death rates during and after the war.

In the 1900s, it became evident that although vital statistics of death and illness were important, following populations over time to ascertain the progression of various diseases and their treatments was also important. As medical scientists discovered and implemented new treatments, the primary causes of death changed over time from predominantly contagious diseases to chronic diseases that were influenced by lifestyle behaviours. For instance, between the 1920s and the 1970s, death rates from health challenges such as cardiovascular and renal diseases rose, while death rates for diseases such as tuberculosis and influenza decreased. In 1949, the first cohort study—the Framingham Heart Study—was begun, followed in 1950 by the publication of the first case-control studies of smoking and lung disease. Four years later, the Salk polio vaccine field trial was conducted. Modern epidemiologic studies have all been developed from these pioneering works.

Basic Building Blocks in Epidemiology

Basic building blocks of the science of epidemiology include the epidemiologic model, the concept of susceptibility, modes of transmission, the natural history or progress of disease, association and causation, and the web of causation. Modern CHNs use these concepts and processes to determine and test appropriate interventions.

Epidemiologic Model The classic epidemiologic model contains the elements of host, agent, and environment. The model is frequently presented as a triangle. The **host** is the human being in which the disease occurs. The **agent** is the contagious or non-contagious force that can begin or prolong a health problem. Agents include bacteria and viruses, as well as "stimuli" such as smoking or the absence of vitamin C. The **environment** is the context that promotes the *exposure* of the host to the agent. The **epidemiologic model** posits that disease is the result of the interaction among these three elements. Harkness (1995) noted that using a **Venn diagram** instead of the classic triangle emphasized the interrelatedness within the model. With the Venn diagram, overlaps do exist (see Figure 11.1).

Epidemiologic Variables In order to completely and accurately describe the patterns of health challenges, the descriptive

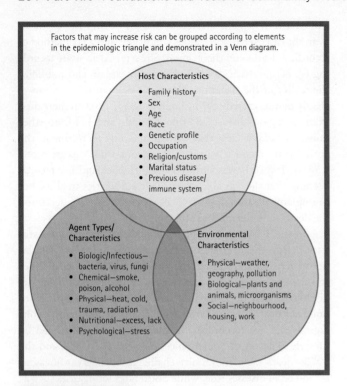

Factors that may increase risk can be grouped according to elements in the epidemiologic triangle and demonstrated in a Venn diagram.

Host Characteristics
- Family history
- Sex
- Age
- Race
- Genetic profile
- Occupation
- Religion/customs
- Marital status
- Previous disease/immune system

Agent Types/Characteristics
- Biologic/Infectious—bacteria, virus, fungi
- Chemical—smoke, poison, alcohol
- Physical—heat, cold, trauma, radiation
- Nutritional—excess, lack
- Psychological—stress

Environmental Characteristics
- Physical—weather, geography, pollution
- Biological—plants and animals, microorganisms
- Social—neighbourhood, housing, work

FIGURE 11.1 Epidemiologic Triangle as a Venn Diagram

variables of epidemiology are used. These are person, place, and time (Friis & Sellers, 2014). Within each variable are factors or characteristics that further describe the event. For instance, under the variable of person, you might look at age differences, sex, ethnicity, genetic predisposition, immune status, marital status, place of birth, and immigration. Other influences for the person such as education level, socioeconomic status, and occupation are also important pieces of information. Lastly, individual lifestyle characteristics such as dietary practices, use of alcohol or tobacco, and physical activity may be helpful.

The variable of time considers such characteristics as cyclic or seasonal variation of a health event, health challenges following specific events (such as postpartum depression), or time trends (increase of chronic disease over time) (Friis & Sellers, 2014). The variable of place can include variation between regions, countries, or continents; population density; rural/urban; or specific geographical characteristics, such as working in a particular building or living close to a cataclysmic event such as Chernobyl (Friis & Sellers, 2014). During the beginning identification of AIDS, careful documentation of person, time, and place assisted health professionals to accurately describe the health challenge.

Susceptibility You might think that if a group of people were all exposed in the same manner to the same disease, all would get the disease to the same degree. However, the combination of characteristics of each individual within that host group, interacting with the factors present or absent in the other elements of the epidemiologic triangle, determines the risk (or

degree of susceptibility) of each person to a particular agent. **Susceptibility** and **risk** can also be described as vulnerability, which determines the individual host response. The answers to the person, place, and time questions, while pointing to group susceptibility, can also point to group protection. For instance, we may discover that one or more of the characteristics studied (such as age or physical activity) may in fact mitigate some of the effects of other characteristics.

Within each element of the epidemiologic triangle are factors or characteristics that may increase or decrease the risk or susceptibility of the host to the disease. Figure 11.1 identifies some of these factors or characteristics. It is evident that some factors (e.g., lifestyle behaviours) may be changed or modified by the individual, whereas others (e.g., age, gender, genetic makeup) are not under the control of the individual.

Modes of Disease Transmission A **mode of transmission** is one way in which a disease moves to a new host. **Direct transmission** involves contact between the person with the disease and another person, such as skin-to-skin contact or sexual intercourse. **Indirect transmission** involves a common vehicle or **vector** that moves the disease to the new host, such as a contaminated water supply or lake. A mosquito can also function as a common vector in disease transmission. Indirect transmission may be airborne (droplets or dust), water-borne, vector-borne, or vehicle-borne (contaminated utensils, hygiene articles, or clothing). Different **pathogens** (microorganisms or other substances that cause disease) are viable under different conditions; therefore, you need to ascertain the potential mode of transmission for each disease.

Because a given disease may have more than one mode of transmission, understanding those modes is central to controlling the disease. When HIV/AIDS first became recognized as a threat to public health, the mode of transmission was greatly misunderstood: it was not known whether the disease could be contracted through everyday contact, such as by using a toilet seat used by someone with HIV/AIDS or by shaking that person's hand, thereby marginalizing and stigmatizing people living with HIV/AIDS. It soon became clear that such minimal contact did not result in disease transmission. However, the fear of HIV/AIDS greatly increased the use of universal precautions by health professionals—a positive outcome. More recently we have seen efforts to ensure our understanding of the spread of Ebola, and strategies to contain it are, in fact, correct and effective.

Natural History/Progression of a Disease A disease in a human host should be observed as a process rather than as a single incident. In 1965, Leavell and Clark plotted the natural progression of the disease process and identified prevention and health promotion strategies that could be employed at each stage. This work is foundational to current strategies. As seen in Figure 11.2, health promotion and prevention are always important. The first stage in the disease process is the **prepathogenesis** or **etiologic** period. During this phase, the human host may be exposed to a variety of agents through

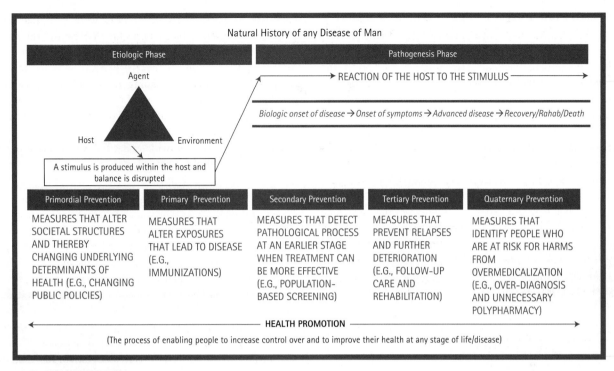

Natural History of any Disease of Man

Etiologic Phase	Pathogenesis Phase

Agent

REACTION OF THE HOST TO THE STIMULUS

Biologic onset of disease → Onset of symptoms → Advanced disease → Recovery/Rahab/Death

Host   Environment

A stimulus is produced within the host and balance is disrupted

Primordial Prevention	Primary Prevention	Secondary Prevention	Tertiary Prevention	Quaternary Prevention
MEASURES THAT ALTER SOCIETAL STRUCTURES AND THEREBY CHANGING UNDERLYING DETERMINANTS OF HEALTH (E.G., CHANGING PUBLIC POLICIES)	MEASURES THAT ALTER EXPOSURES THAT LEAD TO DISEASE (E.G., IMMUNIZATIONS)	MEASURES THAT DETECT PATHOLOGICAL PROCESS AT AN EARLIER STAGE WHEN TREATMENT CAN BE MORE EFFECTIVE (E.G., POPULATION-BASED SCREENING)	MEASURES THAT PREVENT RELAPSES AND FURTHER DETERIORATION (E.G., FOLLOW-UP CARE AND REHABILITATION)	MEASURES THAT IDENTIFY PEOPLE WHO ARE AT RISK FOR HARMS FROM OVERMEDICALIZATION (E.G., OVER-DIAGNOSIS AND UNNECESSARY POLYPHARMACY)

HEALTH PROMOTION

(The process of enabling people to increase control over and to improve their health at any stage of life/disease)

FIGURE 11.2 Natural History of a Disease

several modes of transmission. Depending on the unique characteristics of the prospective host, repeated exposure or a combination of additional stressors may be required for the host to become susceptible to the agent and the disease to begin. **Stressors** are events or situations that cause discomfort to a person, such as chronic fatigue or a poor diet. During the etiologic period, and throughout the continuum, primordial and primary prevention activities, are used by health professionals and the general public alike. In contrast to primary prevention, which tends to focus on actions designed to prevent individual exposure to a risk or disease (e.g., use of sunscreen or bicycle helmets), primordial prevention is focused on broad health issues, as illustrated by the social determinants of health (see Chapter 4). Thus, policy actions such as ensuring safe drinking water, introduction of stop signs or lights at busy intersections, and well-lit streets contribute not only to decreased personal risk but also decreased risk (and greater health) to the whole population.

When the human host begins to react to the agent (or stimulus), the period of **pathogenesis** begins. Depending on the disease, the host may or may not experience symptoms, but microscopic changes take place that indicate the presence of the disease. Pathogenesis ends with recovery, disability, or death. Two categories of health promotion activities are used during the period of pathogenesis. The first category is early diagnosis and treatment, which occurs early in the pathogenesis period. For instance, screening mammography is used for early detection of breast cancer, and the Pap test screens for cervical cancer. The second category, disability limitation, occurs later in the pathogenesis period, when the disease is active or there are recognizable

symptoms. During this period, health promotion activities are aimed at preventing complications; for example, ongoing examination and care of the feet in persons living with diabetes. Early diagnosis and disability limitation may also be called secondary prevention.

Tertiary prevention is the term given to the last health promotion category and occurs during the latter phases of the pathogenesis period. At this stage, health promotion activities might include client and family education to understand the chronicity of the disease, to adapt to sequelae of the disease process, or to maximize the health of the individual through use of aids such as a walker or adapted eating utensils. Figure 11.2 identifies this period as rehabilitation, but it may also be the time when palliative care and assistance for the individual and family to move toward a dignified death would be appropriate. It is important to recognize that the presence of chronic diseases or health challenges in individuals also increases their vulnerability or susceptibility to additional health challenges. This has become increasingly evident as more and more of our population lives longer due to enhanced medical care and health practices. Disease processes that would have ensured a speedy death only a few decades ago are now managed with little ongoing medical care. CHNs can use their knowledge of the progression of a disease and the levels of prevention to plan and implement interventions at the individual, family, aggregate, and population levels.

Finally, quaternary prevention is a term that was first coined in 1995 by Jamoulle and Ronald. This is based on the concept of "over-medicalization" as part of disease diagnosis and treatment. Nurses are concerned with the human response to diagnosis and treatment of disease. Thus, quaternary prevention would posit that each diagnostic and treatment activity should first be examined in light of the whole person to ascertain if the benefit of the activity is outweighed by the potential or actual harm to the patient. Just because we have the science and techniques to engage in certain activities does not mean they should be used in every situation. This is illustrated by the situation where an older adult woman with multiple chronic illnesses collapses at home and is rushed to hospital in an ambulance. The family arrives to find that their loved one is now unconscious, intubated, with IVs running, and many other interventions planned. When the physician talks the family about what should be done next, one family member comments, "I think you have done too much already." Another example is population-based testing for a disease. If there is no possible treatment, or the treatment is not available to the patients who test positive, is it ethical to mandate the test?

Screening and Surveillance

Screening and surveillance are tools that CHNs and other public health officials use to assist them in preventing or controlling certain diseases. These concepts can be difficult for new practitioners to understand. The testing of individuals who do not have symptoms is called **screening** (Merrill, 2013). An example of this is a colonoscopy to look for signs of rectal cancer. Screening or diagnostic tests need to be constantly examined to ensure they have both validity (they test what you want them to test) and reliability (they are consistent in their results over time and populations). As new knowledge about a disease is uncovered, the diagnostic or screening tests or policies may change. An example is the sexually transmitted infection chlamydia. Previously, testing for chlamydia involved swabbing the urethra. Now it is possible to be diagnosed through a urine test. In addition to being more sensitive, this new test is more acceptable to patients. Further, gathering of a sample can be accomplished outside of a clinic visit, making it less stigmatizing and more available to individuals with less access to health care. Finally, given the high rate of positive results in persons who are nonsymptomatic, health care providers can encourage patients who are at high risk (e.g., unprotected sex with multiple partners) to engage in ongoing testing (Public Health Agency of Canada [PHAC], 2017).

Surveillance is the constant watching or monitoring of diseases to assess patterns and quickly identify events that do not fit the pattern. Gathering and analyzing the number and type (age, gender) of individuals of persons diagnosed with influenza in a certain geographic location (province) over time to ascertain if public health interventions need to be initiated is an example of surveillance. Here a sudden spike in the incidence may signal the beginning of an epidemic. In the case of diseases with a genetic component, data may be collected to track the disease through extended family relationships. Using the sexually transmitted infection from the previous paragraph, chlamydia, an increased incidence was noted across Canada

from 2005–2014. The highest rates were in Nunavut and Northwest Territories, although Quebec reported the highest increase. It is still unclear if these rises were actual increases in incidence, increased testing of at-risk individuals through more acceptable and available screening, increased testing of exposed persons, or increased sensitivity of the diagnostic tests (PHAC, 2017). In all cases, the data must be reliable and follow-up testing consistent so that appropriate individual and public health decisions can be made and effective interventions can be planned and implemented.

Association and Causation Before planning interventions that prevent or ameliorate a disease or health problem, you must clearly understand the how and why of the disease or health problem. Two terms are used to describe the relationship between a stressor and a disease: association and causation. An **association** occurs when there is reasonable evidence that a connection exists between a stressor or environmental factor and a disease or health challenge. For example, a CHN might notice that many patients who exhibit a certain condition spent their childhoods in a particular geographic location. Thus, the relationship is first noticed through observation. Based on these observations, the CHN or epidemiologist examines the data to see if the relationship or association is strong or weak—is it all patients or just a few? If the association appears strong from the limited data sample, then a larger, more comprehensive exploration might be conducted. Such investigations often generate data from several sources. When a relationship or association has been confirmed beyond doubt, **causation** (or causality) is said to be present. In other words, causality occurs when you can state that there is a definite, statistical, cause-and-effect relationship between a particular stimulus and the occurrence of a specific disease or health challenge, or that the occurrence could not happen by chance alone.

In some ways, causation was simpler when the majority of diseases were infectious, as they were more likely to have only one cause. For example, streptococcus bacteria produce strep infection. Two important concepts in establishing causality are "necessary" and "sufficient." "Necessary" refers to the notion that a particular stressor *must* be present before a given effect can occur. For example, exposure to *Mycobacterium tuberculosis* is required before a person becomes ill with tuberculosis. "Sufficient" refers to the amount of exposure required to result in the disease. Some people exposed to *Mycobacterium tuberculosis* only once (minimal dose) become ill, and some do not become ill unless exposed several times (larger dose).

In the past 40 years, several authors have identified factors or criteria that researchers and practitioners could use to assess a causal relationship between a stimulus and the occurrence of a disease (Hill, 1965). The most commonly cited criteria of causation are summarized in Table 11.1 (Friis & Sellers, 2014; Gordis, 2014; Merrill, 2013). The criteria may be used for individual health challenges as well as population events.

When reading research that examines a particular nursing practice or new intervention, it is prudent to examine the presented results or recommendations in light of the criteria in Table 11.1. Similarly, when CHNs observe a recurring phenomenon that appears to have a relationship with a human

Table 11.1	Illustrations of Causation Criteria

Temporal relationship – A person does not get the disease until after exposure to the cause.

Strength of association – Exposure to a specific stressor or cause is most likely to bring on the disease.

Dose-response – Persons who are most exposed to the contaminated food (e.g., ate the most) are the most ill.

Specificity – The cause is linked to a specific disease (e.g., *Mycobacterium tuberculosis* does not result in chickenpox).

Consistency – Everyone who eats contaminated food gets the illness. If other food in another time and place is contaminated with the same bacteria, the same illness occurs.

Biologic plausibility – Findings are consistent with the biologic/medical knowledge that is known (new discoveries may precede biologic plausibility).

Experimental replication – Several studies done by different scientists in different places produce the same or similar results.

or environmental factor, a close examination of the data considering the criteria may assist them in planning subsequent observations.

Web of Causation Previous chapters have introduced the concept of the social determinants of health. In contrast to the time when each illness was thought to have a unique and specific cause, it is now recognized that many health problems have multiple causal factors, both direct and indirect. For instance, issues of poverty, education, and environment (e.g., pollution) have been shown to be influential in many health challenges. In looking for the causes of today's health challenges and assessing for the presence or absence of determinants of health, the CHN is well served by partnering with practitioners from a variety of disciplines. For instance, in addition to other health professionals, the CHN looking at population influences might look to the disciplines of sociology, anthropology, genetics, psychology, geography, and economics. As well, working with experts in social trends and public policy could bring additional understanding to the specific issue at hand. A model called a **web of causation** can be helpful to CHNs in visualizing the relationships among the many causes or influences of a given health challenge. Within that model, the relationship between the direct and indirect causes can be hypothesized, at which point research studies can be designed to test the hypotheses suggested by the web of causation.

Figure 11.3 illustrates a web of causation for lead poisoning. Obviously, the most direct causes or factors of lead poisoning are ingestion or inhalation of lead. However, behind those primary causes are several other causal factors possessing various levels of influence. For instance, food grown near high auto traffic or artists' materials can be sources of contamination that may not be quickly identified.

At any one time, each individual is subjected to multiple agents delivered through many modes of transmission. If you compared webs of causation for several common health challenges, some specific health promotion activities would appear to serve more than one purpose. Conversely, there may be a health promotion activity that is helpful for one challenge but contributes to susceptibility for another challenge. CHNs must examine all possible benefits and consequences of an intervention.

MEASUREMENT IN EPIDEMIOLOGY

To determine the extent of a disease process or health challenge and its final effects on a population, data must be collected and analyzed. However, for the resulting measurements to be useful to the CHN, the raw data or crude numbers must be presented in conjunction with other factors, such as population, time frame, or human characteristic (e.g., gender, race, age). These numbers, expressed as fractions, are known as **rates**. The numerator of each fraction is generally the crude count of the disease in question, and the denominator is generally the size of the population in question. In each case, the population or subpopulation of the numerator and denominator of the fraction are the same. For example, a rate of teen pregnancies might look like this:

$$\text{Rate} = \frac{\text{Number of live births delivered to teen mothers in the population}}{\text{Total numbers of teen women in the population}}$$

This fraction, or rate, is usually expressed for a set number of the population (e.g., per 100 000 people, per 100 cases, or per 1000 births) so that different-size populations can be compared. Table 11.2 presents the formulae for commonly used rates, and the following section describes these rates, how they are calculated, and how they might be used by CHNs.

Mortality (Death) Rates

Health care providers are legally required to complete death certificates for all deaths and file them with the government authorities. Thus, death or **mortality rates** are generally complete and easily obtainable. Mortality rates can be crude or specific in nature. **Crude mortality rates** compare the number of deaths from a specific cause within the entire population, whereas **specific mortality rates** compare the number of deaths from a specific cause in a particular subgroup with that whole subgroup. For example, if you examined all deaths from motor vehicle collisions and compared them with the total population, you would have a crude mortality rate. However, if you examined only teenage male deaths from motor vehicle collisions, you would compare that with the number of male teens driving at that time, a specific mortality rate. Mortality rates from a specific cause are often different when different

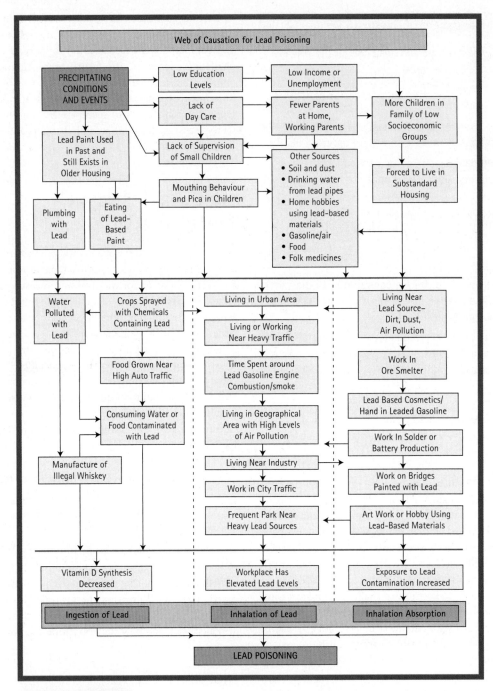

FIGURE 11.3 Web of Causation for Lead Poisoning

Source: Merrill (2013).

subgroups (e.g., teenage males, children aged 4–8, older adults) are examined. For example, Figure 11.4 illustrates the age-specific suicide rates for Canada for 2014, stratified (divided) by gender. Note the bars representing all suicides lay between the male and female bars for each age group, representing the specific total mortality rate for each age group that represents the specific total mortality rate for each age group. If only these bars (data) were presented, it would be statistically correct but fail to inform the reader that the rate for males is significantly higher than for females in each age group. These stratified data would lead you to conclude that males are more susceptible (or at least more successful) than females to death by suicide.

Proportional mortality rates can be used to stratify crude mortality rates. The number of deaths from a specific cause in a given population for a particular time period is compared with the total number of deaths in that same population and time period. A common use of proportional mortality rates is to state that *x*% of the deaths in a given year were due to breast cancer or motor vehicle collisions (see Figure 11.5). Note that two causes of death, cancers and diseases of the heart, account for over half the deaths.

Historically, the health of a population has been exemplified by maternal and infant mortality rates. Families used to have many children, partly because few were expected to live past the first years of life (assuming the mother and child

Table 11.2	Commonly Used Rates in Epidemiology
Rate	**Formula**
Crude mortality rate	Number of deaths from a certain disease during a specified time period / Number of cases of that disease occurring within the same specified time period
Specific mortality rate	Total deaths from a specific cause during a specified time period in a population (subgroup) / Average number of population (subgroup) within the same specified time period
Infant death rate	Total deaths of infants in a population during a specified time period / Total number of live births occurring within the same specified time period
Prevalence rate	Number of people with given disease in given population at one point in time / Total in given population at same point in time
Incidence rate	Number of new cases of given disease in a population during a specified time period / Average total population within the same specified time period
Relative risk	Incidence rate of disease in exposed population / Incidence of disease in unexposed population

survived the birth and neonatal period). With the advent of better hygiene as well as prenatal and postnatal care, maternal and infant mortality rates decreased. CHNs often compare infant mortality rates across developing and developed countries, the assumption being that lower maternal and infant mortality rates are indicative of a healthier population. When looking at these statistics, it is particularly important to determine the stage (e.g., perinatal vs. infant) that has been studied so that the comparisons are accurate. The following definitions are used in maternal and infant mortality statistics. In all but the perinatal rate, the denominator is the number of live births in that year in that population.

- Maternal or puerperal death rate: Any deaths of the mother resulting from pregnancy-related causes.

- Perinatal death rate: Fetal deaths occurring during the last few months of pregnancy and during the first seven days of life. Here the denominator includes both live births and fetal deaths.

- Neonatal death rate: Deaths occurring in infants in their first 28 days of life.

- Infant death rate: Deaths occurring in the first year of life.

A more recent way of presenting mortality statistics is in terms of **potential years of life lost (PYLL)**. This has arisen from the assumption that a person who dies early in life has lost greater potential than has a person who dies much later in life. PYLL statistics give CHNs additional information on which health challenges or diseases result in the greatest lost potential to the population. While this may raise some ethical

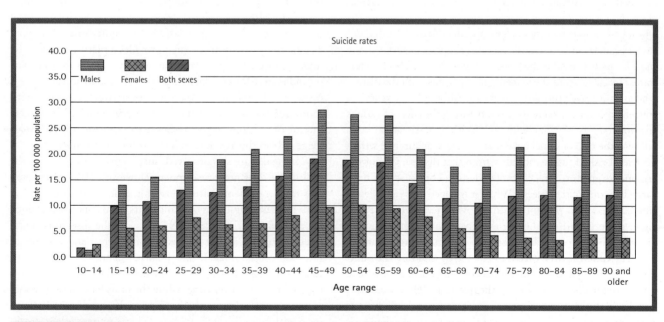

FIGURE 11.4 Suicide Rates by Age and Gender, Canada, 2014

Source: Statistics Canada (2018).

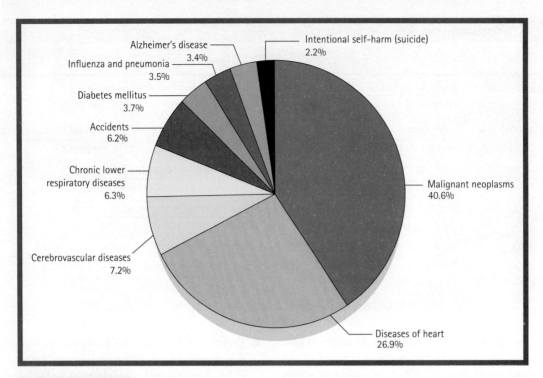

FIGURE   11.5 Top Nine Leading Causes of Death, Canada, 2014

Source: Statistics Canada (2018).

issues in terms of where a society or country chooses to place its resources, PYLL statistics are certainly a part of the picture that must be heeded.

Survival (Prognosis) Rates

Survival rates are often used to describe the effect of a given disease (e.g., cancer) and are also referred to as prognosis rates. Survival rates partially answer the common client question, "How bad is it?" Survival rates can also be used to compare the efficacy of various treatments for a specific disease. For diseases such as cancer, and its treatments, the prognosis or survival rate most frequently used is the five-year survival rate. This is determined by calculating the percentage of persons with the disease who are alive five years after diagnosis. Although five years is a convenient time period to use for comparing the effect of various treatments, it is easy for clients and health professionals alike to fall into the trap of somehow equating five-year survival with a decreased risk of future mortality from that disease. One of the arguments presented in favour of widespread breast screening is early detection of the disease. While it is hoped that early detection coupled with prompt treatment will increase the survival time, there is still conflicting evidence that these actions in fact contribute to decreased mortality rates from breast cancer.

The **case-fatality rate** is calculated by dividing the number of people who die from a disease by the number of people who have the disease, answering the question, "How likely is it that I will die from this disease?" For instance, recent advances have greatly increased the length of time between the diagnosis of a person with HIV and that person's death, but the case-fatality rate for HIV/AIDS remains very high, as most people

will die from the complications of the disease. The case-fatality rate for a person with arthritis, for instance, is much lower.

Morbidity (Illness) Rates

Illness or morbidity rates are valuable for the CHN. **Morbidity rates** give a picture of a population and a disease or health challenge over time, suggesting questions about the susceptibility of the population or subpopulation and the effectiveness of either health promotion or treatment strategies. Two types of rates are commonly used to describe morbidity in a population. The first is **prevalence**, which provides a picture of a specific disease process in a population at one given point in time. The second is **incidence**, which describes the identification of new cases of a disease in a population over time. Together with mortality rates and survival rates, they present a fairly complete picture of the population's response to a disease or health challenge. (Read the Yes, But Why? box for an example.)

If the disease is short-lived, such as measles or the flu, the prevalence does not reveal much. However, CHNs might use this rate in epidemic situations to plan for extra staff to deal with increased inquiries or clinic visits from concerned clients; for example, during the H1N1 crisis. If the disease is short-lived, resulting in few deaths, the incidence and prevalence rates are very similar. If, on the other hand, the health challenge is chronic in nature, the incidence rate (number of new cases) stays static over time, while the prevalence rate increases as more people live with the disease. If the disease is long-term with complications, such as diabetes or multiple sclerosis, the prevalence rate over time informs CHNs about the need for community and institutional support for the future. This is very important in terms of public and community health planning.

The population in question is usually the population at risk for the disease. For instance, when calculating the incidence of prostate cancer, the number of cases is compared with the population of males rather than with the whole population. Incidence rates, when calculated within the same population over several years, show whether the population seems more or less susceptible to the disease in question. For example, the number of motor vehicle collisions in a given year involving teenage drivers might change over time in response to changes in the legal drinking age.

When CHNs test for a specific cause of a health challenge, they compare the incidence of that health challenge in a population exposed to the identified cause with the incidence of the same health challenge in a population not exposed to the same cause. If the suspected cause were indeed a factor, you would expect the incidence rates to be quite different. For example, you would expect the incidence of lung cancer to be much greater in smokers than in non-smokers. If the cause being examined is not the *only* cause of the disease (e.g., lung cancer), you might find the incidence rates are more similar than expected. Such results might lead the CHN to explore other factors (e.g., secondhand smoke) to explain the incidence rates.

One frequently asked question is, "Are some populations more at risk of or vulnerable to a specific disease than others?" To find the answer to that question, a statistic known as **relative risk** is used. This measure divides the incidence of a given problem or disease in a population exposed to a given risk factor by the incidence of the same problem in a population not exposed to the same risk. For example, CHNs might compare the incidence of childhood asthma in a population exposed to a certain air pollutant with the incidence in a population not exposed to that pollutant. If the resulting number is 1.0, it means both groups have the same risk of the health problem, and most likely the risk factor in question makes little or no difference. If the resulting number is >1.0, it indicates that the risk in the exposed group is higher than the risk in the unexposed group, and the risk factor in question is at least one of the significant risk factors for the problem or disease. Should the relative risk ratio be <1.0, the given risk factor is probably not significant for the problem or disease. However, such results may indicate that the factor in question has a protective effect; for example, a population where the physical activity is high may have a lower relative risk for diabetes.

Incidence and prevalence rates can be further stratified to increase the descriptiveness of the statistic. Data are frequently obtained through interviewing members of the population, also known as self-reporting. For instance, the question, "Do you currently smoke?" elicits data that could contribute to a **point prevalence** statistic of smokers in the population. This statistic describes the situation only for that point in time. The question, "Have you smoked within the last six months?" gives us data that could be useful for **period prevalence** statistics. However, asking, "Have you ever smoked?" gives the researcher data that could be used for **cumulative or lifetime incidence** statistics. This demonstrates why it is important for researchers to clearly state their methods and sources of data in journal articles and reports, and why it is equally important for CHNs reading those articles to critically examine the evidence presented.

YES, BUT WHY?

HIV in Indigenous Canadians

What?

In Canada, First Nations, Inuit, and Métis populations are disproportionately affected by HIV (PHAC, 2014). According to Statistics Canada (2017) there were approximately 1.7 million Indigenous people in Canada in 2016, totaling less than 5% of Canada's total population. However, in 2011, 12.2% of new HIV infections (incidence) and 8.9% of individuals living with HIV in Canada (prevalence) were Indigenous people (PHAC, 2014). In 2016, less than half of new HIV cases had a reported ethnicity, of which the proportion of Indigenous people was 21.4% (Bourgeois et al., 2017). In addition, a recent study found that Indigenous people living with HIV in British Columbia have a higher mortality rate when compared to non-Indigenous people living with HIV, including those from other ethnic minority groups (Benoit et al., 2017).

So What?

In Canada, the health status of Indigenous people falls significantly behind that of other Canadians on essentially every measure (Greenwood, Leeuw, Lindsay, & Reading, 2015). Issues specific to Indigenous people further complicate health disparities, including loss of sense of personhood as it relates to community identity, rural-urban migrations, violence against women, and mental health and addictions (King, Smith, & Gracey, 2009). These issues represent the myriad of devastations to Indigenous communities resulting from colonial oppression. However, the reasons for the health status inequities we see with Indigenous populations cannot be attributed to lifestyle, behavioural, political, historical, or cultural factors alone. Racism and the accompanying intersecting forms of discrimination must also be considered (Browne, 2017).

Systemic racism translates into an access issue, where it is more difficult for Indigenous populations than non-Indigenous populations to access the type of health care they require. It should not, then, come as a surprise that Indigenous people are at a higher risk for HIV–hepatitis C co-infection (PHAC, 2014) or that Indigenous people living with HIV are less likely to access antiretroviral therapy (which is known to decrease HIV-related mortality) when compared to non-Indigenous peoples living with HIV (Nowgesic, Meili, Stack, & Myers, 2015). This disgraceful situation is compounded by the fact that services and support for Indigenous community health are fragmented and siloed across different levels of government and different departments with little collaborative efforts (King et al., 2014). The resulting health inequities observed between Indigenous and non-Indigenous populations may be interpreted as the Canadian government's lack of concern for the rights to health care of First Nation, Inuit, and Métis peoples (McCallum, 2017).

Now What?

CHNs are in an ideal position to contribute to decreasing inequities in access to health care for Indigenous communities. CHNs can help other health care providers understand the structural, historical, political, and cultural forces that lead to racial disparities in the health care arena (Goodman et al., 2017). Furthermore, CHNs can mobilize various other health care professionals and stakeholders to identify and correct structural injustices that act as barriers to accessing health care, including racism and its many forms—stigma, stereotyping, discrimination, and oppression (Cameron, Plazas, Salas, Bearskin, & Hungler, 2014). Participating in this type of work will help shed light on access to health issues for Indigenous people and promote social justice. We hope this will lead to additional avenues to increase access for care of HIV/AIDS for Indigenous communities.

Standards of Practice Fulfilled

#2 Prevention and Health Protection
- Participates in surveillance, recognizes trends in epidemiology data, and utilizes this data through population level actions such as health education, screening, immunization, and communicable disease control and management.
- Uses prevention and protection approaches with the client to identify risk factors and to address issues such as communicable disease, injury, chronic disease, and physical environment (e.g. air, climate, housing, work, water, land).

#6 Health Equity
- Understands historical injustices, inequitable power relations, institutionalized and
- interpersonal racism and their impacts on health and health care and provides culturally safe care.
- Advocates for resource allocation using a social justice lens (CHNC, 2019, revised).

RESEARCH IN EPIDEMIOLOGY

Sources of Epidemiologic Data

One of the largest sources of epidemiologic data is the government. Canada has several sources of government or government-funded data, such as the Public Health Agency of Canada (PHAC), Health Canada, Statistics Canada, and the provincial government health ministries. As birth and death statistics are required by law to be filed with the appropriate government agency, they are generally very accurate. Birth and death statistics can be teamed with the census data reported by Statistics Canada for further detail. Statistics Canada data can be found in its daily newsletter (*The Daily*), which reports on recent data and analysis and often provides a historical trend analysis for the disease (e.g., breast cancer) or issue (e.g., family structure in Canada). Statistics Canada also has a website where more detailed information, such as profiles of individual

communities and archived newsletters, can be found. Although Statistics Canada is recognized as an exemplary source of epidemiological data, it must also be recognized that these data are not always well stratified for easy use. For example, to fully grasp health equity (and inequity), data need to be stratified by ethnic or racial groups, small geographic areas, or other characteristics. At a governmental level, this is not always possible. Thus, it is important for individual nurses or community groups to gather, keep, and manage local data for comparison purposes, to identify areas of health inequity, and to ensure interventions are congruent with the target population.

In the wake of Walkerton and SARS, it was recognized that a stronger emphasis on public health by the government was required. In response, the PHAC was formed. Many of the reports and statistics previously reported by Health Canada may now be found at the PHAC website. These include information on surveillance of **reportable diseases** (diseases that are required to be reported by law; for example, tuberculosis, sexually transmitted infections, AIDS) as well as surveillance data on cancer, chronic disease, and cardiovascular diseases. Health Canada remains a source of information on many disease states, including epidemiologic data and links to other sites. All provinces also maintain health websites that provide information for the province in question. Specifically, many of the provincial health ministry websites provide birth and infant mortality statistics. (See Case Study for an example of how data can be used to describe a situation.)

The Canadian Institute for Health Information (CIHI) is also an excellent source for data. A non-governmental organization, CIHI collects and collates information from many sources to provide analyses that can inform policy. The epidemiologic data it reports include data from hospital sources and from the various provincial health plans. In addition, there are agencies that focus solely on specific disease issues. For example, the Canadian Diabetes Association or the Heart and Stroke Foundation of Canada are sources for statistics relative to those diseases. When using information found on the internet, the CHN needs to examine the source of the data to ensure it is from a reputable organization.

For the CHN wanting to compare data between Canada and the United States, the Centers for Disease Control and Prevention website is a valuable resource. For international data, the World Health Organization's website is very helpful. The final source of data is to gather data yourself. Although this can result in accurate data that deal with the specific question being asked, the cost of creating a survey instrument that is clear and understood by all respondents, choosing an appropriate sample (especially a national sample), and gathering the data often is beyond the financial reach of most researchers. If this is the case, researchers may be able to add questions to a survey being conducted by a community health care centre or agency.

Types of Epidemiologic Research

Research is one method of finding answers to questions. It is critical that CHNs have a clear understanding of research methodologies to understand, participate in, and conduct

CASE STUDY

HIV/AIDS continues to be a concern across the country. Surveillance in Canada is undertaken by the PHAC, and data are collected from the national HIV/AIDS Surveillance System (HASS); Immigration, Refugees and Citizenship Canada (IRCC); and the Canadian Perinatal HIV Surveillance Program (CPHSP). In 2016 there were 2344 newly diagnosed cases of HIV, bringing the cumulative total to 84 409 cases since 1985. Of all cases, 28.7% were adults aged 30–39. Similar age distribution of HIV cases was observed between males and females, with the most significant increases noted in people aged 50 years and older over the past five years. The "men who have sex with men" exposure category continued to represent the largest number of all reported HIV cases in adults at 44.1%. With respect to race/ethnicity, White (40.4%), Black (21.9%), and Indigenous (21.2%) categories represented the largest proportions of cases.

Discussion Questions

1. What information would you require to calculate the incidence of HIV in Canada in 2016?

2. What information would you require to calculate the prevalence of HIV in Canada in December 2016?

3. What information would you require to calculate the specific mortality of HIV infection for men who have sex with men in Canada in 2016?

Source: Bourgeois, A. C., Edmunds, M., Awan, A., Jonah, L., Varsaneux, O., & Siu, W. (2017). HIV in Canada—Surveillance Report, 2016. *Canadian Communicable Disease Report, 43*(12), 248–255.

research. This is because the study design is strongly linked to the research question—if an inappropriate study design is chosen, the results will not provide answers.

Different authors categorize types of epidemiologic research in different ways. For example, Grobbee and Hoes (2015) viewed it from a medical perspective and categorized in terms of diagnostic, etiologic, prognostic, and intervention research, each contributing different kinds of evidence to use in clinical practice. Conversely, Bhopal (2008) used the types of research designs as the categories—case series/population case, cross-sectional, case-control, cohort, and trial. The first four can also be termed observational or descriptive research because they are concerned with the variables of time, person, and place and answer the basic questions of who, when, and where. Analytic observational research adds the techniques of comparison and attempts to answer the questions of how and why. Trial or intervention research is considered experimental research, where the researcher manipulates selected variables and, for example, examines the efficacy of a new treatment, tests for causality, or compares communities in terms of a public health intervention. In the following section, each of the research designs is considered.

Case series studies are counts of selected variables within a specific population. Through this data collection,

the researcher determines morbidity and mortality rates, and through analysis of the various factors, looks for evidence of association and causality. Case series studies are often the basis of higher level studies and provide the researcher with data to generate hypotheses to be tested. Examples of research questions that could be answered include the following: Are mortality rates for cardiac disease higher for men than for women? Does age at diagnosis or geographic residence affect survival rates for infants born preterm? What are the current incidence rates for HIV in young gay men compared with 5, 10, or 20 years ago? Frequently, factors that increase risk may be used as a variable of interest; for example, gender may be considered as a risk factor for heart disease.

Cross-sectional studies are snapshots of the present and may also be called prevalence studies. Cross-sectional data may be collected as baseline data for planning and implementing interventions or to measure change. For example, CHNs may be concerned about the age of initiation of smoking behaviours relative to a specific planned health curriculum. The CHNs may work with the community to develop an anonymous survey that asks about smoking behaviours and administer it to students in various grade levels within the school district. The results of the survey may indicate that more than one-third of students in grade 6 have already tried smoking, suggesting that beginning health education about smoking in grade 6 is too late. The CHNs and teachers decide to move their initial anti-smoking education to grades 1 and 2, in which fewer than 3% of the students have tried to smoke. A time series of cross-sectional studies could also be used with a specific group of students to assess the effectiveness of the intervention. After implementing the new curriculum in grades 1 and 2, grade 6 classes would be tested in subsequent years. The data would be compared with those from the present grade 6 students, who did not receive the intervention, to ascertain if the program made a difference in the future smoking behaviours of students.

In **case-control** studies, the individuals in the group with the disease are matched with individuals who are similar in some characteristics (e.g., age, gender, time, geographic residence) but who have not manifested the disease in question. The health histories or characteristics of the individuals in both groups are then obtained. These data are compared, and the common factors and differences between the two populations are identified.

A case-control study of children with type 2 diabetes would include children with the disease in one group and children without the disease in the other group. The two groups would be matched for age and geographic location. The epidemiologist might search for common and different factors such as amount of physical activity, obesity, and family history of diabetes. In each case, the researcher would expect to find some similarities and differences between the two groups that could contribute to theories of causality.

The relative risk ratio compares the risk for a disease between two populations: one exposed to a stressor and one not exposed to the stressor. Case-control studies also involve

Table 11.3	Calculation of Odds Ratio		
Risk Factor	Persons with Lung Cancer	Persons without Lung Cancer	Total
Smokers	35 (*a*)	15 (*b*)	55
Non-smokers	15 (*c*)	135 (*d*)	145
Total	50	150	200

$$\text{Odds Ratio} = \frac{\text{Exposed persons with the disease/unexposed persons with the disease}}{\text{Exposed persons without the disease/unexposed persons without the disease}}$$

$$OR = \frac{a/c}{b/d} = \frac{a/d}{b/c} = \frac{(35)(135)}{(15)(15)} = \frac{4725}{225} = 21$$

The odds ratio for these data is 21. As with the relative risk ratio, a number >1.0 means that the persons exposed to the risk factor are more likely to develop the disease than those who are not exposed. In this example, men who smoke are 21 times as likely to develop lung cancer as men who do not smoke.

two groups: one group composed of individuals who have the disease and one of individuals who do not have the disease. Relative risk cannot be calculated here because neither the incidence nor the prevalence is known. The **odds ratio** provides epidemiologists with an estimate of the relative risk factor. To demonstrate the calculation of this statistic, consider the following example. A hypothetical community health centre practice has 200 male patients between the ages of 45 and 65; 50 of them have lung cancer, and 150 do not. Thirty-five of the patients with lung cancer are smokers, while 15 patients without lung cancer are smokers. Table 11.3 illustrates the calculation of the odds ratio for this example.

In **cohort studies**, the researcher examines the individual histories of a group of people manifesting a certain disease to find out what factors they share and what differences can be discerned. Cohort studies may be retrospective or prospective. **Retrospective studies** are studies that begin in the present and search the past for information to explain the present. **Prospective studies** (or longitudinal studies) begin in the present and follow the subjects into the future or make predictions about the future that can be tested at a later date. These studies focus on individuals exposed to a health problem or potential stressor over time. For a prospective study, it is important to measure the incidence of the problem at various times. For instance, a group of people with high exposure to a stressor (e.g., occupational stress) may be matched with a group of people with low exposure to the problem, and both are followed over time. The incidence levels of the health problem being studied (e.g., hypertension or myocardial infarction) in the two groups are compared at each measuring time.

Prospective studies have several unique issues:

■ The sample size must be very large at the beginning to allow for attrition as people move, die, or lose interest.
■ It is evident that health problems generally increase with increased age. By its very nature, a longitudinal study follows a group of people who are aging. Thus, a method to control for the effects of aging must be applied to any results.

■ Outside factors may affect the different groups differently. For instance, researchers may decide to compare hypertension in Canadian and U.S. executives who live in large cities and experience long commutes to work. The cities chosen are Toronto, Montreal, Chicago, and New York. The time frame is 2000–2020. Might the events of September 11, 2001, have an effect on the data and results?

CANADIAN RESEARCH 11.1

Type 2 diabetes in Canadian Aboriginal adolescents: Risk factors and prevalence (Spurr, Bally, Bullin, Trinder, 2017)

Being of Indigenous descent, among other factors, is recognized as a risk factor for type 2 diabetes. These authors decided to test for prediabetes risk factors in high school students in three Northern communities in Canada. In this cross-sectional study, demographic data, family medical history, body mass index, blood pressure, and hemoglobin A1c were gathered from 160 students who were 13–21 years old, in grades 9–12, and enrolled in high school. Ninety-three percent of the students identified as Indigenous. Sixty percent were of average weight, and almost 90% had normal HbA1c levels. However, when all the data were considered, only 4% of the tested students had no risk factors for type 2 diabetes, while 35% had two and 38% had more than two. These data are congruent with other published studies, underscoring the need for early and frequent screening of populations with known risk factors.

Discussion Questions

1. How might you, as a CHN, use this study in your practice?

2. What kind of interventions might you consider if this were your population?

3. How might you make those interventions culturally safe?

In trials or experimental studies, the researcher manipulates some of the variables to ascertain the effect of the manipulation. **Manipulation** means to change something that is happening to some or all the subjects within the study, rather than only observing what is present. In health care, the manipulation usually involves a new treatment or the encouragement of a new behaviour. The researcher believes that the new treatment or behaviour will positively affect the health of the subjects and uses the research to test that belief or hypothesis.

The "gold standard" of experimental study design is the **randomized controlled trial (RCT)**. In an RCT design, individuals are assigned randomly either to a group that receives the new treatment or to a group that does not receive the new treatment. The latter is known as the control group. After a period of time, specific variables are measured in each group and compared. Frequently, neither the researchers nor the subjects are aware of which group they are part of until the end of the study. This is known as a blind RCT.

In community nursing and health promotion, the treatment or intervention studied may be a new health education or social marketing protocol (e.g., new advertisements for breast screening) or a change in policy (e.g., adding fluoride to drinking water for a community). In the example of new marketing for screening, the outcome examined could be the increase or decrease in the number of persons participating in the screening. In the case of adding fluoride to the drinking water, the outcome measured might be the number of dental cavities found in six-year-olds.

In the examples above, randomized control groups would be almost impossible. One variation of this might be to compare several communities, with one or more serving as treatment groups and the others serving as control groups. Another variation may be that the community might serve as its own control group—measuring the outcome of interest (e.g., participation in screening) before and after the treatment (e.g., advertising for breast screening clinics).

Ethical Concerns Ethical concerns during observational studies such as case, cross-sectional, case-control, or cohort are rare but possible because of the nature of those studies. The researcher is not manipulating the variables but is systematically collecting and analyzing observations to make inferences and predictions. However, CHNs must always remember that most people are interested in participating in any study that they perceive will help someone else with a health problem. If a researcher has no intention of *using* the data (e.g., to plan interventions that are intended to be carried out), it is unethical to collect them. Ethics approval must be sought for any study where data are collected about or from humans. In any trial or experimental study, the competing issues of strong scientific experimental design and ethical considerations must be addressed. The first ethical concern is how the human subjects are approached. Most health care agencies and university research centres have an ethics committee that reviews research proposals to ensure that humans are treated fairly, the information is gathered and used in a confidential manner, and the privacy of the subjects is protected. However, ethical questions also arise about the design of the research. For instance, is it ethical to withhold a treatment that is felt to be beneficial from people who need it because a research design with a control group would be more scientific? Researchers must consider these questions and consult with appropriate sources for advice when designing scientific and ethical research studies.

CONCLUSION

The science of epidemiology is an important one for the CHN. Community health professionals are confronted with increasingly complex health challenges that were unheard of just a few short decades ago, such as type 2 diabetes in children. It is becoming increasingly evident that Hippocrates had it right more than two millennia ago: nurses must look at what the person eats, what the person does, and what the person's habits are. Health practitioners face the task of using the results of epidemiologic research to influence citizens to change or enhance their activities of daily living to actively promote maximum health, while recognizing that the individual and group environment may well influence people in other directions.

KEY TERMS

agent (p. 203)
association (p. 206)
case-control (p. 213)
case series (p. 213)
case-fatality rate (p. 210)
causation (p. 206)
cohort studies (p. 214)
cross-sectional studies (p. 213)
crude mortality rates (p. 207)
cumulative or lifetime incidence (p. 211)
direct transmission (p. 204)
environment (p. 203)
epidemiologic model (p. 203)
epidemiology (p. 203)
etiologic (p. 204)
host (p. 203)
incidence (p. 210)
indirect transmission (p. 204)
manipulation (p. 215)
mode of transmission (p. 204)
morbidity rates (p. 210)
mortality rates (p. 207)
odds ratio (p. 214)
pathogens (p. 204)
pathogenesis (p. 205)
period prevalence (p. 211)
point prevalence (p. 211)
potential years of life lost (PYLL) (p. 209)
prepathogenesis (p. 204)
prevalence (p. 210)
proportional mortality rates (p. 208)
prospective studies (p. 214)
randomized controlled trial (p. 215)
rates (p. 207)
relative risk (p. 211)

STUDY QUESTIONS

1. Identify and define five criteria for causality.

2. Differentiate between mortality and morbidity rates. How does each inform the CHN?

3. Identify the three elements of the epidemiologic triangle, and define each.

4. Differentiate between incidence and prevalence. What does it mean when the incidence and prevalence rates for a given health problem are very different? What does it mean when they are very similar?

5. Describe prospective and retrospective studies, and give two examples of research questions that could be answered with each.

INDIVIDUAL CRITICAL-THINKING EXERCISES

1. Select a health problem. Using Figure 11.2 as a guide, suggest five CHN actions for each of the five levels of prevention. Include actions for individuals as well as populations. How might CHNs collaborate with other health professionals to implement the actions?

2. Discuss the pros and cons of having national registries for disease processes such as tumours, diabetes, and HIV/AIDS. Did your discussion differ according to the statistics available regarding incidence and prevalence? What about possible social stigma?

3. Why are infant and child mortality rates used as a measure of the health of a population? Using the national and provincial infant mortality rates (www.statcan.gc.ca), what do you discern about provincial disparities? Are you surprised? What factors might influence the rates noted? Where might you go to find further evidence?

GROUP CRITICAL-THINKING EXERCISES

1. Select a condition you are familiar with (e.g., type 2 diabetes, asthma, heart attack). From two different provinces' health websites and the PHAC website, compare the mortality and morbidity rates for that condition. Are they similar or different? What factors might influence the rates in those jurisdictions?

2. As a group, discuss the pros and cons of using an epidemiologic approach to planning CHN actions.

3. Physical activity is recognized as a protector of health for all humans, regardless of age and current health status. Using the tables found at www.statcan.gc.ca, consider how you might design a national campaign aimed at increasing physical activity. Which groups would be most important to target? Why?

REFERENCES

Benoit, A. C., Younger, J., Beaver, K., Jackson, R., Loutfy, M., Masching, R., . . . Raboud, J. (2017). Increased mortality among Indigenous persons in a multisite cohort of people living with HIV in Canada. *Canadian Journal of Public Health, 108*(2), e169–e175. doi:10.17269/CJPH.108.5708

Bhopal, R. (2008). *Concepts of epidemiology. Integrating the ideas, theories, principles and methods of epidemiology.* New York, NY: Oxford University Press.

Browne, A. J. (2017). Moving beyond description: Closing the health equity gap by redressing racism impacting Indigenous populations. *Social Science & Medicine, 184,* 23–26. doi: 10.1016/j.socscimed.2017.04.045

Bourgeois, A. C., Edmunds, M., Awan, A., Jonah, L., Varsaneux, O., & Siu, W. (2017). HIV in Canada—Surveillance Report, 2016. *Canadian Communicable Disease Report, 43*(12), 248–255.

Cameron, B. L., Plazas, M. D. P. C., Salas, A. S., Bearskin, R. L. B., & Hungler, K. (2014). Understanding inequalities in access to health care services for Aboriginal people: A call for nursing action. *Advances in Nursing Science, 37*(3), E1–E16. doi:10.1097/ANS.0000000000000039

Cohen, I. B. (1984). Florence Nightingale. *Scientific American, 3,* 128–137.

Community Health Nurses of Canada (CHNC). (2019 revised). *Canadian community health nursing: Professional practice model and standards of practice* (ISBN 978-0-9733774-5-3). Retrieved from http://www.chnig.org/wp-content/uploads/2016/02/chnc-standards.pdf

Friis, R. H., & Sellers, T. A. (2014). *Epidemiology for public health practice* (5th ed.). Sudbury, MA: Jones and Bartlett.

Goodman, A., Fleming, K., Markwick, N., Morrison, T., Lagimodiere, L., & Kerr, T. (2017). "They treated me like crap and I know it was because I was Native": The healthcare experiences of Aboriginal peoples living in Vancouver's inner city. *Social Science & Medicine, 178,* 87–94. https://doi.org/10.1016/j.socscimed.2017.01.053

Gordis, L. (2014). *Epidemiology* (5th ed.). Philadelphia, PA: Elsevier Saunders.

Greenwood, M., Leeuw, S. D., Lindsay, N. M., & Reading, C. (Eds.). (2015). *Determinants of Indigenous peoples' health in Canada: Beyond the social.* Canadian Scholars' Press, Toronto, ON.

Grobbee, D. E., & Hoes, A. W. (2015). *Clinical epidemiology: Principles, methods and applications for clinical research* (2nd ed.). Sudbury, MA: Jones and Bartlett.

Harkness, G. A. (1995). *Epidemiology in nursing practice.* St. Louis, MO: Mosby.

Hill, A. B. (1965). The environment and disease: Association or causation? *Proceedings of the Royal Society of Medicine, 58,* 295–300.

Hippocrates. (400 BCE). *On airs, waters and places.* The Internet classics archive, Part 1. Retrieved from http://classics.mit.edu/Hippocrates/airwatpl.1.1.html

King, M., Smith, A., & Gracey, M. (2009). Indigenous health part 2: The underlying causes of the health gap. *The Lancet, 374*(9683), 76–85.

Jamoulle, M., & Roland, M. (1995). *Quaternary prevention.* Available at http://www.ph3c.org/PH3C/docs/27/000103/0000261.pdf

Leavell, H. F., & Clark, E. G. (1965). *Preventive medicine for the doctor in his community: An epidemiologic approach.* New York, NY: McGraw- Hill.

McCallum, M. J. L. (2017). Starvation, experimentation, segregation, and trauma: Words for reading Indigenous health history. *Canadian Historical Review, 98*(1), 96–113.

Merrill, R. M. (2013) *Introduction to Epidemiology.* Burlington, MA: Jones & Bartlett, page 235, Reproduced with permission.

Nowgesic, E., Meili, R., Stack, S., & Myers, T. (2015). The Indigenous Red Ribbon Storytelling Study: What does it mean for Indigenous peoples living with HIV and a substance use disorder to access antiretroviral therapy in Saskatchewan? *Canadian Journal of Aboriginal community-based HIV/AIDS Research, 7*(1), 27.

Porta, M. S., & International Epidemiological Association. (2008). *A dictionary of epidemiology* (5th ed.). Oxford, UK: Oxford University Press.

Porta, M. (Ed.). (2014). *A dictionary of epidemiology* (6th ed.). Oxford, UK: Oxford University Press.

Public Health Agency of Canada (PHAC). (2014). HIV/AIDS among Aboriginal people in Canada. Centre for Communicable Diseases and Infection Control—2014 HIV/AIDS Epi Updates. Ottawa, ON: Author. Retrieved from https://www.canada.ca/en/public-health/services/hiv-aids/publications/epi-updates/chapter-8-hiv-aids-among-aboriginal-people-canada.html

Public Health Agency of Canada (PHAC). (2017). Report on sexually transmitted infections in Canada: 2013–2014. Ottawa, ON: Author. Retrieved from https://www.canada.ca/content/dam/phac-aspc/documents/services/publications/diseases-conditions/report-sexually-transmitted-infections-canada-2013-14/report-sexually-transmitted-infections-canada-2013-14-eng.pdf

Spurr, S., Bally, J., Bullin, C., & Trinder, K. (2017). Type 2 diabetes in Canadian Aboriginal adolescents: Risk factors and prevalence. *Journal of Pediatric Nursing 36*, 111–117. https://doi.org/10.1016/j.pedn.2017.05.011

Starfield, B. (2001). Basic concepts in population health and health care. *Journal of Epidemiology & Community Health, 55*(7), 452–454.

Statistics Canada. (2018). Deaths and age-specific mortality rates, by selected grouped causes. Retrieved from https://www150.statcan.gc.ca/t1/tbl1/en/tv.action?pid=1310039201

Statistics Canada. (2018). Deaths and age-specific mortality rates, by selected grouped causes. Retrieved from https://www150.statcan.gc.ca/t1/tbl1/en/tv.action?pid=1310039201

Tesser, C. D., & Norman, A. H. (2016). Differentiating clinical care from disease prevention: A prerequisite for practicing quaternary prevention. *Cadernos de saude publica, 32*(10), e00012316.

Vollman, A. R., Anderson, E. T., & McFarlane, J. (2017). *Canadian community as partner: Theory and multidisciplinary practice* (4th ed.). Philadelphia: Wolters Kluwer.

World Health Organization. (1986). Ottawa charter for health promotion. Geneva, CH: Author.

ABOUT THE AUTHORS

Lynnette Leeseberg Stamler, RN, PhD, DLitt, FAAN, is Professor and Associate Dean for Academic Programs at the University of Nebraska Medical Center, College of Nursing. From 1984 to 2012 she taught in Canadian schools of nursing and was a VON nurse prior to her teaching career. She completed her BSN at St. Olaf College, Minnesota, her MEd in health education at the University of Manitoba, and her PhD in nursing at the University of Cincinnati. Her research interests include patient/health education, diabetes education, nursing education, and quality care. She is active in national and international nursing organizations, including Sigma Theta Tau International, and was president of the Canadian Association of Schools of Nursing from 2008 to 2010. In 2011 she was inducted into the American Academy of Nursing.

Aliyah Dosani, RN, BN, MPH, PhD, is Associate Professor in the School of Nursing and Midwifery, Faculty of Health, Community and Education at Mount Royal University in Calgary, Alberta. She is also an Adjunct Associate Professor in the Department of Community Health Sciences, Cumming School of Medicine, at University of Calgary in Calgary. She holds a PhD from the University of Calgary with a specialization in population/public health. Her nursing practice includes instructing students in the Bachelor of Nursing program, population/public health, community health nursing, and legal issues in nursing. Her work focuses on maternal, newborn, and child health. Her research interests include working on health equity and social justice issues through community-based programs and interventions. She also shares a passion for global health issues.

Communicable Diseases

Sarah Alley

LEARNING OUTCOMES

After studying this chapter, you should be able to:

1. Identify and discuss historical strategies that have led to declining morbidity and mortality rates from communicable diseases in the global context.

2. Explain the nature and types of communicable diseases: vaccine preventable diseases; sexually transmitted and blood-borne infections; enteric, food-, and water-borne infections; zoonotic and vector-borne infections; respiratory infections; and health care-acquired infections.

3. Discuss the implications of antimicrobial resistance on the evolution of communicable diseases.

4. Describe the roles of international, national, provincial or territorial, and local authorities in the control, management, and reporting of communicable diseases.

5. Identify and discuss activities community health nurses utilize to implement the levels of prevention in the control and management of communicable diseases.

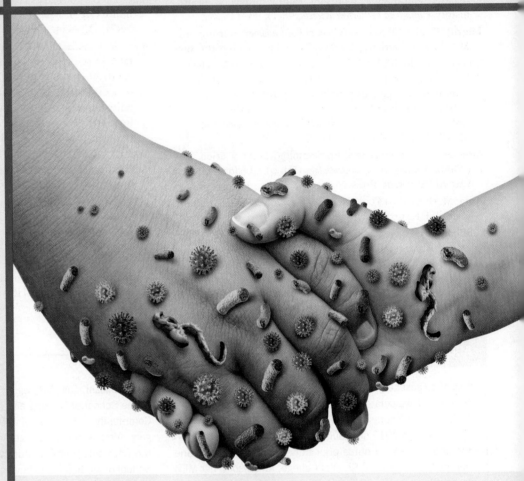

Source: Freshidea/Fotolia

INTRODUCTION

Communicable diseases are illnesses caused by a "specific infectious agent, or its toxic products, that arise through transmission of that agent, or its products from an infected person, animal, or inanimate source to a susceptible host; either directly or indirectly through an intermediate plant or animal host, vector or the inanimate environment" (Heymann, 2015, p. 694). As long as history has been recorded, communicable diseases have been an intricate part of our lives, affecting health outcomes on a global scale. In the early 1900s improvements in sanitation, implementation of infection control procedures and programs, development of vaccines to prevent certain illnesses, and the discovery of antibiotics to treat bacterial infections caused a significant decline in morbidity and mortality rates related to communicable diseases.

Along with advances in technology and modern medicine, the impact and severity of illnesses associated with many of these diseases further declined as society and public health authorities shifted their view of communicable diseases away from a response and treatment focus to one with more emphasis on prevention, control, and early detection. Despite these improvements, communicable diseases are now seen in areas around the world previously untouched as newer challenges have surfaced, including increasing population mobility due to efficient transportation systems as well as lifestyle and environmental changes.

Communicable diseases occur in every society, from rural areas to cities, in all countries, and without discrimination between the rich and poor. The economic and societal consequences of communicable diseases can be enormous, particularly the impact to tourism and trade. This was evident during the SARS outbreak in 2003 when the city of Toronto "shut down" as thousands of people were placed in quarantine and hundreds more were hospitalized. Tourism to the city and the Toronto Stock Exchange were significantly impacted. Globally, 26 countries were affected, 8098 cases were identified, 774 deaths occurred, and economic losses were estimated at almost US$60 billion (United Nations World Tourism Organization, 2009). Another example of how communicable diseases can affect more than just individual health was evident when sales of beef in Canada and the United Kingdom plummeted due to bovine spongiform encephalopathy, or "mad cow disease." Consumers of beef feared acquiring the human form of this disease, called variant Creutzfeldt-Jakob disease. Cattle farming provinces in Canada were severely impacted, although to date only two human cases have ever been identified in Canada, with both appearing to have contracted the disease outside of the country (Public Health Agency of Canada [PHAC], 2011, 2017a).

Given the current challenges in managing communicable diseases, community health nurses (CHNs) must have a solid foundation in communicable diseases to prevent, limit, and protect the health of the public from transmission of these diseases. This chapter offers a historical perspective on communicable diseases, describes the host-agent-environment model, reviews the implications of antimicrobial resistance, and considers the roles of international, national, provincial or territorial, and local governments. The role of CHNs in the field of communicable diseases is also examined in terms of primordial, primary, secondary, tertiary, and quaternary prevention.

COMMUNICABLE DISEASES: A HISTORICAL PERSPECTIVE

For many centuries, communicable diseases such as tuberculosis (TB), smallpox, leprosy, cholera, scarlet fever, typhoid fever, diphtheria, and poliomyelitis have caused many casualties and threatened the health of humankind. The first recorded worldwide threat from a communicable disease, the bubonic plague, also known as the "Black Death," occurred in the 14th century. Half of the cases occurred in Africa and Asia, and the other half in Europe, where one-quarter of the population succumbed—an estimated 50 million deaths (World Health Organization [WHO], 2014). The Spanish influenza pandemic of 1918 was another major threat, spreading globally in less than six months and killing approximately 21 to 50 million people worldwide and infecting an additional 500 million people (Taubenberger & Morens, 2006). Many communicable diseases were brought to Canada with the arrival and migration of early settlers in the 16th century. Indigenous populations, who had never been exposed to infectious or parasitic diseases before, were severely affected, as they had little to no resistance and no opportunity to develop natural immunity.

Since the mid-1800s, advances in scientific and medical knowledge, and in public health measures, have contributed to declining morbidity and mortality from communicable diseases among Canadians. The development of microscopes, germ theories, and vaccines and the improvement of nutrition, sanitation, and living conditions have been instrumental in this decline. In 1967, 60% of the world's population was at risk for contracting smallpox. At that time, health professionals from the World Health Organization (WHO) launched the highly successful smallpox eradication program. The last known case of smallpox was in Somalia in 1977, and in 1980, the world was declared smallpox free (WHO, 2010). The documented success of the smallpox eradication program opened the doors for the WHO's Expanded Program on Immunization in 1974. Initially, the program targeted diphtheria, whooping cough, tetanus, measles, poliomyelitis, and tuberculosis. In 1977, as part of the WHO's strategy to achieve health for all by 2000, global policies for immunization were established with the hope of providing universal immunization for all children by 1990 (WHO, 2013a). By 2016, approximately 86% of infants around the world had received at least three doses of the DTP (diphtheria, tetanus, and polio) vaccine (WHO, 2017a). Hepatitis B, haemophilus influenzae type b (Hib), and pneumococcal conjugate vaccines have also been added by many countries to their routine infant immunization schedules. However, the addition of rotavirus vaccines continues to be a challenge, as global coverage in 2016 was estimated at only 25% (WHO, 2017a). Immunization is accepted as the most successful health intervention. As a result, the Global Vaccine Action Plan (GVAP) was endorsed by 194 member states of the WHO Assembly in May 2012. The GVAP is a framework to improve access to existing vaccines for all people, regardless of where they are born, who they are, and where they live (WHO, 2013b). To further build on the goals of strengthening immunization, a new resolution of the GVAP was endorsed in May 2017. The resolution "urges countries to strengthen the governance and leadership of national immunization programs, and improve monitoring and surveillance systems to ensure up-to-date data guides policy and programmatic decisions to optimize performance and impact" (WHO, 2017a). Moreover, it encourages countries to expand immunization programs beyond infancy.

Public health professionals continue their efforts to combat infectious diseases such as malaria, TB, and parasitic diseases, which can cause lifelong disabilities and have socioeconomic consequences (WHO, 2009a). Recent developments in vaccine production and disease control have lessened the impact on morbidity and mortality in Canada for communicable diseases like influenza and TB. However, newly emerging and re-emerging infectious diseases are increasingly challenging the public health system worldwide. For instance, when treatment protocols to cure TB were developed in 1948, it was anticipated that the disease would be eradicated by 2000. Ironically, TB has now re-emerged as an increased public health threat because of multidrug-resistant (MDR) strains and clients' noncompliance with chemoprophylaxis. Other existing diseases, such as influenza, are less of a threat than was true historically, due to the availability of vaccines and antiviral drugs. However, transmission of other infectious diseases has increased related to global travel and trade, climate change, poverty, inadequate health care resources, inconsistent vector control programs, overuse of antibiotics, and changing lifestyle practices. As such, the WHO has become increasingly vigilant with mechanisms for international disease surveillance, which has reduced the delay in recognizing global communicable disease threats. One of the positive outcomes of increased vigilance was demonstrated in the 2009 H1N1 influenza pandemic. Unlike SARS, there was a relatively short period between the first cases of the 2009 H1N1 pandemic influenza in Mexico and notification of the potential threat to international public health agencies. The Public Health Agency of Canada (PHAC) was a key lead in contributing to this success at the national level. PHAC was established in September 2004 in response to the SARS outbreak by the Government of Canada because there was a need to strengthen Canada's capacity to protect Canadians from infectious diseases and other threats to their health (PHAC, 2014a).

As part of its role, the PHAC publishes a weekly, bilingual, peer-reviewed, open-access online scientific journal called the *Canada Communicable Disease Report* (CCDR). This publication provides timely and practical information on infectious diseases to clinicians, public health professionals, and policy makers to inform various health interventions in terms of practice, program development, implementation, and evaluation, and policy development (PHAC, 2014b).

TRANSMISSION OF COMMUNICABLE DISEASES

"Communicable diseases kill more than 14 million people each year, largely in resource poor countries. In these countries, approximately 46% of all deaths are due to communicable diseases, and 90% of these deaths are attributed to acute diarrheal and respiratory infections of children, AIDS, tuberculosis, malaria, and measles" (Heymann, 2008, p. 12). Preventing transmission is key to controlling the number of people infected with an organism.

There are many ways of classifying communicable diseases, and the categorization varies depending on the purpose and use for the classifications. One way to classify communicable diseases is by the **epidemiologic triangle**, as discussed in Chapter 11. The epidemiologic triangle is used to describe the dynamics of the agent, host, and environment. In order for an infectious disease to be acquired, three elements are needed: an infective agent, a susceptible host, and a supportive environment. To prevent the disease, it is necessary to modify one or more of the elements on the corners of the triangle. For example, you could immunize the host, disinfect a room to eliminate the agent, or develop a protective environment by wearing personal protective equipment, like a mask, when caring for a patient with a respiratory infection. As such, understanding the infectious agent's characteristics is paramount to assisting health care providers to prevent, diagnose, and manage a communicable disease.

Table 12.1 displays the different ways communicable diseases can be classified. The classification is dependent on what you are using the categories for and in what setting. For example, in a hospital setting you may want to categorize the disease by its means of transmission, particularly if you are trying to determine which infection control precautions are needed.

The communicable diseases discussed in the following sections have been categorized into the following classifications: (a) vaccine-preventable diseases, (b) sexually transmitted and blood-borne infections, (c) enteric, food-, and water-borne infections, (d) zoonotic and vector-borne infections, (e) respiratory infections, and (f) health care–associated infections.

Table 12.1	Classification of Communicable Diseases			
Clinical Characteristics Classification	**Microbiologic Classification**	**Means of Transmission Classification**	**Reservoir in Nature Classification**	**Public Health Programs Classification**
Diarrheal	Bacterial	Contact	Human	Vaccine preventable
Respiratory	Viral	Food- or water-borne	Animals (zoonoses)	Respiratory
Central nervous system	Fungal	Airborne	Soil	Enteric, food-borne, and water-borne
Cardiovascular	Parasitic	Vector-borne	Water	Sexually transmitted and blood-borne
Sepsis	Prion	Perinatal		Zoonotic and vector-borne

VACCINE-PREVENTABLE DISEASES

Vaccination is often seen as one of the greatest contributions to global health of any intervention, apart from the introduction of clean water and sanitation (Greenwood, 2014). Vaccines work by creating an immune response by stimulating the body's immune system to make antibodies that provide protection from the infection (Centers for Disease Control and Prevention [CDC], 2017; PHAC, 2013). Immunity to the bacteria or virus can often last a lifetime. Booster doses may be needed for some vaccines (e.g., diphtheria and tetanus every 10 years), and others may require an annual dose (e.g., influenza), as the viruses that cause the disease change, and vaccines protecting against new strains are needed (PHAC, 2013).

Through successful immunization programs, smallpox has been eradicated globally; poliomyelitis has been eradicated in resource-rich countries; and measles, mumps, and rubella have been dramatically reduced in many countries. The goals of the immunization program in Canada are to prevent, control, eliminate, or eradicate vaccine-preventable diseases by directly protecting individuals who receive the vaccine and by indirectly protecting individuals who are vulnerable who may not respond to vaccines or for whom vaccines may be contraindicated (PHAC, 2016a). Comprehensive federal, provincial, and territorial immunization policies, and the ongoing monitoring and evaluation of vaccines and immunization programs, have contributed to a significant decline in the incidence of vaccine-preventable diseases and their associated morbidity and mortality.

The National Advisory Committee on Immunization (NACI) is a group of experts in the fields of pediatrics, infectious diseases, immunology, and public health. The NACI is instrumental in developing guidelines for the use of approved vaccines in Canada in addition to identifying groups at risk for vaccine-preventable diseases for whom vaccination should be targeted and advising on immunization best practices to assist CHNs and other health care providers to critically examine their standards of practice related to immunization. The recommended **immunization** schedules for infants, children (Photo 12.1), adolescents, adults, and older adults vary by each province and territory across Canada based on local information. (See Figure 12.1.)

Community immunity (or **herd immunity**) is "the resistance of a group to invasion and spread of an infectious agent, based on a high proportion of individual members of the group being resistant to infection" (Heymann, 2015, p. 696). As such, when a sufficient proportion of a group is vaccinated, both the vaccinated and unvaccinated are protected from disease. If you are vaccinated, you typically do not contract the disease and therefore do not spread it to others. Even when vaccinated people do become ill, their symptoms are often milder, and they are less likely to spread the infection. In Figure 12.2, the first group is represented by individuals where the majority are not immunized, and as a result an outbreak occurs. The second group is represented by individuals where significantly enough of the population is immunized that they protect many of the other members of that population through community immunity.

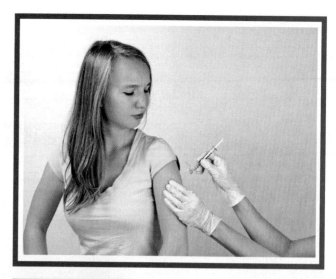

SEXUALLY TRANSMITTED INFECTIONS AND BLOOD-BORNE INFECTIONS

Sexually Transmitted Infections

Sexually transmitted infections (STIs) are passed from one person to another through intimate sexual and non-sexual contact. The majority of STIs, which includes more than 30 different bacterial, viral, and parasitic infections, are transmitted through sexual contact (vaginal, anal, or oral sex); a few can be spread through non-sexual contact via intimate skin-to-skin contact (e.g., viral STIs such as genital herpes and human papillomavirus), contact with blood, or during pregnancy and childbirth (PHAC, 2016b; WHO, 2016). STIs are different from other infections because their risk of acquisition is primarily determined by behavioural factors. Different types of sexual activity result in greater risk of acquisition of an infection. Receptive anal intercourse and vaginal intercourse carry the highest risk of acquiring an STI (PHAC, 2016b; Royce, Sena, Cates, & Cohen, 1997).

In Canada there are four nationally reportable STIs: chlamydia, gonorrhea, syphilis, and human immunodeficiency virus (HIV). Since 2000, the rates of reported cases for chlamydia, gonorrhea, and infectious syphilis have been steadily rising. This phenomenon is not unique to Canada; other regions, including the United States and the United Kingdom, have reported similar trends (PHAC, 2017b). STI incidence is highest among adolescents and young adults, with chlamydia being the most commonly reported notifiable infection in Canada. An estimated 50% of males and 70% of females infected with chlamydia are asymptomatic, so in the absence of screening, an undiagnosed person further contributes to the spread of the infection. Between 2005 and 2014, the chlamydia rate in Canada increased by 49.3% from 206 to 307 per 100 000 persons, the gonorrhea rate increased by 61.2% from 28.4 to 45.8 per 100 000 persons, and the infectious syphilis rate increased by 95.1% from 3.4 to 6.6 per 100 000 persons (PHAC, 2017b).

Canada's Provincial and Territorial Routine (and Catch-up) Vaccination Routine Schedule Programs for Infants and Children

This table summarizes the current routine vaccination schedule for infants and children in all provinces and territories across Canada. Changes to this schedule are updated regularly in collaboration with the Canadian Nursing Coalition for Immunization (CNCI) and the Canadian Immunization Committee (CIC) schedules for each province or territory can be found here. Additional information is available on Canada.ca\vaccines (last update: June 2018).

VACCINES		Provincial & Territorial Vaccination Schedules												
Abbreviations	Description	BC	AB	SK	MB	ON	QC	NB	NS	PE	NL	YT	NT	NU
DTaP-IPV-Hib	Diphtheria, Tetanus, acellular Pertussis, Inactivated Polio Virus, Haemophilus Influenzae type B vaccine	Age: 18 mos	Age: ,18 mos	Age: 2,4,6,18 mos	Age: 2,4,6,18 mos	Age: 2,4,6,18 mos	Age: 6 mos	Age: 2,4,6, 18 mos	Age: 2,4,6, 18 mos	Age: 18 mos	Age: 2,4,6, 18 mos	Age: 18 mos	Age: 2,4,6,18 mos	Age: 2,4,6,18 mos
DTaP-HB-IPV-Hib	Diphtheria, Tetanus, acellular Pertussis, Hepatitis B, Inactivated Polio Virus, Haemophilus Influenzae type B	Age: 2,4,6 mos	Age: 2,4,6 mos				Age: 2,4,18 mos			Age: 2,4,6 mos		Age: 2,4,6 mos		
Tdap-IPV	Tetanus, diphtheria (reduced toxoid), acellular pertussis (reduced toxoid), Inactivated Polio Virus vaccine	Age: 46 yrs	Age: 4-6 yrs	Age: 4-6 yrs	Age: 4-6 yrs	Age: 4-6 yrs	Age: 4-6 yrs	Age: 4 yrs	Age: 4-6 yrs	Age: 4-5 yrs	Age: 4-6 yrs	Age: 4-6 yrs	Age: 4-6 yrs	Age: 4-6 yrs
Tdap	Tetanus, diphtheria (reduced toxoid), acellular pertussis (reduced toxoid) vaccine	Grade 9	Grade 9	Grade 8	Age: 13-15 yrs	Age: 14-16 yrs	3rd year of high school	Grade 7	Grade 7	Grade 9	Grade 9	Grade 9	Grade 7	Grade 6
HB	Hepatitis B vaccine	HB is provided in a 3-dose combination vaccine (DTaP-IPV-Hib) in infancy	(3-dose) Grade 5	(2-dose) Grade 6	(2-dose), Grade 6	(2-dose) Grade 7	HB is provided in a 3-dose combination vaccine (DTaP-HB-IPV-Hib) in infancy / Catch-up (2-dose) 2013/14 to 2022/23 Grade 4[5]	Age: At birth, 2,6 mos	(2-doses) Grade 7	HB is provided in a 3-dose combination vaccine (DTaP-HB-IPV-Hib) in infancy	(2-dose) Grade 6	HB is provided in a 3-dose combination vaccine (DTaP-HB-IPV-Hib) in infancy	Age: At birth,1,6 mos	Age: At birth, 1,9 mos
MMR	Measles, Mumps, Rubella vaccine	Age: 12 mos				Age: 12 mos	Age: 12 mos					Age: 12 mos		
Var	Varicella vaccine	Age: 12 mos	Catch-up (2nd dose) 2015 to 2021 Grade: 6			Age: 15 mos	Age: 4-6 yrs	Catch-up (2nd dose) 2016/17 to 2022/23 Grade 9				Age: 12 mos		Catch-up Grade 6
MMRV	Measles, Mumps, Rubella, Varicella, vaccine	2nd dose Age: 4-6 yrs	Age: 12 mos, 4-6 yrs	Age: 12,18 mos	Age: 12 mos, 4-6 yrs	2nd dose Age: 4-6 yrs	Age: 18 mos	Age: 12,18 mos	Age: 12 mos, 18 mos-6 yrs	Age: 12,18 mos	Age: 12,18 mos	2nd dose Age: 4-6 years	Age: 12, 36 mos	Age: 12, 18 mos
Men-C-C	Meningococcal conjugate (Strain C) vaccine	Age: 2,12 mos	Age: 4,12 mos	Age: 12 mos,	Age: 12 mos[4],	Age: 12 mos	Age: 12 mos, 3rd yr of high school	Age: 12 mos	Age: 12 mos	Age: 12 mos	Age: 12 mos	Age: 12 mos	Age: 2, 12 mos	Age: 2, 12 mos
Men-C-ACYW-135	Meningococcal conjugate (Strains A, C, Y, W135) vaccine	Grade 9	Grade 9	Grade 6		Grade 7		Grade 9	Grade 7	Grade 9	Grade 4	Grade 9	Grade 12[a]	Grade 9
Pneu-C-13	Pneumococcal conjugate (13-valent) vaccine	Age: 2,4,12 mos	Age: 2,4,12 mos	Age: 2,4,12 mos	Age: 2,4,12 mos	Age: 2,4,12 mos		Age: 2,4,12 mos	Age: 2,4,12 mos	Age: 2,4,6 if high risk, 12 mos	Age: 2,4,6 if high risk 12 mos	Age: 2,4,12 mos	Age: 2,4,6,18 mos	Age: 2,4,6,18 mos
Pnue-C-10	Pneumococcal conjugate (10-valent) vaccine						Age: 2,4,12 mos							
Rota	Rotavirus vaccine	Age: 2,4,6 mos	Age: 2,4 mos	Age: 2,4, 6 mos	Age: 2,4,6 mos	Age: 2,4,6 mos	Age: 2,4 mos	Age: 2,4,6 mos		Age: 2,4,6 mos	Age 2,4 mos	Age: 2,4,6 mos	Age: 2,4 mos	Age: 2,4,6 mos
HPV	Human Papillomavirus vaccine	(2-dose) Grade: 6[1]	(3-dose) Grade 5[1] / Catch-up (3-dose) 2014 to 2018 Grade 9[3]	(2-dose) Grade 6[1]	(2-dose) Grade 6[1] / Catch-up (2-dose) Grade: 8,9[3]	(2-dose) Grade 7[1] / Catch-up (2 or 3-dose) Grade 8[1], Grades 9 to 12[2]	(2-dose) Grade 4[1] / Catch-Up (2-doses) Grade 9	(2-dose) Grade 7[1]	(2-dose) Grade 7[1]	(2-dose) Grade 6[1]	(2-dose) Grade 6[1]	(2-dose) Grade 6[1]	(9-14 yrs: 2-dose 15 yrs +: 3-dose) Grade 4-6[1]	(2-dose) Grade 6[1]

[PHAC logo] Public Health Agency of Canada / Agence de la santé publique du Canada   Canada

LEGEND	
Abbreviation/footnote	Definition
yrs	Years (age)
mos	Months (age)
a	If attending post-secondary school out-of-territory
1	Males and Females
2	Females only
3	Males only
4	Starting as early as September 2019, Manitoba's Meningococcal School-Based Immunization Program will be offered at a later grade; no child will miss the opportunity to be vaccinated
5	Students are provided with a combination vaccine that protects against hepatitis A and B
	Vaccine is not publicly funded in this province/territory
	A specific catch-up program is currently underway. A catch-up program is defined as a time-limited measure to implement a new vaccine program to a certain age cohort (e.g. an additional dose of a vaccine is recommended and a targeted program is put in place). It can also be used when a vaccine is added at a younger age (e.g. in infancy) and the existing program continues until that infancy age cohort "catches up" to the current age cohort (e.g. hepatitis b vaccine is added to the infancy program, but the school immunization program continues until those infants reach school aged immunization). With that said, a province or territory can still provide catch-up vaccine at the individual level even if there's no specific program in place.

[PHAC logo] Public Health Agency of Canada / Agence de la santé publique du Canada   Canada

FIGURE 12.1 Canada's Provincial and Territorial Routine (and Catch-up) Vaccination Programs for Infants and Children

Source: Government of Canada (2018).

Blood-Borne Infections

Blood-borne infections are carried and transmitted by blood (PHAC, 2016b). The most common examples of blood-borne infections are HIV, hepatitis B, hepatitis C, and viral hemorrhagic fevers. Diseases that are not usually transmitted directly by blood contact but rather by insect or some other vector are more usefully classified as vector-borne diseases, even though the causative agent can be found in blood. (Vector-borne diseases are discussed as a separate section in this chapter.)

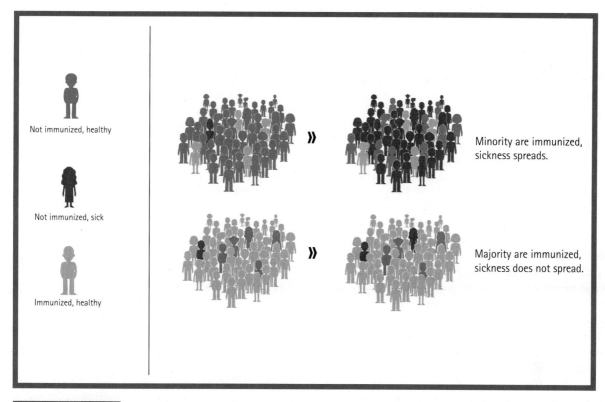

As our scientific knowledge and surveillance abilities have increased, potential indirect contact modes of transmission in some diseases were identified, including the transplantation of donor organs and the transfusion of blood products. Changes to screening practices were subsequently made to organ and blood donor screening and testing practices as well as the clinical use of donated organs and blood. Canadian Blood Services routinely screens all blood products for known infectious diseases such as HIV, syphilis, hepatitis B and C, human T-cell lymphotropic virus, and West Nile virus (Canadian Blood Services, 2016). Please refer to Chapter 31 for more specific information on STIs and blood-borne pathogens.

ENTERIC, FOOD-, AND WATER-BORNE INFECTIONS

Enteric Infections

Enteric infections enter the body through the mouth and intestinal tract and affect the digestive system (CDC, 2013a). This primarily occurs through eating or drinking contaminated foods or liquids. Infections acquired through ingestion of food are called food-borne infections; those by water are called water-borne infections. Direct contact with contaminated feces or vomit is a secondary method of acquiring an infection. Enteric infections acquired through feces can be transmitted from person to person or through a contaminated object to person. For example, hepatitis A infection is typically acquired through the ingestion of fecal-contaminated food (i.e., through a contaminated food handler who does not wash his or her hands after using the washroom) or water source (i.e., ingesting raw or undercooked shellfish from waters polluted with sewage).

Food-Borne Infection and Food-Borne Intoxication

Food-borne infection and **food-borne intoxication** are acquired through the consumption of contaminated food. Riemann and Cliver (2006) noted that *infections* occur when people consume food containing pathogenic microorganisms, which multiply in the gastrointestinal tract; *intoxications* occur when bacteria multiply in food and produce a toxin that is poisonous to the person ingesting the food. The most common causes of food-borne illnesses include the following:

- Toxins released by bacterial growth in food before consumption (e.g., *Clostridium botulism*, *Staphylococcus aureus*, and *Bacillus cereus*) or in the intestines (*Clostridium perfringens*)
- Bacterial, viral, or parasitic infections (brucellosis, campylobacter enteritis, diarrhea caused by *Escherichia coli*, hepatitis A, listeriosis, salmonellosis, shigellosis, toxoplasmosis, viral gastroenteritis, trichinosis)
- Toxins produced by harmful algal species (shellfish poisoning)

Food-borne infections are illnesses that occur within a variable but usually short time frame after a meal. **Food-borne outbreaks** are identified when an illness presents among individuals who have consumed common foods. For example, a community food-borne outbreak of *E. coli* O157:H7 was identified in 2008 in Ontario, when over 350 individuals who all consumed food from the same fast-food establishment became ill. Fifty individuals in this outbreak had lab-confirmed disease (North Bay Parry Sound District Health Unit, 2009). Food-borne outbreaks can be community-based or have a much more widespread impact depending on food distribution patterns. For example, a food-borne outbreak with national impact occurred in 2015 when salmonella associated with raw or undercooked poultry affected 110 people in nine provinces (PHAC, 2017c). Another food-borne outbreak with national impact occurred in 2017 when an outbreak of *E. coli* O121 was linked to various flour and flour products (PHAC, 2017d). Thorough and prompt collection and testing of implicated foods is essential, as is laboratory testing of stool samples obtained from cases. Many food-borne infection cases are unreported to health authorities, and outbreaks are often unrecognized.

Food-borne diseases can be prevented and controlled by avoiding food contamination, destroying contaminants (e.g., meat irradiation is one option), and eliminating spread or multiplication of the contaminants. Ultimately, prevention rests on educating food handlers of proper practices in cooking and storage of food, and personal hygiene. This includes keeping working areas clean, separating raw and cooked foods, cooking foods thoroughly, keeping foods at safe temperatures, and using safe water and raw materials (WHO, 2009b).

Water-Borne Diseases

Water-borne pathogens usually enter water supplies through fecal contamination from animals or humans to cause enteric illnesses (e.g., cholera, typhoid fever, dysentery, some types of salmonella, shigellosis, vibrio, and various coliform bacteria, including *E. coli* O157:H7). An outbreak of water-borne disease is usually defined when two cases that are epidemiologically linked by time and location of water exposure experience similar symptoms after consuming water from a common source (CDC, 2013b). Municipal water systems that have appropriate filtration and chlorination have decreased diseases such as amebic dysentery and giardiasis. However, effective filtration devices are needed for control of protozoa because they do not respond to traditional chlorine treatment. Outbreaks of cryptosporidium in North Battleford, Saskatchewan (PHAC, 2001), and *E. coli* in Walkerton, Ontario (PHAC, 2000) have raised awareness of the importance of safe municipal water systems across Canada.

Parasitic Diseases

Parasitic diseases are categorized with enteric infections since the primary mode of transmission in Canada is typically water, and secondarily is person-to-person through contaminated feces. When associated with water, parasitic diseases tend to be acquired from drinking unfiltered surface-water sources or shallow wells, or swimming in bodies of fresh water. Large community outbreaks have occurred from drinking treated but unfiltered water. Smaller outbreaks have resulted from contaminated food, person-to-person transmission in childcare centres,

and contaminated recreational waters (including swimming and wading pools). An outbreak in 1993 of cryptosporidiosis occurred in the Kitchener-Waterloo area of Ontario and was believed to have affected between 23 900 and 100 000 residents. These residents were drinking from the municipal water system that was likely contaminated during an unusual season of heavy rains, when the stools of cattle leached into rivers that fed the city's water treatment plant. Large supplies of water were pushed through the water system too quickly to allow time for the larger cryptosporidial oocysts to settle, and traditional chlorine disinfection likely did not work. This resulted in the oocysts entering the city's water supply. Residents of the city who used that water supply as their source became ill, whereas residents who had other sources for water did not become ill.

ZOONOTIC AND VECTOR-BORNE DISEASES

Zoonotic Infections

Zoonotic infections are transmitted between animals and humans; however, they do not need humans to maintain their life cycles. Transmission occurs by bites, inhalation, ingestion, direct contact, and arthropod intermediaries. Rabies, hantavirus pulmonary syndrome, salmonellosis, listeriosis, and brucellosis are examples of zoonotic diseases.

Rabies

Rabies has the highest case-fatality rate of any known human infection—essentially 100%. In 2015 the major carriers of rabies in Canada were bats, foxes, raccoons, and skunks (PHAC, 2015a). The virus is transmitted through a bite, scratch, or preexisting open wound and attacks the central nervous system (Government of Canada, 2014a). The best prevention is the vaccination of animals against rabies and pre-exposure vaccination of people working with animals. **Post-exposure prophylaxis (PEP)** is available after an exposure and occurs in consultation with public health officials. Determination of the need for follow-up by a CHN requires critical assessment of the endemic rates. For example, an animal exposure in Newfoundland would require further investigation to determine the history of the animal's habitation (the animal may have been brought from or migrated from a rabies-endemic area) since rabies is not usually present in the animal population in Newfoundland, whereas an exposure in eastern Ontario, where raccoon rabies is prevalent, would require follow-up. Often CHNs recommend or administer rabies immune globulin with the dosage calculation based on client weight and a series of the rabies vaccine. The animal, if located, should be kept in a confined area for a period of 10 days to determine if it was infectious with rabies at the time of the exposure. Most infected animals succumb to rabies within a five-day period, but 10 days is used to avoid any possible exceptions. If the animal exhibits signs and symptoms of rabies or dies during the isolation period, the exposed person is started on PEP as soon as possible. If the animal is deceased immediately following the exposure, rabies testing of brain tissue is conducted at a national laboratory, and the exposed individual is offered PEP based on the findings. If a client is started on PEP and animal testing indicates that the rabies virus was not present, the PEP can be stopped prior to completion (PHAC, 2015a).

Hantavirus

Hantavirus is a viral disease found in the droppings, urine, and saliva of infected rodents. Humans can contract the virus from breathing in airborne particles or from being bitten. In Canada, although the risk of exposure is low, when it happens, the disease can be severe (PHAC, 2009a). Humans can inhale the virus, which may lead to hantavirus pulmonary syndrome (HPS). The earliest documented case of HPS in Canada was contracted in Alberta in 1989 (Alberta Health Services, 2012). Since then there have been over 70 confirmed cases. Most occurred in western Canada (Manitoba, Saskatchewan, Alberta, and British Columbia). Hantavirus infections contracted by Canadians outside the country have also been recognized, including two fatal cases from South America (PHAC, 2009a). HPS is extremely serious; 38% of all cases are fatal (Alberta Health Services, 2012). Primary prevention strategies taken by individuals at risk, such as workers in agricultural or rural settings or hikers and campers, include keeping woodpiles away from dwellings, keeping items off the floor to prevent rodent nesting, trapping rodents, wet-mopping areas where droppings are located to prevent aeration of feces, and not camping near rodent-infested areas.

Vector-Borne Infections

Vector-borne infections are caused by viruses, bacteria, and parasites that living creatures carry and pass on to other living creatures. Disease carriers, called "vectors," are usually mosquitoes, ticks, and mammals. For example, mosquitoes carry the infectious agents that cause malaria, West Nile virus, and Zika virus. Other vector-borne diseases include Lyme disease, avian influenza, and rabies (British Columbia Ministry of Health, n.d.). Climate change has a potential impact on the distribution of various diseases. Malaria and dengue fever, also vector-borne diseases, are seen in travellers who have contracted these diseases in other countries from the bite of an infected mosquito. Vector-borne diseases most commonly seen in Canada include Eastern equine encephalitis, Lyme disease, and West Nile virus.

Lyme Disease

Lyme disease is transmitted by black-legged ticks that carry the bacteria *B. burgdorferi.* (See Photo 12.2.) Transmission occurs as the ticks attach themselves to migratory birds, mice, squirrels, rodents, and other small animals that can carry the bacterium. Although black-legged ticks (also called deer ticks) can be found in all areas of Canada, only about 10% are infected with Lyme disease. Given that localized tick populations can spread, it is difficult to define the geographic limits of the

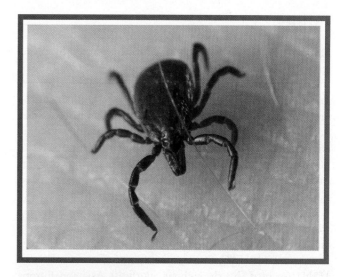

PHOTO 12.2 A close-up of a black-legged tick. Through the bite of an infected tick, Lyme disease can be transmitted to humans.

Source: Steven Ellingson/Shutterstock

tick population. However, the PHAC, in partnership with provincial and territorial public health organizations, has identified the spread of black-legged tick populations in Canada through ongoing surveillance. Parts of the following provinces have been identified as areas of concern: British Columbia, Manitoba, Ontario, Quebec, New Brunswick, and Nova Scotia (Government of Canada, 2017a).

West Nile and Zika Virus

West Nile virus is carried and spread by mosquitoes. It can cause severe neurological complications. Personal protection against this vector and reducing areas where mosquitoes breed are important strategies in controlling the spread. As part of the West Nile virus surveillance program, several provinces and territories conduct mosquito surveillance activities. Planning is also underway to enhance mosquito surveillance to detect new mosquito species into Canada, including species responsible for Zika virus transmission. Zika virus infection has been associated with congenital anomalies, including microencephaly and/or central nervous system malformation (Government of Canada, 2017b).

RESPIRATORY INFECTIONS

In a large percentage of patients with acute respiratory infections, the causative organism is unknown. Viruses cause most infections within the respiratory system; bacterial infections occur at a lesser frequency. Typically, upper viral respiratory infections are caused by rhinoviruses (30–50%) or coronaviruses (5–20%). The remaining infections (30–65%) are due to influenza viruses, parainfluenza viruses, respiratory syncytial virus, adenoviruses, and certain enteroviruses (Berman et al., 1983; Reed, 1981).

Influenza

Human influenza is a respiratory infection caused by influenza virus, which is spread via droplets through coughing or sneezing. Vaccination against influenza, which usually lasts four to six months, is routinely administered annually at the onset of the influenza season, typically starting in October or November in Canada. Each year the influenza vaccine contains three influenza strains predicted by the WHO to be the most common circulating strains. Due to the significant morbidity, mortality, and societal costs associated with influenza, vaccinations are recommended for everyone six months or older, especially individuals with chronic illness, people aged 65 and over, residents in chronic care and nursing homes, health care service providers, and pregnant women (PHAC, 2014c). The spread of avian influenza H5N1 (or bird flu) throughout Southeast Asia and Europe generated much discussion on the implications for human health. However, in April 2009 a novel strain of influenza H1N1 was recognized in Mexico, causing a cluster of illness with the potential to become a pandemic. Following the WHO raising the pandemic alert to level 6, indicating that a novel strain of influenza was rapidly spreading from human to human across international jurisdictions, globally, many nations declared a pandemic. This event moved public health activity from the planning phase to action at local, provincial, and federal levels throughout Canada. With the advent of new strains of influenza, the health care system is taxed during the vaccine development period, with the medical system waiting to obtain strain-specific vaccines for primary prevention.

Tuberculosis

Tuberculosis (TB) is caused by the bacteria *Mycobacterium tuberculosis*, which is transmitted from person to person through the air. TB often affects the lungs; pulmonary TB is the most commonly reported site, accounting for 66% of all cases in Canada in 2015, followed by TB of the peripheral lymph nodes at 13.5% (Gallant, Duvvuri, & McGuire, 2017). Globally, approximately one-quarter of the world's population has latent TB, wherein the disease is dormant, does not affect the infected person, and cannot be transmitted (WHO, 2017b). When a person develops active TB, symptoms may be mild for months and can include cough, fever, night sweats, or weight loss.

In Canada, statistics for active cases of TB are collected nationally through the Canadian Tuberculosis Reporting System (CTBRS). Annually, about 1600 new cases of active TB are reported in Canada (Government of Canada, 2016). Although the incidence of active TB in Canada continues to decrease and is among the lowest in the world (4.6 per 100 000 population), high rates persist among foreign-born and Indigenous populations (Gallant et al., 2017). Foreign-born individuals accounted for 71% of cases, and the incidence among Canadian-born Indigenous people was highest at 17.1 per 100 000 population.

YES, BUT WHY?

High Incidence of Tuberculosis in the Inuit Population

What?

The rate of active TB among the Inuit is more than 270 times higher than in the Canadian-born, non-Indigenous population. In Canada, Nunavut has the highest rate of active TB disease at 0.17% (Gallant et al., 2017).

So What?

The prevention and control of TB is a shared responsibility among all levels of government in Canada. The focus remains on identifying and treating populations most at risk, which include individuals with active TB disease and those with latent TB infection who are at risk of developing active TB disease. Indigenous populations continue to be disproportionately represented among reported cases of active TB disease, particularly communities in Nunavut (Government of Canada, 2014b; PHAC, 2016a). These disproportionately high rates reflect significant health inequalities between this population and the general Canadian population (PHAC, 2014d). Indigenous communities often face numerous challenges. For example, living in substandard conditions with housing that is overcrowded and poorly ventilated can increase an individual's exposure to TB (Hargreaves et al., 2011). Poor nutrition due to lack of access to healthy food, and underlying conditions and co-morbidities such as diabetes and HIV infection, can further increase the risk to individuals with latent TB infection progressing to active TB disease (PHAC, 2016a). Moreover, these factors are exacerbated in remote and isolated communities, such as those in the Arctic, where access to health care services is further limited or delayed. The impact of the social determinants of health on increasing both the risk of exposure to TB and the progression from latent TB infection to active TB disease need to be addressed to prevent and control the TB epidemic evolving in the Nunavummiut.

Now What?

Through developing and maintaining partnerships with communities, CHNs have the ability to improve overall health outcomes by increasing individuals' involvement and engagement in the prevention and control of TB. Building capacity of community members is essential as developing relationships with government and local agencies is key to addressing the socioecological factors that contribute to TB (PHAC, 2014d). Advocacy is another key role for CHNs in partnership with community members and other stakeholders: they can draw awareness to the impact poverty and overcrowding have in the spread of TB, particularly across Inuit populations, where climate is a unique factor that creates additional challenges in containing the spread of the disease. In the community, CHNs can undertake surveillance to monitor epidemiological trends of active TB disease and TB drug resistance, deliver TB services directly to community members through directly observed therapy (DOT), and provide support for TB outbreak management.

Moreover, CHNs should ensure Inuit culture, traditions, and perspectives are reflected in the development of health policies and programming for innovative health promotion and disease prevention strategies to combat TB.

Standards of Practice Fulfilled

#1 Health Promotion
- Uses a collaborative relationship with the client and other partners to facilitate and advocate for structural system change and healthy public policy using multiple health promotion strategies.
- Seeks to identify and assess the root and historical causes of illness, disease and inequities in health, acknowledges diversity and the adverse effects of colonialism on Indigenous people, and when appropriate incorporates Indigenous ways of knowing including connectedness and reciprocity to the land and all life in health promotion.
- Considers the determinants of health, the social and political context, and systemic structures in collaboration with the client to determine action

#2 Prevention and Health Protection
- Participates in surveillance, recognizes trends in epidemiology data, and utilizes this data through population level actions such as health education, screening, immunization, and communicable disease control and management.

#3 Health Maintenance, Restoration and Palliation
- Includes cultural safety and cultural humility approaches in all aspects of health maintenance, restoration and palliation interventions.
- Holistically assesses the health status, and functional competence of the client within the context of their environment, social supports, and life transitions.

#5 Capacity Building
- Uses a comprehensive mix of strategies such as coalition building, inter-sectoral collaboration, community engagement and mobilization, partnerships and networking to build community capacity to take action on priority issues.

#6 Health Equity
- Engages with clients who are marginalized in the coordinating and planning of care, services and programs that address their needs and perspectives on health and illness.
- Participates with community members and advocates for health in intersectoral policy development and implementation to reduce health equity gaps between populations (Community Health Nurses of Canada [CHNC], 2019, revised).

Drug-resistant TB is a growing concern, as resistance to first-line therapies are increasing, and multidrug-resistant TB (MDR-TB) is becoming more common. Drug resistance to traditional TB treatment was seen in 8% of Canadian cases reported in 2015; 7.9% were monoresistant, 1.6% were resistant to two or more drugs, and no cases of extensively drug-resistant TB(XDR- TB) were reported (Government of Canada, 2017c).

HEALTH CARE-ASSOCIATED AND HEALTH CARE-ACQUIRED INFECTIONS

A **health care–associated infection (HAI)** is an infection that a patient acquires in a setting where health care is delivered, such as a hospital, long-term care facility, or home care setting. It is estimated that each year more than 200 000 Canadians acquire an HAI, and almost 8000 of them die as a result (PHAC, 2013). HAIs typically occur in patients who are admitted to a hospital, but others who visit or work in the facility may also be susceptible. HAIs can also be acquired through outpatient clinics, health care facility day treatment programs (e.g., dialysis clinic, doctors' office visit, or outpatient cancer treatments), or home care services. "Routine practices and additional precautions for preventing the transmission of infection in healthcare setting" is one guideline published by the PHAC to assist health care providers in all health care settings develop routine practices and precautions to prevent HAIs (PHAC, 2016c).

Hand hygiene is the most effective way of preventing the spread of HAIs transmitted by direct contact with hands, surfaces, or objects that have been contaminated by an infected person. Routine precautions are taught, and their use encouraged by all health care facility employees. The practice of infection control and familiarity with infection control policies and practices is essential for nurses, as they are the health care professionals with the most "hands on" time with patients and therefore more likely to transmit or acquire these types of infections. Nurses are at the front line of defence against transmission. As such, using routine precautions with every patient is essential to prevent the transmission of organisms that cause infections. Figure 12.3 is a summary of the elements of routine infection prevention and control practices.

CHNs should become familiar with the different infection control and prevention guidelines, and utilize the ones that are most appropriate in their scope of practice. Figure 12.4 displays the elements of **point-of-care practice**, in which every encounter with a patient within the health care system entitles a risk assessment of the patient, the environment, and the interaction within it to determine what appropriate personal protective equipment (e.g., gloves, gowns, masks, etc.) is needed. (See Photo 12.3.)

Effective **surveillance systems**, **infection control** programs, and education for nurses in hospitals and community settings, including long-term care homes, are essential in controlling the spread of infections to clients who are at risk. Screening patients who are at risk for HAIs can ensure early identification and appropriate infection control procedures are in place to mitigate transmission to other patients. Typical health care–associated organisms are identified as either a colonization or an infection. A **colonized patient** is one who is colonized with the organism but shows no signs or symptoms of the infection. This type of person, if swabbed (a specimen sample is taken from the nose, rectum, or peritoneal area), grows the organism. Colonized patients are treated with

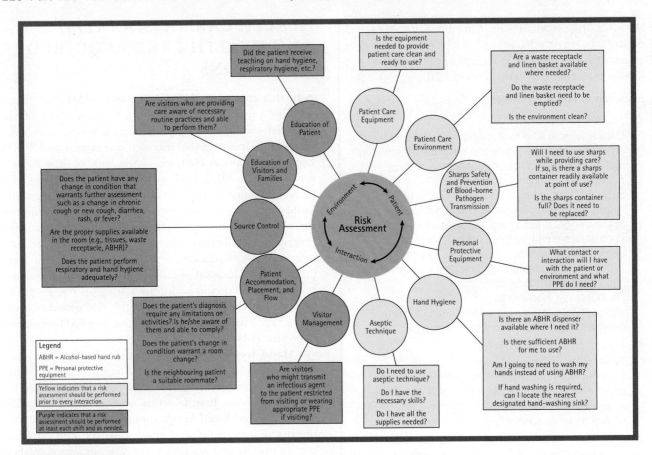

FIGURE 12.3 Elements of Routine Practices Summary

Source: Public Health Agency of Canada. (2014). *Routine practices and additional precautions assessment and educational tools.* Reproduced with permission from the Minister of Health, 2018. © All rights reserved.

appropriate medication as if they had the infection. Colonized and **infected patients** may receive similar care, including appropriate treatment and more stringent infection control practices such as being put in isolation or cohorted with other similar patients.

The Canadian Nosocomial Infection Surveillance Program (CNISP) monitors HAIs in **sentinel hospitals** throughout Canada (PHAC, 2012). CNISP was established in 1994 with the overall objective of providing rates and trends of HAIs in Canadian health care facilities, thus enabling comparison of rates (benchmarks) and provision of data that can be used in the development of national guidelines on clinical issues related to HAIs. At present, 64 sentinel hospitals from 10 provinces participate in the CNISP network (PHAC, 2017e). It has been estimated that approximately 8% of children and 10% of adults in Canadian hospitals have a HAI at any point in time (Gravel et al., 2007a; Gravel et al., 2007b). However, the severity is greatest among vulnerable populations, such as older adults, the very young, individuals with weakened immune systems, or individuals with one or more chronic medical condition (Canadian Institute for Health Information, 2008). More than 50% of HAIs are caused by bacteria that are resistant to at least one type of antibiotic. The four priority antibiotic-resistant organisms found in hospitals in Canada are methicillin-resistant *Staphylococcus aureus* (MRSA), vancomycin-resistant enterococci (VRE), *Clostridium difficile*, and carbapenamase-producing organisms (e.g., enterobacteriaceae).

ANTIMICROBIAL RESISTANCE

Antimicrobial resistance (AMR) is when micro-organisms (bacteria, viruses, fungi, and parasites) change in a way that reduces or eliminates the effectiveness of drugs, chemicals,

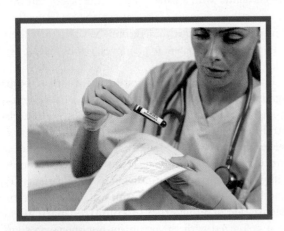

PHOTO 12.3 Using personal protective equipment

Source: Tek Image/Science Source

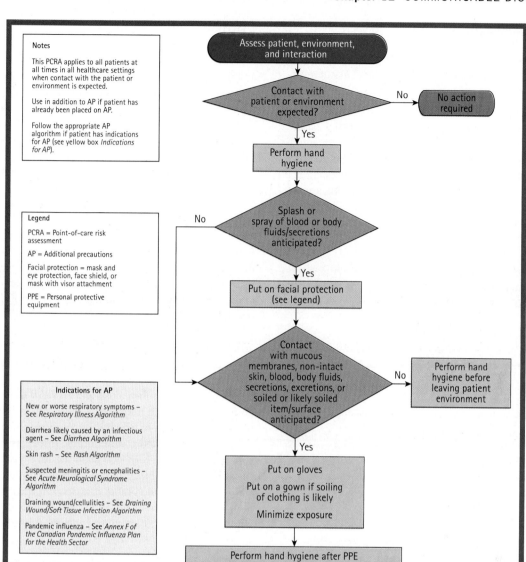

Notes

This PCRA applies to all patients at all times in all healthcare settings when contact with the patient or environment is expected.

Use in addition to AP if patient has already been placed on AP.

Follow the appropriate AP algorithm if patient has indications for AP (see yellow box *Indications for AP*).

Legend

PCRA = Point-of-care risk assessment

AP = Additional precautions

Facial protection = mask and eye protection, face shield, or mask with visor attachment

PPE = Personal protective equipment

Indications for AP

New or worse respiratory symptoms – See *Respiratory Illness Algorithm*

Diarrhea likely caused by an infectious agent – See *Diarrhea Algorithm*

Skin rash – See *Rash Algorithm*

Suspected meningitis or encephalitis – See *Acute Neurological Syndrome Algorithm*

Draining wound/cellulitis – See *Draining Wound/Soft Tissue Infection Algorithm*

Pandemic influenza – See *Annex F of the Canadian Pandemic Influenza Plan for the Health Sector*

Assess patient, environment, and interaction

Contact with patient or environment expected? — No → No action required

Yes ↓

Perform hand hygiene

Splash or spray of blood or body fluids/secretions anticipated? — No →

Yes ↓

Put on facial protection (see legend)

Contact with mucous membranes, non-intact skin, blood, body fluids, secretions, excretions, or soiled or likely soiled item/surface anticipated? — No → Perform hand hygiene before leaving patient environment

Yes ↓

Put on gloves

Put on a gown if soiling of clothing is likely

Minimize exposure

Perform hand hygiene after PPE removal and before leaving patient environment

FIGURE 12.4 Point-of-Care Risk Assessment for Routine Practices Algorithm: Appropriate Use of Personal Protective Equipment

Source: Public Health Agency of Canada. (2014). *Routine practices and additional precautions assessment and educational tools.* Reproduced with permission from the Minister of Health, 2018. © All rights reserved.

or other agents intended to cure or prevent infections and disease caused by the micro-organism (PHAC, 2013). Although antimicrobial resistance is a natural phenomenon as infectious diseases evolve, resistance is greatly increased when drugs are overused or used inappropriately (Heymann, 2015). **Intrinsic resistance** occurs when bacteria become naturally resistant or insensitive to antimicrobial agents, whereas **acquired resistance** occurs when bacteria become resistant after being exposed to antimicrobial agents (PHAC, 2016d).

Antimicrobial resistance is a global issue, present in every country. As medicines become ineffective at preventing and treating infections, "patients with infections caused by drug-resistant bacteria are at increased risk of worse clinical outcomes and death, and consume more health-care resources than patients infected with non-resistant strains of the same bacteria" (WHO, 2017c). Moreover, patients with prolonged illnesses increase the risk of transmitting infections to others. For example, resistance has been extensively noted in the treatment of tuberculosis, malaria, HIV, gonorrhea, and influenza.

In Canada, antibiotic use and resistance are monitored through four surveillance systems: the Canadian Integrated Program for Antimicrobial Resistance Surveillance (CIPARS), the Canadian Nosocomial Infection Surveillance Program (CNISP), the Enhanced Surveillance of Antimicrobial-Resistant Gonorrhea program (ESAG), and the Canadian Tuberculosis Laboratory Surveillance System.

CANADIAN RESEARCH 12.1

How is an international public health threat advanced in Canada? The case of antimicrobial resistance. (Tsegaye et al., 2016)

AMR is a complex issue, not one that can be solved with a single intervention. There is a need for coordinated action, given that many sectors are interconnected and impacted. The One Health framework is a collaborative effort that recognizes the inextricable connection between humans, animals, and the environment. By using antimicrobials more judiciously and responsibly in food (animal and crop) production, there is the potential to minimize resistance and the risk of subsequent transmission to humans via the food chain or the environment. This article examines the work that has been done to develop a coordinated AMR action plan to align Canada's response efforts with the WHO's Global Action Plan.

Discussion Questions

1. Why is it important to utilize an intersectoral collaborative approach when implementing the One Health framework?

2. What are some factors that are contributing to the increasing number and significance of zoonotic diseases?

3. What important clinical practice strategies can be implemented to combat the development of antimicrobial resistance?

NOTIFIABLE/REPORTABLE DISEASES IN CANADA

While some infectious diseases are common and mild (such as the common cold or pediculosis), others are serious enough to be defined as notifiable diseases (such as hepatitis C and HIV/AIDS) and must be reported to the local health authority. Local public health personnel are mandated by the provinces and territories to report all notifiable diseases to their respective ministry or department of health. The terms *notifiable* and *reportable diseases* are commonly used interchangeably. A communicable disease is identified as a **notifiable disease** (or reportable) by experts around the world in infectious diseases who study the morbidity and mortality of an identified disease and then, through consensus, recommend the need for notification. The morbidity and mortality impact may be in a small defined area or on a worldwide scale. Reportable diseases are identified in the public health act of each province or territory. Whenever a case of a reportable disease is identified, the collection of information to further describe the case is necessary. This includes information about the person, symptoms, date of onset of the presenting illness, and his or her travel history. Additional information collected, dependent on the disease, may include social history, sexual history, diagnostic tests done to date, and prescribed treatment. Reporting of some communicable diseases is not only required by provinces and territories within Canada but in some instances may also require international reporting to the WHO.

Legislation

In Canada, both provincial/territorial and national guidelines and legislation dictate which diseases must be reported, who is responsible for reporting them, what the reporting format should be, and what the mechanism for reporting is to the national surveillance system. The list of reportable diseases is mandated by provincial or territorial legislation and, therefore, differs by province or territory, although the recommendations are provided by the PHAC. Currently, some provinces and territories report within the *integrated Public Health Information System (iPHIS),* a database used by public health units to report information on cases of reportable diseases (PHAC, 2007). If there is a requirement for international health reporting, the PHAC reports to the WHO. The International Health Regulations (IHR) (WHO, 2009c) are the only legally binding instrument requiring the reporting of communicable diseases at the international level, and reporting is currently limited to smallpox, poliomyelitis, human influenza caused by a new subtype, and severe acute respiratory syndrome (SARS) (Heymann, 2015). The WHO updates and revises the IHR to address the threat of new and re-emerging infections and to accommodate new reporting sources. A number of diseases *under surveillance* by the WHO (e.g., tuberculosis and HIV/AIDS) are required to be reported at varied frequency, depending on the disease and the geographic area in which it has occurred.

Public health and communicable disease surveillance is a shared responsibility, with local public health departments having the primary responsibility for detecting, monitoring, controlling, and reporting communicable diseases. On the ground, public health nurses and public health inspectors in local public health offices work together to monitor potential public health threats.

Nationally Notifiable Diseases

The list of notifiable diseases at the national level is identified by provincial, territorial, and federal health authorities as an effort to monitor and control priority diseases. The National Notifiable Diseases list helps to ensure consistency among provinces and territories to conform with international reporting requirements and facilitates tracking and control efforts by public health personnel (PHAC, 2009b). Annually, all provinces and territories submit notifiable disease data, which are used to produce national disease rates and allow jurisdictions to explore possible trends. Due to the changing nature and epidemiology of infectious diseases, the National Notifiable Diseases list is reviewed and modified periodically. In 2017, 59 notifiable diseases were reportable to the PHAC. (See Table 12.2.)

SELECT COMMUNICABLE DISEASES IN CANADA BY GROUPINGS

In Table 12.3, selected communicable diseases with high incidence rates in Canada are listed by group. The diseases are grouped into the following categories: enteric, food-, and water-borne diseases;

Table 12.2	Diseases Under National Surveillance (May 2017)	
Acquired Immunodeficiency Syndrome (AIDS)	Hantavirus Pulmonary Syndrome (HPS)	Paralytic Shellfish Poisoning
Acute Flaccid Paralysis (AFP)	Hepatitis A	Paratyphoid
Anthrax	Hepatitis B	Pertussis
Botulism	Hepatitis C	Plague
Brucellosis	Human Immunodeficiency Virus (HIV)	Poliomyelitis
Campylobacteriosis		Rabies
Chickenpox (Varicella)	Influenza, Epidemic	Rubella
Chlamydia	Influenza, Laboratory-Confirmed	Salmonellosis
Cholera	Invasive Group A Streptococcal Disease	Severe Acute Respiratory Syndrome (SARS)
Clostridium difficile Associated Diarrhea	Invasive Haemophilus influenzae type b (Hib) and non-b Disease	Shigellosis
Congenital Rubella Syndrome (CRS)	Invasive Meningococcal Disease	Smallpox
Congenital Syphilis	Invasive Pneumococcal Disease	Syphilis
Creutzfeldt-Jakob Disease (CJD), Classic and New Variant	Legionellosis	Tetanus
Cryptosporidiosis	Leprosy	Tuberculosis
Cyclosporiasis	Listeriosis	Tularemia
Diphtheria	Lyme Disease	Typhoid
Giardiasis	Malaria	Verotoxigenic Escherichia coli Infection
Gonorrhea	Measles	Viral Haemorrhagic Fever
Group B Streptococcal Disease of the Newborn	Mumps	West Nile Virus Infection
	Norovirus infection	Yellow Fever

Source: Public Health Agency of Canada. (2017). *List of nationally notifiable diseases* (May 2017). Reproduced with permission from the Minister of Health, 2015. Retrieved from http://diseases.canada.ca.

diseases transmitted by respiratory routes; health care–acquired infections; vaccine-preventable diseases; sexually transmitted and blood-borne pathogens; and zoonotic and vector-borne diseases.

CONTROL AND MANAGEMENT OF COMMUNICABLE DISEASES

The successful control and management of communicable diseases is integrally tied to using sound principles of epidemiology. (See Chapter 11.) **Surveillance** of a disease consists of "the process of systematic collection, orderly consolidation, analysis, and evaluation of pertinent data with prompt dissemination of the results to those who need to know, particularly those who are in a position to take action" (Heymann, 2015, p. 704). Through data analysis, the investigator may uncover the cause or source of the disease (e.g., investigation of a case of salmonella infection may uncover a contaminated food item in a restaurant).

Surveillance

Monitoring of diseases, investigation of disease outbreaks, and observation of patterns of disease are responsibilities of the local health authorities. **Active surveillance** is the collection of data

utilizing screening tools, interviews, and sentinel systems to identify disease occurrence in the community when individuals present with suggestive symptoms. Such surveillance depends on the creation of surveillance screening tools that heighten the awareness of health care practitioners in relation to a specific disease. Active surveillance may be best illustrated by the screening created in response to the increasing risk across Canada of West Nile virus (WNV), first recognized as a threat in North America in 1999. When WNV was first reported, provincial and federal health authorities applied public health measures to identify the spread of this new communicable disease. WNV was detected for the first time in Canada in 2001, in birds and mosquitoes. In 2002, Canadian health authorities documented 414 human cases of WNV in five provinces: Nova Scotia, Quebec, Ontario, Manitoba, and Saskatchewan. In 2007, more than 2200 human cases were identified in Canada (PHAC, 2017f).

The active surveillance activities during the early days of WNV infections in Canada were conducted partly through the availability of a screening tool. Similarly, a screening tool has been developed by the Ontario Ministry of Health and Long-Term Care for active surveillance of influenza-like illnesses (ILI). The ILI screening tool is utilized in emergency rooms and other acute-care settings to provide consistent and early identification of respiratory illnesses such as influenza and SARS to facilitate the necessary control activities to decrease transmission risks in

Table 12.3	Select Communicable Diseases in Canada					

Enteric, Food- and Water-borne Diseases

Disease	Infectious Agent	Mode of Transmission	Incubation Period	Clinical Presentation	Period of Communicability	Control Measures
12.3.1 CAMPYL-OBACTER ENTERITIS or CAMPYLO BACTERIOSIS	• *Campylobacter jejuni* • Less commonly *Campylobacter coli*	• Ingestion of the organisms in undercooked meat, particularly poultry, other contaminated food, water, or raw milk. • Contact with infected pets, farm animals, or infected infants. • Person-to-person transmission is uncommon.	Usually 2–5 days, with a range of 1–10 days depending on dose ingested.	An acute zoonotic bacterial enteric disease of variable severity characterized by diarrhea, abdominal pain, malaise, fever, nausea, and vomiting.	Throughout the course of the infection; usually several days to several weeks.	• Isolation: Enteric precautions for hospitalized patients. • Concurrent disinfection: Cleaning of areas and articles soiled with stools.
12.3.2 SALMO-NELLOSIS	• Nearly all *Salmonella* isolated from ill persons are serotypes of *S. enterica* subsp. *enterica*. • Approximately 2500 serotypes of *Salmonella* have been identified.	• Ingestion of the organism in food derived from infected animals, contaminated by feces of an infected animal or person.	From 6 to 72 hours, usually about 12 to 36 hours.	A bacterial disease commonly manifested by acute enterocolitis, with sudden onset of headache, abdominal pain, diarrhea, nausea, and sometimes vomiting.	Throughout the course of the infection, extremely variable, usually several days to several weeks.	• Proper handwashing should be stressed. • Enteric precautions when handling feces and contaminated clothing and bed linen: • Concurrent disinfection of feces and articles soiled with stools. • Culture stools of household contacts and individuals who are involved in food handling, direct patient care, or care for young children or older adults in institutional settings.

(continued)

Table 12.3 Continued

Disease	Infectious Agent	Mode of Transmission	Incubation Period	Clinical Presentation	Period of Communicability	Control Measures
12.3.3 GIARDIASIS	*Giardia lamblia* (*G. intestinalis*, *G. duodenalis*), a flagellate protozoan	• Principal mode of transmission is person to person, which occurs by hand-to-mouth transfer of cysts from the feces of an infected individual, especially in institutions and childcare centres. • Anal intercourse also facilitates transmission.	Usually 3–25 days or longer; median 7–10 days.	A protozoan infection, principally of the upper small intestine, it can (a) remain asymptomatic; (b) bring on acute, self-limited diarrhea; and (c) lead to intestinal symptoms such as chronic diarrhea, steatorrhea, abdominal cramps, bloating, frequent loose and pale greasy stools, fatigue, malabsorption (of fats and fat-soluble vitamins), and weight loss.	Entire period of infection, often months.	Enteric precautions • Concurrent disinfection of feces and articles soiled with stools. • Microscopic examination of feces of household members and other suspected contacts, especially if symptomatic.
Diseases Transmitted by the Respiratory Route						
12.3.4 INVASIVE PNEUMOCOCCAL DISEASE OR PNEUMOCOCCAL PNEUMONIA	*Streptococcus pneumoniae* (pneumococcus)	Droplet spread. Person-to-person transmission of the organisms is common, but illness among casual contacts and attendants is infrequent.	Not well determined; may be as short as 1–3 days. Infection is thought to be preceded by asymptomatic colonization.	Includes sudden onset, high fever, rigors, pleuritic, chest pain, dyspnea, tachypnea, and cough productive of "rusty" sputum.	Presumably until discharges of mouth and nose no longer contain sufficient numbers of pneumococci, which usually occurs within 24 hours of initiation of effective antibiotic therapy.	• Respiratory isolation may be warranted for hospitalized patients with antibiotic-resistant infection, who may transmit it to high-risk patients. • Hand hygiene and cough etiquette. • No practical value to investigate contacts or source of the infection.

(continued)

Table 12.3	Continued					
Disease	**Infectious Agent**	**Mode of Transmission**	**Incubation Period**	**Clinical Presentation**	**Period of Communicability**	**Control Measures**
12.3.5 INVASIVE GROUP A STREPTOCOCCAL DISEASE	*Group A Beta-hemolytic Streptococci*	• Large respiratory droplets or direct contact with patients or carriers. • Indirect contact through objects, although extremely rare.	Short, usually 1–3 days, rarely longer.	• Clinical presentation varies and depends on where the invasive disease occurs. Examples of the types of invasive disease include streptococcal toxic shock syndrome (STSS), necrotizing fasciitis (NF), pneumonia, and bacteremia. • Symptoms will vary depending on primary site of infection.	• In untreated, uncomplicated cases, 10–21 days; • In untreated cases, conditions with purulent discharges, weeks or months. • With adequate penicillin treatment, transmissibility of group A streptococcal disease generally ends in 24 hours. • Drainage and secretion precautions may be terminated after 24 hours of effective antibiotic therapy.	• Disinfection of purulent discharges and all soiled articles. • Terminal cleaning. Critical assessment of adherence to infection control practices should be undertaken in group A streptococcal outbreaks in facilities housing highly vulnerable populations (e.g., nursing homes and acute and long-term rehabilitation facilities).

(continued)

Table 12.3	Continued				
Disease	**Infectious Agent**	**Mode of Transmission**	**Incubation Period**	**Clinical Presentation**	**Period of Communicability**	**Control Measures**
12.3.6 PULMONARY TUBERCULOSIS (TB, TB DISEASE)	*Mycobacterium tuberculosis*	Exposure to tubercle bacilli in airborne, aerosolized droplet, produced by persons with pulmonary or high respiratory tract tuberculosis (e.g., laryngeal) during forceful expiratory efforts (e.g., coughing, singing, or sneezing). The droplet nuclei are inhaled by a vulnerable contact into the pulmonary alveoli. Here, the aerosolized particles containing *M. tuberculosis* are ingested by alveolar macrophages, initiating a new infection.	• Two to 10 weeks from infection to demonstrable primary lesion or significant TB skin test (TST) reaction and positivity of interferon-gamma release assays (IGRA). • Latent infection may persist for a lifetime.	Cough, fatigue, fever, night sweats, weight loss, and pleuritic pain are common signs and symptoms associated with pulmonary TB disease. • Most children (less than 5 years) with TB are asymptomatic at presentation. • Older children and adolescents are more likely to experience adult-type disease and often present with a classic triad of fever, night sweats, and weight loss. Degree of communicability depends on number of bacilli discharged, virulence of bacilli, adequacy of ventilation, exposure of bacilli to sun or UV light, and opportunities for aerosolization through coughing, sneezing, talking, singing, or during aerosolized procedures.	• Theoretically, as long as viable tubercle bacilli are discharged in the sputum. • Effective antimicrobial chemotherapy usually eliminates communicability within 2–4 weeks. • Effective antimicrobial chemoprophylaxis usually eliminates communicability within 2–4 weeks.	• Isolation until antibiotic treatment of a minimum of 2 weeks has been completed. • Contact tracing and TB skin testing of all vulnerable contacts. • Screening with tuberculin testing/x-rays among the at-risk populations. • Provide adequate anti-TB chemotherapy and prophylactic treatments. • Patients in a congregated setting should be placed in airborne infection isolation rooms with negative pressure ventilation. Persons entering the room should wear N95 face respirators. • Handwashing and good housekeeping practices must be maintained according to policy. • Recently, with the emergence of highly drug-resistant forms of TB (MDR-TB, XDR-TB), quarantine measures may be warranted to enforce isolation. • Investigation of potentially exposed contacts is recommended at the time of diagnosis. TST or IGRA tests for all household members and other close contacts are recommended.

(continued)

Table 12.3	Continued					

Vaccine-Preventable Diseases

Disease	Infectious Agent	Mode of Transmission	Incubation Period	Clinical Presentation	Period of Communicability	Control Measures
12.3.7 CHICKENPOX/ HERPES ZOSTER (varicella)	Varicella-zoster virus	• Airborne through respiratory secretions. • Direct or indirect contact from vesicle fluid of person with varicella-zoster.	10–21 days	• Low-grade fever, maculopapular rash on trunk, face, scalp, mucous membrane of mouth, then changes to vesicular for 3–4 days. • Herpes zoster is a local manifestation of reactivation of latent varicella infection in the dorsal root ganglia.	From 2–5 days before onset of rash and until skin lesions have crusted.	• Exclude from childcare, school, work, and public places at least 5 days until all vesicles become crusted. • Avoid contact with immunosuppressed persons. • Varicella-zoster immunoglobulin (IG) within 96 hours of exposure in susceptible close contacts of cases.
12.3.8 MEASLES (Rubeola, Hard measles, Red measles, Morbilli)	Measles virus, a member of the genus Morbilli-virus of the family paramyxoviridae	• Airborne by droplet spread. • Direct contact with nasal or throat secretions of infected persons. • Less commonly by articles freshly soiled with nose and throat secretions. • Measles is one of the most highly communicable infectious diseases.	About 10 days, but may be 7–18 days from exposure to onset of fever, usually 14 days until rash appears; rarely, as long as 19–21 days.	• Prodromal fever, conjunctivitis, coryza, cough, and small spots with white or bluish-white centres on an erythematous base on the buccal mucosa (Koplik spots). • A characteristic red blotchy rash appears on the 3rd to 7th day; the rash begins on the face, then becomes generalized, lasts 4–7 days, and sometimes ends in brawny desquamation. • Leukopenia is common. • The disease is more severe in infants and adults than in children.	From 1 day before the beginning of the prodromal period (usually about 4 days before rash onset).	• Children should be kept out of school for 4 days after the appearance of the rash. • Immunization of contacts previously not immunized within 72 hours of exposure.

(continued)

Table 12.3 Continued

Disease	Infectious Agent	Mode of Transmission	Incubation Period	Clinical Presentation	Period of Communicability	Control Measures
12.3.9 INFLUENZA	Influenza A, B, and C viruses	Large droplet is the primary means of transmission through coughing and sneezing by infected person.	Average 2 days (range 1–4).	Fever, cough (usually dry), headache, myalgia, prostration, coryza, and sore throat.	• In adults, 3–5 days. • In children 7–10 days.	• Education about hand hygiene. • Yearly immunization for the immunocompromised, individuals with chronic conditions, older adults, and individuals who might spread the infection (health personnel). • Antivirals available to the unimmunized and to residents in institutions. • Cohort ill persons from well persons in institutions and at home, if possible.
Sexually Transmitted Infections and Blood-Borne Pathogens						
12.3.10 CHLAMYDIA (genital infections)	*Chlamydia trachomatis*	• Sexual contact with the penis, vagina, mouth, or anus of an infected person. • Vertical transmission from mother to infant during childbirth.	Poorly defined, probably 7–14 days or longer.	• In males primarily as a urethritis, this includes moderate or scanty mucopurulent discharge, urethral itching, and burning on urination. • In females as a cervical infection, with symptoms that include mucopurulent endocervical discharge with edema, erythema, and easily induced endocervical bleeding. *Approximately 50% of males and 70% of females infected with chlamydia are asymptomatic.	• Unknown-infected individuals presumed to be infectious. Without treatment, infections can persist for months. • Reinfection is common.	• Health and safer sex education with emphasis on condom use. • Presumptive treatment of sexual partners.

(continued)

Table 12.3	Continued					
Disease	**Infectious Agent**	**Mode of Transmission**	**Incubation Period**	**Clinical Presentation**	**Period of Communicability**	**Control Measures**
12.3.11 HEPATITIS B	Hepatitis B virus (HBV)	• Percutaneous and mucosal exposure to infective blood and blood products. • Sexual or close household contact with an infected person. • Perinatal mother to infant transmission. • Injection drug use with contaminated and inadequately sterilized syringes and needles.	• Range 45–180 days. • Average 60–90 days.	Insidious onset of symptoms, nausea, vomiting, anorexia, lethargy, abdominal discomfort, and jaundice.	• Many weeks before onset of symptoms. • May persist for life.	• Pre-exposure vaccination to at-risk populations; vaccination to susceptible sexual contacts. • Give HBIG treatment to contacts as needed. • Universal precautions to prevent exposure to blood and blood products.
12.3.12 HEPATITIS C	Hepatitis C virus (HCV)	• Parenterally through injection drug use, and through exposure of contaminated and inadequately sterilized syringes and needles. • Perinatal mother to infant transmission and sexual transmission is less common, except for instances of HIV co-infection.	6–9 weeks.	• Insidious, with anorexia, nausea, vomiting, lethargy, abdominal discomfort and jaundice. • Progression to jaundice less frequent than hepatitis B (90% asymptomatic).	• From one or more weeks before onset of symptoms. • Persists in most people indefinitely.	• No available vaccine. • Routinely screen blood products. • Education. • Interferon treatment for active disease.

(continued)

Table 12.3 Continued

Zoonotic and Vector-Borne Diseases

Disease	Infectious Agent	Mode of Transmission	Incubation Period	Clinical Presentation	Period of Communicability	Control Measures
12.3.13 WEST NILE VIRUS	*Flavivirus*	• Transmitted primarily through the bite of an infected mosquito, predominantly *Culex* mosquitoes.	• Ranges from 2–14 days, but can be as long as 21 days in immuno-compromised people. • Usually 2–6 days.	• 70–80% of infections are asymptomatic. • If symptomatic, experience a systemic fever that includes headache, myalgia, or arthralgia. • Less than 1% develop neuroinvasive disease, which typically manifests as meningitis, encephalitis, or acute flaccid paralysis.		• Screening of blood and organ donations. • Use personal protective measures, including mosquito repellents. • Eliminate or treat all mosquito breeding grounds and consider adult mosquito control measures.
12.3.14 LYME DISEASE	*Borrella burgdorferi*	Tick borne	From 3 to 32 days after tick exposure (mean 7–10 days), early stages of the illness may be unapparent and the patient may present with later manifestations.	Characterized by a distinct skin lesion, systemic symptoms and neurological, rheumatological, and cardiac involvements occurring in varying combinations over months to years.		• Avoid tick-infested areas when feasible. • After being in an infested area, examine body for ticks and remove them.

(continued)

Table 12.3	Continued				
Disease	Infectious Agent	Mode of Transmission	Incubation Period	Clinical Presentation	Period of Communicability	Control Measures
12.3.15 BRUCELLOSIS	*Brucella abortus*	• Contact through breaks in the skin with animal tissue, blood, urine, vaginal discharges, aborted fetuses and especially placentas. • Ingestion of raw milk and dairy products from infected animals. • Airborne infection occurs in pens and stables for animals, and in laboratories and abattoirs for humans.	• Variable and difficult to ascertain, usually 5–60 days • 1–2 months is commonplace and occasionally several months.			Educate public about the risk of drinking untreated milk or eating products made from unpasteurized or untreated milk.

Sources: Heymann, D. L. (Ed.). (2015). *Control of communicable diseases manual* (20th ed.).

Government of Canada. (2013). (unpublished report). *Canadian Notifiable Diseases Surveillance System 2009–2011: National number and rate (per 100,000 population/per 100,000 live births) of reported cases by age group and sex.*

Government of Victoria, Australia. (2009). *Red book: 2009 Report of the Committee on Infectious Diseases (28th ed.)*. Elk Grove Village, IL: American Academy of Pediatrics.

hospitals and other settings. It is also utilized to quickly detect and contain clusters and outbreaks and helps to identify any new or virulent microorganism-caused respiratory infections (Ontario Ministry of Health and Long-Term Care, 2009).

Passive surveillance occurs when a health care provider must contact the local health authority to notify it of an identified case of a "reportable" disease. It is said to be "passive" as a case typically presents to a health care provider, and no activities were undertaken searching for cases. Surveillance, whether active, passive, or both, does not end with the notification of the case to the local health authority; rather, it initiates the next steps toward the control and management of the disease. Surveillance also plays a significant role in the management of reports of suspected cases. CHNs provide guidelines to institutions, health care professionals, and others in relation to diagnostic tests and control measures to identify and manage a *suspected* case of disease in terms of transmission risk and potential community impact.

OUTBREAKS AND CONTACT TRACING

A communicable disease may occur as an individual case or as a group of cases known as an outbreak. An **outbreak** occurs when the new cases of a disease exceeds the normal occurrence during a given period of time. For example, TB and invasive pneumococcal disease are common outbreaks in under-housed populations in winter and spring seasons in Canada. **Endemic** refers to the constant presence of a disease or infectious agent within a given geographic area or population group. For example, malaria is always present in some countries. Occasionally, if the occurrence of a disease is in excess of what would normally be expected, this is called an **epidemic**. For instance, while influenza may be a constant presence (endemic), it has the potential to become an epidemic during specific times of the year. More rarely, a **pandemic** occurs over a wide area and usually affects a large proportion of the population (e.g., pandemic [H1N1] 2009 influenza and acquired immune deficiency syndrome [AIDS]) (Last, 1988). **Syndemic** is an uncommon term, but it is significant in today's emerging changes for infectious diseases. Syndemic refers to the synergistic interaction of two or more coexistent diseases and the resultant excess in burden of disease. This became evident in Canada when AIDS was emerging. As AIDS became more prominent, so did the AIDS-indicative disease of TB. TB became a syndemic disease that occurred as a result of an altered immune system, which made individuals infected with HIV vulnerable to TB infections, thereby increasing the incidence of TB (Ofner, 1993). This syndemic effect is also seen with most STIs, where one infection makes an individual more susceptible to other STIs, if they are exposed.

Contact tracing is a response to a communicable disease report. After a communicable disease is reported to the local health authority, the infected person is interviewed by a CHN regarding contacts—specifically, people exposed to the client during the incubation period of the disease. The CHN must know the mode of transmission, incubation period, and infectious period of the particular disease in order to determine

what constitutes a contact in each individual situation. The *initial contact definition* must be formulated based on signs and symptoms and on place and time of exposure. A list of contacts must be collected from the first identified case. With this list, the local health authority proceeds with further assessment and investigation and follows up with recommendations for treatment or post-exposure chemoprophylaxis as deemed necessary.

Contacts are identified based on the possibility of transmission, where the window of risk can be very short or quite long. For example, when investigating a case of measles, the CHN would include in the contact list people who were in contact with the infectious individual seven days prior to the onset of the rash; whereas while investigating a case of TB, the CHN may identify not just recent contacts but contacts as far back as three months. The **degree of exposure** (the time spent with the infected person) and where the exposure took place are also included in the data collected. Not all reportable diseases warrant the same type of contact tracing because of varying degrees of burden of illness (e.g., varicella) or because of the nature of the communicability (e.g., TB). Contact tracing can involve identification of individuals who have not had any proximal contact with the case, and these individuals are called **indirect contacts**. To effectively manage cases of blood-borne disease with possible indirect contact modes of transmission, it is important in contact tracing to recognize that an individual infected with a disease may not be able to provide all contact information, as some contacts may be unknown to them. As noted earlier, blood products and solid organ implantation were historically a significant disease transmission risk for recipients before changes in organ and blood donor screening and testing practices were made. For example, WNV was identified in four clients receiving organs from an asymptomatic donor in 2002 (CDC, 2002). Other emerging diseases, such as Creutzfeldt-Jakob disease (CJD), necessitate that the CHN thoroughly understand modes of transmission in order to perform thorough health histories when completing contact tracing. For example, it would be important to know if instruments used in invasive procedures involving brain or neural tissue on a client diagnosed with CJD may have been contaminated.

Effective contact tracing requires comprehensive assessment of the infected individual and accurate disease reporting. While facilitating this process, the CHN is also assessing the individual as part of the community where they live, work, and play. For example, contact tracing conducted during an outbreak of TB in a homeless shelter requires the local public health unit to be cognizant of the community defined by this unique population. This involves learning about the soup kitchens, drop-in centres, parks, and other areas where individuals congregate. Local public health personnel could not achieve this task without the assistance of the ill individual (who provided information about the likely first case) and the community partners (who work closely with this population). These partners are not limited to health care providers but include all community agencies that provide services to under-housed populations. The resulting partnership develops a more focused and targeted screening of contacts. CHNs who work with marginalized populations, such as in street nursing programs across Canada, develop trusting relationships, which facilitate contact tracing in these populations.

A confidential approach when completing contact tracing is essential, since much of the information is disease- and client-specific. However, an exception to the necessity and practice of confidentiality in contact tracing is occasionally required. For example, during the SARS outbreak in March to May 2003 in Toronto, quarantine acts of the federal and Ontario ministries of health allowed health and safety authorities to conduct contact tracing in a public forum by naming individuals with SARS in the public media. Their purpose was to protect the public as well as to notify the contacts of those first infected persons to allow the contacts to self-identify and come forward for health assessment. Although contact tracing might be viewed as an infringement of a person's right to privacy, it is necessary to contain the spread of disease while providing ethically competent care. (See Chapter 6.)

The ease with which public health professionals are provided with comprehensive and inclusive lists of contacts will depend on how the individual or community comprehends the scope of the issue or an individual's or community's experience with the disease in the past. For example, obtaining contacts from individuals who have had an experience with an adolescent dying from meningococcal disease is easier than obtaining a comprehensive list of contacts from an infected food service worker whose perception is that hepatitis A infection is not a serious disease. The report is only as reliable and accurate as the person relaying the information and the parameters required for reporting. That is, if the health care provider is unsure of the signs and symptoms of the disease, the need for reporting will go unrecognized, and surveillance and contact tracing may be delayed.

Ongoing education of health care professionals helps to ensure detailed disease reporting. The integrated Public Health Information System (iPHIS) is an electronic system of reporting that allows jurisdictions within a province to communicate disease patterns and contacts with one another (PHAC, 2007). As well, the National Enteric Surveillance Program, an outbreak-specific electronic system, has been developed for health care professionals to communicate outbreaks of respiratory or enteric illnesses inter-provincially (PHAC, 2015b). It enables public health professionals to make links in person, place, and time for clients with similar presentation.

Response to Outbreaks An outbreak can be identified when expected symptoms in the population exist at an increased level. These symptoms may exist in the general population or in institutions such as hospitals, long-term care homes, or child-care centres. An outbreak may not necessarily be a reportable disease but may initially be of unknown etiology, suggestive of a communicable disease. An outbreak can be identified when a group of persons present with similar signs and symptoms, such as fever, coughing, and malaise in the case of an outbreak of an influenza-like illness. Generally, **outbreak reports** are communicated to public health authorities as soon as possible to allow investigation into the cause of the illness. In addition, early notification facilitates establishing timely and appropriate control methods, such as separating well and ill clients.

The terms "case" and "index case" are used throughout any discussion of outbreaks. A **case** refers to a single ill individual. When an individual person is identified as the likely first case in an outbreak, this person is referred to as the **index case**. Often, the index case in an outbreak is identified after other persons become ill, and all surveillance data indicate that the outbreak began with the identified individual. The purpose in identifying a common source (contaminated food) or an index case (infectious person) is two-fold: (1) to interrupt further transmission of the disease by identifying the route of transmission, and (2) to understand the cause of the outbreak by identifying the origin of the pathogen. The information that a CHN gathers to understand and define an outbreak is often like pieces of a puzzle and requires the CHN to possess critical-thinking and analytical skills.

Steps in Managing an Outbreak The initial investigation of an outbreak includes review of the signs and symptoms the ill clients have in common, the onset, whether some clients are recovering, the usual course of the illness, and the source of the outbreak (e.g., a contaminated air-conditioning unit in a case of legionella outbreak or an infected person in the case of a pertussis, measles, or mumps outbreak). Heymann (2015) outlines seven essential steps in the management of an outbreak:

1. Confirming the outbreak
2. Establishing a task force and designating an outbreak control team
3. Establishing and maintaining regular communications
4. Managing sick persons
5. Conducting an outbreak investigation
6. Preventing further transmission
7. Monitoring the response

An outbreak report is usually generated after the outbreak is determined to be over, although in large outbreaks, reporting may occur throughout the course of the outbreak. Scientific study and learning is generated after each outbreak, as each presents differently. Debriefing sessions with all involved in any aspect of the outbreak are an important and often missed learning opportunity. Efforts should be made to approach debriefing sessions with a structured format to avoid placing blame on individuals and to ensure behaviour change occurs to prevent similar future outbreaks from happening.

ROLE OF THE COMMUNITY HEALTH NURSE

History has shown that communicable diseases are controlled through changes in practice or the environment. Typhoid and cholera are two communicable diseases that can be transmitted via contaminated water. The sanitation of water is one of the public health triumphs that occurred in the early 1900s. Improved sanitation and the development of vaccines for typhoid and cholera have virtually eliminated these diseases from the developed world; however, these diseases continue to

CASE STUDY

Outbreak Investigation

In a pertussis outbreak, the CHN initially gathered the following information: seven ill children, all in elementary schools, only two children in the same school, all children in the same city. There appeared to be no other common links—they did not know each other, had no common social events or travel, and no shared activities. The CHN could not identify a common source. Then an adult was diagnosed with pertussis, and on investigation the CHN found that the adult was the spouse of a teacher who had been ill for several weeks with pertussis-like symptoms. The teacher was a special education teacher who travelled throughout the city to elementary schools. This teacher had been in every school the ill children attended.

Discussion Questions

1. Who is the index case?
2. Would you do active surveillance or passive surveillance? Why?
3. Outline the steps to control and manage the pertussis outbreak.

plague developing countries where water sanitation and vaccination programs are limited or not available (Heymann, 2008). As such, education strategies have been key in these countries in order to break the chain of infection at the mode of transmission. Today, breaking the chain of infection is achieved through various methods, each one targeted at different links. Through utilizing the nursing process, CHNs can implement primordial, primary, secondary, tertiary, and quaternary prevention activities in controlling communicable diseases.

Levels of Preventive Measures

Primordial prevention measures remove risk factors for a disease from existing, such as the following:

- Ensuring access to a safe water supply and maintaining adequate sewage systems
- Developing healthy public policies to create programs and services to prevent infectious diseases from occurring, such as removing stagnant water to prevent mosquitoes from laying eggs

Primary prevention measures attempt to prevent the disease from occurring by doing the following:

- Promoting and implementing immunization programs, notifying contacts, and making referrals for follow-up diagnosis
- Providing chemoprophylaxis and antitoxins for prevention of disease
- Working with public health authorities and community partners concerning infection control measures for communicable diseases

- Educating the public on safer sexual practices, optimal nutrition, healthy environments for better air quality and sanitation, and the use of preventive measures such as universal precautions

Collaborative relationships between CHNs and other health care providers, schools, childcare agencies, laboratories, the general public, and health care institutions are not only essential in helping CHNs investigate, track, and determine linkages between cases but are also necessary to prevent further disease transmission. Diseases that do not fit one specific mode of transmission, and can therefore make case and contact follow-up complex and multifaceted, are one challenge CHNs encounter. For example, hepatitis A can be transmitted through contaminated food and water or through sexual contact. Therefore, the CHN must identify contacts and recommend post-exposure prophylaxis (PEP) based on all possible modes of transmission, and provide comprehensive education and exclusion to further prevent transmission. Provincial databases, such as the integrated Public Health Information System (PHAC, 2007), are tools that allow tracking of disease occurrence and its source, if known.

Secondary prevention measures detect a disease or condition in a certain population, usually by screening or testing for the disease, and can include the following:

- Screening, case finding, referral, and mass screening for early detection
- Early diagnosis and the interpretation of diagnostic results
- Early treatment, including the provision of antimicrobial medications for newly diagnosed contacts
- Teaching for medication and treatment compliance, including provision of supportive care such as diet, rest, and exercise, and teaching for side effects of medications
- Advocacy for accessible diagnostic and treatment services for socially disadvantaged groups such as people who are under-housed, with low socioeconomic status, or with language and cultural barriers

Screening There are two reasons to test or screen for a communicable disease. The first is in response to the disease being identified in the community; epidemiological reports can reveal or identify a population that is at risk for disease. CHNs screen the population to validate these reports and to identify the at-risk individuals. The individuals being tested have not been identified in contact screening but are part of the population at risk. For example, a student is diagnosed with TB, and all students in his or her school, not just those with close contact to the index student, may be tested for TB. The list of exposures of the case must be analyzed to also identify the *index* or *first case*. As well, the history of the cases may help to determine the *index case*; that is, who first presented with the disease symptoms.

Isolation and Quarantine Isolation and quarantine are also secondary preventive measures. Treatment or management of some infectious agents includes isolation or quarantine to reduce the transmission and break the chain of infection. **Isolation** refers to the separation of an *infectious person* for a period of time to prevent or limit the direct or indirect transmission of the infectious agent. **Quarantine** is the restriction of activities for a *well person* who has been exposed to an infectious agent. Generally, communicable diseases that are transmitted by direct or airborne routes require that the contacts be separated from other people and possibly placed in quarantine. The length of the isolation or quarantine period is specific to the incubation and communicable period of each disease (Heymann, 2008). For example, varicella is considered to be most infectious one to two days before the onset of the rash and remains infectious until all lesions are dried and crusted, whereas hepatitis A is most infectious one to two weeks before the onset of symptoms until one week after the appearance of jaundice. The communicable period is not always known for every disease, especially emerging diseases. SARS is considered to have an incubation period of up to 10 days (Heymann, 2008). During the SARS outbreak, it was uncertain when the infected person was most contagious or when the symptoms displayed by the patient equated to communicability. For this reason, contacts were placed in quarantine for a minimum of 10 days.

Prophylaxis **Prophylaxis**, a secondary preventive measure, is the utilization of chemoprophylaxis or immunoprophylaxis agents to prevent illness from a pathogen or infectious agent following a known or possible exposure. Prophylactic agents may be prescribed for exposed vulnerable hosts such as pregnant women, infants, people who have an immune disorder or transplant, or anyone who had contact with a disease that has a high morbidity and mortality rate or a disease that has significant long-term effects. **Immunoprophylaxis** includes both active and passive immunizing agents. **Active immunizing agents** are vaccines that stimulate the immune system to create antibodies. **Passive immunizing agents** include immune serum globulin, which is of human origin, and immune globulins that contain specific antibodies to a particular organism, such as hepatitis B immune globulin (HBIG) or rabies immune globulin (RIG).

Prophylaxis provides protection to the vulnerable hosts in the general population. The role of the CHN is to identify the vulnerable hosts, monitor the therapy if it is long term, and possibly administer or facilitate the administration of one-time prophylaxis. An example of the use of **chemoprophylaxis** includes the administration of isoniazid (INH) to children younger than six years of age who are identified as contacts in a TB outbreak despite having a negative response to the tuberculin skin test. These children are given this medication daily to prevent the development of TB. If, after a period of eight weeks after the last contact, the repeat TST is negative and the child remains asymptomatic, the INH can be discontinued. It is recognized that young children may not have the ability to fight the TB organism as well as older children or adults. However, the medication provides the child with the ability to fight the organism, reduces bacterial load, and reduces the possibility of disseminated disease. Immunoprophylaxis can be an appropriate choice if, for example, during an outbreak of varicella in the community, contact-tracing reveals that one of the contacts is a pregnant woman; she may be a candidate

for varicella-zoster immune globulin (VZIG). The VZIG will either protect the woman from acquiring varicella or lessen the symptoms if the disease occurs, thereby protecting the fetus.

Tertiary prevention measures aim to reduce the extent and severity of health problems to minimize the complications by:

- Educating and monitoring treatment compliance to prevent complications
- Monitoring effectiveness of treatment and identifying and referring for adverse effects

Education of the public may be carried out at the individual, family, and community levels through community-based programs. Education is not directed at a single stage in the chain of infection; rather, it targets the whole chain and teaches measures that can be adopted into the individual's personal health habits. The goal is to help the client and the community return to baseline functioning or a new state of health. Examples include the administration of **directly observed therapy (DOT)**, which is a mechanism used to ensure TB clients take their prescribed medications. The nurse observes the clients taking the medications on a preset schedule. This is to prevent the risk of non-compliance, thereby reducing the possibility of drug-resistant TB developing, which could place communities at risk.

Quaternary prevention measures identify the over medicalization of interventions to protect a population from unnecessary or unethical treatments, and includes overtreating clients for infectious diseases with antibiotics, leading to their unnecessary use and possible emergence of antimicrobial resistance.

Through various levels of preventive activities, CHNs play major roles in education, health promotion, direct care, community development and mobilization, liaison, research, advocacy, program planning and evaluation, and policy formulation. All are essential skills that contribute to the successful management and control of communicable diseases. Utilizing these skills is essential, as was shown by the role of CHNs in the H1N1 pandemic of 2009. Although the 2009 pandemic was considered to be mild, Canada was one of the few countries that had a pandemic plan in place well in advance of the H1N1 influenza virus outbreak. The overall goals of the Canadian Pandemic Influenza Plan were to minimize serious illness and overall deaths and to minimize societal disruption caused by the pandemic. In the 2009 pandemic, there were 428 deaths and 8678 hospitalizations in Canada due to influenza A/H1N1 (PHAC, 2010). Across the country, the PHAC recommendations for health care workers were followed by acute and community health workers on issues like infection control and occupational health, resource management, clinical care, and the distribution of antivirals and vaccines. Guidelines were followed by CHNs on addressing the outbreak, reinforcing the recommended infection control practices and public health measures. As a result, minimal illness occurred, and societal disruption was kept to a minimum. Effective pandemic preparedness is essential to mitigate the effects of a pandemic, particularly if it becomes severe. CHNs play a pivotal role in planning with community partners to create policies, enhance environmental supports, and provide educational resources.

CONCLUSION

This chapter discussed the basic principles of communicable disease control, including vaccine-preventable diseases and the role of the CHN in dealing with them. The topic of communicable disease control is broad, and each day the world faces a new disease that may or may not find its way into any community. CHNs must be prepared to respond to the unexpected. They must work in partnership with the local, national, and global communities to develop effective surveillance methods and screening tools, enhance emergency response mechanisms, and implement public health measures at the primordial, primary, secondary, tertiary, and quaternary levels. It is imperative that CHNs possess a strong relationship with their community partners, a solid knowledge base of epidemiology, current information on communicable diseases, knowledge of available resources, and strong decision making and research skills. Integration of these skills will help the CHN to be successful in the role of protecting and promoting the health of Canadians.

KEY TERMS

acquired resistance (p. 229)
active immunizing agents (p. 244)
active surveillance (p. 231)
antimicrobial resistance (AMR) (p. 228)
blood-borne infections (p. 222)
case (p. 242)
chemoprophylaxis (p. 244)
colonized patient (p. 227)
communicable diseases (p. 218)
community immunity (p. 221)
contact tracing (p. 241)
degree of exposure (p. 241)
directly observed therapy (DOT) (p. 244)
endemic (p. 241)
enteric infections (p. 223)
epidemic (p. 241)
epidemiologic triangle (p. 220)
food-borne infection (p. 223)
food-borne intoxication (p. 223)
food-borne outbreaks (p. 223)
hand hygiene (p. 227)
health care–associated infection (HAI) (p. 227)
herd immunity (p. 221)
immunization (p. 221)
immunoprophylaxis (p. 244)
index case (p. 242)
indirect contacts (p. 241)
infected patients (p. 228)
infection control (p. 227)
intrinsic resistance (p. 229)
isolation (p. 243)
notifiable disease (p. 230)
outbreak (p. 241)
outbreak reports (p. 242)
pandemic (p. 241)
parasitic diseases (p. 224)

passive immunizing agents (p. 244)
passive surveillance (p. 241)
point-of-care practice (p. 227)
post-exposure prophylaxis (PEP) (p. 224)
prophylaxis (p. 244)
quarantine (p. 244)
sentinel hospitals (p. 228)
sexually transmitted infections (STIs) (p. 221)
surveillance (p. 231)
surveillance systems (p. 227)
syndemic (p. 241)
vector-borne infections (p. 225)
water-borne pathogens (p. 224)
zoonotic infections (p. 224)

STUDY QUESTIONS

1. What are the modes of transmission of communicable diseases?

2. A high school student is diagnosed with tuberculosis. How would you conduct contact tracing?

3. A childcare centre has just notified you, a new CHN, that a child in its care has meningitis. The staff and parents of other children are very anxious. Describe your nursing interventions.

4. The local health authority has just hired you to work on hepatitis A management and control. Being new to the region, what would be your priority tasks?

5. What information would you need from the index case about his or her disease (e.g., HIV) to conduct comprehensive contact tracing?

INDIVIDUAL CRITICAL-THINKING EXERCISES

1. You are working in a downtown clinic that provides services to marginalized and vulnerable persons when a client presents with non-specific ailments. While completing his health history, the client reveals addictions to opioids and other substances, and that he has multiple sexual partners. Your recommendation is to have a full work-up for STIs. The client refuses. Discuss your nursing responsibilities.

2. Refer to Question 1. The client's HIV test shows a positive result. What should be your next steps?

3. You have been assigned a client who has active TB, who has been on treatment in her home country, and who has just arrived in Canada and does not understand English or the purpose of the treatment. How would you ensure an accurate nursing assessment for this client, and how would you facilitate a supportive treatment environment for her?

GROUP CRITICAL-THINKING EXERCISES

1. Large numbers of immigrants come from regions where the prevalence of tuberculosis is high. This has resulted in the importation of a large burden of latent infection that can

be expected to generate future active cases in aging immigrant populations. Discuss the implications for caring for the future active cases. Healthy public policy should be included in the discussion as opposed to local health authority policy.

2. AIDS can manifest after years of HIV-positive status; a positive HIV test may not occur until three months after the contact. Similarly, in TB, the skin test can be negative up to 12 weeks post-exposure, and the manifestations of the disease may occur sometime in a person's life. Discuss the implications of contact tracing for these two diseases.

3. Emerging diseases, changes in antimicrobial resistance, and threats of terrorism with biological agents have heightened the awareness of surveillance needs worldwide. Since September 11, 2001, the threats of smallpox and anthrax have been in the media. Discuss the information needed to control the spread of smallpox.

REFERENCES

Alberta Health Services. (2012). *Public health notifiable disease management guidelines: Hanta Virus Pulmonary Syndrome.* Alberta: Author. Retrieved from http://www.health.alberta.ca/documents/Guidelines-Hantavirus-2012.pdf

Berman, S., Duenas, A., Bedoya, A., Constain, V., Leon, S., Borrero, I., & Murphy, J. (1983). Acute lower respiratory tract illnesses in Cali, Colombia: A two-year ambulatory study. *Pediatrics, 71*(2), 210–218.

British Columbia Ministry of Health. (n.d.). *Vector-borne diseases.* Vancouver, BC: Author. Retrieved from http://www.health.gov.bc.ca/protect/ehp_vector.html

Canadian Blood Services. (2016). *Surveillance report.* Ottawa, ON: Author. Retrieved from https://blood.ca/sites/default/files/Surveillance_Report_2016_EN.pdf

Canadian Institute for Health Information. (2008). *Patient Safety in Ontario acute care hospitals: A snapshot of hospital-acquired infection control practices 2008.* Ottawa, ON: Author. Retrieved from https://secure.cihi.ca/estore/productFamily.htm?pf=PFC1089&lang=en&media=0

Centers for Disease Control and Prevention. (2002, September 6). Public health dispatch: West Nile virus infection in organ donor and transplant recipients—Georgia and Florida, 2002. *Morbidity and Mortality Weekly Report, 51*(35), 790. Retrieved from http://www.cdc.gov/mmwr/preview/mmwrhtml/mm5135a5.htm

Centers for Disease Control and Prevention. (2013a). *Enteric diseases epidemiology branch.* Atlanta, GA: Author. Retrieved from http://www.cdc.gov/ncezid/dfwed/edeb

Centers for Disease Control and Prevention. (2013b, September 6). Surveillance for waterborne disease outbreaks associated with drinking water and other nonrecreational water—United States, 2009–2010. *Morbidity and Mortality Weekly Report (MMWR), 62*(35), 714–720. Retrieved from http://www.cdc.gov/mmwr/preview/mmwrhtml/mm6235a3.htm

Centers for Disease Control and Prevention. (2017). *For parents: Vaccines for your children.* Atlanta, GA: Author. Retrieved from https://www.cdc.gov/vaccines/parents/vaccine-decision/index.html

Community Health Nurses of Canada (CHNC). (2019 revised). *Canadian community health nursing: Professional practice model & standards of practice.* St. John's, NL: Author. Retrieved from https://www.chnc.ca/en/publications-resources

Gallant, V., Duvvuri, V., & McGuire, M. (2017). Tuberculosis in Canada—Summary 2015. *Canada Communicable Disease Report, 43*(3), 77–82.

Greenwood, B. (2014). The contribution of vaccination to global health: Past, present and future. *Philosophical Transactions of the Royal Society B, 369*(1645), 1–9.

Government of Canada. (2014a). *Rabies in Canada.* Ottawa, ON: Author. Retrieved from http://travel.gc.ca/travelling/health-safety/diseases/rabies

Government of Canada. (2014b). *Tuberculosis.* Ottawa, ON: Author. Retrieved from http://healthycanadians.gc.ca/diseases-conditions-maladies-affections/disease-maladie/tuberculosis-tuberculose-eng.php

Government of Canada. (2016). *Surveillance of tuberculosis (TB).* Ottawa, ON: Author. Retrieved from https://www.canada.ca/en/public-health/services/diseases/tuberculosis-tb/surveillance-tuberculosis-tb.html

Government of Canada. (2017a). *Risk of Lyme Disease to Canadians.* Ottawa, ON: Author. Retrieved from https://www.canada.ca/en/public-health/services/diseases/lyme-disease/risk-lyme-disease.html

Government of Canada. (2017b). *Surveillance of Zika virus.* Ottawa, ON: Author. Retrieved from https://www.canada.ca/en/public-health/services/diseases/zika-virus/surveillance-zika-virus.html

Government of Canada. (2017c). *Tuberculosis: Drug resistance in Canada 2015.* Ottawa, ON: Author. Retrieved from https://www.canada.ca/en/public-health/services/publications/diseases-conditions/tuberculosis-drug-resistance-canada-2015.html#a10.2

Government of Canada. (2018). *Canada's provincial and territorial routine (and catch-up) vaccination routine schedule programs for infants and children.* Retrieved from https://www.canada.ca/en/public-health/services/provincial-territorial-immunization-information/provincial-territorial-routine-vaccination-programs-infants-children.html

Gravel, D., Matlow, A., Ofner-Agostini, M., Loeb, M., Johnston, L., Bryce, E., . . . Canadian Nosocomial Infection Surveillance Program. (2007a). A point prevalence survey of health care-associated infections in pediatric populations in major Canadian acute care hospitals. *American Journal of Infection Control, 35*(3), 157–162.

Gravel, D., Taylor, G., Ofner, M., Johnston, L., Loeb, M., Roth, V. R., Stegenga, J., . . . Canadian Nosocomial Infection Surveillance Program. (2007b). Point prevalence survey for healthcare-associated infections within Canadian adult acute-care hospitals. *Journal of Hospital Infection, 66*(3), 243–248.

Hargreaves, J. R., Boccia, D., Evans, C. A., Adato, M., Petticrew, M., & Porter, J. D. (2011). The social determinants of tuberculosis: From evidence to action. *American Journal of Public Health, 101*, 654–662.

Heymann, D. L. (2008). *Control of communicable diseases manual: An official report of the American Public Health Association* (19th ed.). Washington, DC: American Public Health Association.

Heymann, D. L. (2015). *Control of communicable diseases manual: An official report of the American Public Health Association* (20th ed.). Washington, DC: American Public Health Association.

Last, J. M. (1988). *A dictionary of epidemiology*. New York, NY: Oxford University Press.

North Bay Parry Sound District Health Unit. (2009). *Investigative summary of the escherichia coli outbreak associated with a restaurant in North Bay, Ontario: October to November 2008.* (North Bay: NBPSDHU, June 2009). Retrieved from http://www.myhealthunit.ca/en/partnerandhealthprovider-resources/resources/InvestigativeSummaryoftheEcoliOut-breakJune2009.pdf

Ofner, M. (1993). Tuberculosis and AIDS in Ontario—A record linkage. *Public Health and Epidemiology Report for Ontario (PHERO), 4*, 11.

Ontario Ministry of Health and Long-Term Care. (2009). *Screening tool for influenza-like illness in the emergency department.* Retrieved from http://www.health.gov.on.ca/en/pro/programs/emb/health_notices/ihn_screening_tool_042909.pdf

Public Health Agency of Canada (PHAC). (2000). Waterborne outbreak of gastroenteritis associated with a contaminated municipal water supply, Walkerton, Ontario. *Canada Communicable Disease Report, 26*(20), 170–173. Retrieved from http://www.phac-aspc.gc.ca/publicat/ccdr-rmtc/00vol26/index.html

Public Health Agency of Canada (PHAC). (2001). Waterborne Cryptosporidiosis outbreak, North Battleford, Saskatchewan. *Canada Communicable Disease Report 27*(22), 185–192. Retrieved from http://www.collectionscanada.gc.ca/webarchives/20071122093556/; http://www.phac-aspc.gc.ca/publicat/ccdr-rmtc/01vol27/index.html

Public Health Agency of Canada (PHAC). (2007). *Canadian Integrated Public Health Surveillance (CIPHS).* Ottawa, ON: Author. Retrieved from http://www.phac-aspc.gc.ca/surveillance-eng.php

Public Health Agency of Canada (PHAC). (2009a). *Hantaviruses.* Ottawa, ON: Author. Retrieved from http://www.hc-sc.gc.ca/hl-vs/iyh-vsv/diseases-maladies/hantavirus-eng.php

Public Health Agency of Canada (PHAC). (2009b). *National notifiable diseases.* Ottawa, ON: Author. Retrieved from http://dsol-smed.phac-aspc.gc.ca/dsol-smed/ndis/list_e.html

Public Health Agency of Canada (PHAC). (2010). *Surveillance: Deaths associated with H1N1 flu virus in Canada.* Ottawa, ON: Author. Retrieved from http://www.phac-aspc.gc.ca/alert-alerte/h1n1/surveillance-archive/20100128-eng.php

Public Health Agency of Canada (PHAC). (2011). *Frequently asked questions about Variant Creutzfeldt-Jakob Disease (Variant CJD).* Ottawa, ON: Author. Retrieved from http://www.phac-aspc.gc.ca/cjd-mcj/vcjd-faq-03-eng.php#a11

Public Health Agency of Canada (PHAC). (2012). *The Canadian nosocomial infection surveillance program.* Ottawa, ON: Author. Retrieved from http://www.phac-aspc.gc.ca/nois-sinp/survprog-eng.php

Public Health Agency of Canada (PHAC). (2013). *The Chief Public Health Officer's report on the state of public health in Canada, 2013: Infectious disease—The never-ending threat.* Ottawa, ON. Retrieved from https://www.canada.ca/en/public-health/corporate/publications/ chief-public-health-officer-reports-state-public-health-canada/chief-public-health-officer-report-on-state-public-health-canada-2013-infectious-disease-never-ending-threat/healthcare-associated-infections-due-diligence.html

Public Health Agency of Canada (PHAC). (2014a). *About the agency.* Ottawa, ON: Author. Public Health Agency of Canada, 2015. Adapted and Reproduced with permission from the Minister of Health, 2015. Retrieved from http://www.phac-aspc.gc.ca/about_apropos/index-eng.php

Public Health Agency of Canada (PHAC). (2014b). *Canada communicable disease report (CCDR).* Ottawa, ON: Author. Retrieved from http://www.phac-aspc.gc.ca/publicat/ccdr-rmtc/dr-rm-ab-pr-eng.php

Public Health Agency of Canada (PHAC). (2014c). *National Advisory Committee on Immunization (NACI): Statement on seasonal influenza vaccine for 2014–2015.* Ottawa, ON: Author. Retrieved from http://publications.gc.ca/collections/collection_2014/aspc-phac/HP40-114-2014-eng.pdf

Public Health Agency of Canada (PHAC). (2014d). *Tuberculosis prevention and control in Canada: A federal framework for action.* Ottawa, ON: Author. Retrieved from https://www.canada.ca/content/dam/phac-aspc/migration/phac-aspc/tbpc-latb/pubs/tpc-pct/assets/pdf/tpc-pcta-eng.pdf

Public Health Agency of Canada (PHAC). (2015a). *Canada immunization guide.* Ottawa, ON: Author. Retrieved from http://www.phac-aspc.gc.ca/publicat/cig-gci/p01-12-eng.php#tab1

Public Health Agency of Canada (PHAC). (2015b). *National Enteric Surveillance Program.* Retrieved from https://www.nml-lnm.gc.ca/NESP-PNSME/index-eng.htm

Public Health Agency of Canada (PHAC). (2016a). *Tuberculosis in Canada, 2014—Pre-release.* Ottawa, ON: Author. Retrieved from http://healthycanadians.gc.ca/publications/diseases-conditions-maladies-affections/tuberculosis-2014-tuberculose/alt/tuberculosis-2014-tuberculose-eng.pdf

Public Health Agency of Canada (PHAC). (2016b). *Canadian guidelines of sexually transmitted infections.* Ottawa, ON: Author. Retrieved from https://www.canada.ca/en/public-health/services/infectious-diseases/sexual-health-sexually-transmitted-infections/canadian-guidelines/sexually-transmitted-infections.html

Public Health Agency of Canada (PHAC). (2016c). *Routine practices and additional precautions for preventing the transmission of infection in healthcare settings.* Ottawa, ON: Author. Retrieved from https://www.canada.ca/en/public-health/services/publications/diseases-conditions/routine-practices-precautions-healthcare-associated-infections.html

Public Health Agency of Canada (PHAC). (2016d). *Canadian antimicrobial resistance surveillance system report 2016.* Ottawa, ON: Author. Retrieved from https://www.canada.ca/en/public-health/services/publications/drugs-health-products/canadian-antimicrobial-resistance-surveillance-system-report-2016.html

Public Health Agency of Canada (PHAC). (2017a). *Creutzfeldt-Jakob disease: CJD-surveillance.* Ottawa, ON: Author. Retrieved from https://www.canada.ca/en/public-health/services/surveillance/blood-safety-contribution-program/creutzfeldt-jakob-disease/cjd-surveillance-system.html#ref

Public Health Agency of Canada (PHAC). (2017b). *Report on sexually transmitted infections in Canada: 2013–2014.* Ottawa,

ON: Author. Retrieved from https://www.canada.ca/en/ public-health/services/publications/diseases-conditions/ report-sexually-transmitted-infections-canada-2013-14.html

Public Health Agency of Canada (PHAC). (2017c). *Public health notice—Outbreak of salmonella infections under investigation.* Ottawa, ON: Author. Retrieved from https:// www.canada.ca/en/public-health/services/public-health-notices/2015/public-health-notice-outbreak-salmonella-infections-under-investigation.html

Public Health Agency of Canada (PHAC). (2017d). *Public health notice—Outbreak of* E. coli *infections linked to various flours and flour products.* Ottawa, ON: Author. Retrieved from https://www.canada.ca/en/public-health/services/ public-health-notices/2017/public-health-notice-outbreak-e-coli-infections-linked-various-flours-flour-products.html

Public Health Agency of Canada (PHAC). (2017e). *Canadian Nosocomial Infection Surveillance Program (CNISP) summary report for ARO data from January 1, 2011 to December 31, 2015.* Ottawa, ON: Author. Retrieved from https://www .canada.ca/en/public-health/services/publications/science-research-data/canadian-nosocomial-infection-surveillance-program-summary-report-aro-data-2011-2015.html#a5

Public Health Agency of Canada (PHAC). (2017f). *Surveillance of West Nile virus.* Ottawa, ON: Author. Retrieved from https://www.canada.ca/en/public-health/services/diseases/ west-nile-virus/surveillance-west-nile-virus.html

Reed, S. E. (1981). The etiology and epidemiology of common colds and the possibilities of prevention. *Clinical Otolaryngology, 6,* 379–387.

Riemann, C., & Cliver, D. (Eds.). (2006). *Foodborne infections and intoxications* (3rd ed.). New York, NY: Academic Press.

Royce, R. A., Seña, A., Cates, W. J., & Cohen, M. S. (1997). Sexual transmission of HIV. *New England Journal of Medicine, 336*(15), 1072–1078.

Taubenberger, J. K., & Morens, D. M. (2006). 1918 Influenza: The mother of all pandemics. *Revista Biomédica, 17,* 69–79.

Tsegaye, L., Huston, P., Milliken, R., Hanniman, K., Nesbeth, C., & Noad, L. (2016). How is an international public health threat advanced in Canada? The case of antimicrobial resistance. *Canada Communicable Disease Report, 42*(11), 223–226.

World Health Organization (WHO). (2009a). *Communicable diseases: Highlights of communicable disease activities, major recent achievements.* Geneva, CH: Author. Retrieved from http:// www.searo.who.int/EN/Section10.htm

World Health Organization (WHO). (2009b). *Five keys to safer food.* Geneva, CH: Author. Reprinted with permission from World Health Organization. Retrieved from http://www .who.int/foodsafety/publications/5keysmanual/en

World Health Organization (WHO). (2009c). *International health regulations.* Geneva, CH: Author. Retrieved from http://www.who.int/topics/ international_health_regulations/en

World Health Organization (WHO). (2010). *Anniversary of smallpox eradication.* Geneva: CH. Retrieved from http:// www.who.int/mediacentre/multimedia/podcasts/2010/ smallpox_20100618/en

World Health Organization (WHO). (2013a). *Immunization, vaccines and biologicals: The expanded programme on immunization.* Geneva: CH. Retrieved from http://www.who .int/immunization/programmes_systems/supply_chain/ benefits_of_immunization/en

World Health Organization (WHO). (2013b). *Global vaccine action plan 2011–2020.* Geneva, CH: Author. Retrieved from http://www.who.int/immunization/global_vaccine_ action_plan/GVAP_secretariat_report_2013.pdf

World Health Organization (WHO). (2014). *Plague.* Fact Sheet N°267. Geneva, CH: Author. Retrieved from http://www .who.int/mediacentre/factsheets/fs267/en

World Health Organization (WHO). (2016). *Sexually transmitted infections (STIs) {Fact sheet}.* Geneva, CH: Author. Retrieved from http://www.who.int/mediacentre/factsheets/ fs110/en

World Health Organization (WHO). (2017a). *Immunization coverage {Fact sheet}.* Geneva, CH: Author. Retrieved from http://www.who.int/mediacentre/factsheets/fs378/en

World Health Organization (WHO). (2017b). *Tuberculosis.* Geneva, CH: Author. Retrieved from http://www.who.int/ mediacentre/factsheets/fs104/en

World Health Organization (WHO). (2017c). *Antimicrobial resistance.* Geneva, CH: Author. Retrieved from http://www .who.int/mediacentre/factsheets/fs194/en/index.html

United Nations World Tourism Organization. (2009). *Towards a safer world: The travel, tourism and aviation sector.* Madrid, Spain: Author: Retrieved from http://cf.cdn.unwto.org/ sites/all/files/docpdf/unwtotowardasaferworld.pdf

ABOUT THE AUTHOR

Sarah Alley graduated from the University of Toronto with a Bachelor of Science in Nursing and a Master of Public Health with a specialization in health promotion. She has worked in the area of communicable diseases throughout her career and is currently focused on vaccine-preventable infections. She has volunteered with a non-governmental organization exploring HIV/AIDS programming in rural parts of Northern India in addition to working in a number of public health settings in various capacities in both rural and urban communities in Canada. During H1N1 she was a key lead in developing emergency pandemic plans and outbreak control measures in the Kitikmeot Region of Nunavut.

Community Nursing Process

Lucia Yiu

Source: Pongsuwan/Fotolia

INTRODUCTION

Community health nurses (CHNs) care for people where they live, learn, play, worship, and work. Their goal is to improve the health of the community by promoting, preserving, and protecting the health of individuals, families, aggregates, and populations. Their practice includes promoting health, building individual or community capacity, connecting and caring, facilitating health equity, and demonstrating professional responsibility and accountability (Community Health Nurses of Canada [CHNC], 2019, revised). When entering the practice of community health nursing, novice nurses often ask, "What does caring for a community mean?" "Where and how do I begin?" and "What is a healthy community?"

Unlike having clients in hospitals or acute-care settings who actively seek episodic care for their presenting problems, CHNs must determine *who* and *where* their clients are, and *why*, *what*, *when*, and *how* best to promote their health in the community. Today, as a result of early hospital discharges, CHNs must provide complex home care for post-hospital clients

LEARNING OUTCOMES

After studying this chapter, you should be able to:

1. Discuss the concepts of community, community as clients, community as partners, community functions, community dynamics, and healthy communities.

2. Describe the selected common community assessment models and frameworks used in community health nursing practice.

3. Explain the application of community health nursing process in caring for community clients.

4. Explain the importance of population health promotion, health equity, risk assessment, community governance, community engagement, capacity building, community development, and community mobilization.

5. Discuss the purposes and use of selected community participatory tools for community planning.

6. Discuss the role of the nurse in caring for clients in the community.

who now have more acute health problems than ever before. They must also respond to the diversity and changing population demographics; this ranges from providing culturally safe and sensitive care to Indigenous peoples, to responding to chronic illnesses and palliative care of the rapidly aging population. To do so, CHNs work autonomously to build community partnerships that are based on a philosophy of primary health care to achieve health for all. This chapter provides an overview of the community health nursing process, including community assessment, selected community health practice models, population health promotion, community development, and community participatory tools. The role of the nurse in caring for community clients in ethical and socially just manners to reduce health inequities is discussed.

COMMUNITY DEFINED

Community as Clients versus Community as Partners

CHNs have always cared for the *community as their clients*. Historically, CHNs cared for sick and destitute individuals and families. Florence Nightingale cared for the soldiers in the Crimean War by improving sanitation and hygiene conditions to reduce infections and deaths among them. Lillian Wald established the Henry Street Settlement in New York to improve housing, nutrition, and sanitation for impoverished mothers and children (McKay, 2012). Today, CHNs care for their clients in various community settings, healthy or sick, from homes to schools, workplaces, community centres, and clinics.

CHNs also work with the *community as partner*; they collaborate with multidisciplinary teams of health care providers, politicians, community leaders, and the public at large to implement an affordable, accessible, and well-integrated primary health care system to meet the needs of the community. CHNs help strengthen the various social determinants of health and advocate for equity in health.

Developing an understanding of a community is fundamental to providing competent community care. A **community** may be defined as a group of people who live, learn, work, worship, and play in an environment at a given time. They share common characteristics and interests, and function within a larger social system such as an organization, region, province, or nation. The core of any community is its people, who are characterized by their age, gender, socioeconomic status, education level, occupation, ethnicity, and religion.

A community is also defined by its place or geopolitical boundaries, which often are used to determine the location of service delivery (Vollman, Anderson, & McFarlane, 2016). **Geopolitical boundaries** refer to both *geographic* boundaries such as mountains, rivers, or lakes and *political* boundaries such as districts or areas of service delivery that are bounded by legal jurisdictions with real or imagined boundaries. **Aggregate communities** refer to groups of people with common interests, culture, beliefs, or goals. **Virtual communities** such as Facebook, Google Hangout, Snapchat, Instagram, blogs,

Twitter, WeChat, and WhatsApp are places where members tend to share their common interests on the internet.

Community Functions

To sustain the day-to-day livelihood of their residents, all communities provide the following **community functions**:

- Space and infrastructure for housing, schools, recreation, government, and health and social services
- Employment and income, including productivity and distribution through consumption of goods, trading, and economic growth
- Security, protection, and law enforcement to protect the public from crime
- Participation, socialization, and networking for all community members
- Linkages with other community systems for opportunities for growth and capacity building

Community Dynamics

Community functions are supported by three interactive **community dynamics**: effective communication, leadership, and decision making (Clemen-Stone, Eigsti, & McGuire, 2002).

Communication Competent communities have strong and cohesive vertical, horizontal, and diagonal patterns of communication among the community key partners. *Vertical communication* links communities to larger communities or to those with higher decision-making power. *Horizontal communication* connects the community to work collaboratively with its own members, environment, and other service systems. *Diagonal communication* reinforces the cohesiveness of both horizontal and vertical communications.

Leadership Leaders lead their members by influencing the decision-making process using their status and position in the community. *Formal leaders* are elected official politicians, such as mayors, members of parliament, or the prime minister. *Informal leaders* are individuals with prominent positions in the community, such as religious leaders, executives or representatives of community organizations or professionals, elders of community groups, philanthropists, celebrities, or local heroes.

Decision Making Formal leaders use government policies to make decisions for the community, whereas informal leaders use their status to influence community groups and to effect change. Effective leaders collaborate with community groups to advocate for optimal change.

Healthy Communities

Competent community dynamics foster public participation, mutual support, and community action to promote community

WHAT CONSTITUTES HEALTHY COMMUNITIES?

A Healthy Communities Process Involves

- Equitable community engagement
- Intersectoral partnerships
- Political commitment
- Healthy public policy
- Asset-based community development

Qualities of a Healthy Community Include

- Clean and safe physical environment
- Peace, equity, and social justice
- Adequate access to food, water, shelter, income, safety, work, and recreation for all
- Adequate access to healthcare services
- Opportunities for learning and skill development
- Strong, mutually supportive relationships and networks
- Workplaces that are supportive of individual and family well-being
- Wide participation of residents in decision making
- Strong local cultural and spiritual heritage
- Diverse and vital economy
- Protection of the natural environment
- Responsible use of resources to ensure long-term sustainability

Source: Ontario Healthy Communities Coalition. (n.d.). *What makes a community healthy?* Copyright © by Ontario Healthy Communities Coalition. Used by permission of Ontario Healthy Communities Coalition. Retrieved from www.ohcc-ccso.ca

growth and, ultimately, healthy communities. What, then, is a healthy community? **Healthy communities** was a movement that began in the 1980s and became an international effort that promotes the health and well-being of members in the community. The guiding principles of healthy communities are based on the concepts of health and health promotion (see Chapter 8) and of community members from multiple sectors working together to create a sustainable and healthy community. See the box titled "What Constitutes Healthy Communities?"

SELECTED COMMUNITY ASSESSMENT MODELS AND FRAMEWORKS

CHNs use models and frameworks to systematically collect data and analyze the relationships of various data components. They select models or frameworks should be easy to use and reflect their practice philosophy. Most existing nursing models and frameworks focus only on individual and not community

care. (See Chapter 7.) This section briefly describes frameworks commonly used in community nursing practice.

Community-as-Partner Model

Vollman et al. (2016) described community and nursing process as the two main attributes in their community-as-partner model. The *community attribute* is the community assessment wheel, which depicts the components of the community assessment: physical environment, education, safety and transportation, politics and government, health and social services, communication, economy, and recreation. At the core of this community assessment wheel are the community residents.

The *nursing process attribute* reflects Betty Neuman's stress adaptation model, which is derived from the general systems theory. Within the community are the *lines of resistance* or strengths that protect the community from harm or threats. Surrounding the community are the *normal lines of defence* that reflect the normal state of health attained by the community. *Flexible lines of defence* form the outer layer around the community to buffer stressors impacting it. These stressors create tension-producing stimuli and may, in turn, penetrate the various lines of defence surrounding the community, affecting the system equilibrium. CHNs assess and analyze the degree of reaction to the stressors experienced by the community and implement purposeful primary, secondary, and tertiary interventions to promote optimal client health. (See Chapter 7.)

Epidemiologic Framework

The *epidemiologic triangle* (host–environment–agent) may be used to examine the frequency and distribution of a disease (e.g., gonorrhea or tuberculosis) or health and social conditions (homelessness or opioid crisis) in the population being studied. CHNs determine *what* the community is, *who* is affected (host), *where* and *when* the condition occurred (environment), and *why* and *how* (agent) it occurred. They may also use the "web of causation" to study the chains of causation and their effects on a health problem. (See Chapter 11.)

Community Capacity Approaches

Capacity building is a process to *strengthen* the ability of an individual, an organization, a community, or a health system to develop and implement health promotion initiatives and sustain positive health outcomes over time. It involves human resource and skills development, leadership, partnership, resource allocation, and policy formulation. Community capacity building is a continuous process that allows the community members to take responsibilities of their own development (Minkler, 2012; Stuart, 2014).

Youth suicide in Indigenous and non-Indigenous communities, mass killings from school shootings, or disasters after a flood or forest fire can be used to illustrate capacity building.

This can be seen when grief counselling is made available for the people affected to share their collective grief and pain following the tragic event. Partnership with the media, education and service providers, government, and police can help mobilize community resources to rebuild life and maintain and improve the health of the community. Establishment of community gardens to help combat rising food cost is also another example of capacity building.

Community asset mapping is used to outline the assets and capacity of the community, and identify strengths and potential resources for program planning and interventions (Kretzmann & McKnight, 1993). A community assets map may include skills and experiences of individuals and organizations, services, and physical and financial resources within and outside the community. CHNs evaluate the "assets" and build community capacity through activities such as strategic planning, community mobilization, and community development.

Community Health Promotion Model (CHPM)

The goal of the **community health promotion model (CHPM)** is to apply community health promotion strategies to achieve collaborative community actions and to improve sustainable health outcomes of the community. The CHPM (Figure 13.1) incorporates strategies from Epp's (1986) health promotion framework, the Ottawa Charter of Health Promotion (World Health Organization, Canadian Public Health Association, & Health and Welfare Canada, 1986), and primary health care principles (World Health Organization, 1978) to guide community planning, intervention, and evaluation. (See Chapters 8 and 14.) Nursing process and primary health care are an integral part of the CHPM.

The CHPM provides a framework for purposeful and systematic community assessment, planning, implementation, and evaluation. It uses a holistic approach to promoting the health of the population to attain a higher quality of community life and health equity. The CHPM emphasizes the health of the population, which is influenced by the interplay of various social determinants of health. These may include employment, housing, food, education, childhood years, workplace safety, social inclusion, and access to health systems. CHNs examine how people cope with the challenges in their lives, with a goal of reducing health inequities among people of various social positions within and between communities and countries (Public Health Agency of Canada [PHAC], 2011). For example, a young single mother's decision to feed a high-carbohydrate diet to her children may not be her poor

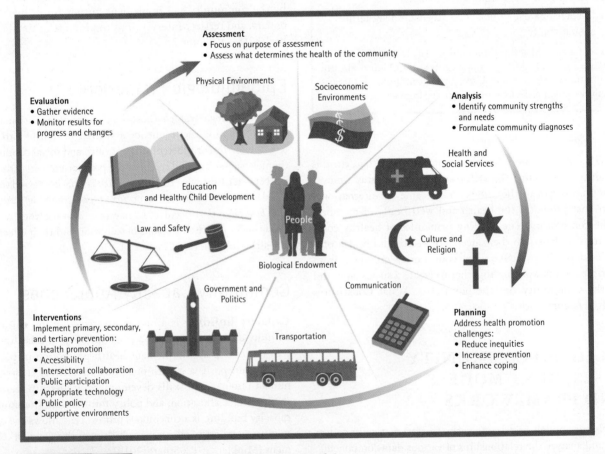

FIGURE 13.1 Community Health Promotion Model

Source: Community Health Promotion Model by Camillia F Matuk. Copyright © by Camillia F Matuk. Used by permission of Camillia F Matuk.

parenting skills but rather her inability to meet her children's nutritional needs as a result of her low income. The community health nursing process using the CHPM is described in the next section.

APPLICATION OF THE COMMUNITY HEALTH NURSING PROCESS

The *process* of community health nursing is continuous and cyclical; it consists of four phases: assessment, planning, implementation, and evaluation. CHNs may enter at any of these phases while focusing on the purpose of their nursing involvement. The *purpose* of community assessment is to gather information of the health needs of community. Such information may include health status, gaps, problems or issues, and community assets. This goal-oriented activity enables CHNs to collect relevant community data, critically analyze the problem or issue, make inferences on the implications of the problems or issues, formulate community nursing diagnoses, plan and implement the interventions, and evaluate the outcomes. The following sections focus on community assessment and common intervention tools.

Community Assessment

Community assessment is an ongoing systematic appraisal of the community. It is a comprehensive process because the health of community clients is affected by the complexity of community functions and dynamics and the various social determinants of health.

Some key questions that guide the beginning steps of community assessment are as follows:

- What is the purpose of my community assessment? Why is it needed? Which social determinants of health are being affected?
- Who, where, and what are the characteristics of my target population? How is my population different from others in the region or the nation?
- Where is my community, and what are its characteristics (e.g., community functions, process, and boundaries)?
- What information about the community do I need to know, and where can I obtain this information?
- What would be the best approaches or techniques to collect my community data? Who, how, and when should I engage the community to do these?
- What are my resources or constraints to complete this community assessment (i.e., time, political environment, expertise, labour, and cost)?

CHNs must be clear on the reasons for conducting their community assessment. There are four types of community assessment that may be used alone or in a combination: environmental scan, needs assessment, problem investigation, and resource evaluation.

Environmental Scan The most preliminary assessment of the community is an **environmental scan**, in which the CHN scans the overall environment through a windshield survey. **Windshield surveys** can be done by driving, riding on public transportation, or walking around the neighbourhood. As with health inspection on individual clients, CHNs use their senses of sight, touch, hearing, and smell to gather information and form their preliminary assessment of the community. They can see the people, the housing conditions, the geography, and the physical layout of various services in the community. During a walking tour, CHNs can listen to what languages people speak and what concerns them during their daily conversations in neighbourhood cafés or markets. They can smell the air quality or taste the water, and they can feel the temperature, humidity, and oppression or friendliness of the people. By scanning the environment, CHNs can familiarize themselves with their work environment and connect people to the resources in the environment in which they live. Windshield surveys are best done at two different times of day and on different days of the week for data comparison purposes.

Needs Assessment Appropriate and cost-effective services that meet the health needs of the population are based on the community's *needs* or deficits, not on its unrealistic *wants* or *desires*. **Needs** are what the community experiences as the gap between its current situation and desired situation. To perform a needs assessment—for example, opening a teen health centre—CHNs must (a) investigate the nature of the needs of these teens, (b) determine the congruence between the teens' expressed needs and those of the community, and (c) determine whether the community is willing and has the resources to take action to bridge the service gaps.

Problem Investigation Problem investigations are conducted in response to a problem or concern. For example, with an *E. coli* or measles outbreak, high suicide rates among Indigenous youth, or honour killings of Muslim women, CHNs investigate the occurrence and distribution of the problems in a community, explore the roots or causes of the problems and their effects, and develop responsive plans with the community for positive change.

Resource Evaluation Resource evaluation involves the assessment and evaluation of existing community resources and services. This includes an examination of the adequacy of human, financial, and physical resources, community partnerships, service utilization, gaps and duplications, affordability, and accessibility to the target populations. Service providers aim to provide cost-effective, efficient, and seamless services through resource allocation and reallocation.

Community assessment must be purposeful and evidence-based, showing the intent of *who* is the population (P), *what* is the intervention (I), *where* is the setting (S) for intervention, and the anticipated intervention *outcome* (O). In short, community assessment begins with a PISO statement. Tables 13.1A and 13.1B illustrate examples of how evidence-based PISO purpose statements or questions are formulated.

Table 13.1A	Formulating a Focus–Evidence–Purpose Statement or Question

In this example, a CHN wants to address risky drinking on university campus by applying a harm reduction strategy. The aim is to decrease the incidence of negative consequences associated with excessive alcohol consumption.

PISO* statement: What **harm reduction strategies** are effective in **decreasing risky drinking and negative consequences** among **campus students** at the **University of Windsor**?

Population	campus students
Intervention	harm reduction strategies
Setting	University of Windsor
Outcome	decreasing risky drinking and negative consequences

*PISO is a term used in Albert, D., & Herrera, C. (2009, November 20). *Getting lost in the evidence? Part 1: Developing an evidence question and search strategy.* Fireside Chat Presentation. Ottawa, ON: University of Ottawa.

Table 13.1B	Examples of PISO* Focus Evidence Questions

Type of Community Assessment	Population	Intervention/ Strategy	Setting	Outcome	Focus Evidence Question
Problem investigation	First Nation youth	Capacity building	Saskatchewan	Improve mental health services to decrease deaths by suicide	What **capacity building strategies** are effective to **improve mental health support and services** for **First Nation youth** in **Saskatchewan**?
Resource evaluation	Clients with low income	Program evaluation	Downtown area in Windsor, ON	Use of methadone clinic from January to June	How well do **low-income clients** living in the **downtown core of Windsor** use the **methadone clinic** from **January to June**?
Environmental scan	Clients with disabilities	Community mapping and surveys	Windsor-Essex County	Transportation services for individuals with disabilities	Based on **community mapping and surveys,** how available are the **transportation services** for **clients with disabilities** living in **Windsor-Essex county**?
Needs assessment	Newcomers	Focus group discussions	Windsor-Essex County	Challenges and barriers to assessing breast health services	Through **focus group discussions,** what are the **challenges and barriers to accessing breast health services** as experienced by **newcomers** living in **Windsor-Essex County**?

*PISO is a term used in Albert, D., & Herrera, C. (2009, November 20). *Getting lost in the evidence? Part 1: Developing an evidence question and search strategy.* Fireside Chat Presentation. Ottawa, ON: University of Ottawa.

Components in Community Assessment

The following are basic components to assess a community.

Community History and Perception Understanding the past allows the CHN to appreciate the root of the problem or issue, build on existing strengths, and avoid repeating the same failures. Areas for examination include the history of the issues or problems and community actions taken in the past; the attitudes of officials and local politicians; and the community's perceptions, attitudes, beliefs, and felt needs for health, education, and health care services. CHNs should explore reasons for any noted discrepancies between their own and their clients' perceptions.

Population The *core* of any community is people. A **population** is a diverse group of people or aggregates residing within the boundaries of a community. A **group** refers to two or more people, whereas an **aggregate** is a group of people with common interests, demographics, cultural heritages, and socio-economic and education levels. Population and aggregates are terms commonly used interchangeably. A **target population** refers to the population for whom nursing intervention is intended. **Population at risk** refers to a group of individuals who have a high probability of developing illness. People who are disadvantaged, susceptible, or vulnerable to health inequity, injury, disease, or premature death are described as a **priority or vulnerable population**.

In addition to biology and genetic endowment, CHNs also examine the composition of the population by age distribution, gender, marital status, social class, occupation, birth rate, employment, religion, education level, family size, and other factors related to their developmental and situational needs. Community data such as trends in mortality rates (e.g., maternal and infant death rates and suicide rates), morbidity rates (e.g., common infectious diseases and chronic conditions), and life expectancy give indications regarding the health status of the population. CHNs study the rate of population growth or decline to examine the population and demographic trends and plan for anticipated services. For example, when noting the aging Canadian population in Figure 13.2 and the most recent hospital admission statistics, where between 20–30% of community-dwelling older adult aged 65 plus fall at least once a year, and about 85% of these unintentional falls account for hospital admissions (PHAC, 2014; Statistics Canada, 2015), CHNs could anticipate chronic health conditions in the aging population will put more demands on home care services; they could also consider fall-prevention programs as priority interventions, especially for frail older adult clients living alone in their homes.

People tend to reside in areas for a variety of reasons: proximity to their employment and extended family, accessibility to education, affordable amenities and recreational facilities, crime rate, political reasons, and climate (Statistics Canada, 2017c). The *density* of the population may shift with time and demographic makeup. For example, an influx of refugees or unemployed workers into a community may be driven by political or economic changes.

Communities are not static. The needs, characteristics, makeup, and health status of the population also change over time within its physical and social environments. For example, a surge in a community's unemployment rate may result in high family stress, a poor economy, and the relocation of many young people to other communities for work; strengthening community and social services for these communities would then become a health priority. Similarly, promoting healthy lifestyles and community support to combat social isolation and poverty is much needed in the remote Northern communities because of their higher rates of smoking, obesity, suicide, and alcohol use compared to the nation's averages (PHAC, 2016).

Boundaries The boundary of the community refers to where the target population lives, works, worships, plays, and learns. Healthy communities do not exist in isolation; they have permeable boundaries for the exchange of services among communities. Communities are separated from or connected to other communities by physical or artificial boundaries. **Physical boundaries** include geographic boundaries, such as mountains, valleys, roads, lakes, rivers, or oceans. **Artificial boundaries** include (a) *political boundaries*, which depict governance of various

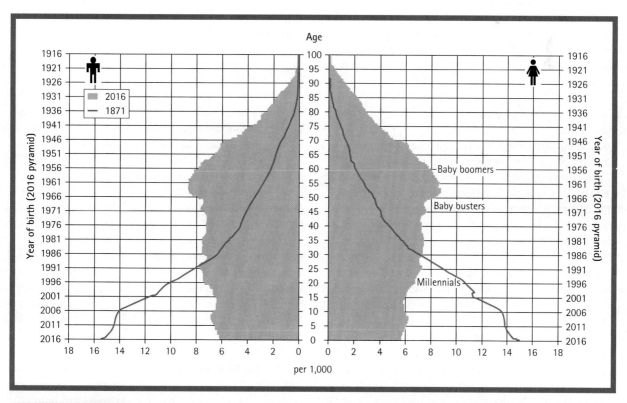

FIGURE 13.2 Age Pyramid of Canada in 1871 and 2016, 150 Years of Demographic History

Source: Statistics Canada. (2017a). *Census of population, 1871 and 2016.* (May 13, 2017). Retrieved from https://www.statcan.gc.ca/daily-quotidien/170503/g-a001-eng.htm

townships, counties, cities, and provinces; and (b) *situational boundaries*, which are governed by specific circumstances such as zoning for schoolchildren, traffic patterns, or smoking areas.

Environments Physical, chemical, biological, social, and psychosocial factors in the environment contribute to our quality of life. Air and water pollution may cause respiratory problems, digestive problems, cancer, and birth defects; geographic isolation may lead to poor access to health services, poverty, and depression (PHAC, 2011). (See Chapter 29.) Physical environments include (1) *biological and chemical characteristics*: vegetation and forestry, animals and insects, bacteria and other microorganisms, food and water supply, chemicals, and toxic substances; and (2) *physical characteristics*: geography, climate, and natural resources such as soil, mountains, valleys, rivers, lakes, oceans, water, air, oil, and designs of buildings and roads.

Socioeconomic Environments The interaction between social and economic conditions of the community affects the health and well-being of individuals and populations. High employment rates, new housing, and business developments are common signs for communities with a healthy economy. In poor economic times, a community must have resources such as social services, affordable housing, and food banks to assist individuals in need. A strong social network within a community allows its residents to build relationships and share resources (PHAC, 2013).

Income and Social Status Income and education are the most important determinants of health (PHAC, 2011). Although income and social status are positively associated with education level, good health, and quality of life, upward or downward mobility can be seen in various social classes during economic turmoil (PHAC, 2013). Many low-income families are working poor with low education; they are in and out of poverty depending on job and housing availability and whether they have health issues. Common health issues they experience include mental illness, diabetes, substance-related disorders, and chronic obstructive pulmonary disease.

Income equality, employment, housing, and food security all affect people's health and their sense of well-being. In 2013, low-income Canadians rated their health as very good or excellent, compared to those in the highest income bracket. Individuals who live in poverty have higher hospital admission rates and shorter life expectancy than those with higher incomes (PHAC, 2013).

Employment and Working Conditions Unemployment, underemployment, economic instability, and stressful or unsafe working conditions significantly affect not only people's physical, mental, and social health and general well-being but also their families and communities. People who are employed and work in a safe workplace experience less stress, live longer, and have fewer health problems (PHAC, 2013; Statistics Canada, 2016b).

Social Supports and Networks Early hospital discharge, an aging population, and rising rates of chronic diseases have led to the need for strong formal and informal social supports and networks from families, friends, and communities. Research shows a positive relationship between social support and health status; this includes happiness, high psychological well-being, life satisfaction, a strong sense of belonging their community, and perceived health (Government of Canada, 2016; PHAC, 2013).

Diversity and Social Inclusion Healthy communities embrace harmony, safety, and diversity as the social norm. For example, schools educate young children by instilling culturally competent and safe materials to reduce racism or bullying; service agencies provide classes to strengthen parenting skills and promote family relationships, which indirectly prevent family violence; and neighbourhood watch programs reduce crime rates. Social inclusion by gender, age, ability, sexual orientation, race, ethnicity, and religion will create a community where people feel safe and treated without prejudice. When people feel they belong, they strive to reach their full potential as contributing members to the society (PHAC, 2013).

Recreation Recreation provides a form of socialization and a means for healthy physical and mental activity for people outside of their family, school, and work life. Healthy communities have accessible and affordable recreational facilities or activities for their residents of all ages to play or to spend time together after school or work.

Education and Healthy Child Development Education provides people the needed life skills and technical skills for their day-to-day living and, therefore, health and prosperity. Canadians with low literacy skills are more likely to be poor and unemployed, suffer from poor health, have low self-esteem, and miss opportunities for learning and community participation than those with higher levels of education (PHAC, 2013).

Healthy physical, cognitive, and emotional development in children is determined by effects ranging from preconception health and prenatal care to the quality of parental nurturing and supervision. (See Chapter 16.) Poor early childhood developmental characteristics, such as low birth weight or poor nutrition, can delay language or brain development and compromise physical and mental health through to adulthood (Letourneau et al., 2015).

Schools are ideal settings in which children can learn to adopt societal norms and health behaviours in their early years. Disadvantaged and low-income children tend to not perform well in school; they are at greater risk for poor health. Youth with positive assets such as parental nurturing and monitoring, school engagement, and peer connections are more likely to have high self-worth and healthy lifestyles (PHAC, 2013). (See Chapter 17.) CHNs can advocate for healthy nutrition, adequate social policy surrounding issues such as parental leaves, national childcare policy, unemployment benefits, and social assistance to meet the health and social needs of families and children.

Culture and Religion Canada is second to Australia in having a vast number of people of different races or ethnic groups, colours, and religions. One in every five Canadians (21.9%) is foreign-born and belongs to a visible minority group, with 58% from Asia and the Middle East; 67.3% are Christians and Catholics, and others are Muslim, Hindu, Sikh, Jewish, or Buddhist (Statistics Canada, 2016a, 2017b). *Religion* offers a form of spiritual support for many people, especially those in crisis; it can also frame individuals' health care practices. For example, Jehovah's Witnesses refuse blood transfusions, and Muslims need adjustment of family, school, and work routines during their religious celebrations and prayers.

Culture is the way we think, live, act, believe, and feel. Various ethnocultural groups strive to preserve their heritage through their own social activities and language classes. Visible minorities and new Canadians with language and cultural barriers are often alienated from mainstream society and experience inequities in health from poverty, social isolation, bullying, and poor access to services (e.g., high unemployment or underemployment rates in newcomers and a high incidence of suicide and diabetes among Indigenous peoples) (George, Thomas, Chaze, & Guruge, 2015; Long & Dickason, 2016). Consequently, many ethnic groups tend to live and work in their own ethnic communities to avoid marginalization.

Culture insensitivity can be seen recently in how Canadian Muslim women wearing niqabs were ostracized, and their face covering became a legal or controversial issue in public places (*CBC News*, 2012). Moreover, generations of Indigenous children sent to residential schools to be assimilated into Euro-Canadian culture are currently reclaiming their language, culture, spiritual beliefs, and identity (Truth and Reconciliation Commission of Canada, 2015). (See Chapter 22.) With the knowledge of various culture groups, their needs, and their health care practices, CHNs can address inequality, cultural competence and safety, and societal acceptance as they work with diverse populations in their community. (See Chapter 9.)

Health and Social Services Most people, whether sick or healthy, seek health services at some time in their lives. *Health services* include primary, secondary, and tertiary care, ranging from promotion and protection of health to hospital, rehabilitative, and palliative care services. *Social services*, including welfare, unemployment benefits, mothers' allowance, and disability pensions, are examples of assistance for single parents, unemployed Canadians, or individuals with physical or mental disabilities.

An infrastructure of a wide range of health and social services can help people emerge from their crises. However, territorialism and unwillingness to share information or resources among community agencies for fear of losing program funding often result in fragmentation or duplication of services. "Spending on social services can improve health" for Canadians (Dutton, Forest, Kneebone, & Zwicker, 2018, p. E71). With escalating health care costs, CHNs must determine how best to refer, re-allocate, and coordinate community resources efficiently to meet their clients' needs. They assess what and how services are used and delivered to their communities and whether service gaps and duplications, unmet needs, and strengths exist. They work with the community to facilitate better coordination and more affordable and accessible services to people in need.

Transportation A reliable and affordable transportation system is necessary for residents to access essential services. CHNs can mobilize and coordinate resources to attend to transportation needs for rural clients, low-income individuals, frail and older adults, and clients with physical limitations (e.g., reduced taxi fare, handi-buses, or volunteer drivers for older adults or clients with disabilities).

Communication Effective and efficient communication is crucial for building supportive and collaborative relationships. CHNs must convey clear messages, the methods, location, and timing of which are pivotal in communicating how to deliver quality care to community members. The common modes of formal and informal communication for community members include newspapers, newsletters, emails, radio, television, flyers, community forums, and social media such as Twitter, Facebook, and Skype.

Governments and Politics Governments set policies to deliver essential services to meet the needs of the community. They provide formal leadership to communities and reinforce compliance to their policies (e.g., smoke-free regulations, service agreements). Although formal leaders hold authority in making decisions, informal leaders and community members often have the power to influence change.

CHNs must be aware of the existing government policies, work with both formal and informal leaders, and be involved in the decision-making process. They assess the relationships and the degree of cooperation or conflict between the community and other agencies or decision-making bodies.

Law and Safety Governments set rules and regulations as law. Crimes such as homicides, assaults, and thefts are symptoms of family and community response to stress (e.g., family violence, unemployment, and drug use). Safety is a prerequisite to quality of life. Communities grow and prosper economically in peaceful times. Peace is achieved when society has law and order. CHNs assess whether residents are feeling safe by examining the occurrences of crimes (i.e., types, rates, and locations) and collaborating with the police on crime prevention to create a safe place for people to live.

Community Data Collection

Communities have multisystem components, and collecting community data can be abundant and overwhelmingly complex. Therefore, CHNs need to be very clear on the purpose of their community assessment and to use credible and appropriate sources and techniques to collect valid community data. One or multiple methods may be used to collect needed community data. Generally, existing data should be examined before gathering new data. New data can be gathered from surveys and meetings with community residents and leaders or other key informants.

There are two main types of community data: (1) *quantitative data*, such as facts and figures shown in population statistics or health status reports, and (2) *qualitative data*, such as statements or opinions gathered from windshield surveys, focus groups, forums, key informants, or public or town hall meetings.

Sources of Community Data

The following are common community data sources:

- Participant observation: Windshield surveys, walking tours
- Literature review: Published studies, including systematic reviews, help validate the community needs and show evidence of best practices for interventions
- Demographic and epidemiologic data: Statistics Canada (e.g., census data, trends, and vital statistics)
- National and local policy data:
  - Public Health Agency of Canada (PHAC) (e.g., diseases, injuries, and other threats to public health)
  - Canadian Institute for Health Information: Statistics related to determinants of health and diseases, health care occupations, spending, and hospitalizations
  - Local, provincial, and federal health departments and municipal planning departments (e.g., local census, housing, and business and industrial developments)
  - Environment Canada (e.g., environmental indices)
  - Local organizations, such as hospitals, school boards, and agencies (e.g., annual reports on services delivered)
  - Municipal traffic departments and provincial transportation departments (e.g., traffic accidents, resulting injuries, and deaths)
  - Workers' Compensation Board (e.g., work-related injuries and deaths)
  - Other social data from Juristat (for crime statistics and trends, victim services, and court statistics) and Citizenship and Immigration Canada (for immigration-related statistics)
- Community surveys:
  - Canadian Community Health Surveys (e.g., health profiles and indicators, mortality, and census information)
  - Key informant surveys (e.g., focus groups, community forums)

Methods for Community Data Collection

The extent of community data collection is often determined by the resources available and the time constraints. This section specifically focuses on community surveys, community forums, and focus groups.

Community Surveys **Community surveys** involve a series of questions addressing the issue(s) or population(s) being studied. They capture a broad range of data from a representative sample population in a short period of time. They can be conducted via regular mail, internet, telephone, or face-to-face interviews. The data collected provide a *snapshot* of the population being studied at that particular time and may be generalized to describe the larger population. National surveys are usually done every five to ten years to examine changes in behaviours over time. The Canadian Community Health Survey was conducted biannually from 2001 to 2007 and now is conducted annually.

Community Forums **Community forums** are public meetings in which community members discuss issues of concern and share their experiences and opinions with their community leaders or decision makers. A community forum is an inexpensive way to collect community data. The people who attend these meetings are either directly involved in or affected by the topic being discussed (e.g., the impact of a school closure, service restructuring in a community, or methadone clinic set up in a neighbourhood). CHNs should note that when opinions are expressed by one person or a few people who dominate the discussions, their opinions may not represent the majority's view, and the purpose of the forum may be derailed. Community forums should be conducted by trained facilitators to elicit maximum public response.

Focus Groups **Focus groups** are small group discussions, conducted by trained facilitators with an average of eight to 12 people (ideally six people), that usually last one to two hours (Office of Quality Improvement, 2007). There may be a series of focus groups on the same topic across the community, region, province, or nation. Similar to the community forums but smaller in scale, the focus group participants are more homogeneous in their characteristics or experience related to the issue or topic being discussed. Focus groups and community forums are useful for collecting more in-depth information such as qualitative data when surveys fail to serve this purpose; they are not a place for debate or confrontation.

CHNs use multiple strategies to collect needed data as no single source or method can provide all the assessment data on a community. Epidemiological and research skills are particularly important for analyzing and interpreting vital statistics and figures. (See Chapters 10 and 11.) Collecting community data can be an overwhelming experience, but it need not be a time-consuming process. The key is to focus on the purpose of the assessment and to understand what determines the health of the community client and where and how to collect meaningful data.

POPULATION HEALTH

Population health builds on the practice of health promotion and public health with a focus on prevention and disease management. **Population health** is "an approach to health that aims to improve the health of the entire population and to reduce health inequities among population groups . . . . it acts upon the broad range of factors and conditions that have a strong influence on our health" (PHAC, 2012, para. 4). Federal, provincial, territorial, and local governments play a leadership role to implement population health policies and set clear program goals and targets (Senate of Canada, 2009).

Healthy populations contribute to the overall productivity and quality of life in the community and to a sustainable and equitable health care system. Based on this belief, the PHAC

(2002) developed a *population health template* with eight key elements and corresponding action steps for health practitioners, educators, and researchers: (1) focus on the health of population, (2) address the determinants of health and their interactions, (3) base decisions on evidence, (4) increase upstream investments, (5) apply multiple strategies, (6) collaborate across sectors and levels, (7) employ mechanisms for public involvement, and (8) demonstrate accountability for health outcomes (Health Canada, 2001).

Risk Assessment

It will be unrealistic and impossible for CHNs to work with every member in the community. Thus, CHNs start with assessing the conditions of risks and benefits that apply to the entire population or to its significant aggregates; they then deliver health services to individuals who are at risk to reduce health inequity caused by various social determinants of health. **Risk** refers to the probability or likelihood that healthy persons

---

CASE STUDY

What Does Health Mean to People Living in a Slum Area?

Study the community scene illustrated in Figure 13.3. List and rank what you think the people in this community would say was needed to improve their health. In a group of four to six students, compare the individual rankings and discuss the following questions.

Discussion Questions

1. Who are the experts in identifying the local needs of a community? By priority, rank the areas you feel would

improve the health of this community, and relate them to the determinants of health.

2. If you were a resident of this community, how would you feel if someone made judgments about your living situation? Why? What do you see as the priority area to improve the health of your community?

3. What data sources and data collection methods would you use to establish a community profile as depicted in this figure?

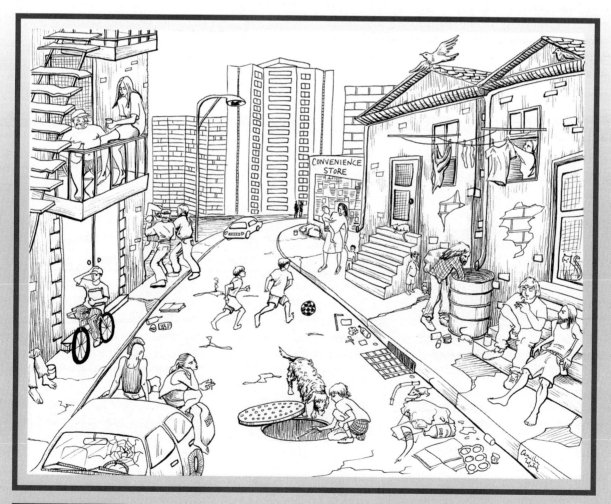

FIGURE 13.3 Slum Area

Source: Slum Area by Camillia F Matuk. Copyright © by Camillia F Matuk. Used by permission of Camillia F Matuk.

exposed to a specific factor will acquire a specific disease. These specific factors, called *risk factors*, can be environmental, lifestyle, and psychosocial factors (e.g., sources of exposure, cultural practices, patterns of behaviour, local concerns, direct impact from the service delivery system), or biological factors (e.g., age, gender, or genetic makeup).

When doing *risk assessment*, CHNs identify and target clients who are most likely to contract a particular disease or develop unhealthy behaviours, and assess attributes that affect or potentially affect their health. For example, teens have a higher risk than adults of contracting sexually transmitted infections or getting pregnant, as they tend to experiment more with their sexuality; similarly, older adults are more likely to have falls than are younger adults due to the aging process.

Community Analysis and Nursing Diagnoses

The purpose of data analysis is to identify *actual* and *potential* community strengths and needs that are relevant to improving the health of the community. Competent *community analysis* relies on a clear conceptual understanding of how social determinants interact and impact on community health, functions, and dynamics. Community data are systematically summarized into categories and compared with other relative community systems for significance; inferences are then made to formulate *community nursing diagnoses*.

Similar to nursing diagnoses, community nursing diagnoses go beyond individual or family nursing diagnoses in that they are broader and address a community or aggregate. All communities have strengths as well as problems. Formulation of community nursing diagnoses must be based on community assessment data collected. *Community nursing diagnoses* may be problem or wellness diagnoses, with statements consisting of the following components:

- Specific aggregate or target group
- Actual or potential unhealthy or healthy response/situation a nurse can change
- Etiology or cause for the unhealthy or healthy response/situation
- Characteristics (i.e., signs and symptoms) or evidence that describe the response or situation

Table 13.2 illustrates examples of nursing diagnoses formulation.

Planning, Implementation, and Evaluation Once the identified community needs are prioritized, the CHN devises interventions to resolve them. The intervention plan should address the *challenges* to achieving health for all: reducing inequalities, increasing prevention, and enhancing community coping (Epp, 1986). The goals and objectives for intervention are derived from the community nursing diagnoses.

Nursing interventions include primary, secondary, and tertiary preventive services that reflect the five principles of

Table 13.2	**Examples of Community Health Nursing Diagnoses**		
Focus Population *(Who is your target group or community?)*	**Problem or Wellness Diagnosis** *(What is the potential/ actual community issue, concern, situation, or response you need to manage or intervene in?)*	**Etiology** *(Why is there this community issue, concern, situation, or response? Identify the causation factors.)*	**Characteristics** *(How did you make this etiologic inference? Give supporting community data/evidence or manifestations— i.e., signs or symptoms.)*
1. Students in high school	Potential for healthy lifestyles	Related to their desire to learn about nutrition and physical activities	As evidenced by integrated school curriculum with an emphasis on healthy lifestyle practices
2. Residents in Kent community	Risk for imbalanced nutrition; more than body requirements	Related to poor optimal lifestyle choices	As evidenced by increased in prevalence of obesity, high consumption rates of fast food, and low physical activity level in the residents
3. First Nation reserve-based peoples in Saskatchewan	Increased number of deaths by suicide	Related to inadequate mental health support and services	As evidenced by 4.3x higher rate of death by suicide than non-Indigenous peoples and lack of mental health experts and resources in these isolated communities
4. Newcomers	Inadequate income and resources and high family stress level	Related to inadequate language and skilled trades programs to prepare newcomers to be employable	As evidenced by high unemployment rates at 25%, inability to find work because of lack of language skills and Canadian work experience/requirements, high anxiety, and stress expressed by family

primary health care: accessibility, health promotion, intersectoral cooperation, appropriate technology, and public participation (WHO, 1978). Population-focused health promotion strategies include but are not limited to advocacy for healthy public policy, the strengthening of community action, and the creation of supportive environments (CHNC, 2019, revised; Epp, 1986). (See Chapter 8.)

Depending on the role and practice settings, CHNs such as home health or community-based nurses focus on direct-care services to individuals and families, whereas public health nurses provide population-focused health protection and health promotion services. Specific public health nursing interventions include consultation, counselling, health teaching, case management, referral and follow-up, screening, outreach, disease surveillance, policy development and enforcement, social marketing, advocacy, community organizing, coalition building, and collaboration (Canadian Public Health Association [CPHA], 2010; CHNC, 2015). (See Chapters 3, 4, and 5.) Nursing interventions are successful when the community is fully engaged and empowered throughout the nursing process.

Subjective and objective community data help form the needed indicators for evaluation of any evidence of success. Community planning and interventions are effective when public policy and supportive environments are addressed and when the community is committed to ongoing monitoring and evaluation of the intended health outcomes. (See Chapter 14.) The following section describes common planning and evaluation tools used in community settings. (See the Yes, But Why? feature.)

YES, BUT WHY?

Building a Healthier Community in a Slum Area

What?

Income inequities exist in many communities. Food banks and shelters serve as support services for the poor and homeless, including Indigenous populations, youth, and drug users. Local residents and businesses often express concerns over the aesthetics (e.g., makeshift shelters) and safety of their neighbourhood when they see scattered litter and discarded syringes in their parks, vacant houses, and alleys.

So What?

The underlying problems seen in slum neighbourhoods often are symptoms of poverty, homelessness, and drug use (Gaetz, Dej, Richter, & Redman, 2016). To promote the health and quality of life for people living in the slum areas, CHNs could address ways to provide a clean and safe *physical environment* (a social determinants of health) so that people can live, work, learn, play, and worship (PHAC, 2011).

Now What?

CHNs must first explore the *roots* of the problems for the exhibiting symptoms in their community. They can collect data (see Table 13.4 on page 264) on who the high-risk and at-risk people are in the neighbourhood and how they perceive their own health. CHNs collaborate with community

partners, which may include the residents, stakeholders (e.g., city counsellors, politicians, government, business community), the homeless and poor, and drug users. Windshield surveys and focus groups may be conducted to further validate information and gain more understanding of the community's perception of their concerns, issues, strengths and needs.

CHNs could explore the following key questions with the community:

1. What would make the community residents feel safe in and proud of their neighbourhood?
2. What can be done with the people in poverty or homeless and drug users in the neighbourhood?

To decrease the vulnerability to any social consequences of ill health to their clients, CHNs aim to promote health equities and social justice by assisting vulnerable clients to attain their social and economic rights and the highest level of health, including education, living wage, affordable housing, and participation in the society (Braveman, 2013).

Standards of Practice Fulfilled

#1 Health Promotion
- Collaborates with client to do a comprehensive, evidence informed, and strength-based holistic health assessment using multiple sources and methods to identify needs, assets, inequities, and resources.
- Uses a collaborative relationship with the client and other partners to facilitate and advocate for structural system change and healthy public policy using multiple health promotion strategies.

#5 Capacity Building
- Uses capacity building strategies such as mutual goal setting, visioning and facilitation in planning for action.
- Helps the client to identify and access available resources to address their health issues (CHNC, 2019, revised).

COMMUNITY PARTICIPATORY TOOLS FOR COMMUNITY PLANNING

A **community participatory approach** is key to community planning. Through dialogue with stakeholders and community members during the process, the community decides what makes a need become a priority, who is to take the action, what the action will be, and when and how it is to be done. Community participatory tools help quantify and qualify the health issues, needs, or concerns they identify. Active participation and sharing of experiences can empower people to take responsibility and ownership in health and to effect change.

Community Needs Matrix Tool

Participants may use the *community needs matrix tool* to discuss, identify, rate, or explain what they perceive to be the most important health problems or the most feasible interventions in

Table 13.3	Example of the Results of a Community Needs Matrix Tool			
Identified Health Need	Not a Concern	Somewhat Concerned	A Concern	Very Concerned
Accidents	*	***	***	****
Nutrition	*	**	**	****
Pneumonia	*	**	***	*
Sexually transmitted infections	*	***	***	*

their community. The degree of concern about each issue is tallied on a blank chart similar to that in Table 13.3, which shows this community is most concerned about accidents. CHNs facilitate the discussion to learn what the community has to say about their lived experiences. Through mutual planning, the CHNs assist the participants to make informed choices of the needed action and, thus, improved client outcomes.

Community Mapping

Community mapping is a schematic map of the community indicating the distribution and occurrence of illness, disease, and health; major resources; environmental conditions; and accessibility and barriers to various services. CHNs use the members' perceptions and experiences of service use to mutually formulate the intervention plans. Figure 13.4 illustrates an example of community mapping on the case distribution of spina bifida.

Present–Future Drawing

CHNs may ask their community clients to draw a *present–future drawing* (see Figure 13.5) to reflect upon their present situation and what resources and constraints contributed to it, and to visualize how the future might appear. This tool allows the nurse and the clients to see where the community wants to go and, hence, to formulate mutual intervention goals and objectives.

Community Governance and Community Engagement

Community governance and community engagement are pivotal to achieving program sustainability and accountability, building community capacity, and building social equity (Nonprofit Quarterly, 2015). **Community governance** is a decision-making process where management and leadership are usually undertaken by a group of community stakeholders to meet the health needs and priorities of the community through community engagement and empowerment (Totikidis, Armstrong, & Francis, 2005). Effective community governance must encompass three community skills: engaging citizens,

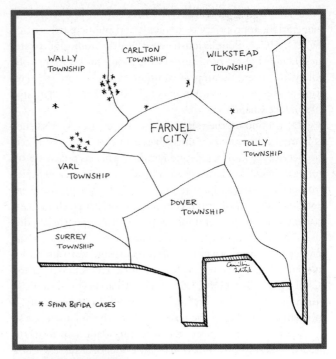

FIGURE 13.4 Community Map Showing Distribution of Spina Bifida

Source: Community Map Showing Distribution of Spina Bifida by Camillia F Matuk. Copyright © by Camillia F Matuk. Used by permission of Camillia F Matuk.

measuring results, and getting things done (Epstein, Coates, Wray, & Swain, 2006).

Community engagement is "a process involving citizens at various levels of participation based on interpersonal communication and trust and a common understanding and purpose" (Ontario Local Health Integration Network, 2011, p. 4). The purpose of community engagement is "to inform, educate, consult, involve, and empower stakeholders [and community members] in both health care [and] health service planning and decision-making processes to improve the health care system" (p. 5). (See Canadian Research 13.1.) This community engagement process can not only build trust but also allow the stakeholders to recognize and respect their differences, values, and interests as they develop a comprehensive understanding of the problem or issue and work collaboratively to find the optimal solutions (Holzer, Ellis, & Merritt, 2014).

Community Development and Community Mobilization

Community development is the "process of involving a community in the identification and strengthening those aspects of daily life, culture life, and political life which support health. This might include support for political action to change total environment and strengthen resources for healthy living" (CPHA, 2010, p. 32). Community development begins with a need or a vision for change. The community member(s) may start with asking (1) where is their community at, (2) what they want their community to be, (3) how they can get there, and (4) who can help in the process of change (Cavaye, n.d.).

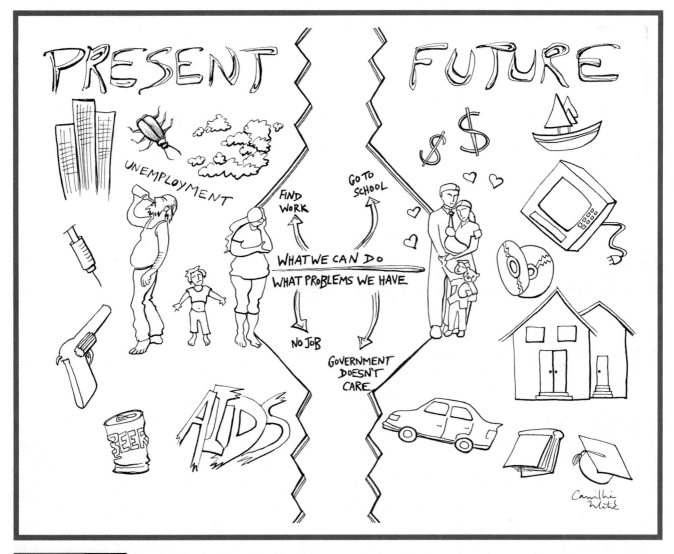

FIGURE 13.5 Present–Future Drawing

Source: Present–Future Drawing by Camillia F Matuk. Copyright © by Camillia F Matuk. Used by permission of Camillia F Matuk.

CANADIAN RESEARCH 13.1

Promoting face-to-face dialogue for community engagement in a digital age. (Scruby, Canales, Ferguson, & Gregory, 2017)

This article describes how community engagement was used in a collaborative research project that aimed to improve access to community health services in the inner city of Winnipeg. Because of cost savings and the availability and convenience of digital technology, most academic researchers and service providers communicated their research needs digitally rather than in face-to-face meetings. This community-based participatory action research used community engagement to promote face-to-face dialogue between four academic health researchers, 21 interdisciplinary inner-city community health and social service agency providers, and five community advisors. All participants met in a one-day meeting to brainstorm what they viewed as their research needs and used coloured tags to rank their priorities. The research

team then met to debrief and begin analyzing the data together.

Findings revealed that community engagement had stimulated dialogue between the researchers and service agencies, and thereby strengthened the academic-agency partnership. The authors concluded that community engagement was a welcomed choice of communication. The agencies also gained an increased understanding of the inner-city service needs and priorities and were interested in building more capacity and collaborations.

Discussion Questions

1. Explain the benefits of using community engagement over digital communication or virtual meetings.

2. What might be the challenges of the methodology in this research study?

3. Explain when and why you would use community engagement when working with your community. Give examples.

These questions reflect the value of the community and provide a framework for the community development process.

The process of community development to bring on the change usually starts with one or a few individuals at a grassroots level, taking collective action to generate solutions to common problems, and it eventually involves the larger community. This process is referred to as **community mobilization**. Community development involves capacity building and community mobilization.

CHNs can engage the community members and work in partnership with their communities as they define their own goals, mobilize resources, and develop action plans for collectively identified issues or problems. Community development focuses on consensus building; improving, strengthening, and sustaining community life and local conditions for people, particularly those in disadvantaged situations; and engaging them in decision making to achieve greater control over their circumstances. One example is Terry Fox's Marathon of Hope, which started in 1980. As a cancer survivor, Fox had a vision to find a cure for cancer, and he began running across the country to raise funds for cancer research. Since then, his one-person dream has become a world movement. Some examples of community development initiatives related to poverty are community gardens, food canning using excess farm produce, and dragon boat races to raise breast cancer awareness. (See also an example in the Yes, But Why? box.)

Community interventions must be evaluated to measure the outcomes, whether or not the expected results were achieved. The steps for *community program evaluation* are (1) determining what needs to be evaluated based on the evaluation criteria; (2) engaging stakeholders throughout the process; (3) determining the appropriate methods of measurement; (4) developing data collection instruments, budget, and timeline for evaluation; (5) collecting and analyzing data; (6) reporting and disseminating the results; and (7) making decisions for action. (See Chapter 14.)

Successes and lessons learned from mistakes or challenges should be shared with the community to benefit other communities. Communities build on successes and work on perfecting problems for future changes and continuous improvement. Interventions should be evaluated and documented to support evidence-based practice.

Table 13.4 provides a summary guide that CHNs may use to assess the *general* health of a community and develop a community intervention plan. The assessment questions should be modified to fit the specific purpose of the assessment.

ROLE OF CHNs

CHNs care for diverse populations in complex social, political, and economic environments. With an in-depth understanding of what makes a community healthy and how social determinants of health can affect the overall population health, competent CHNs use the community health promotion process to implement their primary health care roles as they address health inequities and social justice for the marginalized populations (National Expert Commission, 2012, revised). They engage the community and strategically invest primary, secondary, and tertiary levels of prevention to strengthen individual and community capacity; to identify populations who are at risk; and to provide maintenance, protective care, and palliative care for their clients as needed. CHNs make ethical decisions while advocating for human and equality to achieve optimal health for all (CHNC, 2011, revised). (See Chapter 6.)

Table 13.4	Guide to Community Health Nursing Process	
AREAS FOR ASSESSING A COMMUNITY'S GENERAL HEALTH (Modify these general questions to reflect the specific purpose of your community assessment.)		**DATA/OBSERVATIONS** Gather subjective and objective data, and note discrepancies between the CHN and the clients.
A. ASSESSMENT **1. Purpose of Community Assessment, Target Group, and Location** – Purpose of assessment (e.g., environmental scan, needs assessment, problem investigation, or resource evaluation)? – Rationale for the assessment? – Who is the target group? What are their characteristics? – Boundaries where target group resides? – Supportive evidence for the health needs of the target group? **2. Community Historical and Perception** – Previous history of community actions by local groups or government? – Perceptions of the residents on the community issues, problems, concerns, attitudes, beliefs, felt needs? How are they similar or different from those of the larger community or the nurse?		

Table 13.4	Continued

AREAS FOR ASSESSING A COMMUNITY'S GENERAL HEALTH (Modify these general questions to reflect the specific purpose of your community assessment.)	DATA/OBSERVATIONS Gather subjective and objective data, and note discrepancies between the CHN and the clients.

3. Population
– Total composition and characteristics of the population in the community (e.g., age group distribution, gender, marital status, birth rate, and family size)?
– Density and rate of population growth, increased or decreased?
– Health status
  • Mortality and morbidity rates for age-specific diseases or causes, their incidence and prevalence?
  • Comparison of mortality and morbidity rates with previous years, with regional, provincial, and national rates?
  • Life expectancy and trends?
  • Biologic and genetic endowment?
  • Health status: indicators and influencing factors related to purpose of assessment (e.g., nutrition; immunization; lifestyles; stress; STIs; unplanned pregnancy; prenatal care; emergency care; primary, secondary, and tertiary care; personal health practices) and coping skills (e.g., healthy lifestyle practices, effective or maladaptive coping)?
4. Physical Environments
– Location: boundaries, geography, climate, plants, and animals posing threats to health, percentage of urban or rural area?
– Housing: type, condition, slum areas, sanitation, adequacy, crowding?
– Shopping facilities: types, location, and accessibility?
– Safety: crime rates, types, and where? Feeling safe? Police and relationships with the community?
– Water supply: quality and adequacy?
– Sanitation: sewage and waste disposal?
5. Socioeconomic Environments
– Income: income levels, poverty rate, number receiving social assistance?
– Social status and mobility
  • Percentages for each social class?
  • Patterns and impact of mobility on health needs and health service planning?
– Employment and working conditions
  • Major industries and business establishments?
  • Primary occupations? Employment rate? Unemployment or underemployment?
  • Occupational hazards?
  • Safe and supportive work life?
– Social supports and networks: Social isolation? Any support groups and community group involvement?
– Social inclusion: embrace diversity and share social experience by gender, sexual orientation, race, ethnicity, and religion?
– Recreation: facilities, affordability, accessibility, and appropriateness for all ages?	

(continued)

Table 13.4	Continued

AREAS FOR ASSESSING A COMMUNITY'S GENERAL HEALTH (Modify these general questions to reflect the specific purpose of your community assessment.)	DATA/OBSERVATIONS Gather subjective and objective data, and note discrepancies between the CHN and the clients.

6. Education and Healthy Child Development
– Education: literacy rates, attitudes, and facilities/programs for life skills and technical skills?
  • Available and accessible resources, peer support, and engagement?
– Healthy child development: preconception health, prenatal and parenting class, and daycare?
  • Early identification and intervention programs?
  • Accessible and affordable resources and services?
 	
7. Culture and Religion
– Ethnic and racial group composition and subcultures, culture, and languages spoken?
– Cultural diversity and tolerance, positive and negative influence on health practices?
– Cultural adaptation, perceptions of health?
– Religious affiliations and spiritual support and influence on health practices?
 	
8. Health and Social Services
– Services and community organizations
  • Location, ratios of health workers to rural and urban populations?
  • Number of beds available and type, health service utilization? Wait list? Health budget priorities, amount per capita, and spending?
  • Provision of adequate and quality primary, secondary, and tertiary care?
  • Service coordination, gaps, and duplications?
  • Impact of funding on service delivery?
  • Evidence of community engagement and community governance (e.g., intersectoral cooperation, health promotion, public participation, and appropriate technology used in service delivery)?
  • Available and adequate social assistance to meet community needs in a timely manner?
 	
9. Transportation
– Type, availability, accessibility, affordability, and usage?
 	
10. Governance and Politics
– Communications
  • Methods, timing, and locations of verbal and nonverbal communication (e.g., newspapers, radio, television, flyers, internet, and forums)?
  • Relationships with other organizations, degree of conflict, and collaboration?
  • Evidence of interpersonal relationships, commitment, and partnerships?
– Leadership
  • Who are the formal and informal leaders? What are their visions for the community?
  • Power structure, delegations, politics?
– Decision making: effective and efficient process of decision making (e.g., policy formulation, human resources)?	

(continued)

Table 13.4	Continued	
AREAS FOR ASSESSING A COMMUNITY'S GENERAL HEALTH (Modify these general questions to reflect the specific purpose of your community assessment.)		**DATA/OBSERVATIONS** Gather subjective and objective data, and note discrepancies between the CHN and the clients.
B. ANALYSIS **1. Wellness Nursing Diagnoses** – Potential and actual community strengths? **2. Problem Nursing Diagnoses** – Potential and actual community needs and gaps? **C. PLANNED INTERVENTIONS** – Implementation of primary, secondary, and tertiary preventive care focusing on health promotion challenges such as reducing inequities, increasing prevention, and enhancing coping? – Evidence of incorporation of primary health care principles, public policy, and supportive environments in nursing care planning? – Expected outcomes and target dates clearly defined? **D. EVALUATION** – Monitoring of progress and gathering of evidence of success based on outcomes objectives? – Lessons learned, decision for action, and knowledge transfer?		

CONCLUSION

Promoting the health of the populations is not new to community nursing; it has been the very core of this profession since its origin. (See Chapter 1.) Healthy community does not just happen. Excellence in promoting healthy communities and population health requires CHNs to overcome personal and systemic barriers that impede their care. Confident and conscientious CHNs strive to achieve excellence in promoting the equity and health of the population they serve. Expert CHNs will demonstrate competent leadership in community health promotion and advocate for the importance of population-focused health promotion (Valaitis et al., 2014).

KEY TERMS

aggregate communities   (p. 250)
aggregate   (p. 254)
artificial boundaries   (p. 255)
capacity building   (p. 251)
community   (p. 250)
community assessment   (p. 253)
community asset mapping   (p. 252)
community development   (p. 262)
community dynamics   (p. 250)
community engagement   (p. 262)
community forums   (p. 258)
community functions   (p. 250)
community governance   (p. 262)
community health promotion model (CHPM)   (p. 252)

community mapping   (p. 262)
community mobilization   (p. 264)
community participatory approach   (p. 261)
community surveys   (p. 258)
environmental scan   (p. 253)
focus groups   (p. 258)
geopolitical boundaries   (p. 250)
group   (p. 254)
healthy communities   (p. 251)
needs   (p. 253)
physical boundaries   (p. 255)
population   (p. 254)
population at risk   (p. 255)
population health   (p. 258)
priority or vulnerable population   (p. 255)
risk   (p. 259)
target population   (p. 255)
virtual communities   (p. 250)
windshield surveys   (p. 253)

STUDY QUESTIONS

1. Name four community settings where CHNs work, and describe their role and functions in these settings.

2. What are the characteristics of a healthy community?

3. What nursing process skills will you use to promote the health of the community?

4. What assessment components are used when assessing community health?

5. Define population health, community engagement, community governance, community development, and capacity building.

INDIVIDUAL CRITICAL-THINKING EXERCISES

1. Why is it important for the nurse to provide care to the community?

2. How would you work with your community to identify their health needs and share their community experiences?

3. In developing a health profile for a community, what assessment questions would you ask for each category of the community components? Where and how would you collect the needed data?

GROUP CRITICAL-THINKING EXERCISES

1. Discuss the benefits of community dialogue between CHNs and Indigenous populations or any other population groups.

2. In a group of two to four, spend about an hour visiting and talking to people in your local neighbourhood. Describe your community visit, and explain your impression about the felt needs, real needs, and wants of the community.

   a. Formulate your nursing diagnoses, and propose your actions.

   b. Discuss possible ways to engage your community to meet the identified health needs.

REFERENCES

Albert, D., & Herrera, C. (2009, November 20). *Getting lost in the evidence? Part 1: Developing an evidence question and search strategy.* Fireside Chat presentation. Ottawa, ON: University of Ottawa.

Braveman, P. (2013, September 26). *What is health equity? What are health disparities? And why do the definitions matter?* Slide presentation. Center on Social Disparities in Health. San Francisco, CA: University of California.

Canadian Public Health Association. (2010). *Community health–public health nursing in Canada: Preparation and practice* (4th ed.). Ottawa, ON: Author.

Cavaye, J. (n.d.). *Understanding community development.* Retrieved from http://vibrantcanada.ca/files/understanding_community_development.pdf

CBC News. (2012, December 20). *6 niqab legal controversies in Canada.* Retrieved from http://www.cbc.ca/news/politics/6-niqab-legal-controversies-in-canada-1.1238055

Clemen-Stone, S., Eigsti, D., & McGuire, S. (2002). *Comprehensive community health nursing* (6th ed.). Toronto, ON: Mosby.

Community Health Nurses of Canada (CHNC). (2019, revised). *Canadian community health nursing: Professional practice model & standards of practice.* St. John's, NL: Author. Retrieved from https://www.chnc.ca/en/publications-resources

Community Health Nurses of Canada (CHNC). (2015). *Leadership competencies for public health practice in Canada: Leadership competency statements Version 1.0.* St. John's, NL: Author. Retrieved from https://www.chnc.ca/en/publications-resources

Dutton, D. J., Forest, P-G., Kneebone, R. D., & Zwicker, J. D. (2018). Effect of provincial spending on social services and health care on health outcomes in Canada: An observational longitudinal study. *CMAJ, 190*(3) E66–E71. doi: https://doi.org/10.1503/cmaj.170132

Epp, J. (1986). *Health for all: A framework for health promotion.* Ottawa, ON: Health and Welfare Canada.

Epstein, P. D., Coates, P. M., Wray, L. D., & Swain D. (2006). *Improving communities by engaging citizens, measuring performance and getting things done.* Mississauga, ON: Jossey-Bass.

Gaetz, S., Dej, E., Richter, T., & Redman, M. (2016). *The state of homelessness in Canada 2016.* Toronto, ON: Canadian Observatory on Homelessness Press.

George, U., Thomas, M. S., Chaze, F., & Guruge, S. (2015). Immigrant mental health, a public health issue: Looking back and moving forward. *International Journal of Environmental Research and Public Health, 12*(10), 13624–13648. doi: 10.3390/ijerph121013624

Government of Canada. (2016, May 5). *Measuring mental health in Canada: Social support.* Retrieved from https://www.canada.ca/en/public-health/services/publications/healthy-living/measuring-positive-mental-health-canada-social-support.html

Health Canada. (2001). *The population health template: Key elements and actions that define a population health approach.* Retrieved from http://www.atlantique.phac-aspc.gc.ca/ph-sp/pdf/discussion-eng.pdf

Holzer, J. K., Ellis L., & Merritt M. W. (2014). Why we need community engagement in medical research. *Journal of Investigative Medicine. 62*(6), pp. 851–855.

Kretzmann, J. P., & McKnight, J. L. (1993). *Building communities from the inside out: A path towards finding and mobilising a community's assets.* Chicago, IL: ACTA Publications.

Letourneau, N., Whitty, P., Watson, B., Phillips, J., Joschko, J., & Gillis, D. (2015). The influence of newborn early literacy intervention programs in three Canadian provinces. *Issues in Comprehensive Pediatric Nursing, 38*(4), 245–265. doi: 10.3109/01460862.2015.1065933

Long, D., & Dickason, P. (2016). *Visions of the Heart: Issues involving Aboriginal peoples in Canada* (4th ed.). Don Mills, ON: Oxford University Press Canada.

McKay, M. (2012). The history of community nursing in Canada. In L. Stamler & L. Yiu (Eds.), *Community health nursing: A Canadian perspective* (3rd ed., pp. 1–20). Toronto, ON: Pearson Canada.

Minkler, M. (Ed.). (2012). *Community organizing and community building for health* (3rd ed.). New Brunswick, NJ: Rutgers University Press.

National Expert Commission. (2012, revised). *A nursing call to action.* Ottawa, ON: Canadian Nurses Association. Retrieved from http://www.cna-aiic.ca/~/media/cna/files/en/nec_report_e.pdf

Nonprofit Quarterly. (2015). *Community-engagement governance: Systems-wide governance in action.* Retrieved from https://nonprofitquarterly.org/index.php/governancevoice/12021-community-engagement-governance-systems-wide-governance-in-action

Office of Quality Improvement. (2007). *Focus groups: A guide to learning the needs of those we serve.* University of Wisconsin-Madison. Retrieved from https://oqi.wisc.edu/resourcelibrary/uploads/resources/Focus_Group_Guide.pdf

Ontario Healthy Communities Coalition. (n.d.). *What makes a community healthy?* Copyright © by Ontario Healthy Communities Coalition. Retrieved from http://www.ohcc-ccso.ca/en/what-makes-a-healthy-community

Ontario Local Health Integration Network. (2011). *LHIN community engagement guidelines and toolkit.* Toronto, ON: Author.

Public Health Agency of Canada. (2002). *Summary table of population health key elements.* Public Health Agency of Canada. Reproduced with permission from the Minister of Health, 2015. © All rights reserved. Retrieved from http://www.phac-aspc.gc.ca/ph-sp/approach-approche/pdf/summary_table.pdf

Public Health Agency of Canada (PHAC). (2011). *What determines health?* Retrieved from https://www.canada.ca/en/public-health/services/health-promotion/population-health/what-determines-health.html#What

Public Health Agency of Canada (PHAC). (2012). *What is the population health approach?* Retrieved from https://www.canada.ca/en/public-health/services/health-promotion/population-health/population-health-approach.html

Public Health Agency of Canada (PHAC). (2013). *What makes Canadians healthy or unhealthy?* Retrieved from https://www.canada.ca/en/public-health/services/health-promotion/population-health/what-determines-health/what-makes-canadians-healthy-unhealthy.html#unhealthy

Public Health Agency of Canada (PHAC). (2014). *Seniors' falls in Canada: Second report.* Retrieved from https://www.canada.ca/content/dam/phac-aspc/migration/phac-aspc/seniors-aines/publications/public/injury-blessure/seniors_falls-chutes_aines/assets/pdf/seniors_falls-chutes_aines-eng.pdf

Public Health Agency of Canada (PHAC). (2016, December). *Health status of Canadians 2016: A report of the Chief Public Health Officer.* Cat: 978-0-660-05480-3. Retrieved from https://www.canada.ca/content/dam/hc-sc/healthy-canadians/migration/publications/department-ministere/state-public-health-status-2016-etat-sante-publique-statut/alt/pdf-eng.pdf

Scruby, L. S., Canales, M. K., Ferguson, E., & Gregory, D. (2017). Promoting face-to-face dialogue for community engagement in a digital age. *Canadian Journal of Nursing Research, 49*(4), 170–177. Retrieved from http://journals.sagepub.com/doi/pdf/10.1177/0844562117726939

Senate of Canada. (2009). *A healthy, productive Canada: A determinant of health approach.* The Standing Senate Committee on Social Affairs, Science and Technology. Retrieved from http://nlhfrp.ca/wp-content/uploads/2015/01/Fracking-Panel-Determinants-of-Health-Senate-Report-Keon-Pepein.pdf

Statistics Canada. (2015, November 27, Modified). *Understanding seniors' risk of falling and their perception of risk* (82-624-X). Retrieved from https://www.statcan.gc.ca/pub/82-624-x/2014001/article/14010/mi-rs-eng.htm

Statistics Canada. (2016a, September 15, Modified). *Immigration and ethnocultural diversity in Canada.* Retrieved from http://www12.statcan.gc.ca/nhs-enm/2011/as-sa/99-010-x/99-010-x2011001-eng.cfm#a6

Statistics Canada. (2016b, September 28) *Perceived health* (82-229-x). Retrieved from http://www.statcan.gc.ca/pub/82-229-x/2009001/status/phx-eng.htm

Statistics Canada. (2017a, May 13). Age pyramid of Canada in 1871 and 2016, 150 years of demographic history. *Census of population, 1871 and 2016.* Retrieved from https://www.statcan.gc.ca/daily-quotidien/17

Statistics Canada. (2017b, October 25). *Canada {Country} and Canada {Country}* (table). *Census Profile.* 2016 Census. Statistics Canada Catalogue no. 98-316-X2016001. Ottawa. Retrieved from http://www12.statcan.gc.ca/census-recensement/2016/dp-pd/prof/details/page.cfm?Lang=E&Geo1=PR&Code1=01&Geo2=&Code2=&Data=Count&SearchText=Canada&SearchType=Begins&SearchPR=01&B1=All&TABID=1

Statistics Canada. (2017c, March 30). Population size and growth in Canada: Key results from the 2016 Census. *The Daily.* Retrieved from https://www.ncbi.nlm.nih.gov/pubmed/26368512https://www.ncbi.nlm.nih.gov/pubmed/26368512

Stuart, G. (2014). What is community capacity building? *Sustaining Community.* Retrieved from https://sustaining-community.wordpress.com/2014/03/10/ccb

Totikidis, V., Armstrong, A., & Francis, R. (2005). *The concept of community governance: A preliminary review.* Presented at the GovNet Conference, 28–30 Nov, 2005, Melbourne, Australia. (Unpublished).

Truth and Reconciliation Commission of Canada. (2015). *Honouring the truth: Reconciling for the future.* Retrieved from http://www.trc.ca/websites/trcinstitution/File/2015/Honouring_the_Truth_Reconciling_for_the_Future_July_23_2015.pdf

Valaitis, R., Schofield, R., Akhtar-Danesh, A., Baumann, A., Martin-Misener, R., Underwood, J., & Isaacs, S. (2014). Community health nurses' learning needs in relation to the Canadian community health nursing standards of practice: Results from a Canadian survey. *BMC Nursing, 13,* 31. Retrieved from https://doi.org/10.1186/1472-6955-13-31

Vollman, A. R., Anderson, E. T., & McFarlane, J. (2016). *Canadian community as partner: Theory and multidisciplinary practice* (Canadian 4th ed.). New York, NY: Wolters Kluwer/Lippincott Williams & Wilkins.

World Health Organization. (1978). *Primary health care: Report on the International Conference on Primary Health Care,* Alma Ata, USSR, 6–12, September 1978. Geneva, CH: Author.

World Health Organization, Canadian Public Health Association, & Health and Welfare Canada. (1986). *Ottawa charter of health promotion.* Ottawa, ON: Health and Welfare Canada.

ABOUT THE AUTHOR

Lucia Yiu, RN, BScN, BA (University of Windsor), BSc (University of Toronto), MScN (University of Western Ontario), is Associate Professor Emeritus with the Faculty of Nursing at the University of Windsor and an educational and training consultant in community nursing. Her practice and research include multicultural health, international health, experiential learning, community development, breast health, and program planning and evaluation. Lucia was the recipient of the 2014 Community Health Nurses of Canada Award of Merit. She was also co-editor for the first four editions of *Community Health Nursing: A Canadian Perspective* and for the second and third Canadian editions of Kozier's *Fundamentals of Nursing: Theory to Practice.*

Community Health Planning, Monitoring, and Evaluation

Nancy C. Edwards and Josephine Etowa

SOLUTION STRATEGY PLANNING

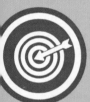 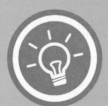 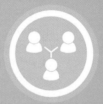 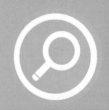

GOAL   PROCESS   INSPIRATION   PLANNING   RESEARCH

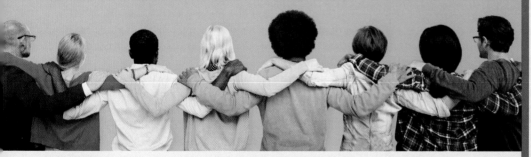

Source: Rawpixel.com/Fotolia

LEARNING OUTCOMES

After studying this chapter, you should be able to:

1. Describe components of the assessment–planning–evaluation cycle, and use a logic model to guide the process.

2. Describe the importance of program planning, monitoring, and evaluation in the practice of community health nursing.

3. Describe elements of the multiple interventions framework and its application to a complex community health issue.

4. Explain how the socio-structural determinants of health and social justice approaches can be reflected in planning, monitoring, and evaluation.

5. Discuss strategies for engaging citizens and stakeholders in the assessment–planning–evaluation cycle.

6. Select indicators for program accountability with consideration of the program's health equity impact.

INTRODUCTION

Planning, monitoring, and evaluating community health programs are fundamental processes used by community health nurses (CHNs) as they work in partnership with the community (Community Health Nurses of Canada [CHNC], 2019, revised). With more scrutiny of how public funds are being expended, increased demands for evidence-based programs, standards of practice, and including national and international interest in population health intervention research, these processes have become even more critical (Commission on Social Determinants of Health, 2008). The Canadian Community Health Nursing Standards of Practice (CHNC, 2011, revised) describe how nurses are expected to plan new programs, redesign existing services, monitor the implementation of programs, and evaluate their impact. Nurses often make important contributions to these processes with the substantial involvement of community representatives, key stakeholders from a variety of service sectors, and colleagues from multiple disciplines.

There are many tools available to assist CHNs in program planning, but their utility will be diminished if underlying sociostructural determinants of health are ignored and programs are developed without considering social justice issues. Thus, while research evidence and theory are important, the authentic engagement of the community is also essential in planning, monitoring, and evaluating community health programs.

PROGRAM PLANNING AND EVALUATION

The planning–evaluation cycle involves several key components. Although various planning frameworks are in common use, all contain similar elements. A classic **planning–implementation–evaluation cycle** (Figure 14.1) involves the following steps:

- conducting a situational analysis or community assessment
- identifying the problems or issues of concern
- considering possible solutions or actions to address the problem
- selecting the best alternative(s)
- designing and implementing the program
- monitoring and evaluating the program

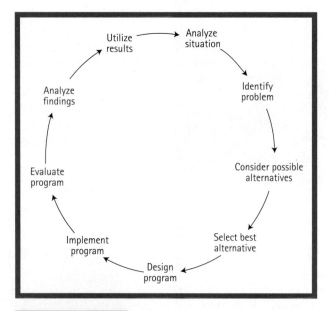

FIGURE   14.1 Planning–Implementation–Evaluation Cycle

Source: Based on Trochim, W. M. K. (2006). The research methods knowledge base (2nd ed.). Retrieved from http://www.socialresearchmethods.net/kb/pecycle.php

- analyzing and interpreting results of the monitoring and evaluation process
- using the results to make modifications to the program or to inform decisions about other programs

The steps in this cycle may need to be repeated as you develop a better understanding of an issue and obtain additional input from partners. It may be necessary to go back to other steps in the planning cycle and try to develop a more complete picture of the factors that are affecting the problem or influencing the community's response to the problem, as these factors shape potential solutions.

Selecting a Program Planning and Evaluation Framework

Many program planning and evaluation frameworks are available. Frameworks provide a guide for the types of information that need to be assembled and for organizing this information into a coherent plan. There are several considerations when selecting a framework for use. First, most community health agencies will have a standard planning framework that is used across departments. Applying a common framework allows for a coherent and consistent approach to planning within an organization. Second, the use of a particular framework may be a requirement of those who fund programs, as this allows them to compare results across funded programs. Third, a framework may be chosen because it helps detail a particular aspect of the planning process that is vexing or challenging. For instance, a framework may be chosen because it is particularly useful in defining the underlying sociostructural determinants of a problem, it guides the choice of theory that will help define program elements, it is more appropriate for addressing the needs of marginalized populations, or it is more consistent with Indigenous peoples' philosophies and ways of knowing. Finally, the selection of a framework may be influenced by a set of underlying values or principles that will guide programs such as participatory development or social justice (Edwards & Davison, 2008).

The **program logic model** is used extensively in many public health agencies in Canada, at both regional and municipal levels, and by provincial and federal government agencies (Morestin & Castonguay, 2013; Porteous, Sheldrick, & Stewart, 2002). Logic models provide a coherent structure for complex health programs, help to expose gaps, and yield an overview of programs with appealing visual clarity. As a support to planning, analysis, and program evaluation preparation, the logic model provides a means of documenting "what the program is supposed to do, with whom, and why" (Porteous et al., 2002, p. 116).

Wooten et al. (2014) note that the logic model is unique among tools for its simplicity in demonstrating program interrelationships and linkages. Logic models should be developed in collaboration with community and academic partners. In this way, both experiential learning and research findings can inform model development. Joint preparation of a logic model will help build consensus about program priorities among the

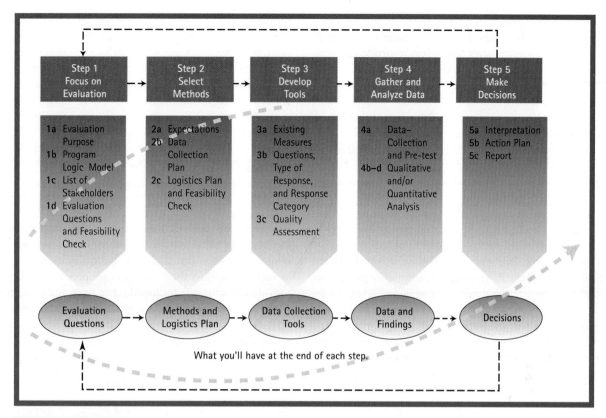

FIGURE 14.2 Public Health Agency of Canada Tool Kit Decision-Oriented Model for Program Evaluation

Source: "Tool kit decision-oriented model for program evaluation." by Public Health Agency of Canada, *2008*. Reproduced with permission from the Minister of Health, 2015. © All rights reserved.

planning team. In using a logic model, you should avoid positioning it as a rigid guideline, which prevents iterative evolution or lateral exploration of the program under review.

Development of a logic model consists of two planning stages, referred to as **CAT (components, activities, and target groups)** and **SOLO (short-term outcomes and long-term outcomes)**. For the CAT stage, activities are first clustered thematically into components for the program under review. For example, a suicide prevention program for youth might include the components of risk assessment, crisis intervention, and peer support. Activities are the specific intervention strategies to be used for each component. The crisis intervention component may include training youth workers in crisis management and developing community supports for youth in crisis. Target groups are the intended recipients of a program. In this example, these might be youth who are homeless or dislocated from their families, immigrants or refugees having difficulty in school, front-line workers for youth in health and social service organizations, or older adults and community leaders working with Indigenous youth.

The purpose of the SOLO stage is to identify program outcomes. Short-term outcomes are the immediate and direct results of the program, and long-term outcomes reflect the ultimate goals of the program. Building the knowledge and skills of youth workers to identify and support youth in crisis would be a short-term outcome; reducing youth suicide rates would be longer term. Many extraneous factors may influence

the achievement of long-term outcomes. Thus, they are more difficult to directly and exclusively attribute to the program.

The **program evaluation tool kit** (Figure 14.2) incorporates the use of a logic model and identifies which evaluation processes may be used to inform decision making during program planning and implementation (National Collaborating Centre for Methods and Tools, 2010). Evaluation is an ongoing, dynamic process that supports further refinement of program activities and helps to identify gaps or flaws in the original program design. It is critical to involve community partners in the evaluation process. They can play key roles in helping with data interpretation and identifying recommendations emerging from program evaluation.

Tools and Processes to Support Planning and Evaluation

Many tools and processes may be used in combination with an organizing framework. However, these tools must be used in conjunction with approaches that build relationships and create opportunities to hear the voices and understand the varying perspectives of disadvantaged groups. Intersectionality is an analytical tool used in equity work. Collins and Bilge (2016) describe intersectionality as "a way of understanding and analyzing the complexity in the world, in people, and in human experiences" (p. 2). It is a theoretical perspective that helps explicate power relations and the intersecting factors that influence how power is used in society (Collins & Bilge, 2016). Intersectionality highlights multiple forms of discrimination and places a clear emphasis on the intersection of contextual factors such as class, religion, culture, race, and gender (Bilge, 2010).

Crosby and Noar (2011) suggest that using tools like the **PRECEDE-PROCEED planning model** enables the community program developer to think logically about the desired end point and work "backward" to achieve that goal. The efficient involvement of community partners is important because those working in service delivery sectors have many demands on their time. Involving them in the planning process helps build commitment to the program and aids the design of a program that reflects the dynamic realities and strengths of the community (Angeles, Dolovich, Kaczorowsk, & Thabane, 2013). There are practical tools available to help engage community partners in a planning process. For example, environmental scans can be used to gather information about community needs and priorities. Key informant interviews and focus groups may be conducted (see Chapter 13), or an analysis of strengths, weaknesses, opportunities, and threats (SWOT) may be undertaken. You should be mindful that tools used need to be an appropriate fit with the social dynamics and cultural norms of a community. Their use should help uncover factors that drive inequities such as underlying power structures and the community's experiences of racism, class, and oppression.

A **SWOT (strengths, weaknesses, opportunities, and threats) analysis** identifies internal strengths and weaknesses of the organization or program, along with external opportunities and threats. It may involve document and policy reviews, community meetings, key informant interviews, and focus groups. It helps individuals planning a program to ensure it will be adequately staffed and resourced, and to customize its fit within the implementation environment (e.g., community) (Helms & Nixon, 2010). A SWOT analysis may also assist in determining the feasibility of initiating or continuing a program and may help identify potential service delivery partners. SWOT analyses are frequently used as part of a strategic planning process when managers are developing long-term plans for their organizations.

Assessing needs through the use of qualitative research strategies such as individual interviews and focus groups elaborates on issues and experiences that are not readily understood through quantitative and statistical tools (Creswell & Poth, 2018). For example, although quantitative evaluation tools may demonstrate that a particular subpopulation is less likely than others to use community health services, they may not be able to explain why and how. Similarly, quantitative data may not shed light on the perceived appropriateness of community health services or underlying community tensions that disadvantage population subgroups. Qualitative research tools not only address these gaps but also assess the meanings of health and care (Pope & Mays, 2013). Qualitative data can increase the relevance and interpretability of quantitative data generated during a needs assessment.

Individual interviews allow for exploration of first-person experiences and prompt interactive discussions that centre on the perspectives of participants (Patton, 2015). The qualitative research interview "elicits the participants' experiences, perceptions, thoughts and feelings" and helps to illuminate the meanings of key themes in the lives of study participants (Moser & Korstjens, 2017, p. 4). Focus group discussion is a commonly applied technique for qualitative research data collection that explicitly uses "group interaction as research data" (Stalmeijer, McNaughton, Vanmook, & Walthern, 2014, p. 923). The composition of focus groups must be carefully planned. Although some diversity of viewpoints is important, you should try to assemble a group where there is not an underlying power structure among its members that may discourage some participants from openly sharing their viewpoints. For example, it may not be appropriate to have a focus group consisting of both front-line workers and their managers because front-line workers may hesitate to discuss issues concerning organizational leadership or conditions when their managers are present. Focus groups provide opportunities for members to share and validate their individual experiences. The discussion may stimulate participant ownership of the program under development and may prompt participants toward action.

Organizing Information and Setting Priorities

The second set of tools help with organizing and understanding data and information, and guide priority setting. (See Chapters 10 and 13 for additional examples.) Analyzing and representing qualitative data involves describing, classifying, and connecting data (Miles, Huberman, & Saldana, 2014). **Content analysis** is a systematic, replicable technique for compressing large volumes of text data into fewer content categories based on explicit rules of coding. This involves assigning codes or labels to the text data. Data are then grouped into categories to reflect emerging patterns of responses. Systematic counting and recording techniques may help identify patterns of responses such as the predominant use of certain kinds of phrases by some respondents but not others. Analyzed qualitative data can be packaged in text, matrix, or figure formats. A text format involves the use of illustrative quotes. Matrices are used to compare major categories of data and highlight differences and similarities among subgroups. For example, a matrix of needs-assessment information may be used to compare responses from homeless men and shelter staff regarding the fairness of the shelter rules; or to compare the perspectives of teachers, parents, and students regarding the acceptability and need for school sexual health clinics. Figures may be a useful visual tool to reflect emerging relationships among categories of coded data.

Many sources of quantitative data may be accessed as you plan a program. These include local and provincial data documenting the magnitude of the problem and contributing factors, and how these differ across social and economic classes. These data are often obtained through special surveys (e.g., school surveys to document patterns of smoking among youth), routinely collected information (e.g., police reports, administrative health utilization data, or air pollution records), and surveillance data (e.g., reports of injuries or communicable diseases). It may be essential to seek data that include vulnerable populations such as Indigenous peoples, immigrants and refugees, or individuals living in homeless shelters who are either excluded from or under-represented in surveys or census data.

Various reporting formats have been developed to display quantitative data. A useful starting point is to examine existing reports (e.g., health status reports) and to enlist the assistance of someone with epidemiological training. Quantitative data may be needed to estimate program costs and the potential return on investments. Costing approaches should take into account variable costs involved in reaching higher risk groups and more isolated or less densely populated communities. Various methods and tools may be helpful, including the balanced score card (Weir, d'Entremont, Stalker, Kurji, & Robinson, 2009), the health impact assessment (McCallum, Ollson, & Stefanovic, 2015), and the application of health economics methods (Shiell, Hawe, & Gold, 2008). Systematic reviews provide an important source of data on the effectiveness of programs. Systematic reviews of quantitative research assemble findings from studies with a common research objective. Individuals undertaking systematic reviews use a thorough and rigorous set of methods both to identify all potentially relevant studies and to review the methodological quality of these studies. Studies deemed to be relevant and of adequate quality are included in the review.

Outcome data are extracted using standard procedures. When possible, the quantitative findings from two or more studies are collapsed into a single estimate of effect. This is done using statistical techniques, and the review process is then called a **meta-analysis**. (See Chapter 10 for more detail.)

An example is provided in Figure 14.3, which summarizes results from 19 studies on the effectiveness of multifactorial fall prevention interventions. There are three important things to understand in this diagram. First, the relative risk or risk ratio is used to indicate whether or not those who received the intervention had a lower rate of falls than those who did not. If there is no difference between the intervention and control groups, the relative risk is one. If the intervention group has a lower rate of falls than the control group, the relative risk or risk ratio will be less than one (indicating a protective effect). Sixteen of the 19 studies had a relative risk ratio less than one, indicating a protective effect. Second, if this intervention effect is statistically significant (indicating that if we repeated the studies, we are 95% certain we would again find a difference between groups), then the confidence interval (CI) around the relative risk ratio will also be less than one. In Figure 14.3, the CI is shown as a horizontal line on the diagram and numerically described in the right-hand column. We can see that only nine of the 19 studies found statistically significant protective effects of the intervention. Third, results are then pooled

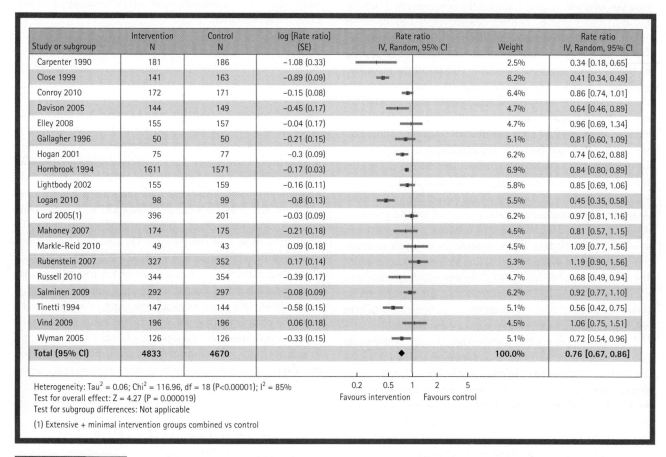

Study or subgroup	Intervention N	Control N	log [Rate ratio] (SE)	Rate ratio IV, Random, 95% CI	Weight	Rate ratio IV, Random, 95% CI
Carpenter 1990	181	186	−1.08 (0.33)		2.5%	0.34 [0.18, 0.65]
Close 1999	141	163	−0.89 (0.09)		6.2%	0.41 [0.34, 0.49]
Conroy 2010	172	171	−0.15 (0.08)		6.4%	0.86 [0.74, 1.01]
Davison 2005	144	149	−0.45 (0.17)		4.7%	0.64 [0.46, 0.89]
Elley 2008	155	157	−0.04 (0.17)		4.7%	0.96 [0.69, 1.34]
Gallagher 1996	50	50	−0.21 (0.15)		5.1%	0.81 [0.60, 1.09]
Hogan 2001	75	77	−0.3 (0.09)		6.2%	0.74 [0.62, 0.88]
Hornbrook 1994	1611	1571	−0.17 (0.03)		6.9%	0.84 [0.80, 0.89]
Lightbody 2002	155	159	−0.16 (0.11)		5.8%	0.85 [0.69, 1.06]
Logan 2010	98	99	−0.8 (0.13)		5.5%	0.45 [0.35, 0.58]
Lord 2005(1)	396	201	−0.03 (0.09)		6.2%	0.97 [0.81, 1.16]
Mahoney 2007	174	175	−0.21 (0.18)		4.5%	0.81 [0.57, 1.15]
Markle-Reid 2010	49	43	0.09 (0.18)		4.5%	1.09 [0.77, 1.56]
Rubenstein 2007	327	352	0.17 (0.14)		5.3%	1.19 [0.90, 1.56]
Russell 2010	344	354	−0.39 (0.17)		4.7%	0.68 [0.49, 0.94]
Salminen 2009	292	297	−0.08 (0.09)		6.2%	0.92 [0.77, 1.10]
Tinetti 1994	147	144	−0.58 (0.15)		5.1%	0.56 [0.42, 0.75]
Vind 2009	196	196	0.06 (0.18)		4.5%	1.06 [0.75, 1.51]
Wyman 2005	126	126	−0.33 (0.15)		5.1%	0.72 [0.54, 0.96]
Total (95% CI)	**4833**	**4670**		♦	**100.0%**	**0.76 [0.67, 0.86]**

Heterogeneity: Tau² = 0.06; Chi² = 116.96, df = 18 (P<0.00001); I² = 85%
Test for overall effect: Z = 4.27 (P = 0.000019)
Test for subgroup differences: Not applicable

0.2 0.5 1 2 5
Favours intervention   Favours control

(1) Extensive + minimal intervention groups combined vs control

FIGURE 14.3 Example of Meta-Analysis Completed for Systematic Review Examining Effectiveness of Multi-Component Interventions to Reduce Risk of Falls

Source: Gillespie, L. D., Robertson, M. C., Gillespie, W. J., Sherrington, C., Gates, S., Clemson, L. M., & Lamb, S. E. © 2015, Cochrane Collaboration. Reproduced with permission of Wiley Publishing Inc,.

across the 19 studies (the meta-analysis part of the exercise). A weighting factor is used in making this calculation so that studies with smaller sample sizes contribute less weight to the pooled estimate than studies with larger sample sizes. In this example, the pooled relative risk ratio is 0.76, and the result is statistically significant (the test for overall effect yields a p value of 0.000019 and a CI that excludes 1). Thus, it follows that the recommendation in the abstract for this review concludes that "multifactorial interventions, which include individual risk assessment, reduced rate of falls (RaR 0.76, 95% CI 0.67 to 0.86; 19 trials; 9503 participants)" (Gillespie et al., 2012, p. 2).

Integrative reviews use findings from both qualitative and quantitative studies to provide theoretical insights that guide program strategies (Mays, Pope, & Popay, 2005). The phases of an integrative review process include (a) problem formulation, (b) data collection or literature search, (c) evaluation of data from studies of diverse research designs, (d) data analysis, and (e) interpretation and presentation of results (Whittemore & Knafl, 2005).

Priority Setting

Setting priorities is a vital step in the planning process. An in-depth examination of a problem in the community may leave you overwhelmed at the thought of narrowing down the possibilities for action or differentiating priorities for target subgroups. The guiding principles for priority setting are buy-in, transparency, and communication. Priority setting inevitably means that you can neither address all the identified needs nor operationalize all the proposed interventions. The first principle, buy-in, needs to be addressed early on. Getting buy-in involves gaining trust; this will inevitably take longer and involve more effort with marginalized populations. Engaging community members and key stakeholders in discussing the problem may help with *buy-in* but runs the risk of backfiring if the priorities selected suggest that their input and ideas were not considered. Thus, it is also important to look at ways to involve the community in the process of setting priorities as you begin to more clearly define program components and activities. While it may not be realistic to involve a community in all phases of a priority-setting process, you can invite input during some critical phases, such as selecting criteria to inform priority setting. Agreement among senior managers on a common priority-setting process for an organization will help ensure managerial support for the priorities identified.

The second principle is transparency, whereby the process for selecting priorities is made apparent to individuals who were not directly involved. In other words, key stakeholders are able to understand how you got from point A (understanding the problem and considering possible intervention strategies) to point B (priority definition of the problem and strategies). Both objective and subjective criteria are important to identify priority interventions. Objective criteria are measurable facets of a problem and its solutions. For example, what is the magnitude (prevalence or incidence) of a problem, disaggregated by socioeconomic quintiles; what are the short- and long-term consequences of the problem; are there effective strategies to address the problem; and how cost-effective are these strategies relative to other approaches? Subjective criteria require judgment calls that are based on underlying organizational and social values about the issue. For instance, will working on the problem lead to new and stronger partnerships with other community agencies? Is tackling the problem within the mandate of our organization? Is there community readiness and capacity to address this problem? Will community elders and political leaders support change?

The third principle is communication. A clear communication strategy needs to accompany efforts to set priorities. Both internal and external communication processes are vital. Internally, the identification of priorities should be directly linked to approval mechanisms for program funding. Communication and collaborative technologies or tools are increasingly influencing the nature of health care interactions and should be used to facilitate internal dialogue. CHNs need to master the use of these tools for a variety of purposes such as debating issues, assessing media coverage, networking with and seeking support from peers or experts, using crowd-source information, providing advice (van de Belt et al., 2013), or designing social marketing campaigns. (See Chapter 8.) Externally, you need to communicate priorities to partners who have provided input on the program and to the public. Citizen engagement approaches are particularly important for marginalized groups. Targeted and well-designed communication will increase buy-in for program implementation.

Planning, Monitoring, and Evaluating Programs

Various resources are available to assist nurses and other public health professionals to plan, monitor, and evaluate programs. **Gantt charts**, depicted in a tabular format, are commonly used to present the sequence and timing of activities that must take place in order to accomplish the specific objectives of the program or project. These charts are particularly helpful when planning activities for a complex program with many components. The Gantt chart provides a good starting point for identifying these main components. The timelines for activities that must be undertaken in a particular sequence and details about these activities are then elaborated. For instance, permission must be obtained for the use of space before focus groups can be held, and these focus groups must take place before members of a planning group convene to consider community input on priorities. One example of a Gantt chart is provided in Figure 14.4. Software packages such as Microsoft Project and Excel can also be used to help develop plans and manage timelines with Gantt charts.

THE SHIFT TO MULTIPLE INTERVENTIONS

Increasingly, community health programs are targeting the complexity and root causes of problems. This requires a socioecological examination of the issue of interest and a

Activities	2011				2012								
	S	O	N	D	J	F	M	A	M	J	J	A	S
Site visit: review of evaluation framework	■												
Identify staff & roles for the project	■												
Develop project-specific timelines/activities	■												
Prepare materials for data collection		■											
Prepare for ethical considerations			■	■									
Prepare software/techinical specifications				■									
Pilot-test data collection procedures					■								
Staff training (if needed)					■								
Collect data; refine measures/procedures						■	■	■					
Analyze data									■	■			
Share preliminary findings											■		
Prepare final report												■	

FIGURE 14.4 Example of a Gantt Chart

Source: From Ontario Centre of Excellence for Child and Youth Mental Health (2013).

planning–intervention–evaluation cycle that addresses these underlying determinants. Raphael (2016) defines social determinants of health as "the economic and social conditions that shape the health of individuals, communities and jurisdictions as a whole" (p. 3). We use the term "sociostructural determinants" to reinforce the fact that some determinants are embedded in social structures such as legislation, standards, and regulations that generate or perpetuate social and health inequities. Sociostructural determinants shape contemporary community health programs. These determinants do not reside in isolation from each other. Rather, determinants are nested; that is, they are interrelated and as one determinant changes, another may shift. Some determinants are deeply embedded, following from historical inequities such as the oppression that Indigenous populations have experienced (Truth and Reconciliation Commission of Canada [TRC], 2016) and stigma faced by marginalized groups such as those living with mental illness or HIV/AIDS (Mill, Edwards, Jackson, MacLean, & Chaw-Kant, 2010). This notion that health is largely influenced by multiple factors beyond biology, genetics, and the health care system provides the foundation for a population health approach. A **population health approach** aims to improve the health of groups of people while reducing health inequalities and their underlying determinants (Health Canada, 2001). Successfully tackling determinants of health requires coherent, multi-level policies in health and other sectors (Commission on Social Determinants of Health, 2008; TRC, 2016). A sociostructural determinants of health approach recognizes the need to implement population health interventions at multiple levels of the system (individual, community, municipal, provincial, federal, and global). Structural barriers such as the one described in the Yes, But Why? box call for a population health approach.

YES, BUT WHY?

Improving Health Care Access for Immigrants and Refugees

What?

Timely health care access is an important determinant of the health and successful integration of new immigrants to Canada. However, a significant number of Canadian immigrants find it difficult to navigate the maze of health and social services available to them, impeding their timely access to quality care (Higginbottom & Safipour, 2015; Wilson-Mitchell, 2014; Woodgate et al., 2017).

So What?

Various classes of immigrants have different migration trajectories. However, some commonalities exist in their post-migration health care experiences. The healthy immigrant effect is a well-documented phenomenon that occurs in many Western countries; immigrants initially report better health outcomes compared to native-born populations (Subedi & Rosengerg, 2014), but this health advantage is not maintained. For instance, within four years, immigrants to Canada report worse health status than Canadian-born populations (Fuller-Thomson, Noack, & George, 2011). A possible explanation for healthier new immigrants is the requirement for "good health" as a criterion for admission. Worsening health may be explained by lack of fluency in one of Canada's official languages, difficulty getting employment, acculturation and its accompanying dietary changes, social isolation, and poor access to appropriate health care (Higginbottom & Safipour, 2015). The decline in the health of recent immigrants to Canada is even more dramatic for women than for men, and more so for women from non-Western countries of origin (Fuller-Thomson et al., 2011). Despite our universal health care system, immigrants still face challenges at individual, institutional, and systemic levels of care, including lack of appropriate services, poor quality care, and systemic discrimination (Guruge & Butt, 2015). In Ontario, only 78% of recent immigrants reported having a family doctor or other primary care provider compared to 88.1% of Canadian-born individuals (Health Quality Ontario, 2016). Even individuals with primary-care providers may face barriers accessing care when they need it (Aery, 2017).

Now What?

CHNs need to have an in-depth understanding of the structural barriers that may limit access to health resources for immigrant people. Although CHNs strive for universality and equity in practice, many structural barriers limit care access, adequacy, and acceptability for immigrant people. A holistic approach to these issues requires providers to move beyond individual-level awareness-raising and education to targeting systemic challenges. Monitoring and evaluation strategies also need to address both personal and systemic-level issues (Higginbottom & Safipour, 2015). Addressing health equity in this context requires CHNs to collaborate with immigrant communities and service organizations to advocate for policies that will reduce structural barriers to health care. Such policies may include funding for multisectoral and context-specific health promotion programs or access to health care navigators who can connect immigrants to health services that are culturally appropriate.

Standards of Practice Fulfilled

#5 Capacity Building
- Uses a comprehensive mix of strategies such as coalition building, inter-sectoral collaboration, community engagement and mobilization, partnerships, and networking to build community capacity to take action on priority issues.

#6 Health Equity
- Advocates for healthy public policy and social justice by participating in legislative and policy-making activities that influence determinants of health and access to services (CHNC, 2019, revised).

The **Multiple Intervention Program (MIP) framework** arises from earlier work by Edwards and Moyer (1999). In Ontario in the late 1980s, there was a shift away from public health programs that predominantly involved home visits and clinically oriented services in schools and workplaces. As evidence on determinants increased, and as considerations of how best to distribute scarce resources in public health were debated, programs increasingly began to focus on interventions targeting multiple layers of the system. Nurses were being asked to expand their repertoire of interventions to include not only those appropriate for individuals and families (such as home visits and primary care clinics) but also those targeted at community, organizational, and policy levels (such as

community action, and policy strengthening and enforcement). Please re-visit Chapter 3 for more in-depth discussion about the CHN scope of practice. With the input of front-line public health nurses and managers in Ottawa, a program framework was developed to reflect the integration of self-care capacity and action, collective care capacity and action, and environmental supports (Edwards & Moyer, 1999).

The next generation of this framework was developed 10 years later (Edwards, Mill, & Kothari, 2004), and further refinements have been made in the intervening years (Edwards, 2018). Its evolution arose from the observations and reflections of practitioners and from research. Managers identified the challenges of trying to plan and evaluate MIPs. Research findings were shedding light on a related set of issues. Through the 1990s, results from some well-designed experimental studies of MIPs were yielding unexpected and disappointing findings (Bauman, Suchindran, & Murray, 1999; Merzel & D'Afflitti, 2003; Sorenson, Emmons, Hunt, & Johnston, 1998). For instance, a seminal study, the COMMIT trial (COMMIT Research Group, 1995a), was a four-year multiple intervention study that targeted tobacco cessation and compared 11 matched pairs of communities in the United States and Canada. Eleven communities were in the control group and received no intervention. Eleven communities received a theory-based intervention that aimed to increase cessation rates among heavy smokers. The intervention program that was designed was considered "state-of-the-art-and-science." It included over 50 strategies that were aimed at various levels of the system, including individual behaviour change strategies, community mobilization, and organizational and policy change. However, the goal of reducing smoking rates among heavy smokers was not reached (COMMIT Research Group, 1995b). Authors have attempted to explain why the COMMIT trial and other multiple interventions did not achieve their expected outcomes (Zanna et al., 1994). Common reasons include failing to involve the community in the planning process, the short duration of programs that did not allow enough time for policy change, not planning for long-term sustainability, and inadequate funding (Edwards, MacLean, Estable, & Meyer, 2006; Merzel & D'Afflitti, 2003; Stirman et al., 2012).

Yet in apparent contradiction to some of the earlier research on MIPs, there have been compelling examples of significant MIP successes in fields such as tobacco control, cervical cancer screening, and injury prevention. Prolonged efforts (often over more than a decade) have yielded substantial improvements in health outcomes from multi-strategy, multi-level, and multi-sector interventions. In the case of injury prevention, for example, MIPs have included a combination of strategies aimed at raising awareness (e.g., public media campaigns), supporting behaviour change (e.g., infant car seat clinics), changing social norms (e.g., it is no longer socially acceptable to drink and drive), and developing regulations or passing legislation and setting up enforcement approaches (e.g., traffic calming strategies and police checkpoints for seat belt use and drunk driving). But we have also learned that health inequities must be explicitly addressed in the design of programs. Socioeconomic gradients reveal marked disparities in the effectiveness of programs. Tobacco use and related disease outcomes, for example, remain highest among the impoverished, Indigenous peoples, and individuals suffering from severe mental illness.

THE MULTIPLE INTERVENTION PROGRAM FRAMEWORK

The MIP framework consists of five main elements (Figure 14.5). Use of the framework involves an iterative cycle whereby emerging lessons from program implementation and new research findings continuously inform program adjustments. Optimal application of the framework should be based on in-depth knowledge of the local community (tacit knowledge), expertise with relevant theories, and up-to-date familiarity with good quality research evidence (both primary studies and systematic and integrative reviews). We describe each element of the framework using the exemplar of preventing falls among older adults. Table 14.1 provides illustrative examples of data and research studies that are relevant to each element of the model.

Identify Health Issue, Burden of Illness, and Inequity Gaps

The first framework element involves identifying the community health issue that is the program focus. Epidemiological

and surveillance data are used to describe the current and shifting patterns of illness within the population. It is important to identify population subgroups that may be disadvantaged because they bear an unequal or inequitable burden of the health problem.

Describe Sociostructural Features

The second framework element involves describing the sociostructural features of the problem. This includes identifying factors that may be directly contributing to or causing the problem, or producing disparities in how the problem manifests or is experienced by different sub-populations. Since factors contributing to the problem are often present at more than one ecological system level, it is important to examine how these determinants are nested or interconnected and what determinants are deeply embedded in the system (e.g., racist policies). An analysis of strengths and capacities at different levels of the system may reveal potential solutions to the problem.

Several types of research inform this element of the framework. Etiological research examines putative causes of health problems. Both qualitative and quantitative studies may reveal the complex relationships among upstream determinants that perpetuate the problem. Laboratory studies may yield insights into biological and environmental factors that are having an

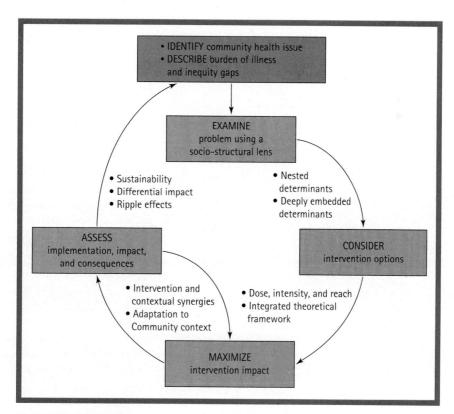

FIGURE 14.5 Multiple Intervention Program Framework

From "Programs of Research Within Programs of Research," by N. Edwards, in N. Edwards (Ed.) & S. Roelofs (Assistant Ed.), *Developing a Program of Research: An Essential Process for a Successful Research Career* (p. 223), 2018, Vancouver, Canada: CHNET Press. Copyright 2018 by Nancy Edwards. CC BY 4.0.

Table 14.1	Assembling the Research Evidence	
Element of Framework	**Types of Research Studies and Examples of Relevant Data**	**Examples from Research on Preventing Falls**
Burden of illness and inequity gaps	Epidemiological studies and surveillance systems provide data on prevalence and incidence of disease and injuries for population subgroups (e.g., age- and gender-specific rates of disease or injury).	*Burden of Illness:* One in three older adults falls each year. Approximately 25% of all falls result in injuries. Falls are the sixth leading cause of death among older adults in Canada. *Inequities:* Higher social inequalities are associated with an increased risk of falling among women (Syddall, Evancrou, Cooper, & Aihie Sayer, 2009).
Sociostructural and socioecological features of the problem	Etiological studies, laboratory studies, integrative reviews, and qualitative and quantitative studies provide insights on micro (individual, family) and meso (community and organizational) factors that are at play, while organizational and policy studies may reveal determinants that operate at a macro level.	Cumulative findings from individual studies and reviews (Gill, Williams, & Tinetti, 2000; Kearney, Harwood, Gladman, Lincoln, & Masud, 2013; Letts et al., 2010; Muir, Gopaul, & Montero Odasso, 2012) indicate that major risk factors for falls among community-dwelling older adults are: • Use of benzodiazepine sedative hypnotics • Polypharmacy (using four or more drugs) • Cognitive impairment • Problems with balance and peripheral neuromuscular dysfunction • Environmental hazards Qualitative and quantitative studies describe the perspectives of older adults on risk factors for falls and identify outcomes that are most important to them (e.g., loss of independence) (Grant, Edwards, Sveistrup, Andrews, & Egan, 2010; McInnes, Seers, & Tutton, 2011). Concept mapping indicates what aspects of the built and social environment influence older adults' outdoor walking (Hanson et al., 2013). Surveillance data identify the location of falls, and laboratory studies identify specific features of the built environment (e.g., configuration of grab bars, height of stairs, dimensions of handrails) that may interact with personal variables (e.g., poor balance, weak hand-grip strength) to increase the risk of falls (Guitard, Sveistrup, Lockett, & Edwards, 2011; King & Novak, 2017). Policy studies examine gaps in and the influence of policies in health and other sectors on the risk of falls (Edwards, 2017; Edwards et al., 2006; Grant, Andrews, Edwards, Sveistrup, & Egan, 2011; Yen & Anderson, 2012).

Table 14.1	Continued	
Element of Framework	**Types of Research Studies and Examples of Relevant Data**	**Examples from Research on Preventing Falls**
Intervention options	Efficacy and effectiveness studies, cost-effectiveness or cost–benefit studies, program evaluation, systematic reviews, best practice guideline documents, and studies that have tested mid-range theories yield evidence to inform intervention options.	Cochrane reviews and primary studies provide evidence of the efficacy, effectiveness, and efficiency of strategies to prevent falls and fall-related injuries (Frick, Kung, Parrish, & Narrett, 2010; Gillespie et al., 2012; Huang, Feng, Li, & Lv, 2017). Best practice guidelines for preventing falls (Registered Nurses' Association of Ontario, 2017) are informed by effectiveness studies.
Optimal blend of strategies	Effectiveness studies of multi-strategy and multi-level interventions. Studies informed by integrated theories and research. Studies that examine contextual influences on intervention strategies yield data on how intervention strategies may be synergistic (working together for positive effect) or antagonistic (working against each other for a poor outcome).	Evidence that multi-factor approaches are more effective in reducing falls than single strategies (Gillespie et al., 2012). Building-code policies have a sustained impact on the built environment due to the long lifespan of homes and other public buildings (Edwards, 2017). Age-friendly cities and aging-in-place policies provide opportunities for synergistic fall prevention programs.
Assess implementation, impact, and consequences	Potential indicators are identified with consideration given to any mandatory reporting requirements or pre-existing accountability frameworks. A **health impact assessment** can be used to examine the potential effects of a policy, including its anticipated impact on health disparities (McCallum, Ollson, & Stefanovic, 2015).	The Ontario Public Health Standards (Ministry of Health and Long-Term Care, 2008) include societal outcomes for injury prevention programs. The Ontario Health Equity Impact assessment tool (Ontario Ministry of Health and Long-Term Care, n.d.) is used to assess the potential for unintended differential impact of a program or policy on population subgroups.

impact on the problem, whereas organizational and policy studies may reveal determinants that operate at a meso or macro level. Individual primary studies may be useful, but systematic or integrative reviews that synthesize the best available evidence should be sought. Evidence on determinants is lined up with relevant ecological levels. (See Table 14.2.) In consultation with the community, priority levels for action are then selected based on community characteristics and knowledge of the policy context.

The nature or scope of different health issues may render some ecological levels more relevant than others. For instance, in the case of injury prevention, features of the built environment are likely to be a central concern, whereas with tobacco control, the accessibility of tobacco products, addiction, and social norms are particularly important. Furthermore, the level(s) of government (municipal, provincial, national, or self-governing) to target is determined by who has budgetary and policy jurisdiction over the problem.

Consider Intervention Options

The third element of the framework specifies intervention options. Here, we consider strategies that have demonstrated effectiveness and are theoretically sound. This knowledge must be coupled with community input on the feasibility of implementing interventions in their setting and the need to adapt interventions to ensure sociocultural and geographic relevance. For instance, while there is solid evidence of efficacy from laboratory studies (Laing & Robinovitch, 2008) and some evidence of effectiveness from studies with nursing home residents that hip protectors will reduce the risk of a hip fracture when a fall occurs, problems with compliance in using hip protectors have been reported (Gillespie, Gillespie, & Parker, 2010). Reasons for not using these protectors are related to the cost of purchasing them, inconvenience when busy nursing staff in long-term care settings have to help residents with dressing, perceptions of a socially unacceptable appearance if hip protectors are

Table 14.2	Socioecological Determinants of Falls among Older Adults
Levels of Socioecological Model	**Examples and References to Supporting Empirical Literature**
Individual	Perceptions of enablers or barriers to physical activity (Grant et al., 2010; Hanson et al., 2013)
	Perceptions of risk of falling (McInnes et al., 2011)
	Personal barriers to use of hip protectors (Blalock, Demby, McCulloch, & Stevens, 2010)
Interpersonal	Active on-line networks where neighbours and friends check on each other to see if anyone has had an injurious fall (Maher et al., 2014).
Community	Coalitions or other organized collectives taking action on preventing falls by raising awareness and addressing policy change (Edwards, 1999).
	Skilled volunteers available in the community to make home modifications such as installing handrails on stairs (Keall et al., 2015; Pega, Kvizhinadze, Blakely, Atkinson, & Wilson, 2016).
Built/Physical Environment	Universal access to grab bars in bathrooms (Aminzadeh, Edwards, Lockett, & Nair, 2001; Guitard et al., 2011)
	Older-adult-friendly, accessible, or walkable environments (Ontario Seniors' Secretariat, 2013; Grant et al., 2011)
Social Environment	Accessibility of esthetically pleasing and safe walking areas near older adults' homes (Grant et al., 2010)
	Intersections of built and social environment (Hanson, Ashe, McKay, & Winters, 2012)
Organizational Policy (e.g., workplace, places of worship, housing)	Organization policies in long-term care settings influencing physical activity (Benjamin, Edwards, Ploeg, & Legault, 2014)
Self-determining (e.g., First Nations) Community Programs and Policy	Access to provincial or federal programs to cover the cost of home modifications
Municipal Policy	Accessibility guidelines used for urban planning
Provincial Policy	Provincial building regulations for private and public housing
National Policy	Model building codes provided by National Research Council and uptake of empirical evidence in modifications to building codes (Edwards, 2017)

bulky under regular clothing, and hygiene problems for older adults with urge incontinence. These adherence factors reduce the effectiveness of hip protectors as a hip fracture reduction strategy.

A mix of studies is required to inform intervention choices. For example, etiological studies consistently indicate that the use of benzodiazepine sedative hypnotics is a risk factor for falls. This suggests that minimizing use of these medications would be a useful fall prevention strategy. For individuals planning a program, however, the question that arises is this: Who is the most effective target, the older adults who use these sedatives or physicians who prescribe the medication? Studies from the field of addictions indicate that it is difficult to wean an individual off this class of drugs following long-term use. However, studies that have targeted changes in prescribing practice suggest that academic detailers (e.g., representatives from pharmaceutical companies who directly market new drugs to physicians) and audit and feedback strategies are effective in modifying physician prescribing (Chhina et al., 2013). This combination of evidence indicates that a public health strategy targeting individual counselling for those who are taking benzodiazepines may be less likely to have a population impact than a public health strategy that either targets prescribing patterns among family physicians, discouraging the unnecessary initiation and long-term use of this class of drugs, or targets nurses and nurse practitioners to help older adult clients try new sleep hygiene strategies.

When selecting intervention options, planning teams also need to pay close attention to the reach, dose, and intensity of strategies that are required (Jilcott, Ammerman, Sommers, & Glasgow, 2007) to have their intended effect. The reach of an intervention concerns what proportion and which particular segments of an intended target population receive the interventions. For example, social marketing approaches (Luca & Suggs, 2013) such as public-service advertisements may be intended for all older adults but will only reach those who are watching television or listening to the radio when the advertisement is run and may not be understood by those who speak neither English nor French. The dose is the amount of intervention required to have an effect. Multiple exposures to a public-service announcement are required to change awareness. The intensity of the intervention refers to its quality and whether it is tailored to the targeted population subgroup. For instance, a media campaign about the importance of walking regularly may have adequate intensity for older adults who have good functional status but is unlikely to provide suitable messages for very frail older adults who are not independently mobile. A note of caution is important here. If strategies that appear promising are watered down due to funding constraints or other limitations on program delivery capacity, the dose and intensity required for the intervention to make a difference may be diluted, and the expected outcome is unlikely to be achieved.

Choosing strategies requires in-depth knowledge of the community characteristics that may influence uptake and effectiveness of the intervention strategies. The readiness and capacity of the community for the intended change is an important consideration that can best be gauged by community partners. The identification of policy windows and policy levers is also important (Kingdon, 1995). **Policy windows** are periods of opportunity to get an issue on the policy agenda. Policy windows may open because of a community crisis, mounting concern about a growing problem among the public and substantial press coverage on this issue, or a period of planned change such as the amalgamation of municipalities. These policy windows can create the momentum and public support required for policy change. Identifying policy levers requires an understanding of the ways in which different kinds of policies (e.g., community health nursing standards, or provincial legislation or bylaw enforcement policies) can be introduced or changed. It is important to involve individuals with expertise in policy change processes such as political science, public administration, or legal practices on your planning team.

In addition to evidence on what works and knowledge of the community, theoretical considerations should also drive the planning process. We are often inclined to apply theories most familiar to us, rather than theories most pertinent for the problem at hand. Since a multiple intervention approach tackles more than one level of the socioecological system (Edwards & Davison, 2015), a mix of theories is required to guide multiple intervention programs. This involves integrating theories from various disciplines (e.g., psychology, sociology, political science, health sciences) and involving individuals who know the theories well. Identifying a range of relevant theories may expand the intervention options to be considered.

Maximize Intervention Impact

The fourth framework element focuses on identifying an optimal set of intervention strategies for maximum impact. That is, how can we increase the likelihood that the combination of interventions works in a well-orchestrated fashion, and how can we adapt our interventions to both historical and contemporary contexts (Edwards & Di Ruggiero, 2011)? Sorting this out requires that we attend to the sequence and combination of strategies and to the ways in which the political, social,

organizational, and policy environments (contexts) are changing. The integrated theory that guides our program should inform decisions on how to blend intervention strategies. Since intervention strategies may work together positively or negatively, questions to consider when discussing how to optimize them include the following:

- What is a particular program trying to achieve, and how can we combine intervention strategies to potentiate this?
- Are there ways in which a particular combination of interventions might nullify each one's effects?
- What is going on in the community that might enhance or reduce the impact of the intervention?
- Who is likely to disproportionately benefit from or be disadvantaged by the program, and how can we mitigate unintended consequences?

Two examples of how selected interventions might be maximized are provided in Table 14.3. The first example, which involves using the media and a risk-counselling approach, illustrates how intervention strategies can be combined to potentiate their effect. The second example shows how a planned intervention strategy can be successfully combined with a contextual influence. Although programs have no direct control over contextual influences, anticipating those that may arise and making program adjustments to reflect contextual influences that do emerge may either enhance the planned intervention strategies or mitigate the influences of negative contextual changes.

Assess Implementation, Impact, and Consequences

In the final element, monitoring and evaluating program implementation; outputs, outcomes, impacts; and expected and unexpected consequences, including program spin-offs and sustainability, are the central concern. Outputs indicate that a program is being implemented as planned. Identifying output indicators involves looking at the critical steps required for the program. For instance, initiating partnerships with other community organizations, engaging community members in a coalition, and getting a health issue on a political agenda would be relevant indicators to assess progress toward ultimately achieving policy change. Outcomes are medium-term changes that can be attributed to the program. Changes in knowledge, attitudes, and behaviours among the target population would be anticipated at several levels. In the case of fall prevention, these outcomes would be assessed among older adults, health professionals (e.g., prescribing practices, assessing patients' risk profile for falls), and individuals responsible for policy change (e.g., awareness of existing policies that increase risk for falls). Impacts are the longer-term results of a program, often taking some years to achieve. As with outputs and outcomes, impacts may be assessed at various ecological levels. Thus, you might expect to see impact indicators of individual health status changes, shifts in social norms, changes to the built environment, or policy change, all depending on the original intent of the program. The impact of a program is rarely uniform.

Table 14.3	Theory Integration to Maximize Interventions	
Examples of Intervention Strategies and Intended Effect	**Underlying Theory and Research to Support Plan for Intervention Strategies**	**Maximize Intervention Impact**
Media campaign to raise awareness about the risk of hazardous stairs and volunteer program to encourage older adults to take action to improve safety of home stairs.	Social marketing theory (Luca & Suggs, 2013), media communication studies (van de Belt et al., 2013), and stages of change theory (Prochaska & Velicer, 1997) indicate that a media campaign can shift a segment of the population from precontemplation to contemplation in a short interval (days or weeks).	Media campaign should be timed to coincide with accessible options for action, such as a help line for older adults to call to obtain volunteer assistance to make modifications to stairs (e.g., installation of handrails).
Collective action by a fall prevention coalition may increase community awareness of the importance of bathroom grab bars and can be used in combination with input to technical committees responsible for reviewing building codes.	Collective action, using participatory principles, is an essential component of programs informed by community development theories (Burke et al., 2013). This approach builds on strengths and resources within the community to promote co-learning and action for the mutual benefit of all stakeholders. Kingdon's (1995) political-science theory on agenda setting indicates that public opinion is a critical influence in the policy change process, both with respect to creating a demand for the change and providing the support necessary for either introducing a new policy or modifying one that already exists.	Effective and strategic application of Kingdon's (1995) theory by a coalition requires an understanding of how the cycles of revising and adopting building codes work, how public input on proposed changes is obtained, and whether other key stakeholders such as the home-building industry support or oppose proposed changes to the codes. The action by fall prevention coalitions through this process will require timely interventions to (a) mobilize public awareness and support, (b) work with key stakeholders to mobilize action by them, and (c) network with other coalitions.

Therefore, consider disaggregating indicators by gender and socioeconomic status to examine disparities in program access or effectiveness.

The selection of impact indicators should be guided by what we know about effective interventions and the "dose" of intervention expected to achieve a particular effect. Programs that are overly ambitious may appear ineffective because their resources are spread too thin. When program managers cannot demonstrate an improvement in program outputs or outcomes, ongoing funding for the program may be threatened. Impact indicators for a multiple intervention program are illustrated in Canadian Research 14.1.

Spin-offs are unintended effects of a program. They may be positive or negative. Ongoing community consultation may provide the first hints of such spin-offs. Formalized plans to assess spin-offs are rare. However, spin-offs may be identified through reflective approaches such as the maintenance of field notes during program implementation or team meeting discussions regarding observed spin-offs, and via mid- or end-of-program interviews with individuals who have participated in the program.

Sustainability concerns the longer-term viability of program interventions (Stirman et al., 2012). Evidence of

CANADIAN RESEARCH 14.1

Two-generation preschool program: Immediate and seven-year-old outcomes for low-income children and their parents. (Benzies et al., 2014)

Poverty and its sequelae are important determinants of health, and their impact is perhaps most injurious for young children and their families. Lack of school readiness and parenting stress may be associated with poverty, inadequate housing, and unemployment. Early interventions can offset these health effects.

This two-generation program is aimed at the needs of low-income preschool children and their parents. Program interventions included early childhood education (20 hours per week provided by the centre), parenting and life skills education (designed and implemented on-site by program staff), and family support provided by a registered social worker during home visits. This MIP was offered to families at no cost. A single group pretest (program intake) and post-test (at program exit) with follow-up (when children were seven years old) design was used to evaluate outcomes. Bioecological theory guided the evaluation. In total,

132 children and 79 parents enrolled in the study. At the time of the study's publication, 95 children who had provided both intake and exit data had reached seven years of age and were eligible to participate in the follow-up portion of the study. Sixty-seven parents (of 79) completed intake and exit data collection, and 38 parents provided data at all three time points.

Parents completed a parenting stress index, community life skills scale, self-esteem scale, and a scale measuring attitudes associated with child maltreatment. Measures were self-completed at the outset of their enrolment in the program, following program completion, and when their child was seven years old. In the portion of the study examining child outcomes, intake and exit data were collected from 109 (of 132) children. Data from all three time points were available for 60 children. A research assistant assessed children's receptive language skills using the Peabody Picture Vocabulary Test and their global development using the Battelle Developmental Inventory-Screening Test at all three time points. Study participants' results were compared to standardized scores for their age or grade.

Parents reported positive differences in self-esteem, use of community resources, parental distress, and parenting attitudes related to corporal punishment and appropriate parent–child roles. Moreover, at seven years, parental distress had continued to decrease. The preschool children demonstrated a statistically significant improvement in receptive language skills that was sustained at age seven. Children's global development scores improved during the program, and improvements in communication, motor, and personal-social domains were sustained up to age seven years. Findings suggest that appropriate and timely supports and services for low-income families can reduce the negative impact of their economic pressures.

Discussion Questions

1. How does poverty affect children living in low-income families?

2. What are the strengths and limitations of the research design used to assess the impact of this program?

3. Were the evaluation measures used examples of output, outcome, or impact indicators?

CASE STUDY

Rachelle is the public health nurse providing pre- and postnatal visits with pregnant and parenting women at an outreach centre for young single parents. The outreach centre is a "one stop" location where mothers under the age of 25 can access health, educational, and social services. Over the past five years, Rachelle and other staff at the centre have noted an increase in the proportion of young pregnant women attending services at the centre who have been diagnosed with, or exhibit symptoms of, mood disorders (e.g., depression, anxiety) or have experienced traumatic childhoods (e.g., violence in the home, parent with addictions). Most of the outreach centre's programming focuses on promoting healthy behaviours, prenatal education, and good parenting practices. Rachelle is concerned about the lack of resources to address the mental health of the young mothers currently accessing the centre's services.

Discussion Questions

1. At what stage in the planning–implementation–evaluation cycle are Rachelle and her colleagues in their work at the outreach centre?

2. Which community partners should be included in the planning–implementation–evaluation cycle, and how can Rachelle engage them?

3. Using a socioecological framework to guide your approach, what sources of literature and community data might help you develop an intervention plan?

---

sustainability at an organizational level may occur when an intervention becomes part of the routine. For instance, the introduction of a new assessment form during a program may become routine when this form becomes part of standard data collection within the agency. Sustainability at a policy level may occur when a policy is established and enforcement strategies are routinely put in place. Sustainability does not necessarily refer to the ongoing funding of a program; nor does it infer that a program will be organized the way it started out or was run by the same organization. Rather, the intent of sustainability is to continue addressing the problem and to evolve strategies to match how the problem is changing.

CONCLUSION

CHNs are key players in health program delivery and must also be integral to the dynamic process of program planning and evaluation. Familiarity with the tools and processes described in this chapter will help you contribute fully as a member of a program planning and evaluation team. As our examples have illustrated, community health programs are often aimed at community issues with a complex set of underlying sociostructural determinants. It is not surprising that the planning process needs to be informed by a diverse set of data and evidence and by a community consultation process. Planning and evaluation should not occur in isolation. Rather, you must pull together an interdisciplinary team with a wide range of experience to help with different facets of this process. By working together, CHNs with program planning experience, academic researchers who are familiar with the theoretical and empirical literature, and community partners who bring important insights and essential experiential learning can substantially strengthen the design and evaluation of MIPs in community health. This in turn will help us meet the complex needs of populations and close the disparity gaps in health status that persist while demonstrating better accountability for the public funds used when programs are delivered.

KEY TERMS

CAT (components, activities, and target groups) (p. 273)

content analysis (p. 274)

Gantt charts (p. 276)

health impact assessment (p. 281)

meta-analysis (p. 275)

Multiple Intervention Program (MIP) framework (p. 278)

planning–implementation–evaluation cycle (p. 272)

policy windows (p. 283)

population health approach (p. 277)

precede-proceed planning model (p. 274)

program evaluation tool kit (p. 273)

program logic model (p. 272)

SOLO (short-term outcomes and long-term outcomes) (p. 273)

spin-offs (p. 284)

sustainability (p. 284)

SWOT (strengths, weaknesses, opportunities, and threats) analysis (p. 274)

STUDY QUESTIONS

1. Are the steps in the planning–implementation–evaluation cycle always followed in a linear fashion? Explain.

2. List four factors that influence the choice of a program planning and evaluation framework.

3. Identify some tools commonly used in planning programs.

4. List three uses of quantitative data in planning and evaluating a program.

5. Identify the three principles of priority setting.

6. List the five main elements of the MIP framework.

INDIVIDUAL CRITICAL-THINKING EXERCISES

1. Your health care agency is collaborating with a community advocacy group to address escalating substance use among youth aged 12 to 17. What are some of the underlying sociostructural determinants of substance abuse in this age group?

2. Using the same substance abuse problem, what types of evidence would you assemble to support the development of the program plan, and why?

3. What are the strengths and weaknesses of each type of evidence you have selected for the substance abuse problem?

4. What are some examples of indicators you can use to assess the impact of the substance abuse program at the individual, organization, community, and policy levels?

5. Identify a community health issue of interest. What are some examples of synergies that might be expected to occur between program strategies and community context?

GROUP CRITICAL-THINKING EXERCISES

1. You are part of a team evaluating a childhood obesity program delivered through the local schools. What information would you need to develop a logic model for this initiative? Describe to the members of your team why it is important to spend time developing the logic model.

2. Locate a good example of a community health program plan that illustrates the integration of several different theories. Do these theories reflect different levels of a socioecological model?

3. You have been asked to develop a multiple intervention program and evaluation plan to address homelessness among older adults. What community partners would you involve in this process, and why? How would you get community partners involved?

REFERENCES

Aery, A. (2017). *Innovations to champion access to primary care for immigrants and refugees.* Retrieved from Think Piece of Wellesley Institute website: http://www.wellesleyinstitute.com/wp-content/uploads/2017/03/Innovations-to-champion-access-to-primary-care-for-immigrant-and-refugees.pdf

Aminzadeh, F., Edwards, N., Lockett, D., & Nair, R. C. (2001). Utilization of bathroom safety devices, patterns of bathing and toileting, and bathroom falls in a sample of community living older adults. *Technology and Disability, 13*(2), 95–103.

Angeles, R. M., Dolovich, L., Kaczorowsk, J., & Thabane, L. (2013). Developing a theoretical framework for complex community-based interventions. *Health Promotion Practice 14*(5), 100–108. doi:10.1177/1524839913483469

Bauman, K. E., Suchindran, C. M., & Murray, D. M. (1999). The paucity of effects in community trials: Is secular trend the culprit? *Preventive Medicine, 28*(4), 426–429.

Benjamin, K., Edwards, N., Ploeg, J., & Legault, F. (2014). Barriers to physical activity and restorative care for residents in long-term care homes: A review of the literature. *Journal of Aging and Physical Activity, 22*(1), 154–165.

Benzies, K., Mychasiuk, R., Kurilova, J., Tough, S., Edwards, N., & Donnelly, C. (2014). Two-generation preschool programme: Immediate and 7-year-old outcomes for low-income children and their parents. *Child & Family Social Work, 19*(2), 203–214. doi:10.1111/j.1365-2206.2012.00894.x

Bilge, S. (2010). Recent feminist outlooks on intersectionality. *Diogenes, 57*(1), 58–72. doi:10.1177/0392192110374245

Blalock, S. J., Demby, K. B., McCulloch, K. L., & Stevens, J. A. (2010). Factors influencing hip protector use among community-dwelling older adults. *Injury Prevention, 16*(4), 235–239.

Burke, J. G., Hess, S., Hoffmann, K., Guizzetti, L., Loy, E., Gielen, A., & Yonas, M. (2013). Translating community-based participatory research principles into practice. *Progress in Community Health Partnerships: Research, Education, and Action, 7*(2), 115–122.

Chhina, H. K., Bhole, V. M., Goldsmith, C., Hall, W., Kaczorowski, J., & Lacaille, D. (2013). Effectiveness of academic detailing to optimize medication prescribing behaviour of family physicians. *Journal of Pharmacy & Pharmaceutical Sciences, 16*(4), 511–529.

Collins, P. H., & Bilge, S. (2016). *Intersectionality.* Cambridge, MA: Polity Press.

Commission on Social Determinants of Health. (2008). *Closing the gap in a generation: Health equity through action on the social determinants of health. Final report of the Commission of Social Determinants on Health.* Geneva, CH: World Health Organization.

COMMIT Research Group. (1995a). Community intervention trial for smoking cessation. (COMMIT). I: Cohort results from a four-year community intervention. *American Journal of Public Health, 85*(2), 183–192.

COMMIT Research Group. (1995b). Community intervention trial for smoking cessation. (COMMIT). II: Changes in adult cigarette smoking prevalence. *American Journal of Public Health, 85*(2), 193–200.

Community Health Nurses of Canada. (2019, revised). *Canadian community health nursing: Professional practice model & standards of practice.* Retrieved from https://www.chnc.ca/en/standards-of-practice

Creswell, J. W., & Poth, C. N. (2018). *Qualitative inquiry and research design. Choosing among five approaches* (4th ed.). Thousand Oaks, CA: Sage.

Crosby, R., & Noar, S. M. (2011). What is a planning model? An introduction to PRECEDE-PROCEED. *Journal of Public Health Dentistry, 71*(S1), S7–S15. doi:10.1111/j.1752-7325.2011.00235.x

Edwards, N. (1999). Prevention of falls among seniors in the community. In M. Stewart (Ed.), *Community nursing: Promoting Canadians' health* (2nd ed., pp. 296–316). Toronto, ON: W. B. Saunders.

Edwards, N. (2017). Knowledge translation for intersectoral action: The case of Canada's building codes. In I. L. Bourgeault, R. Labonte, C. Packer, & V. Runnels (Eds.), *Population health in Canada: Issues, research, and action.* Toronto, ON: Canada Scholars Press.

Edwards, N. (2018). Programs of research within programs of research. In N. Edwards (Ed.) & S. Roelofs (Assistant Ed.), *Developing a program of research: An essential process for a successful research career.* Vancouver, BC: CHNET Press.

Edwards, N., Birkett, N., Nair, R., Murphy, M., Roberge, G., & Lockett, D. (2006). Access to bathtub grab bars: Evidence of a policy gap. *Canadian Journal on Aging, 25*(3), 295–304.

Edwards, N., & Davison, C. (2008). Social justice and core competencies for public health: Improving the fit. *Canadian Journal of Public Health, 99*(2), 130–132.

Edwards, N., & Davison, C. (2015). Strengthening communities with a socio-ecological approach: Local and international lessons in whole systems. In L. K. Hallstrom, N. Guehlstorf, & M. Parkes (Eds.), *Ecosystems, society and health: Pathways through diversity, convergence and integration.* Montreal/Kingston, ON: McGill Queen's University Press.

Edwards, N., & Di Ruggiero, E. (2011). Exploring which context matters in the study of health inequities and their mitigation. *Scandinavian Journal of Public Health, 39*(Suppl. 6), 43–49.

Edwards, N., MacLean, L., Estable, A., & Meyer, M. (2006). *Multiple intervention program recommendations for Mandatory Health Program and Services Guidelines Technical Review Committees.* Ottawa, ON: Community Health Research Unit, University of Ottawa.

Edwards, N., Mill, J., & Kothari, A. (2004). Multiple intervention research programs in community health. *Canadian Journal of Nursing Research, 36*(1), 40–54.

Edwards, N., & Moyer, A. (1999). Community needs and capacity assessment: Critical component of program planning. In M. Stewart (Ed.), *Community nursing: Promoting Canadians' health* (2nd ed., pp. 420–442). Toronto, ON: W. B. Saunders.

Frick, K. D., Kung, J. Y., Parrish, J. M., & Narrett, M. J. (2010). Evaluating the cost-effectiveness of fall prevention programs that reduce fall-related hip fractures in older adults. *Journal of the American Geriatric Society, 58*(1), 136–141.

Fuller-Thomson, E., Noack, A.M., & George, U. (2011). Health decline among recent immigrants to Canada: Findings from a nationally-representative longitudinal survey. *Canadian Journal of Public Health, 102*(4), 273–280. https://doi.org/10.17269/cjph.102.2423

Gill, T., Williams, C., & Tinetti, M. (2000). Environmental hazards and the risk of nonsyncopal falls in the homes of community-living older persons. *Medical Care, 38*(12), 1174–1183.

Gillespie, L. D., Robertson, M. C., Gillespie, W. J., Sherrington, C., Gates, S., Clemson, L. M., & Lamb, S. E. (2012). Interventions for preventing falls in older people living in the community. *Cochrane Database of Systematic Reviews, 12*(9), CD007146. © 2015, Cochrane Collaboration. Reproduced with permission of Wiley Publishing Inc.

Gillespie, W. J., Gillespie, L. D., & Parker, M. J. (2010). Hip protectors for preventing hip fractures in older people. *Cochrane Database of Systematic Reviews, 10,* Art. No.: CD001255.

Grant, T., Andrews, C., Edwards, N., Sveistrup, H., & Egan, M. (2011). Creating walkable places: Neighbourhood and municipal level perspectives on the socio-political process in Ottawa, Canada. *Journal of Urbanism, 4*(1), 81–104.

Grant, T., Edwards, N., Sveistrup, H., Andrews, C., & Egan, M. (2010). Neighbourhood walkability: Older people's perspectives from four neighbourhoods in Ottawa, Canada. *Journal of Aging and Physical Activity, 18*(2), 293–312.

Guruge, S., & Butt, H. (2015). A scoping review of mental health issues and concerns among immigrant and refugee youth in Canada: Looking back, moving forward. *Canadian Journal of Public Health, 106*(2), E72. doi: 10.17269/CJPH.106.4588

Guitard, P., Sveistrup, H., Lockett, D., & Edwards, N. (2011). Use of different bath grab bar configurations following a balance perturbation. *Assistive Technology, 23*(4), 205–215.

Hanson, H. M., Ashe, M. C., McKay, H. A., & Winters, M. (2012). *Intersection between the built and social environments and older adults' mobility: An evidence review.* Retrieved from http://ncceh.ca/sites/default/files/Built_and_Social_Environments_Older_Adults_Nov_2012.pdf

Hanson, H. M., Schiller, C., Winters, M., Sims-Gould, J., Clarke, P., Curran, E., . . . & Ashe, M. C. (2013). Concept mapping applied to the intersection between older adults' outdoor walking and the built and social environments. *Preventive medicine, 57*(6), 785–791.

Health Canada. (2001). *The population health template: Key elements and actions that define a population health approach.* Strategic Policy Directorate of the Population and Public Health Branch, Health Canada. Retrieved from http://www.phac-aspc.gc.ca/ph-sp/pdf/overview_handout_black-eng.pdf

Health Quality Ontario. (2016). *Measuring up 2016: A yearly report on how Ontario's health system is performing.* Retrieved from http://www.hqontario.ca/portals/0/Documents/pr/measuring-up-2016-en.pdf

Helms, M. M., & Nixon, J. (2010). Exploring SWOT analysis—where are we now? A review of academic research from the last decade. *Journal of Strategy and Management, 3*(3), 215–251.

Higginbottom, G., & Safipour, J. (2015). Access to primary health care by new and established immigrants in Canada. *Journal of Family Medicine & Community Health, 2*(5), 1–7.

Huang, Z. G., Feng, Y. H., Li, Y. H., & Lv, C. S. (2017). Systematic review and meta-analysis: Tai Chi for preventing falls in older adults. *BMJ Open, 7*(2), e013661.

Jilcott, S., Ammerman, A., Sommers, J., & Glasgow, R. E. (2007). Applying the RE-AIM framework to assess the public health impact of policy change. *Annals of Behavioural Medicine, 34*, 105–114.

Keall, M. D., Pierse, N., Howden-Chapman, P., Cunningham, C., Cunningham, M., Guria, J., & Baker, M. G. (2015). Home modifications to reduce injuries from falls in the Home Injury Prevention Intervention (HIPI) study: A cluster-randomised controlled trial. *Lancet, 385*(9964), 231–238. doi: 10.1016/S0140-6736(14)61006-0

Kearney, F. C., Harwood, R. H., Gladman, J. R., Lincoln, N., & Masud, T. (2013). The relationship between executive function and falls and gait abnormalities in older adults: A systematic review. *Dementia, Geriatric and Cognitive Disorders, 36*(1–2), 20–35.

King, E. C., & Novak, A. C. (2017). Effect of bathroom aids and age on balance control during bathing transfers. *American Journal of Occupational Therapy, 71*(6), 7106165030p1-7106165030p9.

Kingdon, J. W. (1995). *Agendas, alternatives, and public policies* (2nd ed.). New York, NY: Addison-Wesley.

Laing, A. C., & Robinovitch, S. N. (2008). The force attenuation provided by hip protectors depends on impact velocity, pelvic size and soft tissues stiffness. *Journal of Biomechanical Engineering, 130*(6), 061005. doi:10.1115/1.2979867

Letts, L., Moreland, J., Richardson, J., Coman, L., Edwards, M., Ginis, K. M., . . . Wishart, L. (2010). The physical environment as a fall risk factor in older adults: Systematic review and meta-analysis of cross-sectional and cohort studies. *Australian Occupational Therapy Journal, 57*(1), 51–64.

Luca, N. R., & Suggs, L. S. (2013). Theory and model use in social marketing health interventions. *Journal of Health Communication, 18*(1), 20–40.

Maher, C. A., Lewis, L. K., Ferrar, K., Marshall, S., De Bourdeaudhuij, I., & Vandelanotte, C. (2014). Are health behavior change interventions that use online social networks effective? A systematic review. *Journal of medical Internet Research, 16*(2).

Mays, N., Pope, C., & Popay, J. (2005). Systematically reviewing qualitative and quantitative evidence to inform management and policy-making in the health field. *Journal of Health Services Research & Policy, 10*(S1), 6–20.

McCallum, L. C., Ollson, C. A., & Stefanovic, I. L. (2015). Advancing the practice of health impact assessment in Canada: Obstacles and opportunities. *Environmental Impact Assessment Review, 55*, 98–109.

McInnes, E., Seers, K., & Tutton, L. J. (2011). Older people's views in relation to risk of falling and need for intervention: A meta-ethnography. *Journal of Advanced Nursing, 67*(12), 2525–2536.

Merzel, D., & D'Afflitti, J. (2003). Reconsidering community-based health promotion: Promise, performance, and potential. *American Journal of Public Health, 93*(4), 557–574.

Mill, J. E., Edwards, N., Jackson, R. C., MacLean, L., & Chaw-Kant, J. (2010). Stigmatization as a social control mechanism for persons living with HIV and AIDS. *Qualitative Health Research, 20*(11), 1469–1483.

Miles, M. B., Huberman, A. M., & Saldana, J. (2014). *Qualitative data analysis: A methods sourcebook* (3rd ed.). Thousand Oaks, CA: Sage.

Ministry of Health and Long-Term Care. (2008). *Ontario public health standards 2008.* Retrieved from http://www.health.gov.on.ca/en/pro/programs/publichealth/oph_standards/docs/ophs_2008.pdf

Moser, A., & Korstjens, I. (2017). Series: Practical guidance to qualitative research. Part 3: Sampling, data collection and analysis. *European Journal of General Practice, 24*(1), 9–18. doi: 10.1080/13814788.2017.1375091

Morestin, F., & Castonguay, J. (2013). *Constructing a logic model for a healthy public policy: Why and how?* Retrieved from http://www.ncchpp.ca/172/publications.ccnpps?id_article=898

Muir, S. W., Gopaul, K., & Montero Odasso, M. M. (2012). The role of cognitive impairment in fall risk among older adults: A systematic review and meta-analysis. *Age and Ageing, 41*(3), 299–308. doi:10.1093/ageing/afs012

National Collaborating Centre for Methods and Tools. (2010). *Program evaluation toolkit.* Hamilton, ON: McMaster University. Retrieved from http://www.nccmt.ca/registry/view/eng/68.html

Ontario Centre of Excellence for Child and Youth Mental Health. (2013). *The road to data collection.* Retrieved from http://www.excellenceforchildandyouth.ca/sites/default/files/docs/webinars/_attach/road_to_data_collection_presentation_02092012.pdf

Ontario Ministry of Health and Long-Term Care. (n.d.). *Health equity impact assessment (HEIA).* Retrieved from the Ministry of Health and Long-Term Care website: http://www.health.gov.on.ca/en/pro/programs/heia

Ontario Seniors' Secretariat. (2013). *Independence, activity, and good health: Ontario's action plan for seniors.* Retrieved from http://www.oacao.org/images/ontarioseniorsaction-plan-en.pdf

Patton, M. Q. (2015). The nature, niche, value, and fruit of qualitative inquiry. In M. Q. Patton, *Qualitative research & evaluation methods* (4th ed., pp. 2–13). Thousand Oaks, CA: Sage.

Pega, F., Kvizhinadze, G., Blakely, T., Atkinson, J., & Wilson, N. (2016). Home safety assessment and modification to reduce injurious falls in community-dwelling older adults:

Cost-utility and equity analysis. *Injury prevention, 22*(6), 420–426. doi: 10.1136/injuryprev-2016-041999

Pope, C., & Mays, N. (2013). *Qualitative research in health care.* Toronto, ON: John Wiley & Sons.

Porteous, N., Sheldrick, B., & Stewart, P. (2002). Introducing program teams to logic models: Facilitating the learning process. *The Canadian Journal of Program Evaluation, 17*(3), 113–141.

Prochaska, J. O., & Velicer, W. F. (1997). The transtheoretical model of health behaviour change. *American Journal of Health Promotion, 12*(1), 38–48.

Public Health Agency of Canada (PHAC). (2008). Tool kit decision-oriented model for program evaluation.

Raphael, D. (2016). *Social determinants of health: Canadian perspectives* (3rd ed.). Canadian Scholars' Press.

Registered Nurses' Association of Ontario. (2017). *Preventing falls and reducing injury from falls* (3rd ed.). Toronto, ON: Registered Nurses' Association of Ontario.

Shiell, A., Hawe, P., & Gold, L. (2008). Complex interventions or complex systems? Implications for health economic evaluation. *British Medical Journal, 336*(7656), 1281–1283.

Sorenson, G., Emmons, K., Hunt, J. K., & Johnston, D. (1998). Implications of the results of community intervention trials. *Annual Review of Public Health, 19*, 379–416.

Stalmeijer, R., McNaughton, N., & Vanmook, W., & Walthern, N. (2014). Using focus groups in medical education research: AMEE Guide No. 91. *Medical Teacher, 36*, 923–939.

Stirman, S. W., Kimberly, J., Cook, N., Calloway, A., Castro, F., & Charns, M. (2012). The sustainability of new programs and innovations: A review of the empirical literature and recommendations for future research. *Implementation Science, 7*(17), 1–16.

Subedi, R. P., & Rosenberg, M. W. (2014). Determinants of the variations in self-reported health status among recent and more established immigrants in Canada. *Social Science & Medicine, 115*, 103–110. https://doi.org/10.1016/j.socscimed.2014.06.021

Syddall, H., Evandrou, M., Cooper, C., & Aihie Sayer, A. J. (2009). Social inequalities in grip strength, physical function, and falls among community dwelling older men and women. *Journal of Aging, 21*(6), 913–939.

Trochim, W. M. K. (2006). *The research methods knowledge base* (2nd ed.). Retrieved from http://www.socialresearchmethods.net/kb/pecycle.php

Truth and Reconciliation Commission of Canada. (2016). *TRC final report.* Retrieved from http://www.trc.ca/websites/trcinstitution/index.php?p=890

van de Belt, T. H., Engelen, L. J., Berben, S. A., Teerenstra, S., Samsom, M., & Schoonhoven, L. (2013). Internet and social media for health-related information and communication in health care: Preferences of the Dutch general population. *Journal of Medical Internet Research, 15*(10), e220.

Weir, E., d'Entremont, N., Stalker, S., Kurji, K., & Robinson, V. (2009). Applying the balanced scorecard to local public health performance measurement: Deliberations and decisions. *BMC Public Health, 9*(1), 127.

Whittemore, R., & Knafl, K. (2005). The integrative review: Updated methodology. *Journal of Advanced Nursing, 52*(5), 546–553.

Wilson-Mitchell, K. (2014). Increasing access to prenatal care: Disease prevention and sound business practice. *Health care for women international, 35*(2), 120–126. https://doi.org/10.1080/07399332.2013.810221

Woodgate, R. L., Busolo, D. S., Crockett, M., Dean, R, A., Amalada, M. R & Plour, P. J. (2017). A qualitative study on African immigrant and refugee families' experiences of accessing primary health care services in Manitoba, Canada: "It's not easy." *International Journal for Equity in Health, 16,* 1. https://doi.org/10.1186/s12939-016-0510-x

Wooten, K. C., Rose, R. M., Ostir, G. V., Calhoun, W. J., Ameredes, B. T., & Braiser, A. R. (2014). Assessing and evaluating multidisciplinary translational teams: A mixed methods approach. *Evaluation & the Health Professions 37*(1), 33–49. doi:10.1177/0163278713504433

Yen, I. H., & Anderson, L. A. (2012). Built environment and mobility of older adults: Important policy and practice efforts. *Journal of the American Geriatrics Society, 60*(5), 951–956.

Zanna, M., Cameron, R., Goldsmith, C. H., Poland, B., Lindsay, E., & Walker, R. (1994). Critique of the COMMIT study based on the Brantford experience. *Health and Canadian Society, 2*(2), 319–336.

ABOUT THE AUTHORS

Nancy Edwards, RN, PhD, is Professor Emeritus and Distinguished Professor at the University of Ottawa, School of Nursing. Nancy's research program examines multiple interventions in community health.

Josephine Etowa, RN, PhD, is Professor and Loyer-DaSilva Research Chair in Public Health Nursing at the University of Ottawa, School of Nursing. Her research is in the area of community health, inequity in health, and health care.

The authors would like to acknowledge and thank Wendy Peterson, RN, PhD, and Margaret Ann Kennedy, RN, PhD, for their important contributions to earlier editions of this chapter.

CHAPTER 15

Digital Health

Linda Ferguson and Tracie Risling

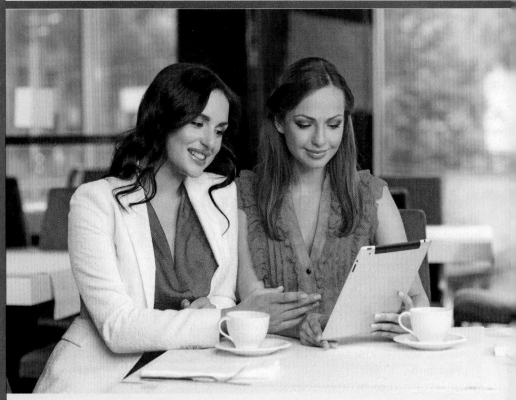

Source: BlueSkyImages/Fotolia

INTRODUCTION

Exponential growth has occurred in the use of internet-based **information and communication technologies (ICTs)** by health professionals and the public. The term "ICT" represents a variety of computer-based technology systems that support gathering, analyzing, archiving, retrieving, processing, and transmitting information and communication. ICTs can empower people to increase control over their health through allowing access to health information, providing social support, facilitating behaviour change, and supporting community mobilization. Primary health care nursing service delivery can be improved through the use of innovative, interactive e-health interventions that are tailored to individual needs. Hebda and Czar (2013) defined **e-health** as a "wide range of health care activities involving the electronic transfer of health-related information on the Internet" (p. 578). **Telehealth** is defined as "the use of telecommunications technologies and electronic information to exchange health care information and to provide and support services such as long distance clinical health care to clients" (Hebda & Czar, 2013, p. 505). Now most commonly referred to as **digital health**, the inclusion of ICTs into patient or client care can assist individuals to track, manage, and improve their health (Topol, 2013). There has been a rapid expansion of digital health application in the last decade. Canada Health Infoway (2015) reported that 72% of family physicians are referring their patients to websites for information about their health care and lifestyle.

Where the integration of ICTs into nursing was once seen as a specific strategy (Canadian Nurses Association [CNA], 2006), nursing informatics is now an essential component of nursing practice in all settings, including community health nursing. **Nursing informatics** is defined in broad terms as the use of information and computer technology to support all aspects of nursing practice, including direct delivery of care, administration, research, and education (Hebda & Czar, 2013). Using the concept of **digitally connected health**, ICTs are used to empower nurses and assist the Canadian health care system to more effectively meet patient needs and ultimately to achieve a primary health care focus (Topol, 2013). The ability of nursing informatics to extend the reach of care is evident in the endorsement of this science as a means "to promote the health of people, families, and communities worldwide" (CNA & Canadian Nursing Informatics Association [CNIA], 2017, p. 1).

The use of nursing informatics can support community health nurses (CHNs) to promote health, prevent illness, enable consultations, educate clients and families, provide service, provide therapy, and support and manage chronic disease. CHNs are expected to meet the Canadian Community Health Nursing standards of practice (Community Health Nurses of Canada [CHNC], 2019, revised), which include specific standards related to nursing informatics. (See Appendix A for the full list of standards.)

In this chapter, you will learn about CHN competencies as they relate to nursing informatics and gain an overview of current research on digital health. You will explore innovations in technology that have shown potential to support health promotion, disease prevention, chronic disease management, and health-related communication. Finally, you will be introduced to ICTs that support professional development and knowledge exchange in community health nursing.

NURSING INFORMATICS COMPETENCIES

Canada Health Infoway (www.infoway-inforoute.ca) is an organization that supports transformation of health care in Canada through the appropriate use of information technology. Canadian Health Infoway is a federally supported organization that facilitates the implementation of health information systems needed to manage Canadians' health and health care information. The organization provides support for clients, health care providers (HCPs), health care managers, and organizations.

Canada Health Infoway supported the Canadian Association of Schools of Nursing (CASN) in identifying expected ICT competencies of graduates of baccalaureate nursing programs (Canadian Association of Schools of Nursing [CASN], 2012) and providing strategies and a toolkit to facilitate the teaching of such competencies (CASN, 2013; 2014). The overarching competency is the use of ICTs to support information synthesis in accordance with professional and regulatory standards in the delivery of patient or client care. Entry-to-practice competencies of ICT have been highlighted in three distinct areas:

1. uses relevant information and knowledge to support delivery of evidence-informed patient/client care;

2. uses ICTs in accordance with professional and regulatory standards and workplace policies; and,

3. uses ICTs in the delivery of patient/client care.

These informatics competencies build on foundational aspects of existing registered nursing professional standards and expectations, such as these CASN (2014) public health competencies:

1. applies health literacy when working with clients;

2. uses social media, community resources, and social marketing techniques appropriately to disseminate health information;

3. documents population health nursing activities; and

4. uses appropriate communication techniques to influence decision makers.

Because of their importance to the health of nations, national-level nursing informatics competencies are being developed in a number of countries by a number of prestigious agencies such as the Centre for Disease Control and Prevention in the United States (Borycki, Foster, Sahama, Frisch, & Kushniruk, 2013; Husting & Gadsden-Knowles, 2011).

Public health informatics is defined as "the systematic application of information and computer sciences and technology to public health practice, research and learning" (Hebda & Czar, 2013). This definition reflects a public health perspective on disease surveillance and management, with an emphasis on population health. The Canadian Community Health Nursing Standards of Practice are based on the principles of primary health care that include the appropriate use of technology and resources, specifically Standard 7, Professional Responsibility and Accountability. The standard states that CHNs are expected to identify variety of information sources and determine which information sources are reliable to support nursing practice (CHNC, 2019, revised). The Canadian Nursing Informatics Association (www.cnia.ca) and the Canadian Nurses Association have also made recommendations concerning basic internet and computer competencies of nursing graduates (CNA & CNIA, 2017). The Canadian Nursing Informatics Association identified a need to build strong links between nursing informatics and evidence-based practice; increase informatics skills of educators, clinicians, and students; identify how informatics is covered in curricula; build stronger human, material, and financial infrastructure for ICT in clinical and academic settings; and strengthen partnerships with the private sector.

USE OF THE INTERNET TO ACCESS HEALTH INFORMATION

Rapid growth has occurred in Canadians' use of the internet, with nearly all Canadians under the age of 45 reporting daily use (Statistics Canada, 2017). This statistic also includes increasing access of health information. According to the

Internet Use Survey, in 2009, 69.9% of individuals searched for medical or health information at home using the internet (Statistics Canada, 2009). The last Statistics Canada report indicated that 97% of Canadian households had internet connections (Statistics Canada, 2013a). Although 98% of high-income households had high-speed internet connections, only 58% of low-income households reported the same, a factor that contributes to effective use of the internet (Statistics Canada, 2013a). More recent Canadian statistics are not available. However, in the United States, the Pew Research Internet Survey (2011) also indicated an existing disparity in internet access. This divide has persisted, and in 2017, although approximately 75% of American adults reported having broadband internet service at home, older adults, racial minorities, rural residents, and individuals with lower levels of education and income were less likely to report this access (PEW Research Center, 2017). According to Horrigan (2015), 73% of adults stated that librarians assist people to find health information, and 42% have used library facilities to access health information online. However, women and individuals with higher levels of education are more likely to use libraries.

Rooks, Wiltshire, Elder, BeLue, and Gary (2012) found that people of color and ethnic minorities were less likely than Caucasians to seek information online or to use internet-accessed information in their discussions with physicians. Compared to individuals who do not seek digital health information, those who frequently use the internet for this purpose were also likely to access health services significantly more often (Suziedelyte, 2012). Certain treatment can prompt internet use. Half of individuals who were prescribed contraceptive medications sought additional information online, suggesting that more health teaching is necessary with these prescriptions (Russo, Parisi, Kukla, & Schwarz, 2013).

Canadians are increasingly using online sources to support their personal health maintenance. In 2009, only 1.4% of Canadian internet users purchased pharmaceuticals online (Statistics Canada, 2010), whereas in 2012, 6% purchased online pharmaceuticals, and 15% purchased health or beauty products online (Statistics Canada, 2013b). Many people are using online sources to address health-related decisions and lifestyle behaviours, or as a supplement to information received from a health professional; it is the third most frequent use of internet information (Ramsey, Corsini, Peters, & Eckert, 2017). There are differences in the use of digital health information. While adults living with disabilities or chronic disease are less likely to use the internet overall, those who do go online search for health information more frequently than those without chronic conditions (Fox, 2007). Persons experiencing a high level of anxiety about their health status searched for online information more frequently and for a longer duration. Significantly, this online search contributed to an increasing anxiety level for these people (Muse, McManus, Leung, Meghreblain, & Williams, 2012). A systematic review found that online information seeking, and subsequent discussion of such with a physician, could improve patient–physician relationships (Tan & Goonawardene, 2017). In 2012, over 72% of people discussed an internet resource with their physicians and found that their relationship with the physician was more positive because

of this action (AlGhamdi & Moussa, 2012). Xiao, Sharman, Rao, and Upadhyaya (2014) identified that individuals who perceive their own health status to be poor, or who have significant anxiety related to their status or lack of diagnosis, use the internet more frequently, regardless of their relationships with their physicians.

Manafo and Wong (2012) found that the accessibility and availability of online nutrition information enabled some older adults, but that the amount of information available online overwhelmed and dis-enabled others. **Health literacy** is generally defined as an individual's ability to obtain and use health information to make decisions and choices about health behaviours and health care, and is related to health status, health care service use, and self-care behaviours. Age, race, ethnicity, and socioeconomic status can influence health literacy levels (Ownby, Acevedo, Waldrop-Valverde, Jacobs, & Caballera, 2014) and contribute to health inequities in various populations. Xie (2011) has demonstrated that health literacy courses can increase older adults' confidence in the information they access online. Overall, Chaudhuri, Le, White, Thompson, and Demiris (2013) confirmed that older adults preferred sources where they were able to discuss the information. Internet information ranked low in their list of trusted sources, along with newspapers and television; health professionals were preferred sources.

Canada Health Infoway is facilitating the implementation of a Pan-Canadian electronic health record (EHR) and more recently has been advocating for patient access to EHR data. In examining the gap between the desire for increased access to digital health solutions and actual use, it found although more than 8 in 10 Canadians wanted online access to their own EHR information, only 4% actually reported having that access (Zelmer & Hagens, 2014). Risling, Martinez, Young, and Thorp-Froslie (2017) highlighted patient portals that provide online personal health information as a significant way to influence patient empowerment and engagement.

Personal empowerment, defined as the development of personal involvement and responsibility, is enhanced by the use of online health resources (Lemire, Sicotte, & Paré, 2008). Through self-report, internet users identified three aspects of empowerment: agreement with expert advice, self-reliance through individual choice, and social inclusion through the development of collective support. Internet users perceived that all three aspects were enhanced by access to online health information (Lemire, Sicotte, & Paré, 2008). Determinants of use of online health information included its perceived usefulness, concern for personal health, specific health issues experienced, importance given to the opinions of physicians and other health care professionals, and trust placed in the online information (Lemire, Paré, Sicotte, & Harvey, 2008).

Khechine, Pascot, and Prémont (2008) demonstrated that people with long-term illnesses were more likely to access websites that were scientific in nature (medical, electronic library, government websites, or foundations). They often accessed online health information at two points in the medical decisional process: identification of possible treatments and treatment follow-up. In this study, only about 25% of respondents frequently used online discussion forums for information, even though Hoffman-Goetz, Donelle, and Thomson (2009) demonstrated that 91% of the advice provided in the forums was congruent with best practice guidelines. Cole, Watkins, and Kleine (2016), using physicians to assess the quality of advice provided on discussion forums, indicated that only a small amount of the advice provided was of poor quality and that participants would not likely be led to inappropriate actions based on this advice. See Canadian Research 15.1.

Recent research has demonstrated that more health-iterate clients rely on online information to prepare for their medical appointments and to engage more fully in health-seeking behaviours (Ramsey et al., 2017). Less health-literate clients and those from rural areas, however, may be less confident in accessing credible resources or discussing the online materials with their HCPs (Dean et al., 2017). Women, as compared to men, are also more likely to use the internet for health information or cancer information, or to use the internet over time for health information (Manierre, 2015). These findings highlight

an important health education role for CHNs, especially when working with internet users. Nurses are cautioned that online health information is only one approach to delivering health messages within myriad other communications media. Some clients may rely more heavily on non-online sources of information, including written materials and professional verbal explanations. Careful assessment of client needs is important.

Internet Access Issues

Although many populations use the internet for health information, access to this resource is not equitable, as has been noted. Tapscott (1998) first identified the **digital divide** as referring to internet users and non-users, resulting in information "haves" and "have-nots," thus identifying segments of the population that may not use the internet for health information. Over the past years, this "divide" has changed. Although youth were early adopters of the internet, older adults are now using it in high numbers, and older adults are currently the fastest-growing group of users. Sixty-nine percent of adults over the age of 65 are using the internet, and over half of those older adults are using the internet to search for health-related information (McMaster Health Forum, 2014). The number of much older adults using the internet is lower, about 21% of older adults over the age of 75 (Statistics Canada, 2010); however, this number continues to grow each year. It is older persons in the lowest income brackets in Canada who account for much of the persistent digital divide (Statistics Canada, 2013a). In 2012, only 28% of Canadians aged 65 years and over with the lowest incomes used the internet in comparison with 95% of those aged 16–24 in similar low-income brackets (Statistics Canada, 2013a). One of the main limitations to internet use is the lack of computers and internet access in the home (McMaster Health Forum, 2014; Statistics Canada, 2013a). Individuals with low income, limited education, living on First Nation reserves or in rural and remote areas, and who are members of minority ethnic groups or recent immigrants may have significant limitations to the use of the internet for health information (Statistics Canada, 2013a). Older adults may also experience limitations in accessing internet information or may have concerns about the credibility of the information they have accessed (Chaudhuri et al., 2013; McMaster Health Forum, 2014).

Despite any challenges associated with use of online resources, people are motivated to use these resources if they are suitable to their needs, fit their life stage and age, create the opportunity for interaction with others with similar interests, allow for self-paced learning or use of the resources, or provide possible interventions (Ammerlaan et al., 2017). These factors should be considered in the development of online resources. Low-income communities, older adults, ethnic groups, and disadvantaged groups have been shown to use and benefit from community-based internet access to empower and build healthier neighbourhoods and populations (Chaudhuri et al., 2013; Lober & Flowers, 2011). These same groups in Canada, however, have lower utilization of online resources and may need significant support and encouragement from HCPs to use them (McMaster Health Forum, 2014). In other instances, the internet has been found to be a poor source of health information for some, including the Chinese immigrant

---

CANADIAN RESEARCH 15.1

Does a website navigation tool facilitate access to health information online? (Haase, Strohschein, Lee, & Loiselle, 2016)

Researchers interviewed HCPs and cancer patients to determine their perceptions of a virtual navigation tool (Oncology Interactive Navigator [OIN]) in assisting oncology clients to access credible digital health information. Providers offered care or service as part of a multidisciplinary colorectal oncology team at a university-affiliated teaching hospital in Montreal, Quebec. In this study, the perceptions of HCPs and patients about the suitability of the virtual navigation tool were compared. Through qualitative analysis, researchers demonstrated that HCPs and patients both viewed the OIN as a highly accessible repository of high-quality and reliable cancer information, a means of enhancement to HCP–patient communication and trust, and a useful catalyst for patient and family communication and support. Patients, however, viewed the tool as a primary resource for health information needs, whereas HCPs viewed the tool as an adjunct to information provided by the HCPs. In addition, HCPs viewed the tool as adding burden to their patient education as they needed to address the quality and nature of information accessed. A person-centred approach, incorporating a tailored approach to the needs and preferences of cancer patients, was the common thread that linked the perceptions of the participants.

Discussion Questions

1. How could nurses assist clients to use a navigation tool to access credible information relative to their needs?

2. What assessments could nurses make to determine client or family limitations to the use of such a navigation tool?

3. As an equity issue, how could nurses support clients who lack computer literacy to use navigation tools to access high-quality oncology information?

YES, BUT WHY?

Human Trafficking of Children in Canada

What?

Human trafficking is a global migration issue frequently connected with the sex trade; it is an issue in Canada. The Criminal Code of Canada defines human trafficking as the recruitment, transportation, or transfer of persons, or the exercise of control over the movement of persons, for the purpose of exploitation of them (Karem, 2016). Although human trafficking is associated with cross-border transportation of persons, it occurs domestically whereby persons, often women or girls, are recruited through acquaintances or the internet, and control is exercised over their actions, often in prostitution or sexual exploitation. Issues of sexual exploitation of children are included under the trafficking section of Canadian Criminal Code of Canada. Individuals from poorer communities, at-risk youth, children in protection, and runaways are most vulnerable (Barnett, 2017). The number of police reports of human trafficking in 2016 was 340 victims. However, this number is notoriously under-reported and has increased significantly over time. Of particular concern, from 2009–2016, more than 25% of victims of trafficking in Canada were under the age of 18, and 45% were between the ages of 18–24 (Ibrahim, 2018).

So What?

The vulnerability of children to recruitment and exploitation via the internet has become increasingly more evident due to their extensive use of social media and their naivety to these risks. Children at greatest risk are those dislocated from their families and social supports, such as children in protection and those who spend extensive time on various social media sites and unmonitored chat rooms. Risks to these children include luring, sexual exploitation, abduction, forcible confinement, cyberbullying, child pornography, or prostitution.

Now What?

CHNs, especially school nurses or individuals working with at-risk youth, may partner with police units to educate youth about risks associated with social media and chat rooms. Classroom presentations identifying possible grooming via the internet could include information about a person online who asks questions about their parental supervision and where their computer is located, explores their interests and hobbies, requests or coerces pictures (some of which may be sexually explicit), offers a "listening ear" about the youth's problems, invites youth to private chat rooms, or threatens youth if they stop responding (Puresight, 2018). Youth may also be subjected to online bullying as part of the process of grooming (Health Canada, 2018). Identifying how youth can address inappropriate situations and providing support for reporting such situations are important to protect children and youth from domestic and global human trafficking and exploitation.

Standards of Practice Fulfilled

#5 Capacity Building
 – Assists the client to make an informed decision in determining their health goals and priorities for action.
 – Supports community-based action to influence policy change in support of health

#7 Professional Relationships
 – Uses culturally safe communication strategies in professional relationships, recognizing
 – communication may be verbal or non-verbal, written or graphic. Communication can occur via a variety of mediums (CHNC, 2019, revised).

population of Vancouver and Seattle (Woodall et al., 2009). Therefore, nurses should not assume that all clients can, or will, access the internet for health information and should address accessibility issues for populations rendered vulnerable.

An issue that has arisen is the circulation of "fake" health information, often from websites promoting specific treatments or approaches, many of them based on limited, faulty, or questionable research evidence. In part, non-evidence based information may be promoted supporting a personal perspective or belief or promoting specific products or services. A good example is websites promoting views on immunization and its relationship to autism, often promoted by individuals with public personas such as movie stars (Specter, 2013). Such websites tend to cite other websites with similar views, thus creating the impression of credibility. A role for CHNs is to bring the weight of good evidence to bear on health decisions, recognizing that many laypeople may have challenges in identifying these questionable websites as inappropriate or profit-driven. Youth have primarily been early adopters of technology; therefore, technology has the significant potential to enhance youth's health decision making and support. Their access issues, however, differ from those of other age groups. In a study of youth use of online resources, specific issues were noted, and Valaitis (2005) advocated for attention to the factors of privacy, gatekeeping, timeliness, and functionality when designing internet-based resources for youth. Youth are often attracted to websites and chat rooms that may address their specific concerns in ways that are relevant and entertaining to them but that may jeopardize their well-being or lead to their exploitation. (See Yes, But Why box about human trafficking of children in Canada.) They may be unaware of privacy needs and the risks of divulging personal information in an unsupervised website. They likely consult friends about websites rather than knowledgeable adults. Again, the importance of providing information about the criteria for credibility of various websites is beneficial.

Access for Populations who are Differently Abled

CHNs often work with populations living with disabilities, recognizing that disabilities take many forms and can be associated with acute and chronic situations. People who are differently abled can benefit from using ICTs, since they can reduce social isolation by helping them reach people with similar experiences, become better informed, increase communication, and enhance access to health information (McMaster Health Forum, 2014). The next section will review accessibility standards that guide the design of health information websites and will provide a basic overview of technology tools to enhance internet access for people who are differently abled.

The World Wide Web Consortium (W3C) (www.w3.org) is an international organization that oversees the standardization and operation of the Web. In 1997, to ensure equitable and universal access to information for all populations, including people who are differently abled, W3C launched the **Web Accessibility Initiative** (W3C, 2017a). Under this initiative, accessibility standards for web content designers and developers were created. The **Web Content Accessibility Guidelines** 2.0 document provides a review of accessibility factors of online resources (W3C, 2017b), and tutorials are available to support designers in making their websites accessible to individuals with disabilities (W3C, 2017c). These guidelines define *accessible* as materials that are usable to a wide range of people with disabilities, including blindness and low vision, deafness and hearing loss, learning difficulties, cognitive limitations, limited movement, speech difficulties, photosensitivity, and combinations of these (W3C, 2017c). Standards are grouped into different priority levels. Disability advocates recommend that websites at a minimum meet the Priority Level One standard.

The principles are related to perceivability, operability, understandability, and robustness of the resource. Guideline One design standards are relatively simple to meet. For example, webpage images need clear text descriptions. HTML code should include "alt tags" (alternative text tags) so that when a user rolls over the image, a text description appears. When browser preferences are set for "text only," the option for viewing images is turned off. This option is useful for people who are visually impaired. Screen readers turn screen text to speech and can read text programmed in the alt tag codes, thereby informing visitors what images are on the page. Another Guideline standard includes the use of contrasting background and text colours. Such standards help to ensure that web documents are navigable. Many government health resources now incorporate these guidelines to ensure accessibility.

Health information websites generally get failing grades with respect to accessibility and usability. Goldberg et al. (2011) indicated that issues of accessibility must be addressed at the onset of development and that although usability is a quality of the website, it is defined in terms of the people using the site. Hardiker and Grant (2011) explored factors that influence public engagement with e-health, identifying improved access and tailored services as necessary conditions for ease of use. Burns, Jones, Inverson, and Caputi (2013) indicated that there is a lack of current research on the usability of websites that are easily accessible to individuals with visual and auditory disabilities. In addition, there is limited access to translation devices to meet the public's needs for accessibility.

CASE STUDY

Testing Website Accessibility

Identify your favourite health information website or your current clinical placement agency website. Once you have located the website, highlight and copy the URL (universal resource locator—a unique identifier that provides an address for an internet site). Then proceed to an accessibility checker website. W3C lists many website accessibility checkers, such as the University of Toronto checker.

Paste in the URL at the site to obtain a report on how well it complied with W3C Web Content Accessibility Guidelines.

Discussion Questions

1. How accessible was your site?
2. Which standards did it fail?
3. Consider how the website could be improved.

Numerous software and hardware devices are available to assist differently abled populations. Some commonly used devices for people who are visually impaired include screen readers, screen magnifiers, Braille displays, voice recognition technologies, data extraction tools that filter content from overly busy webpages, and OCR software to turn a printed page into electronic text for screen reading. Portable note-taking devices can help people with speech communication disorders, and ergonomic adapters, dictation programs, and voice-controlled software can assist people who have mobility impairments. Simple adjustments can be made with most operating systems to enhance accessibility. For example, explore the "Accessibility Options" folder in the control panel of your own computer to adjust settings for hearing, vision, and mobility.

QUALITY OF DIGITAL HEALTH INFORMATION

In recent years, emphasis has shifted from educating people about health issues to educating people to access health information themselves and assisting them to interpret that information as needed. Access to good-quality health information can empower clients to address their health issues; however, increased public access to digital health information has introduced both risks and opportunities. The quality of health information online is highly variable; thus, the public is challenged to determine the quality and credibility of the health information provided. Digital health information includes health promotion information, screening tests, personal accounts of illness, patient testimonials about treatment effectiveness, patient opinions or perspectives on their illness experiences, product advertisers, treatment providers, discussion and support groups, peer-reviewed articles, and decision-making aids. A goal for CHNs includes assisting clients to become knowledgeable consumers of information available to them in this medium as part of their general health management (Anker, Reinhart, & Feeley, 2011).

Nurses can assist their clients to use the Internet with greater confidence, by supporting client skills and by designing patient portals for ease of use. The first step is to identify those clients who need greater assistance, including those with limited computer skills, limited computer access, poor health literacy, or needing assistive devices (Dickerson, 2006). In addition, individuals with lower educational levels or from some ethnic groups may be less likely to use these resources (Sarkar et al., 2011). Individuals in later stages of illness or with advanced symptoms may need greater assistance (Kruse, Argueta, Lopez, & Nair, 2015). The provision of easily-accessible technical support can increase client usage of online resources (Kruse et al., 2015).

Many clients, particularly those using patient portals to access their personal health information, expressed concerns about information security and privacy. Nurses can reassure clients about privacy protection and assist clients to use the internet in a way that protects their information security. Patient portals that use a standard portal format and ease of navigation can facilitate client use (Kruse et al., 2015). In addition, provision of recommended resources within the portal and a health library that explains terminology, test procedures, lab results, medication, and treatments can increase usage. Nurses can participate in the design of patient portals to provide easily understood resources. Where clients are independently seeking resources on the internet, nurses can ensure that clients can evaluate the quality of the resources (Dickerson, 2006) or use a website to assist them (Health on the Net, 2018). Lastly, nurses can promote local resources accessible to clients in their home communities (Dickerson, 2006).

Although some internet users have expressed concern about the credibility of internet-based health information, they continue to access a variety of internet-based health information resources, including health promotion, scientific and medical information, and patient testimonials about their illness experiences (Kivits, 2009; Ramsey et al., 2017). Unfortunately, even though internet users may indicate they use criteria such as source credibility, language, and transparency to determine the value of online health information, they have tended to disregard these criteria when actually conducting a search. In addition, internet users often rely only on the search engine or their own personal experience to judge the usefulness of the information (Eysenbach, 2007) and use correspondence with the content of other websites to judge its accuracy (Kivits, 2009). Users have tended to develop a practical knowledge based on their experience to determine what information and sources of knowledge to select (Kivits, 2009). Kitchens, Harle, and Li (2014) found that search techniques and use of search engines were poor, and that users relied heavily on the first few websites or resources identified by the search.

Comfort and familiarity with the internet does not guarantee the ability to obtain credible online health information. An internet behaviour and preference study of 60 English-speaking Caribbean immigrant women in New York City revealed that although internet use was high in this group, many participants did not know the differences among websites with domain names of .edu, .gov, .com, or .net (Changrani & Gany, 2005). When searching for digital health information, participants used links from the first screen of results displayed by the search engine and rarely refined their search terms or repeated the search. Most searches were concluded within five minutes. If participants repeated a search, they stated it was because they did not trust the source or understand the information. Kivits (2009) reported similar findings.

Tools Available for Rating Digital Health Information

There are many tools available to consumers and HCPs that rate the quality of digital health information. Various dimensions of internet resources can be evaluated, including content, journalistic value, targeted audience, website design, readability and usability, and ethical issues of privacy. These dimensions have changed over time as Web 2.0 technologies, including collaborative, adaptive, and interactive sites, have emerged (Burns et al., 2013). Unfortunately, consumers may have difficulties determining the value of the ratings provided on the health information websites.

Providing clients with clear criteria of credible online information is the best means of enabling them to assess its quality. Using the **HON code** (www.healthonnet.org) (Health on the Net Foundation, 2016) to examine online information with clients is an effective way of teaching the criteria while simultaneously critiquing the online information. In Table 15.1, eight principles are listed and described.

Although health care professionals may be adept at applying HON criteria, most laypersons will not be. The HON website provides a search engine wherein the client can enter a search term that will identify HON-certified websites only. The US National Library of Medicine (https://www.nlm.nih.gov) provides an online tutorial intended for laypersons to empower them to determine the usefulness of online health information. Individuals may need CHN encouragement and support in using these resources.

In Table 15.2, questions that clients may use in assessing digital health information are presented. Assisting clients to interpret and apply these criteria will empower them to use internet health information with greater confidence. HON (Health on the Net Foundation, 2016) also supports a service where health information consumers may submit a URL to the "WRAPIN" service (www.wrapin.org) to determine if the site is accredited or trustworthy (WRAPIN, 2014). Sites are searched in various languages. In addition, clients can be encouraged to download the HON code toolbar into their browser, which helps them search for HON-approved sites.

Table 15.1	HON Code of Conduct for Medical and Health Websites
1. Authoritative	Any medical or health advice provided and hosted on this site will only be given by medically trained and qualified health professionals unless a clear statement is made that a piece of advice offered is from a non-medically qualified individual or organization.
2. Complementarity	The information provided on this site is designed to support, not replace, the relationship that exists between a patient/site visitor and his/her existing physician.
3. Privacy	Confidentiality of data relating to individual patients and visitors to a medical/health website, including their identity, is respected by this website. The website owners undertake to honour or exceed the legal requirements of medical/health information privacy that apply in the country and state where the website and mirror sites are located.
4. Attribution	Where appropriate, information contained on this site will be supported by clear references to source data and, where possible, have specific HTML links to that data. The date when a clinical page was last modified will be clearly displayed (e.g., at the bottom of the page).
5. Justifiability	Any claims relating to the benefits/performance of a specific treatment, commercial product, or service will be supported by appropriate balanced evidence in the manner outlined previously in Principle 4.
6. Transparency	The designers of this website will seek to provide information in the clearest possible manner and provide contact addresses for visitors that seek further information or support. The webmaster will display his/her email address clearly throughout the website.
7. Financial disclosure	Support for this website will be clearly identified, including the identities of commercial and non-commercial organizations that have contributed funding, services, or material for the site.
8. Advertising policy	If advertising is a source of funding, it will be clearly stated. A brief description of the advertising policy adopted by the website owners will be displayed on the site. Advertising and other promotional material will be presented to viewers in a manner and context that facilitates differentiation between it and the original material created by the institution operating the site.

Source: *The HON code of conduct for medical and health websites (HON code)*. Copyright © 2015 by Health on the Net Foundation. Used by permission of Health on the Net Foundation. Retrieved from http://www.hon.ch/HONcode/Pro/Conduct.html. Reproduced with permission.

Table 15.2	Questions for Clients to Use in Assessing Internet Health Information

1. Is the health information provided by a qualified medical practitioner or an organization that is committed to the public's health?

2. Does the website encourage you to discuss the health information with your physician or another health care professional?

3. Is your identity protected on this website?

4. Does the website indicate sources or references for the information provided? Are these sources credible?

5. Are claims of effectiveness of treatments supported by credible evidence?

6. Is the authorship of this website clear to you? Can you contact the webmaster for more information?

7. Is the sponsorship of the website clearly apparent to you?

8. Are the commercial advertisements clearly separated from the health information presented on the website? Is the advertising policy stated on the website?

9. Is there a link to the homepage of the sponsoring organization from the health information webpages?

10. Does the homepage explain the mission, purpose, and objectives; sources of funding; and governance of the organization?

Assessment of Health Information Websites

The usability of health information websites may relate to more than the accuracy of the information provided. Another set of criteria evaluates health information websites on their usability for consumers, including navigation and design (Mitretek Systems Health Summit Working Group, 2017). These criteria include credibility, content, disclosures, links, design, interactivity, and caveats and relate to the presentation of information and ease of use.

Several highly credible sources (Health on the Net Foundation, 2016; McMaster Health Forum, 2014; Mitrek Systems Health Summit Working Group, 2014) provide advice on criteria that can be used to evaluate websites. Credibility of the information provided is critical to the usefulness of the website and is based on the expertise of the authors and sponsoring agency, the currency of the information, and its relevance to the user's perceived health issue. From the perspective of health professionals, the accuracy of the information, and the evidence to support that information, are important and should be disclosed on the website. However, providing information that is targeted to the intended user is important; sources should be indicated and evidence should be understandable to users or explained appropriately. Users value interactivity within websites but privacy issues and security of information thus provided should be clear to users. Health professionals seek reassurances to users of websites that the information should be used in partnership with health professionals rather than replacing such relationships.

Health professionals are also aware that ease of navigation within the website is important to users of those sites. Navigation links should be clear and easily used, indicate when links are to outside sites, and provide links to bring the user back to the original site easily. User frustrations related to navigation issues may result in users seeking other sites. Content maps at the start of the website, the ability to search websites, and ease of navigation facilitate user persistence. When commercial products are available on the website, or links take users to product websites, the relationship of the website to the commercial enterprise should be clearly stated.

Readability of text is an important design aspect of every webpage. Readability is a measure of how easily and comfortably text can be read. People with lower reading skills also use the internet. For websites intended for laypersons, reading levels should be focused approximately at a Grade 9 level (Canadian Public Health Association [CPHA], 2018). Reading experts suggest that the majority of the population prefers written materials three grades below the last grade attended at school (Bastable, 2013). Although this level may seem low, it may still be higher than the reading comprehension level of the general population, which is estimated to be, on average, at a Grade 5–6 level (Bastable, 2013). Within the Canadian population, 89% of the population aged 25 to 64 has completed high school, and 65% has completed post-secondary education (Statistics Canada, 2014). Nonetheless, 42% of the working-age population scored below the functional level in prose literacy scales and 43% below functional level in document literacy (OECD & Statistics Canada, 2011). The Canadian Literacy and Learning Network (2014) indicates that 42% of Canadian adults between the ages of 16 and 65 have low literacy skills, with 55% of this population possessing inadequate health literacy skills. Eighty-eight percent of the population over the age of 65 fall into this category. Unfortunately, most websites have much higher reading levels than can be comprehended by a large portion of the general population. Ache and Wallace (2009) found that internet-based client education materials were generally written at the Grade 7 to 12 levels, with a mean of Grade 11, and Lam, Roter, and Cohen (2013) found that 86% of websites for adolescents failed readability standards of less than Grade 8 level.

Health professionals who are recommending or creating websites for clients can assess the readability of written or internet text using a relatively simple tool, the SMOG (Simple Measure of Gobbledygook) Readability Test (McLaughlin, 1969). (See Table 15.3.) SMOG reading levels correlate well with grade levels identified by other tests of readability (Bastable 2013; Beaunoyer, Arsenault, Lomanowska, & Guitoon, 2017). Because these tests are based on two variables of reading comprehension, word length and sentence length, the reading level of text materials can be reduced by using simple words and shorter sentences (Table 15.4). The CPHA, in its National Literacy and Health Program, published the Directory of Plain Language Health Information to assist health educators in

Table 15.3	SMOG Readability Assessment Tool: Document Assessment for Approximate Grade Level of Reading Skills
Step 1 Sample selection	Select 30 sentences from the text material: 10 consecutive sentences from each of the start, middle, and end of the material. A sentence is a complete idea with a period, question mark, or exclamation mark, a bulleted point, or both parts of a sentence with a colon included.
Step 2 Word count	Count the number of words with more than three syllables (polysyllabic) in the 30-sentence sample. Include all repetitions of a word, proper nouns, full text of abbreviations, and hyphenated words as one word.
Step 3 Short text conversion	For documents of fewer than 30 sentences, multiply the number of polysyllabic words by a factor to simulate a sample of 30 sentences. For example, if the document contained 15 sentences, the factor would be 30 divided by 15 to equal a factor of 2. For documents of 24 sentences, the factor would be 30 divided by 24 to equal 1.25.
Step 4 Calculate	Determine the nearest square root of the number of words in the sample. A square root is a number multiplied by itself to equal a perfect square. For example, 8 multiplied by 8 (square root) equals 64 (perfect square). The number that is a square root is usually between 3 and 15.
Add the constant "3" to the square root obtained in step 4.	Example: A sample is assessed as having 86 polysyllabic words in 30 sentences. The nearest square root is 9 (9 times 9 equals 81). The constant of 3 is added to give an approximate reading level of 12, or more appropriately described as a reading level requiring the reading skills approximately at the Grade 12 reading level.

The result is the approximate grade level of reading skills required to read the document. The resultant grade level is correct within 1.5 grades in 68% of cases.

Source: SMOG (Simple Measure of Gobbledygook) Readability Test. Adapted from McLaughlin, G. H. (1969). SMOG-grading: A new readability formula. *Journal of Reading, 12*, 639–646.

Table 15.4	Examples of Different Reading Levels
Grade 12 reading level*	Include exercise such as walking, biking, swimming, jogging, and active sports, according to your individual preferences. Consider other means of transportation or use stairs instead of elevators. Incorporate physical activities into your interactions with your children. The recommended amount of activity per week is 20 minutes of activity daily, on at least five separate occasions per week. Monitor your pulse rate, keeping it within the recommended target level during your activity. To stay physically fit, keep active and have fun.
Grade 9 reading level*	Include exercise such as walking, biking, swimming, jogging, and active sports, as you prefer. Consider walking to the store or using the stairs instead of elevators. Be active with your children. We recommend 20 minutes of activity daily, at least five times per week. Monitor your pulse rate, keeping it within the target level during your activity. To stay physically fit, keep active and have fun.
Grade 6 reading level*	Include walking, biking, swimming, jogging, and active sports in your daily life. Choose other ways of being active. Take the stairs. Walk to the store. Play with your kids. We suggest at least 20 minutes of exercise per day, 5 times per week. Include more time as you wish. Learn how to take your own pulse rate. Keep your pulse rate within the target level. Stay fit. Keep active. Have fun.

Source: SMOG (Simple Measure of Gobbledygook) Readability Test. Adapted from McLaughlin, G. H. (1969). SMOG-grading: A new readability formula. *Journal of Reading, 12,* 639–646.

*Approximate reading levels based on SMOG assessment

publishing clear and easily understood written materials. Key points are summarized in Table 15.5. CPHA also offers a plain language service for the assessment and clarification of health resources (CPHA, 2018).

Health care professionals may refer clients to well-developed websites specific to their needs. Factors to be considered when judging the utility of online health information include ease of navigation and ease of accessing webpages within the site (Goldberg et al., 2011). Internal links for ease of access are beneficial to users. External links should be assessed for their relatedness and ease of return to the original website. Use of graphics to illustrate concepts enhances usability; however, advertising on the website and irritating pop-ups may interfere. Users also find a pleasing appearance and the opportunity for interactivity, such as calculations of body mass index, daily calorie counters, or self-report progress charts, to be beneficial (Lustria, Cortese, Noar, & Glueckauf, 2009). Inclusion of videos on a website has also been effective in user satisfaction and recall of information (Bol et al., 2013). Ease of usage enhances a user's ability to read and use information contained on a website. Clients can also be referred to government-sponsored health information websites that have high credibility and accuracy of information.

Targeting Specific Users of Digital Health Information

Online health information should be designed for specific users. A combination of health messaging with individual-level participant information permits better targeting. **Targeting** is the development of online resources that allow for personal and direct content presentation based on elements such as preferences, needs, and current health behaviours or behavioural intentions, and that lead to positive outcomes (Lustria et al., 2009). The concept comes from advertising principles that are related to market segmentation.

Research with immigrant populations illustrates that they want health information to make good decisions about maintaining their health and exploring their vulnerability to health risks (Kreps & Sparks, 2008). These individuals need access to culturally relevant, accurate, and timely health information. The information should be specifically designed to be compatible with the cultural beliefs, values, and attitudes of the targeted group. In addition, the health education messages should be pre-tested with representatives of the target group for their cultural sensitivity. Kreps and Sparks (2008) also indicated that such messages should be provided in multiple messaging strategies for reinforcement of the message. Preferences for being able to ask questions and to interact with knowledgeable respondents was also evident.

Because scrolling through a website presents challenges for some older adults, website designs that present one paragraph per webpage are a better alternative. The U.S. National Institute on Aging maintains a website (www.nia.nih.gov/health) with common health concerns where text can be enlarged, and a "talking function" can be activated as needed. The site provides links to other credible websites to assist older adults in making decisions about the value of the information they have accessed. Websites with these characteristics will be more useful to older adults.

Table 15.5	Plain Language Strategies

- Use active voice by stating the subject of the action first, as for example, "You should eat 5 to 10 fruits and vegetables per day," instead of, "5 to 10 fruits and vegetables should be eaten every day."
- Write directly to the reader, using "you" or implying "you" as the subject of the sentence; for example, "Take this medication once per day," instead of "This medication should be taken once per day."
- Maintain a positive tone, stating actions as positive behaviours rather than avoidance behaviours; for example, "Contact your doctor as soon as you feel sick," instead of "Avoid waiting too long to contact your doctor."
- Use common simple terms rather than technical jargon; e.g., "Medicine will relieve your child's pain," instead of "An analgesic will relieve your child's pain."
- Use short words and short sentences.
- Replace more difficult words with simpler words:
  — *drug* or *medicine* in place of *medication*
  — *heart* in place of *cardiac*
  — *doctor* in place of *physician*
  — *take part in* rather than *participate in*
  — *problems* in place of *difficulties*
- When in doubt, ask your learners what words are most meaningful.
- Do not change verbs into nouns. The action word is a stronger depiction; for example, "Decide when to involve your children in meal planning," instead of "Make decisions about your children's involvement in meal planning."
- List important points separate from the text.
  — Use bullets to highlight important points.
  — Keep bullets short.
  — Use boxes to highlight important information.
- Write instructions in the order that you want them to be carried out.
- List items such as nouns or actions in parallel form.
- Keep your writing in a conversational form.
- Test whatever you write with learners before you formalize it.

Source: Public Health Agency of Canada (PHAC). (2017a).

Tailoring Digital Health Interventions

The integration of features that enhance interactivity has long been known to enhance learning (Goldberg et al., 2011; Hardiker & Grant, 2011). **Interactivity** refers to a process where a user is an active participant in using technology and information exchange occurs (e.g., chat rooms, calorie calculators, links). For example, computer programs that integrate social cognitive theory to promote behaviour change for management of weight and physical activity have shown positive results. Combining the concept of behavioural economics with interactive digital health interventions is driving the development of unique health promotion solutions like the Carrot Rewards application. Working from the premise that Canadians respond positively to loyalty programs, where they can earn points for movies, grocery store purchases, gas, or travel, the app rewards points to users for simply downloading it and then "for referring friends, and completing an average of 1 to 2 short educational health quizzes each week

(micro-learning), with the ultimate goal of increasing health knowledge and promoting healthy behaviors" (Mitchell et al., 2017, p. 2). These programs are based on the assumption that participants have access to resources and may neglect social determinants of health that have contributed to obesity. Content related to low cost, healthy, and easily accessible foods may better reflect the participant's needs and life situation.

Features in programs that generate personalized responses can also increase positive attitudes and learning about health issues and have been shown to result in positive health outcomes (Suggs & McIntyre, 2009), as long as anonymity of the user is assured (Hardiker & Grant, 2011). For example, the generation of clear and understandable tailored messages that include the user's name and provide specific information addressing individual health needs is important when designing computer-based health promotion interventions. Compared to the concept of targeting, which focuses on interventions for groups, **tailoring** has been referred to as a process of creating individualized intervention materials. Tailored

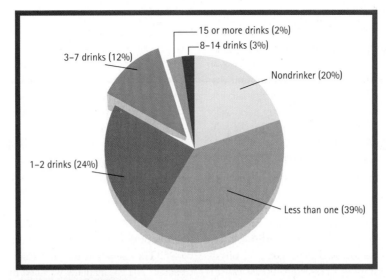

FIGURE 15.1 Portion of a Tailored Final Report for a Fictitious Website User Created from Check Your Drinking

Average drinks per week for females aged 35–44 from Canada.

Source: From V-Alcohol Help Centre. Copyright © by Evolution Health Systems Inc. Used by permission of Evolution Health Systems Inc.

messages are typically "pushed" to the user, as opposed to sites where users "pull" or search for information from fact sheets, booklets, videos, and images. Tailored messages are typically presented with self-comparisons and recommendations based on authoritative research. (See Figure 15.1.) Suggs and McIntyre (2009) found that only 13 of 497 English-language online health resources were tailored messages, in spite of the identified efficiencies of such websites. However, a study of tailored versus targeted computer-based interventions to promote hearing-protection use among construction workers showed that a targeted intervention was preferred and was more cost effective (Kerr, Savik, Monsen, & Lusk, 2007). Overall, tailoring on individual characteristics (age, gender, readiness) has been shown to outperform static health information (Bennett & Glasgow, 2009).

TECHNOLOGY TO SUPPORT HEALTH PROMOTION, DISEASE PREVENTION, AND CHRONIC DISEASE MANAGEMENT

Primordial Prevention The use of ICTs to support e-health promotion interventions has grown. This growth can be attributed to increased internet use by the public, the low cost of delivery, and public willingness to actively manage their health. It has been demonstrated that e-health promotion interventions are effective means of self-education and self-enhancement (Hardiker & Grant, 2011). With current interest in healthy lifestyles, many people are engaged in primordial prevention that involves such strategies as addressing nutrition and exercise, avoiding harmful situations, advocating for healthy

policies in your community, using organic foodstuffs, or incorporating precautions such as child car seats. All these actions address health status. Technology such as wearable fitness devices and internet websites supporting healthy lifestyles are useful adjuncts to these initiatives and are used extensively by the general public.

Primary Prevention Primary prevention is an approach to reduce the incidence of disease by reducing the impact of specific risk factors or interrupting the causal factors related to certain conditions prior to the physiological manifestations of illness. Digital health solutions have proven very useful, particularly in improved lifestyle choices or the avoidance of risky situations.

Secondary Prevention Secondary prevention, the interruption of the chain of causality or reduction of the prevalence of disease conditions, has also been effectively addressed online. Screening for certain conditions or exploring the meaning of symptoms on online information sources such as Health Canada have been used extensively by Canadians. Online interventions for weight management (Bennett & Glasgow, 2009), cancer care (Becker, Mackert, & Kang, 2013), gambling addiction (Mudry & Strong, 2012), smoking cessation (De Ruijter, Smit, de Vires, & Hoving, 2016), asthma care (Letourneau et al., 2012), and hypertension management (Liu et al., 2013), among others, have shown promise.

Tailored messages are particularly appropriate for online screening. Online screening interventions have been implemented with varying degrees of success, including for mental health (Nguyen, Klein, Meyer, Austin, & Abbott, 2015), chlamydia and gonorrhea infection (McRee, Esber, & Reiter, 2015), cervical cancer screening for adolescents (Choma &

McKeever, 2015), HIV/AIDS with adolescents (Ybarra, Biringi, Prescott, & Bull, 2012), fruit and vegetable consumption, fitness levels, problem gambling (Mudry & Strong, 2012), and alcohol intake (Cunningham, Humphreys, Kypri, & van Mierlo, 2006). U.S. researchers (Saitz et al., 2004) found that screening and management of alcohol problems was a successful internet health-promotion intervention. Many users were women reporting hazardous amounts of alcohol intake who might not have otherwise looked for help.

Online counselling interventions can be helpful for people who live in remote areas, value anonymity, belong to a special interest group (Donelle & Hoffman-Goetz, 2008), or have access problems (transportation, scheduling). A systematic review of randomized controlled trials of consumer health informatics interventions (Gibbons et al., 2009) showed that many applications that addressed diet, exercise, physical activity, alcohol abuse, smoking cessation, breast cancer, diabetes, mental health, asthma and chronic obstructive pulmonary disease, and menopause and hormone replacement therapy studies had significant positive impact on at least one intermediate health outcome. No studies identified harm attributed to health informatics interventions. A review of the internet as a delivery platform for public health interventions showed potential for broad population dissemination of primary and secondary prevention interventions, many of which showed positive results (Bennett & Glasgow, 2009). The authors stressed the importance of intervention designs and components. For example, the most effective weight-loss interventions were highly structured, focused on tailored materials, included a counsellor, and promoted frequent web logins.

Tertiary Prevention Tertiary prevention, focused on reducing the persistence of disease, and quaternary prevention, focused on reducing the impact of over-medicalization of the person's condition, are well addressed through a variety of online resources. Web 2.0 technologies and socially oriented sites such as YouTube, Twitter, Facebook, Instagram, and MySpace have gained popularity, especially among youth and others experiencing stigmatization related to their conditions. The general use of social media in Canada is on the rise, with 67% of Canadians who used the internet in 2012 reportedly visiting social networking sites such as Facebook or Twitter, an increase from 58% in 2010 (Statistics Canada, 2013a). Research on the use of these technologies to promote health and provide support is also growing (Antheunis, Tates, & Nieboer, 2013; Griffiths et al., 2012; Househ, Borycki, & Kushniruk, 2014). Social media are generally seen as internet-based applications that allow the creation and exchange of user-generated content (Antheunis et al., 2013). These tools can afford clients an opportunity to gain access to health information, explore care options, and share health experiences (Househ et al., 2014). "Social media provide online platforms for interactions to occur around various health topics related to patient education, health promotion, public relations, and crisis communication" (Househ et al., 2014, p. 51).

Web 2.0 emphasizes the social and participatory nature of web services and empowers users as well as focuses on content generation and the phenomenon of inclusion, factors well aligned to enhance health promotion and various levels of prevention. A Facebook conversation as a health promotion intervention concerning sexual health demonstrated that 93% of the content was generated by users, and 576 users interacted over a five-month period. However, once advertising for the site discontinued, so did user participation (Syred, Naidoo, Woodhall, & Araitser, 2014). Interestingly, and in contrast to concerns of health care professionals, very little information provided by online participants on these discussion forums was deemed potentially harmful to users (Cole et al., 2016). YouTube is also a well-used source of health information. In April 2014, a search of the term "human papillomavirus" on YouTube resulted in about 160 000 video clips, illustrating the growth and potential power of this medium for health information and misinformation. The Canadian Internet Registration Authority reported that in 2011 Canadians watched more online videos than anyone else in the world (Canadian Internet Research Authority [CIRA], 2013). Every second video was viewed using YouTube, resulting in a massive reported overall viewing increase in Canada of 170% (CIRA, 2013).

Digital health interventions that include interactive components have been demonstrated as more effective (Burns et al., 2013; Goldberg et al., 2011). Examples of interactive components are calculators that estimate the cost of smoking, online social support groups where participants communicate with ex-smokers, features that permit posting of personal stories, and email follow-ups before and after "quit dates" for added support. Such programs can supplement face-to-face programs. The growth of online groups for new parents has been rapid; these communities can provide social support to parents who feel psychologically or geographically isolated and can meet the needs of parents with unique interests (e.g., adoption, bereavement, multiple births). A review of internet use by parents showed that many use online sources for information and encouragement as a result of weaker supports from family and friends (Vennick, Adams, Faber, & Putters, 2014). Online support groups are also useful in supporting populations who may experience stigma as a result of their conditions (Royer, Fernandez-Lambert, & Moreno, 2013). Internet users have indicated a preference for social interaction on websites (Goldberg et al., 2011; Lustria et al., 2009). Newer technologies are also being studied. A Cochrane review of cell phone–based interventions, using text messaging in particular, showed short-term positive effects on smoking cessation, although no long-term effects were found (Whittaker, Borland, & Bullen, 2009).

TELEHEALTH

The use of telehealth technology continues to expand across Canada, providing accessibility to health care and community health services that might not be available to clients otherwise, including access to health care professionals, health educators, and specialist services typically concentrated in urban or high-population areas. Although typically used in health care services, CHNs can use the same technology to provide their assessment, health promotion, and educative services to remote populations. In some cases, these services may be available to rural, remote, or disadvantaged populations only through telehealth services. (See Chapter 24 for examples of telehealth with rural clients.) Developments in telehealth technology allow health care professionals to assess clients; review assessment data; and diagnose, treat, and counsel clients at a distance (Godwin et al., 2013). Recent use has involved support of family caregivers in their homes, empowering clients to make decisions about their caregivers and the setting of their care (Stern, Valaitis, Weir, & Jadad, 2012).

POPULATION HEALTH AND TECHNOLOGY

There are many online approaches that can support population health interventions. Technology has long been used to support community empowerment and capacity building (Korp, 2006; Valaitis, 2005; Valaitis & O'Mara, 2005). An evaluation of the use of an interactive website to involve local citizens in driving policy related to a smoking bylaw in Calgary was very successful (Grierson, van Dijk, Dozios, & Mascher, 2006). The website sparked public debate about the issue, provided citizens with information about smoking, suggested messages to communicate to city councillors, and updated citizens on how council voted on the issue. Public response was very positive. The website was an effective community capacity-building tool and mobilization strategy that increased citizen participation in building local policy for a healthier community. A similar finding was demonstrated in an Israeli study that engaged stakeholders in consideration of the health impact of a national hazardous industry on nearby land use (Negev, Davidovitch, Garb, & Tal, 2013).

Social media has become another powerful vehicle for influencing public health. Numerous uses have been identified, including "epidemiologic monitoring and surveillance, situational awareness during emergency response and communication surveillance" (Fung, Tsz Ho Tse, & Fu, 2015, p. 3). These media have proven effective in detecting outbreaks, promoting disease awareness, and gauging the impact of health communication (Fung et al., 2015). Social media monitoring supplements the numerous existing population-based **surveillance** systems within the public health system, which provide valuable data for program planning and evaluation. The Canadian Integrated Public Health Information System combines iPHIS—a client health-reporting surveillance system that supports tracking, follow-up, reporting, and management of cases related to immunization, communicable disease, and population health surveillance—with a laboratory data management system. Panorama, developed by Canada Health Infoway, includes tools to support outbreak identification, vaccine inventory management, case management, and notifications (Mowat

& Butler-Jones, 2007). Panorama data are included in the national EHR. CANSIM (Canadian Socioeconomic Information Management System) tables report social trends impacting the lives of Canadians that can be accessed through E-STAT, which also provides access to Canadian census data. It is available at no cost to students and educators through educational institutions. These data are essential for program planners.

ELECTRONIC DOCUMENTATION FOR COMMUNITY HEALTH NURSING

The use of technology to support electronic documentation systems has been growing across Canada, including in community health organizations (Stonham, Heyes, Owen, & Povey, 2012). Although this technology is currently focused on acute nursing, such as home care nursing, it has potential to be used by CHNs to link their interventions to the person's health record. Three types of electronic documentation systems that have been developed are the electronic medical record (EMR), the electronic patient record (EPR), and the electronic health record (EHR). Nagle (2007) differentiated these terms with respect to access to information, scope of the information included in the documentation, and custodianship of the record. Typically, EMRs are found in primary health care settings and clinics, whereas EPRs are maintained by health care organizations. Access to both of these records is limited to authorized caregivers, and the content typically reflects information that previously was recorded in paper-based systems. The EHR is a more comprehensive record that can incorporate content from the EPR and EMR. It typically includes most information gathered from encounters with the health care system, such as primary care, pharmacies, laboratories, and diagnostic imaging units, and could include immunizations, educative interventions, and health promotion activities embraced by the client. The client controls access to his or her record, which is "owned" by the client but is hosted by a jurisdiction (Nagle, 2007, p. 2). The EHR, which provides a longitudinal record of an individual's health history and care, is currently being tested in numerous provinces by Canada Health Infoway.

Nurses in the community are using mobile devices to view health records, complete documentation, order supplies, make appointments, review medications, and access evidence for practice. With the creation of EHRs, CHNs could link their interventions to the health status of individuals, thus creating the opportunity for integration of health promotion and the health status of the client. Stonham et al. (2012) identified the benefit of being able to document best practice in care and service with clients, and Rutten et al. (2014) identified client expectations of the maintenance of an EMR they could access. For community-based nurses providing care in the home, access to information at the bedside is considered a major advantage (Caligtan, Carroll, Hurley, Gersh-Zaremski, & Dykes, 2012; Luo, Tang, & Thomas, 2012). A challenge for nurses is the use of mobile devices such as cell phones and tablets at the client's bedside, specifically in terms of contamination of devices (Albrecht et al., 2013; Unstun & Cihangiroglu, 2012), especially for nurses who access clients in both acute-care and community-based settings. Unstun and Cihangiroglu (2012) demonstrated that virtually all cell phones belonging to health care workers were contaminated with nosocomial pathogens, 10% with Methicillin-resistant *Staphylococcus aureus* and 11% with *E. coli*, particularly if the health care workers were employed in intensive care units. Albrecht et al. (2013) demonstrated that tablets used in clinical and nonclinical settings could be disinfected effectively through the use of isopropanol wipes.

TECHNOLOGIES THAT SUPPORT KNOWLEDGE EXCHANGE AND PROFESSIONAL DEVELOPMENT

ICTs can greatly benefit CHNs through the provision of access to supports for professional development and evidence-based decision making. These technologies include online **communities of practice**, portals, and repositories of evidence-based community health literature. A community of practice refers to groups of people who share common interests, values, and problems about a topic and interact together to deepen their knowledge (Wenger, McDermott, & Snyder, 2002). Canadian nursing researchers investigated networking needs of community health nursing researchers and decision makers (Edwards & Kothari, 2004; Kothari et al., 2005). They identified a need for a formal community health network to assist decision makers, researchers, and practitioners to debate the management of complex community health problems, supported by relevant research. Although face-to-face networks were preferred, there was willingness to try online networks. Findings resulted in an online networking project, CHNET-Works! Nurses are encouraged to join the asynchronous communication boards and weekly webinars on current community health topics (www.chnet-works.ca).

CHNs can harness the power of social media by creating their own **personal learning network (PLN)**. Gathering online information and resources and organizing these through a PLN can assist with professional development. CHNs unfamiliar with social media should consider adopting one tool, such as Twitter, and begin to explore its use. New users can find how-to resources online for establishing social media accounts. Once the account is in place, the use of hashtags can assist in creating a dynamic and informative PLN. Hashtags (#) are a means of organizing information on social media platforms. CHNs can explore any of these well-established health care hashtags to get a sense of the wealth of information available: #cdnhealth (Canada health care), #CHC (community health

centres), #hcsmca (health care social media Canada), and #rnchat (registered nurses chat).

NurseONE/INF-Fusion, developed by the Canadian Nurses Association, is a personalized interactive Web 2.0 resource designed to assist nurses in Canada to manage their professional development, connect with colleagues, and gain access to current, credible, reliable information resources and tools to support evidence-based nursing practice (www.nurseone.ca; see Figure 15.2). The Public Health Agency of Canada (2017) has a long-established online portal for knowledge exchange: the Canadian Best Practices Portal for Health Promotion and Chronic Disease Prevention (http://cbpp-pcpe.phac-aspc.gc.ca). It aims to enhance knowledge exchange in best practices and provides a central access point for best practices approaches. The Public Health Agency of Canada also provides practitioners with online learning modules to enhance skills in public health practice. Practitioners in public health can register to take the skills enhancement online modules. A reliable source of evidence-based materials relevant to CHNs includes the fully searchable online service Health-Evidence.ca (http://health-evidence.ca). The Effective Public Health Practice Program also provides links to numerous systematic literature reviews and summaries (www.ephpp.ca). The National Collaborating Centre of Methods and Tools (NCCMT) (www.nccmt.ca) provides information and resources about knowledge translation methods and tools relevant for community health students and practitioners. In particular, the NCCMT has collaborated with the Health Communication Unit to develop and disseminate the Online Health Program Planner, an interactive, flexible, and intuitive tool to assist with the development of evidence-informed program plans (Ciliska et al., 2009).

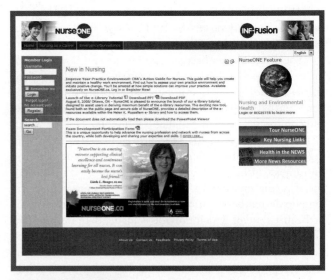

FIGURE 15.2 Screen Capture of NurseONE/INF-Fusion

Source: Screen shot from Canadian Nurses Association. Copyright © Canadian Nurses Association. Reprinted with permission. Further reproduction prohibited.

CONCLUSION

Digital health interventions provide extensive and often targeted information, expand communication, and offer new supports to empower individuals, groups, and communities to take a more active role in their health. CHNs should incorporate appropriate digital health solutions into their plan of care and also have a critical leadership role to play in enabling the public to use online health information resources safely and effectively. CHNs can help ensure accessibility to quality health information for the populations they serve and act as advocates to prevent a widening of the digital divide. The use of digital health solutions to support health promotion, disease prevention, and chronic disease management will play a prominent role in securing a healthier future for all Canadians. Online resources and social media connectivity provide new professional development opportunities for CHNs, including ready access to communities of practice, online learning modules or webinars, and evidence-based materials to support professional growth and practice excellence.

KEY TERMS

communities of practice   (p. 304)
digital divide   (p. 293)
digitally connected health   (p. 291)
digital health   (p. 290)
e-health   (p. 290)
health literacy   (p. 292)
HON code   (p. 296)
information and communication technologies (ICTs)   (p. 290)
interactivity   (p. 300)
NurseONE/INF-Fusion   (p. 304)
nursing informatics   (p. 291)
personal learning network (PLN)   (p. 304)
public health informatics   (p. 291)
readability   (p. 298)
surveillance   (p. 303)
tailoring   (p. 300)
targeting   (p. 299)
telehealth   (p. 290)
Web Accessibility Initiative   (p. 295)
Web Content Accessibility Guidelines   (p. 295)

STUDY QUESTIONS

1. Identify different ways that the "digital divide" has been conceptualized since the term first appeared.

2. Describe three tools that can be used to enhance internet accessibility for disabled populations.

3. What is the HON code, and what is its purpose?

4. Describe three online health promotion interventions that show promise.

5. Where can CHNs get access to evidence-based information on the Web to guide their decision making in practice?

6. What is the nursing role with respect to digital health information?

INDIVIDUAL CRITICAL-THINKING EXERCISES

1. What criteria would you use to evaluate a health promotion intervention, such as a smoking-cessation website?

2. What would you need to consider when working as a CHN with a client who is visually impaired and wants to use the internet?

3. Discuss the merits and drawbacks of the HON code. Review the editorial and the response to it found in the *Journal of Medical Internet Research* by Eysenbach (2001).

4. What would you need to take into account when designing a web-based intervention for an older adult?

5. How can technology help to empower individuals and communities?

6. How would you determine if a health promotion website is appropriate for an Indigenous community with whom you are working?

7. How would you explain privacy protections to a youth who is considering accessing your ethically designed health promotion website but is concerned that his identity will be apparent?

GROUP CRITICAL-THINKING EXERCISES

1. Discuss the informatics core competencies you think a new graduate working in community health is required to have at a high level of proficiency. Use the Community Health Nurses Standards of Practice (Appendix A) to help you.

2. What trends do you anticipate in the use of the internet to promote health by youth, older adult, new immigrant, and disabled populations? What role could Web 2.0 technologies have in promoting health and preventing disease?

3. Should nurses encourage their clients to join online social support groups? Why or why not?

REFERENCES

Ache, K. A., & Wallace, L. S. (2009). Are end-of-life patient education materials readable? *Palliative Medicine, 23*, 545–548. doi:10.1177/0269216309106313

Albrecht, U. V., von Jan, U., Sedlacek, L., Groos, S., Suerbaum, S., & Vonberg, R. P. (2013). Standardized, app-based disinfection of iPads in a clinical and nonclinical setting: Comparative analysis. *Journal of Medical Internet Research, 15*(8), e176. doi:10.2196/jmir/2643

AlGhamdi, K. M., & Moussa, N. A. (2012). Internet use by the public to search for health-related information. *International Journal of Medical Informatics, 81*, 363–373. doi:10.1016/j.ijmedinf.2011.12.004

Ammerlaan, J. W., van Os-Medendorp, H., de Boer-Nijhof, N., Maat, B., Scholtus, L., Kruize, A. A., . . . Geenen, R. (2017). Preference and needs of patients with a rheumatic disease regarding the structure and content of online self-management support. *Patient Education and Counseling, 100*, 501–508. doi: 10.1016/j.pec/2016.10.009

Anker, A. E., Reinhart, A. M., & Feeley, T. H. (2011). Health information seeking: A review of measures and methods. *Patient Education and Counselling, 82,* 346–354. doi:10.1016/j.pec/2010.12.008

Antheunis, M. L., Tates, K., & Nieboer, T. E. (2013). Patients' and health professionals' use of social media in health care: Motives, barriers and expectations. *Patient Education and Counselling, 92,* 426–431. doi:10.1016/j.pec.2013.06.020

Barnett, L. (2017). *Bill C-38: An Act to amend an Act to amend the Criminal Code (Exploitation and Trafficking in Persons)* [*Legislative Summary*]. Government of Canada Publication no. 42-1-C38-E.

Bastable, S. (2013). *Nurse as Educator: Principles of teaching and learning for nursing practice.* Burlington, MA: Jones & Barlett.

Beaunoyer, E., Arsenault, M., Lomanowska, A. M., & Guitton, M. J. (2017). Understanding online health information: Evaluation, tools, and strategies. *Patient Education and Counseling, 100,* 183–189. doi 10.1016/j.pec2016.08.028

Becker, H., Mackert, M., & Kang, S. J. (2013). Using an e-health intervention to promote the health of cancer survivors with preexisting disabling conditions. *Computers, Informatics, Nursing, 31*(3), 107–114. doi:10.1097/nxn.0b013e3182771895

Bennett, G. G., & Glasgow, R. E. (2009). The delivery of public health interventions via the internet: Actualizing their potential. *Annual review of public health, 30,* 273–292. doi:10.1146/annurev.publhealth.031308.100235

Bol, N., Smets, E. M., Rutgers, M. M., Burgers, J. A., de Haes, H. C., Loos, E. F., & van Weert, J. C. (2013). Do videos improve website satisfaction and recall of online cancer-related information in older lung cancer patients? *Patient Education and Counseling, 92*(3), 404–412.

Borycki, E. M., Foster, J., Sahama, T., Frisch, N., & Kushniruk, A. W. (2013). Developing national level nursing informatics competencies for undergraduate nurses: Methodological approaches from Australia and Canada. *Enabling Health and Healthcare through ICT. IOS Press.* doi:10.3233/978-1-61499-203-5-345

Burns, P., Jones, S. C., Inverson, D., & Caputi, P. (2013). Usability testing of AsthmaWise with older adults. *Computers, Informatics, Nursing, 31*(5), 219–226. doi:10.1097/nxn.0b013e31829b0627

Caligtan, C. A., Carroll, D. L., Hurley, A. C., Gersh-Zaremski, R., & Dykes, P. C. (2012). Bedside information technology to support patient-centered care. *International Journal of Medical Information, 81,* 442–451. doi:10.1016.j.ijmed inf.2011.12.005

Canada Health Infoway. (2015). *Report on digital health: Canadians embracing digital health.* Retrieved from https://www.infoway-inforoute.ca/en/component/edocman/resources/reports/2815-infographic-report-on-digital-health-canadians-embracing-digital-health

Canadian Association of Schools of Nursing (CASN). (2012). *Nursing informatics: Entry-to-practice competencies for registered nurses.* Retrieved from http://www.casn.ca/2014/12/casn-entry-practice-nursing-informatics-competencies

Canadian Association of Schools of Nursing (CASN). (2013). *Nursing informatics teaching toolkit: Supporting the integration of the CASN nursing informatics competencies into nursing curricula.* Retrieved from http://www.casn.ca/2014/12/nursing-informatics-teaching-toolkit

Canadian Association of Schools of Nursing (CASN). (2014). *Entry-to-Practice Public Health Nursing Competencies for Undergraduate Nursing Education.* Ottawa ON: Author. Retrieved from http://www.casn.ca/2014/12/entry-practice-public-health-nursing-competencies-undergraduate-nursing-education-2

Canadian Internet Registration Authority. (2013). *CIRA factbook.* Retrieved from http://www.cira.ca/factbook/2013/index.html

Canadian Literacy and Learning Network. (2014). *Literacy statistics in Canada.* Retrieved from http://www.literacy.ca

Canadian Nurses Association (CNA). (2006). *e-Nursing strategy for Canada.* Retrieved from https://www.cna-aiic.ca/en/download-buy/nursing-informatics

Canadian Nurses Association & the Canadian Nursing Informatics Association (CNA & CNIA). (2017). *Joint position statement: Nursing informatics.* Retrieved from https://cnia.ca/standards

Canadian Public Health Association. (2018). *Plain language service.* Canadian Public Health Association. Ottawa, ON: Author. Retrieved from https://www.cpha.ca/search/node?keys=plain+language+health+information

Changrani, J., & Gany, F. (2005). Online cancer education and immigrants: Effecting culturally appropriate websites. *Journal of Cancer Education, 20,* 183–186. doi:10.1207/s15430154jce2003_14

Chaudhuri, S., Le, T., White, C., Thompson, H., & Demiris, G. (2013). Examining health information-seeking behaviors of older adults. *Computers, Informatics, Nursing, 32*(11), 547–553. doi:10.1097/01.NCN.0000432131.92020.42

Choma, K., & McKeever, A. E. (2015). Cervical cancer screening in adolescents: An evidence-based internet education program for practice improvement among advanced practice nurses. *Worldviews on Evidence-Based Nursing, 12*(1), 51–60.

Ciliska, D., Clark, K., Hershfield, L., Jetha, N., Mackintosh, J., & Finkle, D. (2009). *Using an online health program planner: What's in it for you?* Ottawa, ON: Canadian Public Health Association.

Cole, J., Watkins, C., & Kleine, D. (2016). Health advice from internet discussion forums: How bad is dangerous? *Journal of Medical Internet Research, 18*(1), e4. doi: 10.2196/jmir.5051

Community Health Nurses of Canada (CHNC). (2019, revised). *Canadian community health nursing: Professional practice model & standards of practice.* St. Johns, NL: Author. Retrieved from https://www.chnc.ca/en/publications-resources

Cunningham, J. A., Humphreys, K., Kypri, K., & van Mierlo, T. (2006). Formative evaluation and three-month follow-up of an online personalized assessment feedback intervention for problem drinkers. *Journal of Medical Internet Research, 8*(2), e5. doi:10.2196/jmir.8.2.e5

Dean, C. A., Geneus, C. J., Rice, S., Johns, M., Quasie-Woode, D., Broom, K., & Elder, K. (2017). Assessing the significance of health information seeking in chronic condition management. *Patient Education and Counseling, 100,* 1519–1526. doi: 10.1016/j.pec.2017.03.012

De Ruijter, D., Smit, E. S., de Vries, H., & Hoving, C. (2016). Web-based computer tailoring for practice nurses aimed to improve smoking cessation guideline adherence: A study protocol for a randomized controlled effectiveness trial. *Contemporary Clinical Trials, 48*, 125–132. doi 10/1016/k/cct2016/04.007

Donelle, L., & Hoffman-Goetz, L. (2008). An exploratory study of Canadian Aboriginal online health care forums. *Health Communications, 23*(3), 270–281. doi:10.1080/10410230802056388

Edwards, N., & Kothari, A. (2004). CHNET-Works! A networking infrastructure for community health nurse researchers and decision-makers. *Canadian Journal of Nursing Research, 36*(4), 203–207.

Eysenbach, G. (2001). What is e-health? *Journal of Medical Internet Research, 3*(2), e20. doi:10.2196/jmir.3.2.e20

Eysenbach, G. (2007). From intermediation to disintermediation and apomediation: New models for consumers to access and assess the credibility of health information in the age of Web 2.0. *Studies in Health Technology and Informatics, 129*(1), 162–166.

Fox, S. (2007). *E-patients with a disability or chronic disease.* Pew Research Center. Retrieved from http://www.pewinternet .org/files/old-media/Files/Reports/2007/EPatients_Chronic_Conditions_2007.pdf.pdf

Fung, I. C., Tsz Ho Tse, Z., & Fu, K. (2015). The use of social media in public health surveillance. *Western Pacific Surveillance and Response Journal, 6*(2), 3–6. doi: 10.5365/WPSAR.2015.6.1.019

Gibbons, M. C., Wilson, R. F., Samal, L., Lehmann C. U., Dickersin, K., Lehmann, H. P., . . . Bass, E. B. (2009, October). *Impact of consumer health informatics applications* (Evidence Report/Technology Assessment No. 188). (Prepared by Johns Hopkins University Evidence-based Practice Center under contract No. HHSA 290-2007-10061-I.) AHRQ Publication No. 09(10)-E019. Rockville, MD: Agency for Healthcare Research and Quality.

Goldberg, L., Lide, B., Lowry, S., Massett, H. A., O'Connell, T., Preece, J., . . . Shneiderman, B. (2011). Usability and accessibility in consumer health informatics: Current trends and future challenges. *American Journal of Preventative Medicine, 40*(5S2), S187–S197. doi:10.1016/j .amepre.2011.01.009

Godwin, Z. R., Bockhold, J. C., Webster, L., Falwell, S., Bomze, L., & Tran, N. K. (2013). Development of novel smart device based application for serial wound imaging and management. *Burns, 39*, 1395–1402. doi:10.1016/j .burns.2013.03.021

Grierson, T., van Dijk, M. W., Dozois, E., & Mascher, J. (2006). Policy and politics. Using the internet to build community capacity for healthy public policy. *Health Promotion Practice, 7*, 13–22. doi:10.1177/1524839905278590

Griffiths, F., Cave, J., Boardman, F., Ren, J., Pawlikowska, T., Ball, R., . . . Cohen, A. (2012). Social networks—The future for health care delivery. *Social Science & Medicine, 75*, 2233–2241. doi:10.1016/j.socscimed.2012.08.023

Haase, K. R., Strohschein, F., Lee, V., & Loiselle, C. (2016). The promise of virtual navigation in cancer care: Insights from patients and health care providers. *Canadian Oncology Nursing Journal, 26*(3), 238–245. doi:10.5737/23688076263238245

Health Canada. (2018). *Cyberbullying information for teens.* Retrieved from https://www.getcybersafe.gc.ca/cnt/cbrbllng/tns/index-en.aspx

Hardiker, N. R., & Grant, M. J. (2011). Factors that influence public engagement with eHealth: A literature review. *International Journal of Medical Informatics, 80*, 1–12. doi:10.1016/j.ijmedinf.2010.10.017

Health on the Net Foundation. (2016). HON code of conduct (HON code) for medical and health Web sites. *Health on the Net Foundation.* Retrieved from http://www.hon.ch/HONcode/Pro

Hebda, T., & Czar, P. (2013). *Handbook of informatics for nurses & healthcare professionals* (5th ed.). Boston, MA: Pearson.

Hoffman-Goetz, L., Donelle, L., & Thomson, M. D. (2009). Clinical guidelines about diabetes and the accuracy of peer information in an unmoderated online health forum for retired persons. *Informatics for Health and Social Care, 34*(2), 91–99. doi:10.1001/archinte.165.22.2618

Horrigan, J. (2015). *Libraries at the crossroads.* Pew Research Center. Retrieved from http://www.pewinternet .org/2015/09/15/2015/Libraries-at-crossroads

Househ, M., Borycki, E., & Kushniruk, A. (2014). Empowering patients through social media: The benefits and challenges. *Health Informatics Journal, 20*(1), 50–58. doi:10.1177/1460458213476969

Husting, E. L., & Gadsden-Knowles, K. (2011). The Centers of Excellence in public health informatics: Improving public health through innovation, collaboration, dissemination, and translation. *Online Journal of Public Health Informatics, 3*(3). doi: 10.5210/ojphi.v3i3.3897

Ibrahim, D. (2018). *Trafficking in persons in Canada, 2016.* Statistics Canada, Canadian Centre for Justice Statistics. Statistics Canada Catalogue no. 85-005-X.

Kerr, M., Savik, K., Monsen, K. A., & Lusk, S. L. (2007). Effectiveness of computer-based tailoring versus targeting to promote use of hearing protection. *Canadian Journal of Nursing Research, 39*(1), 80–97.

Khechine, H., Pascot, D., & Prémont, P. (2008). Use of health-related information from the internet by English-speaking patients. *Health Informatics, 14*, 17–28. doi:10.1177/1460458207086331

Kitchens, B., Harle, C. A., & Li, S. (2014). Quality of health-related search results. *Decision Support Systems, 57*, 454–462.

Kivits, J. (2009). Everyday health and the internet: A mediated health perspective on health information seeking. *Sociology of Health and Illness, 31*(5), 673–687. doi:10.1111/j.1467-9566.2008.01153.x

Korp, P. (2006). Health on the internet: Implications for health promotion. *Health Education Research, 21*, 78–86. doi:10.1093/her/cyh043

Kothari, A., Edwards, N., Brajtman, S., Campbell, B., Hamel, N., Legault, F., . . . Valaitis, R. (2005). Fostering interactions: The networking needs of community health nursing researchers and decision-makers. *Evidence and Policy, 1*, 291–304.

Kreps, G. L., & Sparks, L. (2008). Meeting the health literacy needs of immigrant populations. *Patient Education and Counseling, 71*, 328–332. doi:10.1016/j.pec.2008.03.001

Kruse, C. S., Argueta, D. A., Lopez, L., & Nair, A. (2015). Patient and provider attitudes toward the use of patient portals for the management of chronic illness: A systematic review. *Journal of Medical Internet Research, 17*(2), e40. doi:10.2196/jamir.3703

Lam, C. G., Roter, D. L., & Cohen, K. J. (2013). Survey of quality, readability, and social reach of websites on osteosarcoma in adolescents. *Patient Education and Counseling, 90,* 82–87. doi:10.1016/j.pec.2012.08.006

Lemire, M., Paré, G., Sicotte, C., & Harvey, C. (2008). Determinants of internet use as a preferred source of information on personal health. *International Journal of Medical Informatics, 77,* 723–734. doi:10.1016/j.ijmedinf.1008.03.002

Lemire, M., Sicotte, C., & Paré, G. (2008). Internet use and the logics of personal empowerment in health. *Health Policy, 88,* 130–140. doi:10.1016/j.healthpol.2008.03.006

Letourneau, N., Stewart, M., Masuda, J., Anderson, S., Cicutto, L., McGhan, S., & Watt, S. (2012). Impact of online support for youth with asthma and allergies: Pilot study. *Journal of Pediatric Nursing, 27,* 65–73. doi:10.1016/j.pedn.2010.07.007

Liu, S., Dunford, S. D., Leung, Y. W., Brooks, D., Thomas, S. G., Eysenbach, G., & Nolan, R. P. (2013). Reducing blood pressure with internet-based interventions: A meta-analysis. *Canadian Journal of Cardiology, 29,* 613–621. doi:10.1016/j.cjca.2013.02.007

Lober, W. B., & Flowers, J. L. (2011). Consumer empowerment in health care amid the internet and social media. *Seminars in Oncology Nursing, 27*(3), 169–182. doi:10.1016/j.soncn.2011.04.002

Lustria, M. L. A., Cortese, J., Noar, S. M., & Glueckauf, R. I. (2009). Computer-tailored health interventions delivered over the web: Review and analysis of key components. *Patient Education and Counselling, 74,* 156–173. doi:10.1016/j.pec.2008.08.023

Luo, G., Tang, C., & Thomas, S. B. (2012). Intelligent personal health record: Experience and open issues. *Journal of Medical Systems, 36,* 2111–2128. doi:10.1007/s10916-011-9674-5

Manafo, E., & Wong, S. (2012). Exploring older adults' health information seeking behaviors. *Journal of Nutrition and Behavior, 44*(1), 85–89. doi:10.1016/j.jneb.2011.05.018

Manierre, M. J. (2015). Gaps in knowledge: Tacking and explaining gender differences in health information seeking. *Social Science & Medicine, 128,* 151–158. doi: 10.1016/j.socscimed.2015.01.028

McLaughlin, G. H. (1969). SMOG-grading: A new readability formula. *Journal of Reading, 12,* 639–646.

McMaster Health Forum. (2014). *Sharing health information with older adults through online resources in Canada.* Retrieved from http://mcmasterhealthforum.org

McRee, A., Esber, A., & Reiter, P. L. (2015). Acceptability of home-based chlamydia and gonorrhea testing among a national sample of sexual minority young adults. *Perspectives on Sexual and Reproductive Health, 47*(1), 3–10, doi: 10.1363/47e2715

Mitchell, M., White, L., Oh, P., Alter, D., Leahey, T., Kwan, M., & Faulkner, G. (2017). Uptake of an incentive-based mHealth app: Process evaluation of the Carrot Rewards app. *Journal of Medical Internet Research Mhealth Uhealth, 5*(5), e70. doi: 10.2196/mhealth.7323

Mitretek Systems Health Summit Working Group. (2017). *Mitretek criteria for evaluating the quality of health information on the internet.* Retrieved from http://www.bmj.com/content/suppl/2001/04/26/322.7293.1035.DC1

Mowat, D., & Butler-Jones, D. (2007). Public health in Canada: A difficult history. *Healthcare Papers, 7,* 31–36.

Muse, K., McManus, F., Leung, C., Meghreblian, B., & Williams, J. M. G. (2012). Cyberchondriasis: Fact or fiction? A preliminary examination of the relationship between health anxiety and searching for health information on the internet. *Journal of Anxiety Disorders, 26,* 189–196. doi:10.1016/j.janxdis.2011.11.005

Mudry, T. E., & Strong, T. (2012). Doing recovery online. *Qualitative Health Research, 23*(3), 313–325. doi:10.1177/1049732312468296

Nagle, L. (2007). Informatics: Emerging concepts and issues. *Nursing Leadership, 20,* 30–32.

Negev, M., Davidovitch, N., Garb, Y., & Tal, A. (2013). Stakeholder participation in health impact assessment: A multicultural approach. *Environmental Impact Assessment Review, 43,* 112–120. doi:10.1016/j.eiar.1013.06.002

Nguyen, D. P., Klein, B., Meyer, D., Austin, D. W., & Abbott, J. M. (2015). The diagnostic validity and reliability of an internet-based clinical assessment program for mental disorders. *Journal of Medical Internet Research, 17*(9), e218. doi:10.2196/jmir.4195

OECD & Statistics Canada. (2011). *Literacy for life: Further results from the adult literacy and life skills survey.* OECD Publishing. doi:9789264091269-en. Retrieved from http://www.statcan.gc.ca/pub/89-604-x/89-604-x2011001-eng.pdf

Ownby, R. L., Acevedo, A., Waldrop-Valverde, D., Jacobs, R. J., & Caballera, J. (2014). Abilities, skills and knowledge in measures of health literacy. *Patient Education and Counselling, 95,* 211–217. doi:10.1016/j.pec/2014.02.002

Pew Research Internet Survey. (2013). *Health information is a popular pursuit online.* Retrieved from http://www.pewinternet.org/2013/01/15/health-online-2013/

Pew Research Center. (2017). *Internet/broadband fact sheet.* Retrieved from http://www.pewinternet.org/fact-sheet/internet-broadband

Public Health Agency of Canada. (2017). *The Canadian Best Practices Portal for health promotion and chronic disease prevention*: About the portal. Retrieved from http://cbpp-pcpe.phac-aspc.gc.ca

Puresight. (2018). *How do online predators operate?* Retrieved from https://puresight.com/Pedophiles/Online-Predators/how-do-online-predators-operate.html

Ramsey, I., Corsini, N., Peters, M. D. J., & Eckert, M. (2017). A rapid review of consumer health information needs and preferences. *Patient Education and Counseling, 100,* 1634–1642. doi: 10.1016/j.pec.2017.04.005

Risling, T., Martinez, J., Young, J., & Thorp-Froslie, N. (2017). Evaluating patient empowerment in association with ehealth technology: A scoping review. *Journal of Medical Internet Research, 19*(9), e329. doi:10.2196/jmir.7809

Rooks, R. N., Wiltshire, J. C., Elder, K., BeLue, R., & Gary, L.C. (2012). Health information seeking and use outside of the medical encounter: Is it associated with race and ethnicity? *Social Science & Medicine, 74,* 176–184. doi:10.1016/j.socscimed.2011.09.040

Royer, H. R., Fernandez-Lambert, K. M., & Moreno, M. A. (2013). Formative research for the development of an interactive web-based sexually transmitted disease management for young women. *Computers, Informatics, Nursing, 31*(9), 430–438. doi:10.1097/01.NCN.0000432123.79452.32

Russo, J. A., Parisi, S. M., Kukla, K., & Schwarz, E. B. (2013). Women's information-seeking behavior after receiving contraceptive versus noncontraceptive prescriptions. *Contraception, 87,* 824–829. doi:10.1016/j.contraception.2012.09.028

Rutten, L. J. F., Vieux, S. N., St. Sauver, J. L., Arora, N. K., Moser, R. P., Beckjord, E. B., & Hesse, B. W. (2014). Patient perceptions of electronic medical records use and ratings of care quality. *Patient Related Outcome Measures, 5,* 17–23. doi:10.2147/PROM.S58967

Saitz, R., Helmuth, E. D., Aromaa, S. E., Guard, A., Belanger, M., & Rosenbloom, D. L. (2004). Web-based screening and brief intervention for the spectrum of alcohol problems. *Preventive Medicine, 39*(5), 969–975. doi:10.1016/j.ypmed.2004.04.011

Sarkar, U., Karter, A. J., Liu, J. Y., Adler, N. E., Nguyen, R., Lopez, A., & Schillinger, D. (2011). Social disparity in internet patient portal use in diabetes: Evidence that the digital divide extends beyond access. *Journal of American Medical Informatics Association, 18*(3), 318–321. doi:10.1136/jamia.2010.006015

Specter, M. (2013). *Jenny McCarthy's dangerous views.* Retrieved from https://www.newyorker.com/tech/elements/jenny-mccarthys-dangerous-views

Statistics Canada. (2009). *Internet use by individuals, by type of activity.* Retrieved from http://www40.statcan.gc.ca/l01/cst01/comm29a-eng.htm?sdi=internet

Statistics Canada. (2010). *Online activities of Canadian Boomers and seniors.* Retrieved from http://www.statcan.gc.ca/pub/11-008-x/2009002/article/10910-eng.htm

Statistics Canada. (2013a). *Canadian internet use survey.* Retrieved from http://www5.statcan.gc.ca/subject-sujet/result-resultat.action?pid=2256&id=2256&lang=eng&type=DAILYART

Statistics Canada. (2013b). *Individual internet usage and e-commerce 2012.* Retrieved from http://www.statcan.gc.ca/daily-quotidien/131028/dq131028a-eng.pdf

Statistics Canada. (2014). *Education indicators in Canada: An international perspective.* Retrieved from http://www.statcan.gc.ca/daily-quotidien/141215/dq141215b-eng.pdf

Statistics Canada. (2017). *The internet and digital technology.* Catalogue no. CS11-627/2017-32E-PDF. Available at http://publications.gc.ca/collections/collection_2017/statcan/11-627-m/11-627-m2017032-eng.pdf

Stern, A., Valaitis, R., Weir, R., & Jadad, A. R. (2012). Use of home telehealth in palliative cancer care: A case study. *Journal of Telemedicine and Telecare, 18*(5), 297–300. doi:10.1258/jtt.2012.111201

Stonham, G., Heyes, B., Owen, A., & Povey, E. (2012). Measuring the nursing contribution using electronic records. *Nursing Management, 19*(8), 28–32.

Suggs, L. S., & McIntyre, C. (2009). Are we there yet? An examination of online tailored health communication. *Health Education and Behavior, 36,* 278–288. doi:10.1177/1090198107303309

Suziedelyte, A. (2012). How does searching for health information on the internet affect individuals' demand for health services? *Social Science & Medicine, 75,* 1828–1835. doi:10.1016/j.socscimed.2012.07.022

Syred, J., Naidoo, C., Woodhall, S. C., & Araitser, P. (2014). Would you tell everyone this? Facebook conversations as health promotion interventions. *Journal of Medical Internet Research, 16*(4), e108. doi:10.2196/jmir.3231

Tan, S. S., & Goonawardene, N. (2017). Internet health information seeking and the patient-physician relationship: A systematic review. *Journal of Medical Internet Research, 19*(1), e9. doi: 10.2196/jmir.5729

Tapscott, D. (1998). The digital divide. In *Growing up digital: The rise of the net generation* (pp. 255–279). New York, NY: McGraw-Hill.

Topol, E. (2013). *The creative destruction of medicine: How the digital revolution will create better health care.* New York, NY: Basic Books.

Unstun, C., & Cihangiroglu, M. (2012). Health care workers' mobile phones: A potential cause for microbial cross-contamination between hospitals and communities. *Journal of Occupational and Environmental Hygiene, 9*(9), 538–42. doi: 10.1080/15459624.2012.697419

Valaitis, R. (2005). Computers and the internet: Tools for youth empowerment. *Journal of Medical Internet Research, 7*(5), e51. doi:10.2196/jmir.7.5.e51

Valaitis, R., & O'Mara, L. (2005). Enabling youth participation in school-based computer-supported community development in Canada. *Health Promotion International, 20*(3), 260–268. doi:10.1093/heapro/dah611

Vennick, F. D., Adams, S. A., Faber, M. J., & Putters, K. (2014). Expert and experiential knowledge in the same place: Patients' experiences with online communities connecting patients and healthcare professionals. *Patient Education and Counselling, 95,* 265–270. doi:10.1016/j.pec.2014.02.003

W3C. (2017a). Web accessibility initiative (WAI). World Wide Web Consortium W3C. Retrieved from http://www.w3.org/WAI

W3C. (2017b). How to meet WCAG 2.0. World Wide Web Consortium W3C https://www.w3.org/WAI/WCAG20/quickref

W3C. (2017c). Web accessibility tutorials. World Wide Web Consortium W3C. Retrieved from http://www.w3.org/WAI/tutorials

Wenger, E., McDermott, R., & Snyder, W. (2002). *A guide to managing knowledge: Cultivating communities of practice.* Boston, MA: Harvard Business School Press.

Whittaker, R., Borland, R., & Bullen, C. (2009). Mobile phone-based interventions for smoking cessation. *Cochrane Database of Systematic Reviews,* Oct. 7 (4): CD006611.

WRAPIN. (2014). *Worldwide online reliable advice to patients and individuals.* European Project-IST-2001-33260. Retrieved from http://www.wrapin.org

Woodall, J., Taylor, V. M., Chong T., Li, L., Acorda, E., Tu, S., & Hislpo, G. (2009). Sources of health information among Chinese immigrants to the Pacific Northwest. *Journal of Cancer Education, 24*(4), 334–340. doi:10.1080/08858190902854533

Xiao, N., Sharman, R., Rao, H. R., & Upadhyaya, S. (2014). Factors influencing online health information search: An empirical analysis of a national cancer-related survey. *Decision Support Systems, 57,* 417–427. doi:10.1016/j.dss.2012.10.047

Xie, B. (2012). Improving older adults' e-health literacy through computer training using NIH online resources. *Library & Information Science Research, 34,* 63–71. doi:10.2196/jmir.1880

Ybarra, M. L., Biringi, R., Prescott, T., & Bull, S. S. (2012). Usability and navigability of an HIV/AIDS internet intervention for adolescents in a resource-limited setting. *Computers, Informatics, Nursing, 30*(11), 587–595. doi:10.1097/NSN.0b013e318266cb0e

Zelmer, J., & Hagens, S. (2014). Understanding the gap between the desire for and use of consumer health solutions. *Healthcare Papers, 13*(4), 9–21. doi: 10.12927/hcpap.2014.23871

ABOUT THE AUTHORS

Linda Ferguson, RN, PhD, is a full professor in the College of Nursing, University of Saskatchewan. Her undergraduate, master's, and PhD degrees are in the field of nursing, and she has a post-graduate diploma in Continuing Education. She has worked extensively in the field of faculty development within the College of Nursing and the University of Saskatchewan. Dr. Ferguson has taught educational methods courses at the undergraduate (nursing and physical therapy), post-registration, and master's levels for the past 28 years. Her research has focused on mentoring and preceptoring nurses, teaching excellence, interprofessional education, and the process of developing clinical judgment in nursing practice. She is past director of the Centre for the Advancement of the Study of Nursing Education and Inter-professional Education within the College of Nursing at the University of Saskatchewan, and she was president of the Canadian Association of Schools of Nursing (2012–2014).

Tracie Risling, RN, PhD, is Associate Professor in the College of Nursing at the University of Saskatchewan and serves as the Communications Director for the Canadian Nursing Informatics Association. Her program of informatics research has two foci: social media and the advancement of professional and patient voice, and the development and implementation of patient-centred technologies. Dr. Risling is exploring the role of technology in supporting patient empowerment and engagement through access to electronic health data and specific application design for health care transition.

Maternal, Newborn, and Child Health

CHAPTER 16

Josephine Etowa, Aliyah Dosani, and Heather Bensler

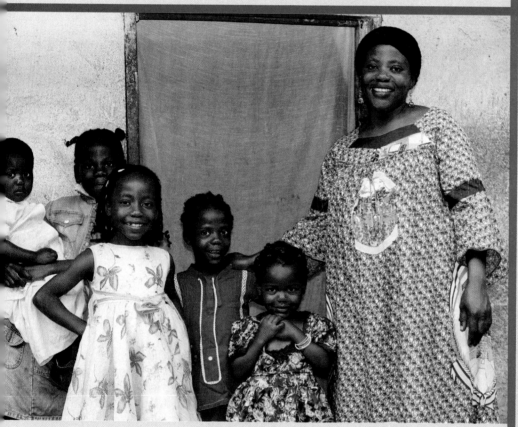

Source: Sylvie Bouchard/Shutterstock

LEARNING OUTCOMES

After studying this chapter, you should be able to:

1. Define key terms, and provide an overview of maternal, newborn, and child health.

2. Discuss perinatal health indicators in Canada.

3. Examine the sociocultural contexts of maternal newborn, and child health in Canada.

4. Identify the trends and issues related to teenage motherhood.

5. Explore perinatal health promotion in terms of reproductive health, rights, and justice.

6. Explore early childhood health indicators and health promotion in Canada.

INTRODUCTION

Maternal health and **maternal health care** generally refer to the health and services provided to women who are of childbearing age (after menses) and include preconception care, pregnancy, childbirth, and the postpartum period (Public Health Agency of Canada [PHAC], 2013). Sometimes this period of time just before conception, during pregnancy, and after labour and delivery is referred to as the **perinatal period**. Globally, the health of women and children is considered a key marker for the overall health status of families, communities, and societies, and it is upheld as an indicator for the overall health of people in Canada. Women, infants, and children around the world face numerous barriers in achieving an optimal health status. The World Health Organization (WHO, 2018) estimates that 830 women die every day around the world from preventable causes related to pregnancy and childbirth.

Canada has historically been a leader in promoting the health of women and children across the globe. Yet even in a country as wealthy as Canada, women and children continue to face barriers to achieving optimal health. Urban and rural women and children in Canada who already face poverty, unemployment, or lower levels of education are at an increased risk of disparities in health status, access to health care, and health promotion initiatives (Angus et al., 2012). Maternal, newborn, and child health challenges are particularly problematic for Indigenous communities in Northern Canada. According to a Health Council of Canada (2011) report, access to maternal, newborn, and child health services in Indigenous communities is compromised by the lack of culturally safe care, limited service providers, and the intergenerational effects of colonialism, racism, and residential schools. Community health nurses (CHNs), physicians, social workers, youth workers, police, and immigration workers all play active roles in identifying and addressing challenges to women and children achieving their best health.

PERINATAL HEALTH INDICATORS

In Table 16.1, specific epidemiologic terms that are often used in discussions about perinatal health are presented. According to Statistics Canada, approximately 97% of mothers with children ages 0 to 11 months receive prenatal care, but it is not known exactly what physical, emotional, or pregnancy-related care and information are provided at prenatal visits (Canadian Institute for Health Information, 2006). Over the past 150 years, Canadian mothers have encountered the medicalization of childbirth, where the biomedical model of being cared for by a physician, often in a tertiary care centre or doctor's office, is considered the "gold standard" of care for women and their children. For mothers who require close medical supervision, physicians, obstetricians, and tertiary care centres are the best choice. **Midwives** support traditional birthing practices—such as water births and the natural delivery of the placenta, for example—which had been lost within the modern medical system (Canadian Association of Midwives, 2014). Receiving medicalized prenatal and birth care, and information about fundamentals of childcare, such as breastfeeding, from medical professionals can send the message to mothers that even though mothering should be a very natural and safe process, it must be monitored by health care professionals.

The Canadian Perinatal Surveillance System is used to capture current information on major maternal, fetal, and infant health determinants and outcomes in Canada. From 2010–2014, there were 1.43 million live births (PHAC, 2017a). The rate of live births to older mothers aged 35–49 years gradually increased from 2005–2014 (PHAC, 2017b). The most pronounced increase was observed in women aged 35–39 years, where the birth rate increased from 44.2 to 53.6 per 1000 women (PHAC, 2017b). Table 16.2 provides information on provincial and territorial differences for live

Table 16.1	Key Epidemiologic Definitions for Perinatal Health
Maternal mortality ratio*	The number of maternal deaths during a given period per 100 000 live births during that same period.
Maternal mortality rate*	The number of maternal deaths in a given period per 100 000 women of reproductive age during the same time period.
Maternal death+	"The death of a woman while pregnant or within 42 days of termination of pregnancy, irrespective of the duration and the site of pregnancy, from any cause related to or aggravated by the pregnancy or its management but not from accidental or incidental causes." Maternal mortality is usually expressed per 100 000 deliveries.
Preterm birth**	An infant born with less than 37 weeks of gestation completed.
Small-for-gestational-age birth**	An infant who falls in the less-than-10th percentile at birth, based on the Canadian Fetal Growth Standard.
Low birth weight**	An infant who weighs less than 2500 grams at birth.
High birth weight**	An infant who weighs more than 4000 grams at birth.
Large-for-gestational-age birth**	An infant who falls in the greater-than-90th percentile at birth, based on the Canadian Fetal Growth Standard.
Neonatal death**	An infant who dies 0–27 days after birth.
Post-neonatal death**	An infant who dies 28–364 days after birth.
Total infant death**	An infant who dies 0–364 days after birth.

Sources: *World Health Organization. (2012). Trends in maternal mortality: 1990 to 2010, WHO, UNICEF, UNFPA and the World Bank estimates. Retrieved from http://www.unfpa.org/sites/default/files/pub-pdf/9789241507226_eng.pdf; +*International statistical classification of diseases 10th revision* (ICD-10); **Luo, Z. C., Wilkins, R., Heaman, M., Martens, P., Smylie, J., Hart, L., Simonet, F., . . . Fraser, W. D. (2010). Birth outcomes and infant mortality by the degree of rural isolation among First Nations and non-First Nations, in Manitoba, Canada. *Journal of Rural Health, 26*(2), 175–181.

Table 16.2	Proportion of Live Births to Mothers Aged 35–39 and 40–49 Years, By Province/Territory (Excluding Quebec), 2010–2014				
	35–39		**40–49**		
Province/territory	**Number of live births**	**Proportion (%) of total live births**	**Number of live births**	**Proportion (%) of total live births**	**Total number of live births****
Newfoundland and Labrador	2,956	13.1	487	2.2	22,558
Prince Edward Island	909	13.1	160	2.3	6,953
Nova Scotia	5,856	13.8	1,120	2.6	42,445
New Brunswick	3,766	10.9	624	1.8	34,638
Ontario	122,653	18.2	27,652	4.1	672,111
Manitoba	9,832	12.4	1,920	2.4	79,267
Saskatchewan	7,370	10.2	1,348	1.9	72,587
Alberta	36,770	14.4	7,359	2.9	256,037
British Columbia	39,909	19.0	9,467	4.5	210,252
Yukon	392	19.4	75	3.7	2,020
Northwest Territories	417	11.6	87	2.4	3,601
Nunavut	263	6.6	47	1.2	3,935
Canada*	**234,852**	**16.4**	**51,350**	**3.6**	**1,430,647**

Source: Canadian Institute for Health Information-Discharge Abstract Database (CIHI-DAD)

*Includes data from unknown provinces and territories
**Excludes live births to mothers aged 50 years and over, and those with unknown maternal age.
Data for Quebec were excluded because they do not contribute to CIHI-DAD.

Source: Perinatal Health Indicators for Canada, 2017.

births for women aged 35–39 and 40–49. Conversely, the rate of live births to mothers aged 15–17 years decreased from 8.4 per 1000 women in 2007 to 5.3 per 1000 women in 2014 (PHAC, 2017b). Similarly, the rate of live births to mothers aged 18–19 decreased from 27.2 per 1000 in 2007 to 18.6 per 1000 in 2014 (PHAC, 2017b). However, as demonstrated in Table 16.3, there is much inequality in the teenage pregnancy rates between provinces. British Columbia boasts the lowest pregnancy rate for individuals aged 10–17 at 1.7 live births per 1000, whereas Nunavut has the highest pregnancy rate for the same age group at 26.8 per 1000 (PHAC, 2017b).

Immigrant and Refugee Perinatal Mental Health Outcomes

Immigrant and refugee women are rendered vulnerable to negative mental health outcomes during the perinatal and postnatal periods due to social determinants of health such as inadequate social support, poverty, and demanding gender roles that reduce a women's self-esteem and perceived power (O'Mahony & Donnelly, 2013). When comparing depression rates at 16 weeks postpartum, asylum seekers have a significantly higher rate of postpartum depression (14.3%) compared with refugee women (11.5%), recent non-refugee immigrant women, (5.1%) and Canadian-born women (2.6%) (Dennis, Merry, & Gagnon, 2017). Dennis et al. (2017) suggest that factors such as vulnerable immigration status, food insecurity, lack of social support, and a sense of not belonging in Canadian society put migrant women at higher risk for postpartum depression. Migrant women are also more likely to experience barriers to health care services exacerbated by language and gender-based cultural issues than Canadian-born women (Khanlou, Haque, Sinner, Mantini, & Kurtz Landy, 2017). Guruge, Thomson, George, and Chaze (2015) suggest that interventions, programs, and services be aimed at improving social networks and structures of support, which are protective factors that build resilience. Further, policies and programs that provide culturally safe support, and inter-sectoral collaboration are needed to reduce barriers and enable access to appropriate care (Guruge et al., 2015). Immigrant and refugee women are at increased risk of negative mental health outcomes, particularly when their immigration status is precarious (Khanlou et al., 2017).

Table 16.3	Proportion of Live Births to Mothers Aged 10–17 and 18–19 Years by Province/Territory (Excluding Quebec), 2010–2014				
	10–17		16–19		
Province/territory	Number of live births	Proportion (%) of total live births	Number of live births	Proportion (%) of total live births	Total number of live births**
Newfoundland and Labrador	373	1.7	868	3.8	22.558
Prince Edward Island	80	1.2	236	3.4	6,953
Nova Scotia	695	1.6	1,641	3.9	42,445
New Brunswick	604	1.7	1,510	4.4	34,638
Ontario	5,764	0.9	14,278	2.1	672,111
Manitoba	1,926	2.4	3,910	4.9	79,267
Saskatchewan	1,861	2.6	3,667	5.1	72,587
Alberta	2,845	1.1	6,576	2.6	256,037
British Columbia	1,594	0.8	3.876	1.8	210,252
Yukon	22	1.1	66	3.3	2,020
Northwest Territories	108	3.0	256	7.1	3,601
Nunavut	335	8.4	423	10.6	3,985
Canada*	**16,349**	**1.1**	**37,767**	**2.6**	**1,430,647**

Source: Canadian Institute for Health Information-Discharge Abstract Database (CIHI-DAD)

*Includes data from unknown provinces and territories
**Excludes live births to mothers aged 50 years and over, and those with unknown maternal age
Data for Quebec were excluded because they do not contribute to CIHI-DAD.

Source: Perinatal Health Indicators for Canada, 2017.

Infant Outcomes

One important key indicator of child health is the **infant mortality rate**. It is worrisome that Canada's infant mortality rate ranked 10th among 24 Organisation for Economic Co-operation and Development countries in 1980 (Robert Wood Johnson Foundation, 2008), and it dropped even further down the list to 27th of 36 countries in 2010 and 30th of 44 countries in 2015, a span of just 35 years (Organisation for Economic Co-operation and Development, 2011, 2017). In the Canadian context, the infant mortality rate ranged from 3.6 per 1000 live births in Prince Edward Island to 17.9 per 1000 live births in Nunavut between 2002 and 2011 (Figure 16.1). Lower socioeconomic status and lower levels of neighbourhood income have been found to be associated with a higher risk of adverse perinatal health outcomes, particularly infant mortality (de Graff, 2013). First Nation, Inuit, and Métis populations have historically had poor health outcomes relative to non-Indigenous Canadians. A similar trend has been observed in infant health. Luo et al. (2010) observed that in urban areas, Indigenous infants fare more poorly than non-Indigenous infants. In contrast, rural residence, regardless of degree of isolation, appears to be a protective factor against preterm birth, small for gestational age, and low birth weight for both Indigenous and non-Indigenous populations.

SOCIOCULTURAL CONTEXTS OF MATERNAL, NEWBORN, AND CHILD HEALTH IN CANADA

Mothering: A Kaleidoscope of Ideologies

Mothering . . .
. . . is fundamental to all beings.
. . . involves nurturing and raising children.
. . . extends far beyond biology and bodies.
. . . is the act and practice of love and the passing on of knowledge.
. . . occurs across multiple times and spaces.
. . . is political.
. . . is life.
(National Collaborating Centre for Aboriginal Health, 2012)

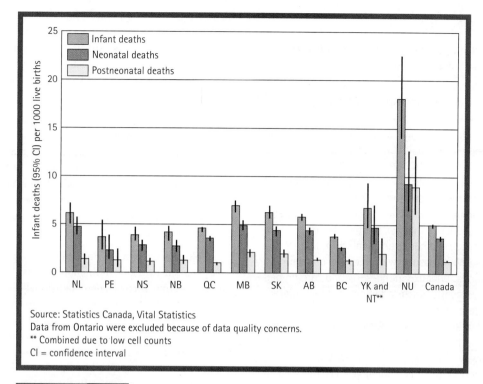

FIGURE 16.1 Crude Mortality Rates by Province/Territory (Excluding Ontario, 2007–2011)

Source: Perinatal Health Indicators for Canada, 2017.

In Western societies, becoming a mother is often exalted and envisioned as a beautiful state that all women should embrace. The reality is that for many women in Canada, mothering can be profoundly different from this. See Research box 16.1. The discussions that societies, communities, families, and individuals have about mothering can both help and hinder the health of women and their families. For example, a positive message of the importance of mothering in Canadian society is the public health policy of a paid maternity and parental benefit that enables many women to stay home with their child up to 18 months after birth (Government of Canada, 2018). Many families benefit from the paid leave as childcare costs can be reduced and children can benefit from time with a parent over their first year of life. However, there are contradictory messages about mothering that can isolate women and set up unrealistic or unfair disconnects. For example, the weekly benefit rate is a mere 55% of the claimant's average weekly insurable earnings up to a maximum amount (Government of Canada, 2018, para 1). In addition, breastfeeding is widely accepted as the best **nutrition** a mother can offer her baby. Yet when mothers across Canada have attempted to breastfeed in public, they have faced discrimination. For example, some mothers have been asked to stop feeding their infant or to continue to feed in a "private" area such as a public bathroom (Photo 16.1). Breastfeeding campaigns across North America are moving to bring this issue to light to promote social justice for mothers and babies and to change the culture of how breastfeeding is viewed.

The Experience of Birthing for Indigenous Communities

The concept of mothering and how to become a mother is not a uniformly held belief across Canada. Many Indigenous cultures hold traditional beliefs about how women become

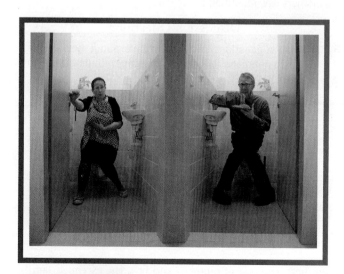

PHOTO 16.1 If you are not willing to eat your lunch in the bathroom, then don't expect me to feed my kid there!

Source: Tamar Shugert Photography

CANADIAN RESEARCH 16.1

Mother's level of confidence in caring for her late preterm infant: A mixed methods study. (Premji et al., 2018)

While public health nurses (PHNs) provide a supportive care environment in the community for mothers during the postpartum period, we know little about the confidence mothers have while caring for a late preterm infant (LPI) and how maternal depression compounds this experience. The purpose of this study was to determine what it means to be a mother of a late preterm infant using a mixed method approach. A convenience sample of 71 mothers of LPIs completed questionnaires on maternal confidence, parenting stress, social support, and postpartum depression. In addition, 11 of these mothers participated in semi-structured interviews. While issues with feeding undermined maternal confidence, prior experiences in child care helped mothers feel more confident. In addition, positive interactions with the infant and adequate social support increased maternal confidence. Confidence for both depressed and non-depressed mothers decreased from 3-4 weeks to 6-8 weeks after delivery. This was due to the inability to grasp the unique attributes of LPIs challenges experienced of caring for their LPI, including the possibility of re-hospitalization and the use of deficit-based approach used by PHNs to educate and guide them. Mothers in our study also noted both positive and challenging interactions with PHNs. Mothers of LPIs who experienced health issues had a higher stress level and lower level of confidence. Of all mothers in the study, 25.4% were depressed. Mothers in this study did not discuss mental health issues. We take note of this because it could be a reflection of the protective effects of social support on emotional stability or an inability to recognize postpartum depression. While PHNs are seen as a postpartum resource, the need for improvement in the development of optimal relationships between PHNs and mothers was identified in the study.

Discussion Questions

1. What suggestions might you have about how PHNs should approach relationship building with mothers who have LPIs?

2. PHNs could interact with families with LPIs prior to discharge from hospital. What changes to the health care system in your region would you propose to ensure that the transition for families with a LPI is seamless from hospital to the community?

3. What do you think community health nurses need to advocate for, in terms of their practice settings, to ensure appropriate care is provided to families with LPIs?

mothers, the role of mothers, and how the extended family community is involved in raising children. Traditionally, in many Indigenous communities, pregnant women and mothers were supported by the entire community, provided with healthy foods, supported to be physically active, and cared for spiritually through prayers and traditional ceremonies that were passed down over generations. The gathering of family members and friends during labour and delivery created a sense of belonging-through-birth and formed cultural and emotional ties to the land (Kornelsen, Kotaska, Waterfall, Willie, & Wilson, 2010).

"A Saulteaux Elder describes how in the past, the whole community celebrated pregnancy: Everybody knew about it. Everybody wanted to be part and parcel of that child within that womb. [The child] had to have a sense of belonging through the mother, and the woman had to have a sense of pride because she was contributing to the life of the community. She was bringing in new life, and she was treated special." (Lavell-Harvard & Lavell, 2006)

Colonization and the dominance of the biomedical model have resulted in many Indigenous women receiving prenatal care and giving birth in non-traditional settings that do not support sacred and traditional practices. Many First Nation communities are isolated, requiring women and families to travel great distances to receive prenatal care or live away from their communities for several weeks to give birth in larger centres (Kornelsen & Grzybowski, 2005). Funding for medical transportation covers only the mother and not a support person, so this means most women travel to the larger birthing centre alone and without any social support (Olson & Couchie, 2013). In Manitoba, it is estimated that as many as 1100 prenatal women relocate temporarily from First Nation communities in rural and remote regions of the province, such as Norway House Cree Nation, to urban centres to give birth each year (Phillips-Beck, 2010). Due to the need to relocate women for care outside the community, birth can be a stressful and disruptive rather than a community-strengthening experience (Society of Obstetricians and Gynaecologists of Canada, 2017).

Traditional, community-based midwives were eliminated due to the imposed belief that giving birth in a hospital and being attended by a physician is safer (Browne, McDonald, & Elliott, 2009). Despite the efforts to provide safer care, birth outcomes are significantly worse for Indigenous than for non-Indigenous populations in Canada, including higher rates of premature birth, large for gestational age, and infant deaths from sudden infant death syndrome (SIDS) (Sheppard et al., 2017). A nation's infant mortality rate is thought to be a significant upstream indicator of the health of the entire population as well as a reflection of underlying social determinants of health (Reidpath & Allotey, 2003). Widespread changes to health services, programs, and policy that includes the participation of Indigenous people in the development, governance, and management of their health are required to improve the health disparities in the social and environmental determinants of Indigenous infant health. Further, the United Nations Declaration on the Rights of Indigenous Peoples (United Nations General Assembly, 2007) article 23 supports Indigenous peoples' right to determine and develop health strategies and programs that affect their health. The inclusion of Indigenous participation in decision making processes is an important factor in improving the health of the population.

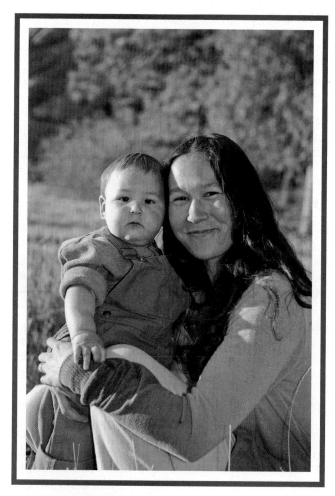

Many communities across Canada are taking up grassroots initiatives and political advocacy to bring social justice to women of childbearing age in Indigenous communities. From the education of a new generation of midwives in these communities to the creation of birthing centres in large urban cities in Canada that enable urban Indigenous women to deliver in a home-like setting, attended by an Indigenous midwife, health-promotion activities are recognizing the importance of supporting a positive, culturally safe transition to motherhood. (See Photo 16.2.) Advocacy by CHNs for an expanded role of Indigenous midwifery care and a return of birth services to rural and remote communities aligns well with the Canadian Community Health Nursing Standards of Practice (Community Health Nurses Canada [CHNC], 2011).

Breastfeeding

Breastfeeding is considered the normal and best method of infant feeding, and the WHO (2014a) recommends that all infants be exclusively breastfed for the first six months of life.

There are numerous benefits, both long and short term, for the mother and her infant. The benefits of breastfeeding for mothers include a measure of protection against breast cancer and ovarian cancer, protection against weak bones later in life, cost effectiveness, and portability, allowing breastfeeding to be done anywhere and supporting mothers to be active as their children grow (PHAC, 2015).

"Breast milk is custom made by each mother for her own baby, and contains the perfect amount of protein, carbohydrate, fat, vitamins and minerals" (PHAC, 2015). As the infant grows, breast milk changes in order to meet the infant's nutritional needs. Breast milk is known to have both short-term and long-term benefits for infants and children. Short-term benefits include protection against various infectious diseases in infancy, including acute otitis media, gastroenteritis and diarrhea, severe lower respiratory infections, and SIDS (Rennick Salone, Vann, & Dee, 2013). Long-term benefits include protection against obesity (Rennick Salone et al., 2013) and enhanced cognitive development (Quigley et al., 2012). Furthermore, breast milk is easier to digest than formula (Gionet, 2015).

The long-term disadvantages of not breastfeeding are becoming increasingly recognized as significant. Yet there are women who either do not initiate breastfeeding or who are not able to continue breastfeeding through to the recommended age of six months. Breastfeeding initiation rates in Canada, in 2012, ranged from 59.3% in Newfoundland and Labrador to 99.2% in the Yukon. The rates of breastfeeding initiation are lower in the east and steadily increase as you move west across Canada (Gionet, 2015). Although the infant benefits of breastfeeding are widely documented, the rates of exclusive breastfeeding at four to six months are suboptimal in many countries, including Canada (Cai, Wardlaw, & Brown, 2012; Gionet, 2015). In 2011–2012, 89% of mothers breastfed their infant, a slight increase from 85% in 2003 (Gionet, 2015). More mothers (26%) were exclusively breastfeeding their infant in 2011–2012 when compared to 17% in 2003 (Gionet, 2015). Furthermore, infants who were exclusively breastfed had mothers who were 30 years or older and had post-secondary education (Gionet, 2015; PHAC, 2015). Across Canada, breastfeeding rates varied widely from 57% in Newfoundland and Labrador to 96% in British Columbia and the Yukon in 2011–2012 (Gionet, 2015). CHNs must actively support initiatives that promote exclusive breastfeeding for the first six months of life. In Newfoundland, a province with low breastfeeding initiation rates, CHNs facilitate breastfeeding support groups to encourage breastfeeding mothers and provide a positive breastfeeding experience (Eastern Health, 2017).

There are many reasons why Canadian mothers discontinue breastfeeding before their infant reaches six months of age, including a belief that they had insufficient breast milk (44%) and difficulties with their breastfeeding technique (18%) (Gionet, 2015). Additionally, babies who consume other liquids and solids before the recommended initiation at six months tend to breastfeed less. In 2011–2012, 76% of mothers who breastfed exclusively for six months (or more) had post-secondary education, compared with the mothers who breastfed less than six months (partially or exclusively) or mothers who did not breastfeed at all (Gionet, 2012). Mothers who are older and have higher education levels are more likely to initiate and continue with breastfeeding. CHNs are in an ideal position to use the information about why mothers may choose not to initiate breastfeeding (or the reasons for discontinuing breastfeeding) to implement various interventions that promote breastfeeding-friendly environments.

CHNs often interact with young families and can provide useful resources and supports to facilitate healthy transitions. Practices such as delayed cord clamping promote uninterrupted skin-to-skin physical contact between mother and infant, facilitate parent–infant attachment, and support early breastfeeding (PHAC, 2017a). CHNs can promote these health practices through educational activities when interacting with expectant families. Further, CHNs can provide evidence-informed educational resources to raise awareness regarding unsafe trends such as placentophagy (the practice of consuming the placenta in various forms).

Smoking in Pregnancy

It is well researched that smoking is harmful to the health of individuals and their family members. Smoking in pregnancy not only impacts the mother but also directly impacts the fetus. When mothers smoke during their pregnancy, their fetus is exposed to dangerous chemicals like nicotine, carbon monoxide, and tar, which can result in the fetus receiving less oxygen and directly impacting growth and development (March of Dimes, 2015). Women who smoke in pregnancy are more likely to be younger, to be of lower socioeconomic status, and not to have attended a post-secondary educational institution (Cui, Shoosthtari, Forget, Clara, & Cheung, 2014). It is important for CHNs to identify women who are ready to quit smoking and provide relevant information about how to access smoking cessation programs. Maternal smoking while breastfeeding has been linked to early weaning, lowered milk production, and inhibition of the milk ejection ("let-down") reflex (La Leche League International, 2013). However, the risks of not breastfeeding even though mother smokes outweigh the risks (to mother and infant) of not breastfeeding at all. It is important to convey the following illness prevention information related to smoking:

- A smoke-free home environment should be encouraged for pregnant and breastfeeding women to avoid exposure to secondhand smoke. During pregnancy and breastfeeding, behavioural and cognitive therapies are recommended as first-line treatment for smoking cessation.
- Partners, friends, and family members should also be offered smoking cessation interventions.
- Nicotine levels in breast milk are halved about 97 minutes after a cigarette. The longer the time between smoking a cigarette and breastfeeding, the less nicotine the baby will be exposed to through breast milk.

- Do not smoke in the house or in the car. Keep the area around baby as smoke-free as possible. Do not allow anyone else to smoke near your infant. (Australian Breastfeeding Association, 2014)

HEALTH PROMOTION AND DISEASE PREVENTION: TEENAGE MOTHERHOOD

Trends in Teenage Pregnancy

Trends in **teenage pregnancy** over time are a significant marker of young women's sexual and reproductive health as well as overall well-being (McKay, 2012). Teenagers in Canada may be more likely to become pregnant if they are of a lower socioeconomic status, are from an Indigenous community, are the children of teen mothers, or experience barriers to accessing education and birth control services (Luong, 2014). Although childbearing is often initiated at an earlier age in other parts of the world, rates of teenage pregnancy in Canada have decreased steadily from 2005 to 2014. (See Table 16.4.) At a basic level, collecting and monitoring trends in teenage pregnancy rates can provide an indication of changing levels of effective contraceptive use among sexually active young women and their partners (McKay, 2012). Levels of effective contraceptive use among adolescents are determined by factors such as access to effective and affordable contraception, reproductive health services, and high-quality sexual health education. At a broader level, monitoring trends in teenage pregnancy rates can also reveal changes in population demographics and community sociocultural, norms, values, attitudes, and beliefs related to adolescent sexuality and teenage childbearing. Pregnant adolescents often experience unique challenges during pregnancy and after childbirth. Pregnant teenagers are at higher risk of obstetric complications, including anemia, toxemia, eclampsia, and hypertension (Al-Sahab, Heifetz, Tamim, Bohr, & Connolly, 2012). Additionally, infants of adolescent mothers are at two times higher risk of being of low birth weight or born premature.

Teenage Motherhood and the Social Determinants of Health

There are a variety of ways in which the social determinants of health impact teen parenthood. This section is meant to provide a general overview. With respect to income and social status, Al-Sahab et al. (2012) examined the prevalence and characteristics of adolescent pregnancy in Canada. They found that when compared to average-aged mothers, adolescent childbearing is more common in teenagers who are of lower socioeconomic status; come from non-immigrant families; have no partner; come from Saskatchewan, Manitoba, and Alberta; and have experienced physical or sexual abuse, or both. In addition, teenage mothers are less likely to complete high school or post-secondary education (Luong, 2014). Last, children of teen mothers have higher rates of becoming teen parents themselves,

Table 16.4	Number and Percent of Live Births in Teenagers by Year across Canada (Excluding Quebec)						
	10–14 years		15–17 years		18–19 years		
Year	Number of Live Births	Percent of Total Live Births	Number of Live Births	Percent of Total Live Births	Number of Live Births	Percent of Total Live Births	Total Number of Live Births**
2005	112	0.04	3819	1.4	8459	3.2	266 874
2006	113	0.04	3973	1.5	8950	3.3	273 101
2007	117	0.04	4272	1.5	9201	3.2	283 328
2008	123	0.04	4174	1.4	9392	3.3	288 519
2009	110	0.04	4120	1.4	9109	3.1	289 639
2010	88	0.03	3849	1.3	8646	3.0	285 215
2011	81	0.03	3448	1.2	8044	2.8	284 599
2012	77	0.03	3313	1.2	7613	2.6	287 294
2013	61	0.02	2913	1.0	6954	2.4	285 170
2014	62	0.02	2457	0.9	6510	2.3	288 369

** Excludes live births to mothers ≥50 years and those with unknown maternal age.

Source: Public Health Agency of Canada (PHAC). (2017a).

perpetuating the cycle of teen pregnancy (Ontario Ministry of Health & Long-Term Care, 2012).

It is important to note that teenage mothers are twice as likely to experience postpartum depression when compared to adult mothers (Kim, Connolly, & Tamim, 2014). Kim, Rotondi, Connolly, and Tamim (2017) found that regardless of age, mothers with lower levels of social support were at higher risk of postpartum depression. In this study, teen mothers reported less social support than their adult counterparts, suggesting social stigma and a lack of connectivity with their own peer group might lead to social isolation. Children of teen mothers are at increased risk of maltreatment and poor health outcomes; however, growing evidence supports public health nurse–led interventions to enhance pregnancy outcomes, child health and development, and social supports (Hovdestad, Shields, Williams, & Tonmyr, 2015; Tonmyr, 2015). Teenage mothers access health information and build emotional support and social capital through social media (Nolan, Hendricks, Ferguson, & Towell, 2017). Bennet et al. (2017) suggest that nurses focus on interventions that promote social connectivity as means of supporting healthy transition to parenthood. CHNs can help to build social capital with teen mothers through the use of social media platforms.

It is well known that children born to teenage mothers are more likely to engage in juvenile delinquency, be less successful in school, be at greater risk of violence and neglect (Sen & Ariizumi, 2014). Not surprisingly, Sen and Ariizumi (2014) discovered a positive correlation between increasing minimum wage and teen pregnancy rates. The higher minimum wage may be associated with greater increases in average earnings in male teens, relative to females, leading to family formation. Sen and Ariizumi (2014) also found that higher minimum wage may result in a higher birth rate for married,

versus unmarried, teenagers. Adolescent mothers are more likely to be smokers before they get pregnant, while they are pregnant, or after they give birth (PHAC, 2009). Researchers suggest women who stop smoking when pregnant are at higher risk of relapse when they lack social support and experience high stress (Constantine, Slater, Carroll, Tamar, & Antin, 2014; Gilbert, Nelson, & Greaves, 2015). Tackling teenage smoking as a CHN requires that the CHN examine the broad social determinants of health and social influences that surround teenage mothers. (See box titled "Tobacco and Alcohol Use by Teenage Girls during Pregnancy and Postpartum Period in Canada.") In summary, there are a variety of ways in which the social determinants of health impact adolescent parents and their children. If this area is of interest to you, we invite you to conduct a review of the literature to help you understand how the social determinants of health impact teenage parents and their offspring.

Teenage Women and Smoking: Health Promotion and Prevention

Although smoking among teenagers in Canada has been on the decline over the past decade, it is interesting to note there is no difference in prevalence of cigarette smoking between male and female youth (Health Canada, 2017). Smoking rates are often found to be significantly higher within specific populations rendered vulnerable. For example, 46% of Indigenous women aged 13 to 18 years reported smoking (Bottorff et al., 2014). Internationally, rural adolescent women who are pregnant have higher rates of smoking than their non-pregnant counterparts, and smoking may increase in the first and third trimesters.

The federal, provincial, and municipal governments in Canada have taken an active role in implementing smoking prevention programs targeting adolescents and young adults. Multifaceted *primary prevention* initiatives include media campaigns and in-school education programs. Additionally, there are active efforts to create the new normal of a tobacco-free lifestyle by preventing the promotion of tobacco at venues and events that appeal to young people, such as organized sports (Canadian Partnership Against Cancer, 2017). Across Canada legislation exists that prohibits smoking in a motor vehicle when a child is present. This is an example of *primordial prevention*. Under this law, any driver or passenger smoking in a motor vehicle while someone under the age of 16 is present is committing an offence and can be fined. The use of modern media tools like Facebook has enabled campaigns such as "Quit the Denial," which compares social smoking at parties to activities such as social farting. Opening space to promote an anti-smoking social marketing campaign in places that are frequented by Canadian youth is intended to prevent young people from taking up smoking in the first place. Various programs are available that are aimed at smoking prevention, reduction, and cessation among teenagers and teenage mothers. The Canadian Paediatric Society has raised concerns regarding the growing popularity e-cigarette products, which it fears is renormalizing public smoking (Stanwick, 2016). CHNs play a pivotal role in identifying, supporting, and connecting teenage women and mothers to the most appropriate primary, secondary, or tertiary smoking cessation programs available.

TOBACCO AND ALCOHOL USE BY TEENAGE GIRLS DURING PREGNANCY AND POSTPARTUM PERIOD IN CANADA

- Teenage girls are more likely than women of older ages to smoke, drink alcohol, and binge drink during pregnancy.

- There are important health-related consequences of smoking and drinking on maternal, fetal, and infant health.

- Teenage girls who smoke cigarettes pre-pregnancy are more likely to relapse during the postpartum period and becoming lifelong smokers.

- Few examples exist of gender-informed prevention and treatment programs to prevent and reduce alcohol and tobacco use among teenage girls, despite this being strongly encouraged.

- There is a clear need for effective and integrated approaches to prevent and reduce alcohol and tobacco use among teenage girls pre-pregnancy, during pregnancy, and postpartum.

- Approaches must consider the influence of partner and friends on cigarette smoking and alcohol consumption in a sensitive and culturally safe manner.

Source: Bottorff et al. (2014).

Cannabis Use in Pregnant Teenagers

Cannabis is the most common illicit drug used by Canadian teenagers, which is concerning given the functional and structural changes to the adolescent that can result (Grant & Bélanger, 2017). In 2015, 21% of youth and 30% of young adults in Canada reported using cannabis within the last year (Government of Canada, 2017b). Planned changes in the Cannabis Act will loosen the restrictions surrounding cannabis possession in Canada, but the sale of cannabis to young people under the age of 18 will remain illegal (Government of Canada, 2017a). The Canadian Medical Association has voiced concerns that the legislative changes will not adequately protect Canada's youth (Kelsall, 2017).

Cannabis is the most frequently used illicit drug during pregnancy, and growing evidence suggests that prenatal cannabis exposure has lasting effects on children's neurocognitive and behavioural functioning (Porath-Waller, 2015). For pregnant teens, care is focused on reducing the use and effects of smoking, alcohol, and substances such as cannabis because pregnancy is often a powerful incentive to stop using them. Knowing the risks of cannabis to teens and their growing fetuses, CHNs who interact with pregnant teens play an important role in reducing the risks of cannabis use in pregnancy through interventions focused on prevention.

PERINATAL HEALTH PROMOTION: REPRODUCTIVE HEALTH, RIGHTS, AND JUSTICE

Reproductive health is understood to address the reproductive processes and functions and the bodily systems impacted throughout all stages of life. The term "reproductive health" implies that every individual has the ability to reproduce and the right to decide when, if, and how this occurs (WHO, 2014b). This means both men and women must therefore have access to health care services and knowledgeable health care providers who can safely support women and their families through pregnancy, labour, and delivery, and the postpartum period. It is of utmost importance that women be able to make decisions about their reproductive health free from coercion and discrimination. One of the main United Nations Sustainable Development Goals is for all women globally to have universal access to safe and reliable sexual and reproductive health services and education (United Nations, 2017).

Reproductive rights are a series of legal rights that were established at the United Nations 1968 International Conference on Human Rights and have been taken up in varying degrees by countries around the world since then. In 1994, reproductive rights were clarified and endorsed internationally in the Cairo Consensus that emerged from the International Conference on Population and Development (United Nations Population Fund,

2012). The rights reaffirmed at that time included the following:

- reproductive health as a component of overall health, throughout the life cycle, for both men and women
- reproductive decision making, including voluntary choice in marriage, family formation, and determination of the number, timing, and spacing of children and the right to have access to the information and means needed to exercise voluntary choice
- equality and equity for men and women, to enable individuals to make free and informed choices in all spheres of life, free from discrimination based on gender
- sexual and reproductive security, including freedom from sexual violence and coercion, and the right to privacy (United Nations Population Fund, 2012, para. 3)

Reproductive justice is a term that was developed to connect the right of reproductive health with the concept of social justice. Reproductive justice acknowledges that although every woman may have reproductive rights, women face barriers every day in accessing those rights, including lower socioeconomic status and lack of political influence and advocacy.

> Reproductive justice is the complete physical, mental, spiritual, political, economic, and social well-being of women and girls, and will be achieved when women and girls have the economic, social, and political power and resources to make healthy decisions about our bodies, sexuality, and reproduction for ourselves, our families, and our communities in all areas of our lives. (Asian Communities for Reproductive Justice, 2005, p. 1)

Experts around the world agree that until these issues, including economic disparities, racial discrimination, and inequalities in power, are addressed, women will never have full control over their reproductive lives and decisions.

reflect this changing demographic in the workforce. This is because the political rhetoric at the time was that families ought to be self-sufficient, and social policies translated into welfare spending, which was viewed as "a drain on the public purse" (Pasolli, 2015; Warner & Prentice, 2011, p. 195).

In 1997 the government in Quebec introduced a new family policy that included a $5 per day daycare rate (later increased to $7 in 2004) for children who required care at least three days per week (Albanese & Rauhala, 2015). Currently, full-time care for children in Quebec amounts to approximately $140/month. However, the same policy does not exist in other provinces, where parents are paying up to $1650/month for full-time care (Racco, 2016)! As a result of these exorbitant childcare costs and the lack of a universal childcare policy across the provinces and territories, only 19% of children who are three years old and younger in Canada have access to regulated childcare (Warner & Prentice, 2011). What this means is that one parent, frequently mothers, are required to leave paid employment after childbirth as childcare costs consume a significantly large portion, if not all, of their wages (Telford, 2016). Yet dual-income households are often required for families to be financially stable. Other complex components of childcare policy related to this discussion are gender, early childhood development, caregiver role-strain, and unpaid work.

Now What?

CHNs can help change the rhetoric around the importance of a universal childcare policy across Canada. One way is to participate in research to produce evidence that documents the benefits of universal childcare, since there is little research evidence on its impact on child development and family outcomes (Kottelenberg & Lehrer, 2013). These data can then be used by CHNs as they participate in policy discussions that will help to untangle current provincial and territorial legislation and create a universal childcare policy (Friendly, 2000). Engaging in this type of work will help advocate for universal childcare as a social right and promote social justice with respect to gender (Warner & Prentice, 2011).

Standards of Practice Fulfilled

#2 Prevention and Health Protection
- Engages in collaborative, interdisciplinary and intersectoral partnerships in the delivery of preventive and protective services with particular attention to populations who are marginalized.

#6 Health Equity
- Advocates for healthy public policy and social justice by participating in legislative and policy-making activities that influence determinants of health and access to services (Community Health Nurses of Canada [CHNC], 2019, revised).

YES, BUT WHY?

Inequality in Access to Universal Child Care

What?
A longstanding inequity exists across Canada with respect to access to universal childcare programs. Residents in Quebec have access to a universal daycare program, whereas populations outside Quebec do not (Kottelenberg & Lehrer, 2013; Stalker & Ornstein, 2014).

So What?
During the World War II era, women entered the paid labour force in Canada to support the war efforts and out of the need to financially support their families (Pasolli, 2015). However, government policies were not modified to

Community Health Nursing and Ethical Practice with Reproductive Health

When CHNs work with women, men, children, adolescents, and families within the context of promoting sexual health and providing access to education or health care services, they may face ethical issues that impact themselves or their clients. Discussing sexual health, sexual health education, and supporting sexual decision making may bring CHNs into environments where their own personal ethics or those of their clients may be challenged. The Community Health Nurses of Canada practice guidelines offer that CHNs should be able to work collaboratively with various stakeholders to determining the best course of action when responding to ethical dilemmas (CHNC, 2019, revised). This includes taking into consideration one individual's rights over societal good that involves allocation of scarce resources. For example, CHNs may use their positions to engage in conversations about the medical necessity of cesarean sections. This is significant because the rate of cesarean delivery increased from 27.3 per 100 hospital deliveries in 2005/2006 to 28.4 per 100 hospital deliveries in 2014/2015 (PHAC, 2017b). When CHNs engage in interventions to shed light on when cesarean deliveries are really required, they enact *quaternary prevention* to educate the public, their clients, and other health care professionals. CHNs may assess their values, attitudes, beliefs, and assumptions about reproductive health to determine when or if ethical tensions may impact their nursing practice. In addition, using critical reflection, seeking help and support, using current evidence, knowing who the experts are in your community, and referring your clients to the other professionals working in reproductive health are all supportive ways in which CHNs can negotiate the ethical tensions that they or their clients may experience.

EARLY CHILDHOOD HEALTH: INDICATORS AND HEALTH PROMOTION IN CANADA

Canada has a population of almost 37 million, 20% of which are children and youth. Surprisingly, Canada is among the more unequal societies for children, ranking 26th of the 35 resource-rich countries in the world (UNICEF, 2016b). In particular, children in Canada do not experience conditions equal in opportunity with respect to income, education, health, and life satisfaction, and the inequality has increased in recent years (UNICEF, 2016a). This is significant given that Canada ranks as the ninth richest country in the world, and the extent of the inequality observed is wider than what we ought to expect. The health of Canada's children when compared with other developed countries "is mediocre at best" (Mikkonen & Raphael, 2010; Raphael, 2014, p. 220). Children and

---

CASE STUDY

You are a CHN working to provide postpartum care services to new mothers and their families. You are visiting the home of a family who has just arrived in Canada from Southeast Asia. Although the mother is friendly and keen to interact with you, you notice there are language barriers. It appears the mother understands what you are saying, but you are unsure if she fully understands the messages you are trying to convey. She tells you she has one cousin in the city but that it takes over an hour to commute to his house by public transportation. In addition, many of her immediate family members do not live in Canada. Although she receives some support over the phone, she indicates that she feels alone much of the time. When you arrive back at your community health centre, in discussions with a few colleagues, you realize this is a pattern you are seeing in one quadrant of the city.

Discussion Questions

1. Which of the determinants of health would you want to consider in your community health nursing interventions?

2. Based on your response to Question 1, what CHN interventions might you consider implementing?

3. Based on the perceived language barriers, how might you ensure that the messages you are trying to convey are received as intended?

---

youth use only 3% of Canada's health care resources (Daneman, Stanwick, & Williams, 2016). One explanation might be that we presume our children and youth are generally healthy and therefore do not require additional attention. We know that if children were to encounter child health specialists at one of Canada's 16 pediatric hospitals, they would receive excellent care. The concern does not lie within the realm of the existing health care system. The issue is that not enough attention is being paid to prevention initiatives. The health of Canada's children is closely linked to their social determinants of health, which are of generally lower quality than those of other developed countries (Raphael, 2014). It is important for children to be healthy and have access to health-promotion strategies, as this sets the foundation for the rest of their lives. Sadly, a child health promotion strategy at the national level, with the aim to improve the health and well-being of children overall, does not exist in Canada (Picard, 2016; Raphael, 2014). As such, there currently is no central Canadian agency responsible for tracking the health of children, leaving independent researchers to take up this challenge (Raphael, 2012). The resulting circumstance is that it is difficult to identify trends (or changes in trends) of early childhood health (up to 4 years) at the population level in Canada. In Table 16.5, indicators of **child well-being** are presented. We will discuss important areas for health

Table 16.5	How We Measure Child Well-Being	
Dimensions	**Components**	**Indicators**
Dimension 1: Material well-being	Monetary deprivation	Relative child poverty rate
		Relative child poverty gap
	Material deprivation	Child deprivation rate
		Low family affluence rate
Dimension 2: Health and safety	Health at birth	Infant mortality rate
		Low birthweight rate
	Preventive health services	Overall immunization rate
	Childhood mortality	Child death rate, age 1 to 19
Dimension 3: Education	Participation	Participation rate: early childhood education
		Participation rate: further education, age 15–19
		NEET rate (% age 15–19 Not in Education, Employment, or Training)
	Achievement	Average PISA (Program for International Student Assessment) scores in reading, math, and science
Dimension 4: Behaviours and risks	Health behaviours	Being overweight
		Eating breakfast
		Eating fruit
		Taking exercise
	Risk behaviours	Teenage fertility rate
		Smoking
		Alcohol
		Cannabis
	Exposure to violence	Fighting
		Being bullied
Dimension 5: Housing and environment	Housing	Rooms per person
		Multiple housing problems
	Environmental safety	Homicide rate
		Air pollution

Sources: Raphael (2014); Innocenti Research Centre (2013).

promotion in children, including nutrition, physical activity, and intended and unintended injuries. While the topic of immunizations is also relevant to this discussion, Chapter 12 presents an in-depth discussion of childhood immunizations.

Nutrition in Children Aged 6–24 Months

Breastfeeding that is continued for up to two years or longer, with appropriate complementary feeding, is important for the nutrition, immunologic protection, growth, and development of infants and toddlers (Health Canada, Canadian Paediatric Society, Dietitians of Canada, & Breastfeeding Committee for Canada 2015). When CHNs promote breastfeeding, they are engaging in *primary prevention*. By

about six months of age, infants are developmentally ready for other foods. The signs of this readiness include the following:

- improved head control
- the capacity to sit up and lean forward
- the ability to let the parent or caregiver know when they are full (e.g., turns head away)
- the ability to pick up food and try to put it in their mouth

From six to 12 months, older infants are able to meet their nutrition requirements with a combination of breast milk and complementary foods (Sanders & Schor, 2014). From 12 to 24 months, an estimated one-third of a young child's energy can come from breastfeeding and the remaining two-thirds from complementary foods. At this stage, infants should be offered nutrient-dense and safe complementary foods along with continued breastfeeding (Health Canada et al., 2015). The first foods introduced should be rich in iron. Unpasteurized cow or goat milk (raw milk) should never be offered to infants and young children due to the risk of food-borne illness from pathogens such as salmonella, *E. coli,* campylobacter, and listeria monocytogenes (Moore, Canadian Paediatric Society, and Infectious Diseases and Immunization Committee, 2008).

Nutrition in Preschool-Aged Children

Preschool-aged children should be following Canada's Food Guide. Health Canada has developed a publication specifically for Indigenous peoples titled "Eating Well with Canada's Food Guide—First Nations, Inuit and Métis." This document considers food items that are culturally appropriate for Indigenous populations, including bannock and wild game (Langlois, Findlay, & Kohen, 2013). Very little information is available on the nutrition of preschool children. Often this type of information for younger children is grouped with that for school-aged children. For instance, one in five children aged one to eight years in Canada have calorie intakes that exceed their daily calorie expenditure (Health Canada, 2012). Surprisingly, a significant portion of children aged one to three years old do not have the recommended fat intake, and there appears to be a general concern that children are not getting enough potassium or fibre (Health Canada, 2012).

The health of Canada's children is closely tied to the health of their parents. Personal identity or **social location**—for example, gender, race, class, Indigenous, immigrant, or disability status—influences our ability to access health care services (Anderson, 2011, as cited in Raphael, 2014). Where you are socially located is related to if, how, or when you may leverage power and influence in order to affect the distribution of economic and social resources that are significant to achieving health (Raphael, 2011). Raphael (2014) views the distribution of economic and social resources as the **social determinants of child health**. Children who come from poorer households are more likely to experience food insecurity (St-Germain & Tarasuk, 2017). Therefore, early identification of children who may be at risk for food insecurity and intervening as appropriate may be viewed as *secondary prevention*. Childhood hunger is an extreme consequence of food insecurity and leads to inadequate dietary intake, resulting in poor health. Some factors related to child hunger include older child age, lone-parent households, large household size, low household income, and poor family dynamics (McIntyre, Bartoo, & Potestio, 2012). It is clear that health promotion programs for childhood nutrition in Canada must focus on the broader determinants of health in order to greatly improve the nutrition, and thus health, of our preschool-aged children.

Physical Activity

The early years represent a critical period for **child development** in terms of growth. It is during this time that active living habits, including healthy eating and physical activity,

are established. Physical activity during the preschool years is associated with improved motor skill development as well as improved psychosocial health, cardiac health, and measures of adiposity (LeBlanc et al., 2012; Timmons et al., 2012). Conversely, high levels of sedentary behaviour, including high levels of screen time, are associated with increased adiposity and lower measures of psychosocial and cognitive development. The new Canadian 24-Hour Movement Guidelines (Figure 16.2) for the Early Years (0–4 years): An Integration of Physical Activity, Sedentary Behaviour, and Sleep are part of a shift in thinking by taking a whole-day approach to physical activity (Tremblay et al., 2017). According to a recent study conducted by Colley et al. (2013), 84% of 3- and 4-year-olds across Canada met the current physical activity guidelines (defined as being active at any intensity for at least 180 minutes every day). However, only 18% of children aged 3 and 4 years met the screen-time recommendation within the sedentary behaviour guidelines, which states that children of this age should accumulate less than one hour of screen time per day. Interestingly, Colley et al. (2013) observed the opposite trend in 5-year-old children, with 14% meeting their age-specific physical activity guideline and the majority (81%) meeting their screen-time recommendation.

Injuries

Childhood injuries represent a significant public health problem in Canada (Soubhi, Raina, & Kohen, 2004). Injuries related to physical activity are the main reasons children present in emergency departments across the country (Molcho & Picket, 2011). There is currently a lack of documented evidence about statistical trends in injuries sustained in the 0–4 years age group. However, Saunders and colleagues (2017) found that immigrant children aged 0–4 years old were more likely to sustain unintentional injuries than their Canadian-born counterparts. For both boys and girls aged 0–4 years, Kang, Emery, Senger, and Meeuwisse (2013) found that injuries were caused by playground equipment, bicycling, trampolines, swimming, and tobogganing. Consumer product–related injuries in young children include hazards associated with bunk beds (risks of falls and strangulation), magnets, baby walkers (falling while in a baby walker), and other household products. Injuries from household products were associated with trampolines, bath seats, dangling blind or curtain cords, furniture, appliances, and televisions (PHAC, 2012). CHNs are well-positioned to engage developing recovery and rehabilitation programs with children who have sustained injuries as a form of *tertiary prevention.*

Injury prevention, an example of primary prevention, must entail a surveillance system (Kang et al., 2013). The Canadian Hospitals Injury Reporting and Prevention Program is a surveillance system currently in place in emergency departments of 16 hospitals in Canada. Surveillance systems give rise to epidemiologic information, which then can quantify the magnitude of injuries across various age groups. This information than may be used to develop and tailor various health promotion and injury prevention programs for specific regions, cities, and communities.

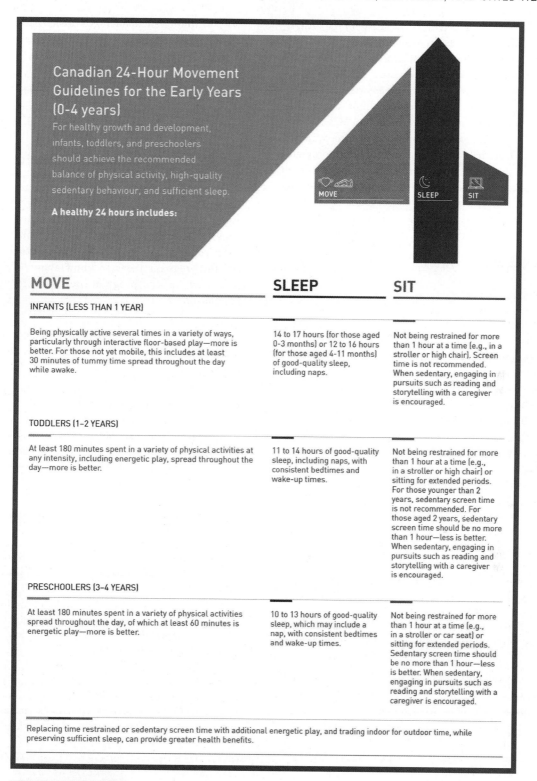

FIGURE 16.2 Canadian 24-Hour Movement Guidelines for the Early Years (0–4 years): An Integration of Physical Activity, Sedentary Behaviour, and Sleep

Source: Tremblay, M. S., Chaput, J. P., Adamo, K. B., Aubert, S.

CONCLUSION

The health of mothers and children is a priority for governments and health care providers globally. CHNs have the opportunity to play an integral role in promoting the health of some of Canada's people who are rendered most vulnerable. CHNs who care for mothers and children in Canada can advocate for evidence-informed health care strategies that promote health versus just mitigating or preventing illness or injury. CHNs are uniquely positioned to care for women and children within the community, enabling them to assess this population with an understanding of the socioenvironmental influences that overtly and subtly shape health. CHNs also have an *ethical* responsibility to advocate for improved access to services that are culturally safe. Maternal newborn and child health services, especially for populations rendered vulnerable like Indigenous communities in Northern Canada, require targeted efforts from CHNs. CHNs need to collaborate with diverse communities and the government, including First Nations, Inuit, and Métis organizations, as well as other health care providers to effectively plan and implement maternal, newborn, and child health programs and the policies that guide them. CHNs across the country can play an active role in advocating for the health and well-being of mothers and children in Canada and beyond. Women and children around the world deserve the same quality and timely care that their counterparts in Western countries receive.

KEY TERMS

breastfeeding (p. 317)

cannabis (p. 320)

child development (p. 324)

child well-being (p. 322)

childhood injuries (p. 324)

infant mortality rate (p. 314)

injury prevention (p. 324)

maternal health (p. 311)

maternal health care (p. 311)

midwives (p. 312)

nutrition (p. 315)

perinatal period (p. 311)

reproductive health (p. 320)

reproductive justice (p. 321)

reproductive rights (p. 320)

social determinants of child health (p. 324)

social location (p. 324)

teenage pregnancy (p. 318)

STUDY QUESTIONS

1. Describe key epidemiologic terms used in perinatal health.

2. What are some of the trends in teenage pregnancy in Canada?

3. Define the difference between reproductive rights and reproductive justice.

4. Name a few benefits of breastfeeding.

5. What are the some of the indicators of child well-being in Canada?

6. By about six months of age, infants are developmentally ready for other foods. What are the signs of this readiness?

INDIVIDUAL CRITICAL-THINKING EXERCISES

1. Visit the Public Health Agency of Canada's Healthy Pregnancy Guidelines online, and compare the recommended guidelines to the resources offered in your local area. Are there differences or similarities? Are there policies or programs in your area that offer unique guidelines based on the population that program or policy is trying to serve?

2. Why are immigrant and refugee women particularly vulnerable to negative mental health outcomes during the perinatal and postnatal periods?

3. What is reproductive justice? What are the resources in your community that would support a client to have access to reproductive justice? What gaps in services exist in your community, and how could a CHN help to fill that void?

GROUP CRITICAL-THINKING EXERCISES

1. Assume your group is a team of CHNs who have been asked to develop a health promotion drop-in program aimed at pregnant teens in your community. What four main topic areas would your group propose as essential for pregnant teens to know about? What may be three barriers your program could face in engaging this population?

2. Consider Table 16.5. Do you agree with the indicators that are being used to measure child well-being? Why do you think these indicators are being used? Discuss with your group any indicators you think should be added or removed and why.

3. Consider the concept of mothering. What responsibilities do CHNs have to ensure women have a positive self-image as mothers? What cultural influences in your communities shape the idea of a "good mother"? What barriers do women face in getting support for positive mothering education and support?

REFERENCES

Al-Sahab, B., Heifetz, M., Tamim, H., Bohr, Y., & Connolly, J. (2012). Prevalence and characteristics of teen motherhood in Canada. *Maternal and Child Health Journal, 16*(1), 228–234. doi:10.1007/s10995-011-0750-8

Albanese, P., & Rauhala, A. (2015). A decade of disconnection: Child care policies in changing economic times in the Canadian context. *International Journal of Child, Youth and Family Studies*, 6(2), 252–274.

Angus, J. E., Lombardo, A. P., Lowndes, R. H., Cechetto, N., Ahmad, F., & Bierman, F. (2012). Beyond barriers in studying disparities in women's access to health services in Ontario, Canada: A qualitative metasynthesis. *Qualitative Health Research, 23*(4), 476–494. doi:10.1177/1049732312469464

Asian Communities for Reproductive Justice. (2005). *A new vision for advancing our movement for reproductive rights, reproductive health, and reproductive justice.* Retrieved from http://strongfamiliesmovement.org/assets/docs/ACRJ-A-New-Vision.pdf

Australian Breastfeeding Association. (2014). *Breastfeeding and smoking.* Retrieved from https://www.breastfeeding.asn.au/bfinfo/breastfeeding-and-smoking

Bennet, C. T., Buchan, J. L., Letourneau, N., Shankar, S. G., Fenwick, A., Smith-Chant, B. & Gilmer, C. (2017). A realistic synthesis of social connectivity interventions during transition to parenthood: The value of relationships. *Applied Nursing Research, 34,* 12–23.

Browne, A. J., McDonald, H., & Elliott, D. (2009). *First Nations urban Aboriginal health research discussion paper: A report for the First Nations Centre, National Aboriginal Health Organization.* Ottawa, ON: National Aboriginal Health Organization. Retrieved from http://www.naho.ca/documents/fnc/english/UrbanFirstNationsHealthResearch-DiscussionPaper.pdf

Bottorff, J. L., Poole, N., Kelly, M. T., Greaves, L., Marcellus, L., & Jung, M. (2014). Tobacco and alcohol use in the context of adolescent pregnancy and postpartum: A scoping review of the literature. *Health and Social Care in the Community, 22*(6), 561–574. doi:10.1111/hsc.12091

Cai, X., Wardlaw, T., & Brown, D. W. (2012). Global trends in exclusive breastfeeding. *International Breastfeeding Journal, 7,* 12. Retrieved from http://www.internationalbreastfeedingjournal.com/content/7/1/12

Canadian Association of Midwives. (2017). *What is a midwife?* Retrieved from http://www.canadianmidwives.org/what-is-a-midwife.html

Canadian Institute for Health Information. (2006). *Giving birth in Canada: The costs.* Ottawa, ON: Author. Retrieved from https://secure.cihi.ca/free_products/Costs_Report_06_Eng.pdf

Canadian Partnership Against Cancer. (2017). *Our work.* Retrieved from http://www.partnershipagainstcancer.ca/what-we-do

Colley, R. C., Garriguet, D., Adamo, K. B., Carson, V., Janssen, I., Timmons, B. W., & Tremblay, M. S. (2013). Physical activity and sedentary behaviour during the early years in Canada. *International Journal of Behavioral Nutrition and Physical Activity, 10,* 54. Retrieved from http://www.ijbnpa.org/content/10/1/54

Community Health Nurses of Canada (CHNC). (2019, revised). *Canadian community health nursing: Professional practice model & standards of practice.* St. John's, NL: Author. Retrieved from https://www.chnc.ca/documents/CHNC-ProfessionalPracticeModel-EN/index.html

Constantine, N. A., Slater, J. K., Carroll, J. A., Tamar, M. J., & Antin, P. H. (2014). Smoking cessation, maintenance, and relapse experiences among pregnant and postpartum adolescents: A qualitative analysis. *Journal of Adolescent Health, 55*(2), 216–221.

Cui, Y., Shoosthtari, S., Forget, E. L., Clara, I., & Cheung, K. F. (2014). Smoking during pregnancy: Findings from the 2009–2010 Canadian Community Health Survey. *PLoS ONE, 9*(1): e84640. doi:10.1371/journal.pone.0084640

Daneman, D., Stanwick, R., & Williams, R. C. (2016). The state of child and youth well-being in Canada: Not even close to good enough! *Paediatrics and Child Health, 21*(5), 236.

de Graaf, J. P. (2013). Living in deprived urban districts increases perinatal health inequalities. *Journal of Maternal-Fetal and Neonatal Medicine, 26*(5), 473–481. doi:10.3109/14767058.2012.735722

Dennis, C. L., Merry, L., & Gagnon, A. J. (2017). Postpartum depression risk factors among recent refugee, asylum-seeking, non-refugee immigrant, and Canadian-born women: Results from a prospective cohort study. *Social Psychiatry and Psychiatric Epidemiology, 52*(4), 411–422.

Eastern Health. (2017). *Breastfeeding support.* Retrieved from http://www.easternhealth.ca/WebInWeb.aspx?d=1535&p=1540

Friendly, M. (2000). *Child care and Canadian federalism in the 1990s: Canary in a coal mine.* Retrieved from http://www.childcarecanada.org/sites/default/files/canaryMFv.pdf

Gilbert, N. L., Nelson, C. R. M., & Greaves, L. (2015). Smoking cessation during pregnancy and relapse after childbirth in Canada. *Journal of Obstetrics and Gynaecology Canada, 37*(1), 32–39.

Gionet, L. (2012). Statistics Canada: *Breastfeeding trends in Canada.* Retrieved from http://www.statcan.gc.ca/pub/82-624-x/2013001/article/11879-eng.htm

Gionet, L. (2013, modified 2015). Breastfeeding trends in Canada. *Health at a Glance.* November. Statistics Canada Catalogue no. 82-624-X.

Government of Canada. (2017a). *Introduction of the Cannabis Act: Questions and answers.* Retrieved from https://www.canada.ca/en/services/health/campaigns/introduction-cannabis-act-questions-answers.html

Government of Canada. (2017b). *Legalizing and strictly regulating cannabis: The facts.* Ottawa, ON: Author. Retrieved from http://www.canada.ca/content/dam/hc-sc/documents/services/campaigns/27-16-1808-Factsheet-The-Facts-eng-03.pdf

Government of Canada. (2018). EI maternity and parental benefits: Overview. Retrieved from https://www.canada.ca/en/services/benefits/ei/ei-maternity-parental.html

Grant, C. N., & Bélanger, R. E. (2017). Cannabis and Canada's children and youth. *Paediatrics & Child Health, 22*(2), 98–102.

Guruge, S., Thomson, M. S., George, U., & Chaze, F. (2015). Social support, social conflict, and immigrant women's mental health in a Canadian context: A scoping review. *Journal of Psychiatric and Mental Health Nursing, 22*(9), 655–667.

Health Canada. (2012). *Do Canadian children meet their nutrient requirement through food intake alone?* Ottawa, ON: Author. Retrieved from http://www.hc-sc.gc.ca/fn-an/alt_formats/pdf/surveill/nutrition/commun/art-nutr-child-enf-eng.pdf

Health Canada. (2017). *Canadian tobacco alcohol and drugs (CTADS): 2015 summary.* Ottawa, ON: Author. Retrieved from http://www.canada.ca/en/health-canada/services/canadian-tobacco-alcohol-drugs-survey/2015-summary.html

Health Canada, Canadian Paediatric Society, Dietitians of Canada, & Breastfeeding Committee for Canada. (2015). *Nutrition for healthy term infants: Recommendations from 6–24 months.* Ottawa, ON: Author. Retrieved from http://www.hc-sc.gc.ca/fn-an/nutrition/infant-nourisson/recom/recom-6-24-months-6-24-mois-eng.php

Health Council of Canada (2011). *Understanding and improving Aboriginal maternal and child health in Canada: Conversations about promising practices across Canada.* Retrieved from http://publications.gc.ca/collections/collection_2011/ccs-hcc/H174-23-2011-eng.pdf

Hovdestad, W., Shields, M., Williams, G., & Tonmyr, L. (2015). Vulnerability within families headed by teen and young adult mothers investigated by child welfare in Canada. *Health Promotion and Chronic Disease Prevention Canada, 35*(8–9), 143–150.

Innocenti Research Centre. (2013). *Child well-being in rich countries: A comparative overview* (p. 5). Florence, Italy: Innocenti Research Centre.

Kang, J., Emery, C. A., Senger, T., & Meeuwisse, W. (2013). Assessing the representativeness of Canadian Hospitals Injury Reporting and Prevention Programme (CHIRPP) sport and recreational injury data in Calgary, Canada. *International Journal of Injury Control and Safety Promotion, 20*(1), 19–26. doi:http://dx.doi.org/10.1080/17457300.2012.656315

Kelsall, D. (2017). Cannabis legislation fails to protect Canada's youth. *Canadian Medical Association Journal, 189*(21), E737–E738. doi: https://doi.org/10.1503/cmaj.170555

Khanlou, N., Haque, N., Sinner, A., Mantini, A., & Kurtz Landy, C. (2017). Scoping review on maternal health among immigrant and refugee women in Canada: Prenatal, intrapartum and postnatal care. *Hindawi Journal of Pregnancy*. Article ID 8783294

Kim, T. H. M., Connolly, J., & Tamim, H. (2014). The effect of social support around pregnancy on postpartum depression among Canadian teen mothers and adult mothers in the Canadian Maternity Experiences Survey. *BioMed Central Pregnancy and Childbirth, 14,* 162. Retrieved from http://www.biomedcentral.com/1471-2393/14/162

Kim, T. H. M., Rotondi, M., Connolly, J., & Tamim, H. (2017). Characteristics of social support among teenage, optimal age, and advanced age women in Canada: An analysis of the national longitudinal survey of children and youth. *Maternal and Child Health Journal, 21*(6), 1417–1427. https://doi-org.ezproxy.lib.ucalgary.c10.100s10995-016-2249-97a

Kottelenberg, M., & Lehrer, S. (2013). New evidence on the impacts of access to and attending universal child-care in Canada. *Canadian Public Policy, 39*(2), 263–285.

Kornelsen, J., & Grzybowski, S. (2005). The cost of separation: The birth experiences of women in isolated and remote communities in British Columbia. *Canadian Women's Studies Journal, 24*(1), 75–80.

Kornelsen, J., Kotaska, A., Waterfall, P., Willie, L., & Wilson, D. (2010). The geography of belonging: The experience of birthing at home for First Nations women. *Health & Place, 16*(4). doi:10.1016/j.healthplace.2010.02.001

La Leche League International. (2013). Breastfeeding and lifestyle choices. Retrieved from http://www.lalecheleague.org/nb/nblifestyle.html

Langlois, K. A., Findlay, L. C., & Kohen, D. E. (2013). *Dietary habits of Aboriginal children*. Statistics Canada Catalogue No. 82-003-X.

Lavell-Harvard, D. M., & Corbiere Lavell, J. (Eds.). (2006). *Until our hearts are on the ground: Aboriginal mothering, oppression, resistance and rebirth*. Toronto, ON: Demeter Press.

LeBlanc, A. G., Spence, J. C., Carson, V., Connor Grober, S., Dillman, C., Janssen, I., & Trembley, M. S. (2012). Systematic review of sedentary behavior and health indicators in the early years (aged 0–4 years). *Applied Physiology, Nutrition, and Metabolism Journal of Public Health, 37*, 753–772. doi:10.1139/H2012-063

Luo, Z. C., Wilkins, R., Heaman, M., Martens, P., Smylie, J., Hart, L., . . . Fraser, W. D. (2010). Birth outcomes and infant mortality by the degree of rural isolation among First Nations and non-First Nations, in Manitoba, Canada. *Journal of Rural Health, 26*(2), 175–181.

Luong, M. (2014). Statistics Canada. Life after teenage motherhood. Retrieved from http://www.statcan.gc.ca/pub/75-001-x/2008105/article/10577-eng.htm

March of Dimes. (2015). Smoking, drugs, and alcohol. Retrieved from https://www.marchofdimes.org/pregnancy/smoking-during-pregnancy.aspx?gclid=CIWf-fm2wr4CFZKCfgodiYUATA

McKay, A. (2012). Trends in Canadian national and provincial/territorial teen pregnancy rates: 2001–2010. *The Canadian Journal of Human Sexuality, 21*(3–4), 161–175.

McIntyre, L., Bartoo, A. C., & Potestio, M. L. (2012). Coping with child hunger in Canada: Have household strategies changed over a decade? *Canadian Journal of Public Health, 103*(6), e428–e432.

Mikkonen, J., & Raphael, D. (2010). *Social determinants of health: The Canadian facts*. Toronto, ON: York University School of Health Policy and Management. Retrieved from http://www.thecanadianfacts.org

Molcho, M., & Pickett, W. (2011). Some thoughts about "acceptable" and "non-acceptable" childhood injuries. *Injury Prevention, 17*(3), 147–148. doi:10.1136/ip.2010.030023

Moore, D. L., Canadian Paediatric Society, and the Infectious Diseases and Immunization Committee. (2008). Food borne infections. *Paediatrics and Child Health, 13*(9), 779–782.

National Collaborating Centre for Aboriginal Health. (2012). *The sacred space of womanhood across the generations: A national showcase on First Nations, Inuit, and Métis women and mothering*. Ottawa, ON: Public Health Agency of Canada. Excerpt from Until Our Hearts Are on the Ground: Aboriginal Mothering, Oppression, Resistance and Rebirth by D.M. Lavell-Harvard and J. Corbiere Lavell in *Journal of Comparative Family Studies*, Vol. 39, No. 2. Published by Journal of Comparative Family Studies, © 2013.

Nolan, S., Hendricks, J., Ferguson, S., & Towell, A. (2017). Social networking site (SNS) used by adolescent mothers: Can social support and social capital be enhanced by online social networks? A structured review of the literature. *Midwifery, 48*, 24–31.

Olson, R., & Couchie, C. (2013). Returning birth: The politics of midwifery implementation on First Nations reserves in Canada. *Midwifery, 29*, 981–987.

O'Mahony, J. M., & Donnelly, T. T. (2013). How does gender influence immigrant and refugee women's postpartum depression help-seeking experiences? *Journal of Psychiatric and Mental Health Nursing, 20*(8), 714–725.

Ontario Ministry of Health and Long-Term Care. (2012). *Teenage pregnancy*. Retrieved from http://www.health.gov.on.ca/en/public/publications/pubhealth/init_report/tp.html

Organisation for Economic Co-operation and Development. (2011). *OECD health data 2011—Frequently requested data*. Paris: Author. Retrieved from http://www.oecd.org

Organisation for Economic Co-operation and Development. (2017). *Health at a glance 2017: OECD indicators*. Paris, France: OECD Publishing. http://dx.doi.org/10.1787/health_glance-2017-en

Pasolli, L. (2015). "I ask you, Mr. Mitchell, is the emergency over?": Debating day nurseries in the Second World War. *Canadian Historical Review, 96*(1), 1–31.

Phillips-Beck, W. (2010). Development of a framework of improved childbirth care for First Nation women in

Manitoba: A First Nation family-centred approach. Unpublished thesis. Retrieved from https://mspace.lib.umanitoba.ca/bitstream/handle/1993/3985/Thesis_wphillips-beck.final.pdf?sequence=1

Picard, A. (2016). Canada needs a vision for child health. *Pediatrics and Child Health, 21*(5), 237–238.

Porath-Waller, A. J. (2015). *Clearing the smoke on cannabis: Maternal cannabis use during pregnancy—An update.* Canadian Centre on Substance Abuse. Retrieved from http://www.ccsa.ca/Resource%20Library/CCSA-Cannabis-Maternal-Use-Pregnancy-Report-2015-en.pdf

Premji, S. S., Pana, G., Currie, G., Dosani, A., Reilly, S., Young, M., . . . & Lodha, A. K. (2018). Mother's level of confidence in caring for her late preterm infant: A mixed methods study. *Journal of Clinical Nursing, 27*(5–6), e1120-e1133. doi:10.1111/jocn.14190

Public Health Agency of Canada (PHAC). (2009). *What mothers say: The Canadian maternity experiences survey.* Ottawa, ON: Author.

Public Health Agency of Canada (PHAC). (2009, revised 2015). Ottawa, ON: Author. Retrieved from https://www.canada.ca/en/public-health/services/health-promotion/childhood-adolescence/stages-childhood/infancy-birth-two-years/breastfeeding-infant-nutrition/10-great-reasons-breastfeed-your-baby.html

Public Health Agency of Canada (PHAC). (2012). *Consumer product related injuries.* Ottawa, ON: Author. Retrieved from http://www.phac-aspc.gc.ca/publicat/cyi-bej/2009/index-eng.php

Public Health Agency of Canada (PHAC). (2013). *Perinatal health indicators for Canada 2013: A report from the Canadian perinatal surveillance system.* Ottawa, ON: Author.

Public Health Agency of Canada (PHAC). (2017a). *Chapter 1: Family-centred maternity and newborn care in Canada: Underlying philosophy and principles.* Ottawa, ON: Author.

Public Health Agency of Canada (PHAC). (2017b). *Perinatal health indicators for Canada 2017: A report from the Canadian perinatal surveillance system.* Ottawa, ON: Author.

Quigley, M. A., Hockley, C., Carson, C., Kelly, Y., Renfrew, M. J., & Sacker, A. (2012). Breastfeeding is associated with improved child cognitive development: A population-based cohort study. *Journal of Pediatrics, 160*(1), 25–32. doi:10.1016/j.jpeds.2011.06.035

Racco, M. (2016). Child care costs in Canada: The most and least expensive cities. Retrieved from http://globalnews.ca/news/3121563/child-care-costs-in-canada-the-most-and-least-expensive-cities

Raphael, D. (2011). Who is poor in Canada? In D. Raphael (Ed.), *Poverty in Canada: Implications for health and quality of life* (2nd ed., pp. 62–89). Toronto, ON: Canadian Scholars' Press.

Raphael, D. (2012). Canadian experiences. In D. Raphael (Ed.), *Tackling health inequalities: Lessons from international experiences.* Toronto, ON: Canadian Scholars' Press.

Raphael, D. (2014). Social determinants of children's health in Canada: Analysis and implications. *International Journal of Child, Youth and Family Studies, 5*(2), 220–239.

Reidpath, D. D., & Allotey, P. (2003). Infant mortality as an indicator of population health. *Journal of Epidemiology & Community Health, 57*, 344–346.

Robert Woods Johnson Foundation. (2008). *Overcoming obstacles to health: Stories, facts and findings.* Princeton, NJ: Robert Woods Johnson Foundation.

Salone, L.R., Vann, W. F., & Dee, D. L. (2013). Breastfeeding: An overview of oral and general health benefits. *The Journal of the American Dental Association, 144*(2), 143–151. doi:10.14219/jada.archive.2013.0093

Sanders, K. M., & Schor, J. (2014). *Introducing baby to solid foods.* The Townsend Letter Group.

Saunders, N. R., Macpherson, A., Guan, J., Sheng, L., & Guttmann, A. (2017). Unintentional injuries in children and youth from immigrant families in Ontario, Canada: A population-based cross-sectional study. *Canadian Medical Association Journal Open, 5*(1), E90–E96. doi:10.9778/cmajo.20160099

Sen, A., & Ariizumi, H. (2014). Teen families, welfare transfers, and the minimum wage: Evidence from Canada. *Canadian Journal of Economics, 46*(1), 338–360.

Sheppard, A. J., Shapiro, G. D., Bushnik, T., Wilkins, R., Perry, S., Kaufman, J. S., . . . Yang, S. (2017). Birth outcomes among First Nations, Inuit and Métis populations. *Statistics Canada Health Reports, 28*(11), 11–16.

Society of Obstetricians and Gynaecologists of Canada. (2010, reaffirmed 2017). Returning birth to Aboriginal, rural and remote communities, *Journal of Obstetricians & Gynaecologists of Canada, 32*(12), 1186–1188.

Soubhi, H., Raina, P., & Kohen, D. (2004). Neighbourhood, family, and child predictors of childhood injury in Canada. *American Journal of Health Behavior, 28*(5), 397–409.

St-Germain, A. A. F., & Tarasuk, V. (2017). High vulnerability to household food insecurity in a sample of Canadian renter households in government-subsidized housing. *Canadian Journal of Public Health, 108*(2), e129–e134. doi: 10.17269/CJPH.108.5879

Stalker, G., & Ornstein, M. (2014). Policy brief no. 15—Quebec, daycare, and household strategies of couples with young children. *Population Change and Lifecourse Strategic Knowledge Cluster Research/Policy Brief, 1*(5), 1–4.

Stanwick, R. (2015, revised 2016). E-cigarettes: Are we renormalizing public smoking? Reversing five decades of tobacco control and revitalizing nicotine dependency in children and youth, *Paediatrics & Child Health, 20*(2), 101–105.

Telford, N. (2016). Can Canadian women have it all? How limited access to affordable child care restricts freedom and choice. *Canadian Journal of Family and Youth, 8*(1), 153–172.

Timmons, B. W., Leblanc, A. G., Carson, V., Connor Gorber, S., Dillman, C., Janssen, I., Tremblay, M. S. (2012). Systematic review of physical activity and health in the early years (aged 0–4 years). *Applied Physiology, Nutrition, and Metabolism Journal of Public Health, 37*, 773–792. doi:10.1139/H2012-070

Tonmyr, L. (2015). The nurse-family partnership: Evidence-based public health in response to child maltreatment. *Health Promotion and Chronic Disease Prevention in Canada, 35*(8–9), 141–142.

Tremblay, M. S., Chaput, J. P., Adamo, K. B., Aubert, S., Barnes, J. D., Choquette, L., . . . Gruber, R. (2017). Canadian 24-hour movement guidelines for the early years (0–4 years): An integration of physical activity, sedentary behaviour, and sleep. *BMC Public Health, 17*(5), 874. doi:10.1186/s12889-017-4859-6

United Nations. (2017). *Report of the secretary-general—Progress towards the Sustainable Development Goals.* Retrieved from http://www.un.org/ga/search/view_doc.asp?symbol=E/2017/66&Lang=E

United Nations General Assembly. (2007). *United Nations Declaration on the Rights of Indigenous Peoples.* Resolution adopted by the General Assembly, 2 October 2007, A/RES/61/295 Retrieved from https://www.un.org/development/desa/indigenouspeoples/declaration-on-the-rights-of-indigenous-peoples.html

UNICEF. (2016a). Fairness for Children. A league table of inequality in child well-being in rich countries, no. 13, Canada Summary. UNICEF Office of Research. Innocenti, Florence. Retrieved from http://www.unicef.ca/sites/default/files/legacy/imce_uploads/images/advocacy/rc/unicef_report_card_13_canada_summary.pdf

UNICEF. (2016b). Fairness for Children. A league table of inequality in child well-being in rich countries,

no. 13, UNICEF Office of Research. Innocenti, Florence. Retrieved from https://www.unicef-irc.org/publications/830/

United Nations Population Fund. (2012). Supporting the constellation of reproductive rights. Retrieved from http://www.unfpa.org/rights/rights.htm

Warner, M. E., & Prentice, S. (2013). Regional economic development and child care: Toward social rights. *Journal of Urban Affairs, 35*(2), 195–217.

World Health Organization. (2014a). *Reproductive health.* Geneva, CH: Author. Retrieved from http://www.who.int/topics/reproductive_health/en

World Health Organization. (2014b). *10 facts on maternal health.* Geneva, CH: Author. Retrieved from http://www.who.int/features/factfiles/maternal_health/en

World Health Organization. (2018). Global health observatory data: Maternal mortality. Retrieved from http://www.who.int/gho/maternal_health/mortality/maternal/en/

ABOUT THE AUTHORS

Josephine Etowa, PhD, MN, BScN, RM, RN, FWACN, FAAN, is Professor and Loyer-DaSilva Research Chair in Public Health Nursing at the University of Ottawa. She is a senior investigator with the Nursing Best Practice Research Centre at the University of Ottawa and a founding member and past president of the Health Association of African Canadians. Her program of research is grounded in over 25 years of clinical practice in maternal newborn and child health and community health nursing with projects funded by local, national, and integrational organizations. She is currently the nominated Principal Investigator for a three-year, three-country study investigating infant feeding practices among Black women is living with HIV/AIDs in Ottawa, Port Harcourt (Nigeria), and Miami.

Aliyah Dosani, RN, BN, MPH, PhD, is Associate Professor in the School of Nursing and Midwifery, Faculty of Health, Community and Education at Mount Royal University in Calgary, Alberta. She is also an Adjunct Associate Professor in the Department of Community Health Sciences, Cumming School of Medicine, at University of Calgary in Calgary. She holds a PhD from the University of Calgary with a specialization in population/public health. Her nursing practice includes instructing students in the Bachelor of Nursing program, population/public health, community health nursing, and legal issues in nursing. Her work focuses on maternal, newborn, and child health. Her research interests include working on health equity and social justice issues through community-based programs and interventions. She also shares a passion for global health issues.

Heather Bensler, RN, MSN, is Director of Indigenous Initiatives (Faculty and Curriculum Development) in the Faculty of Nursing at the University of Calgary. Her nursing practice includes instructing students in the undergraduate nursing program, Indigenous health in South America, community development, and maternal newborn health. She maintains an obstetrics clinical practice. Heather's research interests include knowledge translation, Indigenous health, maternal newborn health, cultural safety, and simulation in undergraduate nursing education.

School Health

Jo-Ann MacDonald and Cheryl van Daalen-Smith

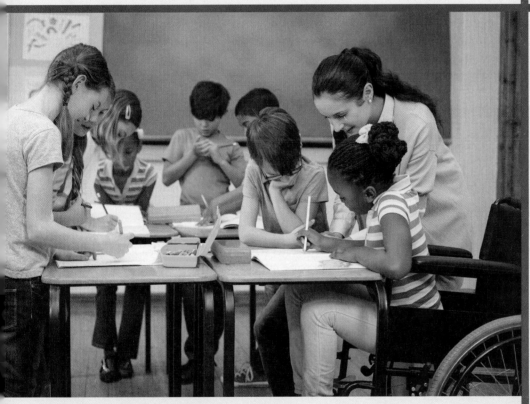

Source: Wavebreak Media Ltd/123RF

LEARNING OUTCOMES

After studying this chapter, you should be able to:

1. Explain the importance of the school as a setting for child and youth health promotion.

2. Understand critical conceptualizations of children, childhood, and children's rights.

3. Through a lens of the social determinants of health, identify pressing health challenges and inequities encountered in the school-aged population.

4. Ensure child health equity efforts are grounded in intersectionality.

5. Discuss how concepts and strategies from population health, comprehensive school health, Indigenous community-based school health, and primary health care are relevant to school-based health promotion.

6. Examine the roles and functions of the public health nurse within a comprehensive school health approach.

INTRODUCTION

Just over 5 million Canadian children and adolescents attend school every day (Statistics Canada, 2017). Schools are settings where children and youth learn, play, and relate; where adults work to support young people; and where families and neighbourhoods gather to engage in various educational and community activities. Although many factors influence the physical, social, and emotional well-being of children and youth, research has shown that school settings have a positive impact on most of the health outcomes of this population (DeBell & Buttigieg, 2016; Joint Consortium for School Health [JCSH], 2014a).

We commence this chapter with an historical overview of school health nursing. For over a century, public health nurses (PHNs) have long been a trusted presence in Canadian schools, supporting, counselling, screening, partnering, educating, and advocating for the health and quality of life of young people. In some communities, especially in rural Canada, the PHN may be the only health professional providing service on an ongoing basis in schools. Concerns regarding an erosion in the depth and breadth of the role of the school nurse in Canada have been raised, but less is discussed regarding how childhood and, by default, children are viewed. As a partner working in a shared-power model of nursing, Canada's community health nurses (CHNs) serve as exemplary health professionals whose practice is rooted in an emancipatory and nonhierarchical approach to health promotion. In order to ensure that this same approach is employed with a population often considered immature and incapable of full participation, we present some thoughts regarding the lenses placed on children and how school health nurses (SHNs) can lead by example in a model of practice that sees children as full citizens, with rights of full participation in any and all health promotion efforts concerning them. We will discuss various health outcomes in this population, including the experience of inequitable access to the social determinants of health for various marginalized young people. Current socio-environmental frameworks for comprehensive health promotion in schools, including a framework for Indigenous school health (National Collaborating Centre for Aboriginal Health [NCCAH], 2010), are also presented. Finally, the diverse roles and activities of school-based PHNs in promoting the health of students, staff, families, and school communities is discussed.

Historical Perspectives on School Nursing in Canada

With the emergence of public health nursing at the turn of the 20th century, schools became one of the initial settings for the provision of health education and preventive programs. (See Chapter 1.) Medical inspection programs were initiated in most schools to counteract absenteeism of children due to communicable disease. Public health officials proposed that poor health inhibited a child's academic performance and could potentially have harmful effects on that child's future economic and social well-being. In several Canadian cities, boards of education initially established school health programs in which PHNs moved between school and home providing preventive health teaching, screening, and counselling, in addition to their primary role in communicable disease control.

For most of the 20th century, PHNs in school settings primarily focused on individual and family counselling, classroom health teaching, screening, case-finding programs, immunization programs, and advising school staff about student health problems. (See Chapters 1 and 4.) Interventions were based on a biomedical model where the emphasis was on the prevention and control of disease. Schools were one of the settings in a district or neighbourhood that received the services of the generalist PHN. District nursing created opportunities for the nurse to really know the community, where regular communication and collaboration with local family physicians, pharmacists, businesses, and other health professionals occurred. School children and their families were often known to the nurse through home visiting or clinic work in the district. With the emergence of health promotion in the mid-1970s, PHNs addressed "lifestyle" issues through health education, health communication campaigns, and individual or group counselling, in addition to the traditional screening and immunization programs.

With the integration of children with complex health needs into publicly funded schools during the 1980s, many jurisdictions developed special nursing services within their home care program or community and social services to provide treatments in the school setting and consultation on health issues related to individual students (see Chapter 5). While these nursing services still play a valuable role in supporting students with special health needs, PHNs focus on promoting the overall health of the whole school population. The 1986 Ottawa Charter for Health Promotion introduced a new way of thinking about health promotion, and PHNs incorporated its principles of equity, social justice, meaningful participation, empowerment, and collaboration in their practices. (See Chapter 1.)

In the 1990s, the shift to population health and program-based delivery of public health programs led to the troubling reduction or elimination of PHNs in schools. **Comprehensive school health (CSH)** was being introduced in many jurisdictions, but fiscally driven constraints often caused school-based nurses to be removed from their weekly presence. Not surprisingly, this resulted in an erosion of the relationships that PHNs had built with principals, teachers, students, and their families, and diminished their overall visibility in the community (Cohen & McKay, 2010; Crouch & Chalmers, 2010). There remains much variation now in the scope of practice, visibility, and impact of school-based PHNs across the country, and as of late, it has garnered attention, especially by the Mental Health Commission (2016), which asked, where are the school health nurses?

To address these challenges, the nursing profession in Canada advocates strongly for school-based PHNs working to their full scope of practice within a CSH approach (Canadian Nurses Association [CNA], 2014; Community Health Nurses Initiatives Group [CHNIG], 2015; Ordre des infirmières et infirmiers du Québec, 2015). Progress in Practice Webinars hosted by the Canadian CNA have addressed important school nursing issues, including school nursing around the world (CNA, 2016). Most recently, CNA has included PHNs in schools as part of its national policy platform, "Caring Ahead: A New Approach to Health Care" (CNA, n.d.). The *Healthy Schools, Healthy Children: Maximizing the Contribution of Public Health Nursing in School Settings* paper released by the CHNIG in 2015 describes the critical issues in school health nursing and outlines a scope of practice for PHNs working in schools. Not only does the CHNIG paper emphasize the broader health issues that impact children and youth, such as social determinants of health and conducive school environments, but it also captures the preventative approach that all PHNs strive for in supporting this population in their practice. Advocacy work within the CHNIG has resulted in the establishment of the National Network of School-Based PHNs to share practice concerns and remain current of new developments. Since 2015, the network has convened on an annual basis and communicates via a school health form hosted on the Community Health Nurses of Canada (CHNC) website. Internationally, there is a growing call for expanding the role of school nurses to include a multidimensional and multisectoral approach to the health promotion and health protection of school-aged children (Department of Health, 2014; National Association of School Nurses [NASN], 2017). (See Canadian Research 17.1.)

Barriers to providing school-based health care: International case comparisons. (Seigart, Dietsch, & Parent, 2013)

Exploring barriers to providing school-based health care, this research used a case-study approach to gather data from in-depth interviews with key stakeholders, on-site observations, agency reports, and the literature. Forty school nurses or CHNs who worked in schools were interviewed, and additional interviews were conducted with 33 parents, teachers, administrators, nursing faculty, and other community leaders in two states or provinces in Australia, Canada, and the United States. Grounded theory approaches such as analysis of interview transcripts, field notes, and records of observations for emerging themes were used in the data analysis.

Common concerns expressed in all three countries included high student-to-nurse ratios, especially in Australia and Canada; limited knowledge of the roles and benefits of school nurses and school-based health care; and a lack of timely access to primary-care services. Canadian and Australian CHNs tended not to engage in hands-on care but to focus on surveillance, health education, infection control, vaccinations, and staff education. U.S. school nurses provided more primary-care services, such as medication administration, health education and promotion, staff education, counselling, referrals, and networking with other health professionals. Another difference observed in Canada and Australia was the lack of school nurse practitioners and school-based health centres as compared to the United States, where both are more common. In all three countries, funding was the most common barrier mentioned to expanding school health services. Australia and Canada also reported an increase in teacher stress due to taking on responsibilities for monitoring the health of children.

Discussion Questions

1. What are some of the unique features associated with providing health services in schools?

2. From the findings discussed, what might explain the differences or similarities among the three jurisdictions in this study?

3. How might provincial and national nursing leadership help SHNs in Canada to perform within the scope of practice identified in Table 17.2 (on page 342)?

The Importance of School Years

Over a period of 12 to 15 years, school-aged young people experience dramatic physical, cognitive, emotional, and social transformations that can create uncertainty and anxiety (DeBell & Buttigieg, 2016). **Middle childhood** extends from age 6 to the onset of puberty at 10 to 12 years, when children shift from seeing themselves as the centre of the world to realizing that the world is a complex environment in which they must find a place (Davies, 2011). **School-aged children** seek opportunities to master and demonstrate new skills, make independent decisions, control their own behaviour, and form positive relationships with peers and adults outside the family. Nearing the end of this period, well-supported children who have successfully mastered these developmental tasks are capable of increasingly complex reasoning, looking at situations from multiple perspectives, and using many adaptive strategies of self-regulation (Davies, 2011).

Adolescence begins with puberty and ends with the beginning of adulthood. The transition to this life stage involves a balance of school, extracurricular activities, and engagement in the workforce. The developmental tasks associated with adolescence include achieving independence, adjusting to sexual maturation, establishing cooperative relationships with peers, preparing for meaningful work or a career, establishing intimate relationships, and developing a core set of values (Registered Nurses Association of Ontario, 2010). Adolescents begin to develop greater autonomy and a stronger sense of who they are and who they want to become.

A child's family and home environment are the most important and influential settings during the school-age years. During these formative years, the school and home interact with each other as determinants of child and youth health (DeBell & Buttigieg, 2016) and this includes the context of children who do not have families or who are homeless, precariously housed or living in institutions. During this time, many young people unfortunately experience stressors that impact their health, emotional and social well-being, and capacity to learn. Many child-serving professionals are significantly concerned about what has been coined *toxic stress* -understood to be prolonged exposure to familial-based turmoil including addiction, depression, and violence. In fact, according to Letourneau (2012), experiences stemming from neglect, abuse, unpredictability or chaos trigger chemical releases in infants' and children's maturing brains that when persistent, become neurotoxins. Stressors that are frequent become dangerously cumulative and leave a 'biological fingerprint of damage' on a child's brain. This increasingly studied phenomenon has garnered so much interest that research now demonstrates how chronic stress can lead to a wide range of neural, immunological, and metabolic problems including asthma, obesity, anxiety, and so on.

The school provides the second most important social and physical environment where significant efforts are made to provide young persons with nurturance and care outside the family. Conversely, schools are increasingly a source of distress for young people, especially those considered to be on the margins of what society considers normal or valuable. Bullying has become epidemic in Canada, and the school nurse is often consulted regarding best practices to decrease the prevalence of bullying incidents in classrooms and online. According to Prevnet (2017), one in three Canadian youth report experiencing online bullying, and the experiences of being bullied and of bullying others are serious. See the box on page 4 for more information (Prevnet, 2017).

THE EXPERIENCE OF BEING BULLIED OR BULLYING OTHERS

Dangers for Children and Adolescents Who Are Bullied:

- Depression (low mood, a sense of hopelessness)
- Social anxiety, loneliness, isolation
- Stress-related health problems (e.g., headaches, stomachaches)
- Low self-esteem
- School absenteeism and academic problems
- Aggressive behaviours
- Contemplating, attempting, or committing suicide

Dangers for Children and Adolescents Who Bully Others:

- Not knowing the difference between right and wrong
- Delinquency and substance use
- Academic problems and increased school dropout rate
- Aggression
- Sexual harassment and dating aggression
- Gang involvement and criminal adulthood
- Difficulties in their relationships with others
- Being bullied at the hands of others

CRITICAL CONCEPTUALIZATIONS OF CHILDREN, CHILDHOOD, AND CHILDREN'S RIGHTS

Dominant Western ideology views children as passive, dependent beings in need of protection. This view, in combination with hegemonic characterizations of childhood suggesting homogeneity, is a social construct that did not exist prior to the Middle Ages (Aries, 1962) and additionally fails to recognize differences across young people related to gender, race, class, ability, Indigenous ancestry, and gender identity.

One of the key barriers to fulsome participation by young persons in their schools in general and in health promotion efforts more specifically arguably could be linked to "pervasive notions found in child development and health literature where young people are viewed as problems to be solved, defined, and evaluated through conceptual lenses of dysfunction and of deficit" (Mitchell, 2011, p. 515). Matthews (2007) argues that young persons are in fact competent social actors with impact, as opposed to incomplete noncitizens in need of protection from themselves. As long as professionals, including those based in schools, view children as what Woodhead (2009) and Matthews (2007) call "not yet members of their societies," true participation rights will be trumped by developmental and protectionist policies and practices. School-based nurses, as social justice activists, are called to advocate for young persons' rights by first calling into question how "strict developmental thinking that homogenizes children . . . regardless of social location or context" (Matthews, 2007, p. 325), which contributes to tokenistic participation and adults-know-best health promotion programming. School-based health promotion must be child- and youth-centred, and the only way to do that is to embrace a rights-based approach.

Article 12 of the 1989 United Nations **Convention on the Rights of the Child (UNCRC)** states that young people have a right to participate in matters that concern them. Canada ratified the convention in 1991, yet like many other UN countries, there remains a reluctance to adopt policies that allow children to have a voice concerning matters that affect them, and this includes (in this case) their health and related health promotion strategies implemented in their schools. "Arguably, this is largely because the notion that children have the capacity to make rational decisions is a concept that challenges the generally accepted 'nature' of young people as dependent, incapable, and immature. However, if we assume that childhood is a construct, and also consider alternative understandings of children, we might want to question if excluding children from the decision-making process is in fact in their best interest" (Johnny, 2006, p. 23).

A very promising development has direct application to school-based nurses. The Canadian Association of Pediatric Nurses (2017) recently developed national standards of practice based in part on the UNCRC that include explicit mention of children's rights and Article 12. In identifying key competency requirements, including knowledge of the UNCRC, Canada's Pediatric Nursing Standards of Practice behoove practitioners to ensure the voice and participation of young people in all aspects of health care.

We challenge Canada's school-based nurses to embrace an anti-oppressive lens to children, childhood, and PHN practice with young people. We recommend a practice model guided by a view that (a) recognizes children are citizens now, and not at some arbitrary date; and (b) replaces ageist assumptions of inherent incompetence or immature viewpoints with a capacity-based approach that considers children as citizens with rights including those affiliated with participation in school-based health promotion.

HEALTH DETERMINANTS AND OUTCOMES

The health and quality of life of young people is shaped by multiple determinants and prerequisites to health (DeBell & Buttigieg, 2016). Contexts and environments where young people learn, live, and play can have a significant impact on health status. Social exclusion and poorer socioeconomic circumstances create conditions that place children's and youth's health at risk (Davison et al., 2013; DeBell & Buttigieg, 2016).

Over 1.2 million (17.4%) of Canadian children and youth under 18 live in poverty, with increased rates for Indigenous youth at 37.9% (Campaign 2000, 2017). Child poverty rates are also very high for new immigrants, visible minorities, and children with disabilities. In 2017, of the more than 860 000 Canadians who used food banks, one in three were children less than 18 years of age (Food Banks Canada, 2017). Children and youth living in poverty are disadvantaged in almost every way, and the health effects last a lifetime. They are more likely to live in unsafe neighbourhoods where exposure to violent and illegal activity occurs. These conditions also create fewer opportunities for them to be physically and socially active and increase their chances of being overweight or obese compared to children living in higher socioeconomic groups. More importantly, inadequate nutrition impacts a child's ability to learn and to develop physically (Chaudry & Wimer, 2016).

Although most Canadian children and youth are in good health, in a primary prevention approach, school-based nurses traditionally address health outcomes related to unintentional injuries, communicable diseases, nutrition/weight obsession, and behaviours that place school-aged young persons at risk. These are briefly discussed in the following section.

Unintentional Injuries

Unintentional injuries due to motor vehicle collisions (67%) and drowning (6%) are the leading causes of death for children and youth aged 10–19 (Statistics Canada, 2011). Sports and recreational activities such as running, biking, and skating are the leading causes of nonfatal injury (Pickett, 2011). For Indigenous children and youth, the unintentional injury rate is three to four times higher than the rate for other children in Canada (Banerji, 2012). Youth who reside in rural areas experience more injuries per capita than their urban counterparts. Rural boys are also more likely to drive a motor vehicle while drinking alcohol or using drugs, and rural girls are more likely to drive while impaired compared to youth in large urban centres (Davison et al., 2013).

Communicable Diseases

Just 100 years ago, infectious diseases were the leading cause of death around the world. Immunization against vaccine-preventable communicable diseases is one of the most cost-effective public health interventions. Public health units are mandated by provincial health legislation to collect and review immunization information on students related to measles, mumps, rubella, tetanus, diphtheria, pertussis, polio, and varicella, and, in some jurisdictions, hepatitis B, human papilloma virus, and meningitis, as well as annual influenza immunization. Routine childhood immunization without cost to the child is, for the most part, accepted as standard practice in Canada (Public Health Agency of Canada [PHAC], 2013). According to Statistics Canada (2015) a large majority of parents choose to get their children vaccinated, and immunization rates are less affected by socioeconomic factors.

Unhealthy Weights/Weight Preoccupation

The prevalence of overweightness and obesity among Canadian children has not changed in the last decade. Approximately one-third (31.5%) of 5- to 17-year-olds are overweight or obese; the percentage of boys who are obese (19.5%) is three

times greater than the percentage of girls (6.3%) (PHAC, 2011). For First Nations children, the numbers are of great concern, with 55% of on-reserve children and 41% of off-reserve children being either overweight or obese (Roberts, Shields, de Groh, Aziz, & Gilbert, 2012). The question here is why. It is not simply a matter of eating "right" and getting exercise. For many Indigenous young people, food insecurity means healthy foods are cost prohibitive. For example, in the northern Ontario community of Moosonee, three bags of milk cost as much as $12. Combined with low income or unemployment rates, many parents and grandparents can only afford the less expensive items such as processed foods that are minimally nutritious and high in fat, sugar, and salt (Ferris, 2011). School-based nurses need to find a balance between supporting healthy eating without reinforcing troubling size and shape expectations, particularly for girls and young women. Further, equipped with the knowledge that healthier foods are cost-prohibitive, the SHN needs to work upstream to advocate for equitable access to healthy food.

Of continuing concern is the prevalence of weight preoccupation and nutritional restriction, primarily by girls and young women. The school nurse is often asked to address the links between body image, social media, and self-esteem in health education classes or small group work. Overweight and obese young people, particularly young girls, are more likely to have mental health problems than young people with a healthy weight, and they often suffer from low self-esteem, social isolation, and depression (Freeman, King, & Pickett, 2011). Of additional concern for the school nurse is the demonstrated relationship between increased internet use and resultant body dissatisfaction (Carter, Forrest, & Kaida, 2017).

Risk-Taking Behaviours

Although risk-taking is an expected behaviour in adolescence, nurses who approach school health from a critical perspective recognize that failure to debunk the belief that health is simply an outcome of an individual's "choices" can preclude an approach to working with children and youth that considers inequities. Further, the school-based nurse understands that **risk-taking behaviours** are associated with a need to be liked or fit in and be seen on social media. Indeed, much concern has been raised regarding the amount of time young people devote to creating and maintaining an online personal brand, which at times includes documenting risky scenarios. Risk-taking behaviours can include alcohol and drug use, smoking, and unprotected sexual activity.

The reported rate of youth aged 15 to 17 having sex has not significantly changed over a decade, but 35% of youth reported having multiple partners, and 20% of 15- to 17-year-olds and 26% of 18- to 19-year-olds reported having sex without a condom (Rotermann, 2012). These patterns of sexual activity have contributed significantly to increasing cases of chlamydia and gonorrhea among young people, particularly women. When compared to other age groups, Canadian youth have the highest reported rates of sexually transmitted infections (PHAC, 2017).

Alcohol and cannabis are the most common substances used by students in grades 7 to 12 in Canada (Government of Canada, 2016). Alcohol use has not changed significantly since the last survey in 2012/13 and remains at a reported rate of 40%. Approximately 24% of students reported binge drinking (i.e., five or more drinks for males and four or more drinks for females), which has decreased from a high of 39% in 2008/2009 (Government of Canada, 2016). (See Yes, But Why box regarding cannabis use.)

YES, BUT WHY?

Cannabis Use in Youth: What Lies Ahead in a Neo-Liberal Policy Environment?

What?

Approximately 21% of Canadian youth reported use of cannabis in 2014/15. The reported rate of past 12-month use was 16%. Boys have consistently reported greater use and access to cannabis than girls, although this difference has contracted over time, and in 2014/15 girls were as likely to report cannabis use in the past 12 months. Approximately half of Canadian youth report it is easy to access cannabis. Self-identified Indigenous youth were more likely to report easy access to cannabis (Government of Canada, 2016).

So What?

Despite the fact that most recent estimates of past 12-month cannabis use show a much lower use than any point since 2006/2007, we know that youth (15–24 years of age) may be vulnerable to substantiated cannabis risks related to, for example, brain development during an important time of transitioning to adulthood and adult-level decision-making (Canadian Paediatric Society, 2017). In addition, there is concern that many Canadian adolescents, especially in grades 9 and 10, perceive that smoking cannabis is less risky than smoking tobacco (Government of Canada, 2016). The lack of sex differences in reported use of cannabis may be indicative of a cultural shift regarding its use among female youth in a Canadian context that is in the process of liberalizing cannabis policies. According to a study conducted by the Canadian Centre on Substance Abuse (2017), youth reported reasons for cannabis use include (a) wanting to be liked and connected to peers, (b) fitting in or taking on an identity, (c) rebelling due to parental disapproval, (d) boredom with life, (e) availability and acceptability, and (f) perceiving it as healthier than tobacco. Youth also reported they completed research and self-diagnosed a need to use cannabis for (a) chronic pain, (b) mental illness, (c) cancer, (d) arthritis, and (e) seizures. Cannabis use is also reported to (a) help increase appetite, (b) promote sleep, and (c) reduce stress and worry. Youth report fewer reasons for not using cannabis, including (a) fearing consequences from parents or legal authorities, (b) avoiding harmful effects such as lung cancer, (c) being changed as a person, (d) triggering mental illness or anxiety, (e) being stigmatized as a stoner or a loser, and (f) being contradictory to their innate values. It is important to note that the potential health, social, and legal impacts of cannabis use among youth, particularly youth who experience health inequities, are yet to be fully understood.

Now What?

SHNs can work to help change the inequities that may be further experienced by Canada's youth in the current federal policy context regarding the legalization and regulation of nonmedical cannabis. SHNs can assist youth-led coalitions to develop a strength-based approach to education interventions that are youth-centric and help them understand the complex issues related to cannabis use. SHNs can work with intersectoral partners in a primordial prevention approach to ensure policies are in place to verify that cannabis does not get into the hands of children, its use is delayed, and retail outlets are a reasonable distance from schools to deter easy access.

Standards of Practice Fulfilled

#1 Health Promotion
- Considers the determinants of health, the social and political context, and systemic structures in collaboration with the client to determine action.

#6 Health Equity
- Advocates for healthy public policy and social justice by participating in legislative and policy-making activities that influence determinants of health and access to services (CHNC, 2019, revised).

These risk-taking behaviours are mostly responsible for the morbidity and mortality in adolescence. But what are the causes of risk-taking for young people? Individual capacity and coping skills, such as personal competence and a sense of control over one's life, also play an important role in supporting mental and physical health (Government of Canada, 2011), but the school nurse understands that many factors come into play that prevent some young people from gaining the strength and self-confidence to say no to risky activities.

A Caution Although it is important to monitor the outcomes of risk-taking behaviours, a critical social theory lens cautions that children and youth are not merely problems to be solved; nor is the SHN's role to simply teach them "right behaviour." Such a focus on studying individual characteristics, deficits (rather than strengths), and risk-taking behaviour contributes to victim-blaming and fails to analyze the belief that health is an outcome of an individual's choices. Shoveller and Johnston (2006) argued that by proceeding with such an approach, "we may be unwittingly committed to an unarticulated and unrealistic set of assumptions about the level of agency and control that is afforded to many young people (p. 48)." In the case of sexual risk-taking behaviours, significant interest has been on the "problems" of youth sexual behaviour and the mostly negative sexual health outcomes (e.g., sexually transmitted infections and teenage pregnancies). Providing approaches that are child- and youth-centred while addressing broader societal issues related to youth sexual health offers critical understandings into the social composition of sexual risk as well as the possibilities for sexual health promotion among young people (MacDonald et al., 2011).

THINKING INTERSECTIONALLY ABOUT CHILD HEALTH EQUITY

As some school populations experience inequitable access to the social determinants of health, a child- and youth-centred social justice and rights-based approach to school health nursing practice must be adopted. Addressing equity issues and the determinants of children's health and well-being was a focus at the 2015 World Health Organization (WHO) meeting in Bangkok called "Global School Health Initiatives: Achieving Health and Education Outcomes." Several key intersectional-based agendas in school health programming were identified, including a need for increased services in schools for students of low socioeconomic status, students who are geographically isolated in low-resource countries, students from an Indigenous community, and students from disadvantaged communities in high-resource countries. In addition, a call was made for inclusive school health environments that are strengthened by concerted and sustained programming in order to respond to growing mental health issues experienced in a wide variety of regions and countries (WHO, 2015).

If all Canada's schoolchildren are to flourish in the 21st century, SHNs must pay particular attention to societal injustices that create health outcome inequities. When it comes to Indigenous youth in particular, equitable services must be a part of Canadian school nurse practice. Aside from understanding the impact of ageism on children's quality of life, an upstream approach is required to address the root causes of health inequities experienced by young people who face attitudinal, structural, and systemic marginalization in the form of racism, ableism, classism, and sizeism. Three populations of young people shed light on the impact of inequities on health and quality of life.

Indigenous Children

One in two First Nation (FN) children live in poverty and face daily food insecurity. Twenty-eight to 34% of shelter users, including family shelters, are Indigenous, and one in seven are children (Campaign 2000, 2017). Indigenous children are at a substantively higher risk of unintentional injuries, communicable diseases, obesity, mental health struggles, suicide, and repeated experiences of grief and loss. Indeed, the prevalence of hopelessness and death by suicide of Indigenous youth in Canada has reached a crisis point. (See Chapters 22 and 23.) Indigenous children and teens face serious discrepancies in their experience of health and health care, with racism as the core causal factor. A long-term initiative called Many Hands, One Dream (First Nations Child and Family Caring Society of Canada [FNCFCS], 2016) brings together multiple health professions in order to reduce the health inequities facing First Nation, Inuit, and Métis youth in Canada. One of the goals of the Many Hands, One Dream initiative is "to integrate traditional medicine practices into the health care of Aboriginal children and youth, to respect it as an asset rather than see it as a barrier" (FNCFCS, 2016).

First Nation schools receive less funding per student than provincial and territorial schools, and no funding for fundamental resources such as libraries, computers, Indigenous language programs, or extracurricular activities. In addition to failing to provide a safe and appropriate learning environment, the conditions of some schools actually cause severe health threats, including exposure to mould contamination, high carbon dioxide levels, rodent infestations, sewage, lack of drinkable water, and inadequate or lack of heating. Shannen Koostachin, a youth education advocate from of the Attawapiskat FN in Ontario (FNCFCS, 2016), is famous for her advocacy of "safe and comfy" schools grounded in culturally based education for First Nation children and youth (FNCFCS, 2016). See Shannen's Dream (https://fncaringsociety.com/shannens-dream).

Newcomer Children and Youth

Of the nearly 1 million food-bank users annually in Canada, nearly half are newcomers, including children. One in five racialized families lives in poverty, in comparison to one in twenty nonracialized families (Campaign 2000, 2017). Adjusting to the Canadian education system causes negative impacts on learning, especially when combined with inadequate educational bridging. When asked, newcomer youth find the barriers faced by their parents, especially those related to perceived employability, to be the most profoundly impactful, and many newcomer children avail themselves of breakfast programs as well as food banks because of it (Food Banks Canada, 2017). The impact of acclimating to Canadian culture can have long-lasting health and social impacts on newcomer children, with every social determinant of health being implicated (Shakya, Khanlou, & Gonsalves, 2010).

'Dis'abled Children and Youth

Aside from being viewed as a burden or as irrevocably immature and incapable, persons with disabilities are twice as likely to live below the poverty line, and children with disabilities are twice as likely to live in households relying on social assistance (Campaign 2000, 2017). According to the Canadian Paediatric Society (CPS), children and youth living with a disability or chronic health condition are more likely to experience sexual abuse (CPS, 2011). The CPS further stresses that young people with "children living with disability often find themselves in settings or situations where they are dependent on the unsupervised care of others … with little control over decisions directly affecting them, particularly those relating to health care and education. There also may be a reluctance by responsible individuals and institutions to hear what they have to say. Young persons with a disability may grow up with the sense that their body is controlled, even 'owned' by others. If abuse occurs, they are more likely to perceive it as a continuation of how they are usually treated" (CPS, 2011, para. 3).

A recent study found that the health-related quality of life of children with physical disabilities was significantly less than typically developing children. Quality of life was impacted by not only the disability itself but also by societal attitudes, barriers, inadequate supports, and the resultant overall strain placed on families trying to cope. Measures of quality of life included physical functioning, role functioning, parental relations, pain, family cohesion, and general health, and all were adversely impacted (Law et al., 2014). Additionally, according to a report by Surry Place (2017), children with developmental disabilities are more likely to:

- Have been exposed to a greater variety of adverse life events, including abuse, serious accidents, bereavement, and domestic violence;
- Be brought up by a single parent;
- Live in poverty;
- Live in a poorly functioning family characterized by disharmony;
- Have a mother who is in poorer health or with mental health needs;
- Live in a family with higher rates of unemployment; and
- Have fewer friends.

For Indigenous or newcomer children living with disability, these issues are further compounded by numerous systemic and societal barriers, including a Western (or settler) way of looking at disability that is incongruent with Indigenous or transcultural lenses. Disabilities within Indigenous communities tend to be addressed by the extended family, whereas in mainstream Canadian society, there tends to be a dependency upon institutional care.

A critical lens assists school-based nurses to avoid the pitfalls of health promotion aimed at merely attempting to prevent flawed choices at the individual level in child and youth populations. The Ottawa Charter for Health Promotion (WHO, 1986) lists seven prerequisites to health, including peace, shelter, education, food, stable ecosystem, sustainable resources. Social justice and equity are most instructive. When applying these as a lens, the school nurse is better able to address issues of health equity, particularly for populations most impacted by structural injustices.

Mental Health

Although mental health issues are significant for mainstream youth, they are particularly grave for marginalized young people, including 'dis'abled, newcomer, and Indigenous children and youth. Many young people living with disability experience significant physical and emotional health problems. Conditions like autism spectrum disorder and Asperger's syndrome make it hard for children and youth to understand and relate to other people, thus exacerbating feelings of aloneness and difference. Other conditions involving sensory and auditory processing problems can also make it hard for children and youth to cope with day-to-day living, often resulting in further isolation and, at times, in-school segregation. Children and youth with these conditions have a greater chance of developing other mental health problems (Children's Hospital of Eastern Ontario, 2018). Newcomer youth face settlement-related stressors, most often related to experiences of discrimination and racism, resulting in stress, anxiety, low self-esteem, worry, sadness, and depression (Shakya et al., 2010). The experience of being viewed as an "other" or as abnormal and of less value has been shown to have significant impacts on youths' sense of self-worth and agency (Shakya et al., 2010).

A promising youth-centred initiative is important for school-based nurses to be aware of. Over the course of two years, the Mental Health Commission of Canada's (MHCC) Youth Council (YC) translated the 2012 Mental Health Strategy for Canada using a critical youth lens (MHCC, 2015). YC members are representative of age and gender, province or territory of residence, cultural background, Indigenous ancestry, linguistic background, siblings or family members of persons with mental illness, experience with the child welfare system, sexual orientation or gender identities, or youth at risk with issues in housing, addictions, or the justice system. It is entirely possible that never before has a group of Canadian youth undertaken a project of this scale or developed a knowledge translation product of an existing policy document written principally for, and by, adults. The youth perspective "builds on the recommendations of the original strategy and others in order to advance the dialogue among mental health advocates, activists, students, community mental health workers, policy makers, or anyone interested in transforming Canada's mental health system" (MHCC, 2015, p. ii) with the specific intent of making the strategy reflect the perspectives and lived experiences of Canada's young people.

SCHOOL-BASED HEALTH PROMOTION MODELS

The term *comprehensive school health* was coined in the 1980s to describe a socioecological approach to school-based health promotion in Canada and the United States. In essence, this comprehensive approach was undertaken when it became evident that an educational approach alone was inadequate for changing student health and quality of life. Students require a social environment, physical environment, and school policies that reinforce educational messages. They also require school partnerships to improve access to programs and services supporting the messages. CSH and the "**health promoting schools**" approaches integrate the principles of primary health care and the strategies of the Ottawa Charter for Health Promotion (WHO, 1986) and support the foundation for a health equity approach in schools. CSH is a health-promotion approach that empowers individuals and school communities to take action for health where the school nurse is a partner who facilitates rather than an assumed expert who attempts to change student behaviour by health teaching alone. It respects children's rights and respects and facilitates their agency. When fully enacted, CSH ensures fulsome and meaningful participation of both young people and the staff who support them.

In Canada, CSH gained momentum following a national conference in 1990 that produced a consensus statement on CSH subsequently endorsed by more than 20 national organizations. In 2007, the consensus statement was revised to reflect a unifying vision for educators, health professionals, policy makers, parents, and youth (Canadian Association for School Health [CASH],

2007). Health Canada, CASH, the PHAC, and Physical and Health Education Canada have played important roles in promoting CSH through research, education, project development, and networking activities. An increasing emphasis on school improvement and school effectiveness has resulted in schools linking student health and academic success. Since its establishment in 2005, the Pan-Canadian Joint Consortium for School Health (JCSH) has facilitated federal–provincial or territorial cooperation and interministerial coordination to promote the wellness and achievement of children and youth in the school setting.

According to the JCSH, comprehensive school health encompasses the *whole* school environment that supports students in becoming healthy and productive members of society, through actions illustrated in four distinct but interrelated pillars (see Figure 17.1): social and physical environment, teaching and learning, healthy school policy, and partnerships and services. Internationally and within Canada, the pillars and terminology may vary, but the essence of the models (e.g., Health Promoting Schools, Coordinated School Health Program, Healthy Schools, and Healthy School Communities) is the same. For clarity, we use the term "comprehensive school health" (CSH) in the remainder of this chapter. Table 17.1 outlines the key components of CSH.

Indigenous School Health Framework

In 2010 the National Collaborating Centre for Aboriginal Health (NCCAH) created a **framework for Indigenous school health** reflecting wide consultation and a deep respect for Indigenous ways of knowing. Of central importance to the

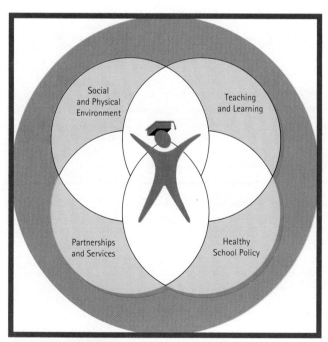

FIGURE **17.1** The Pan-Canadian Joint
Consortium for School Health Model for Comprehensive School Health

Source: Pan-Canadian Joint Consortium for School Health (2014).

school nurse committed to reconciliation are Indigenous ways of practice rooted in consensus-building, respect, a commitment to the well-being of the collective over the self, open and transparent communications, and the importance of individual and collective identities. Further, rather than focusing on assumed weaknesses or shortcomings, the school nurse committed to reconciliation focuses on the strengths of Indigenous communities most often articulated in traditional teachings or through the gift of storytelling. (See Figure 17.2.)

Practice Guidelines for School Nurses Embracing the Indigenous School Health Framework

1. Attending to Fundamental Principles

   - Interconnectedness and relationships
   - Cultural identity and worldview

2. Acknowledging Key Indigenous Cultural Concepts, Knowledge, and Practices

   - Indigenous ways of knowing
   - Indigenous ways of being

3. Affirming and Incorporating the Strengths of the Community

   - Cultural strengths
   - Collective/community strengths
   - Individual strength
   - Resiliency factors

4. Addressing Health, Social, and Educational Issues Most Relevant to Indigenous Communities

   - Healing/reconciliation programs
   - Redefining academic success
   - Suicide prevention and addressing wellness issues rooted in loss
   - Resiliency programs
   - Reduction in the incidence of fetal alcohol syndrome disorder and other substance abuse prevention programs
   - Provision of inclusive programs
   - Family- and student-centred programs
   - Provision of culturally defined parental programs
   - Determinants of health (housing, poverty, unemployment)

ROLES OF THE SCHOOL-BASED PUBLIC HEALTH NURSE

In Canada, PHN practice is guided by the Canadian Health Nurses of Canada (CHNC) Professional Practice Model and Standards of Practice (CHNC, 2011, revised), the Public

Table 17.1	Components of a Comprehensive School Health/Health Promoting Schools Approach
Supportive Social and Physical Environment	Welcoming and positive environment
	Supportive relationships
	Clear expectations and limits
	Inclusive environment that celebrates diversity and ensures *equity*
	Collaborative, partnership approach with input from students, parents, administration, teachers, and local community agencies
	Establishment of **sustainable structures** *and processes (e.g., school health committee/team) to identify and address health issues and* **measure success**
	Democracy/*involving students in decision making/active student participation (e.g., in setting classroom rules, on a school health committee, on a student council, in peer leadership)*
	High degree of staff participation
	Encouragement of staff and student autonomy
	Role modelling by parents, teachers, peers
	Mentoring programs
	Promotion of social-emotional learning and positive mental health
	Clean and hygienic *environment*
	Acceptable air quality and ventilation
	Safe water
	Adequate lighting
	Low-allergen environment
	Safe playground equipment and injury prevention measures in the school
	Universal, nonstigmatizing student nutrition/food programs
	Media reinforcing healthy behaviours
Teaching and Learning	K–12 health and physical education *curriculum*
	Relevant, high-quality teaching/learning materials
	Commitment to *teacher preparation*: pre-service and in-service training
	Empowerment approaches that consider individual and social contexts, promote **action competence,** *and:*
	• use active and cooperative learning techniques
	• develop health knowledge, attitudes, and behaviours
	• emphasize generic skill development (e.g., information seeking, decision making, problem solving, refusal skills, critical thinking, media awareness, coping, personal goal setting, social skills, building relationships, conflict resolution)
	• encourage students to participate in local *community action*
	Cross-curriculum support for health
Healthy School Policy	Government, school board, and school policies/guidelines supporting health
	Funding and agreements facilitating access to services, including partnership policies
	Smoke-free policy enforcement
	Availability of healthy food choices
	Safe food-handling practices
	Daily physical activity policies
	Injury prevention policies
	Sun safety policies
	Mental health and well-being policies
	Safe and healthy school policies/guidelines (e.g., prohibiting harassment)

(continued)

Table 17.1	Continued
Partnerships and Services	Health services (e.g., physical, mental, public health)
	Guidance and career education
	Social work
	Psychology
	Child protection
	Police services
	Early identification, assessment, referral, treatment, and follow-up
	Parks and recreation/Boys' and Girls' Clubs/YMCAs and YWCAs
	Access to community-based services
	"Healthy school" coordinators (provincial, school board, and local school levels)

Note: The words in bold italics refer to the 10 key principles of the Health Promoting School concept as identified at the First Conference of the European Network of Health Promoting Schools in Greece, 1997: (1) Democracy, (2) Equity, (3) Empowerment and Action Competence, (4) School Environment, (5) Curriculum, (6) Teacher Training, (7) Measuring Success, (8) Collaboration, (9) Communities, and (10) Sustainability.

Source: WHO (1997).

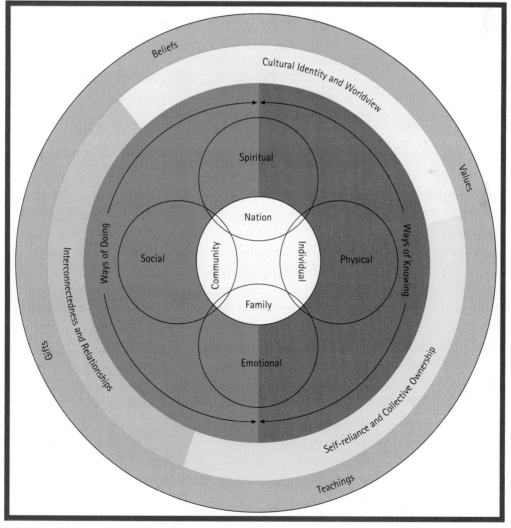

FIGURE 17.2 Indigenous School Health Framework

Source: National Collaborating Centre for Aboriginal Health (2010), p. 33.

Health Nursing Discipline Specific Competencies (CHNC, 2009), and the roles and activities described by the Canadian Public Health Association (2010). (See Chapter 4.)

Within schools, PHNs simultaneously plan and deliver care at multiple levels: individual students or staff, families, groups, classrooms, the entire school population, the community, or the whole school board or jurisdiction. Table 17.2 summarizes a recommended scope of practice for school-based PHNs in Ontario (cited in CHNIG, 2015, pp. 41–42).

Table 17.2	Recommended Scope of Practice for School-Based Public Health Nurses

Goal: To enable all children and youth to attain and sustain optimal health and development, and learning potential ("health" refers to physical, mental/emotional, and social health)

Philosophy: Strengths based/solution focused

Clients: Students and families/school staff/school board/community

Promoting Health with Individuals

- Assessment, supportive counselling, and referral of students to needed services
- Health education and skill development with students, families, school staff
- Provision of some clinical services per locally identified need
- School-based health or wellness clinics or youth health centres in secondary schools
- Consultation and coordination with school staff
- Participation in case conferences
- Communication and coordination with families via school visits, home visits, phone calls
- Coordination with other service or care providers

Promoting Health with Small Groups or Classrooms

- Small group programming with students in areas of identified need (e.g., healthy relationships, self-esteem, communication, social skills, anger management)
- Staff education on health and development issues and on youth engagement
- Parenting education
- Training of groups of peer leaders in various topic areas (e.g., playground activity leaders, nutrition, mental health leaders, healthy school committees)
- Providing or recommending curriculum materials to teachers
- Classroom education sessions on health topics

School-Wide Health Promotion

- Assessment, surveillance, and data analysis to identify strengths and priority needs in school populations
- Ensuring a group to address school health or school improvement issues is established, and that it includes significant student participation and leadership
- Supporting the group in creating comprehensive action plans (i.e., the plans should include the components of teaching and learning; partnerships and services; social and physical environment; healthy school policies)
- Encouraging youth across the school to become involved in health action
- Working with school staff, students, and communities to develop and implement healthy school policies and to create supportive school environments
- Ensuring equitable access to health and social services for the school population

Board- or District-Wide and Community-Level Health Promotion

- Contributing to health policy development on school board working groups
- Participating on board/inter-agency committees related to school services or coordination of care to ensure equitable access
- Engaging young people in the development and implementation of health-related communications/campaigns (including ensuring connection with appropriate health unit staff and maintaining website information)
- Acknowledging school successes at board or community events
- Collecting statistics to identify trends and prevailing issues
- Conducting evaluations as indicated

Source: Community Health Nurses Initiatives Group (2015). Used with the permission of CHNIG and Carol MacDougall.

Working with Individuals: Primary and Secondary Prevention

Today, school-based PHNs provide clinical services that may include immunization, sexual health services, vision and hearing screening, and health counselling and referral. The counselling role of PHNs in schools, especially high schools, contributes to successful adolescent health programs, along with personal skill training in learning life and social skills and dealing with peer pressure and peer influences (Brooks, Kendall, Bunn, Bindler, & Bruya, 2007). PHNs provide this initial assessment, support, and referral as they practise from a solution-focused, strengths-based approach that optimizes the problem-solving and coping abilities of young people and families. PHNs communicate and coordinate care with a student's family and school staff and serve as a consultation resource for school staff.

In Canada and other countries, there is great variability within mandated public health services regarding the provision of individual counselling to students. (See Canadian Research 17.1.) Most PHNs take additional training in solution-focused counselling to augment their roles in listening, **supportive counselling**, and providing information regarding relevant community resources. Even in jurisdictions that encourage the supportive counselling role, most PHNs are on-site only a few hours per week, so it is important to set up a system where students can make appointments with the nurse confidentially and are provided a slip to get out of class. Most PHNs would need to work with the school's guidance and administrative team to set up this sort of process; doing so would reduce barriers to young people working with their nurse on issues they identify as important. Additionally, it is important that access to counselling services by other professionals such as social workers, guidance counsellors, and psychologists be provided. Collaborative partnerships among public health, school boards and districts, and community agencies can share responsibility for funding these types of support services in schools. Delivery of school-based counselling by PHNs yields a high degree of satisfaction among staff, students, and parents (Moynagh & Singleton, 2011; Saewyc, Roy, & Foster, 2014; Trim, 2011).

The school-based health clinic (e.g., teen health clinic) is another model that has gained acceptance and is used in many areas of the country. Health services offered in a school setting that integrate clinical care with public health interventions and environmental change strategies offer an opportunity to address multiple determinants of health (Clayton, Chin, Blackburn, & Echeverria, 2009; Saewyc et al., 2014). In Nova Scotia, the Youth Health Centre (YHC) model operates in high schools, where youth access comprehensive, confidential, and nonjudgmental programs and services, including health education, health assessment and intervention, referral, support, and follow-up by PHNs and other health providers (Nova Scotia Department of Health Promotion and Protection, 2009). Additionally, the YHC coordinators support student action teams, provide health curriculum support through classroom presentations, and coordinate immunization clinics in the school. The Nova Scotia model integrates individual-focused services as well as opportunities for group work and peer-led student action teams that address whole-school issues.

Working with Small Groups: Primary Prevention

Group learning and group discussion co-facilitated by youth leaders and the school-based PHN are an effective approach to actively engage young people in creating peer support and formal or informal learning. Topics should be collaboratively chosen in consultation with the young people themselves as well as with school staff. They may include smoking cessation, healthy relationships, sexual health and sexuality, parenting, understanding emotions, self-esteem, decision making, birth control methods, or puberty. It can involve the training of peer leaders to lead a variety of activities during lunch, at recess, or after school. Such group learning is particularly valuable because it enables a peer group as a whole to experience a shift in social norms and collectively increase its awareness, knowledge, and critical-thinking and advocacy skills in a caring, supportive, and nonjudgmental environment.

Working with Whole Schools, Boards, School Districts, and Communities: Primordial Prevention

School-based PHNs also serve in key consultancy roles for school staff, boards, and their wider communities. As sought-after experts regarding current issues impacting the health and quality of life of young people, CHNs often suggest that for some health concerns that arise during individual or small-group work, school-wide health promotion initiatives may prove most beneficial. Take, for example, the U.S.-based #NeverAgain movement or the nationally successful by youth-for-youth North American movement of Gay-Straight Alliances, whose aim is the prevention of homo- and transphobic attitudes in schools. PHNs can facilitate the implementation of a youth-centred structure and process to address health in schools. (See Photo 17.1.) Engagement of a critical mass of students is essential for the success of healthy school initiatives (MacDougall & Laforêt-Fliesser, 2009). When youth are engaged in decisions concerning their health and their school, they feel more connected to their school and are better able to build relationships with peers and other adults. Such a participatory approach respects and facilitates Article 12 of the UNCRC (UN General Assembly, 1989). Meaningful youth participation on a school health committee or student action team ensures that issues that are central to young people are front and centre and provide students with an opportunity to share ideas, be involved with planning and implementing new programs or policies, and learn new skills in consensus building, project planning, and communication (JCSH, 2014b).

The CSH process is, in essence, the nursing process applied in collaboration *with* a school community. The core nursing skills of mutual respect, caring, listening, assessing, enabling, and empowering are critical to the PHN's work with school communities and school boards. A PHN's practice in school can be complex and challenging because relationships with school staff, parents, students, superintendents, or community partners occur within a complex, changing, and

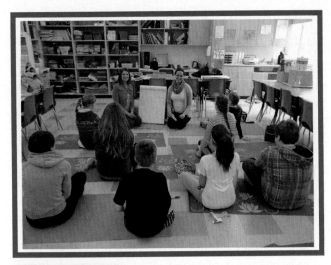

PHOTO 17.1 A PHN and public health promoter co-facilitating a healthy school committee at an elementary school.

Source: Photo courtesy of Carol Arnott, for the Perth District Health Unit.

often ambiguous environment that may present conflicting circumstances for the PHN (Athwal et al., 2014). In addition to meeting the needs of individuals, families, or groups, a PHN uses a macroscopic approach in assessing and planning interventions that address the broader determinants of health within a community. The use of community development principles is particularly relevant when building capacity in school communities. This is often called a grassroots approach, where the needs and concerns to be addressed by the PHN are determined in consultation with a community that in turn prioritizes the issues. PHNs draw on several health promotion strategies first outlined in the Ottawa Charter for Health Promotion (WHO, 1986), including building capacity, strengthening community action, creating supportive environments, re-orienting health services, and developing personal skills. These strategies are initiated through enabling, facilitation, and advocacy.

In facilitating CSH, it is important to determine the school community's level of readiness, its strengths or assets, and the areas that they themselves identify to be of interest or concern. Some school communities may have a **health champion** who can easily facilitate the school's participation in health-promotion activities. Other school communities may be immersed in their academic focus, and the PHN has a role in assisting them to see the value of collaborative school-based health promotion before any action is possible. The PHN can support the initiation of a **health action team** in using the CSH framework to examine how health promoting the school is overall. A PHN can engage a school in reflecting on the following questions:

- What are the steps involved in a comprehensive consultation with all members of the school community? Who do I need to consult with? Am I able to partner with youth during this consultation in a shared leadership approach?
- Is the school aware of and able to access support services from the board and local community to support the health of students, staff, and families in the school community?

- Does the school have a democratic and supportive social environment with shared decision making that enables the voices of young people to be heard and considered?
- How effective is the health, physical education, and other curriculum delivery? Is the physical environment supportive of the health curriculum being taught in the classroom?
- Does the school implement and enforce health-supporting policies? (MacDougall, 2004)

Health promotion programs in schools are often adult-driven, well-intended, and frequently focus on increasing students' awareness about healthy eating, active living, safety issues, avoiding substance use, and developing healthy relationships, including sexual health and violence prevention. But according to the CHNC (2011) standards of practice, health education is but one of many roles of the PHN. School nurses are well-advised to avoid narrowing their role to solely that of health teaching, for not only does it assume that most of these complex issues are within the control of the individual child or young person with just the right information, but also this approach fails to address the source of the issue in the first place. The "school health committee" or "action team" creates a place to discuss and build upon a school's strengths or assets while addressing health concerns and planning appropriate action. When formulating a plan to address an identified health issue, the PHN can support the action team in identifying strategies or activities within each of the four component areas to achieve a degree of comprehensiveness that is more likely to have a meaningful impact on the school community. For example, if student nutrition is the priority concern of the school, then the components of the plan might look like this:

- Supportive social and physical environment—Assist students to run a healthy tuck shop; engage youth in finding solutions for healthier high school cafeteria menus; encourage parents to reinforce healthy eating in the purchases they make for lunches and home meals.
- Teaching and learning—Ensure the provision of in-service for teachers so they are better prepared to deliver the nutrition curriculum.
- Healthy school policies—Establish universal student nutrition programs, such as breakfast, snack, or lunch programs; establish healthy school nutrition policies that address foods offered at school events and for fundraising.
- Partnerships and services—Consult with a public health nutritionist, dietitian, or nurse to explore the many ways student nutrition could be addressed throughout the school and suggest community agencies that could assist students who may have significant nutritional issues, such as weight-preoccupation nutritional restriction.

PHNs can also support school board or district-wide and community-wide health promotion. The formation of strong partnerships between boards or districts of education and public health agencies at the local level enables sustainable implementation of CSH. Examples of effective partnerships include joint committees for curriculum and policy development, which support the health of students and the school environment

(MacDougall & Laforêt-Fliesser, 2009). (See the Case Study that follows.) Joint development of a local CSH initiative or adoption of a provincial initiative greatly increases the commitment of principals and school staff, as their participation becomes part of expected school improvement efforts and is actively recognized by school board leaders (Ontario Ministry of Health Promotion, 2010). As school-based nurses are community-embedded, meaningful participation of PHNs on interagency community planning tables enables coordination of efforts to address youth health trends; for example, self-harm and suicide.

CASE STUDY

High school nurses have the privilege of exposure to the innermost secrets of adolescent life. Although they provide a range of nursing interventions for all levels of prevention, high school nurses are seen as the confidantes for students with serious relationship issues or conflicts at home. In 2010, Mae Katt, an Ojibwe nurse practitioner at Dennis Franklin Cromarty High School in Thunder Bay, realized her students were intimately involved in the opioid crisis that killed almost 2500 Canadians in the previous year. Katt observed that a number of the students were presenting at the clinic with profiles of restlessness, aches, and pains, and asking for medication. She recognized that the students' health concerns were actually representative of experiencing withdrawal from opioid drugs. More than 40% of the students in her high school were addicted to opioids. Many of the students came to Thunder Bay from fly-in communities in northern Ontario with high addiction rates and grew up exposed to ongoing youth mental health crises and suicides. By 2011, Katt had helped develop a program to treat opioid addiction at the school. The program provided a medication called suboxone with grief counselling and other psychosocial interventions. Katt's efforts did not stop there, and along with her colleagues she also successfully lobbied to expand the program into students' home communities in northern Ontario. Treatment is now provided at 22 sites in northern communities. Katt also notes that addiction rates have dropped significantly among students in her high school. The complete radio interview with Katt is available at www.cbc.ca.

Discussion Questions

1. When creating an interest in working together, it is important to recognize what the focus of action will be and how others perceive it. How can the school-based PHN be sure there is support for this collaborative action from the community, other organizations, and the individuals who are to benefit most by it?

2. Name two ways the Indigenous school health framework (NCCAH, 2010), provided in this chapter, is reflected in the approach taken by the SHN in the example.

3. Community capacity influences readiness for community action. Define community capacity in the context of this case study.

Promoting Positive Mental Health

Vancouver-based PHN Fara Lambing (2015) reflected recently on the necessity for her and her team to create a Mindful Kindness Program to counter the negative impact of media, technology, and cyber communications on their physical emotional and educational well-being. Her work, entitled "You Matter to Me, I Care about You," seeks to counter these negative influences by fostering self-esteem through facilitated kindness conversations and role modelling of kind ways of being with others in order to foster inclusionary ways and attitudes. Like this program, research supports the importance of moving beyond a problem-focused approach to embrace a positive mental health view, where there is recognition that the assets within individuals and their social settings can contribute to healthy growth and development (Morrison & Peterson, 2013). A youth-informed view describes good mental health as "a state of wellbeing in which you can realize your own potential, cope with the normal stresses of life, work productively, and make a contribution to your community" (MHCC, 2015, p. 4). The key concepts that describe the nature of positive mental health approaches include social-emotional learning, positive youth development, resiliency, protective factors, diversity, acceptance and understanding of student mental health needs, connectedness, strength-based perspectives, mental fitness, and self-efficacy (JCSH, 2014a). These approaches create supportive environments that promote and sustain positive mental health for all individuals. The development of mental health skills is especially important during the school years as they can help youth cope with the challenges of growing up (Weare, 2015).

In order to promote positive mental health, the school nurse needs to understand the causes of emotional distress first and then seek to prevent them in the first place. Paying attention to patterns in the various stories the nurse hears when working with individuals, groups, teachers, and parents gives rise to trends that the PHN then seeks to address or prevent. Addressing mental health through a health equity lens compels the PHN to ask what forces are contributing to emotional distress; what subgroups of young persons are disproportionately represented in depression, anxiety, and other mental health statistics; and how the school can as a collective address them.

Promoting positive mental health through schools provides another opportunity for PHNs to use their clinical knowledge and expertise in prevention and health promotion. The characteristics of effective *mental health promotion programs* in schools include the following:

- providing a backdrop of universal, multidimensional, coherent programs and services that promote the mental health of all and then effectively targeting those with special needs;
- creating supportive climates that promote warmth, empathy, positive expectations, and clear boundaries;
- tackling mental health problems early when they first manifest themselves and then taking a long-term approach that considers the child's development over time;

- identifying and targeting vulnerable and at-risk groups and helping people acquire the skills and competencies that underlie mental health; and
- involving end users and their families in ways that encourage a feeling of ownership and participation and providing effective training for those who run the programs, including helping them to promote their own mental health (Morrison & Peterson, 2013; Weare, 2015).

CONCLUSION

This chapter describes the importance of the school years and the role of school-based PHNs in promoting the health and quality of life of young people through a health equity approach. It describes CSH and the role of PHNs in partnering with young people, enacting the role of advocate, facilitator, and consultant while building committee structures, initiatives, and processes within schools. CSH offers PHNs the opportunity to work within a broad scope of practice that incorporates one-on-one, small group, and school-, board-, and community-wide health-promotion strategies. By virtue of their presence in schools, PHNs work within the cultures of education and health and bring unique insight that combines both an individual and a population health perspective (CHNIG, 2015). The significant health concerns in this population identified at the beginning of the chapter reinforce the need for an expanded health-promotion role for the PHN in schools that is in keeping with a child-centred, rights-based approach.

Although CSH has gained momentum in this country, PHNs strive to enact a rights-based socioenvironmental and upstream approach to health inequities faced by diverse young people in Canada. Further, the 21st-century school nurse proactively embraces reconciliation with Indigenous communities, paying particular attention to the role of colonization and its impact on health, opportunities, and quality of life of SN children. The CNA continues to assert that PHNs are well positioned to significantly influence the health and education outcomes of Canada's school-age population. Efforts are ongoing to develop a national strategy that clearly defines the roles and contributions of PHNs within a CSH approach. Canada's school-based PHNs are leaders, and as such they have the fortitude and veracity to role-model a rights-based emancipatory practice that affirms young people's status as Canadians and ensures their participation is meaningfully respected.

KEY TERMS

adolescence   (p. 333)
Convention on the Rights of the Child (UNCRC)
    (p. 334)
comprehensive school health (CSH)   (p. 332)
framework for Indigenous school health   (p. 339)
health action team   (p. 344)
health champion   (p. 344)
health promoting schools   (p. 338)
middle childhood   (p. 333)
risk-taking behaviours   (p. 335)
school-aged children   (p. 333)
supportive counselling   (p. 343)

STUDY QUESTIONS

1. Compare and contrast health promotion work with individuals versus school communities.

2. Discuss the challenges for PHNs working in school settings.

3. Research the various comprehensive school-based health promotion models, and describe the commonalities among them; for example, comprehensive school health, health promoting schools, coordinated school health program.

4. List the potential partners on a school health committee or action team.

5. Identify some key principles of effective youth or student engagement, and discuss the importance of using these in a PHN's daily practice.

6. List common health concerns or problems found in school settings.

INDIVIDUAL CRITICAL-THINKING EXERCISES

1. What are the main assumptions underlying comprehensive school health work, in particular work with school health committees?

2. Think of a school you attended in your past, and identify an issue you believe would have benefitted from a CSH approach. Devise a comprehensive action plan.

3. How might a PHN in a school promote the health of families who have disadvantaged children in the school, such as newcomer children, Indigenous children, or children living with disability?

4. What are the benefits of a CSH approach for students, teachers, and the entire school community?

5. Analyze your level of comfort, knowledge, and skill base in facilitating a CSH approach. What would increase your comfort, knowledge, and skill with the structure and process?

GROUP CRITICAL-THINKING EXERCISES

1. Imagine a high school has a sudden increase in the number of teens becoming pregnant, or imagine an elementary school is experiencing a high incidence of cyberbullying. Describe how you would work with the school community to assist it to address this issue.

2. Review current provincial or territorial legislation to determine what health services are provided in schools.

3. In developing a health profile for a school community, what assessment questions would you ask for each component of CSH? What methods might you use for various stakeholders: students, parents, teachers, administration, and community members?

4. A high school administrator wants to find ways to prevent substance use and abuse among the school's students. What are your first three steps, and why? Who will you involve?

5. Discuss the meaning of a "strengths-based approach" and how a school-based PHN could operationalize this in working with students and schools.

REFERENCES

Aries, P. (1962). *Centuries of childhood: A social history of family life.* New York, NY: Vintage Books.

Athwal, L., Marchuk, B., Laforêt-Fliesser, Y., Castanza, J., Davis, L., & LaSalle, M. (2014). Adaptation of a best practice guideline to strengthen client-centred care in public health. *Public Health Nursing, 31*(2), 134–143. doi:10.1111/phn.12059

Banerji, A. (2012). Preventing unintentional injuries in Indigenous children and youth. *Paediatric Child Health, 17*(7), 393. Retrieved from http://www.cps.ca/documents/position/unintentional-injuries-indigenous-children-youth

Brooks, F., Kendall, S., Bunn, F., Bindler, R., & Bruya, M. (2007). The school nurse as navigator of the school health journey: Developing the theory and evidence for policy. *Primary Health Care Research and Development, 8*, 226–234.

Campaign 2000. (2017). *A poverty-free Canada requires federal leadership.* Retrieved from https://campaign2000.ca/wp-content/uploads/2017/11/EnglishNationalC2000Report-Nov212017.pdf

Canadian Association for School Health (CASH). (2007). *Comprehensive school health: Canadian consensus statement* (revised). Retrieved from http://www.albertahealthservices.ca/SchoolsTeachers/if-sch-csh-canadian-consensus-statement-on-comprehensive-school-health.pdf

Canadian Association of Pediatric Nurses. (2017). *Canadian pediatric nursing standards.* Retrieved from https://ken.caphc.org/xwiki/bin/download/Other+Resources/Canadian+Paediatric+Nursing+Standards/FINAL-Paediatric%20Nursing%20Standards.pdf

Canadian Centre on Substance Abuse. (2017). *Canadian youth perceptions on cannabis.* Retrieved from http://www.ccsa.ca/Resource%20Library/CCSA-Canadian-Youth-Perceptions-on-Cannabis-Report-2017-en.pdf

Canadian Nurses Association. (2014). *CNA decision support policy synthesis: Public health nursing in schools.* Ottawa, ON: Author.

Canadian Nurses Association. (n.d.). *Public health nurses in schools.* Retrieved from https://www.cna-aiic.ca/~/media/cna/page-content/pdf-en/phns%20in%20schools%20webinar%20en%20jan2014.pdf?la=en

Canadian Nurses Association. (2016). *CNA webinar series. School nursing around the world.* Retrieved from https://canadian-nurse.com/~/media/cna/page-content/pdf-en/school-nursing-around-the-world_results-of-an-international-survey.pdf?la=en

Canadian Paediatric Society. (2011). *The sexual abuse of young people with a disability or chronic health condition.* Retrieved from https://www.cps.ca/en/documents/position/sexual-abuse-youth-disability-chronic-condition

Canadian Paediatric Society. (2017). Cannabis and Canada's children and youth. *Pediatrics & Child Health, 22*(2), 98–102. doi:10.1093/pch/pxx017

Canadian Public Health Association. (2010). *Public health–community health nursing practice in Canada: Roles and activities.* Ottawa, ON: Author. Retrieved from http://www.cpha.ca/uploads/pubs/3-1bk04214.pdf

Carter, A., Forrest, J., & Kaida, A. (2017). Association between internet use and body dissatisfaction among young females: Cross-sectional analysis of the Canadian community health survey. *Journal of Medical Internet Research, 19*(2), e30. doi:10.2196/jmir.5636

Children's Hospital of Eastern Ontario. (2018). *Mental health and mental illness in children and youth fact sheet for parents and caregivers.* Mental Health Information Committee. Retrieved from http://www.cheo.on.ca/uploads/13389_Mental_Health_and_Illness_Overview.pdf

Chaudry, A., & Wimer, C. (2016). Poverty is not just an indicator: The relationship between income, poverty, and child well-being. *Academic Pediatrics, 16*, S23–S29.

Clayton, S., Chin, T., Blackburn, S., & Echeverria, C. (2010). Different setting, different care: Integrating prevention and clinical care in school-based health centers. *American Journal of Public Health, 100*, 1592–1596. doi:10.2105/AJPH.2009.186668

Cohen, B. E., & McKay, M. (2010). The role of public health agencies in addressing child and family poverty: Public health nurses' perspectives. *The Open Journal, 4*, 60–71.

Community Health Nurses of Canada (CHNC). (2009). *Public health nursing discipline specific competencies Version 1.0.* St. John's, NL: Author. Retrieved from http://www.chnc.ca/documents/competencies_june_2009_english.pdf

Community Health Nurses of Canada (CHNC). (2019, revised). *Canadian community health nursing: Professional practice model & standards of practice.* St. John's, NL: Author. Retrieved from http://www.chnc.ca/documents/chnc-standards-eng-book.pdf

Community Health Nurses Initiatives Group (CHNIG). (2015). *Healthy schools, healthy children: Maximizing the contribution of public health nursing in school settings Version 2.0.* Toronto, ON: Author. Retrieved from http://draftohsc.files.wordpress.com/2014/05/policy-paper-school-health-pdf.pdf

Davies, D. (2011). *Child development: A practitioner's guide* (3rd ed.). New York, NY: Guilford Press.

Davison, C. M., Russell, K., Piedts, S., Pike, I., Pickett, W., & the CIHR team in Child and Youth Injury Prevention. (2013). *Injury among young Canadians: A national study of contextual determinants.* Vancouver, BC: CIHR team in Child and Youth Injury Prevention.

DeBell, D., & Buttigieg, M. (2016). The school as location for health promotion (2nd ed.). In D. DeBell (Ed.), *Public health for children* (pp. 133–167). Boca Raton, FL: CRC Press, Taylor Francis Group.

Department of Health. (2014). *Maximising the school nursing team contribution to the public health of school-aged children.* Retrieved from https://www.gov.uk/government/uploads/system/uploads/attachment_data/file/303769/Service_specifications.pdf

Ferris, M. (2011). Preventing obesity in Canada's Aboriginal children: Not just a matter of eating right and getting active. *The International Indigenous Policy Journal 2*(2), 1–10. Retrieved from http://ir.lib.uwo.ca/iipj/vol2/iss1/2

First Nations Child and Family Caring Society of Canada (FNCFCS). (2016). *Who we are.* Retrieved from https://fncaringsociety.com

Food Banks Canada. (2017). *Hunger in Canada: The more you know.* Retrieved from https://www.foodbankscanada.ca/getmedia/d0ea5ea2-158f-4746-9529-912b5d351d3e/Hunger-Week-infographic-FINAL.pdf.aspx

Freeman, J. G., King, M., & Pickett, W. (2011). *The health of Canada's young people: A mental health focus.* Retrieved from http://www.phac-aspc.gc.ca/hp-ps/dca-dea/publications/health-young-people-sante-jeunes-canadiens/assets/pdf/health-young-people-sante-jeunes-canadiens-eng.pdf

Government of Canada. (2011). *The well-being of Canada's young children.* Ottawa, ON: Author. Retrieved from http://www.dpe-agje-ecd-elcc.ca/eng/ecd/well-being/sp_1027_04_12_eng.pdf

Government of Canada. (2016). *Summary of results: Canadian Student Tobacco, Alcohol and Drugs Survey (CSTADS).* Retrieved from https://www.canada.ca/en/health-canada/services/canadian-student-tobacco-alcohol-drugs-survey/2014-2015-summary.html

Johnny, L. (2006). Reconceptualising childhood: Children's rights and youth participation in schools. *International Education Journal, 7*(1), 17–25.

Joint Consortium for School Health. (2014a). *Annual report.* Retrieved from http://www.jcsh-cces.ca/upload/JCSH_AnnualReport_Eng_Sept14.pdf

Joint Consortium for School Health. (2014b). *Youth engagement toolkit.* Retrieved from http://www.jcsh-cces.ca/ye-book

Lambing, F. (2015). You matter to me. I care about you. *Canadian Journal of Nursing, 11.* Retrieved from https://www.cna-aiic.ca/en/canadian-nurse-home/articles/issues/2015/november-2015

Law, M., Hanna, S., Anaby, D., Kertoy, M., King, G., & Xu, L. (2014). Health-related quality of life of children with physical disabilities: A longitudinal study. *BMC Pediatrics. 14,* 26. doi:10.1186/1471-2431-14-26

Letourneau, N. (2012). Relationships are the antidote to toxic stress. *The Canadian Nurse, 108*(3), 48.

MacDonald, J., Gagnon, A., Mitchell, C., Di Meglio, G., Rennick, J., & Cox, J. (2011). Asking to listen: Towards a youth perspective on sexual health education and needs. *Sex Education, 11*(4), 443–458. doi:10.1080/14681811.2011.595268

MacDougall, C. A. (2004). School health committees: Making "healthy schools" happen. *Canadian Association for Health Physical Education Recreation and Dance Journal, 70*(2), 27–29.

MacDougall, C. A., & Laforêt-Fliesser, Y. (2009). Canada: The evolution of healthy schools in Ontario, Canada: Top-down and bottom-up. In C. Vince Whitman & C. Aldinger (Eds.), *Case studies in global school health promotion: From research to practice* (pp. 143–157). New York, NY: Springer.

Matthews, S. (2007). A window on the "new" sociology of childhood. *Sociology Compass, 1*(1), 322–334.

Mental Health Commission of Canada (MHCC). (2015). *The mental health strategy for Canada: A youth perspective.* Retrieved from https://www.mentalhealthcommission.ca/sites/default/files/2016-07/Youth_Strategy_Eng_2016.pdf

Mitchell, R. (2011). R. C. "Human rights and health promotion: A Canada fit for children?", *International Journal of Child, Youth and Family Studies, 3/4:* 510–526.

Morrison, P., & Peterson, W. (2013). *Schools as a setting for promoting positive mental health: Better practices and perspectives* (2nd ed.). Ottawa, ON: Joint Consortium for School Health. Retrieved from http://www.jcsh-cces.ca/upload/JCSH%20Best%20Practice_Eng_Jan21.pdf

Moynagh, K., & Singleton, M. (2011). *Mental health liaison program evaluation: Client outcomes and satisfaction with services.* Halton, ON: Halton Region Health Department.

National Association of School Nurses. (2017). The role of the 21st-century school nurse. *NASN School Nurse, January,* 56–58. doi:10.1177/1942602X16680171

National Collaborating Centre for Aboriginal Health. (2010). *A framework for Indigenous school health: Foundations in cultural principles.* Retrieved from https://www.ccnsa-nccah.ca/docs/health/RPT-FrameworkIndigenousSchoolHealth-Tagalik-EN.pdf

Nova Scotia Department of Health Promotion and Protection. (2009). *An evaluation of Youth Health Centres in Nova Scotia: Executive summary.* Retrieved from http://novascotia.ca/dhw/healthy-development/documents/Youth-Health-Centres-in-Nova-Scotia-An-Evaluation.pdf

Ontario Ministry of Health Promotion. (2010). *School health guidance document.*

Ordre des infirmières et infirmiers du Québec. (2015). *Standards de pratique pour l'infirmière en santé scolaire* (2nd ed.). Montreal, QC: Author. Retrieved from https://www.oiiq.org/sites/default/files/SanteScolaire-Abrege-Final%20Web.pdf

Pan-Canadian Joint Consortium for School Health (JCSH). (2014). *Annual report.* Used by permission of Joint Consortium for School Health. Retrieved from http://www.jcsh-cces.ca/upload/JCSH_AnnualReport_Eng_Sept14.pdf, p. 7.

Pickett, W. (2011). Injuries. In J. G. Freeman, M. King, & W. Pickett (Eds.), *The health of Canada's young people: A mental health focus.* Retrieved from http://www.phac-aspc.gc.ca/hp-ps/dca-dea/publications/health-young-people-sante-jeunes-canadiens/assets/pdf/health-young-people-sante-jeunes-canadiens-eng.pdf

Prevnet. (2017). *The dangers of bullying.* Retrieved from http://www.prevnet.ca/bullying/dangers

Public Health Agency of Canada (PHAC). (2011). *Our health our future: A national dialogue on healthy weights dialogue report.* Ottawa, ON: Ascentum. Retrieved from http://www.phac-aspc.gc.ca/hp-ps/hl-mvs/ohof-nsna/index-eng.php?utm_source=VanityURL&utm_medium=URL&utm_campaign=ourhealthourfuture.gc.ca

Public Health Agency of Canada (PHAC). (2013). *The Chief Public Health Officer's report on the state of public health in Canada: Infectious disease—the never-ending threat.* Retrieved from http://www.phac-aspc.gc.ca/cphorsphc-resp-cacsp/2013/index-eng.php

Public Health Agency of Canada (PHAC). (2017). *Report on sexually transmitted infections in Canada: 2013–14.* Retrieved from https://www.canada.ca/en/public-health/services/publications/diseases-conditions/report-sexually-transmitted-infections-canada-2013-14.html#s3

Registered Nurses Association of Ontario. (2010). *Nursing best practice guideline: Enhancing healthy adolescent development.* Toronto, ON: Author.

Roberts, K. C., Shields, M., de Groh, M., Aziz, A., & Gilbert, J. (2012). Overweight and obesity in children and adolescents: Results from the 2009 to 2011 Canadian health measures survey. *Health Reports 23*(3). Statistics Canada, Catalogue no. 82-003-XPE.

Rotermann, M. (2012). Sexual behaviour and condom use of 15- to 24-year-olds in 2003 and 2009/2010. *Health Reports, 23*(1). Statistics Canada, Catalogue no. 82-003-XPE.

Saewyc, E., Roy, J., & Foster, S. (2014). *An evaluation of North Shore public health nurses' child and youth school-linked practice.* Vancouver, BC: Vancouver Coastal Health. Retrieved from http://www.saravyc.ubc.ca/files/2014/11/NorthShore-PHN-Evaluation.pdf

Seigart, D., Dietsch, E., & Parent, M. (2013). Barriers to providing school-based health care: International case comparisons. *Collegian, 20,* 43–50. Used by permission of Elsevier Inc.–Health Sciences Division. http://dx.doi.org/10.1016/j.colegn.2012.03.003

Shakya, Y., Khanlou, N., & Gonsalves, T. (2010). Determinants of health for newcomer youth: Policy and service implications. *Canadian Issues, Summer,* 98–102.

Shoveller, J., & Johnston, J. (2006). Risky groups, risky behaviour, and risky persons: Dominating discourses on youth sexual health. *Critical Public Health, 16*(1), 47–60. doi:10.1080/09580590600680621

Statistics Canada. (2011). *Table 102-0551: Deaths and mortality rate by selected group causes, age group and sex, Canada, annual.* CANSIM database. Retrieved from http://www5.statcan.gc.ca/cansim/a26?lang=eng&retrLang=eng&id=1020551

Statistics Canada. (2015). *Childhood national immunization coverage survey, 2013.* Retrieved from http://www.statcan.gc.ca/daily-quotidien/150721/dq150721c-eng.htm

Statistics Canada. (2017). *Table 1: Number of students in public elementary and secondary schools, Canada, provinces and territories, The Daily, November 3,* 1. Retrieved from https://www150.statcan.gc.ca/n1/daily-quotidien/171103/t001c-eng.htm

Surry Place. (2017). *Improving health outcomes for children and youth with developmental disabilities: A literature review in the health status of children and youth with developmental disabilities within a population health framework.* Retrieved from http://www.surreyplace.on.ca/documents/Resources/Children's%20Forum%20Literature%20Review_final(web).pdf

Trim, K. (2011). *Perth District Health Unit and Avon Maitland District School Board: 2006–2010 school-based public health nurse program evaluation.*

Truth and Reconciliation Commission of Canada. (2015). *Honouring the truth, reconciling for the future: Summary of the final report of the Truth and Reconciliation Commission of Canada.* Canada: McGill-Queen's University Press.

United Nations General Assembly. (1989). *Session 44, Resolution 25. Convention on the rights of the child.* United Nations Convention on the Rights of the Child. Retrieved from https://treaties.un.org/pages/ViewDetails.aspx?src=IND&mtdsg_no=IV-11&chapter=4&lang=en

Weare, K. (2015). *What works in promoting social and emotional well-being and responding to mental health problems in schools.* London, UK: National Children's Bureau.

Woodhead, M. (1999). Reconstructing developmental psychology—Some first steps. *Children & Society, 13*(1), 3–19.

World Health Organization (WHO). (1986). *The Ottawa charter for health promotion.* Retrieved from https://www.canada.ca/en/public-health/services/health-promotion/population-health/ottawa-charter-health-promotion-international-conference-on-health-promotion.html

World Health Organization (WHO). (2015). *Global school health initiatives: Achieving health and education outcomes.* Retrieved from http://apps.who.int/iris/bitstream/10665/259813/1/WHO-NMH-PND-17.7-eng.pdf?ua=1

ABOUT THE AUTHORS

Jo-Ann MacDonald, RN, BScN, MN, PhD (McGill University), is an associate professor in the Faculty of Nursing, University of Prince Edward Island, with over 30 years of progressive experience in public health and community nursing, academia, and management. As a volunteer, she has served on a number of boards and committees, including the Community Health Nurses of Canada and the NB/PEI Public Health Association. Dr. MacDonald is the co-principal investigator for the Comprehensive School Health Research Unit in Prince Edward Island, has conducted participatory research with youth on sexual health education in schools, and is a co-investigator for the Canadian Student Tobacco Alcohol and Drug Survey.

Cheryl van Daalen-Smith, RN, BScN, M.A., PhD (University of Toronto), is an associate professor in the School of Nursing at York University. A long-time pediatric and school-based public health nurse whose practice embraces children's rights and social justice, Dr. van Daalen-Smith was the first nurse to serve on the Canadian Coalition on the Rights of Children and is the only nursing scholar on the Canadian Child Rights Academic Network. Founder of the Pediatric Nurses Interest Group of Ontario and the Canadian Association of Pediatric Nurses, Cheryl is thrilled to see the UNCRC embedded in Canada's new Pediatric Nursing Standards of Practice. She is the founder and co-editor of *Witness: The Canadian Journal of Critical Nursing Discourse.* Her "spare" time is spent with a menagerie of cast-away and rescued farm animals in rural Ontario.

CHAPTER 18

Family Nursing

Lisa Underhill, Debbie Sheppard-Lemoine, and Megan Aston

LEARNING OUTCOMES

After studying this chapter, you should be able to:

1. Define family nursing and discuss its importance.

2. Identify current demographic trends in Canadian families.

3. Describe the definition of family and its roles and responsibilities.

4. Discuss the theories, models, frameworks, and tools that inform family assessment.

5. Outline the process of family assessment when conducting a family home visit.

6. Situate family nursing within national policy and standards within a health equity and social justice lens, including the Community Health Nurses of Canada's Standards of Practice.

7. Discuss future research and challenges for community health nurses working with families.

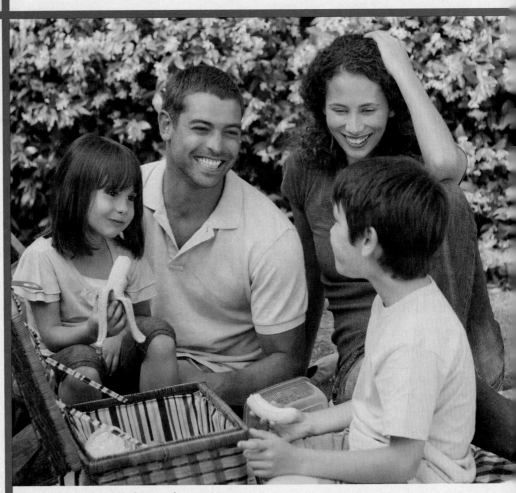

Source: ESB Professional/Shutterstock

INTRODUCTION

Families are a foundation of society and create life routines while also providing emotional, psychological, and informational support for their members. We all begin life as a newborn in relation to someone who is our caretaker including biological, adoptive or foster parents/guardians. Traditional views of the Western family include mothers, fathers, sisters, brothers, grandparents, grandchildren, nieces, nephews, or cousins. However, the traditional heterosexual nuclear family is being challenged and reshaped to include other formations. For many, friends and pets are also treated as family members. We all play many different roles within our family and in the lives of our significant others.

Community health nurses (CHNs) practising family nursing find personal rewards when they can make a difference in promoting not only physical, mental, and emotional health but also health equity and social justice in the lives of their clients. Through conducting family health assessments, CHNs continually ask the questions: "But why does this occur? What is the root cause?" This chapter describes the upstream societal and cultural context of the family and provides a brief overview of theoretical frameworks that guide family nursing practice, family case management, and family-centred care. Opportunities and challenges for CHNs are also discussed.

FAMILY NURSING

Family nursing has evolved considerably since the early 1980s and is now a specialty practice in nursing (Wright & Leahey, 2013). **Family nursing** is a provision of care where the nurse uses nursing processes to assist the family and its members in achieving their highest potential health through adapting to various health and illness situations. A strength-based focus on families is the guiding principle of this chapter. Wright and Leahey (2013) stressed that when working with families, besides developing a therapeutic relationship with the family, the nurse needs to view the family as a system, working to achieve optimal health at all times. Any changes introduced to any parts of the family will cause changes in other parts of the family system.

The meaning of family will influence the way CHNs provide family health nursing care. The health of one family member affects the health of the rest of the family. Your personal experiences may frame perceptions of family composition and interactions. Social stereotypes as to what constitutes the ideal family may also inform perceptions and practice. The dominant Western discourse on families is usually heteronormative, white, middle-class, and nuclear, most often including two parents and two children. Thus, it is critical for CHNs to be aware of the impact of social stereotypes as well as their own values and beliefs about family and how these may shape their approach to providing family nursing care.

Family nursing practice is guided by the Community Health Nurses of Canada (CHNC) (2019, revised) and the Canadian Nurses Association (CNA) (2013), both of which state that CHNs care for families as clients in their practice and that nurses must act in ways to improve social determinants of health to promote family health. Some of these social determinants of health can impact the health of individuals, families, and populations, and result in inequity in the health status of populations.

TRENDS IN CANADIAN FAMILIES

Family compositions are continually evolving in Canada. Understanding trends in family diversity is important when working with families and developing community-based programming that is relevant to the evolving tapestry of Canadian families. A total of 1.7 million Canadians self-identified as Indigenous in 2016, encompassing 4.8% of our population (Statistics Canada, 2018). The most recent Statistics Canada (2017) data reveal that married couples comprise the predominant family structure (66%), more Canadians are living

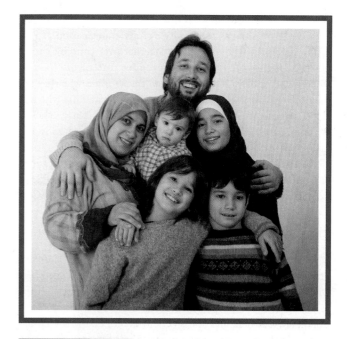

PHOTO 18.1 **Family Diversity**

Source: ZouZou/Shutterstock

alone (28.2%), and fewer households are comprised of a "mom, dad, and kids" family. A significant change impacting **family composition** is the large cohort of aging baby boomers (born between 1946 and 1964) now entering their older adult years. Many of these older adults now are living with their adult children, forming multigenerational households that typically consist of children less than 14 years of age, their parents, and at least one grandparent. **Multigenerational households** were the fastest-growing type of household between 2001 and 2016 (+37.5%). (See Photo 18.1.)

The percentage of couples with (51.1%) and without children (48.9%) (Statistics Canada, 2017) represents a shrinking family size, but the number of Canadian households has increased. This phenomenon is largely due to the aging population and the higher rates of separation and divorce, leading to a growing number of non-traditional families. CHNs should note that the current low fertility rate is below the expected population replacement rate; there will be fewer children available to share the caregiving responsibilities for aging parents. Both trends will have economic and health-care impacts on society. The percentage of one-person households in Canada increased from 7% in 1951 to 28% in 2016. This dramatic shift is due to numerous societal trends, including separation, divorce, longer life expectancy, and increased presence of women in the workforce. Of note for CHNs doing home visits with older adults in particular, more women live alone than any other age group (Statistics Canada, 2017).

WHAT IS FAMILY?

The definition of *family* has changed significantly over the last five decades. Traditional definitions have used the legal concepts of relationships, such as genetic ties, adoption, guardianship, or marriage (Stanhope & Lancaster, 2014). Today, the definitions of family are more encompassing. The Vanier Institute of the Family (2018) defines the family as "any combination of two or more persons who are bound together over time by ties of mutual consent, birth and/or adoption or placement" (p. xii). Wright and Leahey (2013) state that "the family is who they say they are" (p. 55). Some families, especially older adults who live alone, consider their pet a valued family member. Nurses should ask families who they consider to be members of their family and include them in health-care planning (Hunt, 2013).

Family forms refer to how the family is structured or composed, as families can take various forms: nuclear, extended, lone parent, blended, heterosexual, and LGTBQ2S families. In Canada, same-sex marriages have been legalized since July 2005 with the enactment of the Civil Marriage Act (Government of Canada, 2015).

Family structure refers to the characteristics and demographics (i.e., gender, age, and number) of individual members who make up the family. The structure of a family defines the roles and positions of its members (Stanhope & Lancaster, 2014). Friedman, Bowden, and Jones (2003) examine how the family is organized, and they stress four structural dimensions: family power and decision making, roles, values, and communication. For example, a father unilaterally decides where the family will go on vacation. He communicates this decision to his wife with the expectation that she will inform the children. Here we see a patriarchal family where power and decision making reside with the father, who has indirect communication patterns with his children.

Family functions are defined as "behaviours or activities performed to maintain the integrity of the family unit and to meet the family's needs, individual members' needs, and society's expectations" (Stanhope & Lancaster, 2014). How well the family fulfills its functions or attains its goals is related to family structure. Thus, these two concepts are intimately connected (Freistadt & Strohschein, 2012).

The Vanier Institute of the Family (2018) described the following roles or responsibilities characterized by **healthy families**:

- physical maintenance and care of group members
- addition of new members through procreation or adoption
- socialization of children
- social control of members
- production, consumption, and distribution of goods and services
- affective nurturance—love (para 3)

With the use of these guidelines, it is believed that healthy families have clearly defined roles and responsibilities and division of labour for each member. The power structure and communication system for the family are clear and orderly, which enhances the family's relationships, problem-solving or coping skills, and socialization of the family unit with the community. When working with childbearing and childrearing families, CHNs have many opportunities to work with these families to strengthen the family system by promoting healthy parent–child relationships and healthy child development. KidsFirst is a voluntary program in Saskatchewan that helps vulnerable families to become the best parents they can be

Table 18.1	Family Life Cycle Stages and Tasks	
Stages	**Task**
Launching of the single young adult	Differentiation from family of origin
	Financial independence
Marriage: The joining of families	Commitment to and establishing a new family
Families with young children	Adjustment to parenthood and new family members
	Meeting age-appropriate developmental needs of children
	Maintaining supportive relationships with children and across generations
Families with adolescents	Adjustment to needs of young adults leaving or re-entering the family
Launching children and moving on	Adjusting to changes in the partner relationship
Families in later life	Adjustments to retirement, end of life

Source: Based on Wright, L. M., & Leahey, M. M. (2012).

and to have the healthiest children possible (Government of Saskatchewan, 2018).

All families experience many developmental and situational crises throughout their family developmental stages. (See Table 18.1.) Healthy families cope with these crises as they acquire new skills and confidence to cope with other **developmental tasks**. Some families lack problem-solving skills and resources to deal with crises, which results in the buildup of stressful life situations. A family experiencing multiple challenging life situations or stresses is one with "needs in several areas simultaneously, difficulty achieving developmental tasks, illness or loss, inadequate resources and support, or environmental stressors" (Smith, 2013a, p. 374). An example of a family dealing with multiple challenges would be a single, unemployed mother with limited support who has just given birth to an infant with Down syndrome. The intensity and multiplicity of stressors associated with life events can put a family like this at increased risk and vulnerability (Smith, 2013a).

To effectively work with families experiencing challenging life situations or stresses, CHNs must consider four key factors. First, the CHN must understand that situations such as poverty, unemployment, isolation, and lack of support systems can shape the family biologically, psychological, and interpersonally. Second, the CHN can support the family by discussing how they can anticipate risks and subsequently mobilize resources to mitigate risks and promote health. Third, the CHN must work collaboratively with the family in a trusting, respectful, and nonjudgmental environment (Browne, Doane, Reimer, MacLeod, & McLellan, 2011).

Finally, cultural safety is key when working with Indigenous families (Ward, Branch, & Fridkin, 2016) and families with diverse ethnic and racial backgrounds (Richardson, Yarwood, & Richardson, 2017). This way of practising "involves developing an ongoing personal practice of critical self-reflection, paying attention to how social and historical contexts shape health and health care systems, and being honest about one's own power and privilege, especially as these relate to Indigenous people" (Ward et al., 2016).

Family as Context of Care

Viewing the family as context of care is the traditional focus of nursing. There are five ways of viewing the family (Friedman et al., 2003) (see Figure 18.1 and Canadian Research 18.1):

- The first level is to view the family as context to the client. The CHN focuses nursing care on the individual, with the family as a secondary focus. For example, the CHN might provide counselling for teenagers experiencing depression in a clinic setting or care for hospitalized clients.
- In the second level, the family is viewed as the sum of its individual members or parts. The focus of care is on the individual family member, and members are seen as separate entities rather than interacting units. For example, the CHN might provide counselling to each member of a family facing divorce.
- In the third level of family nursing practice, family dyads, triads, and other family subsystems are the focus of care. For example, a CHN might focus on the care of the new mother and her baby during a home visit.
- Viewing the family as client is the fourth level of family nursing practice. It is the most unique type of family nursing. Here the entire family is the unit of care. The nurse provides care for the individual and the whole family and society simultaneously and provides health care for all family members. The focus is placed on internal family dynamics, relationships, family structure, and functions. The CHN assesses the interactions among the family subsystems within its own family system and its external environment. An example is a nurse caring for a family with a family member experiencing cancer or a chronic or acute illness.
- A fifth level of family nursing conceptualizes family as a component of society. The family is seen as one of society's basic institutions.

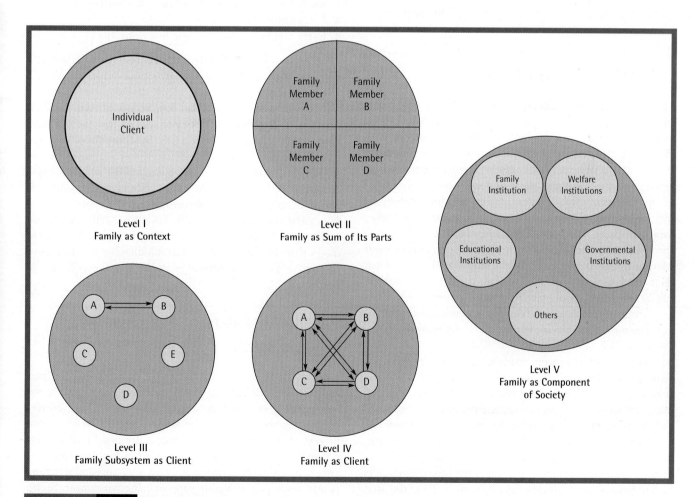

FIGURE 18.1 Five Ways of Viewing the Family

Source: Reproduced with permission from Friedman, M. M., Bowden, V. R., & Jones, E. G. (Eds.). (2003). *Family nursing: Research, theory, and practice* (5th ed.). Upper Saddle River, NJ: Prentice Hall, p. 37. © Reprinted by permission of Pearson Education, Inc. Upper Saddle River, NJ.

CANADIAN RESEARCH 18.1

The power of relationships: Exploring how public health nurses support mothers and families during postpartum home visits (Aston et al., 2015)

Public health nurses (PHNs) work with families postpartum to offer support and information during the transition to parenting. In their research study, Aston et al. (2015) found that building trusting relationships with family members was foundational to facilitating therapeutic conversations and positive health outcomes. Mothers in the study described the importance of PHNs interacting with them in a nonjudgmental, kind, and caring manner. These attributes combined with implementation of complex assessments and interventions were appreciated by all mothers and their families. Relationships created by PHNs with families through supportive strengths-based practices are key to attaining successful outcomes.

Discussion Questions

1. Discuss your thoughts on the level of family nursing addressed in this study.
2. What social determinants of health would you want to examine?
3. What policies within public health should be addressed?

FAMILY ASSESSMENT

The purpose of **family assessment** is to identify and understand family roles, communication, division of labour, decision making, power structure, boundaries, styles of problem solving, coping abilities, and health promotion practices (Friedman et al., 2003; Wright & Leahey, 2013). During the assessment process, the nurse facilitates the family in discovering and articulating the assumptions, context, and expectations underlying their perception of reality. The family assessment process takes time, sensitivity, and flexibility, and requires the CHN to have effective interviewing skills. The nurse conducts the assessment starting from the perspective of the family at the time when the nurse begins to work with the family. Competent holistic family assessment should take place in an atmosphere of openness, awareness, mutual collaboration, and relationship building. The nurse uses relevant family assessment tools to address the purpose of the assessment.

Regardless of the theory, framework, model, or tools used, a comprehensive family assessment uses open-ended and circular questions and is detailed and inclusive. Nursing assessments are an ongoing process. An assessment is not "done to" the family; rather, it is a process that the nurse facilitates and works through with the family over time (Leahey & Wright, 2016). The assessment process is the first phase of the family nursing process. The nurse first assesses the health and role of each individual family member and then the health of the overall family system in terms of its roles and how it supports the needs of individual members. Family assessment data provide the foundation for planning, interventions, and evaluation of nursing care. Both family strengths and weaknesses will be identified during the assessment. However, the CHN focuses on how to assist the family to recognize their own strengths and use various resources to achieve family goals.

Family Assessment Theories

Theories help us to "make sense" of our world, and they guide our nursing practice. Family social science theories, family therapy theories, and nursing models and theories all contribute to the emerging field of family nursing theories. No one theory or conceptual model, however, is sufficient for describing the multifaceted nature of family processes and relationships (Wright & Leahey, 2013). CHNs will need to be competent in knowledge and skills to integrate multiple theories to fully understand the perspectives on families. CHNs then design effective nursing interventions within the contexts of health promotion and the social determinants of health.

Although every family is unique, all families share some universal characteristics. Drake (2014) lists five important characteristics of a family:

- Every family is a small social system.
- Every family moves through stages in its life cycle.
- Every family has its own cultural values and rules.
- Every family has structure.
- Every family has certain basic functions. (p. 571)

These universal **family characteristics** reflect the importance of culture as well as structural–functional theory, systems theory, and theories of family development—all theories from the social sciences that have been applied to families. **Structural–functional theory** focuses on how the structure of the family affects family functions. **Systems theory** focuses on the interactions within and among family subsystems as well as the interaction with extended families and larger systems such as the community, world, and universe (Stanhope & Lancaster, 2014). **Family developmental theory** refers to stages and tasks, as presented in Table 18.1. This family life cycle approach refers to the generally predictable sequence of stages that most North American middle-class families move through despite their cultural or ethnic variations (Wright & Leahey, 2013).

Family Assessment Frameworks, Models, and Tools

It is not a case of "one size fits all" or of designing the "perfect" model. (See Table 18.2.) The theories, frameworks, and assessment models and tools discussed in this chapter all recognize that the CHN and the family are engaged in a social process of exploration, negotiation, and mutual goal setting, centred within the family–nurse relationship. Interventions are grounded in the contexts of family structure and function, family development, family support and environment, health work and potential health promotion, education and advocacy, the social determinants of health, and the principles of primary health care.

Table 18.2	Components of Family Assessment Models	
Friedman Family Assessment Model	**Calgary Family Assessment Model**	**McGill Model**
Aboriginal Ways of Knowing	Developmental stage and history of family	The family as the subsystem
Identifying data		Health as the focus of work
Developmental stage and history of family	Structural	Learning as the process through which health behaviours are acquired
Environmental data	Developmental	
Family structure	Functional	Family collaborates with the nurse in the learning process
Family functions		
Family coping		

Source: Adapted from Registered Nurses Association of Ontario. (2006). *Supporting and strengthening families through expected and unexpected life events* (rev. suppl.). Toronto, ON: Registered Nurses' Association of Ontario.

Indigenous Ways of Knowing The **Ways Tried and True Aboriginal Methodological Framework** (Figure 18.2) is a conceptualization of family, self, and community and was developed by the Public Health Agency of Canada for the Canadian Best Practices Initiative (Public Health Agency of Canada, 2014). This holistic framework identifies a distinct set of criteria that are associated with good practice in Indigenous settings: community-based, holistic, integration of Indigenous cultural knowledge, partnership and collaboration, built on community strengths, sustainable, and effective. All interventions have been assessed using a culturally relevant, inclusive, and validated framework.

Friedman Family Assessment Model The **Friedman Family Assessment Model** has six broad categories (Friedman et al., 2003). Identifying data include family composition, cultural background, religious identification, social class status, and recreational activities. The developmental stage is assessed along with the family's history and the history of both parents' families of origin. Environmental data include characteristics of the home, neighbourhood, and community; the family's geographic mobility; associations with the community and use of community resources; and the family's social support system. Family structure looks at communication patterns, power structure, role structure, and family values. Affective,

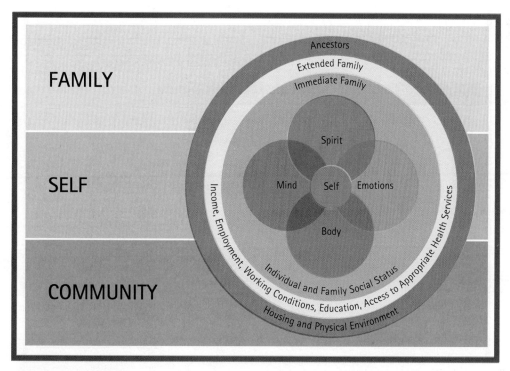

FIGURE   18.2   Ways Tried and True Aboriginal Methodological Framework

Source: Public Health Agency of Canada (2014).

socialization, and health care functions are assessed in the family functions category. The sixth category, family stress and coping, includes assessment of stressors and strengths along with coping strategies. Each category has many subcategories. The nurse and the family decide which areas need in-depth exploration based on the focus for nursing intervention.

Calgary Family Assessment Model Wright and Leahey (2013) first developed the **Calgary Family Assessment Model (CFAM)** in 1983 at the University of Calgary (Figure 18.3). The CFAM has been conceptualized as a branching model with three major categories: structural, developmental, and functional. The nurse decides which subcategories should be explored and to what extent, and assesses each family accordingly. The nurse and the family move back and forth across the branches to integrate all relevant data and build a holistic picture of the family's strengths, problems, and current situation. Although this model was originally developed within a Western context, it has been used by nurses globally in countries such as Japan, India, and Qatar. The model incorporates a variety of theories, including postmodernism, that challenge the nurse to consider multiple truths and diversity of experience. This could be why the concepts in the model are transferable globally. In a recent article Leahey and Wright (2016) personally reflected on the global application of the model they created.

Interventions conceptualized in the **Calgary Family Intervention Model (CFIM)** provide a framework for family functions in three domains: cognitive, affective, and behavioural, and these interventions focus on promoting, improving, and sustaining effective family functioning. Interventions that affect changes in family's beliefs and values (cognition domain) provide the most significant and lasting changes. A change in cognition can, in turn, influence the affective and behavioural domains (Wright & Leahey, 2013).

McGill Model The **McGill Model** has been developed and refined over time by faculty and students at the McGill University School of Nursing (Gottlieb & Gottlieb, 2007; Gottlieb & Rowat, 1987). This model emphasizes family,

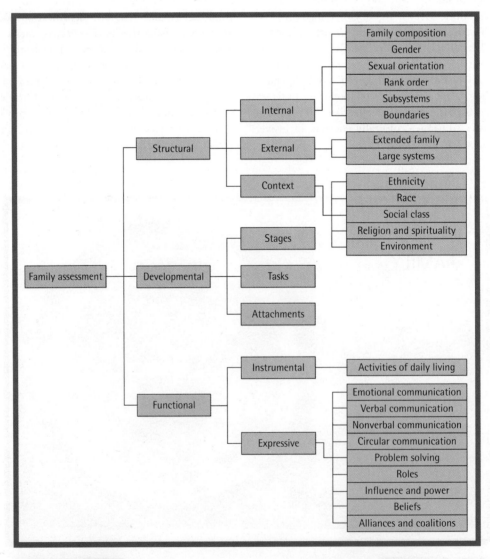

FIGURE 18.3 Branching Diagram of Calgary Family Assessment Model

Source: Wright and Leahey (2013). Used by permission of F. A. Davis & Company.

health, collaboration, and learning; and health consists of processes that are dynamic and multidimensional, especially the processes of coping and development. The family is an active participant throughout the health-care process. In this model, one of the nursing goals is to help families use the strengths of the individual members and of the family as unit, as well as resources external to the family system, to cope, achieve their goals, and develop.

The assessment phase of the McGill Model requires the nurse to explore and create a supportive environment so that the family's perceptions and strengths can emerge. Learning needs are identified, and the initiative for planning can be with the nurse or the family (Gottlieb & Rowat, 1987). During the implementation phase, the family becomes an active learner in collaboration with the nurse. The nurse, as an empowering partner, fosters families to reach a potential for positive growth.

The ABCX Model All families encounter stressful events. While some families can overcome these stressful events and maintain family cohesion and function, other families cannot. The **ABCX model**, developed by Rueben Hill (1958), is used to explain "the crisis-proneness and freedom from crisis among families" (p. 143). Also known as the stress model, Hill's ABCX model focuses on the interaction of four common factors faced by families in any crisis state: A (a crisis or precipitating event/stressor) interacting with B (the resources available to the family during the crisis), interacting with C (family's perception of the event or stressor) to produce X (the crisis state experienced by the family).

In the ABCX model, the stressor encountered by a family may be a life event or transition that impacts the family system, thereby affecting the roles and functions of various members in it. **Stressors** may be normative changes experienced along the life cycle, unpredictable challenges, or catastrophic events. A positive stressor might be a job promotion or winning a lottery, whereas a negative stressor might be an illness in a family member (e.g., spouse, child, or grandparent) or a job loss. Strains are additional demands and hardships placed on the family as a direct result of the stressor. Families with good problem-solving and coping skills will learn to adapt and accept life stressors or events in a positive way by using available resources to manage changes or hardships, thereby navigating the crisis in a productive way. Families who view their life events negatively are likely to be reluctant to seek help and will live in crisis or dysfunctional mode (McCubbin & McCubbin, 1993). (See Case Study.)

Genogram Genograms are a visual sketch providing a picture of family structure, relationships, and boundaries. Usually, the nurse constructs a three-generational genogram (or more, as needed) to examine the patterns and relationships of family events. Effective family assessment skills specific to communication and interviewing are essential to constructing meaningful genograms. A **genogram** is a tool that can help the nurse uncover the roots of significant family problems related to intergenerational health and social problems (e.g., alcoholism, diabetes, heart problems, cancer, hereditary diseases, and critical family events such as births, divorces, twin births, and miscarriages).

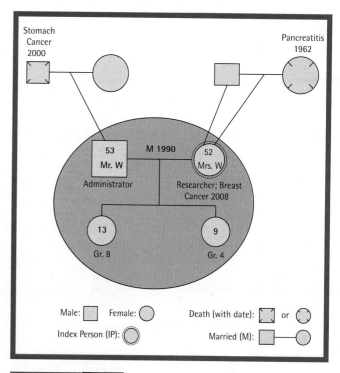

FIGURE 18.4 Genogram

The genogram illustrated in Figure 18.4 shows the family of Mr. and Mrs. W., who were married in 1990. Mrs. W. is 52 years of age and lives with her 53-year-old husband and their two children, who are 9 and 13 years. The oldest daughter is in Grade 8, and the younger daughter is in Grade 4 at the local elementary school. Mr. W.'s father died of stomach cancer in 2000, and Mrs. W.'s mother died of pancreatitis in 1967. Mrs. W. did not know her father. Mrs. W. was diagnosed with locally advanced breast cancer in 2008. Mrs. W. works as a researcher, and Mr. W. works as an administrator.

Ecomap An **ecomap** is a visual representation of a family's connections and the nature and degree of its relationships with the larger community, such as schools, friends, workplace, social and health workers or agencies. The nurse constructs a family ecomap to assess the family strengths, such as available resources and support systems, including strains or conflicting relationships experienced by the family (Wright & Leahey, 2013). (See Figure 18.5.)

THE FAMILY HOME VISIT

Historically, CHNs cared for the sick and the poor and visited families in their homes (see Chapter 1); thus, the **family home visit** is seen as the "root" of community health nursing practice. Family home visits allow the nurse to observe and interact with a family in their natural environment. It also allows nurses to better understand the needs of the collective family in addition to the individual family members (Aston et al., 2014; Sheppard-LeMoine, 2015; Wright & Leahey, 2013). The key benefit of the home visit is supported by a

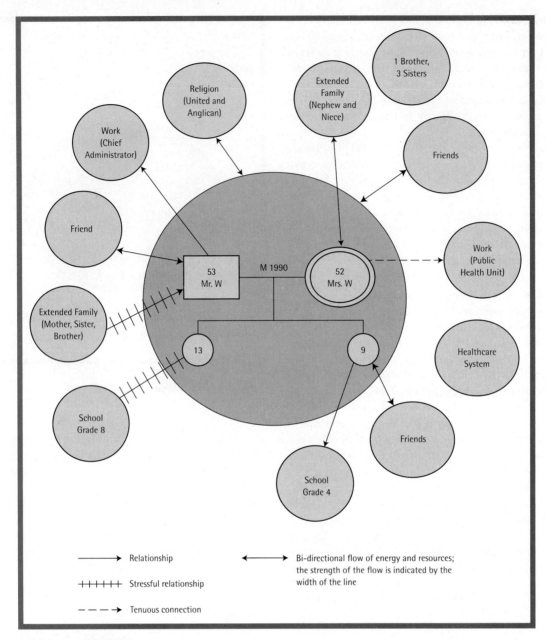

FIGURE 18.5 Ecomap

recent randomized clinical trial conducted in Memphis, Tennessee, from 1990 to 2011. This study examined the effect of prenatal and child health home visiting program on a total of 1238 mothers and their first-borns until the child reached age two. The findings showed that home visits by nurses can reduce mortality among mothers and their infants and toddlers living in highly disadvantaged settings (Olds et al., 2014).

Overview of Conducting a Home Visit

Prior to scheduling a home visit, the CHN must clearly articulate the purpose of the visit. The nurse collects and reviews all pertinent data about the family, and based on this information, the nurse then proceeds to formulate hypotheses

and tentative plans as part of the preparation for the home visit. This is done before phoning the family to schedule an appointment. Drop-in visits are not encouraged, would be unprofessional, and would not be time or cost effective if the family is not home. However, it may be done depending on the situation, such as if the client is well-known to the nurse, has no phone connection, or agrees to the nurse doing drop-in visits. Obtaining consent and openly negotiating the context for the visit is especially important when working with families who have experienced undue trauma, judgment, and resulting distrust with persons in authority. The Truth and Reconciliation Commission of Canada (2015) recommends that health care professionals reflect on their personal biases and stereotypes about survivors and family members affected by residential schools; this is similarly critical for marginalized and racialized people such as LGBTQ2S and Black Canadians.

Active listening and attending to the family's needs are crucial throughout the home-visiting process. The initial home visit should be scheduled by phone as soon as possible. Over the phone, the nurse begins to establish rapport with the family client by introducing her- or himself and stating the reason and anticipated length of visit. The visit usually is no longer than an hour. This first contact to the family, usually by phone, is of prime importance as the nurse enters a working relationship with the family. The CHN conducts a skillful assessment of the family's needs during the phone interview, hypothesizes what the nursing diagnoses might be, and plans for the visit to meet the client's needs accordingly.

The nurse uses the first few minutes of the home visit to gain rapport and put the family at ease. The nurse clarifies their role and informs the family of the agency policies, including confidentiality. The CHN restates the purpose of the home visit to set a focus or to ensure that the family situation has not changed since the last phone contact or scheduled home visit. The family interview usually is carried out in the living room or kitchen, usually as determined by the client.

When the family assessment begins, priority is given to the important needs as identified by the family. Ideally, the whole family should be present at the home visit. If not possible, and at times not all family members need to be present at the family interview, the nurse would interview the person who needs to be visited as determined by the family. Each family member is given an opportunity to provide input where appropriate. Families have the right to terminate the nursing visit anytime. CHNs must use effective interviewing skills, including active listening, when conducting a home visit.

Nurses plan for mutually set goals with the family according to its members' desires and needs. Developing contracts concerning the plan of care and frequency of visits is a way to clearly identify roles and expectations. If the situation arises, it is important for the CHN to discuss with the family their professional and legal responsibility to report to authorities such as Children's Aid Society or the police (Stanhope & Lancaster, 2014; Wright & Leahey, 2013).

When the visit comes to a close, it is important for the nurse to summarize what was discussed or accomplished at the visit, to review mutually agreed-upon roles and actions, to discuss referrals if needed, and to schedule the next visit or terminate the visits where appropriate. Over the course of the working relationship with the family, the nurse works on assisting the family to develop needed knowledge and skills and acquire resources to sustain the progress made. The CHN acts as a helper and not as a rescuer (Stanhope & Lancaster, 2014; Wright & Leahey, 2013). When the goals are achieved, the nurse plans for termination of the visits. If achieving the goals is beyond the nurse's ability or scope of practice, referrals must be made for continuity of care for the family.

Clinical notes should be documented after each visit to record the assessment data, the plan of care, the implementation of the interventions, and an evaluation of any progress toward the goals. When the care for the family is beyond the CHN's scope of practice or ability to care, the nurse will initiate a referral to ensure that the family will receive the right care by the right personnel in a timely fashion. Professional nursing home visits must be purposeful and goal-oriented.

CHNs must pay particular attention to their personal safety. When home visiting, CHNs are most likely going into unknown environments. This is one of the reasons for nurses to be knowledgeable about the neighbourhoods in the community. Nurses could attend to their personal safety by sharing their visiting schedules with the agency, including the location of the visits. A plan of action should be in place in case of emergencies. Once in the home, nurses can quickly determine an exit route and sit in a barrier-free location near the door. If nurses feel uncomfortable or encounter a dangerous situation, they leave at once and notify their supervisor (Stanhope & Lancaster, 2014). CHNs use their judgment and follow the College of Nurses guidelines when accepting gifts from their family clients.

CASE STUDY

Nursing students are exposed to diverse family situations requiring family assessment and intervention. A nurse and a nursing student went to the home of a multi-generational Indigenous family who were living together on a First Nations reserve. Living on the reserve gave this family access to both a health centre where they could drop in and a nurse who would go to their home. The new mom in the family was breastfeeding and needed support as she was getting tired and frustrated that her infant would not settle for sleep. At the same time the grandfather was having vision problems that gave him difficulty seeing and, as a result, was not accurately administering his insulin.

The nursing student and RN spent time getting to know the family and completing an initial assessment that lasted one hour. During the visit they learned that the grandfather felt it was time for him to die. The new mom (granddaughter) was also the primary caregiver for her grandfather. Based upon their first conversation and how the family shared that they were feeling tired from caring for each other, the student and nurse planned another home visit to explore a deeper understanding with the grandfather and new mom. Their plan during the follow-up visit was to not restrict their time spent with the family so they could learn more about the family's story.

Initially, the nurse focused on the strength of the family to support each other. Afterward, when discussing these strengths, the nursing student observed how the family members smiled and nodded their heads in a way she believed demonstrated appreciation. However, she also believed the family was being polite to their guests. The student was left with questions after her home visit and said she wasn't sure what to say or how to initiate conversation with the Indigenous family in their home.

Also, the student talked about culture and her need to better understand what this meant while supporting the Indigenous family in this case.

Discussion Questions

1. What are the priorities for this family visit?

2. What would a strengths-based approach include with this multigenerational Indigenous family?

3. What does cultural safety mean within the context of working with Indigenous families in their homes and community?

YES, BUT WHY?

Targeted and Universal Family Care

What?

The World Health Organization (WHO, 2013) states that all mothers and their families should have access to appropriate pre- and postpartum care. In Canada, formal antenatal care, including support and information, has been provided collaboratively by PHNs, primary care doctors, nurse practitioners, and midwives. However, changes in the delivery of pre- and postpartum public health services from face-to-face support to online forums has created concerns about accessibility of care. Mothers state that while they appreciate online forums, they would prefer to have face-to-face interactions (Aston et al., 2018).

So What?

The Government of Canada mandated public health to provide more targeted services to "at-risk" populations. Therefore, over the past 5–10 years, different public health units have shifted pre- and postpartum programming to focus more on populations who were assessed to be "targeted" or "high risk" due to various determinants of health, including lower socioeconomic status, increased risk for mental health, and lack of support systems. Much research supports a focus on targeted programming (Hedges, Simmes, Martinez, Linder, & Brown, 2005; Jack, DiCenso, & Lohfeld, 2005; Olds, 2006). Labelling mothers and families can be helpful, but it can also be stigmatizing. Mothers may feel judged and not want to have a PHN visit them in their homes (Aston et al., 2018). This population of mothers, along with PHNs, have expressed concern that they have not been able to access public health services to help them with their confidence, breastfeeding, and postpartum depression (Aston et al., 2014). The tensions between targeted, secondary prevention programming and universal programs considered primary prevention programming are a global health issue that affects the practice of PHNs (Appleton & Cowley, 2003; Elkan, Robinson, Williams, & Blair, 2001).

Now What?

CHNs have historically been and continue to be supportive of all mothers through home visits, drop-in clinics, and phone calls. In Nova Scotia, PHNs told us that although they have a "high-risk" Enhanced Home Visiting Program, they also continue to work with "lower-risk" families to ensure all mothers are supported regardless of their situation. Universal support is an upstream approach that can empower and support mothers and families whether they are high or low risk or universal. It is important for PHNs to understand how different populations are socially and institutionally constructed so that programs and systems can be created in ways that are accessible to all mothers and families. PHNs can then practise as excellent advocates who provide evidence to government to ensure best practices and care are available for mothers and families.

Standards of Practice Fulfilled:

#6 Health Equity
  - Advocates for healthy public policy and social justice by participating in legislative and policy-making activities that influence determinants of health and access to services.

#8 Professional Responsibility and Accountability
  - Uses available resources to systematically evaluate the achievement of desired outcomes for quality improvement in community health nursing practice (CHNC, 2019, revised).

Professional Relationships, Responsibility, and Accountability

Nurse–client interaction begins with **relationship building** (Aston et al., 2015; Porr, 2015). Successful family home visits require the nurse to establish mutuality, respect, and trust with the family. This is especially necessary if the family fears that family members will be judged. When the nurse can establish a collaborative, respectful relationship with the family, they can facilitate an assessment of family strengths; gain an understanding of the family's fears, issues, and concerns; and identify opportunities to collaboratively plan, intervene, and evaluate the desired goals.

Family Interview Each family member's perceptions of an event or a situation need to be validated through active listening and patience. CHNs need to skillfully ask meaningful questions to elicit the family's current level of knowledge on the health issues and its desired approaches toward change prior to providing advice (Eddy & Doutrich, 2014; Eggenberger & Regan, 2010; Rowe Kaakinen, Padgett Coehlo, Steele, Tabacco, & Harmon Hanson, 2014). Examples of family interview questions are listed in Table 18.3. These interview questions serve to promote family healing through reflection. For example, the question "What worries you the most?" can provide family members with an opportunity to identify their fears and concerns.

Table 18.3	Examples of Family Interview Questions

1. How can I be most helpful to you and your family (or friends) during your care? (Clarifies expectations and increases collaboration.)

2. What has been most and least helpful to you and your family in past health care experiences? (Identifies past strengths, problems to avoid, and successes to repeat.)

3. What is the greatest challenge facing your family right now? (Identifies actual or potential suffering, roles, and beliefs.)

4. With which of your family members or friends would you like us to share information? With which ones would you like us not to share information? (Indicates alliances, resources, and possible conflictual relationships.)

5. What do you need to best prepare you or your family for _____? (Identifies appropriate community resources.)

6. Who do you believe is suffering the most in your family right now? (Identifies the family member who has the greatest need for support and intervention.)

7. What is the one question you would like to have answered during our meeting right now? I may not be able to answer this question at the moment, but I will do my best or will try to find the answer for you. (Identifies most pressing issue or concern.)

8. How have I been most helpful to you today? How could we improve? (Shows a willingness to learn from families and to work collaboratively.)

Source: Adapted from Wright, L. M., & Leahey, M. M. (2012). *Nurses and families: A guide to family assessment and intervention* (6th ed.). Philadelphia, PA: F. A. Davis. (p. 271). Used by permission of F. A. Davis & Company.

Wright and Leahey (2013) identified three common errors when working with families: (1) failure to establish the context for change, (2) taking sides, and (3) giving too much advice prematurely. CHNs can avoid making these errors by ensuring that they obtain a clear understanding of the family's most pressing concern while validating each family member's perspective. Each family member needs equal time to acknowledge the suffering in the family and the sufferer. CHNs need to remain engaged, not take sides, and seek mutual understanding of the situation.

CHNs should not offer advice or guidance until a thorough assessment has been completed and after they have established that the advice "fits" with the family's perspective of a possible solution. CHNs should always be aware of their own personal experiences and biases, including cultural, ethnic, and gendered positions. This type of insight can lead to being effective allies and advocates with the family. Finally, the intervention needs to be evaluated from the family's perspective and adapted according to the family's response. The decision to end the family visits should be mutual. The CHN reviews and summarizes the family's strengths and lists the strategies used for health promotion, healing, and building capacity at the termination of the visits.

Family Caregiving With the rise of chronic illness, individuals living with chronic illness at home are mainly cared for by family caregivers. CHNs also play a key role to help family members acquire the necessary resources or capacity for the care they require. (See Chapter 5 for the role of the home health nurse.) While the ill family member is the focus of care, the caregivers often are the forgotten clients. The majority of caregivers tend to be women, often mothers (Paulson & Lichtenberg, 2011; Statistics Canada, 2012). The term **caregiver** refers to an individual "who provides a broad range of financially uncompensated care to . . . family members in need due to physical, cognitive or mental health condition" (Duxbury, Higgins, & Smart, 2011, p. 30). A family caregiver may be an older adult caring for many family members.

Interdisciplinary Practice and Case Management

Gathering a team of health care providers to provide care will yield quality health outcomes (Creemers et al., 2014). CHNs need to ensure that their clients will receive the right care by the right people and at the right time to yield optimal health outcomes. **Case management** is a collaborative approach used by CHNs to coordinate and facilitate the delivery of health care services. A CHN case manager works with individuals, families, and other health care providers to facilitate all necessary services for care provided in community settings during times of illness or for other health care conditions requiring nursing intervention. Often these clients are marginalized, powerless, and rendered vulnerable, and they lack experience in navigating the health care system. CHNs, acting as case managers, identify and assess clients' needs, plan care, provide or delegate care, and follow up with an evaluation of care. The goal of case management is to arrive at quality, cost-effective client outcomes (Smith, 2013b).

For example, in Nova Scotia registered nurses, licensed practical nurses, and non-licensed community home visitors collaborate to support family health in homes and communities (Sheppard-LeMoine, 2015). Case management involves accountability and facilitating the coordinated and timely delivery of appropriate planned services, while monitoring and responding to changes in the client's needs and abilities. It must also ensure provision of care that reflects cultural safety, respect, problem-solving strategies, and spiritual and religious considerations (National Case Management Network, 2012).

FUTURE RESEARCH DIRECTIONS AND CHALLENGES

Progress in family nursing research has been made over the years. The First International Family Nursing Conference was hosted in May 1988 by the University of Calgary's Faculty of Nursing under the leadership of Dr. Lorraine M. Wright (Bell, 2014). On the international scene, the International Family Nursing Association (2018) disseminates a collection of family research studies in areas such as conceptual and methodological issues, underpinnings of family research, nature and purpose of research, intervention research, family dyadic studies, and synthesis research. The Canadian Family Practice Nurses Association (2014) was established by a group of seven dynamic nurses in 2008. Both the conference and association brought nursing researchers, educators, practitioners, and nursing students together to share their vision, experiences, and new knowledge in family nursing practice. Family nursing researchers must advance their research and foster utilization of their findings. They play an advocacy role in health policy and health legislation to improve the care of families. Although there has been progress in family nursing research and the related practice, gaps remain in the application of theory.

CONCLUSION

This chapter is an overview of family nursing care in community settings. It is not all encompassing, but it provides a glimpse into this nursing specialty. The changing demographics of the family and the key conceptual frameworks for family assessment were presented. How CHNs could adhere to the CHNC standards of practice when providing family nursing care was outlined, as well as the importance of case management and the challenges and future directions for family nursing. With this understanding, CHNs will provide family care with more confidence and will continue to advance their skills in promoting family health.

KEY TERMS

ABCX Model   (p. 357)
Calgary Family Assessment Model (CFAM)   (p. 356)
Calgary Family Intervention Model (CFIM)   (p. 356)
caregiver   (p. 361)
case management   (p. 361)
developmental tasks   (p. 352)
ecomap   (p. 357)
families   (p. 350)
family assessment   (p. 354)
family composition   (p. 351)
family characteristics   (p. 354)
family developmental theory   (p. 354)
family forms   (p. 352)
family functions   (p. 352)
family home visit   (p. 357)
family nursing   (p. 351)
family structure   (p. 352)
Friedman Family Assessment Model   (p. 355)
genogram   (p. 357)
healthy families   (p. 352)
McGill Model   (p. 356)
multigenerational households   (p. 351)
relationship building   (p. 360)
stressors   (p. 357)
structural–functional theory   (p. 354)
systems theory   (p. 354)
Ways Tried and True Aboriginal Methodological Framework   (p. 355)

STUDY QUESTIONS

1. Define the concept of family, and identify some common family functions.
2. Describe the demographic shifts that are changing the composition of Canadian families.
3. What are the levels of conceptualizing the family in family nursing theory?
4. Describe the key differences between a genogram and an ecomap.
5. Identify the components of a family home visit.
6. Define case management and its role in family-centred care.

INDIVIDUAL CRITICAL-THINKING EXERCISES

1. Draw your family genogram and ecomap. Describe the roles of family members, the quality of the intra-family relationships, and the strengths of your family.
2. Identify some factors that make a family vulnerable.
3. Describe a crisis experience in your family and the family resilience factors that assisted your family to cope with the crisis.
4. Compare your beliefs about your family with those of a romanticized or a stigmatized family.
5. What impact could your values and beliefs about family have on your nurse–family relationships?

GROUP CRITICAL-THINKING EXERCISES

1. Differentiate between viewing the family as client and the family as context. Drawing on your experiences, provide an example to illustrate each concept (family as client and family as context).
2. Reflect on your biases regarding people outside the cultural group you identify with. How might your biases and stereotypes influence the way you assess a family?
3. Describe an approach to the assessment of a family for each of the CCHN standards: promoting health, building capacity, building relationships, facilitating access and equity, and demonstrating professional responsibility and accountability. Provide concrete examples to illustrate the application of each standard in family nursing.
4. Role play a family–nurse situation. Practise the family interview questions listed in Table 18.3.

REFERENCES

Aston, M., Price, S., Etowa, J., Vukic, A., Young, L., Hart, C., . . . & Randel, P. (2014). Universal and targeted early home visiting: Perspectives of public health nurses and mothers. *Nursing Reports, 4*(3290). doi: 10.4081/ nursrep.2014.3290

Aston, M., Price, S., Etowa, J., Vukic, A., Young, L., Hart, C., . . . & Randel, P. (2015). The power of relationships:

Exploring how public health nurses support mothers and families during postpartum home visits. *Journal of Family Nursing, 21*(1), 11–34.

Aston, M., Price, S., Monaghan, J., Sim, M., Hunter, A., & Little, V. (2018). Navigating and negotiating information and support: Experiences of first-time mothers. *Journal of Clinical Nursing, 27*(3–4), 640–649.

Appleton, J. V., & Cowley, S. (2003). Valuing professional judgement in health visiting practice. *Community Practitioner, 76*(6), 215.

Bell, J. M. (2014). *The history of the International Family Nursing Conferences*. Retrieved from http://janicembell.com/2009/09/history-of-the-international-family-nursing-conferences

Browne, A. J., Doane, G. H., Reimer, J., MacLeod, M. L., & McLellan, E. (2011). Public health nursing practice with "high priority" families: The significance of contextualizing "risk." *Nursing Inquiry, 17*(1), 26–37.

Canadian Family Practice Nurses Association. (2014). *History*. Retrieved from http://www.cfpna.ca/history.cfm

Community Health Nurses Association of Canada (CHNC). (2019, revised). *Canadian community health nursing standards of practice*. St. John's, NL: Author. Retrieved from http://www.chnc.ca/documents/chnc-standards-eng-book.pdf

Canadian Nurses Association (CNA). (2013). *Social determinants of health*. Retrieved from http://www.cna-aiic.ca/PositionStatement

Creemers, H., Veldink, J. H., Grupstra, H., Nollet, F., Beelen, A., & van den Berg, L. H. (2014). Cluster RCT of case management on patients' quality of life and caregiver strain in ALS. *Neurology, 82*(1), 23–31. doi:10.1212/01.wnl.0000438227.48470.62

Drake, M. A. (2014). Theoretical bases for promoting family health. In J. A. Allender, C. Rector, & K. Warner (Eds.), *Community health nursing: Promoting and protecting the public's health* (8th ed., pp. 568–583). Philadelphia, PA: Wolters Kluwer/Lippincott, Williams & Wilkins.

Duxbury, L., Higgins, C., & Smart, R. (2011). Elder care and the impact of caregiver strain on the health of employed caregivers. *Work, 40*(1), 29–40.

Eddy, L. L., & Doutrich, D. (2014). Families and communities/public health nursing. In J. Rowe Kaakinen, V. Gedaly-Duff, D. P. Coehlo, & S. M. Harmon Hanson (Eds.), *Family health care nursing: Theory, practice and research* (5th ed., pp. 470–489). Philadelphia, PA: F. A. Davis.

Eggenberger, S. K., & Regan, M. (2010). Expanding simulation to teach family nursing. *Journal of Nursing Education, 49*(10), 550–558.

Elkan, R., Robinson, J., Williams, D., & Blair, M. (2001). Universal vs. selective services: The case of British health visiting. *Journal of Advanced Nursing, 33*(1), 113–119.

Friedman, M. M., Bowden, V. R., & Jones, E. G. (Eds.). (2003). *Family nursing: Research, theory, and practice* (5th ed.). Upper Saddle River, NJ: Prentice Hall.

Freistadt, J., & Strohschein, L. (2012). Family structure differences in family functions: Interactive effects of social capital and family structure. *Journal of Family Issues, 34*(7), 952–974.

Gottlieb, L. N., & Gottlieb, B. (2007). The developmental/health framework within the McGill Model of Nursing: "Laws of nature" guiding whole person care. *Advances in Nursing Science, 30*(1), E43–E57. PMID: 17299275.

Gottlieb, L., & Rowat, K. (1987). The McGill model of nursing: A practice-derived model. *Advances in Nursing Science, 9*(4), 51–61.

Government of Canada. (2015). *Civil Marriage Act*. Retrieved from http://laws-lois.justice.gc.ca/eng/acts/c-31.5/page-1.html

Government of Saskatchewan. (2018). KidsFirst. Retrieved from https://www.saskatchewan.ca/residents/family-and-social-support/child-care/kidsfirst

Hedges, S., Simmes, D., Martinez, A., Linder, C., & Brown, S. (2005). A home visitation program welcomes home first-time moms and their infants. *Home Healthcare Now, 23*(5), 286–289.

Hill, R. (1958). Generic features of families under stress. *Social Casework, 49*, 139–150.

Hunt, R. (2013). Family care. In R. Hunt (Ed.), *Introduction to community-based nursing* (5th ed., pp. 77–118). Philadelphia, PA: Lippincott.

International Family Nursing Association. (2014). *Research, bibliography/seminal works*. Retrieved from http://internationalfamilynursing.org/resources-for-family-nursing/research/research-bibliography

Jack, S. M., DiCenso, A., & Lohfeld, L. (2005). A theory of maternal engagement with public health nurses and family visitors. *Journal of Advanced Nursing, 49*(2), 182–190.

Leahey, M., & Wright, L. M. (2016). Application of the Calgary Family Assessment and Intervention Models: Reflections on the reciprocity between the personal and the professional. *Journal of Family Nursing, 22*(4), 450–459.

McCubbin, H. I., & McCubbin, M. A. (1993). Families coping with illness: The resiliency model of family stress, adjustment, and adaptation. In C. B. Danielson, B. Hamel-Bissel, & P. Winsted-Fry (Eds.), *Families, health and illness: Perspectives on coping and intervention* (pp. 21–63). St. Louis, MO: Mosby.

National Case Management Network. (2012). *Canadian core competency profile for case management providers*. Retrieved from http://www.ncmn.ca/Resources/Documents/NCMN%20VALIDATION%20DRAFT%20July%202012.pdf

Olds, D. L. (2006). The nurse–family partnership: An evidence-based preventive intervention. *Infant Mental Health Journal, 27*(1), 5–25.

Olds, D. L., Kitzman, H., Knudtson, M. D., Anson, E., Smith, J. A., & Cole, R. (2014). Effect of home visiting by nurses on maternal and child mortality: Results of a 2-decade follow-up of a randomized clinical trial. *JAMA Pediatrics, 68*(9), 800–806. doi:10.1001/jamapediatrics.2014.472

Paulson, D., & Lichtenberg, P. A. (2011). Effect of caregiver family status on care recipient symptom severity and caregiver stress at nursing home intake. *Clinical Gerontologist, 34*, 132–143.

Porr, C. J. (2015). Important interactional strategies for everyday public health nursing practice. *Public Health Nursing, 32*(1), 43–49. doi:10.1111/phn.12097

Public Health Agency of Canada. (2014). *Aboriginal ways tried and true*. Retrieved from http://cbpp-pcpe.phac-aspc.gc.ca/aboriginalwtt

Richardson, A., Yarwood, J., & Richardson, S. (2017). Expressions of cultural safety in public health nursing practice. *Nursing Inquiry, 24*(1). doi: 10.1111/nin.12171

Rowe Kaakinen, J., Padgett Coehlo, D., Steele, R., Tabacco, A., & Harmon Hanson, S. M. (2014). *Family health care nursing: Theory, practice, and research* (5th ed.). Philadelphia, PA: F. A. Davis Company.

Sheppard-LeMoine, D. (2015). *Within vulnerability: Understanding the practices and experiences of enhanced home visiting public health nurses and community home visitors. Unpublished thesis.* Retrieved from http://dalspace.library.dal.ca/bitstream/handle/10222/59083/Sheppard-LeMoine-Debbie-PhD-NURS-July-2015.pdf?sequence=3&isAllowed=y

Smith, C. M. (2013a). Multiproblem families. In F. A. Maurer & C. M. Smith (Eds.), *Community/public health nursing practice* (5th ed., pp. 372–391). St. Louis, MO: Saunders.

Smith, C. M. (2013b). Family case management. In F. A. Maurer & C. M. Smith (Eds.), *Community/public health nursing practice* (5th ed., pp. 340–371). St. Louis, MO: Saunders.

Stanhope, M., & Lancaster, J. (2014). *Foundations of nursing in the community: Community-oriented practice* (4th ed.). St. Louis, MO: Mosby Elsevier.

Statistics Canada. (2012). *Portrait of caregivers, 2012.* Statistics Canada Catalogue no. 89-652-X2011003. Retrieved from http://www.statcan.gc.ca/pub/89-652-x/89-652-x2013001-eng.pdf

Statistics Canada. (2017). Families, households and marital status: Key results from the 2016 census. *The Daily,* Catalogue no. 11-001-X. Retrieved from https://www150.statcan.gc.ca/n1/en/daily-quotidien/170802/dq170802a-eng.pdf?st=AO2ecm83

Statistics Canada. (2018). *National Indigenous peoples day . . . by the numbers.* Retrieved from https://www.statcan.gc.ca/eng/dai/smr08/2018/smr08_225_2018

Truth and Reconciliation Commission of Canada. (2015). *Calls to action.* Retrieved from http://www.trc.ca/websites/trcinstitution/File/2015/Findings/Calls_to_Action_English2.pdf

Vanier Institute of the Family. (2010). *Families count: Profiling Canada's families IV.* Ottawa, ON: Author.

Vanier Institute of the Family. (2018). *Definition of family.* Retrieved from http://vanierinstitute.ca/definition-family

Ward, C., Branch, C., & Fridkin, A., (2016). Indigenous people. *Visions Journal, 11*(4), 29.

World Health Organization. (2013). *WHO recommendations on postnatal care of the mother and newborn.* Geneva, CH: World Health Organization. Retrieved from http://www.who.int/maternal_child_adolescent/documents/postnatal-care-recommendations/en

Wright, L. M., & Leahey, M. M. (2013). *Nurses and families: A guide to family assessment and intervention* (6th ed.). Philadelphia, PA: F. A. Davis.

ABOUT THE AUTHORS

Lisa Underhill (MN, PHC, NP) is an advanced practice nurse with a diverse career path in federal public health policy and programming at the Public Health Agency of Canada and most recently providing primary health care services for refugees in her capacity as a nurse practitioner in Ottawa. She is passionate about holistic, client-centred care and lifelong learning. Ms. Underhill brings a unique skill set, incorporating a macro big-picture critical analysis grounded in day-to-day primary health care clinical work.

Debbie Sheppard LeMoine, RN, PhD, is the assistant director and assistant professor at StFX Rankin School of Nursing. Her research has focused on working with vulnerable families in collaboration with public health nurses and family resource centres for over 20 years in Nova Scotia. She is completing an international funded study on innovative teaching strategies to support interprofessional family assessment in diverse settings. A passionate teacher with extensive curriculum development and implementation experience in Canada and internationally, Debbie teaches community and family nursing, research, leadership, and master of nursing students.

Megan Aston, RN, PhD, is Full Professor at Dalhousie University School of Nursing. She teaches qualitative health research and family and community health nursing. Her program of research focuses on family, maternal, child, and newborn health. She uses feminist poststructuralism informed by discourse analysis to examine how nurses and clients negotiate beliefs, values, and practices that have been socially and institutionally constructed through relations of power. She has secured provincial and national funding to support research studies focused on maternal and newborn health in Nova Scotia and Tanzania; mapping mothers' social networks; postpartum home visits; hospital experiences of children with intellectual disabilities, their parents, and nurses; queer women's birthing experiences; and nurses' bereavement support experiences at the Victorian Order of Nurses and a children's hospital.

Gender and Community Health

Cheryl van Daalen-Smith and Aliyah Dosani

CHAPTER 19

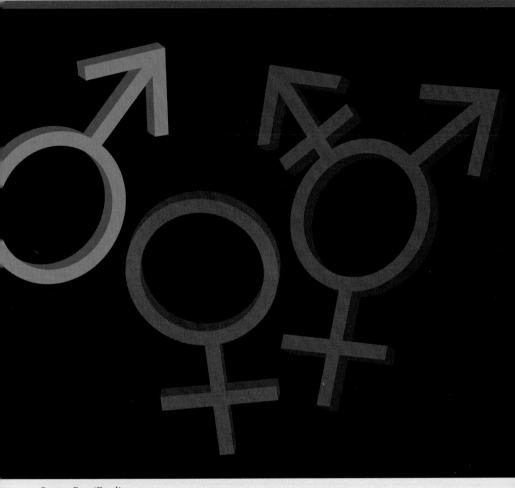

Source: Paw/Fotolia

INTRODUCTION

"Gender equality is more than a goal in itself. It is a precondition of meeting the challenge of reducing poverty, promoting sustainable development, and building good governance" (Kofi Annan, as cited in UNICEF, 2006). Yet gender is a concept that is often taken for granted, with a one-size-fits-all approach that often fails to truly explore how gender-based expectations limit boys and girls, men and women. Sometimes we design health programs and interventions without asking whether they are specifically well suited to the needs of men, women, or transgender individuals. Think about the ways your own gender influences your life. Consider how it influences the way you dress, what you talk about, with whom you are friends, when and where you may feel unsafe, and to whom you go for help. While we often think about gender as something that is not within our control, gender is a concept that we as individuals cultivate, develop, and understand based on what society reinforces through social relations and institutional norms. This can mean that in our society men and women are thought of, live their lives, and are treated as different kinds of people with different bodies and different roles, responsibilities, and opportunities (Jackson, Pederson, & Boscoe, 2009). When we really begin to think about gender, we realize that it influences, overtly and subtly, many aspects of our lives. Indeed, it has been recognized as a key social determinant of health (World Health Organization [WHO], 2008).

When we consider **health inequities**—the unfair and preventable differences in health status seen within and between people or communities—an exploration of the social determinants of health is most helpful. The World Health Organization (WHO) established the Commission on Social Determinants of Health (CSDH) in 2005 to provide advice on how to reduce them (WHO, 2008). One of the chapters in the report focuses on gender equity and health. The authors of this report argue that gender inequities damage the health of women and girls throughout the world, particularly in low- and middle-income countries. As a result, girls and women have less power, privilege, and access to resources than do men. In some countries girls are valued less, receive less education, are fed less, and are restricted in what they can do. In many areas of the world, transgender individuals may be forced to live on the edges of mainstream society, leaving them isolated, facing discrimination and bullying (WHO, 2010). The topic of gender and health is now widely recognized and continues to be discussed at the global level. This difference in how gender is taken up by societies inevitably influences their health outcomes. Is the same true in Canada, where it is often assumed that women and men have equal opportunities, or that people who do not "fit" as either male or female have equal access to health care and employment opportunities?

In this chapter we will explore the many ways that gender is prescribed and how this influences health outcomes and quality of life for men, women, and transgender individuals. Community health nurses (CHNs) in Canada incorporate intersectional analyses, exploring how social and health inequities exist not only based on gender but also on additional layers of social privilege and oppression. We will discover the various roles that CHNs can play to challenge assumptions about gender that create health inequity.

HOW WE UNDERSTAND HEALTH OUTCOMES OF CANADIAN MEN AND WOMEN

As demonstrated in Table 19.1, disparity in life expectancy between males and females varies by country, although Canada's life expectancy ranks among the top in the world. However, the data we have available to us suggest that Indigenous populations in Canada have a lower life expectancy at birth than non-Indigenous populations. (See Table 19.2.) Women in Canada tend to live longer than men and have done so for nearly a century (Nagunar, 2011). In Canada, women are expected to live an average of 4.7 years longer than men (Greenberg & Normandin,

Table 19.1	Life Expectancy at Birth (Years) for Males and Females, Selected Countries, 2015	
Country	**Men**	**Women**
Afghanistan	59.3	61.9
Australia	80.9	84.8
Austria	79.0	83.9
Canada	80.2	84.1
China	74.6	77.6
Costa Rica	77.1	82.2
Cuba	76.9	81.4
Democratic People's Republic of Korea	67.0	74.0
Democratic Republic of the Congo	58.3	61.5
Egypt	68.8	73.2
Ethiopia	62.8	66.8
France	79.4	85.4
Ghana	61.0	63.9
Haiti	61.5	65.5
India	66.9	69.9
Iraq	66.2	71.8
Ireland	79.4	83.4
Japan	80.5	86.8
Kenya	61.1	65.8
Mexico	73.9	79.5
New Zealand	80.0	83.3
Nigeria	53.4	55.6
Pakistan	65.5	67.5
Panama	74.7	81.1
Philippines	65.3	72.0
Saudi Arabia	73.2	76.0
Sierra Leone	49.3	50.8
Singapore	80.0	86.1
South Sudan	56.1	58.6
Switzerland	81.3	85.3
Syrian Arab Republic	59.9	69.9
Trinidad and Tobago	67.9	74.8
Turkey	72.6	78.9
Uganda	60.3	64.3
Ukraine	66.3	76.1
United Arab Emirates	76.4	78.6
United Kingdom	79.4	83.0
United States of America	76.9	81.6
Vietnam	71.3	80.7
Zimbabwe	59.0	62.3

Source: Based on WHO (2017). Annex B Tables of health statistics by country, WHO Region, and globally. *World Health Statistics 2017: Monitoring health for the SDGs.*

Table 19.2	Life Expectancy (Years) at Birth of Indigenous Populations in Canada (Projections for 2017)	
	Men	**Women**
First Nations	73	78
Métis	74	80
Inuit	64	73
Canada (total)	79	83

Source: Statistics Canada (2015). *Aboriginal Statistics at a glance*, 2nd edition. Ottawa, Ontario: Statistics Canada.

2011). The discrepancy in life expectancy between males and females varies across Canada from 3.2 years to 7.5 years (Greenberg & Normandin, 2011). The gap is generally smaller among regions with higher life expectancy and greater among regions with lower life expectancy (Greenberg & Normandin, 2011). These regional differences also reveal important variances with respect to the social determinants of health. Parts of Canada facing the lowest life expectancy also hold some of the highest rates of smoking, obesity, and heavy drinking (Greenberg & Normandin, 2011). In rural or remote regions, we see high long-term unemployment rates, lower levels of education, small immigrant populations, and relatively large Indigenous populations (Greenberg & Normandin, 2011). Conversely, higher neighbourhood income is associated with longer life expectancy. Important to note is a concern for men's lower life expectancy and the general lack of specific focus on men's health as it relates to the social determinants of health (Goldenberg, 2014).

This degree of difference in life expectancy between men and women is clearly complex. Many health care professionals believe that gender-based health differences are due to hormonal differences, simplistically suggesting men and women are different because women give birth and men do not. This is an example of **essentialist thinking**—that women and men have a "true essence" that is entirely related to sex organs, hormones, and their role in reproduction. Essentialist thinking has further been used to reinforce a viewpoint known as "**biology as destiny**," erroneously suggesting that women are naturally caring, relational, and emotional, whereas men are (and should be) naturally assertive, logical, risk-takers, and relationally distant (Hankivsky, 2012). Biology-as-destiny thinking has further given way to lifespan approaches to understanding women's health, in particular categorizing women's health as pubescent, child-bearing, and menopausal, again tying (in this case) a woman to her reproductive capacity and nothing else.

Although we can see how narrow and flawed such approaches to understanding gender as a determinant of health are, it is important to recognize that men and women are not monolithic categories but groups of individuals with multiple and intersecting identities connected to all social determinants of health. Even as Canadians enjoy a publicly funded health system and generally good health, access to and utilization of health care services are not equal. Men have been shown to delay accessing health care, and this can be linked to gender-based expectations to be invulnerable (Goldenberg, 2014). Canada ranks well internationally in terms of life expectancy and quality of life for its citizens, but not every Canadian's health reflects this. It is important to note that differing social locations impact Canadians' health in important ways. Health is not "one size fits all." Not all women experience the same opportunities or limitations, and the same is true for men. Systemic racism, ageism, classism, and heterosexism all impact the opportunities experienced by persons of colour, older adults, individuals experiencing poverty, Indigenous populations, individuals with different abilities, or transgender individuals. Assessing differences and disparities in health status, quality of life, and the experience of health care services based on sex and gender is one step toward ensuring that all Canadians benefit equally from Canada's public health system and enjoy a positive quality of life.

GENDER AS A DETERMINANT OF HEALTH: GETTING CLEAR ON CONCEPTS

Gender is a social determinant of health—that we know, but what does it really mean? To start with, sex is not the same as gender. The differences between the concepts of sex and gender are often misunderstood. Although these terms are related, they are *not* synonymous. CHNs must be mindful of the implications of both "sex" and "gender" as programs and interventions are collaboratively planned, delivered, and evaluated. Further, CHNs must be equally mindful of their own beliefs and assumptions regarding sex, gender, and what constitutes "normal" gender expression. **Sex** is commonly understood to mean chromosomal makeup and is determined by X or Y chromosomes. Sex refers to the biological and physiological characteristics that define men and women (WHO, 2013a, para. 2). Sex differences result from the classification of organisms based on genetic constitution at the cellular level as well as the anatomy and physiology of reproductive organs (Jenkins, Kemnitz, & Tortora, 2010). Obvious examples of sex-specific diseases are cervical cancer and prostate cancer. However, increasing evidence indicates that cells beyond those involved in reproduction have sex differences, and these sex differences can create distinctive patterns of morbidity and mortality in men and women. For instance, Ghandi et al. (2002) found that women have lower levels of human immunodeficiency virus (HIV) RNA than do men at similar stages of HIV infection. This finding is significant because viral loads are often used to guide the initiation and adjustment of antiretroviral therapy. Furthermore, Soldin, Chung, and Mattison (2011) found that males and females differ in drug pharmacokinetics and pharmacodynamics. Therefore, it is imperative that we understand sex differences to ensure interventions are relevant, community-informed, and effective.

Gender "refers to the socially constructed roles, behaviours, activities, and attributes that a given society considers appropriate for men and women" (WHO, 2013a, para. 3). Gender is the expression of one's sex in terms of masculinity and femininity and is rooted in culture and history. Men and women and boys and girls are often treated differently by society, have different life experiences based on what is expected of or denied from them, and therefore have different health outcomes. For example, while women in Canada drive vehicles, up until recently, women in Saudi Arabia were expressly prohibited. More men in Vietnam smoke, as it is customary for men to smoke but not women (WHO, 2013b). Further to the way in which men and women are permitted to live their lives, when differences in life stressors, including violence, oppression, and sizeism, are accounted for, we can clearly see that the health outcomes of males and females are different based on gender. Additionally, transgender individuals face enormous societal judgement and misunderstanding, and correspondingly experience higher-than-average unemployment, depression, addiction, and death by suicide (Bauer & Scheim, 2015). When we consider traditional Indigenous notions of gender, the binary of masculine and feminine may become blurred, and ways of expressing sexual identity are more fluid.

While **Cisgender** refers to a person whose gender identity matches their biological sex, **transgender** refers to "a person whose gender identity is different from his or her biological sex, regardless of the status of surgical and hormonal gender reassignment processes" (Rainbow Health Ontario, n.d., para 3). It is important to note that the term "transgender" does not relate directly to sexuality and that transgender individuals self-identify as straight, gay, lesbian, bisexual, or with any other label they choose to use to define themselves.

Gender identity describes how we see ourselves as women, men, neither, or both, and this affects our feelings and behaviours. "Gender identity is linked to an individual's intrinsic sense of self and, particularly, the sense of being male, female, or somewhere in between and may not conform to a person's birth assigned sex" (Edmonds, 2012, p. 2). Women and men develop their gender identity in the face of strong societal messages about the "correct" gendered role for their presenting sex. Gender identities are actively constructed over time and within cultures (Greco, 2013).

Often closely tied to gender identity are the concepts of masculinity and femininity, both of which are **social constructs**. A social construct is a thought or idea that has been created and reinforced by societies over time and as such are not necessarily rooted in truth or fact. For example, traditionally, men have been viewed as reluctant to seek professional help for depression because the illness and their actions in seeking help suggest weakness, and as such seeking help is supposedly non-masculine. Masculinity theories suggest that men's performance, perceptions, and practices around health and illness may be informed and influenced by **gender norms** (Tyler, 2012). As a result, prescribed masculine "ideals," including self-reliance, stoicism, and emotional control, can be lost and negatively impact many men's self-perceptions about their masculinity (Oliffe & Phillips, 2008). Likewise, traditional femininity can be thought of as the gender norms that are expected and reinforced for girls and women. These include being quiet, nice, selfless, passive, emotional, thin, heterosexual, and defining one's self through relationships above all else (Jack & Ali, 2010). In the context of health, women have been socialized to seek treatment for themselves as well as be the primary health provider to the men and children in their lives (Lee & Owens, 2002). Gender role pressures leave women vulnerable to dissatisfied lives, depression, and denied authenticity (Jack & Ali,

2010). Expectations to be quiet have far-reaching quality-of-life consequences for women, including chronic fatigue syndrome, irritable bowel syndrome, disconnection from one's true self, and living life as a chameleon (van Daalen-Smith, 2009).

Despite many societies and organizations entrenching **binary** notions of sex and gender—in other words, suggesting there is either male or female and "therefore naturally" only masculine or feminine—a binary or either/or construction of sex and gender is being challenged in some societies. For example, the Harvard University application process enables students to choose male, female, or enter in the words that best describe their gender (or nothing at all). The University of Victoria, York University in Toronto, and Mount Royal University in Calgary have renovated several washroom facilities throughout the campus to be gender neutral, enabling individuals who do not identify themselves as men or women to use bathrooms they feel safe to access. CHNs must be aware of the debate and dialogue that is happening around changing notions of the concept of gender to best serve the diverse members of the communities in which they work.

Gender roles are defined as the social *and* cultural expectations that different societies assign to and powerfully expect of boys and girls, and men and women (WHO, 2013b). Although gender roles of men and women have changed slightly, there exist formidable consequences for breaking out of the expected ways of being. Being transgender may not be accepted in some societies, and this form of attitudinal hatred and marginalization results in adverse health and quality of life outcomes. Furthermore, gender is relational and refers not simply to women or men but also to the relationship that exists between them (WHO, 2013a). In all societies, gender role expectations impact the ways individuals see themselves or others and provide or limit opportunities to access resources and societal benefits, thus greatly impacting health.

Gender roles are expressed and enacted in a range of ways, from how we dress or talk, to what we may aspire to do as a career, to what we are made to believe are valuable contributions to make as a woman or a man. These roles are not necessarily rooted in freedom of choice; many social forces exert pressure on us from a very early age, reinforcing, expecting, or denying women and men from certain tasks, jobs, opportunities, ways of being, and spaces. Gender roles often categorize and control individuals within institutions such as the family, community, labour force, and educational systems. For example, a woman may not receive required health care because norms in her community expect that she be accompanied when travelling (WHO, 2013c). In addition, in many cultures men are expected to be the "breadwinner" in the heterosexual family, whereas women are expected to fulfill more nurturing and caretaking roles that include domestic chores, childcare, and the emotional work of relationships. Societies continue to discuss women in "non-traditional jobs," thereby giving recognition to the fact that there is a pattern in which certain forms of paid employment are viewed as men's jobs and others as women's. These differences in gender roles are associated with social status: in almost every society, higher power and prestige is conferred on individuals occupying masculine gender roles (WHO, 2013b).

Gender relations refer to how we interact with or are treated by people in the world around us based on our ascribed gender. They affect us at all levels of society and can restrict or make available various opportunities. Gender relations interact with our race, ethnicity, class, and other identities. In most societies, gender relations reflect differential power between women and men and often disadvantage women (WHO, 2013a). Gender not only affects our personal relationships with others but also guides our interactions within larger social units, including family and the workplace. (See Canadian Research 19.1.)

CANADIAN RESEARCH 19.1

"He's more typically female because he's not afraid to cry": Connecting heterosexual gender relations and men's depression (Oliffe, Kelly, Bottorff, Johnson, & Wong, 2017)

Depression is often underreported in men because it is frequently conceptualized as a women's health issue. We know very little about how heterosexual couples respond when the male partner is depressed. Within the context of men's depression, couples may be challenged to make life adjustments that impact their gender relations. The findings detailed in this article are drawn from qualitative study of 26 Canadian heterosexual couples. Each participant completed individual, semi-structured interviews that focused on exploring how masculinities and femininities intersect to shape and create particular heterosexual gender relations in the context of men's depression. Data analysis revealed three couple patterns: trading places, business as usual, and edgy tensions. Trading places refers to couples who traded typical masculine and feminine roles to compensate for the men's depression-induced losses (e.g., men as homemakers and women as breadwinners). Women partners in this group adopted masculine ideals in how they provided partner support by employing tough-love strategies for self-protection and a means of prompting the men's self-management of their depression. Couples involved in business as usual co-constructed men's alignment with masculine workman ideals and women's support of their partner to counter and conceal men's depression-induced so-called deficits. Couples in the edgy tensions group identified that mismatch of gender expectations fueled resentment and dysfunction that threatened the viability of some relationships. Opportunities for couples to assess their relationship dynamics within a broad range of gender relations might support couples' connectedness and life quality amid the challenges that accompany men's depression.

Discussion Questions

1. In your view, what beliefs do people living in Canadian society have about how men and women ought to behave in relationships?

2. How can CHNs better understand men's depression and advocate for societal acceptance of sadness in men?

3. What is the responsibility of a CHN in promoting gender relations for all people regardless of how they negotiate gender relations in various family and social contexts?

INDIGENOUS NOTIONS OF GENDER

According to Bear (2018), Indigenous cultures across North America have different definitions and expressions of gender than are found in Western cultures. Indigenous cultures have long recognized that gender is a much more fluid notion than just being a man or a woman. The term "Two Spirit," which was recognized at the Third Annual Spiritual Gathering of Gay and Lesbian Native People in 2001, refers to Indigenous people who were born with masculine and feminine spirits in one body (Sheppard & Mayo, 2013). Multiple genders and a wide variance of gender roles existed in many tribal societies and communities. For example, **gender variance** is a concept used to refer to the cultural construction of multiple genders that exists in many communities. Cross-gendered people experience reverence rather than stigma, often holding special roles within their communities. Sometimes individuals took up opposite gender roles and responsibilities creating a third or fourth gender category, neither male or female, and were seen to hold an important role of bridging the genders. Bear (2018) explains that Indigenous children were and sometimes are still raised in flexible ways that allow them to discover their gender identity, thus giving them the freedom to express their own authentic personalities free from expectations or binary notions of male and female. Prior to colonization, gender relations in many Indigenous communities were far more equal and rooted in mutuality and, in some cultures, matriarchal. Traditional Indigenous societies valued gender variance where individuals were free to express varying degrees of masculine and feminine spirit and shame-free sexuality. This way of life only came under attack through Christian-based colonialism (Anderson, 2016).

SOCIETAL CAUSES OF GENDER-BASED INEQUITIES

Institutionalized gender reflects the distribution of power between genders in the political, educational, religious, media, medical, and social institutions in any society. These powerful institutions shape the social norms that define, reproduce, and often justify different expectations and opportunities for women and men and girls and boys. Indeed, it is institutionalized gender that most restricts the way men, women, and transgender individuals are viewed, judged, and related to. This may translate into job segregation, job limitations, dress codes, vulnerability to violence, housing security, experiences in health care settings, and different access to resources such as money, food, or political power. Institutions in society often impose social controls through the ways in which they organize, regulate, and uphold differential values for men and women. Although pay equity is viewed as a fundamental human right and is outlined clearly in section 11 of the Canadian Human Rights Act (Government of Canada, 2013a), it is important to acknowledge how employers often enforce institutionalized gender and power differentials by providing higher rates of pay to men

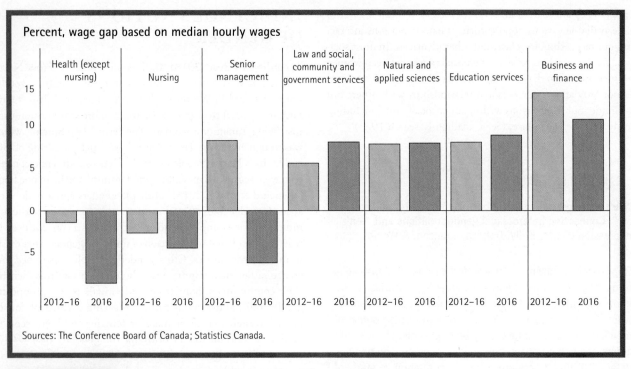

FIGURE 19.1 Gender Wage Gap Varies by Occupation

Source: Conference Board of Canada (2018). Used by permission of the Conference Board of Canada.

for performing similar jobs as women. Statistics Canada (2017) estimates that most Canadians believe men and women are earning an equal salary for equal work, but there is still a significant gap in income between men and women, with women earning $0.87 for every dollar earned by men. Women face deficits in pay ranging from 10.7% to as high as 28.5% (Conference Board of Canada, 2018a). This varies by occupation. (See Figure 19.1.)

The pay equity gap is even wider for women who are older, Indigenous, belong to racialized groups, and live with different abilities. For instance, in Canada, university-educated people of color who were born in Canada earn $0.87 for every dollar earned by their White peers (Conference Board of Canada, 2018b). When gender is factored in, there is up to a 20% female racial gap in Canada (Conference Board of Canada, 2018b). Taking immigration status into consideration, despite having higher levels of education, Canadian immigrants have higher unemployment rates and lower wages than Canadian-born workers, with hourly wages one-fifth lower than those of their Canadian-born peers (Conference Board of Canada, 2018c). Gender-based bias impacts the perceived employability of transgender individuals most profoundly. According to a study of 433 transgender adults in Ontario, a mere 37% were employed full time, and one out of every five were unemployed (Bauer & Scheim, 2015)—despite impressive credentials, work history, and job search effort. Eighteen percent said they had been turned down for a job because of their gender, and 13% said they had been fired or constructively dismissed for being transgender (Bauer & Scheim, 2015).

As demonstrated in this discussion, prescribed gender roles infiltrate institutions and relationships alike and often adversely impact health and quality of life. In fact, how gender is valued, understood, and translated into behaviours in any given time, place, and space can be one of the most significant barriers to improving the overall health and well-being of men, women, and transgender individuals. Gender norms and values are not static; they evolve over time, differ considerably from place to place, and are subject to change. Thus, the poor health consequences resulting from gender differences, biases, and inequities are not fixed. With ardent community-driven advocacy efforts by socially minded CHNs, these, too, can be modified and transformed (WHO, 2013d).

The valuation of men and masculine ideals over women and feminine ideals is one way that "gender is a part of all human interactions" and "is a 'stable' form of structured inequality" (Ettorre, 2004, p. 329). These experiences and cultural values may constrain our everyday life decisions and thereby affect income, employment, housing, safety, inclusion, and overall quality of life. **Gender inequity** occurs when individuals are not provided the same opportunities in society *because* of their gender or gender-identity. Increasingly, governments and other agencies are using **gender-based analyses** to ensure that the programs and policies they develop are equitable. The Government of Canada (2013b) suggests the following factors be considered when examining policies and programs through a gender-based analysis process:

■ Access: The ability for *all* people to have equal access to policy, program, and legislative activities.
■ Inclusion: Representation of diverse groups of men and women throughout the policy or program process.

■ Benefits: The intended advantages of any program or policy are equally available to both men and women of diverse cultures, socioeconomic status, and various levels of identity.

■ Equity: Ensuring that Government of Canada programs and health promotion strategies identify the unique elements, opportunities, and challenges that men, women, and transgender individuals face.

Gender, Sex, and Health Outcomes

Sex and gender are powerful determinants that influence the health of individuals, families, communities, systems, and populations. Biologically and sociologically, male, female and trans-identified individuals differ in terms of the diseases they develop, the symptoms or stressors they experience, and the ways in which they are offered or respond to medicines and other treatments. Although women generally live longer than men, women commonly experience poorer health (WHO, 2013b). Women have higher levels of depression and distress, are more commonly diagnosed with psychiatric 'dis'orders, and experience a variety of chronic illnesses than men. Furthermore, not all women experience life in Canada similarly – other intersecting factors impact the health and quality of life of women. For instance, newcomer women find themselves working part-time with poorer pay and a lack of benefits. They are relied upon to hold their families together yet face social isolation and at times a lack of familiarity with how to navigate societal structures to advocate for the health of their families. Although men have more life-threatening health conditions (WHO, 2013c), again a gender-based analysis of this finding may yield that it still is not safe for boys or men to come forward and seek health care until it is too late. The fact that men die early and often in risky or violent situations deserves national attention.

The effects of sex and gender sometimes combine and lead to particular health outcomes. For example, research has found that women are more likely to experience depression. Many would prefer to suggest the cause is hormonal, as discussed earlier with regard to essentialism, but there are many other reasons for this finding. One explanation for the statistical difference in depression is that men are not socialized to be seen as vulnerable, nor to ask for help. Many argue that the statistics do not adequately capture the suffering of boys and men and that different approaches to men's mental health are necessary. In addition, factors such as poverty, reduced access to education, social isolation, and lack of power can increase the risk for depression and are often unequally distributed among men and women. Additionally, women's expected, yet often devalued, roles within work and family settings can result in work overload and adversely affect women's mental health (Senie, 2014).

Although men and women develop and experience diseases differently, they share the 10 leading causes of death (Table 19.3). A limitation in many of the studies examining gender differences in health is the use of only a dichotomous classification of diseases (i.e., fatal and non-fatal). A clearer depiction of gender differences in health may require a more complex paradigm to gain a stronger understanding of the interplay between sex and gender and their respective contributions to morbidity and mortality. This may be further compounded by the fact that little is known about the health outcomes of people who self-identify as transgender, two sex, or intersex (Health Canada, 2001). Although gender-variant individuals may not experience different disease processes, the institutional nature of recognizing only male or female requires consideration "to avoid the potential for isolation and inequities in service" (Health Canada, 2007, para. 42).

How we account for these gendered differences must not revert back to essentialist thinking. For example, we understand that men are hesitant to seek out help, health care, or support; this reluctance stems from powerful gender-based expectations to be invulnerable. Girls and women experience significant body dissatisfaction because girls and women are persistently judged against impossible standards. Suicide factors more for boys and men than it does for girls and women, not due to "natural tendencies" but rather because of societal messages to handle things on your own and never show any form of weakness. Table 19.3 begins to illuminate how gender impacts men, women, boys, and girls differently, but when we consider additionally powerful factors, such as geography, race, class, ability, and Indigenous status, we see that it is not a one-size-fits-all analysis. For example, lesbian girls and girls living with different abilities are at far

Table 19.3	Leading Health Issues for Boys, Girls, Men, and Women		
Men	**Women**	**Boys**	**Girls**
Cardiovascular disease	Violence, abuse	Stress, depression, anxiety	Depression, self-loathing
Respiratory disorders	Anxiety, depression, stress	Loneliness, isolation	Violence, harassment, abuse
Stress, depression	Body dissatisfaction	ADHD/Ritalin-dependence	Stress, smoking
Suicide	Getting older/poverty	Risk-taking, accidental injuries	Body dissatisfaction
Accidental injuries	Musculoskeletal disease		Education impacted by harassment and bullying
Addiction/substance misuse	Autoimmune diseases	Substance misuse	
	Cardiovascular disease	Violence	

Sources: Goldenberg, S. L. (2014). Status of men's health in Canada. *Canadian Urological Association Journal*, 8(7) 142–144; Bustreo, F. (n.d.). *Top ten issues for women's health*. World Health Organization. Retrieved from: http://www.who.int/life-course/news/commentaries/2015-intl-womens-day/en/; Turcotte, M. (2011). *Women and health*; Bowering, D. (2011). *Where are the men? Chief Medical Officer's report on the health and wellbeing of boys and men in Northern BC*; Northern Health. (2011). *Men's health matters because men matter*; Girls Action Foundation. (2013). *Beyond appearances: Brief on the main issues facing girls in Canada*.

greater risk of bullying than heterosexual or able-bodied girls. In addition, suicide rates for Indigenous girls and boys far surpass those of their non-Indigenous counterparts. Newcomer men have higher rates of emotional distress than do Canadian born men. This is why a gender-based analysis (GBA) is not enough. The "plus" in GBA+ is to signal the necessity to take an intersectional approach when considering health risks and outcomes.

Leading Health Issues for Transgender Individuals

Presently, Statistics Canada does not collect health statistics specifically pertaining to transgender individuals. The census to date collects data reflective of the binary male/female, leading to a lack of national information regarding transgender individuals. Statistics Canada is undergoing national consultations to ameliorate this oversight. In Ontario, an organization called Trans PULSE collects data and uses the social determinants of health as its guide. According to Bauer and Scheim (2015), the Trans PULSE Project explored the social determinants of health among trans people in Ontario. The study revealed that transgender individuals experience substantive barriers to the social determinants of health, including discrimination in employment opportunities, discrimination in health care, overt and covert violence, and loss of family, friends, and social support networks. Widespread experiences of violence and discrimination result in "exclusion from social spaces, unemployment, avoidance of health care and poor mental health" (p. 5). If this is not your own lived experience, imagine for a moment then, how life would be if you felt you had to avoid public spaces out of fear for your own safety. Worse, and very important for the CHN to understand, is that past experiences of discrimination in health care settings lead many transgender individuals to avoid seeking out or participating in any health care programming. The experience of being

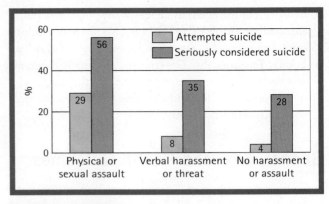

FIGURE 19.2 Proportions of Trans Ontarians Reporting Past-Year Suicidality from Experiences of Transphobic Assault or Harassment

Source: Bauer, G. & Scheim, A. (2015). *Transgender People in Ontario, Canada: Statistics from the Trans PULSE Project to Inform Human Rights Policy.* Technical Report, Reprinted with permission.

viewed as unemployable creates economic marginalization and a life of food and housing insecurity. Transgender individuals experience high levels of depression and suicidality, stemming entirely from the culmination of multiple experiences of violent societal exclusion and hatred. (See Figure 19.2.)

All social determinants of health are impinged upon for transgender individuals, but perhaps it is the determinant of social inclusion that is impacted most. When asked, all respondents in the Trans PULSE Project experienced structural, societal, and familial exclusion, especially young persons aged 16–24 (Bauer & Scheim, 2015). Consider Figure 19.3, which explains how housing, life satisfaction, self-esteem, depression, and suicidality drop as parental support increases.

The UK government recently appointed a Minster of Loneliness, whose key role is to reach out and support the over 9 million individuals experiencing loneliness secondary to,

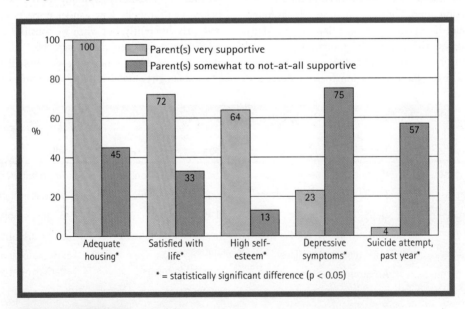

FIGURE 19.3 Proportion of Trans Youth Aged 16–24 in Ontario Experiencing Selected Conditions

Source: Bauer, G. & Scheim, A. (2015). *Transgender People in Ontario, Canada: Statistics from the Trans PULSE Project to Inform Human Rights Policy.* Technical Report, Reprinted with permission.

among other things, social exclusion. Prime Minister Theresa May has called this the reality of modern times. Inclusion is a determinant of health and is key to the role of the Canadian CHN. Above all else, for transgender individuals, belonging, mattering, and being loved are fundamental. CHNs can lead the way in ensuring that all individuals enjoy a life free from judgment and discrimination, and can champion the human rights of transgender individuals.

A GENDER-BASED LENS AND COMMUNITY HEALTH NURSING PRACTICE

The use of a **gender-based lens** is an essential way to ensure that policies, programs, services, and interventions are appropriate for men and women, boys and girls, and transgender individuals. Using a gender-based lens sheds light on the particular constraints and opportunities that men, women, and transgender individuals face. The application of a gender-based lens can be likened to putting on eyeglasses, which enable you to see how differently male, female, and transgender individuals all experience life differently. A gender-based plus (GBA+) lens further enables the CHN to consider race, class, ability, sexual orientation, and Indigenous status when considering the strengths

and barriers faced by the communities they serve. According to Status of Women Canada (2017), health care professionals do not always acknowledge the impact of gender. The organization invites us to ask ourselves these important questions:

1. Do I believe that the issues I work on are gender neutral? Or culturally neutral? Ability neutral? Is this based solely on my own experience?

2. Is it possible that my assumptions prevent me from asking questions and hearing or understanding answers that are outside my own experience?

3. How might attitudes and norms—my own, those of my organization, and those of the institutions and society that surround me—limit the range of policy options I consider and propose?

Acknowledging the necessity to be gender responsive, the WHO (2011) developed a Gender Responsive Assessment Scale that is highly relevant to the work of Canadian CHNs who wish to be appropriate, responsive, and **gender transformative** in their practice. In reflecting on the degree to which programs are gender-blind, aware, exploitative, accommodating, or transformative, CHNs can ask wide-reaching questions, consult with diverse groups, and ensure that the programs and services are gender-appropriate and reflect an intersectional approach. (See Figure 19.4.)

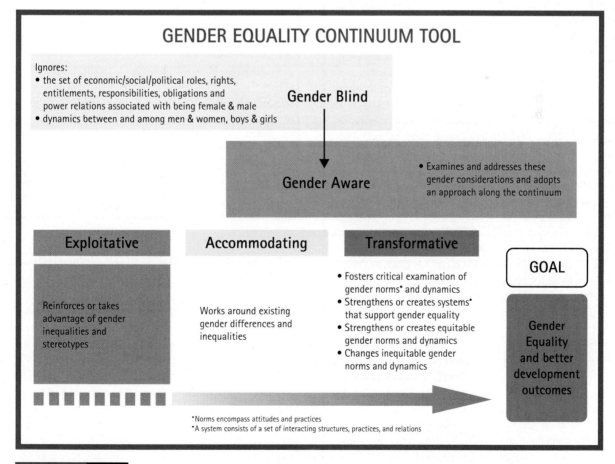

GENDER EQUALITY CONTINUUM TOOL

Ignores:
- the set of economic/social/political roles, rights, entitlements, responsibilities, obligations and power relations associated with being female & male
- dynamics between and among men & women, boys & girls

Gender Blind

Gender Aware — • Examines and addresses these gender considerations and adopts an approach along the continuum

Exploitative

Reinforces or takes advantage of gender inequalities and stereotypes

Accommodating

Works around existing gender differences and inequalities

Transformative

- Fosters critical examination of gender norms* and dynamics
- Strengthens or creates systems* that support gender equality
- Strengthens or creates equitable gender norms and dynamics
- Changes inequitable gender norms and dynamics

GOAL

Gender Equality and better development outcomes

*Norms encompass attitudes and practices
*A system consists of a set of interacting structures, practices, and relations

FIGURE 19.4 Gender Equality Continuum Tool

Source: The General Integration Continuum user's guide developed with assistance from United States Agency for International Development Bureau for Global Health (Washington DC:IGWG, 2017). Used by permission. All rights reserved.

Health Inequities Experienced by Lesbian, Gay, Bisexual, Transgender, Two Spirit, and Other Gender-Variant Individuals

What?

Approximately 3% of the Canadian population self-identified as lesbian, gay, or bisexual in the 2014 Canadian Community Health Survey (Statistics Canada, 2015). Lesbian, gay, and bisexual participants in the survey had consulted with a family physician or specialist physician in the past 12 months—about the same rate as heterosexual participants—but they were less likely to have a regular medical doctor. However, they were more likely to consult a psychologist and to need, but not receive, health care in the past 12 months compared to heterosexuals (Statistics Canada, 2015). Professionally diverse community and home care service providers have limited and uneven access to education to provide equitable care to LGBTQ2S individuals (Daley & MacDonnell, 2015; Daley et al., 2017).

So What?

Despite social gains to improve equality for LGBTQ2S individuals, challenges remain. Within the LGBTQ2S community, "there is a broad spectrum of persons who do not identify with conventional social norms of gender, sex, and sexuality" (Lee & Kanji, 2017, p. 80). LGBTQ2S individuals represent all demographic categories, including age, race, and socioeconomic status. The diversity of sexual orientations and gender identities that exist is not adequately captured in national survey data, nor do the data provide an adequate understanding of the complexity of health issues encountered by LGBTQ2S individuals living in Canada. As a result, some LGBTQ2S individuals, especially transgender individuals, are systematically erased from national-level data (Bauer et al., 2009; Kellett & Fitton, 2017), a factor that results in adverse health outcomes and disproportionate funding to programs and services needed by these populations. Among the transgender population, there is growing evidence that suggests these individuals forego medical care because of previously experienced stigma and discrimination (Clark, Veale, Greyson, & Saewyc, 2017; Sallans, 2016).

Heteronormative assumptions contribute to adverse health outcomes for gay, bisexual, and heterosexual men. Because early research into the lives of LGBTQ2S individuals emphasized disease states (primarily HIV), there is limited published research into the healthy aging of these members of society and what their end-of-life needs are beyond the terminal stages of HIV disease (Stinchcombe, Smallbone, Wilson, & Kortes-Miller, 2017). On November 28, 2017, Canada's Prime Minister Justin Trudeau delivered an apology to LGBTQ2S individuals who were affected by state-sponsored laws and policies that resulted in discrimination and violence that ruined the lives of many LGBTQ2S Canadians (Harris, 2017). This action gives hope to LGBTQ2S communities that Canada will treat its LGBTQ2S population in a more inclusive and socially just manner. Additionally, it serves as a beacon of hope to LGBTQ2S individuals who seek refugee status in Canada because they experience life-threatening persecution in their home country (Kahn, Alessi, Woolner, Kim, & Olivieri, 2017; Keuroghlian, McDowell, & Stern, 2017). Tragically, LGBTQ2S relationships are still considered criminal offences in 73 countries and carry the death penalty in 13 countries (Lee & Kanji, 2017).

Now What?

CHNs can help change the health inequities experienced by LGBTQ2S individuals across Canada. One way to do this is to apply strengths-based approaches to interventions that promote the health of LGBTQ2S individuals (Gahagan & Colpitts, 2017). CHNs can also participate in research that documents the needs of the full spectrum of sexual orientations and gender identities. Additionally, CHNs can advocate for policy change to use strategies to collect psychosocial and health data that are inclusive of all LGBTQ2S individuals. Nurse educators can critically examine the structures within their organizations that perpetuate cis-normativity (e.g., privileging gender binary norms) that render gender diversity invisible through informational erasure (Bauer et al., 2009; Kellett & Fitton, 2017). CHNs can work with members of LGBTQ2S communities to gain the knowledge necessary to challenge transphobia, homophobia, and heterosexism (Clark et al., 2017; Kellett & Fitton, 2017; Knight, Shoveller, Oliffe, Gilbert, & Goldberg, 2012; Sallans, 2016). Finally, Kellett and Fitton (2017) argue for integrating cultural safety into care delivery with LGBTQ2S individuals so to be intersectional in approach.

Standards of Practice Fulfilled

#1 Health Promotion
 – Considers the determinants of health, the social and political context, and systemic structures in collaboration with the client to determine action.

#6 Health Equity
 – Advocates for healthy public policy and social justice by participating in legislative and policy-making activities that influence determinants of health and access to services (CHNC, 2019, revised).

Source: J. Craig Phillips.

Sex, Gender, and Cardiovascular Disease: An Example

Although cardiovascular disease (CVD) is the second leading cause of death for Canadian men, it is the leading cause of premature death for Canadian women. (Heart & Stroke, 2018) Research has demonstrated widespread differences in terms of clinical profiles, presentation, experiences with health care providers, and outcomes (Dey et al., 2009; Norris, Dasgupta, & Kirkland, 2007). In 2018 the Canadian Heart and Stroke Foundation (2018) put out powerful assertions regarding women's unnecessary deaths stating heart disease and stroke claim the life of a woman in Canada every 17 minutes. With conviction, they now state that due to sex and gender blindness in diagnostic tools, research and treatment, too many women's lives are preventably cut short. Two-thirds of heart disease and stroke clinical research still focuses on men, making it difficult to draw conclusions about the effects or risks of the diagnostic tools and therapies on women (Heart and Stroke Canada, 2018). Sex differences in anatomic, physiologic, and biologic characteristics may explain some of the differences in symptoms of acute coronary syndrome, but chronic stress linked to the myriad impossible gender-based expectations placed on women is the key risk factor for women's heart disease (O'Neill, Scovelle, Milner, & Kavanagh, 2018). Many women report being provided with a prescription for a mood-altering medication rather than having their symptoms worked up for possible CVD. Differences exist in heart disease risk among diverse groups of women, with non-White ethnic minority and low-income women having a higher risk for CVD. Indigenous women are at particular risk. This is linked to food insecurity, diminished access to employment, lower income, living on toxic lands, pervasive experiences of violence, and chronic stress (Halseth, 2013).

Gender Considerations in Secondary and Tertiary Prevention It is important to note that women experience and cope with stress in distinctive ways. Women are known to be reluctant to involve family members in lifestyle changes required by their

health problems (Bjarnason-Wehrens, Grand, Loewel, Voller, & Mittag, 2007). Conversely, men may place responsibility for necessary lifestyle changes on their spouses. This may be related to women's expected role as the primary caregiver in the home, which often means women sacrifice their own health and personal preventative health practices to improve those of other family members.

Secondary and tertiary prevention strategies are important, since recent evidence suggests that women receive less information about their cardiovascular illness than men, receive different treatments for their cardiac symptoms, are more likely to experience delayed diagnosis and treatment when compared to men, and receive less information about rehabilitation options and support groups (Genesway, 2001; Kristofferzon, Lofmark, & Carlsson, 2003; Norris et al., 2007). These differences may be the result of institutionalized gender. By using the population health-promotion model (see Chapter 8), a CHN can strengthen community action by bringing together a community of health care professionals involved in cardiovascular health to explore how to address these differences across the continuum of the health care system, particularly in the community setting. CHNs can work with communities of health care professionals to explore potential solutions to reduce such gender-based health and health care differences when and where they exist.

COMMUNITY HEALTH NURSING PRACTICE AND GENDER ADVOCACY—A FORM OF PRIMORDIAL AND PRIMARY PREVENTION

CHNs have wide-ranging and far-reaching roles and responsibilities. One key function of the Canadian CHN is that of advocating for social justice, informed by making links between health and illness experiences and various advocacy efforts aimed at reducing health inequities. Said efforts, at times, are aimed further upstream at changing attitudes, values, beliefs, and perspectives (primordial). At other times, CHNs focus on changing practices (primary) or developing healthy public policy (primordial prevention). Indeed, it takes courage to speak the truth in meetings that are inadvertently gender-blind. CHNs therefore require well-honed relational skills to assist individuals and groups to think critically about gender and health.

Gender considerations are relevant to *all* community health nursing practice. By applying a gender-based lens, informed by an intersectional awareness, we can start to consider the ways in which policies, programs, services, and interventions can better meet the needs of diverse men, women, gender variant, and transgender individuals. CHNs adhere to standards of practice that guide their professional responsibilities (Canadian Nurses Association & CHNC, 2010; CHNC, 2019, revised). Within these standards is an explicit requirement to speak out and advocate. This includes advocacy for gender transformative public policies as well as ensuring that gender norms and relations do not impede access to health and quality of life (Canadian Nurses Association & CHNC, 2010).

CASE STUDY

Recent research indicates more girls than boys experience bullying, with 31% of girls and 25% of boys reporting being victimized (Boak, Hamilton, Adlaf, & Mann, 2017). Cyberbullying and the non-consensual distribution of intimate images is a growing concern in Canada, particularly among youth. The Ontario Student Drug Use and Health Survey reported that online bullying, or cyberbullying, is experienced more by girls, with 28% of girls surveyed reporting this form of targeting compared to 15% of boys.

Cyberbullying GBA+ questions (Status of Women, 2017)

Relevant questions to ask include the following:

- Are there gender differences in cyberbullying behaviour and victimization?
- Are there other identity factors that affect cyberbullying behaviour and victimization (e.g., geography, socioeconomic status)?
- Are the long-term impacts of cyberbullying the same for boys, girls, and gender-diverse youth?
- In consulting with youth, have you considered boys and girls with varied backgrounds? (Status of Women, 2017)

On the surface, it appears that boys get along better than girls, but this assumption is lacking a gender-based analysis. Given how gender-role expectations punish girls for assertiveness and punish boys for being viewed as weak, vulnerable, or "feminine," are these statistics surprising?

Discussion Questions

1. What prevents boys from reporting bullying?
2. How might girls' experiences of societal body shaming impact how they relate?
3. Why has cyberbullying steadily increased, with girls primarily being the target?

Therefore, CHNs must practise from a social justice perspective, asking questions about who benefits and who loses from practices, approaches, erroneous assumptions, or critical research. Firmly planted upstream, the CHN seeking gender transformative primordial and primary prevention would:

- challenge essentialist lenses used to explain sex and gender differences
- strive to reduce and eliminate gender-based inequities, flawed assumptions, and non-critical approaches to community health nursing practice
- advocate for all CHNs to participate in GBA+ training
- think upstream and call into question powerful gender role prescriptions that limit, silence, and oppress humans from living an authentic life
- join with transgender and all gender-variant individuals to eliminate their invisibility, their experiences of harassment and transphobia, and their societal exclusion
- strive to ensure a gender-based lens in health promotion planning while factoring in an intersectional approach that considers additional barriers to quality of life, such as sexism, racism, heterosexism, transphobia, sizeism, xenophobia, classism, ableism, and ageism

CONCLUSION

It is clear that one size does not fit all when it comes to the health and quality of life of diverse individuals and communities. According to the WHO (2013d) nursing strategies in community health need to be gender responsive, appropriate, and transformative. **Gender-appropriate community health nursing interventions** are tailored approaches that ensure the unique needs of men, women, and gender-variant individuals are met. Assessing differences and disparities in health status, human rights, and quality of life grounded in an intersectional view of gender is an important step in ensuring that all Canadians equitably experience positive health and quality of life.

KEY TERMS

binary   (p. 368)
biology as destiny   (p. 367)
cisgender   (p. 368)
essentialist thinking   (p. 367)
gender   (p. 367)
gender-based analyses   (p. 370)
gender-based lens   (p. 373)
gender identity   (p. 368)
gender inequity   (p. 370)
gender norms   (p. 368)
gender relations   (p. 368)
gender roles   (p. 368)
gender transformative   (p. 373)
gender-appropriate community health nursing
    interventions   (p. 376)
gender variance   (p. 369)
health inequities   (p. 366)

institutionalized gender   (p. 369)
sex   (p. 367)
social constructs   (p. 368)
transgender   (p. 368)

STUDY QUESTIONS

1. What distinguishes sex from gender?

2. What is a gender-based lens, and how is it used?

3. How do Canadian men's and women's life expectancy and causes of death differ?

4. When should GBA+ considerations be made in community health nursing?

5. Why is it important to consider gender as part of community health nursing practice?

6. What impacts the health and quality of life of transgender individuals?

INDIVIDUAL CRITICAL-THINKING EXERCISES

1. Imagine a world without gender—what would the world be like?

2. Are there countries that are trying to reduce gender disparities? Do a search online to see how gender disparities are being reduced around the world. Do you believe that any of the strategies you have discovered could be applied in Canada?

3. How do you, as a CHN, improve the health of your clients from a gender-based perspective? In what ways are your expectations different for men and women in your practice?

4. Why is an intersectional approach to gender-informed community health nursing practice necessary? What does it do?

5. What barriers do CHNs face to create spaces where gender diversity is acknowledged and welcomed within the institutions where they work?

GROUP CRITICAL-THINKING EXERCISES

1. Stand up and position yourself on a continuum from one side of the room to another. On one side of the room is feminine; on the other side of the room is the most masculine. After placing yourself on the continuum, look around and see where everyone else is. Discuss why you placed yourself where you did. How do your observations inform your understanding of gender?

2. In 2011, a news story was published about a couple in Canada who opted to raise their baby gender-free. What are our thoughts about this? In groups, have a debate in favour or opposition to this.

3. Now that you understand the health inequities experienced by transgender individuals, what are some specific ways in which CHNs can serve as activists to improve the quality of life of this marginalized population?

REFERENCES

Anderson, K. (2016). *Traditional and Indigenous knowledge: Wiley Blackwell encyclopedia of gender and sexuality studies.* Retrieved from https://onlinelibrary.wiley.com/doi/abs/10.1002/9781118663219.wbegss118

Bauer, G. R., Hammond, R., Travers, R. Kaay, M., Hohenadel, K. M., & Boyce, M. (2009). "I don't think this is theoretical; this is our lives": How erasure impacts health care for transgender people. *Journal of the Association of Nurses in AIDS Care, 20*(5), 348–361. Doi:10.1016/j.jana.2009.07.004

Bauer, G., & Scheim, A. (2015). *Transgender people in Ontario, Canada: Statistics from the Trans PULSE Project to inform human rights policy.* Technical Report. Retrieved from https://www.rainbowhealthontario.ca/wpcontent/uploads/woocommerce_uploads/2015/09/Trans-PULSE-Statistics-Relevant-for-Human-Rights-Policy-June-2015.pdf

Bear, T. (2018). Indigenous Canada: Indigenous concepts of gender. University of Alberta. Available at: https://www.coursera.org/learn/indigenous-canada/lecture/ckZ0u/indigenous-concepts-of-gender

Boak, A., Hamilton, H., Adlaf, E., & Mann, R. (2017). *Drug use among Ontario students: Detailed findings from the Ontario Student Drug Use and Health Survey.* (CAMH Research Document No. 46.) Toronto, ON: Centre for Addiction and Mental Health.

Bjarnason-Wehrens, B., Grand, G., Loewel, H., Voller, H., & Mittag, O. (2007). Gender-specific issues in cardiac rehabilitation: Do women with ischaemic heart disease need specially tailored programmes? *European Journal of Cardiovascular Prevention and Rehabilitation, 14*(2), 163–171. doi:10.1097/HJR.0b013e3280128bce

Canadian Nurses Association and Community Health Nurses of Canada (CHNC). (2010). *Assessment of current CHNC programs, policies, and products using the CAN social justice gauge.* Retrieved from http://www.chnc.ca/documents/SocialJusticeGaugeAssessmentofCommunityHealthNursesofCanadaCHNCMarch312010.pdf

Clark, B. A., Veale, J. F., Greyson, D., & Saewyc, E. (2017). Primary care access and foregone care: A survey of transgender adolescents and young adults. *Family Practice, 35*(3), 302–306. doi:10.1093/fampra/cmx112/4644938

Community Health Nurses of Canada (CHNC). (2019, revised). *Canadian community health nursing: Professional practice model & standards of practice.* St. John's, NL: Author. Retrieved from https://www.chnc.ca/documents/CHNC-ProfessionalPracticeModel-EN/index.html

Conference Board of Canada. (2018a). *Gender income gap.* Retrieved from http://www.conferenceboard.ca/hcp/provincial/society/gender-gap.aspx

Conference Board of Canada. (2018b). *Racial wage gap.* Retrieved from http://www.conferenceboard.ca/hcp/provincial/society/racial-gap.aspx?AspxAutoDetectCookieSupport=1

Conference Board of Canada. (2018c). *Immigrant wage gap.* Retrieved from http://www.conferenceboard.ca/hcp/provincial/society/immigrant-gap.aspx

Daley, A., & MacDonnell, J. A. (2015). 'That would have been beneficial': LGBTQ education for home-care service providers. *Health and Social Care in the Community, 23*(3), 282–291. doi:10.1111/hsc.12141

Daley, A., MacDonnell, J. A., Brotman, S., St. Pierre, M., Aronson, J., & Gillis, L. (2017). Providing health and social services to older LGBT adults. *Annual Review of Gerontology and Geriatrics, 37*(1), 143–160. doi:10.1891/0198-8794.37.143

Dey, S., Flather, M. D., Devlin, G., Brieger, D., Gurfinkel, E. P., Steg, P. G., . . . Eagle, K. A. (2009). Sex-related differences in the presentation, treatment and outcomes among patients with acute coronary syndromes: The global registry of acute coronary events. *Heart, 95*(1), 20–26. doi:10.1136/hrt.2007.138537

Edmonds, R. (2012). *Ontario's human rights code amendments: Deconstructing "gender identity" and "gender expression."* Sexual Orientation and Gender Identity Section. Retrieved from http://www.oba.org/en/pdf/sec_news_sog_dec12_gen_edm.pdf

Ettorre, E. (2004). Revisioning women and drug use: Gender sensitivity, embodiment, and reducing harm. *International Journal of Drug Policy, 15*(5), 327–335. doi:10.1016/j.drugpo.2004.06.009

Gahagan, J., & Colpitts, E. (2017). Understanding and measuring LGBTQ pathways to health: A scoping review of strengths-based health promotion approaches in LGBTQ health research. *Journal of Homosexuality, 64*(1), 95–121. doi:10.1080/00918369.2016.1172893

Gesensway, D. (2001). Reasons for sex-specific and gender-specific study of health topics. *Annals of Internal Medicine, 135*(10), 935–938.

Ghandi, M., Bacchetti, P., Miotti, P., Quinn, T. C., Veronese, F., & Greenblatt, R. M. (2002). Does patient sex affect human immunodeficiency virus levels? *Clinical Infectious Disease, 35*(3), 313–322.

Goldenberg, S. L. (2014). Status of men's health in Canada. *Canadian Urological Association Journal, 8*(7), 142–144.

Government of Canada. (2013a). *Introduction to pay equity.* Retrieved from http://www.labour.gc.ca/eng/standards_equity/eq/pay/intro.shtml#links

Government of Canada. (2013b). GBA+. Ottawa, ON: *Status of Women Canada.* Retrieved from http://www.swc-cfc.gc.ca/gba-acs/overview-apercu-en.html

Greco, J. (2013). Gender: A social construction. *Sociological Imagination: Western's Undergraduate Sociology Student Journal, 2*(2). Retrieved from http://ir.lib.uwo.ca/si/vol2/iss2/8

Greenberg, L., & Normandin, C. (2011). *Health at a glance: Disparities in life expectancy at birth.* Retrieved from http://www.statcan.gc.ca/pub/82-624-x/2011001/article/11427-eng.htm#a3

Halseth, R. (2013). *Aboriginal women in Canada: Gender, socio-economic determinants of health and initiatives to close the wellness-gap.* National Collaborating Centre for Aboriginal Health. Prince George, BC.

Hankivsky, O. (2012). Women's health, men's health and gender and health: Implications of intersectionality. *Social Science and Medicine, 74*(11), 1712–1720.

Harris, K. (2017, November). "Our collective shame": Trudeau delivers historic apology to LGBT Canadians. *CBC News: Politics.* Retrieved from http://www.cbc.ca/news/politics/homosexual-offences-exunge-records-1.4422546

Health Canada. (2001). *"Certain circumstances": Issues in equity and responsiveness in access to health care in Canada.* Ottawa, ON: Author. Retrieved from http://www.hc-sc.gc.ca/hcs-sss/pubs/acces/2001-certain-equit-acces/index-eng.php

Health Canada. (2007). *Chronic disease prevention and management.* Ottawa, ON: Author. Retrieved from http://www.hc-sc.gc.ca/hcs-sss/pubs/prim/2006-synth-chronic-chroniques/index-eng.php

Heart and Stroke Canada. (2018). *Time for Women to Stop Dying Unnecessarily.* News Release, Toronto. Available from: http://www.heartandstroke.ca/what-we-do/media-centre/news-releases/time-for-women-to-stop-dying-unnecessarily

Jack, D. & Ali, A. (2010). *Silencing the self across cultures: Depression and gender in the social world.* New York, NY: Oxford University Press.

Jackson, B. E., Pederson, A., & Boscoe, M. (2009). Waiting to wait: Improving wait times evidence though gender-based analysis. In P. Armstrong & J. Deadman (Eds.), *Women's health: Intersections of policy research and practice* (pp. 35–52). Toronto, ON: Women's Press.

Jenkins, G. W., Kemnitz, C. P., & Tortora, G. J. (2010). *Anatomy and physiology: From science to life* (2nd ed.). Hoboken, NJ: John Wiley & Sons, Inc.

Kahn, S., Alessi, E., Woolner, L., Kim, H., & Olivieri, C. (2017). Promoting the wellbeing of lesbian, gay, bisexual and transgender forced migrants in Canada: Providers' perspectives. *Culture, Health & Sexuality, 19*(10), 1165–1179. doi:10.1080/13691058.2017.1298843

Kellett, P., & Fitton, C. (2017). Supporting transvisibility and gender diversity in nursing practice and education: Embracing cultural safety. *Nursing Inquiry, 24*(1), e12146. doi:10.1111/nin.12146

Keuroghlian, A. S., McDowell, M. J., & Stern, T. A. (2017). Providing care for lesbian, gay, bisexual, and transgender immigrants at health centers and clinics. *Psychosomatics.* Online ahead of print 2017. doi: 10.1016/j.psym.2017.10.008. Retrieved from http://www.sciencedirect.com/science/article/pii/S0033318217302190

Knight, R., Shoveller, J. A., Oliffe, J. L., Gilbert, M., & Goldberg, S. (2012). Heteronormativity hurts everyone: Experiences of young men and clinicians with sexually transmitted infection/HIV testing in British Columbia, Canada. *Health, 17*(5), 441–459. doi:10.1177/1363459312464071

Kristofferzon, M. L., Lofmark, R., & Carlsson, M. (2003). Myocardial infarction: Gender differences in coping and social support. *Journal of Advanced Nursing, 44*(4), 360–374.

Lee, A., & Kanji, Z. (2017). Queering the health care system: Experiences of the lesbian, gay, bisexual, transgender community. *Canadian Journal of Dental Hygiene, 51*(2), 80–89.

Lee, C., & Owens, R. (2002). *The psychology of men's health.* Philadelphia, PA: Open University Press.

Nagunar, D. (2011). Longevity and historical life tables (for 1920–1922 through 1980–1982); Statistics Canada Catalogue no. 84–537, Life Tables (for 1985–1987 and 1990–1992); Statistics Canada, Vital Statistics, CANSIM Table 102–0512, Life expectancy (for 1995–1997 through 2005–2007). Retrieved from http://www.statcan.gc.ca/pub/82-624-x/2011001/article/chart/11427-02-chart2-eng.htm

Norris, C., Dasgupta, K., & Kirkland, S. (2007). Differences in cardiovascular presentation in women and men. *Canadian Medical Association Journal, 176*(6), S22–S23. Published by Canadian Nurses Association.

Oliffe, J. L., & Phillips, M. (2008). Depression, men and masculinities: A review and recommendations. *Journal of Men's Health, 5*(3), 194–202. doi:10.1016/j.jomh.2008.03.016

Oliffe, J. L., Kelly, M. T., Bottorff, J. L., Johnson, J. L., & Wong, S. T. (2017). "He's more typically female because he's not afraid to cry": Connecting heterosexual gender relations and men's depression. *Social Sciences and Medicine, 73*(2011), 775–782.

O'Neill, A., Scovelle, A., Milner, A., & Kavanagh, A. (2018). Gender/sex as a social determinant of cardiovascular risk. *Circulation, 137*(8), 854–864. https://doi.org/10.1161/CIRCULATIONAHA.117.028595

Rainbow Health Ontario (n.d.) *Glossary of terms.* Retrieved from https://www.rainbowhealthontario.ca/wp-content/uploads/Introduction-to-LGBT/story_content/external_files/Glossary.pdf

Sallans, R. K. (2016). Lessons from a transgender patient for health acer providers. *American Medical Association Journal of Ethics, 18*(11), 1139–1146.

Senie, R. T. (2014). *Epidemiology of women's health.* Burlington, MD: Jones and Bartlett.

Sheppard, M., & Mayo, J. B. (2013). The social construction of gender and sexuality: Learning from two spirit traditions. *The Social Studies, 104*(6), 259–270.

Soldin, O. P., Chung, S. H., & Mattison, D. R. (2011). Sex differences in drug disposition. *Journal of Biomedicine and Biotechnology.* doi:10.1155/2011/187103

Statistics Canada. (2015). *Same-sex couples and sexual orientation . . . by the numbers.* Ottawa, ON: Author. Retrieved from https://www.statcan.gc.ca/eng/dai/smr08/2015/smr08_203_2015

Statistics Canada. (2017). *Women in Canada: A gender based statistical report. Pain and unpaid work.* Ottawa, ON: Minister of Industry. Retrieved from http://www.statcan.gc.ca/pub/89-503-x/2015001/article/14694-eng.pdf

Status of Women Canada. (2017). Gender-based analysis plus: Applying GBA+ to your work. Retrieved from http://www.swc-cfc.gc.ca/gba-acs/apply-appliquez-en.html

Stinchcombe, A., Smallbone, J., Wilson, K., & Kortes-Miller, K. (2017). Healthcare and end-of-life needs of lesbian, gay, bisexual, and transgender (LGBT) older adults: A scoping review. *Geriatrics, 2,* 13. doi:10.3390/geriatrics2010013

Tyler, R. E. (2012). Adolescent and young adult male health: A review. *Pediatrics, 132*(3), 535–546. doi:10.1542/peds.2012-3414

UNICEF. (2006). *Statement on International Women's Day.* Retrieved from http://www.unicef.org/media/media_35134.html

van Daalen-Smith, C. (2009). Whispers and roars: A feminist analysis of the anesthetization of girls' and women's anger. *Journal of Radical Psychology, 9*(1), 6–10.

World Health Organization (WHO). (2008). *Closing the gap in a generation: Health equity through action on the social determinants of health.* Geneva, CH: Author. Retrieved from http://www.who.int/social_determinants/thecommission/finalreport/en/index.html

World Health Organization (WHO). (2010). *Gender, women and primary health care renewal*. Discussion Paper. Geneva, CH: Author.

World Health Organization (WHO). (2011). *Gender mainstreaming for health managers: A practical approach*. Department of Gender, Women and Health. Retrieved from http://www.who.int/gender-equity-rights/knowledge/health_managers_guide/en

World Health Organization (WHO). (2013a). What do we mean by gender and sex? *Gender, women, and health*. Geneva, CH: Author. Retrieved from http://www.who.int/gender/whatisgender/en

World Health Organization (WHO). (2013b). *Trade, foreign policy, diplomacy, and health*: *Gender*. Geneva, CH: Author. Retrieved from http://www.who.int/trade/glossary/story032/en

World Health Organization (WHO). (2013c). *Gender and women's mental health*. Geneva, CH: Author. Retrieved from http://www.who.int/mental_health/prevention/genderwomen/en

World Health Organization (WHO). (2013d). *Why gender and health?* Geneva, CH: Author. Retrieved from http://www.who.int/gender/genderandhealth/en

ABOUT THE AUTHORS

Cheryl van Daalen-Smith, RN, PhD, is Associate Professor in the School of Nursing, Faculty of Health at York University. She is cross appointed to the School of Gender, Sexuality and Women's Studies and to the Children's Studies Program, where she teaches a course on children's health and quality of life and a course on girlhood. Her nursing practice includes community health/public health nursing and pediatric nursing, with research exploring girls' and women's mental health, women and anger, women and self-esteem, and an exploration of men's and women's experiences of psychiatric hospitalization in Canada. She is the founder and co-editor of *Witness: The Canadian Journal of Critical Nursing Discourse*.

Aliyah Dosani, RN, BN, MPH, PhD, is Associate Professor in the School of Nursing and Midwifery, Faculty of Health, Community and Education at Mount Royal University in Calgary. She is also an Adjunct Associate Professor in the Department of Community Health Sciences, Cumming School of Medicine, at University of Calgary. She holds a PhD from the University of Calgary with a specialization in population/public health. Her nursing practice includes instructing students in the Bachelor of Nursing program, population and public health, community health nursing, and legal issues in nursing. Her work focuses on maternal, newborn, and child health. Her research interests involve working on health equity and social justice issues through community-based programs and interventions. She also has a passion for global health issues.

CHAPTER 20

Lesbian, Gay, Bisexual, Transgender, Queer, and Two Spirit Clients

Elizabeth M. Saewyc

LEARNING OUTCOMES

After studying this chapter, you should be able to:

1. Describe the developmental processes and dimensions that are part of sexual orientation and gender identity.

2. Recognize different sexual orientations and gender identities generally found within Canadian communities, including Indigenous communities.

3. Identify the shifting societal attitudes and current stressors for lesbian, gay, bisexual, transgender, queer, and Two Spirit (LGBTQ2S) people.

4. Understand the social determinants of health that influence health inequities experienced by LGBTQ2S clients in communities and health care settings.

5. Describe challenges and potential consequences of disclosing sexual orientation to family, peers, and health care providers.

6. Reflect on and identify your own assumptions, values, beliefs, and judgments related to LGBTQ2S people and on how these influence your approach to community health nursing with LGBTQ2S populations.

7. Identify community health nursing interventions for promoting the health of LGBTQ2S people.

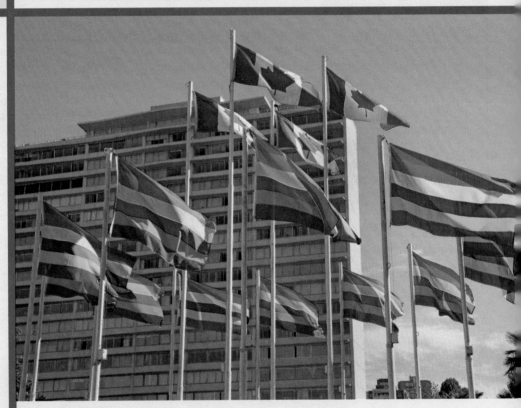

Source: Maxdigi/Fotolia

INTRODUCTION

Sexual orientation and gender identity are two major characteristics that develop during childhood and adolescence. Sexual orientation can be defined as romantic and sexual attractions toward people of one or more genders (Saewyc, 2011). Other dimensions of sexual orientation include sexual relations with people of one or more genders as well as self-labelling as heterosexual, gay, lesbian, bisexual, queer or "questioning," or, in some Indigenous communities, Two Spirit. **Homosexuality** refers to romantic and sexual attractions toward individuals of the same gender, and people with this orientation are commonly referred to in Canada as gay men and lesbian women, as the term "homosexuality" or calling someone "homosexual" can be perceived as negative in LGBTQ2S communities. **Heterosexuality** refers to romantic or sexual attractions to another gender, such as men attracted solely to women or women attracted solely to men. Such people are called heterosexual men or women. **Bisexuality** refers to romantic or sexual attractions to more than one gender, and such people may identify as bisexual men or bisexual women, **pansexual** (attracted to all genders), mostly heterosexual, or other terms. (See Photo 20.1.) Some sexual minority

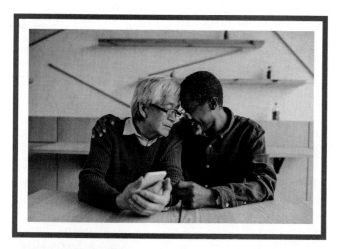

PHOTO 20.1 Cisgender and transgender men in relationships with each other may identify as gay or as bisexual.

Source: LightField Studios/Shutterstock

people prefer the term **queer** as a label for a non-heterosexual orientation. However, this term used to carry strongly negative connotations, and older lesbian, gay, or bisexual people may be offended by its use, so it should generally be used only when someone has self-identified using that term. Some people may be unsure of their orientation, especially adolescents, and may identify as "questioning" their orientation. Since society tends to assume a "default" orientation of heterosexual for most people (see "heterosexism" discussed later in this chapter), when LGBTQ2S people disclose their orientation publicly to others, it is termed **coming out**.

Gender identity is a complex development of your sense of self as a gendered person, with the attributes and social traits assigned in your culture to a particular gender role. This commonly means identifying as a man or woman, as masculine or feminine. However, the traits, appearance, and behaviours associated with various genders may differ across cultures, and a growing number of people identify beyond the binary of man or woman. Gender identity is not the same as **physiological sex**, which is based on chromosomes and phenotypic expression in the body and is most commonly labelled as male or female, even though physical bodies do not always fit neatly into these two categories. Some chromosomal variations lead to differences in physiological development that manifest at birth, or during or after puberty, and although only 1% to 2% of people may have these variations globally, they total more than twice the population of Canada (Saewyc, 2017). Most of the time, gender identity aligns with physiological sex, also identified by the term "cisgender."

Transgender or **gender diverse** people may experience their gender identity as not fitting what others think it is or should be (e.g., their gender assigned at birth might have been male, but they identify as a woman) or as not fitting within a binary model of man and woman (e.g., they identify as non-binary, gender queer, gender fluid, or another label). Some might feel as though their physical bodies do not accurately reflect their gender identity. Transgender or

gender diverse individuals may also see their gender as being more fluid. Transgender people may want to dress and act in line with their gender identity rather than according to others' expectations of how they should look or behave based on their gender assigned at birth. Some may also choose to take puberty blockers, take hormones, or undergo surgery to help align their external body and appearance with their gender identity. In the same way the term "heterosexual" is an acknowledgement that everyone has an orientation, not just gay, lesbian, and bisexual people, the term **cisgender** has emerged in some health and social circles referring to the majority of people whose internal gender identity matches their external body appearance and gender expression (Schilt & Westbrook, 2009). Some Indigenous people, in particular First Nations people, prefer the term **Two Spirit**, or two-spirited, as a cross-cultural term referring to gender identity or sexual orientation, or a combination of both (Hunt, 2015). Please refer to Chapter 19 for an in-depth discussion of gender and its implications on health.

Theories about the nature of sexual orientation and gender identity vary, but most scientific evidence currently suggests a genetic basis influenced in part by environment, culture, and societal attitudes (Mustanski, Chivers, & Bailey, 2002). There is evidence of genetic and prenatal hormonal influences on gender identity development, as well as cultural norms and influences. Studies of monozygotic and dizygotic twins have found enough concordance in sexual orientation to suggest a genetic basis for orientation, but specific genes have not been identified. The variety of cultural meanings and practices around the world for sexual orientation and gender identity suggest people's expression of their romantic attractions and their gender are influenced by culture.

SEXUAL ORIENTATIONS AND GENDER IDENTITIES FOUND WITHIN CANADIAN COMMUNITIES

According to the 2014 Canadian Community Health Survey (CCHS), 1.7% of adults aged 18 to 59 identify as gay or lesbian, and another 1.3% identify as bisexual (Statistics Canada, 2015). Studies of adolescents and adults that include more measures of orientation than just self-labelling suggest a larger percentage of people report same-gender or multiple-gender attractions—between 4% to 7%. Among adolescents, those reporting bisexual attractions outnumber exclusively same-gender attractions by three to one or more. Sexual behaviour is less common than attractions among adolescents, in part because most Canadian adolescents are not sexually active until the later teen years or young adulthood (Saewyc, Poon, Homma, & Skay, 2008). Among adults, identifying as lesbian, gay, or bisexual is less common than attractions or behaviour, so the CCHS data are likely undercounts the population of **LGBTQ2S** people in Canada.

Most Canadian nurses will encounter at least some lesbian, gay, bisexual, Two Spirit, and, less commonly, transgender, and non-binary clients in all age groups. The numbers will reflect regional variation and type of health service, with large metropolitan cities having more LGBTQ2S residents than smaller cities or rural towns. This chapter describes the social context and health issues of LGBTQ2S people in Canada and strategies that community health nurses (CHNs) use in reducing health inequities and promoting their health.

SOCIETAL ATTITUDES AND STRESSORS FOR LGBTQ2S PEOPLE

Some LGBTQ2S clients choose to not disclose their sexual orientation or gender identity, or to limit disclosure to people they trust. This reluctance to disclose can be explained by several essential concepts: homophobia, biphobia, transphobia, heterosexism, and cissexism. **Homophobia** describes a fear or hatred of gay men and lesbian women (*Oxford English Dictionary*, 1993). This prejudice is not usually based on knowledge of actual gay or lesbian people but on myths and assumptions. It is often demonstrated through derogatory language, jokes, or discrimination against individuals perceived to be gay or lesbian. Similarly, **biphobia** is an extreme prejudice toward bisexual people (Eliason, 1997), and **transphobia** is hatred of transgender people (Norton, 1997). At their worst, these prejudices can involve extreme violence toward those perceived to be LGBTQ2S. More often it shows up as bullying or harassment in schools and work, negative comments on social media, and discrimination or social exclusion.

Being surrounded by negative and rejecting messages, hostility, and discrimination can create significant stress in LGBTQ2S people's lives. This stress can contribute to challenges with coping and long-term stress-related health issues. Some LGBTQ2S individuals may accept negative societal views about people like them and, thus, experience a loss of self-worth (Herek, Cogan, Gillis, & Glunt, 1998), known as **internalized homophobia** (or biphobia or transphobia). It can manifest as low self-esteem, reduced self-care, and health-compromising activities, such as substance abuse or high-risk sexual activities, to cope with distress.

Heterosexism, in contrast, refers to the assumption that heterosexuality is the norm and a perspective that other orientations or genders are not "normal." This is acted out constantly in society through behaviours that presume everyone is heterosexual, or should be. Heterosexism in health care systems include asking clients about their marital status or sexual relationships using gendered terms, such as asking a man, "Do you have a wife?" This implies you expect a man would marry only a woman, even though in Canada it is legal for a man to marry another man. Likewise, asking all women what type of contraception they use without first checking they are sexually active and whether their sexual partners are women, men, or another gender assumes that woman only have sexual partners with penises, and they can get pregnant. Heterosexism alienates LGBTQ2S people, and although not as threatening as homophobia, it can lead them to avoid or delay needed health care. **Cissexism** privileges cisgender identities and bodies over trans identities and trans bodies. Cissexism may be evident, for example, through medical forms that offer options for male or female but not other genders or sexes. Gender-segregated spaces, such as public washrooms, change rooms, sports leagues, shelters, and prisons, can become inaccessible to trans people due to transphobia and violence.

HEALTH INEQUITIES AMONG LGBTQ2S PEOPLE

Because of the smaller size of the population of LGBTQ2S people in our society, their health issues and health care needs may not be as visible. Until the mid-1970s, homosexuality was classified as a mental illness, and attention was focused on "curing" LGBTQ2S people (Brotman, Ryan, Jalbert, & Rowe, 2002). This usually involved intensive psychiatric therapy, including classical aversion therapy using electric shock. Today, this type of "conversion" or "reparative therapy" is considered unethical by most professional health organizations because there is no credible evidence of its effectiveness and significant evidence that it is harmful, especially for adolescents when parents force them into therapy to try to change their orientation. This practice has been condemned by the World Health Organization (WHO), which has called on governments to ban reparative therapy (Pan American Health Organization/World Health Organization, 2012).

LGBTQ2S people face a number of health inequities in Canada, and while the causes of these greater risks are complex, a key component is the health-related effects of societal stigma and discrimination. Although laws in Canada are changing, attitudes are slower to shift. Population-based studies have shown LGBTQ2S youth in school still face high levels of discrimination and harassment (Taylor & Peter, 2011) as well as higher rates of physical and sexual abuse (Friedman et al., 2011). LGBTQ2S adults may also face hate crimes and assault in the community, discrimination in the workplace, and rejection within their families.

The stress LGBTQ2S experience as a result of stigma and discrimination has been termed "minority stress" (Meyer, 2003), and it contributes to health problems and poorer self-rated health (Saewyc, 2011; Steele, Ross, Dobinson, Veldhuizen, & Tinmouth, 2009). LGBTQ2S people may face negative attitudes within some communities, witnessing or even experiencing hostility and violence. These experiences may lead people to hide or conceal relationships and identity, and struggle to cope with distress from unsafe environments without social support.

What are these significant health inequities? Population-based research in Canada has documented higher rates of mental health issues, including depressive symptoms and anxiety, self-harm, suicidal thoughts, and suicide attempts among both adolescents and adults (Brennan, Ross, Dobinson, Veldhuizen, & Steele, 2010; Saewyc, 2011; Steele et al., 2009; Rotondi Khobzi et al., 2011a; Rotondi Khobzi et al., 2011b). These studies and others also document higher rates of tobacco use, alcohol use (including binge drinking), and substance use and abuse among LGBTQ2S youth and, to a lesser extent, among adults. Researchers have found that lesbian and bisexual adolescent girls have higher overweight and obese body-mass index (BMI) compared to heterosexual peers (Saewyc, Homma, Hitchcock, & Prior, 2012). Gay and bisexual boys and men have lower BMI and increased risk of eating-disordered behaviours compared to their heterosexual peers (Brennan et al., 2010). Similar patterns are found for transgender youth (Watson, Veale, & Saewyc, 2017) and for LGBTQ2S adults (Calzo, Blashill, Brown, & Argenall, 2017).

Sexual health is another important area of health inequities among LGBTQ2S people. Although most health care providers are aware of the higher risk for HIV/AIDS among men who have sex with men, lesbian, and bisexual women in Canada have also reported higher prevalence of sexually transmitted infections (STIs) (Steele et al., 2009). Similarly, LGBTQ2S adolescents in western Canada have reported higher levels of sexual risk-taking behaviours than heterosexual students, including early sexual intercourse (before age 14), a higher number of sexual partners, unprotected sex, and sex while intoxicated (Saewyc et al., 2006). These high-risk behaviours may be explained, in part, by higher rates of sexual abuse history (Saewyc et al., 2006). As a result, LGBTQ2S youth are also more likely to become pregnant or cause a pregnancy during adolescence (Saewyc et al., 2008; Veale, Watson, Adjei, & Saewyc, 2016). Pregnancy may be used as a way to deflect discrimination and heterosexism (Travers, Newton, & Munro, 2011). Pregnancy among lesbian and bisexual women is also increasingly common (see Photo 20.2), through sexual relationships with men or through assisted reproductive technologies, and many fertility clinics in Canada provide services for lesbian and bisexual women (Corbett, Frecker, Shapiro, & Yudin, 2013).

LGBTQ2S people from racialized ethnocultural backgrounds, such as Indigenous or South Asian heritage, and those with visible or invisible disabilities, face additional challenges. They may experience rejection and stigma both from larger society and within the wider LGBTQ2S community (Balsam,

Huang, Fieland, Simoni, & Walters, 2004; Parks, Hughes, & Matthews, 2004). The intersection of sexual orientation, gender, and ethnocultural background creates varying levels of health inequity as it can lead to multiple levels of discrimination, which are linked to higher health risks (Poon, Saewyc, & Chen, 2011; Saewyc, Clark, Barney, Brunanski, & Homma, 2013; Steele et al., 2009; Veenstra, 2011).

COMING OUT, OR DISCLOSURE OF LGBTQ2S IDENTITY

Disclosing a non-heterosexual sexual orientation or transgender identity can be difficult no matter when it occurs during the lifespan. The amount of difficulty relates to the nature of the relationship (e.g., telling a parent), the age of the individual (e.g., adolescent versus adult), and the value placed on the relationship (e.g., friend, relative, or stranger). Hiding sexual orientation or gender identity can be stressful and lead to poor health outcomes and health-compromising behaviours. LGBTQ2S adolescents' increased risk for depression and suicidal ideation may be highest just before disclosure within important relationships, such as to parents (Igartua, Gill, & Montoro, 2003). The response to that disclosure can also be an important predictor of suicidal ideation and attempt as well as of long-term coping responses (Ryan, Huebner, Diaz, & Sanchez, 2009). Parents' negative responses can include violence or forcing the young person out of home; a disproportionate number of homeless and street-involved youth are LGBTQ2S (Frederick, Ross, Bruno, & Erickson, 2011). Even parents' neutral responses are often interpreted by youth as rejection and are still linked with suicide attempts, problem substance use, and other challenges into young adulthood. In contrast, parents' supportive responses, such as continuing to state their love and acceptance of their child, can improve self-esteem and help buffer the stress of other negative reactions in school or among peers (Ryan, Russell, Huebner, Diaz, & Sanchez, 2010).

Transgender youth face additional challenges, as society does not easily accept individuals who do not fit into traditional masculine or feminine gender presentations. Gender-diverse behaviour is less accepted among school-age children and adolescents than among young children, and trans and gender-diverse youth may experience adversity at school, in their family, and in the wider community (Veale et al., 2015). They may run away or be kicked out, experience homelessness, and may need to exchange sex for food, shelter, money, or drugs (survival sex), which puts them at significant risk for adverse health outcomes (Grossman & D'Augelli, 2006). Fear of the consequences of disclosing transgender identity is a major factor in mental health and affects their personal safety in many social as well as family situations (Rotondi Khobzi et al., 2011a; Rotondi Khobzi et al., 2011b).

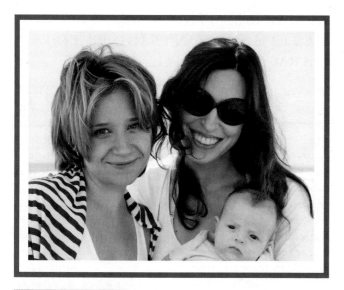

PHOTO 20.2 Lesbian and bisexual women may have children together through assisted reproductive technologies.

Source: Dubova/Fotolia

Disclosing to Health Care Providers

Coming out can support good health and appropriate health care for LGBTQ2S people. However, in health care and community settings it can be a constant process—with each new care provider encountered, the process must be repeated, and the same fears and concerns about providers' reaction are experienced over again (Brotman et al., 2002). Not disclosing (being "closeted") is associated with shame and hiding and can lead to physical and psychological health challenges. LGBTQ2S people may have to educate their health care providers who lack knowledge or comfort in providing appropriate care. They may experience unethical and unprofessional treatment from health care providers who have homophobic, biphobic, or transphobic attitudes, misinformation, and prejudiced assumptions (Bauer, Scheim, Deutsch, & Cassarella, 2014). Previous negative experiences with health care may lead them to avoid care even when it is needed, risking worsening health (Clark, Veale, Greyson, & Saewyc, 2017).

CANADIAN RESEARCH 20.1

Homeless and street-involved Indigenous LGBTQ2S youth in British Columbia: Intersectionality, challenges, resilience, and cues for action. (Saewyc et al., 2017)

This study involved data from a homeless and street-involved youth health survey in 13 communities across British Columbia, including small towns. More than half of the participants aged 12–19 identified as Indigenous, and of these, one in three indicated they were LGBTQ2S. Compared to heterosexual cisgender Indigenous peers, Two Spirit homeless youth reported health inequities and challenging contexts. They were more likely to be on the street because of family conflict, including conflict about their sexual orientation. More than two-thirds had been in foster care, and a similar majority reported at least one close relative was a residential school survivor. They reported much higher rates of sexual and physical violence, and one in three had been sexually exploited, compared to 15% of heterosexual Indigenous youth. They also reported living in more precarious housing, such as abandoned buildings, cars, tents, or on the street. They were twice as likely to report self-harm in the past year (69% versus 31%) as well as higher rates of suicidal ideation and attempts. They were also more likely than Indigenous heterosexual youth to say they had missed needed health care in the past year (36% versus 21%).

Despite these health inequities, there were areas of resilience linked to better health for Two Spirit Indigenous homeless youth. Connections to culture, such as speaking an Indigenous language, were linked to better mental health; about one in five Two Spirit youth spoke an Indigenous language. Those who were involved with cultural activities, such as traditional dance or artistic practice, were also less likely to have self-harmed or attempted suicide. While the Truth and Reconciliation Commission of Canada report did not specifically mention Two Spirit people, some of the Commission's recommendations may be relevant for Two Spirit youth, such as the recommendations to reduce the number of youth in care of child welfare services and to keep children and youth in culturally appropriate settings where possible. Reconnecting homeless Indigenous Two Spirit youth to their culture and families may have significant health benefits.

Discussion Questions:

1. Why do you think Two Spirit homeless youth might experience more health inequities than other Indigenous homeless youth? How might the intersection of racism and stigma contribute to their health issues?

2. This research identifies key resilience factors among Two Spirit youth linked to culture and family connectedness. If you are not Indigenous, how might you, as a CHN working with homeless Two Spirit youth, support their cultural safety in your practice?

3. If you were providing community health nursing care with homeless Indigenous youth, and one of the young people disclosed they were Two Spirit, what are some of the health risks you might assess and need to address?

Many health care providers describe themselves as being "neutral" in their practice around the sexual orientation or gender identity of their clients. This is based on the belief that health care should be accessible to all, not based on the particular needs of any one group or population (Brotman et al., 2002). Such health care providers might not ask about sexual orientation when meeting a new client, or ignore disclosures. It is more appropriate to acknowledge the disclosure and reflect acceptance and caring, which will further encourage the client to share sensitive information that may influence care (Williams-Barnard, Mendoza, & Shippee-Rice, 2001). Acting in a "neutral" or unresponsive manner may in fact be read as a rejecting or negative response (Boehmer & Case, 2004).

RESPONSES THAT PROMOTE HEALTH OR CONTRIBUTE TO HARM FOR LGBTQ2S PEOPLE

How can nurses provide safe and inclusive care for LGBTQ2S people? The first step is to address our own assumptions, beliefs, values, and attitudes about sexual orientation and gender diversity. These may reflect the attitudes we absorbed growing up in our own families. We may not ever have explored our attitudes about homosexuality, bisexuality, or gender diversity, and may not be aware of how heterosexist we are. Think about what you believe about sexual orientation and gender identity, and where those beliefs came from. Have they changed over time? How many different people do you know who are lesbian, gay, bisexual, or transgender? Can you recall caring for a self-identified LGBTQ2S client and what that was like? Did you recognize any assumptions or attitudes that got in the way of providing non-judgmental care?

Reflect whether you regularly use inclusive language when taking a history from a new client. Do you ask if the client has a partner and if that partner is a man, woman, or other gender?

Most heterosexual clients will readily tell you that their partner is a man (or woman), and even if LGBTQ2S clients do not disclose to you at that point, or say they are not partnered at present, you have shown by your word choices that you know that more than just heterosexual relationships exist. This may help the LGBTQ2S client to be more open at this or a future appointment. If a client does identify as LGBTQ2S, do not ignore the comment, but rather thank them for sharing this and indicate how knowing this can be important to providing the right care. Another way of assessing is to ask whether the client is sexually active, and if so, whether their partners are men, women, trans, or some combination. This avoids the assumption that sex only happens in relationships and also shows you recognize the diversity of people's relationships. Directly asking if the client is gay, lesbian, or bisexual can be a problem because social stigma or previous negative experiences with health care providers may make the client reluctant to disclose. As well, the client may not self-identify by those labels but still be having sexual relations with people of the same gender or more than one gender.

Consider the forms we ask clients to complete. Is the language contained in these forms inclusive or exclusive? Think about advocating for a change in the options for gender identity, beyond just male and female. Consider whether the section usually marked as "marital status" is really necessary for health care, and if so, is it as appropriate as asking about "relationship status" and having a space for "name of partner" if the answer is yes, rather than the usual "single, married, separated/divorced, or widowed." Since same-gender relationships can also be legal or common-law marriages in Canada, just having a box to check the usual single, married, separated, or widowed options are relevant, but it may send the implicit message of heterosexual relationships only.

It is also important to be clear about the level of confidentiality that is possible in the clinical and public health agency charting. As with most people, LGBTQ2S clients, especially adolescents, are very concerned about this. Though complete confidentiality is an important standard in health care and usually a requirement under Canadian privacy laws and provincial health system policies, there are some circumstances where it is not possible, usually related to imminent safety concerns. Clients need to know what information about them may be accessible to others and when you might be required to break confidentiality (e.g., when a minor discloses abuse or suicidal intent), and to tailor their disclosure and health-related information accordingly.

Think about the educational material you give to clients, and look to see if there are any images of same-gender couples or gender-diverse people used as illustrations. The same goes for posters displayed on the walls of clinics and hospitals. These seemingly minor details can speak volumes to LGBTQ2S clients attending the clinic or hospital about their safety in disclosing sexual orientation. Familiarize yourself with resources in the community that are LGBTQ2S friendly; know the names and contact information of supportive counsellors and other health care providers. Have information on hand to give out to clients, including websites and other resources that provide information for LGBTQ2S individuals.

ROLES FOR CHNs IN PROMOTING THE HEALTH OF LGBTQ2S POPULATIONS

CHNs have a vital role to play in both modelling and encouraging respect and support in all aspects of daily life, and especially in the various arenas where they work with members of the community. Nurses who work in schools have a particularly important role to play in affecting the health and physical and mental safety of lesbian, gay, bisexual, or transgender youth. It is vitally important that the needs of this invisible population, often rendered vulnerable, are identified and addressed, both on an individual and a school-based level. There is much work to be done in sensitizing teachers, coaches, aides, and other youth to the challenges facing these youth every day in our schools and on playgrounds. This needs to occur within the context of the community's cultural and religious affiliations. Where cultural norms or religious beliefs have problems with sexual minority orientations, there may be resistance, misinformation, or heightened concern about creating safer, more supportive environments. There may be significant challenges for the individual who wants to come out but also wants to maintain ties with family and members of the community.

Though it is important to consider our own attitudes, values, beliefs, and practices, it is also important to challenge discriminatory attitudes and actions among fellow students, coworkers, and colleagues. You may be LGBTQ2S positive, but other people you encounter in class, in clinics, and in the community may not be, and in their opportunities to interact with LGBTQ2S clients they may potentially cause harm through their words or actions. Including fellow students in an exploration of attitudes, knowledge, values, and beliefs will give you a good idea of how easy or difficult it may be to change homophobic or heterosexist attitudes and practices.

Community health nursing interventions for working with LGBTQ2S people do not end with advocacy to shift societal attitudes, reduce stigma, and foster respect, although this is an example of primordial prevention of a primary cause of health inequities. Other primordial prevention interventions might include helping to prevent harassment and violence, and focus on the structural environments of laws and policies. CHNs can recommend policies in workplaces, schools, and health care environments that foster community inclusion and connectedness for LGBTQ2S people and address bullying or harassment.

Since many of the health issues of LGBTQ2S people are also those of the general population, nurses will likewise use primordial, primary, secondary, tertiary, and quaternary prevention interventions to help reduce health inequities in this group. The interventions may need to be adapted to be appropriate and culturally relevant to LGBTQ2S groups. In designing or adapting these health-promotion interventions, CHNs should engage with community members regularly and listen closely, to ensure their views and needs are considered.

Primary prevention interventions around healthy living and stress management are salient for all people. Creating groups or classes for LGBTQ2S people to learn stress coping techniques, or healthy nutrition and physical activity, could be useful strategies for helping them deal with the distress caused by stigma and discrimination. Primary prevention might also include home visits for lesbian, bisexual, and transgender first-time parents as part of a community's maternal home visiting program, or parenting classes for gay, bisexual, and transgender fathers advertised through the LGBTQ2S community newspapers and community groups. LGBTQ2S-inclusive sexual health education for secondary school students, as well as for young adults, that includes accurate information specific to sexual practices of LGBTQ2S youth may help prevent unintended pregnancy and STIs (Doull et al., 2017).

YES, BUT WHY?

Stigma, Violence, and Mental Health Inequities for Transgender Youth

What?

Transgender youth in Canada experience much higher prevalence of stress, depressed mood, self-harm, suicidal ideation, and suicide attempts than similar-age populations of cisgender adolescents (Veale, Watson, Peter, & Saewyc, 2017). For example, in a national survey of transgender youth aged 14–18 across Canada, 65% reported serious suicidal thought in the past 12 months, compared to only 13% of cisgender adolescents the same age, and 36% of trans youth reported at least one suicide attempt compared to 6.5% of cisgender youth.

So What?

Stigma and discrimination play a key role in the health of transgender youth. When most of society is structured around gender and expectations about what boys and girls, men and women are like, those who do not fit those expectations, whether transmen, transwomen, or non-binary people, face stigma, rejection, and even violence (what has been called *enacted stigma*). The same national Canadian Trans Youth Health Survey found that in the past year, 70% had experienced sexual harassment, 69% said someone had said something negative about their gender identity, one in three had been cyberbullied, and 36% had been threatened or physically assaulted (Veale et al., 2015). A history of exposure to violence is strongly linked to emotional distress and mental health problems, including suicide attempts in the general population; one study of adolescents in British Columbia suggested that if we could eliminate all forms of violence and abuse, we could reduce suicide attempts by 75% (Saewyc & Chen, 2013). Part of what explains the higher rates of mental health issues is not just violence exposure but lack of social support: transgender youth often have lower levels family acceptance and support, school belonging, or supportive friends. Without these, trans youth who report high levels of enacted stigma have a 72% probability of suicide attempt; but when they have high levels of these social supports, even when they are experiencing violence, their probability of suicide attempt drops to 25%. If they do not experience violence and bullying but have high levels of family and friend support, their risk of suicide attempt drops to 7%.

Now What?

Reducing enacted stigma *and* promoting supportive families, safe and inclusive schools, and helpful friends for transgender youth are key strategies to promote better mental health. The Canadian Human Rights Code recently added protection from discrimination because of gender identity and expression to the list, and most of the provinces and territories have similar protections in their provincial human rights law. CHNs can help educate communities, transgender youth, and their families about their rights and can work to reduce stigma and discrimination toward transgender individuals in communities. They can work with families to increase their support for their trans or non-binary adolescent through facilitating access to gender-affirming health care as well as providing important information on the link between family rejection and mental health issues. To create safer and more inclusive schools, and foster increased peer support, nurses can advocate for LGBTQ2S-inclusive policies. They can also sponsor gender and sexuality alliances, which are school-based social justice and social support clubs for LGBTQ2S students and their heterosexual and cisgender allies. Both of these strategies are linked to lower rates of suicidal ideation and attempts for LGBTQ2S youth (Saewyc, Konishi, Rose, & Homma, 2014).

Standards of Practice Fulfilled

#6 Health Equity
- Advocates for healthy public policy and social justice by participating in legislative and policy-making activities that influence determinants of health and access to services (CHNC, 2019, revised).

At the secondary prevention level, CHNs might screen for hypertension among older LGBTQ2S people at a local LGBTQ2S community centre or provide counselling and testing for STIs, including HIV, for men, women, and trans people. Given transgender people's expressed concerns about stigmatizing health care, they may not get regular screening for health issues. CHNs could engage in outreach to the transgender community with information about mammograms and Pap smears or testicular and prostate exams, using trans-sensitive language, and offer referrals to trans-friendly service providers. Smoking cessation programs for LGBTQ2S youth and young adults may help prevent cardiovascular problems or cancers later in life. Screening for family violence or intimate partner violence, for suicidal ideation, or for substance use and abuse can be incorporated into any confidential health care interactions, although it would be important to have a list of referrals for LGBTQ2S-welcoming services for these issues.

Tertiary prevention approaches can include interventions to help HIV-positive LGBTQ2S people with medication adherence, as well as referrals to appropriate healthcare services to manage the side effects from some HIV medication regimens.

Locating LGBTQ2S-specific substance abuse treatment programs that attend to societal stigma and unaddressed trauma may be needed for effective support. If the community does not have such services, CHNs may need to advocate for the development of appropriate programs. Many of the tertiary prevention interventions for chronic health conditions—such as supporting effective self-care among people with diabetes, or strategies for managing depression, or exercise programs for people with arthritis or after cardiac bypass surgery—would all be relevant for older members of the LGBTQ2S community. However, outreach for services may need to take place within LGBTQ2S venues. By offering services to targeted groups, CHNs may encourage access to health information and care that otherwise may be missed due to stigma.

Quaternary prevention is relevant for CHNs supporting transgender clients because there is a definite risk of over-medicalization. For example, when very young children express persistent gender non-conforming behaviours, some parents may bring them to their primary-care clinic out of worry. However, until puberty, there is no recommended clinical treatment, just reassuring parents and supporting the child in gender exploration, including possible social transition, which does not require medical care. Likewise, in some regions, transgender youth and adults are required to complete gender-affirming surgery (including sterilization) to change their legal documents such as passports or driver's licences, but if given the choice, some will not want surgery. Nurses can help advocate to change laws and policy to better support trans people.

CASE STUDY

You are a CHN in a child and youth health service, and you are assigned as a school nurse in a local high school. During a school health committee meeting, the vice-principal says some students want to start a gender-sexuality alliance (GSA). They want to make the school climate safer, and they need a staff sponsor for their club. The health committee thinks you would be the best professional to support the GSA. However, the committee's parent representative voices a concern about opposition to a GSA from some parents; some believe this would cause distress for heterosexual students. She notes that a nearby school district had public protests when it adopted an LGBTQ2S inclusive policy and started GSAs in its schools. The principal, vice-principal, and other committee members look to you expectantly.

Discussion Questions

1. What support or assistance might you want to request from the school health committee, or the vice-principal and principal, in taking on this role?

2. What health information and skills-building support do you think the students starting the GSA will want or need?

3. How would you suggest engaging with parents before a GSA becomes a controversy? Or after there is opposition?

CONCLUSION

The diverse populations of LGBTQ2S people in Canada experience an array of health inequities that may be addressed with improved outreach and LGBTQ2S-inclusive approaches. Culturally safe care that respects and acknowledges sexual orientation and gender diversity, and is sensitive to clients' prior experiences of stigma in health care, can promote the health of LGBTQ2S people across the lifespan. It is imperative that CHNs engage with LGBTQ2S populations in a culturally safe way, not only to reduce inequities in health status but also to actively work to promote the health of this population.

KEY TERMS

biphobia (p. 382)
bisexuality (p. 380)
cisgender (p. 381)
cissexism (p. 382)
coming out (p. 381)
gender diverse (p. 381)
gender identity (p. 381)
heterosexism (p. 382)
heterosexuality (p. 380)
homophobia (p. 382)
homosexuality (p. 380)
internalized homophobia (p. 382)
LGBTQ2S (p. 381)
pansexual (p. 380)
physiological sex (p. 381)
queer (p. 381)
transgender (p. 381)
transphobia (p. 382)
Two Spirit (p. 381)

STUDY QUESTIONS

1. How are homophobia, biphobia, or transphobia usually enacted?

2. What are some of the risks of being neutral about sexual orientation or gender identity as a nurse or other health care provider?

3. Why is internalized homophobia a threat to general well-being?

4. What are some of the special health inequities experienced by LGBTQ2S adolescents?

5. When is the time of highest risk of suicide for LGBTQ2S youth?

6. What are some of the health issues of LGBTQ2S adults?

7. How can we make health care settings safer and more supportive for their gay, lesbian, bisexual, transgender, and Two Spirit clients?

8. How can nurses work within their communities to support LGBTQ2S populations?

9. What can you as a school nurse contribute to the health and well-being of LGBTQ2S youth?

10. What are issues for LGBTQ2S youth of colour or of minority social groups?

INDIVIDUAL CRITICAL-THINKING EXERCISES

1. What is your belief about sexual orientation? Do you think it is genetic or a learned phenomenon (i.e., nature or nurture)? What factors in your life may have influenced your thinking?

2. A client discloses to you that she is a lesbian. Do you enter this into her chart or tell other members of the health team about this? Why or why not?

3. How would you address a transgender client who has male genitalia but dresses as a woman?

4. What are your feelings regarding caring for a patient with HIV/AIDS? What are your ethical responsibilities regarding caring for such a patient? You may find it helpful to draw upon the CNA Code of Ethics when thinking about these questions.

5. What, if any, ethical issues can arise from refusing to care for a patient with HIV/AIDS?

6. Do you think that LGBTQ2S people should have access to specialized clinics for their health care? Why or why not?

GROUP CRITICAL-THINKING EXERCISES

1. Identify homophobic, biphobic, transphobic, or heterosexist attitudes that you have witnessed as a student at the university and during your clinical experiences. How did you deal with these?

2. Do you think that a LGBTQ2S should be "out" in the workplace? Why or why not?

3. A client expresses discomfort with being cared for by one of your colleagues who is LGBTQ2S. How do you think you and the clinical setting should respond? Would your response be different if the patient had expressed discomfort with being cared for by a nurse of colour? Or a nurse who is Jewish, Muslim, or Sikh?

REFERENCES

Balsam, K., Huang, B., Fieland, K., Simoni, J., & Walters, K. (2004). Culture, trauma, and wellness: A comparison of heterosexual and lesbian, gay, bisexual, and two-spirit Native Americans. *Cultural Diversity and Ethnic Minority Psychology, 10*(3), 287–301.

Bauer, G. R., Scheim, A. I., Deutsch, M. B., & Cassarella, C. (2014). Reported emergency department avoidance, use, and experiences of transgender persons in Ontario, Canada: Results from a respondent-driven sampling survey. *Annals of Emergency Medicine, 63*(6), 713–720. http://dx.doi.org/10.1016/j.annemergmed.2013.09.027

Boehmer, U., & Case, P. (2004). Physicians don't ask, sometimes patients tell: Disclosure of sexual orientation among women with breast carcinoma. *Cancer, 101*(8), 1882–1889.

Brennan, D. J., Ross, L. E., Dobinson, C., Veldhuizen, S., & Steele, L. S. (2010). Men's sexual orientation and health in Canada. *Canadian Journal of Public Health, 101*(3), 255–258.

Brotman, S., Ryan, B., Jalbert, Y., & Rowe, B. (2002). The impact of coming out on health and health care access: The experiences of gay, lesbian, bisexual and Two-Spirit people. *Journal of Health and Social Policy, 15*(1), 1–29.

Calzo, J. P., Blashill, A. J., Brown, T. A., & Argenal, R. L. (2017). Eating disorders and disordered weight and shape control behaviors in sexual minority populations. *Current Psychiatry Reports, 19*(8), 49.

Clark, B., Veale, J., Greyson, D., & Saewyc, E. (2017). Primary care access and foregone care: A survey of transgender adolescents and young adults. *Family Practice, 35*(3), 302–306. doi:10.1093/fampra/cmx112

Community Health Nurses of Canada (CHNC). (2019, revised). *Canadian community health nursing: Professional practice model and standards of practice* (ISBN 978-0-9733774-5-3). Retrieved from http://www.chnig.org/wp-content/uploads/2016/02/chnc-standards.pdf

Corbett, S. L., Frecker, H. M., Shapiro, H. M., & Yudin, M. H. (2013). Access to fertility services for lesbian women in Canada. *Fertility and Sterility, 100*(4), 1077–1080.

Doull, M., Wolowic, J., Saewyc, E., Rosario, M., Prescott, T., & Ybarra, M. (2017 online in advance of print). Why girls choose not to use barriers to prevent STI transmission during female-to-female sex. *Journal of Adolescent Health.* doi: 10.1016/j.jadohealth.2017.10.005

Eliason, M. J. (1997). The prevalence and nature of biphobia in heterosexual undergraduate students. *Archives of Sexual Behavior 26*(3), 317–326.

Frederick, T. J., Ross, L. E., Bruno, T. L., & Erickson, T. G. (2011). Exploring gender and sexual minority status among street-involved youth. *Vulnerable Children and Youth Studies, 6*(2), 166–183.

Friedman, M. S., Marshal, M. P., Guadamuz, T. E., Wei, C., Saewyc, E., Wong, C. F., & Stall, R. (2011). A meta-analysis to examine disparities in childhood sexual abuse, parental physical abuse, and peer victimization among sexual minority and non-sexual minority individuals. *American Journal of Public Health, 101*(81), 1481–1494. doi:10.2105/AJPH.2009.190009

Grossman, A., & D'Augelli, A. (2006). Transgender youth: Invisible and vulnerable. *Journal of Homosexuality, 51*(1), 111–128.

Herek, G. M., Cogan, J. C., Gillis, J. R., & Glunt, E. K. (1998). Correlates of internalized homophobia in a community sample of lesbians and gay men. *Journal of the Gay and Lesbian Medical Association, 2*(1), 17–26.

Hunt, S. (2015). Embodying self-determination: Beyond the gender binary. In M. Greenwood, S. de Leuw, N. M. Lindsay, & C. Reading (Eds.), *Determinants of Indigenous peoples' health in Canada*. Toronto, ON: Canadian Scholars' Press.

Igartua, K., Gill, K., & Montoro, R. (2003). Internalized homophobia: A factor in depression, anxiety, and suicide in the gay and lesbian population. *Canadian Journal of Community Mental Health, 22*(2), 15–30.

Meyer, I. (2003). Prejudice, social stress, and mental health in lesbian, gay, and bisexual populations: Conceptual issues and research evidence. *Psychological Bulletin, 129*(5), 674–697.

Mustanski, B. S., Chivers, M. L., & Bailey, J. M. (2002). A critical review of recent biological research on human sexual orientation. *Annual Review of Sex Research, 13,* 89–140.

Norton, J. (1997). "Brain says you're a girl, but I think you're a sissy boy": Cultural origins of transphobia. *Journal of Gay, Lesbian and Bisexual Identity, 2*(2), 139–164.

Oxford English Dictionary, 2nd Edition. (1993). Oxford University Press.

Pan American Health Organization/World Health Organization. (2012). *"Cures" for an illness that does not exist. Purported therapies aimed at changing sexual orientation lack medical justification and are ethically unacceptable.* Retrieved from http://www.paho.org/hq/index.php?option=com_content&view=article&id=6803&Itemid=1926

Parks, C., Hughes, T., & Matthews, A. (2004). Race/ethnicity and sexual orientation: Intersecting identities. *Cultural Diversity and Ethnic Minority Psychology, 10*(3), 241–254.

Poon, C., Saewyc, E., & Chen, W. (2011). Enacted stigma, problem substance use, and protective factors among Asian sexual minority youth in British Columbia. *Canadian Journal of Community Mental Health, 30*(2), 47–64.

Rotondi Khobzi, N., Bauer, G. R., Travers, R., Travers, A., Scanlon, K., & Kaay, M. (2011a). Depression in male-to-female transgender Ontarians: Results from the Trans PULSE Project. *Canadian Journal of Community Mental Health, 30*(2), 113–133.

Rotondi Khobzi, N., Bauer, G. R., Scanlon, K., Kaay, M., Travers, R., & Travers, A. (2011b). Prevalence of and risk and protective factors for depression in female-to-male transgender Ontarians: Trans PULSE Project. *Canadian Journal of Community Mental Health, 30*(2), 135–155.

Ryan, C., Huebner, D., Diaz, R. M., & Sanchez, J. (2009). Family rejection as a predictor of negative health outcomes in white and Latino lesbian, gay, and bisexual young adults. *Pediatrics, 123*(1), 346–352.

Ryan, C., Russell, S. T., Huebner, D., Diaz, R. M., & Sanchez, J. (2010). Family acceptance in adolescence and the health of young adults. *Journal of Child and Adolescent Psychiatric Nursing, 23*(4), 205–213. doi:10.1111/j.1744-6171.2010.00246.x

Saewyc, E. M. (2011). Research on adolescent sexual orientation: Development, health disparities, stigma and resilience. *Journal of Research on Adolescence, 21*(1), 256–272.

Saewyc, E. M. (2017). Respecting variations in embodiment as well as gender: Beyond the presumed "binary" of sex. *Nursing Inquiry, 25,* e12184. doi: 10.1111/nin.12184

Saewyc, E., Homma, Y., Hitchcock, C., & Prior, J. (2012). Sexual orientation, stigma, and menarche among adolescent girls in Canada. *Journal of Adolescent Health, 50*(2), S28.

Saewyc, E., & Chen, W. (2013). To what extent can adolescent suicide attempts be attributed to violence exposure? A population-based study from Western Canada. *Canadian Journal of Community Mental Health, 31*(1), 72–94. doi:10.7870/cjcmh-2013-007. PMC4690726.

Saewyc, E., Clark, T., Barney, L., Brunanski, D., & Homma, Y. (2013). Enacted stigma and HIV risk behaviors among sexual minority Indigenous youth in Canada, New Zealand, and the United States. *Pimatisiwin: A Journal of Aboriginal and Indigenous Community Health, 11*(3), 411–420. PMC4716820.

Saewyc, E., Konishi, C., Rose, H., & Homma, Y. (2014). School-based strategies to reduce suicidal ideation and attempts among lesbian, gay, and bisexual, as well as heterosexual adolescents in western Canada. *International Journal of Child, Youth and Family Studies, 5*(1), 89–112.

Saewyc, E. M., Poon, C., Homma, Y., & Skay, C. L. (2008). Stigma management? The links between enacted stigma and teen pregnancy trends among gay, lesbian and bisexual students in British Columbia. *Canadian Journal of Human Sexuality, 17*(3), 123–131. PMC2655734

Saewyc, E., Richens, K., Skay, C. L., Reis, E., Poon, C., & Murphy, A. (2006). Sexual orientation, sexual abuse, and HIV-risk behaviours among adolescents in the Pacific Northwest. *American Journal of Public Health, 96*(6), 1104–1110. doi:10.2105/AJPH.2005.065870

Saewyc, E., Mounsey, B., Tourand, J., Brunanski, D., Kirk, D., McNeil, J., . . . Clark, N. (2017). Homeless and street-involved Indigenous LGBTQ2S youth in British Columbia: Intersectionality, challenges, resilience, and cues for action. In I. A. Abramovich & J. Shelton (Eds.), *Where am I going to go? Intersectional approaches to ending LGBTQ2S youth homelessness in Canada & the U.S.* Toronto, ON: Canadian Observatory on Homelessness, York University.

Schilt, K., & Westbrook, L. (2009). Doing gender, doing heteronormativity: "Gender normals," transgender people, and the social maintenance of heterosexuality. *Gender & Society, 23,* 440–464.

Statistics Canada. (2015). *Same sex couples and sexual orientation . . . by the numbers.* Ottawa, ON: Author. Retrieved from https://www.statcan.gc.ca/eng/dai/smr08/2015/smr08_203_2015

Steele, L. S., Ross, L. E., Dobinson, C., Veldhuizen, S., & Tinmouth, J. M. (2009). Women's sexual orientation and health: Results from a Canadian population-based study. *Women & Health, 49*(5), 353–367. doi:10.1080/03630240903238685

Taylor, C., & Peter, T. (2011). "We are not aliens, we're people, and we have rights." Canadian human rights discourse and high school climate for LGBTQ students. *Canadian Review of Sociology, 48*(3), 275–312.

Travers, R., Newton, H., & Munro, L. (2011). "Because it was expected": Heterosexism as a determinant of adolescent pregnancy among sexually diverse youth. *Canadian Journal of Community Mental Health, 30*(2), 65–79.

Veale, J., Saewyc, E., Frohard-Dourlent, H., Dobson, S., Clark, B., & the Canadian Trans Youth Health Survey Research Group. (2015). *Being safe, being me: Results of the Canadian Trans Youth Health Survey.* Vancouver, BC: Stigma and Resilience Among Vulnerable Youth Centre, School of Nursing, University of British Columbia.

Veale, J., Watson, R. J., Adjei, J., Saewyc, E. (2016). Prevalence of pregnancy involvement among Canadian transgender youth and its relation to mental health, sexual health, and gender identity. *International Journal of Transgenderism, 17*(3–4), 107–113. doi:10.1080/15532739.2016.1216345

Veale, J., Watson, R., Peter, T., & Saewyc, E. (2017). Mental health disparities among Canadian transgender youth. *Journal of Adolescent Health, 60*(1), 44–49. doi:10.1016/j.jadohealth.2016.09.014

Veenstra, G. (2011). Race, gender, class, and sexual orientation: Intersecting axes of inequality and self-rated health in Canada. *International Journal of Health Equity, 10*(3), 1–11. doi:10.1186/1475-9276-10-3

Watson, R. J., Veale, J. F., & Saewyc, E. M. (2017). Disordered eating behaviors among transgender youth: Probability profiles from risk and protective factors. *International Journal of Eating Disorders. 50*(5), 512–522. doi:10.1002/eat.22627

Williams-Barnard, C., Mendoza, D., & Shippee-Rice, R. (2001). The lived experience of college student lesbians' encounters with health care providers. *Journal of Holistic Nursing, 19*(2), 127–142.

ABOUT THE AUTHOR

Elizabeth M. Saewyc, RN, PhD, PHN(Minn.), FSAHM, FCAHS, FAAN, is Professor and Director of the School of Nursing at the University of British Columbia in Vancouver. She held a Canadian Institutes of Health Research/Public Health Agency of Canada national Chair in Applied Public Health Research focused on youth health. She has worked as a public health nurse in both the United States (in Seattle and Minnesota) and Canada, and has taught community health nursing for more than 15 years. She also heads the UBC Stigma and Resilience among Vulnerable Youth Centre for research. Dr. Saewyc conducts research about the health issues of vulnerable populations, including LGBT2S youth, and she has been consulted about school nursing and public health nursing roles provincially, nationally, and internationally, including most recently with the World Health Organization.

Older Adult Health

Christine McPherson and Karen Curry

CHAPTER 21

Source: Sirtravelalot/Shutterstock

INTRODUCTION

Community health nurses (CHNs) play a vital role in promoting the health and well-ness of older adults. The varied and complex needs of this sector of the population bring CHNs in contact with older persons across settings. In this chapter, the role and competencies of the CHN are discussed in relation to key issues that affect the health of older persons. Recognition is given to the broader social, cultural, and politi-cal context that shapes the health and well-being of older persons, with an emphasis on equity in health and health care using a social-justice lens. Particular attention is given to the intersect between older adults and other sectors within society, such as the Indigenous sector and other populations that, because of their circumstances, may be vulnerable. The chapter concludes with a discussion of capacity building, including empowerment, research, policy to promote equity in health and health care for older adults, and future challenges and opportunities. Throughout this chapter, the terms "older adult or adults" or "older person or persons" are used interchangeably rather than terms such as "elderly," "old," and "pensioners" that may diminish the value of older persons.

DEMOGRAPHIC TRENDS IN AGING

Increased life expectancy and lower fertility rates have resulted in a global trend toward **population aging**. Though there are country and regional variations in the rates of growth, most countries have witnessed a substantial increase in the numbers of older people (United Nations, 2017). Current estimates, as shown in Figure 21.1, indicate that Europe and North America have the highest proportions of people 60 years and over, and these figures are predicted to increase over the next few decades. According to the World Population Prospects: The 2017 Revision, the number of

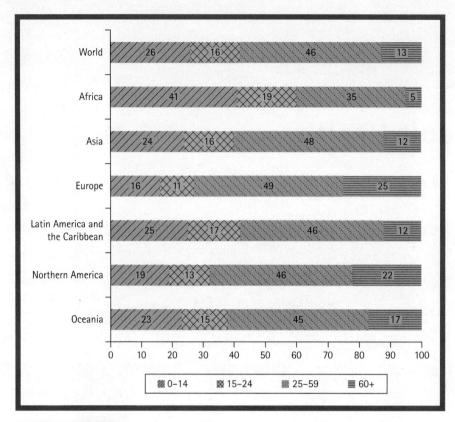

FIGURE 21.1 Percentage of Population in Broad Age Groups for the World and by Region, 2017

Source: Adapted from Figure 8, Page 10 of United Nations, Department of Economic and Social Affairs, Population Division (2017). *World Population Prospects: The 2017 Revision.* New York, NY: United Nations.

persons 60 years and above is set to double, rising from 962 million in 2017 to 2.1 billion in 2050 (United Nations, 2017). The cohort of individuals 80 years and over is one of the most rapidly growing sectors; numbers of this population are expected to triple from 137 million in 2017 to 425 million in 2050 (United Nations, 2017). In Canada, about 750 000 individuals are aged 85 and older, and that number rose by almost 20% from 2011 to 2016 (Statistics Canada, 2017a).

The growth in the numbers of older persons is fuelled in part by the entry into retirement age of the cohort born during the post-war boom (1945–1965), referred to as the "**baby boomers.**" In Canada, the baby boomers currently account for two out of every five Canadians aged 65 and older (40.9%) (Statistics Canada, 2017b), and this will increase as the baby boomers continue to move into retirement age. As of July 2017, there were 6 195 544 Canadians, or one out of every six people in the population, 65 years or older (Statistics Canada, 2017b). By the year 2036, this number is expected to increase to 10.4 million; that is, one in four Canadians will be over the age of 65 (Statistics Canada, 2015). In spite of this, the migration of people to Canada has kept the country relatively "young" compared to other developed countries (Statistics Canada, 2017b), and there is considerable variation in the distribution of older persons across the county. The Atlantic provinces have the highest percentage of people 65 years and older and Alberta one of the lowest.

THE SOCIAL CONTEXT OF AGING

Societal Attitudes toward Aging

Understanding demographic patterns and trends in population aging is crucial for health care planning and policy development to ensure the health and social needs of the older segment of the population are met. At the same time, these demographic trends have prompted catastrophic predictions about out-of-control health care expenditure and limited resources, based on the premise that older persons are frail and excessive users of health care services. Such views perpetuate negative stereotypes of older adults as a homogenous group whose dependency on the rest of the population makes them a burden (Ontario Human Rights Commission, 2013). Negative stereotypes permeate across all levels of society and are ever present in modern media, serving to discriminate against individuals based solely on their age (referred to as **ageism**) (Angus & Reeve, 2006). Although physiological changes occur over time (referred to as **biological aging**) and increase the prevalence of chronic disease, functional, and sensory deficits in older adults (Masoro & Austad, 2005), dependency and frailty do not define this population. Many older adults rate their health as good or excellent (Public Health Agency of Canada [PHAC], 2017a). At the same time, the notion of baby boomers as healthier than previous generations due their increased prosperity, education, and lower smoking rates has to be tempered against the health risks associated with increases in body mass index and levels of obesity (Badley, Canizares, Perruccio, Hogg-Johnson, & Gignac, 2015). Further, not all "baby boomers" have profited from the same access to the social determinants of health. Stereotypes, though positive, do not reflect the experiences of older persons and are unhelpful. CHNs must reflect on their own beliefs about aging and advocate for the rights of older adults.

Diversity and the Social Equity

Chronological age is typically the sole defining marker distinguishing older persons. Global differences in what constitutes old age reflect variations in life expectancy. Canada, like much of the Western world, defines old age as 65 years from birth. This is a time when Canadians typically retire, and pensions become accessible. However, age is a crude marker for functional abilities and health. It is clear that biological aging occurs, and its effects become more evident in advanced age. Individuals over 85 years, for example, are more likely to have multiple chronic illnesses and experience greater functional limitations than older adults under the age of 85 (Denton & Spencer, 2010). However, it is important to note that within the older population there is considerable variability in health and functioning. Nowhere is this more evident than in individuals who are homeless or incarcerated, where biological aging is increased (**accelerated aging**) by 10–15 years due to substance abuse, poor diet, and unhealthy lifestyle (Brown et al., 2017; Office of the Correctional Investigator, 2013).

Viewing older adults as a homogenous group does little to acknowledge the diversity with respect to their identities (e.g., ethnicity, culture, gender, sexual orientation, language) and socioeconomic status in society. For the most part, older adults reflect the heterogeneity observed in adults below the age of 65. It is only at an advanced age that gender differences emerge, as women over 85 outnumber men in the same age group (Statistics Canada, 2017a). Canada's older population is ethnoculturally diverse, and this is expected to increase (National Advisory Council on Aging [NACA], 2005). Older persons from ethnocultural minorities may face barriers to health and access to care because of cultural and language differences that can marginalize them (NACA, 2005). The unique needs of official language minorities, immigrants, and First Nation, Métis, and Inuit populations are discussed later in this chapter.

COMMUNITY GERONTOLOGICAL PRACTICE AND COMMUNITY HEALTH NURSING

Gerontological nursing is a complex specialty of nursing care. CHNs must have competencies in the care of older persons and appreciate how health and illness can impact the quality of life of older adults and their families. The Canadian Gerontological Nursing Association's competencies and standards of practice for nurses, states,

> Gerontological nursing is a dynamic interaction between the client and nurse to achieve health and well-being. The client and the nurse both contribute to the interaction. Clients bring their unique experiences, personal knowledge, and expertise about themselves whereas nurses bring their specific body of knowledge of gerontology and geriatrics, their skills and the art and science of nursing. The historical and current social and cultural climates, political influence and values of the community and society also influence the interaction. (Canadian Gerontological Nursing Association, 2010, p. 7)

The community context is unique to tertiary settings (discussed in Chapter 5). CHNs' scope of practice in the community spans the continuum of care and embraces public health nursing (see Chapter 4) and home health nursing (see Chapter 5) competencies and approaches to care.

CHNs collaborate with older adults and communities to achieve optimal health and well-being by integrating complex knowledge sources such as the social determinants of health, the Population Health Promotion Model, the Community Health Nurses of Canada (CHNC) Standards of Practice (2018), the principles of primary health care, and evidence-informed practice. Using a social-justice lens, CHNs aim to address social and environmental factors that can impact health at various levels (individual, family, and community). For example, CHNs create and support **age-friendly communities** to make environments inclusive of older adults, increase access to the determinants of health, and redress inequity.

A home health nursing approach focuses on maintenance of health, restoration, and palliation. The CHNC Home Health Nursing Competencies (2010) incorporate core home care competencies. CHNs provide home visits to older adults, support family members, or focus on a community's health. CHNs use a strength-based approach to promote independence and autonomy to engage older adults in decision making and self-management of their health and illness (Rapp, Pettus, & Goscha, 2006).

HEALTH PROMOTION, DISEASE PREVENTION, CHRONIC ILLNESS MANAGEMENT, AND CARE AT THE END OF LIFE

Health care for older adults in the community spans the continuum of care, incorporating health promotion, illness and injury prevention, maintenance, rehabilitation, chronic disease management, and end-of-life care. CHNs help older adults and their families to navigate the health care system and facilitate their access to health care determinants and services.

Age-Friendly Communities and Aging-in-Place

Age-friendly communities (see Figure 21.2) facilitate **aging-in-place** by providing an environment that supports older persons to remain independent and at home. The majority of older adults reside in the community; only 8% live in institutions (Statistics Canada, 2012a). CHNs can help support older persons to remain independent and to live in the place they prefer by assessing their needs and identifying services. With changes in older adults' health and functioning or circumstances, needs can alter over time. In-home services such as home care and day hospital care can support individuals to remain in their homes. (See Chapter 5.) Facility-based long-term care may be another option. (See Chapter 25.) CHNs working in home care have a central role in coordinating and providing services to older persons and families.

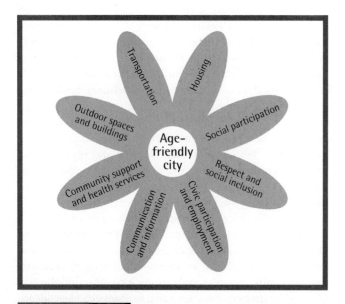

FIGURE 21.2 Eight Domains of Age-Friendly Communities

Source: Reprinted from *Global Age-friendly Cities: A Guide.* Copyright © 2007 with permission of World Health Organization.

Transportation Is One of Older Adults' Greatest Community-Based Needs (Canadian Home Care Association [CHCA], 2016)

What?

In both rural and urban communities, older persons who want to remain in their homes and be active in their communities need transportation to access services and activities. Driving gives older people independence to take part in activities outside the home, shopping, and access to health and community care services. The type and frequency of the use of transportation are shown to impact older adults' level of engagement in social activities and community programs (Turcotte, 2012). Although age is not a determinant of a person's ability to drive, chronic and acute health conditions, medication side effects, and functional limitations can be (Turcotte, 2012). Public transportation, volunteers, family members, friends, and neighbours can be alternatives when driving or access to a vehicle is not possible.

So What?

Exploring alternative modes of transportation and services to serve Canada's aging population is a priority for creating age-friendly communities and supporting policies for older adults to age-in-place. Affordable transportation is not available in an equitable manner across Canada. Public transportation is more readily available in urban centres and can include bus, rail, subway, and taxi services. However, options for older adults in rural settings are limited and services less frequent (Turcotte, 2012). As health care budgets grow, many provinces are looking to work collaboratively across sectors to fund community services to help older adults remain in their homes. The integration of home and community services is a critical area identified in the Canadian Home Care Association's *Better Home Care Now* report (CHCA, 2016).

Now What?

To support access to transportation programs, CHNs need to be aware of the transportation services in their communities. CHNs can explore options with individuals such as public transport and volunteer services to support their needs. At the community, provincial, and national levels, CHNs can facilitate intersectoral collaborations to develop, implement, and evaluate innovative solutions to address issues of access. Research and environmental assessments can inform CHNs, advocacy and strategies to address transportation needs. Engaging older adults and advocacy groups when planning new transportation initiatives or programs will ensure policies and services are relevant (Lehning, 2012).

Physical Activity and Fall Prevention

Being physically active can increase mobility and help maintain functional independence, bone health, an overall feeling of well-being, and decrease the risk of premature death (Canadian Society of Exercise Physiology [CSEP], 2013). The CSEP (2013) recommends that adults over 65 include 150 minutes of moderate or vigorous activity/week in at least 10-minute time frames, with guidelines adapted to suit people with specific needs such as those with Parkinson's disease and multiple sclerosis. An understanding of barriers to physical activity is critical in the development of health promotion strategies (Physical Activity Resource Centre [PARC], 2013):

- Barriers at the individual level: Health (e.g., chronic conditions, symptoms, and functional limitations), motivation, and time
- Barriers to access: Limited resources, lack of opportunities, cost, and environmental factors (e.g., weather, transport, and safety)

CHNs can promote physical activity in older adults by providing information on the benefits of exercise and facilitating environments to encourage them to be physically active. CHNs need an awareness of events and programs in their communities and those suited to older adults with particular needs, such as aquafit classes for individuals with arthritis or rehabilitation needs following cerebrovascular accident (Photo 21.1). To promote physical activity, CHNs can partner with other health professionals and community organizations to develop opportunities for active living for older adults. (See Canadian Research 21.1.) The Physical Activity Promotion for Older Adults: A Step-by-Step Guide is a helpful tool to assist CHNs in their efforts (PARC, 2013).

A benefit of physical activity in older persons is fall prevention. Falls are the leading cause of injury and injury-related hospitalizations in older persons and can have devastating effects on their health and well-being (PHAC, 2014). The consequences of falls also create a significant burden on the health care system. Fall prevention strategies are assessed as part of the Qmentum Accreditation Program (Accreditation Canada, 2014), and CHNs must follow evidence-informed practices for fall prevention (Registered Nurses Association

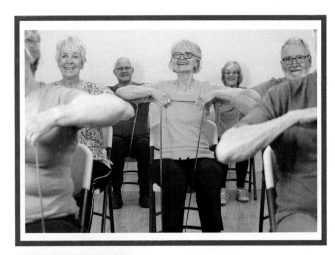

PHOTO 21.1 Group fitness can increase physical activity and social engagement in older adults

Source: SpeedKingz/Shutterstock

CANADIAN RESEARCH 21.1

Better strength, better balance! Partnering to deliver a fall prevention program for older adults (Taing & McKay, 2017)

In this research paper, two CHNs describe their experiences implementing and evaluating the Better Strength, Better Balance! (BSBB) program, a fall prevention exercise and education program. The BSBB program was developed to promote regular physical activity in older adults as recommended by Canadian Physical Activity Guidelines, to increase awareness of behaviours to reduce the risk of falls, and to address barriers to participation in exercise using an equity framework. Working in partnership with community recreation, cultural, and facility services, the BSBB program was delivered to 1539 older adults over two 12-week cycles. Community uptake indicated a keen interest in participation, with high registration rates reflecting an awareness of the BSBB and its accessibility. Evaluation of the BSBB indicated that of the 415 participants surveyed, 94% (n = 389) felt they had better strength and balance, 86% (n = 348) were less worried about falling, 98% (n = 405) intended to continue exercising after the program, and 73% (n = 269) stated they would adopt at least one or more new fall prevention behaviours. All BSBB instructors in the exercise classes noticed a difference in participants' strength, balance, and fitness.

Discussion Questions

1. Identify barriers to physical activity at the personal (individual) level.

2. Identify barriers older adults may face in their access to physical activity.

3. What are the benefits of the approach used by CHNs in the BSBB program?

of Ontario [RNAO], 2017). Fall assessment includes the following:

- Individual risk assessment: History of falls, medication, balance and mobility evaluation, and medical history
- Environmental risk assessment: Identification of hazards (e.g., unattached carpets, inadequate lighting, pets)

Recommendations may include a personal safety device system that can be used to call for help in an emergency—especially important if the older person lives alone. At the community level, CHNs can raise awareness of fall risk and partner with agencies to ensure that environments are age-friendly. (See Canadian Research 21.1.)

Healthy Eating

The *Eating Well with Canada's Food Guide* (Ministry of Health Canada, 2011) provides evidence-informed guidelines on healthy eating. Despite older adults' knowledge of dietary recommendations, they may not be followed (Payette & Shatenstein, 2005). Cost, low vision, altered taste, poor dentition, widowhood, and loneliness are among the factors that contribute to unhealthy food choices (Conklin, Maguire, & Monsivais, 2013; Payette & Shatenstein, 2005). To promote healthy eating, CHNs can perform a nutritional assessment that includes the following:

- Amount and types of food consumed, including what was eaten in the last few days and what meals are planned for the coming days
- Individual preferences, including tastes and cultural and religious food choices
- Accessibility (e.g., transportation to the grocery store, food options, financial costs)
- Knowledge of healthy options, and meal planning and preparation
- Restrictions due to health (e.g., oral health, dietary constraints)

CHNs can tailor advice and resources based on the nutritional assessment. In some instances, referral to a dietitian or a dental visit may be recommended to ensure that issues that impact proper nutrition are addressed. *The Guide to Healthy Eating for Older Adults* provides tips and recipes (Eat Right Ontario, 2012). If access is an issue, home delivery of meals or groceries, group meals at a local older adults club, food banks, and other community services are options. In rural and some Indigenous communities where access to such programs is limited, CHNs can collaborate with community groups to offer group meals and food delivery. Community garden participation and joint programs with youth are new ways to engage older adults in preparing culturally appropriate food.

Medication Safety

Almost all older persons in long-term care facilities and over three-quarters of those living at home consume at least one type of medication (Canadian Institute of Health Information

[CIHI], 2014). In fact, 66% of older persons consume five or more types of medication, known as **polypharmacy** (CIHI, 2014). Polypharmacy increases the risk of non-adherence to prescribed drugs, which can result in adverse drug effects, drug interactions, frequent visits to a primary care provider, and hospitalization (CIHI, 2014). Medication use in older adults is, therefore, a safety concern. CHNs must assess older clients' medication management. An awareness of sensory or cognitive impairments or difficulties with understanding medications is part of this assessment, as are the goals of care, since non-adherence may be a personal choice. To assess medication management, questions should be asked about the time of day a medication is taken, what is done about a missed dose, fear of addiction, adverse effects, and costs. CHNs can organize individual or group sessions to provide information on safe medication use, suggest blister packs or medication organizers, discuss the importance of discarding unused medications, recommend maintenance of an accurate list of drugs, and offer referral to a community pharmacist, as needed.

An essential formal process in medication safety is **medication reconciliation**. The process of medication reconciliation involves the consistent communication of accurate and comprehensive information on medications with individuals, families, and care providers across transitions of care (Institute for Safe Medication Practices Canada [ISMPC], 2014). Medication reconciliation is recognized as a fall prevention strategy (ISMPC, 2014) and is a required organization process for Accreditation Canada (2014), where documentation must demonstrate that this process is followed. (See the following Case Study.)

CASE STUDY

Mrs. McNeil is 80 years old and lives alone in her own two-storey home. Her family lives nearby and helps with maintenance of the house and transportation to medical appointments. Mrs. McNeil has a history of heart disease and congestive heart failure and has been self-managing her medications. She is on five medications, including two metered dose inhalers. After a recent hospital admission for exacerbation of her congestive heart failure, Mrs. McNeil has some forgetfulness and anxiety about her medications. Home care services are referred to help her with medication management. When the CHN arrives for a visit, she finds Mrs. McNeil is very hesitant to accept her help. She states, "I have taken care of myself all my life. I just had a few forgetful spells. I don't think I need nurses interfering with my business."

Discussion Questions

1. What is the first issue the CHN should discuss with Mrs. McNeil?

2. Why is medication self-management important to promote?

3. What resources in the community could the CHN collaborate with to support Mrs. McNeil in managing her medications?

Immunizations

CHNs have an important role in immunization planning and implementation. (See Chapter 12.) CHNs advise older adults on the importance of routine immunizations against vaccine-preventable diseases. Many older adults and health care professionals neglect the need for immunizations in advanced age; yet chronic illness and a weakened immune system may make older adults susceptible to severe illness and death (Fleming & Elliot, 2005). The Public Health Agency of Canada (PHAC, 2017b) recommends that individuals 60 years and over be immunized against diphtheria, tetanus, pertussis, and against herpes zoster (shingles). Individuals 65 years and older should have the pneumococcal vaccine, and specific vaccines may be recommended based on a person's health condition. Regardless, all older adults should be advised to have a yearly influenza vaccination.

Sexual Health

Sex is a normal and healthy part of life. Intimacy may involve sexual intercourse, touch, hugging, holding hands, and emotional closeness. Negative stereotypes about older persons can render them asexual, and issues regarding sexual health can be overlooked (Wilson, 2006). Many older adults enjoy sexual activity more than when they were younger because of feelings of closeness, privacy, and less stress in their lives (Health Canada, 2012; Lindau et al., 2007). Increasing incidence of sexually transmitted infections (STIs) are reported in older adults (PHAC, 2014). Cases of chlamydia and gonorrhea have the highest relative rate increase among women aged 60 years and over. Also, STIs can have long-term impacts, and some, like HIV, are becoming chronic conditions. Older adults often lack information about prevention methods and transmission modes (Canadian AIDS Society, 2013). Underlying health problems more common in older persons, such as diabetes, hypertension, incontinence, arthritis, and the use of certain medications, can alter sexual desire and performance. Older adults may be reticent to talk about sex, especially lesbian, gay, bisexual, transgender, Two Spirit, queer, and questioning individuals, for fear of discrimination. (See Chapter 20.) CHNs should provide advice on sexual health and services in the community using a nonjudgmental approach to facilitate open communication.

Mental Health and Functioning

Depression is the most common mental health condition affecting the older population and can have a detrimental effect on a person's quality of life and those around them (Canadian Coalition for Seniors' Mental Health [CCSMH], 2009). Knowledge of risk factors for depression such as life events (e.g., bereavement, illness, being a family caregiver, and social isolation), previous history of depression, disease, and functional limitations can help in screening, assessment, and treatment (CCSMH, 2009). CHNs need to be aware of how depression is manifested and of barriers to assessment and treatment. CHNs should integrate evidence-informed guidelines specific to older persons in preventing and managing depression (CCSMH, 2009).

Although cognitive impairment in older adults is not inevitable, the prevalence of dementia and the estimated global increase in people expected to develop the disease has led to what is called the *dementia epidemic* (Alzheimer Society of Canada [ASC], 2010). According to the ASC (2010), 15% of older adults have Alzheimer's disease, and the number of Canadians with dementia will double between 2011 and 2031. For the person with dementia, there can be a loss of **personhood** as the gradual decline in cognitive functioning—typical of the most common forms of dementia—can diminish independence and autonomy (Sabat & Harré, 1992). CHNs can promote autonomy by the communication of decisions about care and treatment when the person is competent to make informed decisions through **advance directives**. CHNs have a role in the prevention, early detection, and ongoing support for older adults with dementia and their family caregivers. Preventative efforts focus on risk factors such as healthy eating (Shatenstein et al., 2012), physical activity (Bherer, Erickson, & Liu-Ambrose, 2013), and brain exercises (Nagamatsu, Handy, Hsu, Voss, & Liu-Ambrose, 2012). Identification of individuals most at risk and indicators of cognitive decline such as loss of memory, language, attention, or behavioural or psychological symptoms can signal the need for a physician referral and possible cognitive screening (Canadian Task Force on Preventive Health Care, 2016). CHNs can assist older persons with dementia and their families to navigate and coordinate care options and implement evidence-informed interventions and referrals for appropriate supports such as psychological therapy, peer-led support groups, and educational interventions.

Social Isolation

Social isolation is a significant problem among older adults living in the community and can impact health, quality of life, and well-being. It can lead to depression, loneliness, falls, and hospitalization in about 20% of older adults (Miedema, 2014). The causes of isolation vary from vision and hearing loss, cognitive impairment, and incontinence, to life events such as bereavement (Nicholson, 2012). Research on the impact of social isolation and loneliness identifies that the issues are related but need to be addressed with different interventions (Masi, Chen, Hawkley, & Cacioppo, 2014). Therefore, it is essential for CHNs to be precise in their assessment of older adults' psychosocial functioning for interventions to be effective. To alleviate feelings of isolation, CHNs can provide a link to community resources, local social activities, and support group meetings. (See Chapter 23.) Technology and social media can be a source of social support, especially for individuals who are less mobile or in rural areas. See Photo 21.2. (See Chapter 15.) Half of all older adults are online, and 43% of social media users are adults over the age of 65 (Zickuhr, 2014).

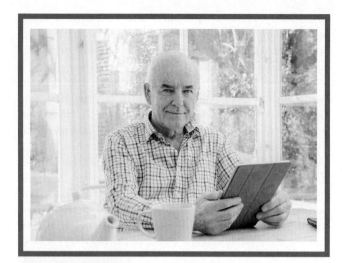

PHOTO 21.2 Technology and social media can be a source of social support and health information for older adults in the community

Source: JohnnyGreig/E+/Getty Images

Elder Abuse

Elder abuse affects up to 10% of older adults in Canada, but very few incidents are reported due to fear of retribution (RNAO, 2014). Forms of elder abuse include physical, sexual, financial, and emotional abuse, and neglect (Government of Canada, 2013). All forms of elder abuse have a negative impact on a person's quality of life (Government of Canada, 2013; RNAO, 2014). CHNs must recognize the signs of elder abuse, including differences in a person's behaviour or appearance, depression, physical injuries or deterioration, and changes in financial resources. Abusers often have power or control over the older adult and can be a partner, family member, friend, or care provider, which can put older persons who are frail, isolated, and dependent at highest risk (RNAO, 2014). CHNs have a responsibility to identify and report any suspicions or confirmed cases of elder abuse to the local police. (See Chapter 28.)

Emergency Preparedness

According to the Canadian Disaster Database, between 2000 and 2017, Canada experienced 136 significant disasters, including floods, wildfires, ice and tropical storms, terrorist incidents, and rioting (Public Safety Canada, 2017). Disruptions to infrastructure and power outages can create difficulties for people to access care and services. (See Chapter 32.) Older adults at highest risk are those with limited functioning, without a caregiver, and receiving intensive treatments such as dialysis, ventilation, intravenous infusions, and oxygen therapy. For these individuals, a plan for supplies and equipment is required to ensure timely intervention. Strategies to support older adults who are at risk include identifying those most vulnerable and developing emergency response plans in collaboration with community agencies and emergency responders to provide care,

equipment, supplies, and services. As a general strategy to help prepare older adults for emergencies, CHNs can advise on the importance of an emergency kit containing bottled water, blankets, a change of clothes, nonperishable foods, cash, and at least a two-week supply of medications (Public Safety Canada, 2012).

Family Caregivers

Family caregivers are family and friends who provide regular unpaid care to support individuals with health and functional limitations that require assistance. The most common reasons for older adults to need family caregiving are **frailty**, dementia, cancer, cardiovascular disease, mental health, neurological conditions, and injury (Statistics Canada, 2012b). Family caregivers provide various types and levels of support, including physical, tangible, emotional, and social support. Canadian health care fiscal restraint and human resources shortages have placed pressure on family caregivers to assume greater responsibilities concerning care (Chappell & Funk, 2011). Although family caregiving can be a rewarding experience, it can also be extremely challenging, negatively impacting family caregivers' mental and physical health (Bookwala, Yee, & Schulz, 2000). CHNs must assess family caregivers' willingness to take on the role. Frank conversations about the nature and extent of the role need to conducted. Preparation to take on the role and an assessment of the family caregiver's ability to cope should be made regularly as he or she adapts to the changing demands of the situation. CHNs can assist with coordination of care and navigation of the health care system and help with accessing resources such as respite services, family caregiver support groups, and equipment. (See Chapter 25.)

Chronic Illness

Chronic diseases such as cardiovascular disease, cancer, respiratory illnesses, and diabetes are prevalent and the primary causes of 60% of mortality (PHAC, 2017a). CHNs must recognize the impact of chronic illness on older adults, such as loss of independence, disengagement, social isolation, immobility, depression, and poor self-esteem. An emphasis of models of care that promote self-management can facilitate independence in chronic disease management. (See Chapter 25.) By adopting preventative and health promotion approaches, CHNs can support older persons with chronic conditions by teaching and providing advice on self-management and preventative and maintenance strategies that can enhance their quality of life. A significant issue facing older persons is **multi-morbidity**, which can render them particularly vulnerable, reducing functioning and quality of life (Denton & Spencer, 2012). A multidisciplinary approach to care is required to ensure that care is comprehensive and coordinated. CHNs have a crucial role in identifying, organizing, and providing care and services in the home and assisting with transitions across settings to optimize continuity in care.

Care at the End of Life

Care at the end of life is an integral part of CHNs' practice in home care with older adults. Meeting the often complex and multifaceted needs of older persons with life-limiting illness and their families requires CHNs to be highly skilled. Multi-morbidity, functional limitations, and the life-limiting diseases that affect older persons such as dementia and frailty can be particularly challenging. Older adults with life-limiting illnesses can benefit from a palliative approach to care where the emphasis is on comfort and support rather than cure. (See Chapter 25.)

In 2016, changes in legislation came into effect with Bill C-14 to make medical assistance in dying (MAiD) legal in Canada. Under the MAiD legalization, individuals meeting specific criteria can request medical assistance to end their lives (Department of Justice, 2016). This change in legislation has resulted in new roles and scopes of practice for CHNs. CHNs need to be aware of their legal and ethical responsibilities concerning MAiD to ensure they respect their clients' autonomy in making this decision and support their care needs and those of family members (Canadian Nurses Association, 2017).

POPULATION GROUPS

Older adults are a heterogeneous group of individuals with different experiences and circumstances. It is critical that CHNs respect individuality by considering the defining factors of culture and the wide range of experiences and contexts in which older adults and CHNs interact.

Official Language Minority

French-speaking older adults living outside the province of Quebec and English-speaking older adults living in Quebec are considered citizens residing in official language minority communities. Many older adults in these communities experience difficulties accessing services and support in their language, thereby augmenting the risk of social isolation (Dupuis-Blanchard, Simard, Gould, & Villalon, 2013; Office of the Commissioner of Official Languages, 2013). Older adults may fear not being able to express themselves correctly during times of health care needs when faced with language and cultural barriers. As a result, older adults may forgo home services and health consultations and delay seeking help. CHNs recognize the importance of language for older adults' health and the need for care to be culturally safe. (See Chapter 9.) CHNs can advocate for the preparation of nurses competent in the official languages and the translation of materials and resources in both official languages.

Rural

Rural, isolated, and remote locations can present certain challenges to older adults. (See Chapter 24.) These challenges, as Keating, Swindle, and Fletcher (2011) identify, are complex and variable across rural communities. Issues related to geographical location in terms of proximity to urban areas and the availability of rural services can limit older adults' access and use of health and social services (Keating et al., 2011). The intersect between location and other issues of rurality such as poverty can render some individuals particularly vulnerable to health disparities and health problems, such as Indigenous peoples living in remote and isolated areas with limited access to the social determinants of health. Research indicates that despite similarities in the general rates of diseases across conditions (e.g., dementias) between urban and rural older adults, there are some significant differences in the rates of depressive symptoms, obesity, and related conditions (e.g., diabetes), with higher rates in rural older adults (Keating et al., 2011). Unhealthy behaviours such as smoking and obesity contribute to higher rates of mortality in rural communities. Living alone, functional limitations, occupational concerns related to financial viability, and inadequate income are associated with depression in rural-dwelling adults (Keating et al., 2011). An appreciation of how community-level influences can affect the health and well-being of older adults, including their inclusion and access to the social determinants of health, is vital for CHNs working with older adults in rural communities. CHNs can foster the opportunities that being part of small communities brings, such as a sense of belonging by encouraging older adults to participate in their communities and by connecting the community and volunteers to provide services such as transport and companionship to older persons. Technologies such as telehealth can be implemented to facilitate access to health, and social media can offer a source of support. (See Chapter 15.)

Indigenous Peoples

Many Indigenous older adults face difficulties in staying healthy. First Nation, Inuit, and Métis older persons live on lower incomes, in less-than-adequate housing, and in poorer health with multiple chronic conditions and disabilities as compared to their non-Indigenous counterparts (Wilson, Rosenberg, Abonyi, & Lovelace, 2010). Obesity, diabetes, and heart disease are prevalent, as are mental health issues. Access and equity remain at the forefront of the problems facing Indigenous peoples as they age (Health Council of Canada, 2013). Addressing the health care needs of older persons who are First Nation, Inuit, and Métis requires an appreciation of their current circumstances and the cultural, historical, and political context in which they are situated. (See Chapter 22.) Being receptive to learning about the experiences of older Indigenous individuals is critical to providing culturally competent care (Richmond & Cook, 2016). Traditional knowledge and medicines in health and healing are an integral part of the culture; however, individual practices may vary. Through open dialogue with older adults and their caregivers, CHNs can provide a therapeutic environment in which to discuss their beliefs and the traditions they follow. Many older First Nation adults live on reserves in remote locations and need to travel to access health care services (Health Council of Canada, 2013). CHNs can advocate for improvements to the environmental and social circumstances of older persons from Indigenous communities to address issues of equity and access.

Immigrants

In general, immigrants are healthier when they arrive in Canada, though this health advantage declines over time (Ng, Wilkins, Gendron, & Berthelot, 2005). There is, however, considerable variation in the health of immigrants depending on their current situation and previous circumstances in their home country, reflecting their access to the social determinants of health and cultural and language barriers once in Canada (National Advisory Council on Aging, 2005). According to Statistics Canada (2010), 50% of new immigrant older adults in the years 2001 to 2009 were unable to speak one of the official languages. Oftentimes, they have had a different life course from older non-immigrants, including poor socioeconomic conditions and life histories involving difficulties such as trauma or torture that contribute to poorer health (Durst, 2005; Edmonston, 2013). In a review of services available to support older adult immigrants, Kilbride (2014) found that mental health, depression, and social isolation were significant issues. Navigating a new society without the necessary language skills left recent older adult immigrants isolated.

Recent older immigrants do not benefit from Old Age Security as they do not meet the legal status and residency requirements of the federal government. Without a private pension or health insurance, they may be disadvantaged in their access to some health services, including prescriptions for medications. Lack of official language skills and access to culturally safe care adds to the challenges faced by some older adults when settling in Canada. CHNs support older adult immigrants by providing guidance on navigating social and health services and how to apply for income supplements if required. Using health promotion and preventive care approaches, CHNs work with individuals, groups, and communities to support immigrants. (See Chapter 9.)

BUILDING CAPACITY

As the first line of contact for older adults and their families, CHNs are well-positioned to identify the needs of the older population. Building capacity means tackling the root causes of health disparities and ensuring that services meet the needs of the community. In this section, empowerment, research, and policy are discussed with an emphasis on capacity building for the future.

Empowerment

Empowerment is a process by which capacity and competence are built. The CHNC defines empowerment as "an actively involved process where people, groups, and communities move towards increased individual and community control, political efficacy, improved quality of community life and social justice" (2008, p. 7). Empowerment is embedded in community partnerships, self-care, self-management, and person- and family-centred care discussed in this chapter, where the philosophy of care and services moves toward persons having greater control over decisions that affect their lives. To do this, older adults need the knowledge, skills, and attitude to feel empowered, and CHNs play an essential role in providing opportunities, mentoring, and leadership to facilitate this process. CHNs must first understand the needs and motivations of older adults, families, and communities to enable goal development, identify opportunities for engagement, and provide sufficient information and skills development. Volunteering in activities such as support groups or advocacy roles on committees are ways of capitalizing on older persons' knowledge and experience. Participation in volunteer work can be meaningful for older persons and promote active aging while at the same time contributing to society.

Research

Research on aging is vital for appreciating heterogeneity in the older population, identifying issues that affect their health and well-being, and informing health care decision making and policies. At the national level, the Canadian Institutes of Health Research (CIHR) remains a major funder of research on aging. The CIHR has an Institute on Aging that focuses on health and wellness of older Canadians, but research relevant to older adults is conducted across the 13 institutes. Current CIHR Institute on Aging research priorities include cognitive impairments, mobility, and healthy and productive work (Canadian Institutes of Health Research, 2017). The CIHR is funding the largest and most comprehensive study on aging— the Canadian Longitudinal Study on Aging (CLSA). The CLSA will follow a random, stratified sample of 50 000 Canadians between 45 and 85 over a 20-year period. The study design will permit researchers to collect information on various aspects of aging that are important for understanding aging and experiences of Canadians as they age (Canadian Longitudinal Study on Aging, 2017). Besides the CIHR, research on aging also occurs at the national, provincial, and local levels through provincial governments (e.g., Ontario Ministry of Health and Long-Term Care), disease-specific associations (e.g., Canadian Cancer Society and Alzheimer Society of Canada), and health care organizations and universities. Researchers use various approaches to the study of aging, but to ensure that the research is relevant and addresses the needs of older persons, it is vital that the voices of older adults be captured. Participatory approaches to research with older persons that incorporate participant–researcher engagement throughout the research process and health care stakeholder involvement enhance the relevance of the research. CHNs are consumers of research as their practice is evidence-informed (see Chapter 10); they are also producers of research, leading research, acting as experts, or collaborating with research teams on projects relevant to community health. CHNs' expertise is also applied in the dissemination of research in knowledge translation to move research into practice.

Public Policy

The Government of Canada has identified three public policy priorities related to aging: public pensions, health care, and caregiving (Echenberg, Gauthier, & Leonard, 2011). Other priorities include community planning, such as age-friendly communities, reframing the labour market for an aging workforce, and affordable medications (Elgersma, Simeone, Roy-César, & Theckedath, 2012; Martin-Matthews, Tamblyn, Keefe, & Gillis, 2009). In fact, the Canadian Public Health Association (2010) identifies policy development as an activity of CHNs for health promotion. (See Chapter 2.) CHNs must voice their opinions to shape public policy development. Examples of CHNs' involvement in policy making include the national strategy plan: *Better Home Care in Canada* and *The Way Forward National Framework*, which aims to make palliative care accessible to all Canadians (Canadian Hospice Palliative Care Association, 2016). Policies impacting older adults include changes in legislation to better support family caregivers (Change Foundation, 2016) and Canada's National Strategy for Alzheimer's Disease and Other Dementias Act (ASC, 2017).

FUTURE CHALLENGES AND OPPORTUNITIES

Population aging creates many challenges and opportunities. Particular attention must be given to address health disparities and ensure that care is culturally safe for the growing ethnocultural diversity in Canada's older population (Légaré, Picard, Martel, & Carrière, 2016). Key issues for CHNs moving forward from a primary health care approach are prevention and maintenance aimed at healthy eating and physical activity to reduce body mass index and associated risks. Other important challenges to older persons' health include fall prevention, emergency response and preparedness, housing, and older workers (Employment and Social Development Canada, 2013). Aging-in-place is likely to remain popular but may necessitate a shift to include other types of housing such as apartment living in older-adult-designated buildings.

The rise in chronic illnesses and multi-morbidity creates situations of complex care in the community. CHNs will need to be knowledgeable and highly skilled in gerontological nursing and home care to meet the demand. Key issues facing older persons, their families, and home care are chronic conditions such as dementia and frailty that restrict a person's independence and compromise autonomy. Aging-in-place for older persons can make them vulnerable to social isolation, mental health issues, and elder abuse, and puts their family caregivers at risk for mental and physical health problems. Measures to support family caregivers such as Employment Insurance Compassionate Care Benefits are limited; moving forward, government will need to develop policies and invest in strategies to assist family caregivers in their role. CHNs play a significant part in the development of innovative solutions to meet growing demand. CHNs have embraced technologies as one solution. Telehealth and e-home care transcend distance and improve access to rural and underserved populations (Ontario Telehealth Network, 2017).

The organization of the health care system remains a significant challenge for an aging population as care is uncoordinated and in silos among acute, chronic, long-term, and home care settings (International Federation on Ageing, 2012). In Canada, home care is absent from the Canada Health Act; therefore, provinces and territories have the responsibility of allocating resources to this sector, resulting in different types of home care programs across the country. Building partnerships across the continuum of care and project management are valued skills for CHNs in their practice as the provincial governments strive to break down silos of care and create evidence-informed, efficient care and services to meet the needs of their communities. Although there are regional variations in the scope of CHNs' practice based on provincial nursing legislation and regulatory body policies, Canada has seen the development and expansion of the scopes of practice of nurse practitioners, registered nurses, and licensed practical nurses/registered practice nurses. The implementation of nurse-practitioner-led clinics and community-based nurse practitioners and registered nurses with prescription rights has improved older adults' access to care. Nurses' advanced practice roles in areas such as gerontology, palliative care, and community health nursing have provided older clients, families, health care providers, and communities with specialists who can build capacity to meet the growing demands on the health care system.

CONCLUSION

This chapter is an overview of community health nursing for older adults. It is not all-encompassing but presents key issues affecting the health and well-being of older adults. Reference is made to specific chapters in the text that provide greater detail on the issues discussed. As the chapter illustrates, community health nursing for older adults incorporates gerontological nursing with public health nursing and home health nursing to meet the diverse needs of the older population across the continuum of care. CHNs working with older adults face many challenges to meet the growing demands on health services. In a health system in constant change, CHNs will need to address issues of inequity in older adult health care in times of fiscal restraint and capitalize on their competencies to adapt to the changing needs of an aging population.

KEY TERMS

accelerated aging   (p. 393)
advance directives   (p. 397)
age-friendly community   (p. 393)
ageism   (p. 393)
aging-in-place   (p. 394)
baby boomers   (p. 392)
biological aging   (p. 393)
elder abuse   (p. 398)
empowerment   (p. 400)
family caregivers   (p. 398)
frailty   (p. 398)
medication reconciliation   (p. 396)
multi-morbidity   (p. 398)
personhood   (p. 397)
polypharmacy   (p. 396)
population aging   (p. 391)

STUDY QUESTIONS

1. Describe sociodemographic trends in aging in Canada.

2. Explain why a social equity approach is important to meet the diverse needs of older adults.

3. Outline the CHN's role from both a public health nursing and a home health nursing approach to the care of older adults.

4. Identify a key issue affecting older adults and the CHN's role in addressing this issue.

5. Explain why knowledge and awareness of the impact of history is essential when working with older First Nation, Inuit, or Métis individuals.

6. List three future challenges or opportunities related to population aging.

INDIVIDUAL CRITICAL-THINKING EXERCISES

1. Arrange a visit with an older adult, and discuss the health care system of the past and how the system has changed. Does the individual have any advice for you as a future nurse?

2. Observe how older people are portrayed in the media. Is ageism evident? How? Why? Reflect on your own feelings about older persons and aging.

3. Examine your surroundings. What barriers do you see to older adults with limited mobility? What might facilitate access?

4. Investigate the community support programs in your community. Are they easily located? Are the referral process and cost easily identified? What barriers are there to accessing the programs?

5. Visit the Alzheimer's Society of Canada website, and identify what information would be useful to a CHN preparing to meet with a group of family caregivers.

GROUP CRITICAL-THINKING EXERCISES

1. Discuss your findings from the Individual Critical-Thinking Exercises with other students.

2. Find out about your province's policy regarding older drivers. Discuss if the policy is appropriate and how it is enforced. What are the implications of an older adult losing her or his driver's licence?

3. Arrange to speak with a CHN who works with older adults to discuss her or his role. After the meeting, as a group, discuss the CHN's perspective on the role. Is it what you expected? Why or why not?

REFERENCES

Accreditation Canada. (2014). The Qmentum Accreditation Program. Retrieved from https://accreditation.ca/accreditation/qmentum

Alzheimer Society of Canada (ASC). (2010). *Rising tide: The impact of dementia on Canadian society*. Toronto, ON: Author. Retrieved from http://www.alzheimer.ca/~/media/Files/national/Advocacy/ASC_Rising_Tide_Full_Report_e.ashx

Alzheimer Society of Canada (ASC). (2017). *Guide to the National Strategy for Alzheimer's Disease and Other Dementias Act*. Retrieved from http://www.alzheimer.ca/en/Home/Get-involved/Advocacy/National-dementia-strategy/Alzheimers-Act

Angus, J., & Reeve, P. (2006). Ageism: A threat to "aging well" in the 21st century. *Journal of Applied Gerontology, 25*(2), 137–152.

Badley, E. M., Canizares, M., Perruccio, A. V., Hogg-Johnson, S., & Gignac, M. A. (2015). Benefits gained, benefits lost: Comparing baby boomers to other generations in a longitudinal cohort study of self-rated health. *The Milbank Quarterly, 93*(1), 40–72.

Bherer, L., Erickson, K., & Liu-Ambrose, T. (2013). A review of the effects of physical activity and exercise on cognitive and brain functions in older adults. *Journal of Aging Research, 2013*, 657508.

Bookwala J., Yee, J. L., & Schulz, R. (2000). Caregiving and detrimental mental and physical health outcomes. In G. Williamson, D. R. Shaffer, & P.A. Parmelee (Eds.), *Physical illness and depression in older adults: A handbook of theory, research, and practice* (The Plenum series in social/clinical psychology) (pp. 93–134). New York, NY: Kluwer Academic/Plenum.

Brown, R., Hemati, K., Riley, E., Lee, C., Ponath, C., Tieu, L., . . . Kushel, M. (2017). Geriatric conditions in a population-based sample of older homeless adults. *The Gerontologist, 57*(4), 757–766.

Canadian AIDS Society. (2013). *HIV and aging in Canada: Prevention*. Toronto, ON: Author.

Canadian Coalition for Seniors' Mental Health (2009). *Tool on depression: Assessment & treatment for older adults*. Markham, ON: Author. Retrieved from https://ccsmh.ca/projects/depression/#

Canadian Gerontological Nursing Association. (2010). Excerpt from *Gerontological Nursing Competencies and Standards of Practice 2010*. Copyright © 2010 by Canadian Gerontological Nursing Association. Used by permission of Canadian Gerontological Nursing Association.

Canadian Hospice Palliative Care Association. (2016). *The way forward national framework: A roadmap for an integrated palliative approach to care*. Ottawa, ON: Author.

Canadian Home Care Association. (2016). *Better home care in Canada: A national action plan*. Ottawa, ON: Author. Retrieved from https://www.cna-aiic.ca/search#q=better%20home%20care&f:cna-website-facet=[cna]

Canadian Institute for Health Information (CIHI). (2014). *Drug use among seniors on public drug programs in Canada (revised)*. Ottawa, ON: Author. Retrieved from https://secure.cihi.ca/free_products/Drug_Use_in_Seniors_on_Public_Drug_Programs_EN_web_Oct.pdf

Canadian Institutes of Health Research. (2017). *Canadian research centres on aging & other associations*. Retrieved from http://www.cihr-irsc.gc.ca/e/30794.html/2017

Canadian Longitudinal Study on Aging (CLSA). (2017). Retrieved from https://www.clsa-elcv.ca

Canadian Nurses Association. (2017). *National nursing framework on medical assistance in dying in Canada* (MAiD). Retrieved from https://cnia.ca/cna-releases-national-nursing-framework-medical-assistance-dying-canada/#

Canadian Public Health Association. (2010). *Public health–community health nursing practice in Canada: Roles and activities.* Ottawa, ON: Author. Retrieved from http://www.cpha.ca/uploads/pubs/3-1bk04214.pdf

Canadian Society of Exercise Physiology. (2017). Canadian Society of Exercise Physiology physical activity guidelines for adults age 65 years and older. Retrieved from http://www.csep.ca/CMFiles/Guidelines/CSEP_PAGuidelines_older-adults_en.pdf

Canadian Task Force on Preventive Health Care, Pottie, K., Rahal, R., Jaramillo, A., Birtwhistle, R., Thombs, B. D., . . . Tonelli, M. (2016). Recommendations on screening for cognitive impairment in older adults. *Canadian Medical Association Journal, 188*(1), 37–46.

Chappell, N. L., & Funk, L. M. (2011). Social support, caregiving, and aging. *Canadian Journal on Aging 30*(3), 355–370.

Change Foundation. (2016). *Legislation supporting family caregivers in Canadian jurisdictions and selected international jurisdictions.* The Change Foundation.

Community Health Nurses of Canada (CHNC). (2008). *Canadian community health nursing standards of practice.* Toronto, ON: Author.

Community Health Nurses of Canada (CHNC). (2010). *Home health nursing competencies.* Toronto, ON: Author. Retrieved from https://www.chnc.ca/en/competencies

Community Health Nurses of Canada (CHNC). (2019, revised). *Canadian community health nursing professional practice model & standards of practice.* St. Johns, NL: Author. Retrieved from https://www.chnc.ca/en/standards-of-practice?lang=switch1

Conklin, A. L., Maguire, E. R., & Monsivais, P. (2013) Economic determinants of diet in older adults: Systematic review. *Journal of Epidemiology and Community Health, 67,* 721–727.

Department of Justice. (2016). Legislative background: Medical Assistance in Dying (Bill C-14, as Assented to on June 17, 2016). Retrieved from http://www.justice.gc.ca/eng/rp-pr/other-autre/adra-amsr

Denton, F. T., & Spencer, B. G. (2010). Chronic health conditions: Changing prevalence in an aging population and some implications for the delivery of health care services. *Canadian Journal on Aging, 29*(1), 11–21.

Dupuis-Blanchard, S., Simard, M., Gould, O., & Villalon, L. (2013). La perception des aînés francophones en situation minoritaire face aux défis et aux enjeux liés au maintien à domicile en milieu urbain néo-brunswickois. *Canadian Journal of Public Health, 104*(6), S71–S74.

Durst, D. (2005). Aging amongst immigrants in Canada: Population drift. *Canadian Studies in Population, 32*(2), 257–270.

Eat Right Ontario (2012). Healthy eating for older adults: Tips and Idea for healthy eating to make it enjoyable. Retrieved from https://www.eatrightontario.ca/EatRightOntario/media/ERO_PDF/en/Seniors/Older-Adult-Guide.pdf

Echenberg, H., Gauthier, J., & Leonard, A. (2011). *Some public policy implications of an aging population.* Ottawa, ON: Parliament of Canada. Retrieved from http://www.parl.gc.ca/content/lop/researchpublications/cei-07-e.htm

Edmonston, R. (2013). Life course perspectives on immigration. *Canadian Studies in Population, 40*(1–2), 1–8.

Elgersma, S., Simeone, T., Roy-César, E., & Theckedath, D. (2012). *Canada's aging population and public policy.* Ottawa, ON: Parliament of Canada. Retrieved from http://www.parl.gc.ca/content/lop/researchpublications/2012-07-e.pdf

Employment and Social Development Canada. (2013). *Addressing the challenges and opportunities of ageing in Canada.* Ottawa, ON: Government of Canada. Retrieved from http://www.esdc.gc.ca/eng/seniors/reports/aging.shtml

Fleming, D., & Elliot, A. (2005). The impact of influenza on the health and health care utilization of elderly people. *Vaccine, 23,* S1–S9.

Government of Canada. (2013). *Elder abuse: It's time to face the reality.* Ottawa, ON: Author. Retrieved from http://www.seniors.gc.ca/eng/pie/eaa/elderabuse.shtml#b

Health Canada. (2012). *Seniors and aging – sexual activity.* Ottawa, ON: Government of Canada.

Health Council of Canada. (2013). *Canada's most vulnerable: Improving health care for First Nations, Inuit and Métis seniors.* Ottawa, ON: Author. Retrieved from http://healthcouncilcanada.ca/content_ab.php?mnu=2&mnu1=48&mnu2=30&mnu3=55

Institute for Safe Medication Practices Canada. (2014). *Medication reconciliation in home care: Getting started kit.* Ottawa, ON: Author. Retrieved from http://www.patientsafetyinstitute.ca/en/toolsResources/Documents/Interventions/Medication%20Reconciliation/Home/Medication%20Reconciliation%20in%20Home%20Care%20Getting%20Started%20Kit.pdf

International Federation on Ageing. (2012). *Current and emerging issues facing older Canadians.* Toronto, ON: Author. Retrieved from http://www.ifa-fiv.org/wpcontent/uploads/2012/12/current-and-emerging-issues-facing-older-canadiansfinal-report-30-march-2012.pdf

Keating, N., Swindle, J., & Fletcher, S. (2011). Aging in rural Canada: A retrospective and review. *Canadian Journal on Aging/La Revue Canadienne Du Vieillissement, 30*(3), 323–338.

Kilbride, K. M. (2014) *Immigrant integration: Research implications for future policy.* Toronto, ON: Canadian Scholars Press.

Légaré, J., Picard, J-F., Martel, L., & Carrière, Y. (2016). *Insights on Canadian society—The contribution of immigration to the size and ethnocultural diversity of future cohorts of seniors.* Statistics Canada. Minister of Industry. Catalogue no. 75-006-X.

Lehning, A. J. (2012). City governments and aging in place, community design, transportation and housing innovation adaptation. *The Gerontologist, 52*(3), 345–356.

Lindau, S. T., Schumm, L. P., Laumann, E. O., Levinson, W., O'Muircheartaigh, C. A, & Waite. L. J. (2007). *A study of sexuality and health among older adults in the United States.* New England Journal of Medicine, 357, 762–774.

Martin-Matthews, A., Tamblyn, R., Keefe, J., & Gillis, M. (2009). Bridging policy and research on aging in Canada: Recognizing an anniversary, realizing an opportunity. *Canadian Journal on Aging, 28*(2), 185–193.

Masi, C. M., Chen, H. Y., Hawkley, L. C., & Cacioppo, J. T. (2011). A meta-analysis of interventions to reduce loneliness. *Journal of Personality and Social Psychology, 15*(3), 219–266.

Masoro, E., & Austad, S. (2005). *Handbook of the biology of aging.* Burlington, ON: Academic Press.

Miedema, D. (2014). Among Canadian seniors, a social isolation epidemic. *eReview, 14*(7), 1–2.

Ministry of Health Canada. (2011). Eating well with Canada's Food Guide: A guide to healthy eating for adults. Retrieved from http://www.eatrightontario.ca/en/Articles/Seniors-nutrition/A-Guide-to-Healthy-Eating-for-Older-Adults.aspx

Nagamatsu, L., Handy, T. C., Hsu, L., Voss, M., & Liu-Ambrose, T. (2012). Resistance training promotes cognitive and functional brain plasticity in seniors with probable mild cognitive impairment. *Archives of Internal Medicine, 172*(8), 666–668.

National Advisory Council on Aging. (2005). *Seniors on the margins: Seniors from ethnocultural minorities.* Minister of Public Works and Government Services Canada.

Ng, E., Wilkins, R, Gendron, F., & Berthelot, J. M. (2005). *Dynamics of immigrants' health in Canada: Evidence from the National Population Health Survey, Healthy Today, Healthy Tomorrow? Findings from the National Population Health Survey*, Statistics Canada, Ottawa, Canada.

Nicholson, N. (2012). A review of social isolation: An important but underassessed condition in older adults. *Journal of Primary Prevention, 33*, 137–152.

Office of the Commissioner of Official Languages. (2013). *Enjoying your senior years in your own language, culture and community.* Ottawa, ON: Minister of Public Works and Government Services Canada. Retrieved from http://www.ocol-clo.gc.ca/sites/default/files/stu_etu_112013_e.pdf

Office of the Correctional Investigator. (2013). *Summary of issues and challenges facing older and aging offenders in federal custody.* Ottawa, ON: Minister of Public Works and Government Services Canada. Retrieved from http://www.oci-bec.gc.ca/cnt/comm/presentations/presentationsar-ra0911info-eng.aspx?texthighlight-aging

Ontario Human Rights Commission. (2013). *Ageism and age discrimination.* Toronto, ON: Author. Retrieved from http://www.ohrc.on.ca/en/time-action-advancing-human-rights-older-ontarians/ageism

Ontario Telehealth Network. (2017). How is Ontario Telehealth network making a difference in transforming health care. Retrieved from https://otn.ca/how-is-otn-making-difference-in-ontario/transforming-health-care

Payette, H., & Shatenstein, B. (2005). Determinants of healthy eating in community dwelling elderly people. *Canadian Journal of Public Health, 96*(3), S27–S31.

Physical Activity Resource Centre. (2013). *Physical activity promotion for older adults: A step-by-step guide.* The Ontario Physical and Health Education Association. Retrieved from http://parc.ophea.net/resource/older-adults-promotion-guide

Public Health Agency of Canada (PHAC). (2014). *Reporting on sexually transmitted infections in Canada: 2011.* Ottawa, ON: Author. Retrieved from http://www.positivelivingbc.org/files/64-02-14-1200-sti-report-2011_en-final.pdf

Public Health Agency of Canada (PHAC). (2017a). *How healthy are Canadians? A trend analysis of the health of Canadians from a health living and chronic disease perspective.* Ottawa, ON: Author. Retrieved from https://www.canada.ca/en/public-health/services/publications/healthy-living/how-healthy-canadians.html

Public Health Agency of Canada (PHAC). (2017b). Immunization schedule for adults over 60. Retrieved from https://www.canada.ca/en/public-health/services/provincial-territorial-immunization-information/routine-vaccination-healthy-previously-immunized-adult.html

Public Safety Canada. (2012). *Your emergency preparedness guide.* Ottawa, ON: Author. Retrieved from http://www.getprepared.gc.ca/cnt/rsrcs/pblctns/yprprdnssgd/yprprdnssgd-eng.pdf

Public Safety Canada. (2017). *The Canadian disaster database.* Ottawa, ON: Author. Retrieved from https://www.publicsafety.gc.ca/cnt/rsrcs/cndn-dsstr-dtbs/index-en.aspx

Rapp, C. A., Pettus, C. A., & Goscha, R. J. (2006). Principles of strengths-based policy. *Journal of Policy Practice, 5*(4), 3–18.

Registered Nurses' Association of Ontario (RNAO). (2014). *Preventing and addressing abuse and neglect in older adults.* Toronto, ON: Author. Retrieved from http://rnao.ca/bpg/guidelines/abuse-and-neglect-older-adults

Registered Nurses' Association of Ontario (RNAO). (2017). *Preventing falls and reducing injury from falls* (4th ed.). Toronto, ON: Author Retrieved from http://rnao.ca/bpg/guidelines/prevention-falls-and-fall-injuries

Richmond, C. A., & Cook, C. (2016). Creating conditions for Canadian Aboriginal health equity: The promise of healthy public policy. *Public Health Reviews, 37*(1), 2.

Sabat, S. R., & Harré, R. (1992). The construction and deconstruction of self in Alzheimer's disease. *Ageing and Society, 12*(4), 443–461.

Shatenstein, B., Ferland, G., Belleville, S., Gray-Donald, K., Kergoat, M. J., Morais, J., . . . Greenwood, C. (2012). Diet quality and cognition among older adults from the NuAge study. *Experiential Gerontology, 47*(5), 353–360.

Statistics Canada. (2010). *A portrait of seniors in Canada: Immigrant seniors.* Ottawa, ON: Author. Retrieved from http://www.statcan.gc.ca/pub/89-519-x/2006001/4122094-eng.htm

Statistics Canada. (2012a). *Population and dwelling counts.* Ottawa, ON: Author. Retrieved from https://www12.statcan.gc.ca/census-recensement/2011/dp-pd/hlt-fst/pd-pl/index-eng.cfm

Statistics Canada. (2012b). *Portrait of caregivers.* Ottawa, ON: Author. Retrieved from https://www.statcan.gc.ca/pub/89-652-x/89-652-x2013001-eng.htm

Statistics Canada. (2015). *Population projections for Canada (2013 to 2063), provinces and territories (2013 to 2038).* Ottawa, ON: Author. Catalogue no. 91-520-X. Retrieved from https://www.statcan.gc.ca/pub/91-520-x/91-520-x2014001-eng.htm

Statistics Canada. (2017a). *A portrait of the population aged 85 and older in 2016 in Canada.* Catalogue no. 98-200-X2016004 Retrieved from http://www12.statcan.gc.ca/census-recensement/2016/as-sa/98-200-x/2016004/98-200-x2016004-eng.cfm

Statistics Canada. (2017b). *Annual demographic estimates: Canada, provinces and territories, 2017.* Catalogue no. 91-215-X. Retrieved from http://www.statcan.gc.ca/pub/91-215-x/91-215-x2017000-eng.htm

Taing, D., & McKay, K. (2017). Better Strength, Better Balance! Partnering to deliver a fall prevention program for older adults. *Canadian Journal of Public Health, 108*(3), e314–e319.

Turcotte, M. (2012). *Profile of seniors' transportation habits.* Ottawa, ON: Statistics Canada. Retrieved from http://www.statcan.gc.ca/pub/11-008-x/2012001/article/11619-eng.pdf

United Nations. (2017). *World population prospects: The 2017 revision, key findings and advance tables.* Working Paper No. ESA/P/WP/248. Department of Economic and Social Affairs, Population Division.

Wilson, K., Rosenberg, M. W., Abonyi, S., & Lovelace, R. (2010). *Aging and health: An examination of differences between older Aboriginal and non-Aboriginal people.* Hamilton, ON: SEDAP Research Program.

Wilson, M. (2006). Sexually transmitted diseases in older adults. *Current Infectious Disease Reports, 8*(2), 139–147.

World Health Organization. (2007). *Global age-friendly cities: A guide.* Geneva, CH: Author.

Zickuhr, K. (2014). *Older adults and technology.* New York, NY: Pew Research Center.

ABOUT THE AUTHORS

Christine McPherson, RN, PhD, is Associate Professor in the School of Nursing at the University of Ottawa. Her clinical experience includes care of older adults in tertiary and community settings. Her research for the past 18 years has focused on chronic disease, palliative care, and family caregiving. She collaborates with local community organizations on projects to improve home care services to older clients at the end of life. She was the development lead on the Registered Nurses' Association's best practice guideline on end-of-life care and is currently revising and updating the guideline. Her undergraduate and graduate teaching includes social and cultural aspects of aging, palliative care, community care, and research.

Karen Curry, RN MN CCHNc, is a practice educator for VON Canada. She has held a variety of roles in the home care setting, and project management and collaborative practice education are her main areas of focus. As a practice educator, Karen is an advocate for practice change initiatives to develop community health nurse capacity. Karen has been actively involved with the CHNC and promotes CHNs to become involved in professional development and the CHNC.

Indigenous Health

Dawn Tisdale and Gwen Campbell McArthur

LEARNING OUTCOMES

After studying this chapter, you should be able to:

1. Identify how cultural safety supports the community health nurse's practice to deliver care for Indigenous peoples and communities.

2. Describe how colonization, assimilation policies, and loss of culture negatively impact the health and well-being of Indigenous peoples.

3. Describe Indigenous peoples' health care delivery systems, including funding implications.

4. Discuss the social determinants of health in relation to the health of Indigenous peoples and communities.

5. Discuss how culture, self-governance, and current policies impact the health of Indigenous communities.

6. Recognize the important role of Traditional Knowledge and medicines in health and healing for Indigenous peoples and how community health nurses can support client-centred holistic health care.

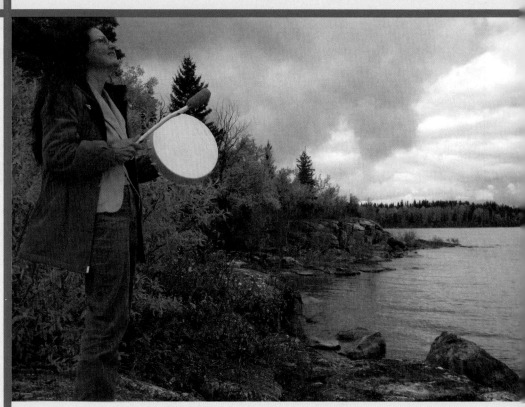

Source: Courtesy of Gwen Campbell McArthur

ELDER BLESSING AND RECOGNITION OF ANCESTORS AND LAND

The blessings for this chapter echo from the voices of the ancestors who have lived through unimaginable hardship and inextricable change. The spirit of many generations come to teach us that life, love, family, and community are sacred as is the land, the water, the air, and each living thing that remains. May you find the wonder of inquiry in these written words on the pages and may they bring you to your own place of health and healing so you too can begin relationships with the wisdom of those indentured to your care. Take only what you need, leave what you do not, and above all consider the possibilities of the meaning of each message herein. The words were created for you, to feed your spirit of curiosity now and as you go forward. *Meegwich, kukstem, haihai, wela'lin.* Thank you, Creator, for all things good and for gifting me this opportunity. With this I say, All My Relations.

—Gwen Campbell McArthur

INTRODUCTION

This chapter provides contexts and resources to community health nurses (CHNs) working in Indigenous communities and with Indigenous peoples to build reflective, culturally safe practices grounded in a strength-based approach that honours Indigenous peoples' cultures and health. Indigenous peoples in Canada have Traditional Knowledge, medicines, and healing practices to support spiritual, physical, mental, and emotional health and well-being. Many Indigenous communities' health is inextricably linked to their distinct culture and worldview that all beings are connected to each other and to the land. The UN's Declaration of the Right of Indigenous Peoples (UNDRIP) Article 24 states, "Indigenous peoples have the right to their traditional medicines and to maintain their health practices, including the conservation of their vital medicinal plants, animals and minerals" (UN General Assembly, 2007). Indigenous individuals also have the right to access, without any discrimination, all social and health services. The role of the CHN is to support these rights and the health and well-being of Indigenous peoples in Canada through nursing practice that respects the dignity of culture and community. This chapter provides the CHN with foundational concepts that support care for Indigenous peoples and communities through understanding the historical, sociocultural, geographic, and economic contexts that impact health.

In this chapter, the history of Indigenous peoples is outlined from pre-contact (prior to colonization) to contemporary times. It is important for CHNs to recognize how colonization, past and present policies of assimilation, and loss of culture have resulted in overwhelmingly negative impacts on the health and well-being of Indigenous peoples and have led to the Truth and Reconciliation Commission of Canada's (TRC) Calls to Action that support peoples' rights and health. The historical and colonial context, as well as Canada's reconciliation mandate, encourage CHNs to practise in a culturally safe way that best supports the communities they serve. While it is important to examine the inequities Indigenous peoples face and understand these inequities as the root cause of the devastating impacts on the health and well-being of Indigenous peoples, the focus of this chapter is not about disparities but rather the inherent strength and holistic approach to health of Indigenous peoples. Describing Indigenous peoples as vulnerable populations perpetuates stigmas of dependency and weakness. CHNs can play a key role in stopping this colonial narrative and the inequities created by continued stigmatization.

An overview of legislation and policy, as well as a description of how services are typically delivered to Indigenous peoples in a distinctly different system, will be explained. We discuss reconciliation, decolonizing health policy, self-determination, and connection to culture and how they can restore and uphold the health of Indigenous peoples in Canada. CHNs working in Indigenous communities and with Indigenous peoples can strengthen their relational practice by learning how Indigenous Knowledge and ways of knowing can help build trusting relationships with the people they serve.

Through sharing our personal stories, legends and traditional teachings, we found that we are interconnected through the same mind and spirit. Our traditional teachings speak to acts such as holding one another up, walking together, balance, healing, and unity. (Reconciliation Canada, n.d.)

HISTORY OF INDIGENOUS PEOPLES IN CANADA

The term **Aboriginal** is a colonial term created by the Canadian federal government that encompasses all First Nation, Métis, and Inuit peoples. **Colonial** refers to the power exerted by the dominant culture of settlers over the Indigenous peoples to maintain authority with the intention to replace the original population. Section 35 of the Constitution Act (1982) defines, recognizes, and affirms *Indian, Inuit,* and *Métis* peoples as "Aboriginal peoples of Canada" along with their existing treaty rights, including land claim agreements. **Indigenous** refers to the original peoples of a land and their descendants and is used by the United Nations (UN) in its aims to uphold the human rights of Indigenous peoples across the world (UNDRIPUN General Assembly, 2007). As part of the decolonizing process, and in safeguarding the rights of Indigenous peoples through the UNDRIP's UN Declaration on the Rights of Indigenous Peoples' mandate, *Indigenous* is now used in lieu of "Aboriginal," "Native," and "Indian," which are colonial terms and typically considered derogatory. **First Nations** refers to the original nations of inhabitants located below the Arctic in modern-day Canada, representing great diversity between nations. Members of a First Nation are legislated as either "status Indians" or "non-status Indians" under the Indian Act. Indigenous peoples of the Arctic are **Inuit**, which means "the people" in Inuktitut. Initially, the **Métis** were identified as mixed-race descendants of early unions between First Nation and colonial-era European settlers during the 18th and 19th centuries. Within generations, a distinct Métis culture emerged, and in 1982 the Canadian Constitution recognized the unique Métis culture, traditions, language, and strong nationhood (Métis National Council, 2011, p. 2). In Canada there is a rich diversity of Indigenous peoples from different linguistic groups, histories, traditions, and cultures. The best nursing practices respect these differing identities, cultures, and nations as specified by each person and community.

Pre-Contact

Indigenous communities hold stories that are intrinsic to their history, culture, and peoples. "From time immemorial, the lands that are now known as Canada and the United States of America have been and continue to be the sacred home of Indigenous Peoples and Nations; Others' hands have drawn boundaries between Canada and the United States. These arbitrary lines have not severed, and never will, the ties of kinship among our peoples" (Assembly of First Nations and National Congress of American Indians, 1999). *Immemorial* is a term used by various Indigenous peoples to describe a relationship to these lands that extends beyond the reach of memory and mores. Anthropologists have often undermined traditional recounts of Indigenous histories as "legends" versus facts, contributing to the predominate colonial lens that depicts the history of these lands before Confederation (Lord & Lewis, 1997).

Before the arrival of Europeans on this continent, an estimated 18 million inhabitants and more than 2200 languages flourished (Lord & Lewis, 1997). Every First Nation and Inuit society in Canada had long-established names, language, spirituality, traditional healing practices, art, deep connections to the land, and culture that contributed to its community's health and well-being (Indigenous and Northern Affairs Canada, 2018). This **Indigenous Knowledge (IK)**, often referred to as Traditional Knowledge, was and continues to be passed down through storytelling, Elders, ceremonies, rituals, songs, and language. IK is rooted in theories, beliefs, and lived experiences that are held by everyone in a community because of its collective nature (Crowshoe, 2005). These customary laws, medicinal practices, protocols, ideologies, dances, art, and spirituality are symbiotic with culture, wellness, and the relationships between them, which are demonstrated through the rich history and health of Indigenous peoples in Canada.

Contact and Colonization

Initial contact was with Norse explorers in the 11th century followed by the arrival of Europeans in the 1500s. Over a significant period of time, colonial settlers arrived on the east coast as far as the area now known as Hudson Bay, and eventually they arrived on the west coast. Explorers, fur traders, and missionaries made their way west, fuelled by the fur trade and Christian doctrine. Settlers brought diseases such as smallpox, TB, and measles, which decimated Indigenous populations by as much as 90%, resulting in the devastation and fragmentation of Indigenous cultures. Furthermore, resources that had sustained Indigenous livelihoods, such as the buffalo and the beaver, were depleted by settlers, thus escalating susceptibility to depopulating epidemics.

Colonization, the process of establishing colonies and settlements in Canada, resulted in negotiations with the original inhabitants. Subsequent establishment of reserves, whereby historically free and independent peoples were forced into restricted areas of land, created further problems, including malnutrition, starvation, and death. At the time of European contact, there were an estimated 60 different languages spoken across what is now Canada. Due to colonization and policies of assimilation, many of those languages are lost and others endangered (Waldram, Herring, & Young, 2006), further contributing to the decimation of Indigenous cultures (Brown, McPherson, Peterson, Neuman, & Cramner, 2012).

Colonialism and Legislation

Though there were about 500 distinct nations in the early 1600s, the land was legally deemed empty by Europeans and therefore claimable (Fleet, 1997). Britain developed **treaties** to appropriate the land that was occupied by First Nations. The British North America Act of 1867 gave Canada its birth as a country, but the Royal Proclamation, 1763, specified that only the British government could buy "Indian lands" or negotiate treaties. In contrast, First Nations entered the treaties with the understanding that it was land sharing, not land cession (Office of the Treaty Commissioner, 2013). Private individuals or other nations (including Canada) were not permitted to go into Indigenous territories to buy land directly (Dickason, 2002). The **Indian Act** of 1876 was passed to ensure the management of reserve lands and communal monies. The intention of the Indian Act was to "civilize the Indian" through **assimilation** into colonial culture. Indigenous peoples were viewed as wards of the state upon whom restrictions were imposed to eliminate their cultures and prohibit their rights. Indian residential schools and reserves were implemented. Women were denied status, and First Nations people were prohibited from voting, forming political organizations, practising spiritual and cultural ceremonies, as well as infringed upon with many other life-limiting policies.

In 1879, Sir John A. MacDonald made the following statement referring to the Indian Act (Moore & Maguire, 1978, as cited in the TRC, 2012, p. 6):

> When the school is on the reserve, the child lives with its parents, who are savages, and though he may learn to read and write, his habits and training mode of thought are Indian. He is simply a savage who can read and write. It has been strongly impressed upon myself, as head of the Department, that Indian children should be withdrawn as much as possible from the parental influence, and the only way to do that would be to put them in central training industrial schools where they will acquire the habits and modes of thought of white men.

Due to the treaties, First Nation peoples were relegated to living on **reserves**. Nations were reduced to small plots of land, some as small as a few acres, and in many cases the land was of no economic value. The Indian reserves were governed by the federal government under the Indian Act (Venne, 2002). Up until the 1960s, **Indian agents**, hired and paid by the federal government, were individuals assigned to carry out the terms of the Indian Act. They typically lived on the reserve or in very close proximity. The government developed a pass system where First Nation people required written permission from the Indian agent to leave the reserve, and every aspect of daily life, including growing their own food or raising livestock, was controlled by the agent. A quote from Deputy Superintendent General of Indian Affairs Duncan Campbell Scott in 1920 sums up the lens placed on Indigenous people and the assumed role of the state: "I want to get rid of the Indian problem . . . Our objective is to continue until there is not an Indian that has not been absorbed into the body politic, and there is no Indian question, and no Indian Department" (Moore & Maguire, 1978, as cited in TRC, 2012, p. 6). Federally governed reserves were implemented to segregate and control First Nation people. Reserves are situated in all of Canada's provinces and territories (Aboriginal Affairs and Northern Development Canada, 2013). The Indian Act imposed the governance structure of First Nation reserve-based communities, including present-day band councils, which are very different from traditional Indigenous governance systems.

Policies of Assimilation

Indigenous peoples' physical, mental, spiritual, and social well-being has been adversely impacted by ongoing colonial and assimilative policies. Canada's history has been written predominantly through a settler lens; therefore, it is important to critically examine the widespread impact these policies have had on Indigenous health in the past and today. The assimilative and segregating policies of Indian residential schools, Indian hospitals, and the child welfare system have left an enduring and pervasive impact on the health and well-being of Indigenous peoples and the status of their community health (TRC, 2015a).

Indian Residential Schools **Indian residential schools (IRSs)** were first established by missionaries in the late 1800s in various locations across Canada and, later, in partnership with the federal government. Children as young as four were forcibly taken from their homes and relocated to schools. With the clear intent of assimilation, they were often separated from siblings and relatives, deliberately placed far from their communities; they were not permitted to speak their language, practise their culture, or form the relationships critically important

in formative years. The premise of the IRS was to absorb the children into the general settler population through a process of education and religious indoctrination. Instead, it caused cultural degradation. Children were taught to be ashamed of their heritage, their people, and themselves.

Parents were legally required to send their children to IRSs. Failure to do so meant punishment, including incarceration, at which point children would become wards of the state and sent to IRSs in any case. Photo 22.1 is a letter from an Indian agent to a store clerk requesting the discontinuation of the J. B. Gambler monthly rations as punishment for the removal of his children from the Wabasca Residential School in 1935.

Although Canada's policies involving Métis children attending Indian Residential Schools (IRSs) were conflicted between federal and provincial jurisdictions, many Métis children were also forced to attend as a means to equally "civilize and assimilate" what government officials considered a "dangerous" population (TRC, 2015a). Physical, emotional, and sexual abuse were rampant in the schools, and little was done to mitigate the situation. Children were provided substandard education and food, often going hungry. Some survivors report being forced to steal food from the kitchens (Aboriginal

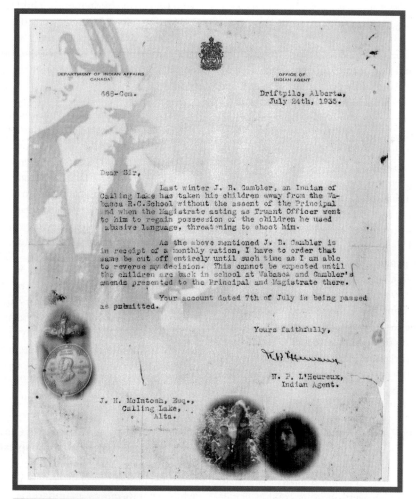

PHOTO **22.1** It would be unfair to the spirit of J.B. Gambler not to point out that he defied the priests and the government and acted with the full authority of a parent. His decision to pull his children out of school was his best judgment as a father, and in the best interests of his family.

Source: Courtesy of Chuck Watson and Gwen Schmidt

Healing Foundation, 2006). As late as the 1950s, more than 40% of the teaching staff at the schools had no professional training (Aboriginal Healing Foundation, 1999). Cultural degradation practices included physical and emotional abuse for speaking a traditional language, cutting of hair (hair has strong cultural and spiritual significance), imposing foreign religious practices, and intentional separation from parents wanting to visit. Children found trying to escape were harshly punished. Disciplinary practices included corporal punishment, solitary confinement, food restrictions, shaming, thrashings, and denial of home visitations (TRC, 2015b). The predominant themes captured in the stories of survivors are "the loneliness, the isolation, the hunger, the homelessness, the hard work, the harsh discipline, the imposition of an alien language and culture, and the poor health, disease and death that haunted many schools" (TRC, 2015b). The following account from a survivor demonstrates the depth of spiritual abuse and the resulting trauma that occurred for many children who attended an IRS:

> In keeping with the promise to civilize the little pagan, they went to work and cut off my braids, which, incidentally, according to the Assiniboine traditional custom, was a token of mourning—the closer the relative, the closer the cut. After my haircut, I wondered in silence if my mother had died, as they had cut my hair close to the scalp. (TRC, 2015b)

Despite poor record keeping, mortality rates were high by all accounts, and thousands of children did not survive due to poor care, illness, and suicide, while even more were injured and traumatized (TRC, 2015c). The IRS system operated 135 schools over the span of 150 years, with the final school closing in 1996. An estimated 150 000 children were sent to these institutions—more than the number of soldiers who died in World Wars I and II combined.

The legacy of IRSs continues to have severe impacts on Indigenous communities through generational and **intergenerational trauma**. The trauma experienced by many IRS survivors often resulted (and continues to result) in poor health, addictions, despair, and depression, impacting not only the survivors but also their parents, families, children, and communities (TRC, 2015d). Many survivors' children also identify as survivors due to the lasting impact of IRSs on their childhoods. It is critical for Canadian CHNs to understand that the violence, abuse, addictions, suicide, incarceration rates, and child welfare apprehension that continue to afflict Indigenous communities are either directly or indirectly related to the IRS experience (TRC, 2015d).

Justice Murray Sinclair summarized the findings of the TRC as follows:

> The residential school system established for Canada's Indigenous population in the nineteenth century is one of the darkest, most troubling chapters in our nation's history. While some people regard the schools established under that system as centers of education, they were, in reality, centers of cultural indoctrination. The most alarming aspect of the system was that its target and its victims were the most vulnerable of society: little children. Removed from their families and home communities, seven generations of Indigenous children were

denied their identity through a systematic and concerted effort to extinguish their culture, language, and spirit. These schools were part of a larger effort by Canadian authorities to force Indigenous peoples to assimilate by the outlawing of sacred ceremonies and important traditions. It is clear that residential schools were a key component of a Canadian government policy of cultural genocide. (TRC, 2015e)

Child Welfare System—60s Scoop IRSs additionally served as state-run orphanages, aiding the child welfare system's increased apprehension of children considered to be suffering from "neglect" at home. In 1960 an estimated 50% of children attending IRSs had been apprehended by child welfare agencies (TRC, 2015f). The intent was to sever all ties to family and culture rather than supporting family reunification. Foster homes and mass transracial adoption followed from 1960–1990. Children were placed with non-Indigenous families, causing a complete disconnect from their culture, customs, language, and spirituality. Adoption rate statistics of this era were highlighted in a 1980 study by the Canadian Council on Social Development, exposing that approximately 15 000 Indigenous children were in care by 1977, representing 20% of all Canadian children in the child welfare system (Johnston, 2016). The **60s Scoop** was coined by Patrick Johnston in his 1983 book, *Native Children and the Child Welfare System*. It is now commonly used in reference to the widespread apprehension of Indigenous children and the policies, or lack of, that prompted it.

> The prior impacts of colonial policies under the Indian act, residential schools, loss of culture and systemic racism in the child welfare system all contributed to break down of community, family and parents increasing child apprehension creating a vicious circle for Indigenous communities. Apprehension was driven by colonial models which perpetuated the rhetoric that Indigenous peoples were culturally inferior in their ability to care for their children and was marked as such in media with economic incentive. (Justice Murray Sinclair; as cited in the TRC, 2015a)

Despite decades of activism to reform the child welfare system and improve outcomes for children and their families, Indigenous children continue to be markedly overrepresented in today's foster care system. Many consider this phenomenon as a continuation of the IRS system in modern times along with its disintegration of culture and the continued neglect and abuse of Indigenous children (McKenzie, Varcoe, Browne, & Day, 2016; First Nations Caring Society, 2005).

Indian Hospitals In the context of Canada's health care system, Lux (2010) examined **Indian hospitals** as places for the intersection of race, medicine, and public policy. Hospitals operating exclusively for Indigenous patients further segregated while attempting to assimilate, and they existed in several forms for over a century, ending in the late 20th century. Similar to IRSs, the establishment of Indian hospitals was through the work of missionaries, later formalized and continued by the Canadian government, peaking during the 1960s with

22 institutions nationwide with more than 2200 beds (Lux, 2016). Colonial policies of the early 1900s led to social, health, and economic inequities for Indigenous peoples, contributing to devastatingly high rates of tuberculosis (TB) during this era. Prior to 1945, many Indigenous people were turned away from provincially run hospitals due to segregation policies and limited budgets. Only those most likely to recover were selected for care, leaving the most sick in their communities (Lux, 2016). Policies isolating the epidemic to reserves, combined with inadequate resources, further contributed to the growing rhetoric and fear of the "diseased Indian" and "Indian TB," giving rise to a culture of segregation and forcing the government to "address" the health crisis by creating sanitariums and hospital wards specifically for Indigenous peoples seen as less worthy of care (Lux, 2016). Sanitariums were later converted to Indian hospitals, which expanded in numbers. Many worked closely with IRSs. The 1950s Communicable Disease Control Act, along with amendments to the Indian Act, allowed authorities to apprehend and forcibly hold Indigenous people in Indian hospitals against their will. Patients were subjected to forced medical examinations and treatment (Lux, 2010). Survivor recounts of Indian hospitals include segregation, poor care, multiple abuses, medical experimentation, and sterilization without knowledge or consent (Lux, 2010). The forced imposition of biomedical treatment in a colonial model of care was another tactic to assimilate Indigenous peoples away from their own cultures and healing practices.

The impact of assimilation policies and colonialism on the health and well-being of Indigenous peoples cannot be understated. The inequities stemming from these policies must be recognized not as issues of the past but as a present-day Canadian health crisis requiring urgent and immediate action by all citizens. It is important for CHNs to understand how ongoing colonial practices impact Indigenous peoples' health, the communities they partner with, and how they provide care.

POLICY ISSUES AFFECTING COMMUNITY HEALTH NURSING IN INDIGENOUS COMMUNITIES

In this part of the world we have had 150 years of colonial rule, where everything from birth to death was ruled by government legislation, and specifically with health it's time we just took control of our own lives again. The introduction of our own traditional medicines, our traditional healing practices, those things that were forced underground by legislation, to bring those back after 150 years of oppression, that's what this is all about. (Chief Kukpi7 Wayne Christian, as cited in First Nations Health Authority, 2015)

An understanding of how treaty status is acquired and defined is indispensable to understanding the health care of Indigenous peoples. The status of being a "treaty Indian" in Canada is not only acquired by birth but also legislated by the Indian Act. A **registered or status Indian** is recognized under the Indian Act and has a unique registration or treaty number.

Non-status Indians are Indigenous, but because they were not registered, or their nation's leaders did not sign a treaty, or their status was lost through deliberately discriminatory Indian Act policies of assimilation, they are not recognized as status Indians by the federal government. There were several ways an individual could lose status, otherwise known as enfranchisement, such as by entering the armed forces; obtaining a university education; becoming a Christian minister, doctor, or lawyer; gaining access to vote; or, for a woman, marrying a non-status man (Furi & Wherrett, 2003). Inuit were put in a separate category because no treaties were signed in the Far North, but they are treated in the same manner as registered Indians by the federal government (Waldram et al., 2006). The isolation and the cold, inhospitable environment are the likeliest reasons the registration process and treaty signing did not occur in the Far North; that is, settlers were unlikely to have wanted the land. Métis are legally considered the same as non-status Indians—in other words, with no recognized rights. Under the Canadian Constitution, Métis are considered Indigenous peoples. They continue to negotiate and acquire rights, such as hunting rights. Certain Métis communities acquire services through the Office of the Interlocutor at the federal government level. Having Indian status, living on or off reserve, or living in the Far North determines how Indigenous people access health care, which significantly differs from the experience of non-Indigenous Canadians.

In 1982, the rights of Indigenous peoples in Canada were given recognition in the Canadian Constitution. Several attempts have been made to define "Aboriginal rights"; however, disagreements over governance and changes in government departments have resulted in confusion and setbacks. Continued Indigenous activism over harmful policies in the Indian Act has brought changes in legislation such as the abolishment of IRSs; addressing discriminatory, gender-based policies; honouring the rights of the Métis; and gaining the right to vote in 1960 (nearly 40 years after Canadian women were granted this right). Despite these changes, there remain many policies entrenched in assimilative intent. Continued advocacy calls on the federal government to further reform and amend wrongdoings of the past and present through the implementation of respectful, equitable policies for Indigenous peoples in Canada.

First Nation Health Care

Working with First Nation communities requires overarching knowledge of the larger system that enacts policy that establishes practices and standards for First Nation health care systems. First Nations health care delivery and other social services such as education fall under different government branches than those of non-Indigenous Canadians. Health care provision is considered a treaty right by First Nation and Inuit peoples; however, government policy states that health care provided to First Nation peoples is benevolence by the federal government. Twenty years ago Dr. George Deagle (1999), a Canadian physician, called out Canada's health care system for operating under a three-tier system, with Indigenous populations ranking the lowest in funding and provision of service. The question is, how much has actually changed?

For decades, the federal government has managed and delivered health services and support for First Nation individuals living on reserves and Inuit people through different departments such as the First Nations and Inuit Health Branch (FNIHB) and Indigenous Northern Affairs Canada (INAC). In 2017, the federal government merged FNIHB and INAC under Indigenous Services Canada with the vision to streamline services and work collaboratively with Indigenous communities to support self-governance (Government of Canada, 2018). First Nation communities are increasingly assuming local control through the transfer of health services to their nation (National Collaborating Centre for Aboriginal Health [NCCAH], 2011). Métis peoples receive health care services through the provincial health care system, whereas First Nation individuals living off reserve and Inuit access care through the same provincial system; then, the province seeks reimbursement from the federal government. The territories assume responsibility for their Indigenous populations through agreements with the federal government. Government relations for First Nation, Métis, and Inuit peoples are done through national organizations that represent their interests in Ottawa. For example, the Assembly of First Nations elects a Grand Chief who negotiates with federal officials for program funding for First Nation health care. The Inuit organization Tapiriit Kanatami similarly negotiates on behalf of 60 000 Inuit across 53 communities throughout the Inuit Nunangat region. The Métis National Council represents Métis from Ontario westward through the democratically elected leadership of the Métis Nation's government. It is essential that CHNs understand how governments function and especially how policies and priorities affect health care delivery to Indigenous populations on a daily basis. Adding to concerns regarding health care provision to First Nation communities is the instability created when the governing party changes. Too often agreements that have been put in place are altered, deleted, or replaced by new legislation.

For acute-care services, First Nation health care systems interface with the greater Canadian health care system, primarily because hospitals are a provincial responsibility. The degree of interfacing required with surrounding communities depends on the type and scope of health services existing on reserves. The more remote or isolated the reserve, the more likely health care services include comprehensive care, including short-term acute-care services. The federal government is now moving toward tripartite agreements between the Federal Ministry of Health, the provinces, and First Nation governments to allow for partnerships in health services governed by and for Indigenous peoples. Examples include the Fort Qu'Appelle All Nations Healing Hospital (Saskatchewan) and the First Nations Health Authority (British Columbia). The governance for health services within a First Nation community is determined by Chief and Council, the governing authority of each Nation. To establish health services in accordance with the Indian Act, a Band Council Resolution (BCR) between a First Nation and the federal government is required. Once a BCR is initiated, a health committee can be formed to determine the health service needs of its membership. First Nation health authorities were established to support the transfer of control of health services to First Nations, and a variety of funding arrangements are available to communities wanting to administer their own health programs (NCCAH, 2011).

INDIGENOUS PEOPLES AND HEALTH INEQUITIES

The overall health status of Indigenous peoples has been greatly impacted by colonialism and assimilation policies, as discussed in this chapter. Colonialism and racism mutually work together, creating health **inequities** in relation to the social determinants of health (Allan & Smylie, 2015; Richmond & Cook, 2016). Barriers in accessing health services, racism, poverty, and social exclusion are forms of interrelated inequities that, in turn, reinforce further oppression and poor health outcomes (Browne et al., 2011). When considering how policies in the Indian Act separately and cumulatively impact every determinant of health, it is easily understood why Indigenous peoples' health is in crisis. CHNs must reflect on how previous acts of colonialism, such as IRSs, have impacted related outcomes of education, employment, and mental health. They must consider the complexities involved in how Indigenous peoples access health care and social services when examining data on personal health status. Inequities related to the determinants of health and critical disruption of Indigenous peoples' cultures, families, and communities have resulted in poorer health outcomes.

It is often easier to access statistical data on a member of a First Nation due to the unique identifying number on the individual's health card; finding data about Métis and Inuit populations is more difficult. Information presented here is as current and comprehensive as possible; however, the reader is encouraged to keep in mind the limitations inherent in missing or unavailable data.

CANADIAN RESEARCH 22.1

Understanding inequalities in access to health care services for Aboriginal people: A call for nursing action
(Cameron, del Pilar Carmargo Plazas, Salasa, & Hungler, 2014)

This study applied Indigenous, interpretive, and participatory research methodologies in partnership with Indigenous peoples to understand inequalities in service access and their relation to health disparities and outcomes. The aims of the research were to reduce health disparities and promote equitable access to care for Indigenous peoples in Canada. The research undertook three qualitative exploratory projects to investigate Indigenous peoples' access to health care services in urban, rural, and inner city settings. The approach was foremost conversational, using hermeneutic phenomenology as a key methodological strategy to describe and interpret the findings. An Indigenous Advisory Committee led by an Elder and comprised of Indigenous stakeholders, community members, health care professionals, and researchers established the design and data collection tools (digitally recorded, semi-structured questions for interviews), adapted approaches to increase cultural sensitivity, and provided feedback and interpretation of the results, including its dissemination.

Significant findings of the study are as follows:

- Participants reported stories of racism, stigmatization, language difficulties, intimidation, harassment, and deep fear.
- Participants described going to the emergency department for a variety of health needs such as access to specialists, lab tests, and immediate treatments. In their search for care they described limited access to comprehensive and specialized care, long waiting times, communication barriers due to medical jargon, and interactive barriers with health care professionals.
- Findings showed that participants described health care professionals as judgmental, were provided inadequate assessments, and reported that their health care needs were not well addressed.

Research to date has shown that access to health services has been identified as essential to improve the health of Indigenous populations. The study's findings indicate that participants had distrust and inhibitions in seeking care because of accumulated past negative experiences. The findings of the study highlight the significance of personal, social, and prior health care experiences in influencing Indigenous peoples' access to emergency services. The nursing implications are to address the inequities of Indigenous peoples in an ethical and political appeal for action. To affect equity, nurses need to cast their gaze toward the conditions and systems that perpetuate inequities.

Discussion Questions

1. As a CHN, how might these findings influence your practice and approach when providing care to Indigenous clients?

2. How would you address the complex reasons of participants resistant to accessing care, including stigma related to their Indigeneity, discourses of blame, poverty, and lack of system capacity? What attention is required to address structural injustices acting as barriers to health care services?

3. What would you do if you witnessed stigma or discrimination against an Indigenous client?

Population Data

According to the 2016 census, the population of Indigenous peoples in Canada was 1 673 785, or 4.9% of total population (Statistics Canada, 2016). The majority of Indigenous peoples reported a single Indigenous identity, although some reported having more than one. First Nations make up 58.4%, Métis

35.1%, and Inuit 29.1% of Indigenous peoples in Canada. (Statistics Canada, 2016). Indigenous peoples are dispersed throughout the country, with Ontario, Quebec, and the four western provinces having the highest numbers. The highest proportion of Indigenous peoples to the total population is found in Nunavut (85.9%), Northwest Territories (50.7%), and the Yukon (23.3%) (Statistics Canada, 2016). There are 618 First Nation communities, otherwise known as reserves, in Canada (Aboriginal Affairs and Northern Development Canada, 2013), and 44.2% of First Nation populations live on these reserves (Statistics Canada, 2016). Ontario has the largest Métis population, which grew by 64.3% from 2006 to 2016. In the western provinces, the Métis population grew by 32.9% in the same time period (Statistics Canada, 2016). Statistics Canada reports that 62.6% of Métis peoples live in the metropolitan areas of Winnipeg, Edmonton, Vancouver, and Calgary (Statistics Canada, 2016). The majority of Inuit continue to live in settlements throughout the North, with 72.8% found in Inuit Nunangat (Statistics Canada, 2016). Indigenous peoples are the fastest-growing population in Canada, experiencing growth of 42.5% between 2006 and 2016 (Statistics Canada, 2016). Indigenous peoples are the youngest population in the country with a median age of 32.1 years compared to 40.9 in the non-Indigenous population (Statistics Canada, 2016). The youngest age category of 0–14 years has the highest rate among Indigenous peoples at 26.8%, whereas non-Indigenous peoples have the highest rate in the 45–54 age group (16.4%) (Statistics Canada, 2016).

There were more than 70 distinct Indigenous languages reported in the census, and the number of people who could speak these languages increased by 3.1% from 2006–2016 (Statistics Canada, 2016). The most common spoken languages are Cree, Inuktitut, Ojibway, Oji-Cree, and Dene (Statistics Canada, 2016).

Socioeconomic Status

Low socioeconomic status can be found in all Indigenous populations, regardless of rural, urban, or remote locations; the median total income of the Indigenous population aged 25–54 in 2005 was just over $22 000, compared to over $33 000 for the non-Indigenous population in the same age group (Statistics Canada, 2010), and more than 50% of Indigenous children live in poverty (Chansonneuve, 2005). Métis have the highest median income at $28 000, followed by Inuit at $25 000, First Nations people living off-reserve at $22 500, and First Nation people living on-reserve at $14 000 (Statistics Canada, 2010). To help put these figures into perspective, Canada's low income cut-off (LICO) for 2012 was $30 945 (Statistics Canada, 2016).

Education Levels

Education, as one of the health determinants, is often seen as a marker for the ability to earn sufficient income. The legacy of the IRS affects all education levels, with 25.6% of the Indigenous population having less than high school education, compared to 13% of the non-Indigenous population (Statistics Canada, 2016), but there is improvement in other areas.

The rate of Indigenous post-secondary school graduates is estimated at 48%: 14% with trade credentials, 21% with a college diploma, and 10% with a university degree (Statistics Canada, 2011). This is an increase from 44% in 2008 and 38% in 2001 (Statistics Canada, 2011). Looking at the figures from the three categories of Indigenous peoples, 59% of Inuit aged 25–64 do not have a high school education; however, 36% had a post-secondary certificate (Statistics Canada, 2011). Among the Métis, 54% had a post-secondary education, while 26% had less than a high school education (Statistics Canada, 2011). Within First Nation populations, 45% indicated post-secondary education as the highest level attained, compared to 40% with less than high school accreditation (Statistics Canada, 2011). First Nation communities have been reclaiming their own education, including the development of culturally relevant curricula and the training of Indigenous teachers, and this movement is becoming evident in the statistics. A teaching degree was the most common university degree obtained by First Nation (27%) and Inuit individuals at 39% (Statistics Canada, 2008).

Employment Indicators

Employment indicators are closely related to education levels and socioeconomic status, so it is not surprising that employment rates among Indigenous peoples continue to be below non-Indigenous population rates. Overall, the employment rate of Indigenous peoples was 62% in the 2011 census (First Nations, 57%; Métis, 71%; Inuit, 59%), compared to 71% in the non-Indigenous population (Statistics Canada, 2011). As stated, many reserves are located in remote or rural areas where job opportunities are often scarce. First Nation individuals living on reserve have an employment rate of 51.8%, slightly lower than First Nation individuals who live off reserve, at 66.3% (Statistics Canada, 2010). There is improvement in the labour participation and employment rates of Indigenous peoples. The employment rate gap decreased from 15.8% in 2006 to 11% in 2011. The employment gap decrease was seen in Métis and First Nation populations; however, it remained unchanged between Inuit and non-Indigenous populations (Statistics Canada, 2011).

Physical Environment

Health determinants cite physical environment as one of the factors that determine the health of individuals in an Indigenous community. One in five (19.4%) participants of the 2016 census lived in homes that were in need of major repairs, a decrease from 2011–2016 (Statistics Canada, 2016). On-reserve housing is often subpar by Canadian standards. Indigenous peoples living on reserve with dwellings in need of major repair went up to 24.2% (Statistics Canada, 2016). The number of individuals with Métis ancestry living in houses that needed major repairs decreased (13.2–11.3%), as did the numbers of houses needing major repair of First Nation people (26.2–24.2%) and Inuit (29.8–26.2%) (Statistics Canada, 2016). Utilities considered essential in urban homes, such as electricity, heating, and indoor plumbing, are not always available to First Nation community homes. Furthermore, urban-based Indigenous peoples are often found in poorer areas of town, such as the inner city, typically rampant with substandard rental housing. Forty-two percent of First Nation people living off-reserve reported residing in houses that needed major repairs (Statistics Canada, 2016) and 18.3% of Indigenous peoples lived in overcrowded housing considered not suitable for the number of people living there (Statistics Canada, 2016).

Trauma and Injury

Risk factors inherent with unsafe physical environments affect health. This is demonstrated in high rates of mortality and morbidity from injury, trauma, chronic illness, depression, and family violence (Sebastian, 2000). Illnesses such as TB and respiratory diseases, exacerbated by crowded housing, continue to be a health threat. For example, the rate of TB in Indigenous populations is six times higher than in non-Indigenous populations, with the highest rate found among Inuit, at 38 times the national average (Public Health Agency of Canada [PHAC], 2013). Respiratory diseases in Indigenous children are among the leading causes of hospitalization and death (Smylie & Adomako, 2009). Burns caused by fires are another area of concern. First Nations and Inuit Health (2009) reports that nearly half of the Indigenous communities under its jurisdiction lack adequate fire protection services. The CHN must be a client and community advocate for the improvement of housing standards and safety for Indigenous communities.

Trauma and injury, whether accidental or intentional, are also related to physical environments and are high on the list of health issues besetting Indigenous populations. Communities that practise hunting and gathering may be prone to injuries related to their particular lifestyle, such as from firearms, boats, ATVs, snowmobiles, or other hunting equipment. Alcohol is often a contributing factor to injuries and death, both accidental and intentional.

In the area of personal health practices and coping skills, lifestyle illnesses caused by drug and alcohol abuse, such as organ damage and fetal alcohol spectrum disorder, are overrepresented among Indigenous populations. Smoking rates continue to be very high—60% among people living on First Nation reserves and 48% among Inuit in the North. The majority of these individuals started smoking between the ages of 12 and 18 (PHAC, 2016). Obesity, which was recently classified as a disease by the American Medical Association, has higher rates among Indigenous populations than non-Indigenous populations. The obesity rates are similar for Inuit, Métis, and off-reserve First Nation populations (23.9%, 26.4%, and 26.1%, respectively) (PHAC, 2011b). Obesity among children and youth (aged 6–14) is also high, ranging from 16.9% among the Métis, to 20.0% among off-reserve First Nation people, to 25.6% among Inuit (PHAC, 2011). Therefore, it is not surprising that diabetes, for which being overweight is a common risk factor, has reached epidemic proportions in Indigenous communities. First Nation people living on reserve have the highest prevalence of diabetes at 16%. First Nation people living off reserve have a prevalence of 6%, and Métis are at 4%, compared to the prevalence rate for the general population of 4% (PHAC, 2016).

Mortality rates from diabetes for Indigenous women living in First Nation communities are five times higher than the national average. Diabetes is being diagnosed at a younger age, with increasing rates among youth and children (PHAC, 2011). Rates of amputation, blindness, and kidney failure are also higher among Indigenous populations. Cancer, which has been relatively uncommon in Indigenous populations, is on the rise, and certain issues are common in relation to cancer screening, diagnosis, and treatment. Screening programs have generally received a low uptake in Indigenous communities, diagnosis is often at advanced stages, and remote locations hamper cancer treatment, which typically takes place in larger urban centres (Shahid & Thompson, 2009).

INDIGENOUS DETERMINANTS OF HEALTH

Although there are many ways to consider factors that influence the overall health and well-being of specific populations, drawing on a critical anticolonial analysis of the determinants of health is central to community health nursing practice rooted in social justice. Figure 22.1 provides examples of proximal determinants of health such as high suicide rates, diabetes, and addictions. Like the leaves on a tree, these "issues" are apparent for everyone in society to see and may be perceived without deeper consideration for the greater context of the person or root causes. As mentioned, unchecked, you might stop here and attempt to address these issues in a downstream approach. Instead, CHNs can counter hegemonic thinking, focusing rather on the strengths of Indigenous peoples and seeking to understand the larger structures, policies, and racism at play.

Intermediate determinants, including inadequate housing, poverty, and economic insecurity, reveal a broader view of the contributing factors that influence the proximal determinants of health. The most upstream lens is through the distal determinants of health, far-reaching systemic factors impacting the health of Indigenous peoples. The Indian Act, colonialism, IRSs, and political decision making are listed in Figure 22.1 to better situate the discussion and provide a broader context to the root causes of the determinants depicted in the tree. Many Indigenous scholars suggest that colonization is indeed a determinant of health and have suggested replacing "Aboriginal status" with colonization in Canada's official listing of the social determinants of health. By taking a critical anticolonial lens and adopting a strength-based approach, CHNs can support the inherent capacity within Indigenous communities and disrupt the colonial health care structures that continue to cause harm. When CHNs shift the settler lens of nurse as expert to client as expert, we stop the continued colonization of health care delivery and instead adopt an authentic client-centred approach to Indigenous community health. Long and Dickason (2007) provide another means to decolonize the determinants of health in their proposed list of Indigenous-specific determinants:

- Participation in traditional activities
- Balance

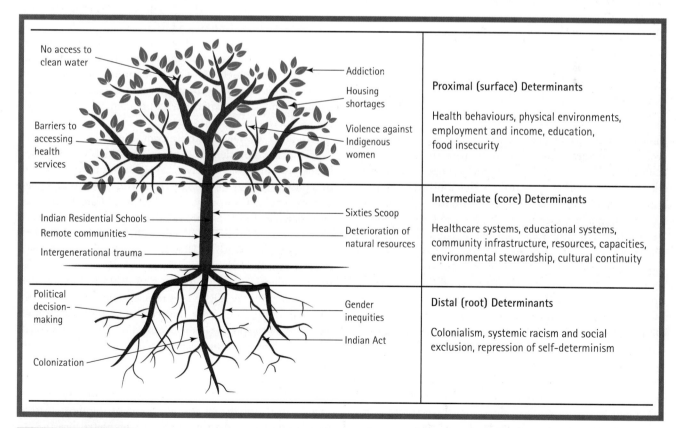

Health behaviours, physical environments, employment and income, education, food insecurity

No access to clean water
Addiction
Housing shortages
Barriers to accessing health services
Violence against Indigenous women

Proximal (surface) Determinants

Health behaviours, physical environments, employment and income, education, food insecurity

Indian Residential Schools
Remote communities
Intergenerational trauma
Sixties Scoop
Deterioration of natural resources

Intermediate (core) Determinants

Healthcare systems, educational systems, community infrastructure, resources, capacities, environmental stewardship, cultural continuity

Political decision-making
Colonization
Gender inequities
Indian Act

Distal (root) Determinants

Colonialism, systemic racism and social exclusion, repression of self-determinism

FIGURE 22.1 Proximal, Intermediate, and Distal Determinants of Aboriginal Health

Source: Reading (2009)

- Life control
- Environmental education
- Material resources
- Social resources
- Environmental and cultural connections

RECONCILIATION, DECOLONIZATION, AND SELF-DETERMINATION

CHNs hold an important role in Canada's journey toward reconciliation, particularly in the context of supporting individual, family, and community health. The National Narrative on Reconciliation Report (Reconciliation Canada, 2017) reveals that Indigenous and non-Indigenous Canadians believe that the current relationship between populations is notably more negative than positive, stemming from relationships entrenched in inequalities, mistrust, stereotypes, and absence of dialogue. They mutually agree that healing relationships through reconciliation efforts is a priority for Canada and identified key factors of reconciliation as building capacity through equity, reducing barriers, and moving away from dependency on government systems (Reconciliation Canada, 2017). Acknowledging the truth of past and present-day traumas resulting from colonization, assimilative policies, and systemic racism is a first step toward reconciliation. As CHNs, knowing and understanding long-hidden historical truths of Canada that contextually impact Indigenous health is fundamental to providing care with humility rooted in social justice while promoting the health of Indigenous peoples.

The Road to Reconciliation

As recently as 1967, when Indigenous peoples in Canada gained the right to vote, non-Indigenous Canadians remained profoundly unaware of the social realities that impact the health and well-being of Indigenous populations. The Oka Crisis of 1990 in Montreal became a pivotal point for municipal and federal authorities confronted by individuals defending and preserving their ancestral burial grounds. During the crisis, the Canadian public consciousness bore witness to overt acts of racism and violence against Indigenous people. Kirmayer, Simpson, and Cargo (2003) suggest that this led directly to the 1991 Royal Commission on Aboriginal Peoples (RCAP). The public hearings held by the RCAP uncovered widespread abuses of the IRSs. In 1993, the RCMP (the federal police force long involved with law enforcement in remote regions, including Indigenous settlements) established a Native Residential School Task Force to investigate IRSs from 1890 to 1984. The RCAP addressed many dimensions of Indigenous health and included special reports on suicide as well as volumes on the needs of urban Indigenous peoples and on healing. The RCAP Final Report included *Breaking the Silence*, a volume that detailed the myriad of abuses in the IRS system. In 1998, the government

responded with *Gathering Strength: Canada's Aboriginal Action Plan,* intended to begin a process of reconciliation and renewal from which the Institute for Aboriginal Peoples Health (one of 13 Canadian Institutes for Health Research, replacing the Medical Research Council) and the National Aboriginal Health Organization were developed. More critical was the establishment of the Aboriginal Healing Foundation (AHF), a federally funded, Indigenous-run, non-profit organization created in March 1998 to support community-based healing initiatives of Indigenous people affected by physical and sexual abuse in IRSs, including intergenerational impacts ("the Legacy"). The AHF received $350 million over 10 years to fund projects to address the legacy of the IRSs. The projects funded have included community services; conferences, workshops, and gatherings; cultural activities; healing services; material development; planning; research; traditional activities (e.g., living-on-the-land programs); and training or educational programs.

The Truth and Reconciliation Commission of Canada (TRC)

Indigenous peoples have sought other avenues for reconciliation and reparation. By February 2002, there were over 4500 claims representing 9000 claimants for damages related to IRSs. Many have now been settled. Legal proceedings often involved re-traumatization, so Indigenous organizations continue to explore alternative dispute resolution methods, including establishing the **Truth and Reconciliation Commission of Canada (TRC)**, similar to the process developed in post-apartheid South Africa. Efforts at reconciliation are consonant with the values in many Indigenous communities, which emphasize maintaining family and community ties and repairing breaches of trust by a public ritual of confession, expiation, and re-commitment to healing (Kirmayer et al., 2003).

In 2005, the federal government signed the Indian Residential Schools Settlement Agreement, which was intended to acknowledge every survivor's experience and was followed by a public apology in 2008 by then Prime Minister Stephen Harper. The TRC's mandate is to inform all Canadians about what happened in IRSs through documentation of the truth of survivors, families, and communities (TRC, 2015c). Uncovering the truth of IRSs has resulted in an acknowledgement of the intergenerational pain and trauma resulting from residential schools, giving way to 94 Indigenous-led Calls to Action. The TRC views reconciliation as establishing and maintaining mutually respectful relationships through awareness of the past, acknowledgment of the harm inflicted, atonement for the causes, and action to change behaviours (TRC, 2015).

Health care systems and professionals, including Canadian nurses, contributed to many assimilative policies that harmed Indigenous peoples. Perhaps the most glaring were segregated Indian hospitals. As regulated health care professionals, Canadian nurses practise according to an internationally revered Code of Ethics. As such, nurses hold an irrefutable responsibility and a key role in supporting the Calls to Action in reconciliation in order to facilitate healing. The TRC's 94 Calls to Action holistically support healing for survivors, communities, and Canadians' overall relationship with Indigenous peoples. Calls to Action pertain to education, justice, child welfare, culture, language, and health. The TRC, 2015d Call to Action 24 specifically addresses health and nursing, stating:

> We call upon medical and nursing schools in Canada to require all students to take a course dealing with Indigenous health issues, including the history and legacy of residential schools, the United Nations Declaration on the Rights of Indigenous Peoples, Treaties and Indigenous rights, and Indigenous teachings and practices. This will require skills-based training in intercultural competency, conflict resolution, human rights, and anti-racism.

Missing and Murdered Indigenous Women and Girls

Another devastating example of trauma brought to light by the TRC is Canada's **missing and murdered Indigenous women and girls**. Violence against women is a global issue; in Canada this is particularly true for Indigenous women. This has not always been the case. Prior to colonization, many Indigenous worldviews of gender were seen as fluid, and concepts of male and female were seen as complementary to one another's strengths and grounded in respect. Loss of culture, implementation of a patriarchal society, and prevalent racialized violence has greatly impacted Indigenous families, men, and, most notably, women (Bourassa, McKay-McNabb, & Hampton, 2004).

Chief Commissioner Marion Buller, Commissioner Michèle Audette, Commissioner Brian Eyolfson, and Commissioner Qajaq Robinson said the following about the issue (as cited in National Inquiry into Missing and Murdered Indigenous Women and Girls [MMIWG], 2017)

> There is no doubt that the loss of Indigenous women and girls to all forms of violence is a national tragedy. It has traumatized generations of families, and it will continue to traumatize communities if we do not commit to action and change. Shining a light on all the causes of violence, murders, and disappearances is a daunting task. But it is a necessary one. We are exposing hard truths about the devastating impacts of colonization, racism and sexism—aspects of Canada that many Canadians are reluctant to accept. In the face of violence suffered since colonization began, Indigenous women in Canada remain determined to reclaim their identities, cultures, languages, and land. They are taking their rightful place in their communities and Nations, and we are ready to support them. This is our collective responsibility to future generations. We can and must act together to create a better future for our women and girls.

The following Yes, But Why? feature explores this issue further.

YES, BUT WHY?

Missing and Murdered Indigenous Women in Canada

What?

To date, over 1000 Indigenous girls and women have been murdered or have gone missing at a rate four times higher than the national average of the Canadian population (Inter-American Commission on Human Rights, 2014). This is particularly concerning given Indigenous women represent only a small percentage of the Canadian population (Inter-American Commission on Human Rights, 2014). Not only do Indigenous women and girls experience higher numbers of violent incidents, but also the severity and frequency is disproportionately higher than the national average (Native Women's Association of Canada, 2016). Amnesty International and the UN have identified the discrimination and violence against Indigenous women in Canada and resulting disappearances and murders as a human rights violation (Amnesty International, 2004; UN Human Rights Office of the High Commissioner, 2018).

So What?

The overrepresentation of violence toward Indigenous women and girls is rooted in gendered, sexualized, and racial discrimination (Native Women's Association of Canada, 2016). Canada's policies have targeted Indigenous women's disenfranchisement through loss of title, land, culture, and community. Colonization and racism have specifically created a legacy of ongoing harm toward the health and well-being of Indigenous women. Their social and economic marginalization have resulted in increased vulnerability to exploitation based on the disproportionate number of Indigenous women living in dangerous situations of poverty, homelessness, and sex work (Amnesty International, 2004). Systemic racism and sexualized objectification has created a societal indifference that has invited perpetrators to seek out Indigenous women for harm (Amnesty International, 2004; Women's Association of Canada, 2016). This violence is compounded by biased and prejudiced systems, agencies, and policies that continuously fail to protect them (Amnesty International, 2004; MMIWG, 2017).

Now What?

Canada has been called upon to address the human rights violation of Indigenous women and the violence against them (Amnesty International, 2004; Native Women's Association of Canada, 2016). Recommendations to address these deep-rooted issues are to examine the root cause of the failures of the Canadian justice system; address the violation of human rights of Indigenous people and women through governmental public acknowledgment and condemnation of violence toward Indigenous women and girls; and provide funding and resources, specifically the acute, primary, and community support needed for the protection and well-being of Indigenous women, including healing for families and communities (MMIWG, 2017).

For decades, the Native Women's Association of Canada has committed to the inquiry and documentation of violence impacting Indigenous women while bringing the issue of missing and murdered Indigenous women and girls to the forefront in Canada through stories of families and calls for action. In 2013 an RCMP report confirmed decades of work revealing 1181 cases of missing and murdered Indigenous women and girls in Canada (MMIWG, 2017). In light of overwhelming statistics of violence, and through relentless efforts of activists, the MMIWG began in 2016. While the inquiry is ongoing, the interim report has identified key issues contributing to missing and murdered Indigenous women and girls as longstanding colonial policies, systemic racism, and sexism combined with the roles of the police, justice system, courts, coroners, corrections, and media in perpetuating racism and injustices against Indigenous women (MMIWG, 2017).

Standards of Practice Fulfilled

#4 Professional Relationships
- "Acknowledges that the current state of Aboriginal health in Canada is a direct result of previous Canadian government policies" in working with Indigenous people as stated in the Truth and Reconciliation Commission of Canada: Calls to Action (CHNC, 2019, revised).

UN Declaration on the Rights of Indigenous Peoples

The **UN Declaration on the Rights of Indigenous Peoples (UNDRIP)** is the universal framework of minimum standards for the survival, dignity, and well-being of Indigenous peoples of the world and is seen by many as the most comprehensive fundamental instrument on the rights of Indigenous peoples (UN General Assembly, 2007). The UN General Assembly adopted the UNDRIP in 2007 by a majority vote of 144 states, with the exception of Canada, Australia, New Zealand, and the United States. Since then all four countries reversed their position in support of the Declaration, with Canada adopting the UNDRIP in 2010. In 2013 the UN Special Rapporteur on the Rights of Indigenous Peoples in Canada concluded that despite ranking near the top among countries with respect to human development standards, wealth, and prosperity, Canada's "aboriginal people live in conditions akin to those in countries that rank much lower and in which poverty abounds." The report speaks to alarming disparities between on-reserve services and those available to other Canadians and highlights the Canadian Human Rights Commission as identifying the conditions of Indigenous peoples as the most serious human rights problem in Canada (UN General Assembly, 2014).

The UNDRIP affirms that Indigenous peoples are equal to all other peoples and in exercise of their rights should be free from discrimination of any kind. Through self-determination and control over developments affecting them and their lands, territories, and resources, the UNDRIP supports the strength of their institutions, cultures, traditions, IK, and well-being. Many articles within the UNDRIP address discrimination, oppression, genocide, and inequities concerning the violations of human rights of Indigenous peoples across the world. The UNDRIP also outlines the inherent rights of Indigenous peoples and communities, providing a foundation for principles of care for CHNs. The UNDRIP proclaims that Indigenous peoples have the right to self-determination in developing and determining health, housing, and other economic and social programs affecting them and, as far as possible, to administer such programs through their own institution. Article 24 declares Indigenous peoples have the right to their traditional medicines and to maintain their health practices, including an equal right to the enjoyment of the highest attainable standards of physical and mental health (UN General Assembly, 2007).

CHNs are often the primary resource for remote Indigenous communities and as such are instrumental in building relationships with community members through respecting and supporting self-governance and **self-determination** involving health and healing practices. Research in protective factors related to self-determination show that community-led health services grounded in a collective sense of history and culture contribute to better mental health outcomes in First Nation communities (Kielland & Simeone, 2014). CHNs supporting self-determination and community-led care are actively participating in reconciliation while working toward improved health outcomes. Understanding and incorporating reconciliation in the practice of community health nursing is integral to building relationships with Indigenous peoples and changing the way other professionals think about, and work alongside, communities.

INDIGENOUS HEALTH AND COMMUNITY HEALTH NURSING

The **decolonization** of nursing practice is an interactive process to expose, resist, and transform colonial processes within nursing and health care. Decolonization disrupts the continued colonization and oppression of Indigenous peoples and instead affirms and supports the strength and knowledge within Indigenous cultures (McGibbon, Mulaudzi, Didham, Barton, & Sochan, 2014). **Cultural humility** supports the continual self-reflection of beliefs by acknowledging personal and systemic biases while adopting a philosophy as a learner in relation to another's experience (First Nations Health Authority, 2015). Cultural humility allows CHNs to come to know a community as expert, with recognition and regard for health and healing practices meaningful to the community and its peoples, supporting mutual trust. **Cultural safety** in nursing practice is not focused on understanding specific details and adopting "Indigenous culture" but rather reflecting upon your own beliefs, practices, and history and how they impact the people you serve (Ward, Branch, & Fridkin, 2016). Transcultural communication was previously adopted in nursing in an attempt to learn about "diversity." The assumption is that by learning specific practices and customs of a people outside the dominant white settler culture would create safe nursing practice. Problematically, this approach runs the risk of perpetuating generalizations and stereotypes about certain groups, deviating nurses from coming to know each client and community individually in a culturally safe way (Bourque Bearskin, 2014). In understanding that people construct and live *their* culture in their own unique way, it is therefore important to inquire into individual spiritual, cultural, and physical health and wellness practices without assumptions. This approach is parallel to patient-centred care. The shift in nursing consciousness and the practice of cultural safety foster a lifelong discussion toward moving from a strictly western or colonial perspective on other cultures to embracing IK and a **Two-Eyed Seeing** approach (Kurtz, Mahara, Cash, Nyberg, & Moller, 2017).

Two-Eyed Seeing is a concept to describe an approach of using two worldviews to "see" community care. Out of one eye we see with Western knowledge and out of the second eye we consider Indigenous ways of knowing centred in the practices and healing traditions of the community. This approach provides a more holistic approach to nursing practice that honours the inherent expertise within these two paradigms.

> "Two-Eyed Seeing is learning to see from one eye with the strengths of (or best in) Western knowledge and ways of knowing . . . .and most importantly, using both eyes together for the benefit of all."
>
> (Bartlett, Marshall, Marshall, et al., 2015, pp. 17–18)

Two-Eyed Seeing calls on health care providers to bring together these two ways of knowing not only to broaden nursing practice in a more holistic way, but to ensure CHNs are always on a journey of looking for different perspectives in pursuit of finding better ways of providing care (Bartlett, Marshall, Marshall, et al., 2015). An example of Two-Eyed Seeing was aptly described by an Indigenous advocate from the Urban Indigenous Opioid Task Force during a 2017 forum on best practices for addictions services in light of the Canadian opioid crisis. He highlighted that clients accessing addictions services currently have to choose between services; either they access treatment in a facility/hospital and lose contact with their traditional healing methods or they can stay within

their community but lose the benefits of medical treatment such as opioid agonist therapy. He advocated that clients should have the benefits of both bio-medicine and traditional healing methods such as Elder support, sweat lodges, and ceremony to support their healing journey in a holistic way.

As a CHN, nursing knowledge supports your practice in many ways, such as decision making, ethics, professional standards, empirical knowledge, and more. IK supports a holistic view of health and wellness through culture, relationships, history, community, oral traditions, land-based knowledge, mutual-respect, and more. The Canadian Indigenous Nursing Association (CINA) works to improve the health of Indigenous peoples by supporting Indigenous nurses and by promoting the development and practice of Indigenous health nursing. To this aim, the CINA provides support and frameworks of care to Indigenous and non-Indigenous nurses practising in Indigenous communities that can be accessed on its website (www.indigenousnurses.ca). CHNs can support the community they are partnering with and caring for by ensuring they are incorporating IK, led by their Indigenous clients, family, and community, deemed meaningful to their care. Browne and Stanfield (2013) explain that nurses must practise cultural safety when incorporating IK and that its use requires consultation, permission, and compensation. IK is considered something that is shared by knowledge holders in Indigenous communities and not "given" to or ever "owned" by those who share or receive it. CHNs must seek guidance from the communities they are visiting, especially regarding protocols and respecting the people and traditions of the nations they serve.

CHNs have the opportunity to disrupt the continued colonization of community health care that has resulted in mistrust, poor health outcomes, and the dominant narrative that Indigenous communities are inept and in need of others to determine their care services. Instead, CHNs can adopt culturally safe practices that honour the inherent strengths within each community and provide meaningful services for this generation, and the next, that are inclusive, respectful, and collaborative.

CASE STUDY

Coyote: Keeper of Memories
by D. Wilson, G. Campbell-McArthur, W. Hulko, S. Mahara, J. William, C. De Rose, & E. Patrick Moller

Traditionally, Secwepemc peoples used storytelling as a means of teaching about their environment, social structures, and beliefs. Coyote is a key figure in Secwepemc storytelling and often represents the trickster. As we learned in previous research with Secwepemc Elders (Hulko et al., 2010) that stories related to memory loss in later life or culturally safe dementia care (whether Coyote stories or not) do not exist, it was recommended that we create new stories based on our research findings (Hulko et al., 2014). Two of the four stories we wrote as a team are included in this book with the permission of the CSDC Elder advisors. Jean William, Cecelia de Rose, and Estella Patrick Moller are the keepers of this new knowledge (the four teaching stories) and plan to use these teaching tools to educate nurses as

well as members of their communities. Below is our teaching story *Coyote: Keeper of Memories*.

Coyote was sitting atop of Mount Paul one day. He was asking the Sun for help with his children. He had many children and they were always making so many demands on him, day and night. Coyote was very tired. He asked:

> Sun, I am tired because of all my children. They are endless in their demands on how to catch fish, to show them how to make pit houses, how to make the fire. Can you help me?

Sun is quiet for a few minutes and says:

> Coyote, you have not helped your children to be self-sufficient. You are doing everything for your children and you have to teach them how to feed, house and care for themselves. After that, you will find your peace. But I must let you know . . .

Coyote is very impatient with Sun—she is old and talks slow and pauses often between words. So Coyote listens as long as he can to Sun and he decides he heard enough. Coyote interrupts Sun:

> Thanks Sun, that is a great idea and I will do just as you say.

Coyote forgets to be patient and listen to the wisdom of Sun. Coyote is anxious to show his children how to feed, house and care for themselves. He starts the very next morning. Coyote teaches the men how to gather Fish from the rivers, how to hunt Deer and Rabbit from the forests. He shows the women where to gather Berries and Asparagus from the earth, how to make clothes for themselves. Coyote shows all his children how to build pit houses and the best places to build them. He teaches his children how to make fire for themselves and how to keep it well.

Coyote is very happy with his teachings. He now has time to sit back and watch his children. But as the sun sets and rises, he is getting bored. He misses the attention from his children. But most troubling is his children are becoming very greedy, they are taking too much Berries and Fish from Bear, not enough trees are left for Beaver to use for his home. Sun watches over the days and sees all this happening.

Coyote decides to talk to his children about this. He says to them:

> My Children, you are not being fair to the other creatures, you are taking everything for yourselves and others are suffering because you are taking too much yourselves. Bear and Beaver are hungry and cold, they need some Fish and Trees for themselves too.

The Children listen to Coyote and they don't think they are being unfair. They feel that Coyote's teachings are enough to lead them down their own paths and that they are wise enough to manage all that they have learned. They say to Coyote that they don't want to share the food and trees with others, they are afraid that they will not have enough for themselves.

Coyote is stuck, he doesn't know what to do. He decides he needs to talk to Sun again, maybe Sun has more to tell him. So Coyote climbs up Mount Paul to talk to Sun. He says to Sun:

> Sun, I don't know what to do. My children are thriving from my teachings but they are taking too much for themselves, so much that other Creatures are suffering because of their greediness. What can I do?

Sun was waiting for impatient Coyote to come back to her. Sun slowly says:

> Coyote, you only listened to half of what I was going to say. Teach your Children to thank the Creator before they take what they need, to take only what they need and to return those parts back to the Creator. Your teachings must be balanced with the giving and taking, Coyote.

Coyote now understands his mistake and wishes he had remembered to be more patient with Sun the first time he talked to her. Coyote knows that his Children are very greedy and don't want to share the food and trees. Coyote knows what he needs to do now.

So Coyote says to his Children:

> My Children, you make me so proud—I have taught you well and you are thriving. You have Fish and Berries for many feasts, even in the cold winter months, you will be well fed. Your homes are sturdy and warm from the fires. You never go hungry or cold. You have learned very well.

Coyote's Children feel their chests swell from the compliments from Coyote. Coyote continued:

> But my Children, you are not doing as good as Eagle. I taught Eagle to build his own nest and catch his own food all by himself. He doesn't have to share with brother or sister Eagle. Everything he catches, he keeps it to himself and his nest is never crowded. Do you want to learn how to be like Eagle?

The Children talk among themselves. How much easier that each Child would like to keep all the Fish and Berries that they catch and gather to stock for their own use? And to have a pit house all for one person? The Children want to learn the Eagle's way because Coyote's Children are greedy and want more and they want to do better than Eagle. Coyote says to them:

> For me to teach you Eagle's ways, you must give back my teachings. I will put those teachings in this grass basket and keep them here beside me. When you give back my teachings, I will give you Eagle's teachings so that you won't have to share anything with your brothers and Sisters.

Coyote's children are eager for Eagle's teachings and they forget that Coyote can be a trickster and speaks only half truths. They give their teachings back to Coyote. Coyote says:

> I need to teach you about giving and taking, my Children. You have taken too much and not given back enough. You are not sharing what you catch and build with your own Brothers and Sisters. Bear and beaver are going hungry and have no shelters for themselves. You are not eagles. I am going to keep my teachings in this basket, I will let you use what I think you need. No longer will I let you use all my teachings for yourselves. I will watch over each of you and take back the teachings that I need.

Coyote's Children were tricked to give back their teachings. Coyote places the memories in his grass basket beside him. He feels proud of himself for restoring the balance again.

But Coyote forgot about the precious balance of memories in his Children. His Children now forget too many things, they forget where their pit houses are, Brothers and Sisters forget each other. Coyote needs to help them with all their daily chores again and he is getting exhausted again. It is like his Children have come full circle to infants. Exhausted Coyote climbs back up Mount Paul to speak to Sun again.

Sun, please help me. I listened patiently to you last time and heard all that you said but my Children are not any better, they are worse than before and I am so tired. What have I done? How can I change things to be better?

Sun nourishes the berries and trees, wakes up Bear from hibernation and warms the land. She is life giving and wants Coyote and his Children to survive. So she says:

Coyote, listen to me well. In taking back your teachings, you took back too many memories by accident. Coyote, you did not realize that other memories are attached to your teachings. Memories are all connected like the grass weaved in a grass basket, you can't pull one piece of grass out without affecting the other grass threads. You have to be careful in what memories you take back.

Again, Coyote sees his mistake—in taking away the traditional teachings of Sun and Eagle, he took away memories important for survival of his Children. Coyote needs to remember the sacred teachings and the precious balance of all living things. Coyote needs to be mindful of his own memories basket.

So Coyote reaches into his grass basket and gives back his teachings to his Children. And he watches closely over his Children to make sure they only take their share of food and trees. When his Children start to become forgetful, they know it is because of Coyote and his grass basket. His children understand that Coyote controls the Basket of Memories and takes them back when he wants to and from whom he wants. Sometimes he keeps the memories for a short time, other times he keeps the memories for a long time, it all depends on how full his grass basket is at the time.

Discussion Questions

1. What are the pearls of wisdom that stand out for you in this story?

2. How would you apply these teachings to your community health nursing practice with Indigenous communities?

3. How would you honour the Indigenous Knowledge from this story's teachings?

CONCLUSION

The chapter outlined the history, diverse cultures, traditional knowledge, and worldviews of Indigenous peoples in Canada. Colonization, colonial and assimilative policies, and systemic racism have had profound negative impacts on the health and well-being of Indigenous populations in Canada. Health systems are complex and distinct between First Nation, status and non-status, Métis, and Inuit peoples. CHNs must stay informed as policies continue to change in order to adopt service models led by and for Indigenous peoples that promote self-determination. Uncovering the truth about Canada's history with Indigenous peoples is critical for CHNs seeking to understand health challenges, inequities, and intergenerational trauma that impact clients and communities today. Enacting reconciliation and practising nursing grounded in cultural humility and cultural safety will support CHNs to build relationships and support communities in leading their health and wellness journey. As nursing shifts its collective consciousness to one of reconciliation, through decolonizing practices and Two-Eyed Seeing, we must acknowledge and embrace the challenges and evolving nature of this important journey through collaborative relationships that benefit all.

KEY TERMS

Aboriginal (p. 407)
assimilation (p. 408)
colonial (p. 407)
colonization (p. 408)
cultural humility (p. 418)
cultural safety (p. 418)
decolonization (p. 418)

First Nations (p. 407)
Indian Act (p. 408)
Indian agents (p. 408)
Indian hospitals (p. 410)
Indian residential schools (IRSs) (p. 409)
Indigenous (p. 407)
Indigenous Knowledge (IK) (p. 408)
Inequities (p. 412)
intergenerational trauma (p. 410)
Inuit (p. 407)
non-status Indians (p. 411)
Métis (p. 407)
Missing and murdered Indigenous women and girls (p. 417)
registered or status Indian (p. 411)
reserves (p. 408)
self-determination (p. 418)
60s Scoop (p. 410)
treaties (p. 408)
Truth and Reconciliation Commission of Canada (TRC) (p. 416)
Two-Eyed Seeing (p. 419)
UN Declaration of the Rights of Indigenous Peoples (UNDRIP) (p. 418)

STUDY QUESTIONS

1. Describe five effects of the residential school legacy that continue to impact Indigenous communities today.

2. What are the health impacts of the 60s Scoop, and how long have they spanned?

3. Describe how colonization is ongoing in today's health care system.

4. What are the rights that the UNDRIP protects in relation to community health?

5. Provide examples of proximal, intermediate, and distal determinants of health.

INDIVIDUAL CRITICAL-THINKING EXERCISES

1. What is the difference between cultural safety and cultural humility, and how do these concepts improve health outcomes?

2. What TRC Calls to Action specifically apply to nursing? How will you incorporate the TRC's Calls to Action into your nursing practice?

3. What does reconciliation mean to you? How will your understanding of reconciliation apply to your nursing practice?

4. Reflect on your own culture and what practices you cherish most. Food, family, language, customs, and spirituality are all elements that make up your own unique culture. Imagine you were no longer able to connect with your culture. How would you feel? What would be some of the impacts on your life and well-being?

GROUP CRITICAL-THINKING EXERCISES

As a class, watch the film *Colonization Road* (available at www .cbc.ca).

1. What are the causes of the disproportionately high adverse health outcomes for Indigenous populations in Canada when compared to non-Indigenous populations?

2. How has enforced geographical isolation contributed to issues related to the quality of life of Indigenous peoples?

3. What are three ways that CHNs can decolonize health promotion practice?

REFERENCES

Aboriginal Affairs and Northern Development Canada. (2013). First Nations in Canada map. Retrieved from http://www.aadnc-aandc.gc.ca/DAM/DAM-INTER-HQ-AI/STAGING/texte-text/ai_mprm_fnc_wal_pdf_1344968972421_eng.pdf

Aboriginal Healing Foundation. (1999). *Annual report 1999.* Retrieved from http://www.ahf.ca/about-us/annual-reports

Aboriginal Healing Foundation. (2006). *Métis history and experience and residential schools in Canada.* Retrieved from http://www.ahf.ca/downloads/metiseweb.pdf

Allan, B., & Smylie, J. (2015). *First Peoples, second class treatment: The role of racism in the health and well-being of Indigenous peoples in Canada.* Toronto, ON: The Wellesley Institute. Retrieved from http://www.wellesleyinstitute.com/wp-content/uploads/2015/02/Summary-First-Peoples-Second-Class-Treatment-Final.pdf

Amnesty International. (2004). *Stolen Sisters: Discrimination and violence against Indigenous women in Canada.* Ottawa, ON: Amnesty International.

Assembly of First Nations and National Congress of American Indians. (1999). *Declaration of kinship and cooperation among the indigenous peoples and nations of north America.* Retrieved from http://www.afn.ca/about-afn/national-congress-of-american-indians/

Brown, H., McPherson, G., Peterson, R., Neuman, V., & Cramner. B. (2012). *Canadian Journal of Nursing Research, 44*(2), pp. 44–63.

Browne, A. J., Smye, V., Rodney, P., Tang, S., Mussell, B., & O'Neil, J. (2011). Access to primary care from the perspective of Aboriginal patients at an urban emergency department. *Qualitative Health Research, 21*(3), 333–348.

Browne, A., & Stanfield, D. (2013). The relevance of Indigenous Knowledge for nursing curriculum. *International Journal of Nursing Education Scholarship, 10*(1), 1–9. doi:10.1515/ijnes-2012-0041

Bourassa, C., McKay-McNabb, K., & Hampton, M. (2004). Racism, sexism, and colonialism: The impact on the health of Aboriginal women in Canada. *Canadian Woman Studies, 24*(1), 23–29. Retrieved from http://www.yorku.ca/cwscf

Bourque Bearskin, L. (2014). *Mâmawoh kamâtowin: Coming together to help each other: Honouring Indigenous nursing knowledge.* Dissertation. Retrieved from https://era.library.ualberta.ca/files/zp38wc706/Bourque_Raymonde_Lisa_L_201409_PhD

Cameron, B. L., del Pilar Carmargo Plazas, M., Salas, A. S., & Hungler, K. (2014). Understanding inequalities in access to health care for Aboriginal people: A call for nursing action. *Advances in Nursing Science, 37*(3), E1–E6.

Chansonneuve, D. (2005). *Reclaiming connections: Understanding residential school trauma among Aboriginal people.* Ottawa, ON: Aboriginal Healing Foundation.

Community Health Nurses of Canada. (2019, revised). *Canadian community health nursing professional practice model and standards of practice.* Revised March 2011. St. John's, NL: Author. Retrieved from https://www.chnc.ca/en/standards-of-practice?lang=switch1

Constitution Act (1982). Schedule B to the Canada Act 1982. Retrieved from http://laws-lois.justice.gc.ca/eng/Const/page-16.html#h-52

Crowshoe, C. (2005). *Sacred ways of life: Traditional knowledge toolkit.* Prepared for the First Nations Centre, National Aboriginal Health Organization.

Deagle, G. (1999). The three-tier system [Editorial]. *Canadian Family Physician, 247*–249.

Dickason, O. P. (2002). *Canada's First Nations: A history of founding peoples from earliest times* (3rd ed.). Don Mills, ON: Oxford.

First Nations and Inuit Health. (2009, February). *A statistical profile on the health of First Nations in Canada: Determinants of health, 1999 to 2003.* Retrieved from http://www.hc-sc.gc.ca/fniah-spnia/pubs/aborig-autoch/2009-stats-profil/index-eng.php

First Nations Caring Society. (2005). *Wen: De The journey continues.* Ottawa, ON. Retrieved from https://fncaringsociety.com/sites/default/files/docs/WendeJourneyContinues.pdf

First Nations Health Authority. (2015) *#itstartswithme; FNHS's policy statement on cultural safety and humility.* Vancouver, BC.

Retrieved from http://www.fnha.ca/Documents/FNHA-Policy-Statement-Cultural-Safety-and-Humility.pdf

Fleet, C. (1997). *First Nations firsthand: A history of five hundred years of encounter, war, and peace inspired by the eyewitnesses.* Edison, NJ: Chartwell.

Furi, M., & Wherrett, J. (2003). *Indian status and band membership issues.* Retrieved from http://www.parl.gc.ca/content/lop/researchpublications/bp410-e.htm#aregistrationtx

Greenwood, M., De, L. S., Lindsay, N. M., & Reading, C. (2015). *Determinants of indigenous peoples' health in Canada: Beyond the social.*

Government of Canada. (2018). *Indigenous health.* Retrieved from https://www.canada.ca/en/services/health/aboriginal-health.html

Hulko, W., Wilson, D., Mahara, S., William, J., Patrick Moller, E., De Rose, E., . . . & Parkscott, A. (2014, October). Culturally safe dementia care; Building the capacity of nurses to care for First Nation Elders with memory loss. Workshop presentation at INIHKD NEAR conference, Winnipeg, MB.

Hulko, W., Camille, E., Antifeau, E., Arnouse, M., Bachynksi, N., & Taylor, D. (2010). Views of First Nation Elders on memory loss and memory care in later life. *Journal of Cross Cultural Gerontology, 25,* 317–342. Online First, 1 July 2010. doi:10.1007/s10823-010-9123-9.

Indigenous and Northern Affairs Canada. (2018). *Indigenous peoples and communities.* Retrieved from https://www.aadnc-aandc.gc.ca/eng/1100100013785/1304467449155

Inter-American Commission on Human Rights. (2014). *Missing and murdered Indigenous women in British Columbia, Canada.* Retrieved from http://www.oas.org/en/iachr/reports/pdfs/Indigenous-Women-BC-Canada-en.pdf

Johnston, P. (2016, June 26). *Revisiting the "Sixties Scoop" of Indigenous children.* Retrieved from http://policyoptions.irpp.org/magazines/july-2016/revisiting-the-sixties-scoop-of-indigenous-children/

Kielland, N., & Simeone, T. (2014). *Current issues in mental health in Canada: The mental health of First Nations and Inuit communities.* Library of Parliament, Ottawa. Retrieved from https://mail.google.com/mail/u/1/#inbox/163716e42642ac5b?projector=1&messagePartId=0.1

Kirmayer, L. J., Simpson, C., & Cargo, M. (2003). Healing traditions: Culture, community and mental health promotion with Canadian Aboriginal peoples. *Australas Psychiatry, 11* (suppl. 1): S15–23. Retrieved from http://www.indiaenvironmentportal.org.in/files/Indigenous%20health%20part%202.pdf

Kurtz, D., Mahara, S., Cash, P., Nyberg, J., & Moller, E. P. (2017). Indigenous methodology in understanding indigenous nurse graduate transition to practice. *The International Indigenous Policy Journal.* Retrieved from https://mail.google.com/mail/u/0/#inbox/16181dfc8386d545?projector=1&messagePartId=0.1

Long, D., & Dickason, P. O. (2007) *Visions of the heart. Canadian Aboriginal issues* (3rd ed.). Oxford University Press.

Lord, L. (1997, August 18). How many people were here before Columbus? *U.S. News and World Report,* 68–70.

Lux, M. K. (2010). Care for the racially careless: Indian hospitals in the Canadian west, 1920–1950s. *Canadian Historical Review.* https://doi.org/10.3138/chr.91.3.407

Lux, M. K. (2016). *Separate beds: A history of Indian hospitals and Aboriginal health.* Toronto, ON: University of Toronto Press.

Maher, S. (2015, June 4). Letter found in shed reveals suffering and anguish residential schools created. *National Post.* Retrieved from http://nationalpost.com/opinion/stephen-maher-a-1935-letter-found-in-shed-reveals-suffering-and-anguish-residential-schools-created

Marshall, M., Marshall, A., Bartlett, C., Greenwood, M., de Leeuw, S., Lindsay, N. M., & Reading, C. (2015). *Two-Eyed Seeing in medicine. Determinants of Indigenous peoples' health in Canada: Beyond the social.* Toronto, ON: Canadian Scholars' Press. 16.

McGibbon, E., Mulaudzi, F. M., Didham, P., Barton, S., & Sochan, A. (2014). Towards decolonizing nursing: The colonization of nursing and strategies for increasing the counter-narrative. *Nursing Inquiry, 21*(3), 179–191.

McKenzie, H., Varcoe, C., Browne, A. J., & Day, L. (2016). Disrupting the continuities among residential schools, the sixties scoop, and child welfare: An analysis of colonial and neocolonial discourses. *International Indigenous Policy Journal, 7,* 4. Retrieved from https://ir.lib.uwo.ca/cgi/viewcontent.cgi?referer=https://scholar.google.ca/&httpsredir=1&article=1260&context=iipj

Métis National Council. (2011). *The Métis nation.* Ottawa, ON: Author. Retrieved from http://www.metisnation.ca/index.php/who-are-the-metis

Moore, J. L., & Maguire, R. (1978). *The historical development of the Indian Act.* Ottawa, ON: Treaties and Historical Research Centre, Indian and Northern Affairs, p. 114.

National Collaborating Centre for Aboriginal Health (NCCAH). (2011). *The Aboriginal health legislation and policy framework in Canada.* Retrieved from https://www.ccnsa-nccah.ca/docs/context/FS-HealthLegislationPolicy-Lavoie-Gervais-Toner-Bergeron-Thomas-EN.pdf

National Inquiry into Missing and Murdered Indigenous Women and Girls (MMIWG). (2017). *MMIW interim report: Our women and girls are sacred,* 30 Retrieved from http://www.mmiwg-ffada.ca/files/ni-mmiwg-interim-report-en.pdf

Native Women's Association of Canada. (2016). The national inquiry on murders and disappearance of Indigenous women and girls: Recommendations from the symposium on planning for change: Towards a national inquiry and an effective national action plan. *Canadian Journal of Women and the Law.* Retrieved from https://www.nwac.ca/wp-content/uploads/2016/02/NWAC-FAFIAsymposium_22reccommendations_2016_EN.pdf

Office of the Treaty Commissioner. (2013). *Aboriginal rights and title.* Retrieved from http://www.otc.ca/pdfs/aboriginal_rights.pdf

Public Health Agency of Canada (PHAC). (2011a, June 23). *Prevalence among Aboriginal peoples.* Retrieved from http://www.phac-aspc.gc.ca/hp-ps/hl-mvs/oic-oac/abo-aut-eng.php

Public Health Agency of Canada (PHAC). (2011b, December 15). *Diabetes among First Nations, Inuit, and Métis populations.* Retrieved from http://www.phac-aspc.gc.ca/cd-mc/publications/diabetes-diabete/facts-figures-faits-chiffres-2011/chap6-eng.php

Public Health Agency of Canada (PHAC). (2013). *TB and Aboriginal people.* Retrieved from Control of Infectious Diseases: http://www.cpha.ca/en/programs/history/achievements/02-id/tb-aboriginal.aspx

Public Health Agency of Canada (PHAC). (2016). *Health status of Canadians 2016*. Retrieved from http://healthycanadians.gc.ca/publications/department-ministere/state-public-health-status-2016-etat-sante-publique-statut/alt/pdf-eng.pdf

Reading, C. (2009). Social determinants of health: The case of Aboriginal women and HIV/AIDS. Research Lecture, University of Victoria.

Richmond, C. A., & Cook, C. (2016). Creating conditions for Canadian Aboriginal health equity: The promise of healthy public policy. *Public Health Reviews, 37*(1): 2. Retrieved from https://publichealthreviews.biomedcentral.com/articles/10.1186/s40985-016-0016-5

Reconciliation Canada. (n.d.). Elder's statement; A shared tomorrow. Retrieved from http://reconciliationcanada.ca/about/history-and-background/elders-statement/

Reconciliation Canada. (2017). *National narrative report*. Retrieved from http://reconciliationcanada.ca/staging/wp-content/uploads/2017/05/NationalNarrativeReport-ReconciliationCanada-ReleasedMay2017_3.pdf

RCMP. (2015). Missing and murdered Aboriginal women: A national operational overview.

Sebastian, J. G. (2000). Vulnerability and vulnerable populations: An overview. In M. Stanhope & J. Lancaster, *Community and public health nursing* (pp. 638–661). Toronto, ON: Mosby.

Shahid, S., & Thompson, S. C. (2009). An overview of cancer and beliefs about the disease in Indigenous people of Australia, Canada, New Zealand and the US. *Australian and New Zealand Journal of Public Health*, 109–118. doi:10.1111/j.1753-6405.2009.0035.x

Sinclair, R. (2007). Identity lost and found: Lessons from the sixties scoop. *First Peoples Child and Family Review, 66*.

Smylie, J., & Adomako, P. (2009). *Indigenous children's health report: Health assessment in action*. Retrieved from http://www.stmichaelshospital.com/pdf/crich/ichr_report.pdf

Statistics Canada. (2008, March). *Educational portrait of Canada, 2006*. Retrieved from http://www12.statcan.ca/census-recensement/2006/as-sa/97-560/pdf/97-560-XIE2006001.pdf

Statistics Canada. (2010, June 21). *Income*. Retrieved from http://www.statcan.gc.ca/pub/89-645-x/2010001/income-revenu-eng.htm

Statistics Canada. (2011, August 23). *Low income cut-offs*. Retrieved from http://www.statcan.gc.ca/pub/75f0002m/2011002/lico-sfr-eng.htm

Statistics Canada. (2016). *Aboriginal peoples in Canada: First Nations people, Métis and Inuit*. Retrieved from http://www12.statcan.gc.ca/census-recensement/2016/as-sa/98-200-x/2016022/98-200-x2016022-eng.pdf

Truth and Reconciliation Commission of Canada (TRC). (2012). Canada, Aboriginal peoples, and residential schools: They came for the children. Winnipeg, MN, p. 6. Retrieved from http://www.myrobust.com/websites/trcinstitution/File/2039_T&R_eng_web%5B1%5D.pdf

Truth and Reconciliation Commission of Canada (TRC). (2015a). Canada's residential schools: The Métis experience. Retrieved from http://www.myrobust.com/websites/trcinstitution/File/Reports/Volume_3_Metis_English_Web.pdf

Truth and Reconciliation Commission of Canada (TRC). (2015b). Canada's residential schools: Missing children and unmarked burials. Retrieved from http://www.myrobust.com/websites/trcinstitution/File/Reports/Volume_4_Missing_Children_English_Web.pdf

Truth and Reconciliation Commission of Canada (TRC). (2015c). Canada's residential schools: The history, part 1, origins to 1939. Retrieved from http://www.myrobust.com/websites/trcinstitution/File/Reports/Volume_1_History_Part_1_English_Web.pdf

Truth and Reconciliation Commission of Canada (TRC). (2015d). Honouring the Truth, reconciling for the future. Retrieved from http://www.trc.ca/websites/trcinstitution/File/2015/Honouring_the_Truth_Reconciling_for_the_Future_July_23_2015.pdf

Truth and Reconciliation Commission of Canada (TRC). (2015e). The legacy. Retrieved from http://www.myrobust.com/websites/trcinstitution/File/Reports/Volume_5_Legacy_English_Web.pdf

Truth and Reconciliation Commission of Canada (TRC). (2015f). What is reconciliation? Retrieved from https://vimeo.com/25389165

UN General Assembly. (2007). *United Nations Declaration on the Rights of Indigenous Peoples: Resolution/adopted by the General Assembly*. Retrieved from http://www.refworld.org/docid/471355a82.html

UN Human Rights Office of the High Commissioner. (2018). *End of mission statement by Dubravka Šimonović, United Nations Special Rapporteur on violence against women, its causes and consequences: Official visit to Canada*. Retrieved from http://www.ohchr.org/EN/NewsEvents/Pages/DisplayNews.aspx?NewsID=22981&LangID=E

UN General Assembly. (2014). *Report of the Special Rapporteur on the rights of Indigenous people, James Anaya*. Retrieved from http://unsr.jamesanaya.org/docs/countries/2014-report-canada-a-hrc-27-52-add-2-en.pdf

Venne, S. (2002). Treaty-making with the crown. In J. Bird, L. Land, & M. Macadam, *Nation to nation: Aboriginal sovereignty and the future of Canada* (pp. 45–52). Toronto, ON: Irwin.

Waldram, J. B., Herring, D. A., & Young, T. K. (2006). *Aboriginal health in Canada: Historical, cultural and epidemiological perspectives*. Toronto, ON: University of Toronto Press.

Ward, C., Branch, C., Fridkin, A. (2016). What is Indigenous cultural safety—and why should I care about it? *Indigenous People, Visions Journal, 11*(4), 29. Retrieved from http://www.heretohelp.bc.ca/visions/indigenous-people-vol11/what-is-indigenous-cultural-safety-and-why-should-i-care-about-it

Dawn Tisdale, RN, BSN, MSN in progress, is of Mi'kmaq and European ancestry. Dawn started nursing in medical and palliative care before moving into nursing policy and advocacy with a specific focus on Indigenous health and nursing initiatives. Dawn's work includes advocacy for Indigenous nursing leadership, student mentorship, and adopting cultural safety within health care systems and nursing education. Dawn has served as president of the Canadian Nursing Students' Association (CNSA) and on the board of directors of the Canadian Nurses Association (CNA), and in 2017 she received CNA's Award for the Top 150 Nurses. Dawn's passion and continued advocacy efforts are to support Indigenous nursing leadership, promote the rights of Indigenous-led health care, and create culturally safe health systems in order to improve the health and well-being of the Indigenous peoples of Turtle Island.

Gwen Campbell McArthur, Elder

Indigenous Elders as identified by communities, clans, bands, or tribal groups have been leading Indigenous culture for millennia. It is only recently that the literature in Canada has validated the roles and significance that Elders bring to every facet of Indigenous lives of the people who honour them. As complex as each cultural language and dialect, Indigenous Elders are eclectic in their birth as they are in their apprenticeship. Age is not a factor, but it is the essence of spiritual understanding, respect for Mother Earth and all she represents, and how an Elder lives his or her life as an example for others. Often identified by their nations, community, or people, Elders each bring their lived experience. It is in this sacred way that teachings of the ancestors continue to live. The ancestors continue to inform generations of Indigenous peoples though Elders who are chosen to hold their traditional language, stories, ceremonies, teachings, spiritual leadership, and sharing of their gifts.

My name is Gwenline Campbell McArthur of Ojibwe/Saulteaux Métis and Ukrainian ancestry. I was born in the Adhesion to Treaty 5 territory at Kississing, Manitoba. I was raised on the land, fishing, hunting, trapping, and gathering along with teachings of my paternal grandmother; my father, Bob Campbell, master hunter and fisherman; and my auntie Mae Louise Campbell, Indspire Laurate for her work with vulnerable Indigenous women and families across Canada. As a psychiatric mental health nurse, my work has spanned five decades, and my practice has been guided by Indigenous Elders and other spiritual leaders. It was during a meeting with a practice advisor from my nursing college in BC that the issue of spiritual cultural practices was raised. After attempting to explain my work, it was suggested that I would have to have insurance to do this work and otherwise had to cease and desist using my registered professional status. Reeling from shock and dismay, I left the meeting feeling as if my world had shifted on its axis. It was only then I searched in earnest for the answers.

My Elder Auntie was the first one I turned to. She was also horrified that someone would suggest I could not practise what I had been born to do. You see, I feel like I have been an Elder in training all of my life from the age of three when I remember sitting on my granny's knee and listening to her stories. As a little girl, I remember falling asleep on the bottom of the little fishing boat my father used on the lake and being lulled by sounds of the water. Being the youngest of five and still not school age, I would go with my dad to bring in moose meat from a kill site miles away from our home. I'd walk with snowshoes that were taller than me, but after a day on the snow, we would at least have meat to eat for supper. Then there were times on a huge dog sled pulled by four sleigh dogs I would go on rounds of my dad's trap line. Skinning muskrat, mink, beaver, and stretching them were valuable lessons I learned from a very young age. The abject poverty of lean years of hunting or trapping left me with an inner strength that survival was more than just eating three meals a day. It was the perseverance of living life true to land and to your family. It left me with a fierce ambition to use these tools in every way.

As I sat with my Elder Auntie in that September of 2017, she said, "No one can tell you what you already know. You lived the life on the land and have more wisdom than any school can tell you. You have so much knowledge. See you went to the white man's school and learned what you had to be a nurse, but they couldn't teach you what you know now about our culture, about the spirit that lives in you from my mom (your granny) and from all the old people you listened to since you were a little girl . . . You are of an age now, you've work really hard, and now I know you are an Elder. You have studied with Elders where you live. You have prayed with them, talked with them, and followed all their ways. That's what an Elder is, my girl. You carry so much knowledge and have healed so many people. Ask the Elders where you live if you need to do an Elder induction ceremony. That should satisfy them." Auntie was referring to "those white women," the nurses at the college office.

An Elder will always tell you, "I don't feel like an Elder because I don't know enough yet." And that is exactly how I feel as well. There is so much to learn about life, about the land, and from our ancestors. They visit us all the time and bring messages we don't yet know. And we don't know what is in the future. We are guided by our spirit, what other Elders teach us, and the people we encounter every day. It is the ways of other people that we have to pay attention to. Sometimes it is just being present, here and now. Solitude and listening to the soul messages of your body, your mind, and how the spirit brings it to the surface are important things to learn.

All My Relations,

Gwen

Community Mental Health

Amélie Perron and Dave Holmes

After studying this chapter, you will be able to:

1. Describe the historical context and challenges underlying current understandings of mental illness and approaches to care in Canada.

2. Analyze the effects, impact, and risk factors for mental illness and how they affect different groups.

3. Examine the causes of suicide, at-risk groups, and related assessment, intervention, and prevention strategies.

4. Identify appropriate approaches to provide mental health nursing care to the most vulnerable populations.

5. Discuss the organization of mental health services and selected models of care.

6. Consider nurses' roles in community mental health and future directions for practice.

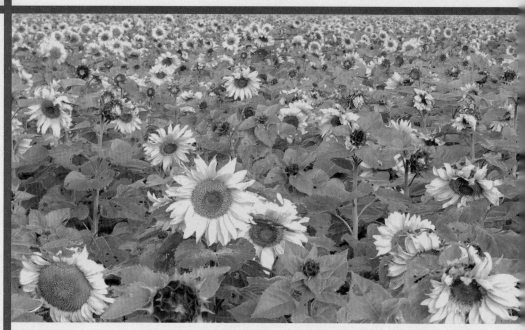

Source: Courtesy of David C. Satcey

INTRODUCTION

Experiences of emotional distress, which are often labelled as mental illness, affect the life trajectory of individuals, disrupt family processes, and impact communities and society through suffering, marginalization, lost productivity, and costly (and at times damaging) treatment. Stigma and discrimination can both cause mental health issues and influence the identification and treatment of people with mental illness and their families. Services are often neither timely nor adequate to facilitate recovery. Realizing that community services must incorporate mental health promotion, prevention, treatment, and rehabilitation, **community mental health nurses (CMHNs)** must strive to establish best practices when working with this population. Mental health impacts the ability of all individuals to enjoy life and deal with its challenges. This chapter discusses some key aspects of what is understood as "mental illness" and "psychiatric treatment," and the challenges faced by persons who experience mental health issues (PMHI). The chapter further promotes a shift in thinking that recognizes mental health issues as the outcome of sociopolitical and economic factors (e.g., poverty, trauma, violence, sexism, racism, trans/homophobia, and discrimination) rather than the result of individual deficits (e.g., brain disease and dysfunction). This shift spells a need for alternative approaches to mental health promotion and service design and delivery in the community, in which PMHIs can play an active part.

MENTAL HEALTH AND ILLNESS

Mental health is the capacity to think, feel, and act in ways that enhance the enjoyment of life and ability to face life's challenges. "It is a positive sense of emotional and spiritual well-being that respects the importance of culture, equity, social justice, interconnections, and personal dignity" (Government of Canada, 2006, p. 2). **Mental illness (MI)** refers to a group of diagnosable conditions that include combinations of altered thinking, mood, behaviour, or will that can be linked with distress or impaired functioning (Mental Health Act, 1990, amended 2010). Throughout this chapter the term *person with a mental health issue* is used in order to focus on the individual rather than his or her condition.

By the year 2041, it is estimated that the number of Canadians living with mental health issues will reach 1 million people. Some estimates indicate that children and adolescents between the ages of 9 and 19 with MI could number over 1.2 million. It is believed that one in four Canadian seniors over the age of 65 suffers from depression, anxiety, or dementia, and it is likely that many do not get diagnosed. (See Figure 23.1.)

Serious and Persistent Mental Illness

Serious and persistent mental illness (SPMI), formerly described as chronic mental illness, is a term used to describe a nonspecific diagnosis, usually schizophrenia, bipolar disorder, substance misuse, personality disorder, or severe depression, resulting in social and functional disability, a prolonged illness, and long-term treatment. Pervasive stigma and fragmented services impede health care delivery (Lawrence & Kisley, 2010).

People with SPMI are disproportionately represented in the Canadian homeless population, with estimates that anywhere between 25% and 50% of homeless individuals could suffer from MI (Mental Health Commission of Canada [MHCC], 2012). Poverty, lack of affordable housing, and inadequate discharge planning from hospitals exacerbate this problem. (See Chapter 29.) The recent national multisite At Home/Chez Soi Housing First project demonstrated that supportive housing based on recovery principles can increase quality of life for people with SPMI (MHCC, 2013a).

HISTORICAL CONTEXT AND CHALLENGES

Mental Health Care in Canada—A Brief History

Historically, mental health care in Canada has taken place within a context of culture, gender, and sociopolitical attitudes. Formal management of PMHIs began in poorhouses and jails that provided little but containment. In the mid-19th century, large institutional hospitals or asylums were built to provide

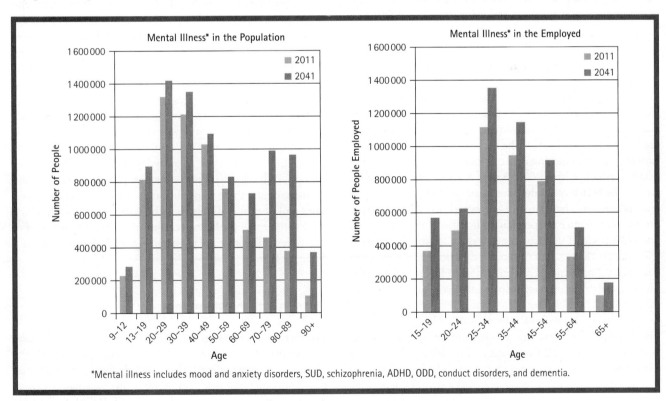

FIGURE   23.1 Estimated Number of People with Mental Illness in the Canadian Population and Employed Population

Source: Smetanin, P., Stiff, D., Briante, C., Adair, C. E., Ahmad, S., & Khan, M. (2011). *The life and economic impact of major mental illnesses in Canada 2011–2041.* Risk Analytica, on behalf of the Mental Health Commission of Canada 2011, p. 7. Used by permission of the Mental Health Commission of Canada.

more humane care. Hospitals were first built in Quebec, New Brunswick, Nova Scotia, Prince Edward Island, Manitoba, and British Columbia, followed by Saskatchewan and Alberta. Although isolated from their homes and families, PMHIs were believed to be in safe, healing environments where they followed structured therapeutic routines (Sussman, 1998). However, asylums became overcrowded and understaffed (Nolan, 1993). The resultant inhumane care evoked public outcry demanding humane treatment and educated caregivers.

Efforts to establish psychiatry as a science (which was introduced in 1846) and to find a cure for MIs prevailed. In the 1960s, a philosophical shift proposed that humane treatment would be best achieved in the community. Concurrently, the discovery of the psychotropic medications chlorpromazine and lithium and cost-containment measures associated with large institutions contributed to deinstitutionalization. Deinstitutionalization resulted in a decrease in bed capacity in provincial mental hospitals from 47 633 beds in 1960 to 15 011 beds in 1976, and a rise in general hospital psychiatric beds from 844 to 5836 (Goering, Wasylenki, & Durbin, 2000). The resources that former residents needed to live in the community were underestimated. People discharged from the institutions were marginalized, with families lacking adequate resources to assist them (Davis, 2006). As a result, many former patients became homeless, with limited means to secure food, housing, and employment, and to manage these new stressors. This in turn exacerbated their symptoms and increased their vulnerability. Many were subsequently criminalized for panhandling, sleeping in public spaces, stealing, and using drugs (Stall, 2013).

Current Developments in Canada

Today, several important trends influence mental health services: the consumer and family movements, the recovery model, and more recently, the national mental health strategies developed by the MHCC (2012). The Kirby report was Canada's first national report addressing deficiencies and inequities of mental health services (Kirby, 2008; Kirby & Keon, 2006). Concurrently, the recovery model identified life beyond symptom management; it is based upon a collaborative, consumer-driven process that challenges previous conceptions of intervention goals (Anthony, 2000). Consumers expect active collaboration with care providers rather than passive participation in dictated treatment. These trends are influencing changes within the Mental Health Act, service delivery, research, policy development, and relationships between service providers, PMHIs, and families. In 2012, a national mental health strategy for Canada was developed. This strategy aims to improve both the mental health outcomes for all Canadians and to rectify inadequacies within the current mental health system (MHCC, 2012).

While most PMHIs receive services within their communities, poor integration of services and alienation among psychiatric hospitals, community mental health programs, and private practitioners continue to fragment service delivery. Rural and remote areas lack access to appropriate and timely mental health services (Ryan-Nicholls & Haggarty, 2007). Comprehensive services that address socioeconomic factors such as housing, income, and supportive resources to facilitate living in the community are required to assist PMHIs and their families (Kirby & Keon, 2006). Recognition of the impact of the social determinants of health, the need for consumer involvement in policy development, the value of self-help groups and peer consultations, and the importance of recovery-oriented policy will help PMHIs live more satisfying and productive lives.

The Deployment of the Advanced Psychiatric Society

Mental illness is often assumed to only affect specific individuals in society. Yet the language of MI and psychiatry suffuses our everyday lives in such a way that every individual can be subject to a psychiatric evaluation of their thinking and functioning. The ability to do math, sadness, a fondness for nicotine, a lack of interest in sex, insomnia due to caffeine, shyness, and excessive video gaming are all amenable to a psychiatric diagnosis (Holmes, Jacob, & Perron, 2014; Wakefield, 2016). In other words, every unease and every difficulty brought on by the struggles (or pleasures) of life can become a symptom to be clinically managed and treated in order to re-establish what is deemed "normal."

Everyday language reflects this social concern for normal and reasonable behaviours: school-aged children are expected to exhibit "normal" emotional responses and social skills and "appropriate energy levels"; teenagers must show "good judgment," face "reality," and should be monitored for "unexplained outbursts"; adults must remain "rational" at all times and "keep their emotions in check"; and older adults must be able to "stay adjusted and functional," "set goals," and remain "positive and hopeful" when facing changes and loss.

This thinking has become difficult to question and challenge. It determines the way we perceive ourselves, our capacities and decisions, how we resolve problems, and how we categorize our responses to everyday occurrences (normal or abnormal). It also changes the way we perceive others around us, in particular those who think and act outside social expectations and norms. CMHNs must be wary of this trend, which can facilitate the **pathologization** of normal life and lead to the overestimation of the prevalence of MI in society (Holmes, Jacob, & Perron, 2014).

Psychiatric Science

Psychiatry is a contested area of clinical practice and the subject of several controversies; this is in large part due to the absence of a robust scientific basis and the historical shifts that have re-oriented the field. For example, over the past 70 years, psychiatrists have shifted from a psychoanalytical model, to a biomedical model, to a biopsychosocial model, to a neurogenetic model of MI, all of which provide very different explanations of mental health issues and approaches to treating them. The sociocultural and political context plays an influential role in the way we define "normal." For example, in 1851, Dr. Cartwight hypothesized the existence of a psychiatric illness called *drapetomania*, which purportedly described the "irrational" tendency of black slaves attempting to flee from their white owners in the Southern United States. In his view, this desire to escape was pathological because black people were born to be enslaved; any desire to change this "natural fact" was therefore a sign of gross insanity.

In Canada and the United States, psychiatrists rely mostly on the *Diagnostic and Statistical Manual of Mental Disorders* (DSM) to diagnose patients. Yet the DSM has been criticized for gender bias, cultural insensitivity, and reliance on nonempirical evidence. It has also been the subject of many disputes, due to its growing tendency to pathologize normal behaviours and occurrences. For example, in its earlier versions, the DSM included homosexuality as a psychiatric category. It was finally removed in 1973 after it was recognized that diverse sexual orientations do not constitute psychiatric disorders. In 2013, premenstrual disorder was included in the fifth edition under the name "premenstrual dysphoric disorder" despite poor scientific evidence. Changes to the DSM are largely based on changes in sociocultural norms and expectations, and do not necessarily reflect scientific discoveries. There have been longstanding attempts to establish MIs as biological diseases, and in particular as the result of chemical imbalances in the brain, abnormal brain activation, or abnormal brain structure. Yet the scientific evidence available to date remains inconclusive (Fried & Kievit, 2015; Müller et al., 2017; Sprooten et al., 2017). Other issues that underlie the DSM include the way diagnostic criteria may oversimplify some conditions such as depression and schizophrenia; and since the publication of its first edition in 1952, the DSM has expanded from 106 to 312 diagnoses, which points to the pathologization of a growing number of (normal) life experiences rather than an explosion of scientifically confirmed, brain-based psychopathologies (Wakefield, 2016). Of concern, clinical guidelines neither address these scientific shortcomings nor do they question the evidence being used to promote the use of medications in the treatment of certain diagnoses, despite inconsistent data regarding their efficacy, safety, and long-term benefits in youth, adult, and older adult populations (Le Noury et al., 2016; United Nations, 2017).

"Psychiatry Inc."

Like other health care fields, mental health is vulnerable to various priorities that may not be centred on the best interests of PMHIs but may instead prioritize the financial interests of corporations. This is visible for example when a new illness is promoted in order to "match" a particular drug. Through the "invention" of an illness, a niche of patient-consumers is also created, which ensures a steady flow of revenue for that medication. Old drugs with expiring patents can be rebranded as a "new" product designed for the "new" illness. Examples of such illnesses include premenstrual dysphoric disorder, female hypoactive sexual desire disorder (Jutel, 2010), and attention deficit disorder, all of which depend on the interpretation of subjective reports according to particular sociocultural norms. Consistent scientific evidence in support of both the existence

and treatment of these disorders is difficult to locate. This is compounded by the fact that drug inserts and websites funded by the pharmaceutical industry tend to present information that is biased in favour of the industry, to the detriment of balanced and accurate information about the etiology and treatment of mental health issues (Read & Cain, 2013). CMHNs must use their critical thinking to ensure that the evidence they use to provide care is sound and free from commercial influence.

The Psychiatric Survivors Movement and the Mad Movement

The **Psychiatric Survivors movement** began in the late 1960s in the wake of the civil rights movement, during which multiple stories of abuse and trauma experienced by current and former psychiatric patients surfaced. The movement, which came to be known as the **Mad Movement** in the early 2000s, expanded through the work of numerous grassroots activists and supporters (including many mental health professionals and scholars) who advocated for PMHIs' rights, self-determination, dignity, and safety following negative experiences with involuntary committal, forced treatment (with neuroleptic medications and electro-convulsive therapy), and discrimination. Numerous psychiatric practices described as "patient-centred" do not take into account individuals' own knowledge about their situation and their ability to make decisions. The Psychiatric Survivors movement and the Mad Movement (also known as consumer or ex-patient movements) work to depathologize distress and diverse mental health states, challenge reductionist views of MI (e.g., brain imbalance), and challenge authoritarian treatment structures. The development and expansion of the recovery movement and user-led philosophies have helped PMHIs reclaim their "mad" identity as a source of pride rather than shame. This has helped shift social, political, and professional discourses and stereotypes about PMHIs, depicting them not simply as people who are ill, powerless, hopeless and victimized but as resilient, resourceful, and creative individuals. These movements promote solidarity, social change, and justice, bringing to light the multiple injustices and hardships faced by PMHIs, in particular in regards to employment opportunities, custody rights, housing and homelessness, criminalization of behaviours, and access to health, social, and legal services (LeFrançois, Menzies, & Reaume, 2013). Given CMHNs' role in advocating for people with mental health issues, it is important for them to understand the purpose and the achievements of such movements with regards to PMHIs' rights, identity, and agency.

RISK FACTORS

The aetiology of mental health issues is not fully understood. However, certain populations are at higher risk of mental health issues because of greater exposure and vulnerability to adverse sociopolitical, economic, environmental, and biological circumstances, all of which can generate risk factors. Risk

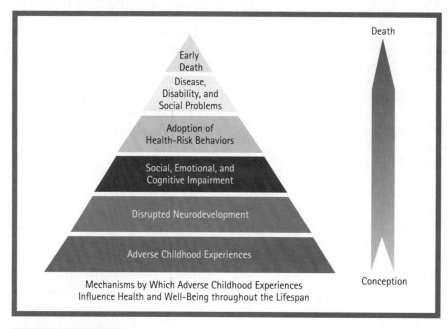

FIGURE 23.2 Effects of Adverse Childhood Events Across the Lifespan

Source: Center for Disease Control and Prevention (2016) Retrieved from https://www.cdc.gov/violenceprevention/acestudy/index.html

factors do not, on their own, predict or cause mental health issues, and a disorder usually involves a complex combination of multiple risk factors that may differ from person to person.

Experiences across the lifespan, such as trauma, violence, poverty, and discrimination, have a fundamental impact on mental health. This was made evident as early as the 1990s by the ACEs study (Felitti et al., 1998), which recruited participants in order to assess childhood experiences, then followed them in the long term to record their health outcomes as adults. The study, and many others since, confirmed that adverse childhood events (ACEs) are linked to multiple physical and mental health problems across the lifespan (see Figure 23.2), such as anxiety, mood disorders, substance misuse, and a range of acute and chronic conditions like diabetes, cancer, Crohn's, arthritis, fibromyalgia, lung disease, and stroke (Afifi et al., 2014; Tonmyr & Shields, 2017).

The ACEs study makes clear that the root causes of mental health issues can be considered through a systemic lens that identifies that people who live with chronic oppression embedded within a social system will develop both physical and mental health issues. Women; Indigenous persons; visible minorities; individuals who identify as lesbian, gay, bisexual, transgender, queer, and Two-Spirit (LGBTQ2S); homeless persons; refugees; and persons with disabilities are particularly vulnerable to such experiences. Many women and children in Canada experience domestic violence, which can lead to accumulative complex trauma situations. Housing and proper nutrition also constitute critical elements of mental health (McGibbon, 2012). Lack of affordable, stable, safe, and sanitary housing and access to food may jeopardize a person's development; cognitive, emotional, and physical health; and ability to manage stressors. It may also expose the person to high levels of contaminants (e.g., toxins, carcinogens, pesticides, heavy metals) that increase the risk of mental health issues, especially

in children and youth (National Collaborating Centre for Environmental Health and National Collaborating Centre for Determinants of Health, 2017).

The circumstances just described disproportionately affect certain groups, such as low-income and First Nation, Inuit, and Métis individuals and families. McGibbon (2012) emphasizes that mental health issues must be viewed beyond the biomedical model; etiologies should therefore reflect societal and systemic factors. CMHNs must take such factors into account during their assessments, as they may spell the need for specific mental health promotion and protection strategies.

Risk factors may be biological in nature. Chronic illness, traumatic brain injury, short- and long-term use of medications (both psychotropic and nonpsychotropic), and medical conditions (e.g., stroke, metabolic disturbances, infectious disorders) can lead to the development of acute and chronic cognitive and emotional symptoms. Genetic vulnerability may also play a role. For example, there is growing evidence that genetic factors may be at play in Alzheimer's disease. However, the evidence regarding other conditions, such as mood and psychotic disorders, remains unclear; while certain genes are suspected of predisposing someone to a particular disorder, not everyone with these genes develop the disorder, which suggests that socioenvironmental factors have an important role in the development of incapacitating cognitive and emotional symptoms.

All of these risk factors can be understood through a social determinant approach, which helps capture the multiple circumstances within which people are born, grow, live, and work. These conditions impact the distribution of resources (e.g., income, education, social and health services, affordable food and housing) and therefore their ability to care for themselves. Figure 23.3 illustrates the **social determinants of mental health**. It is important to note that the social determinants of health may not impact all individuals equally. For example, it has been shown

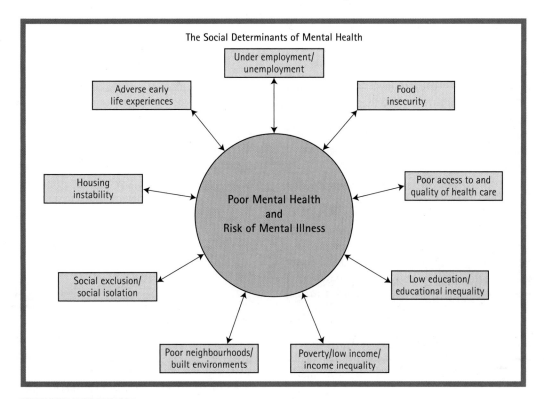

FIGURE 23.3 The Social Determinants of Mental Health

Source: Shim, R., Koplan, C., Langheim, F. J. P., Manseau, M. W., Powers, R. A., & Compton, M. T. (2014). The social determinants of mental health: An overview and call to action. *Psychiatric Annals, 44*(1), 22–26.

that social isolation and loneliness particularly affect youth, men, and older individuals, and can significantly impact their psychological well-being (Luanaigh & Lawlor, 2008).

Gender Considerations

There are differences in the way mental health issues develop in girls and boys, and women and men. As discussed earlier, types of risk factors and specific mental health issues are not gender neutral. Gender, for instance, plays a determining role in the way women and men seek help. Women seeking help are often portrayed as passive, dramatic, even hysterical, while men are perceived as weak and unfit to assume the socially constructed "strong gender" role. As a result, women and men often refrain to ask for assistance, and this has an impact in the way they interact (or not) with the health care system. When they finally reach out, their behaviour is understood through a gendered lens, and their distress and behaviour are pathologized based on gender roles. For instance, society expects today's women to (over)perform in both the domestic and professional spheres. Although these social expectations are unrealistic for most people, those who fail are often portrayed as unable to conform or cope. Rather than challenge the social structures that set these unfair expectations, women are left to feel as though their struggle is their own personal fault. As a result, many suffer from anxiety and depression and seek professional help in order to "adapt." Similar gender expectations apply to children (Abraham, 2010) and men (Ogrodniczuk, Oliffe, Kuhl, & Gross, 2016). Practising

CMHNs should always consider additional aspects related to gender and mental health during their assessments.

YES, BUT WHY?

Challenges Experienced by Men Who Experience Mental Health Issues

What?

Mental health issues among men have been identified as a public health concern (Ogrodniczuk et al., 2016). This is due to the confluence of high rates of completed suicide, lack of help-seeking by boys and men, toxic socialization processes that devalue and ridicule boys' and men's emotional needs, and poor screening of depression and other mental health issues among males by health care professionals. Yet men's mental health needs are evident in official statistics on suicide, alcohol and drug dependence, violence (domestic and other), and homelessness, where men continue to be overrepresented.

Men's presentations of mental health issues often differ from those of women. For example, early manifestations of depression often include irritability, anger, hostility, aggression, substance misuse, and risk-taking behaviours (Ogrodniczuk et al., 2016). These responses differ from "expected" symptoms of depression, including crying, feelings of sadness, guilt or shame, powerlessness, and disruptions in eating habits and sleep patterns. Many men do not recognize signs of mental health problems and do not relate certain physical symptoms (e.g., headaches, abdominal cramps, chest or back pain, palpitations) to potential emotional issues.

So What?

When health care professionals overlook men's mental health needs, focusing instead on physical health, this leads to missed opportunities to initiate a dialogue with men who may be uncomfortable doing so themselves. Furthermore, lack of tailored, accessible, and affordable mental health supports in the community restricts men's ability to seek help before crises occur (Kirby & Keon, 2006). Because men are socialized to and therefore more likely to exhibit behaviours such as anger, hostility, and aggression, especially when experiencing a mental health crisis, they are more likely to come to the attention of law enforcement rather than health care professionals (Coleman & Cotton, 2010). In Canada, such encounters have led to multiple escalations and confrontations wherein distressed men, and in particular homeless men, have been victims of excessive force resulting in injury or death, including high-profile cases such as Lester Donaldson, Sammy Yatim, Edmond Yu, Donald Meyer, Martin Charles Ostopovich, Kevin Geldart, Reyal Jardine-Douglas, Michael Eligon, Laurent Parrouty, Robert Dziekanski, Mario Hamel, Farshad Mohammadi, and Alain Magloire.

Now What?

CMHNs play an important role in challenging gender-limiting, stigmatizing, or dismissive attitudes in the community and among health care professionals. They can work to raise awareness among men and communities about men's vulnerabilities and mental health needs. CMHNs must enact a gender-relevant screening for mental health issues during assessments and reach out to men who may be experiencing emotional difficulties. They can also ensure that the language used does not perpetuate stigma; for example, "getting help," which is perceived by many men as "being weak," can be reframed as an effort to act, problem solve, and regain control (Ogrodniczuk et al., 2016). When interacting with law enforcement, CMHNs can educate officers about men's and women's differing presentations during a crisis. Many Canadian cities now have joint initiatives between police services and community or outreach mental health crisis services. CMHNs can advocate for the creation of such partnerships where they do not yet exist. Finally, CMHNs can advocate for policies that support the implementation and sustained funding of community mental health services, including programs that are specifically tailored to men.

Standards of Practice Fulfilled

#1 Health Promotion
- Uses a collaborative relationship with the client and other partners to facilitate and advocate for structural system change and healthy public policy using multiple health promotion strategies.

#6 Health Equity
- Advocates for healthy public policy and social justice by participating in legislative and policy-making activities that influence determinants of health and access to services (CHNC, 2019, revised).

THE IMPACT OF MENTAL ILLNESS

The global burden of disease attributable to MI and substance misuse has increased by 37% since 1990, and the largest proportion of the population affected is between the ages of 10 and 29, representing a significant loss of well-being, quality of life, potential, and productivity. It is estimated that one in five Canadians will experience a mental health issue (MHCC, 2012). This demonstrates a significant amount of disruption to personal and family life, lost potential, and costs of treatment. Population mental health promotion strategies are urgently needed to prevent this growing problem upstream (Degenhardt et al., 2013).

Stigma and Discrimination

Stigma, discrimination, and mental health are closely linked. As stated earlier, such experiences are important risk factors for the development of cognitive and emotional difficulties that can greatly affect a person's quality of life and ability to function socially and professionally. Youth and adults who are part of marginalized groups are at particular risk.

Similarly, stigma and discrimination can significantly affect a PMHI. The 10-year anti-stigma campaign "Opening Minds" initiated by the MHCC addresses the fact that stigma and discrimination are a reality facing PMHIs. Cultural beliefs, superstitions, and poor understanding of MI contribute to fear, stereotyping, and avoidance of these individuals. Furthermore, while it is widely believed that framing MI as "brain disease" or a disease "like any other" will reduce stigma, evidence shows that it can in fact *increase* stigma (Canadian Health Services Research Foundation, 2013).

Youth with MI identified stigma as the major barrier to their reintegration to society and experienced feelings of exclusion related to their perceived loss of social status (Leavey, 2015). People with co-morbid mental health issues and physical disabilities are doubly jeopardized by stigma from society and health care professionals. Stigma causes people to conceal their illness and delay or refuse treatment and follow-up care.

Efforts to reduce stigma toward MI in Canadian society include the following target groups:

- Youth—many mental health issues begin before age 18; early intervention can make an important difference in quality of life.
- Health care providers—care providers can exhibit stigmatizing attitudes of PMHI.
- Media—it plays an important role in shaping public opinion.
- Workforce—employees avoid treatment for fear of stigma and discrimination from their employers and coworkers (MHCC, 2013b). (See Table 23.1.)

The language used to address or describe PMHIs deserves special consideration. While expressions such as *lunatic, nuts, crazy, retard, drama queen, junkie,* and *hysterical* are obviously damaging because of their highly negative connotation, clinically derived terms such as *depressed, manic, disordered,*

Table 23.1	Anti-Stigma Initiatives		
Youth	**Health Care Providers**	**Media**	**Workplace**
Iris the Dragon series, *He Shoots He Scores!* One of a series of books addressing children's mental health challenges; used with school children in Perth, Ontario. Durham, Talking about Mental Illness (TAMI). Five-class teaching curriculum for Grades 7–12, with professional development workshop. Stigma Summit—Mind your Mind Youth website provides information, personal stories, coping tools; used in London, Ontario.	Practice Support Program for physicians Central Local Health Integrated Network (LHIN) for hospital and support workers with stories from people with mental illness; DVD for discussion points. University programs with specific curriculum content.	Mindset: Reporting on Mental Health: Contract with Canadian Journalism Forum on Violence and Trauma to develop a media resource guide; Canadian Broadcasting Corporation is a partner. Media monitoring project on mental illness issues (McGill University).	Programs for government employees: Mental Health Works (MHW) is a national program created by the Canadian Mental Health Association; Mind Matters, a program for business leaders developed by Mood Disorders Ontario, creates healthy workplaces. Department of National Defence: Road to Mind Readiness aims to increase resiliency and mental health in soldiers and civilians. Economic analysis of the impact of mental illness in the workplace.

Source: Mental Health Commission of Canada, (2013b). *Interim report on opening minds*. Retrieved from http://www.mentalhealthcommission.ca/English/system/files/private/document/opening_minds_interim_report.pdf.

handicapped, and *psychotic* can be equally problematic because they can reduce a person to their condition or diagnosis. Shifting language shifts perceptions. Using a **person-first approach** acknowledges the person first, then the condition. It is more humanizing and recognizes that a person is more than a set of symptoms. Nurses must be sensitive to the terminology they use and respect the language that PMHIs prefer.

Bullying and Harassment

PMHIs often experience harassment and bullying from acquaintances and strangers alike. Youth can also be bullied by peers online or at school. Bullying and harassment have been confirmed as significant contributors to poor short- and long-term mental health outcomes in youth and adults (Wolke & Lereya, 2015). Importantly, these negative outcomes impact both the victims and the perpetrators (Sigurdson, Undheim, Wallander, Lydersen, & Sund, 2015).

Feelings of harassment, humiliation, and intimidation can be caused by the way health care providers speak to and treat PMHIs (Nyttingnes, Ruud, & Rugkåsa, 2016). CMHNs must be mindful of the power differential with care recipients, which often underpins poor relational techniques and communication.

Violence and Trauma

A complex relationship exists between violence and MI. As discussed earlier, many individuals who experience distressing mental health symptoms have experienced abuse, trauma, and exclusion at some point in their lives. As research on the social determinants of mental health has shown, poor mental health is a complex product of various social, political, cultural, and economic factors. Studies focused on social determinants show that MI is better explained by the intergenerational transfer of social and economic inequities, including violence (World Health Organization [WHO], 2014).

It is a common misconception that PMHIs are more likely to be violent, yet compared to the general population they do not present a higher risk. Where they differ is in their experiences of victimization. PMHIs are highly vulnerable to violence because of altered cognitive or emotional functioning, precarious living conditions, socioeconomic deprivation, uncivil treatment by both known and unknown persons, and reduced social supports. For those who use drugs, risk of victimization significantly increases. Violent crimes against PMHIs include rape, sexual assault, physical assault, and mugging, with victimization rates ranging from 5% to 35% (2 to 140 times higher than the general population, depending on the study design) (Maniglio, 2009). Such experiences can induce feelings of fear, anxiety, and insecurity, and exacerbate psychological distress and feelings of powerlessness.

Reporting criminal victimization is highly difficult for PMHIs because they often fear they will not be treated as credible victims, especially if they exhibit cognitive impairment or delusions. They may also fear retaliation from the perpetrator. As a result, current figures of victimization of this population are likely underestimated. It is important for nurses to provide compassionate support to a PMHI who reports experiences of victimization. A supportive attitude may reduce suffering and stigmatization, and promote the person's well-being, social participation, and sense of empowerment.

SUICIDE IN CANADA

Suicide is a critical public health concern affecting all ages, races, abilities, gender identities, and socioeconomic classes. In 2015, the prevalence of suicide in Canada was 12.3 per 100 000, with men completing suicides at a significantly higher rate than women (18.4% versus 6.3%) (Statistics Canada, n.d.). For every completed suicide, it is estimated that there are 20 suicide attempts. Although these figures are concerning, they do not take into account the much higher suicide rates affecting Indigenous communities, a reality poignantly captured in the documentary *Third World Canada* (Cazabon, 2010).

Suicide does not impact everyone equally. For example, suicide is one of the leading causes of death in Canadian youth and is highest in the age group 40 to 59 years with an increased trend in late life for men (MHCC, 2015b). Youth suicide is particularly concerning, with such high incidence in some First Nations and Inuit communities that some communities have declared states of emergency following spates of suicide among their teenagers (Phippen, 2016). A significant number of Canadian college students (6.6%) reported self-harm behaviours indicative of emotional distress and increased potential for suicide (MHCC, 2015b). Post-secondary students represent a population with significant mental health challenges, particularly stress, anxiety, and depression. They struggle with negative feelings and may require significant supports to manage transitions in their lives. (See Table 23.2.)

Stigma surrounding suicide prevents populations at risk and their families from seeking help. Survivors of suicide often feel isolated and experience complex emotions; they need encouragement to attend self-help groups where they

Table 23.2	Percentage of Canadian Post-Secondary School Students with Mental Health Indicators in the Past 12 Months
Mental Health Indicators	**%**
Exhausted	88.2%
Overwhelmed	89.5%
Hopeless	59.6%
Anxiety	64.5%
Self-injured (intentionally cut, burned, bruised, or injured self)	8.7%
Seriously considered suicide	13%

Source: Based on American College Health Association (2016). *Canadian Reference Group Executive Summary, Spring 2016.* Hanover, MD: American College Health Association.

Forty-one Canadian post-secondary institutions self-selected to participate in the Spring 2016 ACHA National College Health Assessment, and 43 780 surveys were completed by students on these campuses. For the purpose of forming the reference group, only Canadian institutions that surveyed all students or used a random sampling technique were included in the analysis.

may benefit from discussion with other group members who have experienced suicide deaths. The Government of Canada recently developed a Federal Framework for Suicide Prevention (Government of Canada, 2016), and several federal initiatives address suicide, including cluster suicides among youth.

Contributing Factors to Suicide

Suicidal behaviours are classified as suicidal ideation, suicide attempt, and completed suicide. **Suicidal ideation** refers to thoughts about suicide; 13.4% of people have seriously thought about suicide during their lifetime. As suicide attempts are not always reported, their incidence is likely underestimated. Statistics indicate that 3.1% of the population over 5 years of age has attempted suicide, with women attempting more than men. However, mortality due to completed suicides is four times higher among men. Men often choose more fatal methods and are reluctant to seek help. This trend is changing, with some women choosing more lethal suicide methods. A significant proportion of people with suicidal ideation and attempts do not perceive a need for or do not access mental health care prior to the event. Community outreach and educational programs for suicide prevention may help decrease this trend.

Youth are vulnerable to suicidal thoughts and attempts due to important life transitions, which may be compounded by intergenerational trauma, abusive experiences, social pressures, and low self-esteem (Schissel, 2011). Indigenous youth aged 15 to 24 are at increased risk, with suicide and self-inflicted injuries the leading cause of death for youth and adults under the age of 45. Inuit youth have one of the highest suicide rates in the world (MHCC, 2012). Older adults often face multiple losses of friends and family, health problems, and diminished capacity. When facing their own mortality, traditionally, they would face the choice to end their life. (See Chapter 21.)

Due to the stigma associated with their sexual identity, LGBTQ2S youth are also at increased risk for suicide. People who "come out" may face increased harassment, while not "coming out" may lead to extreme isolation. LGBTQ2S youth require sensitive assessment to determine their suicide risk.

Several medications used to treat mental health issues can also cause suicidal ideations and attempts. Antidepressants in particular have seen this serious adverse effect underreported in clinical trials, in particular those conducted or funded by pharmaceutical companies. Although it is routinely assumed that people taking antidepressants were at risk for suicide to begin with, systematic reviews show that selective serotonin reuptake inhibitors and serotonin-norepinephrine reuptake inhibitors increase aggression and suicidality among children and teenagers (Sharma, Guski, Freund, & Gøtzsche, 2016) and adults (Bielefeldt, Danborg, & Gøtzsche, 2016).

Indigenous Persons

Some First Nation communities experience low suicide rates, and others experience alarmingly high rates. Suicide among Inuit youth in Canada is 11 times the national average, among the highest in the world (Health Canada, 2015). The rate for First Nation youth (15–24 years) across Canada is five to six times higher than for non-Indigenous Canadians, and rates for adult women and adult men are seven times and five times higher than for non-Indigenous Canadians, respectively (Shulman & Tahirali, 2016). Canada led an international study on how to prevent youth suicide across eight countries with Indigenous Arctic populations (Nunavut Bureau of Statistics, 2015). The high incidence of youth suicide in many communities represents a significant loss of potential years of life for the nation. For many First Nation youth, home is not a haven but may be a place where they are exposed to violence, intergenerational trauma, and multisystemic problems, including structural barriers to every single social determinant of health.

Hardships caused by a long history of oppression, societal exclusion, trauma, loss of cultural pride, inequitable resource and wealth distribution, and compromised social determinants of mental health are significant factors (Bell, 2013; Elias et al., 2012). (See Chapter 22.) These issues typically create critical mental health issues that traditional healing therapies never addressed prior to colonization. Suicide prevention efforts need to be culturally coordinated and holistic in their approach (Health Canada, 2015). Despite a high proportion of mental health problems, conventional services are under-used by Indigenous people. This is due to the fact that mental health services based on a Western way of healing do not consider traditional Indigenous understandings of well-being. In the treatment of individual mental health problems, CMHNs must consider the impact of collective identities and the political realities of Indigenous peoples and their importance in building resilience.

Military Personnel and Veterans

The mental health needs of armed forces personnel and veterans have been acknowledged as an important issue since the 1990s as a result of difficult deployment conditions in conflict zones like Somalia, the Persian Gulf, and Rwanda. Veterans in particular are vulnerable to psychological distress due to reduced supports, difficult transitions back into civilian life, disability due to physical injury, and post-traumatic stress disorder (Thompson et al., 2016). A mental health survey conducted in 2013 among Canadian Forces found that one in six full-time regular members reported symptoms consistent with major depressive episode, post-traumatic stress disorder, chronic anxiety, panic disorder, or alcohol abuse (Statistics Canada, 2014). Although the suicide rate among members of the regular force is similar to that of the general population, numbers for veterans are difficult to obtain, but the rate appears to be higher (Canadian Armed Forces and Veterans Affairs Canada, 2017). Mental health nurses, including those working outside of military institutions, play a key role in identifying and supporting PMHIs who have served in the military.

CARING FOR THE MOST VULNERABLE

Earlier in the chapter we outlined the various ways that societal inequities collude to create fertile ground for the development of emotional distress or MI. For populations either ignored or blamed for their circumstances, the layered ways that they are forgotten plays out not only in their experience of emotional pain but further in the inequitable access to appropriate mental health supports. The following section covers just a few of the most denigrated, forgotten, and misunderstood populations for whom CMHNs must care and advocate.

Indigenous Persons

Testimonies provided by numerous Indigenous individuals during the Truth and Reconciliation Commission (2015) hearings highlight the way mental and emotional pain continues to affect the lives of many people who experienced trauma in residential schools. (See Chapter 22.) However, conventional (Western) approaches to Indigenous mental health have been described as culturally inappropriate, oppressive, and retraumatizing due to their capacity to isolate individuals from their communities. Foreign approaches for foreign ailments result in a further re-colonization of minds and bodies, increasing stigma and marginalization (Health Canada, 2015). Given the history of trauma of this population, a **trauma-informed approach** should be exercised: it views trauma as injury and prioritizes survivors' safety, choice, and sense of ownership and control over their situation. Rather than viewing an individual's "coping skills" as flawed, it highlights the relationship between trauma and emotional distress.

Furthermore, a framework that respects Indigenous understandings of wellness, community, and traditional teachings can help provide culturally sensitive, supportive, and compassionate care. For example, the strengths-based First Nations Mental Wellness Continuum Framework (Health Canada, 2015) describes mental wellness as a balance between the mental, physical, spiritual, and emotional dimensions, achieved through the promotion and protection of a sense of purpose, identity, kinship, and meaning grounded in Indigenous values and traditional knowledges. (See Figure 23.4.) Whenever possible, traditional healers and community Elders should be involved when caring for Indigenous PMHIs.

Homeless Persons

Risks associated with homelessness (e.g., acute and chronic illnesses, deterioration of mental health, violence) make homeless individuals one of the most vulnerable populations and homelessness a public health emergency. (See Chapter 29.) This vulnerability is often compounded by various activities like panhandling, sex work, and stealing in order to meet basic needs. Such activities should be seen as survival strategies rather than strictly antisocial behaviours. The goals of homeless persons may differ significantly from the CMHN's goals. While CMHNs can offer support and links to community resources, they must work in partnership with de-housed persons in order to help them manage their health in ways that

work for them. Although it is widely thought that homeless individuals exploit health and social services for personal gain (e.g., access to a bed or painkillers), research indicates that they tend to distrust these services for fear of being judged, mistreated, and reported to law enforcement (Zakrison, Hamel, & Hwang, 2004). To the extent possible, nurses should link these individuals with existing housing, health, mental health and social services, and food banks. They can also support the development of housing-first approaches, which have been shown to better support homeless PMHIs, making them more likely to exit homelessness and less likely to make substantial and sometimes inappropriate use of health care, social services, and judicial resources (MHCC, 2013a).

Persons Who Use Drugs

Substance misuse is often interpreted as involving illicit street drugs. However, more individuals are addicted to medications that are legally dispensed (e.g., painkillers, anxiety and sleep

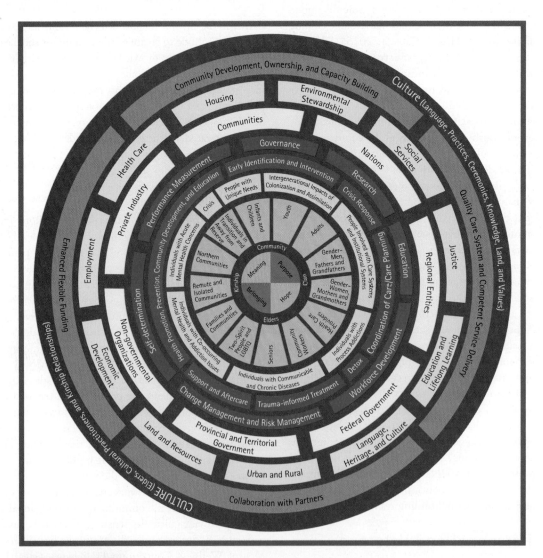

FIGURE 23.4 Mental Wellness Continuum Framework

Source: © All rights reserved. *First Nations Mental Wellness Continuum Framework.* Health Canada, 2015. Adapted and reproduced with permission from the Minister of Health, 2018.

medications) than "hard" drugs. Substance misuse can develop following stressful or traumatic events (e.g., loss of employment, sexual violence), accidents that have caused painful injuries (e.g., car or work-related), or chronically stressful situations (e.g., poverty, homophobia, domestic violence). CMHNs can play a vital role in the care of these highly stigmatized individuals. They must recognize substance use as a coping strategy; as a result, recovery is a long-term process often punctuated with unsuccessful detox attempts and frequent relapses. Working with individuals to get at the core source of their pain is central to their recovery. (See Chapter 30.)

Refugees and Immigrants

The 2011 National Household Survey indicated that one in five people living in Canada is a visible minority, with 20.6% of the Canadian population being born outside of Canada. Current high-priority conditions in recently arriving immigrants and refugees include domestic violence, abuse, anxiety, adjustment struggles, depression, torture, and post-traumatic stress (Swinkels, Pottie, Tugwell, Rashid, & Naraslah, 2011). Often, newcomers to Canada are uncomfortable discussing these concerns with health care professionals. The use of cultural brokers and interpreters should be considered (Kirkmayer et al., 2011).

Accessing mental health services is often problematic due to language barriers and because newcomers often find services are not culturally comfortable (Shakya, Khanlou, & Gonsalves, 2015). For example, immigrant and refugee Iranian and Sri Lankan Tamil women who experienced current and pre-immigration domestic abuse reported their experiences as physical symptoms and were silent on mental health symptoms. If practitioners inquire only about physical health, there is a danger that mental health issues will not be revealed (Guruge, Roche, & Catallo, 2012). Mental health services should respect the principles of **culturally safe care**. (See Chapter 9.)

COMMUNITY MENTAL HEALTH SERVICE DELIVERY

CMHNs work with individuals, families, and populations affected by mental health issues across the lifespan. They support population-wide interventions and have a unique opportunity to advocate on issues that impact the mental well-being and care of Canadians. Discussion regarding resource allocation for an adequate balance of mental health services in institutional and community sectors continues. Three main problems affect service orientation. First, while the move from institutions to intersectoral community services is expected to ultimately reduce costs, currently both systems must be operated with continued community services investment. Public funding of physician- and hospital-centred services disadvantages people with limited incomes seeking alternative services. In remote and rural regions, adequate mental health services are lacking. Second, comprehensive services

must be inter-sectoral and address the basic determinants of health such as housing. Third, stigma and discrimination are formidable barriers preventing people from accessing services. The principles of recovery, which challenge society's assumptions regarding MI, are beginning to be implemented into policy and services.

Mental health resources are organized around primary, secondary, and tertiary prevention. Primary prevention aims to promote positive mental health, psychological well-being, and supportive living and working environments. Primary prevention is achieved through mental health promotion and the prevention and mitigation of stressors known to negatively impact mental health. Anti-bullying strategies in schools are one example. Secondary prevention seeks to lower the prevalence of mental health issues through early screening, healing strategies, and the health promotion of individuals, families, and communities. Its goal is to reduce the frequency and intensity of acute distress and symptoms. Tertiary intervention aims to reduce the severity of the illness and associated disability, assist people in recovery, and prevent relapses (WHO, 2004) by focusing on treatment and case management of PMHIs, with emphasis on recovery through tangible resources, psychoeducation, and rehabilitative strategies.

Organization of Services

Emergency Services Consisting of admissions to hospital and crisis stabilization units, emergency services are initiated through general hospitals' emergency wards, where services are organized for medical emergencies, not psychiatric emergencies. General or psychiatric hospitals provide services for serious acute illness, while **crisis stabilization units** provide services to less acutely ill people, generally judged by indicators of self-harm or homicide. Additional services include 24-hour mobile crisis response teams and professional and peer support telephone crisis lines.

Outpatient clinics and specialized programs, for example, as well as eating-disorder programs and child and adolescent treatment clinics, may be offered as follow-up services in the form of day hospitals, day treatment, and daycare settings. Community mental health workers follow people with MI in the community but often carry large caseloads that leave little time for consistent intervention.

Case Management Case management assists PMHIs and families to navigate the mental health system. Case managers coordinate long-term care, providing and negotiating services for holistic needs related to physical health, leisure, education, and housing. Case management fosters continuity and coordination of care.

Assertive Community Treatment **Assertive community treatment** is a comprehensive, long-term intensive case management approach to treating persons who have a SPMI, struggle with functional impairment, and are intensive users of the health care system. **Functional impairment** refers to an inability to look after hygiene, nutritional needs, and finances, and to develop or sustain support systems. Outreach services decrease hospitalizations by addressing compliance issues and improving the quality of community life.

Primary Health Care Services These services include a wide range of services, and the first contact is often a general practitioner with little time and limited expertise in MI. This can result in overprescribing of medications and fewer people being assessed by mental health specialists. Integrating mental health practitioners with primary health care providers is a goal of the collaborative care movement. This shared care could involve telephone access to psychiatrists or on-site psychiatrists at clinics.

Early Intervention Programs Early intervention programs arose in response to treatment delays. These programs attempt to intervene prior to a full-blown episode of MI to mitigate its effects. The early psychosis intervention program addresses the stigma and demoralization associated with MI, supports family, and actively seeks timely treatment and follow-up (Thomas & Nandrha, 2009).

Co-Occurring Disorder Programs These programs were created to support individuals struggling with a mental health issue as well as substance misuse. People experiencing anxiety and depression have higher rates of substance dependence than the general population. Co-occurring disorder programs accept that the recovery of persons who struggle with mental health issues and substance misuse can be a prolonged process and that relapses are likely (Bartlett, Brown, Shattell, Wright, & Lewallen, 2013).

Self-Help and Peer Support Self-help and support from peers are an integral part of services for PMHIs and their families and allow them to share their lived experiences with one another. Recommendations to fund these programs from public funding attest to their value. Current discussion suggests increasing the number of paid peer support helpers and peer counsellors. Research in this area is new but shows promise for innovation (Cyr, McKee, O'Hagan, & Priest for the MHCC, 2016).

Mental Health Promotion **Mental health promotion** emphasizes positive mental health and recognizes the personal, social, economic, and environmental factors that contribute to mental health. It is becoming increasingly prominent in the mental health and public health systems, and various frameworks have been proposed to incorporate mental health promotion at a policy level for the general population (MHCC, 2012) but also for specific groups such as Inuit, First Nation, and Métis peoples (Health Canada, 2015) and children and youth (Kutcher & McLuckie, 2010). Mental health promotion interventions that recognize and address social determinants of mental health are finally becoming more commonplace, and CMHNs have been identified as playing an important role in this regard (Lauder, Kroll, & Jones, 2007; WHO, 2014). In particular, mental health can be protected and promoted through upstream policies that improve social inclusion, freedom from discrimination and violence, and access to economic resources (WHO, 2014).

The Mental Health Act in Community Mental Health Nursing

The **Mental Health Act** (2010) is a legal document meant to safeguard and ensure humane and just care to PMHIs, while protecting society and PMHIs from harm. It is evoked when acute treatment services are needed on an involuntary basis. PMHI and family members often have diverse opinions when an involuntary admission is enacted, with PMHIs feeling that their rights are violated and family members feeling their loved ones require treatment. While the Mental Health Act covers multiple details on the rights of PMHIs, this discussion focuses on two central issues: committal and compulsory treatment orders.

Committal Mental health act across provinces vary in their wording and criteria for curtailing individual freedoms, but there is general consensus that harm to others or self-harm are key deciding factors, with some provinces adding the criteria of potential physical and mental deterioration. Manitoba, Alberta, and British Columbia include potential physical and mental deterioration, whereas Ontario has specified this may be a criterion only when there is evidence of past successful psychiatric treatment. CMHNs need to be familiar with the mental health act in their province.

Compulsory Treatment Orders Compulsory treatment orders (CTOs) decree that PMHIs must be compliant with treatment, or they must return to the hospital. Laws vary among provinces, with Saskatchewan, Ontario, and British Columbia having statutes for CTOs. CTOs are meant to allow individuals to remain within the community in the least restrictive way while receiving mandated psychiatric treatment. However, in the decade and a half since they were implemented, research has failed to find significant positive outcomes for individuals under CTOs. Large randomized trials have not established a correlation between CTOs and outcome markers such as re-hospitalization rates, symptomatology (including aggression), social functioning, and quality of life (Kisely & Campbell, 2014), despite significant curtailment of individual freedom and impact on social and familial relations.

Mental Health Service Delivery Models

Recovery Model The **recovery model** rests on basic principles such as hope, empowerment, inclusion, respect for personhood and lived experience, and ownership over life. It promotes "living a satisfying, hopeful and contributing life, even when there are ongoing limitations caused by mental health problems" (MHCC, 2015a, p. 11). The assumptions of recovery challenge the status quo to re-examine mental health service delivery. Essential services include crisis intervention, case management, rehabilitation, enrichment, rights protection, basic support, self-help, and prevention. The Canadian Mental Health Association, Ontario (2014) describes recovery as a personal process

Table 23.3	Recovery Principles

Recovery is unique. There is no one path.

Recovery occurs even though symptoms reoccur. Recovery occurs within MI.

Recovery increases control, meaning, and purpose while living with a mental illness.

Recovery orientation to services emphasizes the person is central to planning care.

WRAP—Wellness Recovery Action Plans help people self-manage their condition, connect with helpers, and become empowered and optimistic.

Source: Based on CMHA (2004). A Framework for Support, 3rd ed. CMHA Ontario. Retrieved from: https://cmha.ca/wp-content/ uploads/2004/01/ Framework_for_Support-1.pdf, Canadian Mental Health Association, Ontario.

where some people may live with psychological symptoms in recovery and others look to being symptom free, but both experience more control and optimism about their condition. (See Table 23.3.)

Collaborative Mental Health Care Model This model consists of PMHIs, family and caregivers, and multidisciplinary health care providers from mental health and primary care services to provide more meaningful, coordinated, and effective service. It delivers mental health promotion, prevention, detection, and treatment of MI. In addition, it provides rehabilitation and recovery support that ensures the voice, goals, and strengths of the PMHI are at the centre. The Canadian Collaborative Mental Health Initiative has created a body of evidence-based research papers and toolkits in support of this model (www.ccmhi.ca).

NURSING ROLES IN COMMUNITY MENTAL HEALTH

Case Finding and Referral

Early identification and treatment of MI reduces its severity and promotes quicker recovery. CMHNs providing mental health promotion programs will have opportunities to assess people at risk or who are not receiving appropriate services. CMHNs can assess children living with a parent with MI and ensure their needs are met. CMHNs may also refer parents to parenting programs to assist them with parenting skills.

Advocacy is needed to negotiate the mental health system (Kirby & Keon, 2006). Finding services when you are stressed is difficult. CMHNs ease this tension for PMHIs and their families, ensuring their concerns are represented, their rights are protected, and appropriate services are available. CMHNs advocate for funding for new community programs based on needs and evidence, serve on advisory boards, and lobby to influence healthy public policy. They play a significant advocacy role in reducing social inequities that impede mental health and recovery from MI.

Education and Counselling

CMHNs provide education to the general public, targeted groups, and individuals and families. Within therapeutic relationships, CMHNs promote self-care, coping abilities, and social support networks. In crises, they work with PMHIs and families to find appropriate resources. Individual and group educational counselling promotes discussion of the signs of MI, treatment options, and the recovery model. CMHNs support peer and self-help recovery-based programs, facilitate cognitive behavioural therapy groups, and organize educational programs to promote mental health and reduce risk factors, including programs to inform schools and children of ways to reduce the risk of abuse, which is a precursor to mental health problems.

Prevention: Thinking Upstream

Given the lifelong and intergenerational effects of adverse events such as violence, trauma, discrimination, and poverty, it is critical that policies tackle inequities upstream, in particular through mental health promotion and the prevention of mental health issues. Addressing the social determinants of mental health is also critical. The Canadian Mental Health Association, Ontario (2008) has identified the three main determinants as social inclusion, freedom from discrimination and violence, and access to economic resources. Addressing the reasons why individuals develop mental health issues in the first place is key. Collective, upstream action across society can help reduce disparities and inequities that underpin much of the distress experienced by PMHIs. The Canadian Nurses Association (2012) has taken a longstanding position on the role that mental health nurses play in supporting such policies.

FUTURE DIRECTIONS AND IMPLICATIONS FOR NURSING

Reports on mental health services in Canada demonstrate the need for continued support for PMHIs and families, as well as strategies aimed at preventing the traumas that contribute to emotional distress and MI. Increased recognition of peer and family support programs, self-help, and the principles of recovery are beginning to change service delivery. Listening to PMHIs is an important strategy in understanding what works and what does not. Changes in the community mental health system call for comprehensive funding to address societal barriers that impede PMHIs to live a fulfilling life. Populations societally rendered vulnerable (e.g., children, adolescents, Métis, First Nations, Inuit, people who are homeless, immigrants, and refugees) require specific mental health promotion strategies.

CMHNs are called on to ensure that persons with lived experience are consulted and involved in shaping practices, policies, and reforms. They can prepare themselves to address gaps in mental health services by thinking "outside the box" and mobilizing alternative forms of knowledge and nursing practices based on critical analyses and nursing research in mental health. CMHNs play a key role in facilitating peer programs, self-help groups, and family advocacy and support groups, which they must do in a nonpatronizing way. The recovery model constitutes a sound alternative to the all-too-present biomedical model, for it outlines approaches to working *with* PMHIs while acknowledging the support structures required to live successfully in the community. Future directions require focused nursing efforts to affect policy and the social determinants of mental health and to work collaboratively outside taken-for-granted approaches.

CASE STUDY

You are a community health nurse working with inner-city youth struggling with poverty, racism, substance misuse, and trauma. For the past six months you have been conducting weekly "Ask the Nurse" health clinics at Youth Power, an organization that assists youth with counselling, educational supports, and housing. You have frequently worked with Gary, a 24-year-old man who is a well-liked peer counsellor who encourages youth to return to school, set goals, and establish links to meaningful supports. Gary has had many personal challenges related to substance misuse, poverty, and homelessness. He is a role model for youth who come to the program. On Monday, the program director tells you that Gary committed suicide on the weekend after experiencing a setback. You feel an overwhelming sense of sadness and discouragement.

Discussion Questions

1. What resources can help you to process your feelings in order to practise self-care and continue to work with the youth?

2. How will you assist the youth to understand Gary's suicide and process their emotions?

3. How can CMHNs support peer support workers who may be struggling with their personal circumstances?

CONCLUSION

When working with persons with mental health issues, their families, and their communities, nurses are practising in a system that is subject to unrelenting metamorphosis. New models propose reconfigurations of care that honour personal narratives of PMHIs and families, and that change the nurse–person relationship to one of shared power without pathologizing responses to traumatic experiences. This reconfiguration of nursing care will challenge nursing to examine current practices and assess nurses' openness to radical changes and innovations. As colonialism's effects on mental health are recognized, and traditional wisdom is incorporated into therapies for Indigenous peoples, nurses are also challenged to understand the effects of historical oppression on health and incorporate new ways to promote healing. As cultural diversity increases within Canadian society, nurses will consider alternative ways of understanding psychological distress and MI. The recovery model and the integration of a true collaborative model of mental health care will help nurses to focus on PMHIs' abilities to

build meaningful lives and will strengthen nurses' resolve to think and act upstream to change the inequities that impede the mental well-being of people in the first place.

KEY TERMS

assertive community treatment (ACT) (p. 437)
community mental health nurses (CMHNs) (p. 426)
crisis stabilization units (p. 437)
culturally safe care (p. 437)
functional impairment (p. 437)
Mad Movement (p. 429)
mental health (p. 427)
Mental Health Act (p. 438)
mental health promotion (p. 438)
mental illness (MI) (p. 427)
pathologization (p. 428)
person-first approach (p. 433)
Psychiatric Survivors movement (p. 429)
recovery model (p. 438)
serious and persistent mental illness (SPMI) (p. 427)
social determinants of mental health (p. 430)
suicidal behaviours (p. 434)
suicidal ideation (p. 434)
trauma-informed approach (p. 435)

STUDY QUESTIONS

1. Knowing the history of the mental health system in Canada can help nurses understand current issues. From what you have read about deinstitutionalization, how do you think this has impacted the current problems in the mental health system?

2. Suicide continues to be a troubling problem in Canadian society. Identify groups who are at risk for suicide. Explain four strategies you might use in your community nursing practice to decrease suicide in these groups.

3. Define mental health promotion, and consider how you would implement strategies to promote mental health in the frail older adults living in the community, new immigrant mothers, and suburban high school students.

4. Consider the risk factors for mental illness. How can CMHNs reduce risk factors within their practice communities?

5. Identify and discuss four recommendations from the national report on the state of mental health services in Canada.

INDIVIDUAL CRITICAL-THINKING EXERCISES

1. What strategies might a CMHN use to promote the mental health of elementary-school-age children?

2. How would a CMHN implement the recovery model with a person who suffers from depression and that person's family?

3. What issues are important to consider in designing mental health services for diverse cultural groups?

4. What are the unique challenges that face Indigenous people in restoring mental health and healing to their communities?

5. Why do you think "person-first" language is important?

6. Reflect on each of the following sets of statements:

> Madison is mentally ill.
> Madison has a mental health issue.
> Madison is experiencing psychological distress.
>
> Brian is a drug addict.
> Brian uses drugs.
> Brian struggles with substance misuse.
>
> Anthony is schizophrenic.
> Anthony has schizophrenia.
> Anthony lives with schizophrenia.

a) What are the differences between each statement? Does the phrasing of each statement impact how you perceive these individuals?

b) How would you prefer to be described if you were Madison, Brian, or Anthony?

GROUP CRITICAL-THINKING EXERCISES

1. How might CMHNs ensure that the physical and mental health needs of PMHIs are met within a primary health care clinic?

2. How might CMHNs influence and develop a national suicide prevention strategy?

3. How can the principles of recovery be implemented and researched within the mental health system?

REFERENCES

Abraham, C. (2010). Are we medicating a disorder or treating boyhood as a disease? *The Globe and Mail* (18 October). Retrieved from https://www.theglobeand-mail.com/news/national/time-to-lead/part-3-are-we-medicating-a-disorder-or-treating-boyhood-as-a-disease/article4330080

Afifi, T. O., MacMillan, H. L., Boyle, M., Taillieu, T., Cheung, K., & Sareen, J. (2014). Child abuse and mental disorders in Canada. *Canadian Medical Association Journal, 186*(9), E324–E332.

Anthony, W. A. (2000). A recovery service system: Setting some systems level standards. *Psychiatric Rehabilitation Journal, 24*(2), 160–166.

Bartlett, R., Brown, L., Shattell, M., Wright, T., & Lewallen, L. (2013). Harm reduction: Compassionate care of persons with addictions. *Medsurg Nursing, 22*(6), 349–358.

Bell, J. (2013). *Suicide in Nunavut: Child abuse, pot smoking, mental disorders the biggest factors. Nunatsiaq News* (June 6). Retrieved from http://www.nunatsiaqonline.ca/stories/article/65674suicide_in_nunavut_child_abuse_pot_smoking_mental_disorders_the_bigges

Bielefeldt, A. Ø., Danborg, P. B., & Gøtzsche, P. C. (2016). Precursors to suicidality and violence on antidepressants: systematic review of trials in adult healthy volunteers. *Journal of the Royal Society* of *Medicine, 109,* 381–392.

Canadian Armed Forces and Veterans Affairs Canada. (2017). *Joint suicide prevention strategy.* Retrieved from https://www.canada.ca/content/dam/dnd-mdn/documents/reports/2017/caf-vac-joint-suicide-prevention-strategy.pdf

Canadian Health Services Research Foundation. (2013). Myth: Reframing mental illness as a "brain disease" reduces stigma. *Journal of Health Services Research & Policy, 18*(3), 190–192.

Canadian Mental Health Association, Ontario. (2008). *Mental health promotion in Ontario: A call to action.* Retrieved from http://ontario.cmha.ca/documents/mental-health-promotion-in-ontario-a-call-to-action

Canadian Mental Health Association, Ontario. (2014). *Recovery.* Retrieved from http://ontario.cmha.ca/mental-health/mental-health-conditions/recovery

Canadian Nurses Association. (2012). *Position statement on mental health services.* Retrieved from https://www.cna-aiic.ca/-/media/cna/page-content/pdf-en/ps85_mental_health_e.pdf?la=en&hash=638E0CBA8037C88BF14DEED764CB54D9E832DE77

Cazabon, A. (2010). Third World Canada. Retrieved from http://www.thirdworldcanada.ca/

Coleman, T., & Cotton, D. (2010). *Police interactions with persons with a mental illness: Police learning in the environment of contemporary policing.* Retrieved from https://www.mentalhealthcommission.ca/sites/default/files/Law_Police_Interactions_Mental_Illness_Report_ENG_0_1.pdf

Community Health Nurses of Canada (CHNC). (2019, revised). *Canadian community health nursing: Professional practice model & standards of practice.* Retrieved from https://www.chnc.ca/documents/CHNC-ProfessionalPracticeModel-EN/index.html

CMHA (2004). A Framework for Support, 3rd ed. CMHA Ontario. Retrieved from: https://cmha.ca/wp-content/uploads/2004/01/Framework_for_Support-1.pdf

Cyr, C., McKee, H., O'Hagan, M., & Priest, R. for the MHCC. (2016). *Making the case for peer support: Report to the peer support project committee of the Mental Health Commission of Canada* (2nd ed.). Retrieved from https://www.mentalhealthcommission.ca/sites/default/files/2016-07/MHCC_Making_the_Case_for_Peer_Support_2016_Eng.pdf

Davis, S. (2006). *Community mental health in Canada: Policy, theory, and practice.* Vancouver, BC: UBC Press.

Degenhardt, L., Whitford, H. A., Ferrari, A. J., Baxter, A. J., Charlson, F. J., Hall, W. D., . . . Vos, T. (2013). Global burden of disease attributable to illicit drug use and dependence: Findings from the Global Burden of Disease Study 2010. *The Lancet, 382*(9904), 1564–1574.

Elias, B., Mignone, J., Hall, M., Hong, S., Hart, L., & Sareen, J. (2012). Trauma and suicide behaviour histories among a Canadian Indigenous population: An empirical exploration of the potential role of Canada's residential school system. *Social Science and Medicine, 74*(10), 1560–1569.

Felitti, V. J., Anda, R. F., Nordenberg, D., Williamson, D. F., Spitz, A. M., Edwards, V., . . . Marks, J. S. (1998). Relationship of childhood abuse and household dysfunction to many of the leading causes of death in adults: The Adverse Childhood Experiences (ACE) study. *American Journal of Preventive Medicine, 14*(4), 245–258.

Fried, E., & Kievit, R. A. (2015). The volumes of subcortical regions in depressed and healthy individuals are strikingly similar: a reinterpretation of the results by Schmaal et al. *Molecular Psychiatry—Nature, 1*–2.

Goering, P., Wasylenki, D., & Durbin, J. (2000). Canada's mental health system. *International Journal of Law and Psychiatry, 23*(3–4), 345–359.

Government of Canada. (2006). *The human face of mental health and mental illness in Canada 2006* (Cat. no. HP5-19/2006E). Ottawa, ON: Minister of Public Works and Government Services.

Government of Canada. (2016). *Working together to prevent suicide in Canada. The federal framework for suicide prevention.* Retrieved from https://www.canada.ca/content/dam/canada/public-health/migration/publications/healthy-living-vie-saine/framework-suicide-cadre-suicide/alt/framework-suicide-cadre-suicide-eng.pdf. Government of Ontario (1999, amended 2010). Mental Health Act, R.S.O, c. M7. Retrieved from : https://www.ontario.ca/laws/statute/90m07

Guruge, S., Roche, B., & Catallo, C. (2012). Violence against women: An exploration of the physical and mental health trends among immigrant and refugee women in Canada. *Nursing Research and Practice,* 434–592.

Health Canada. (2015). *First Nations mental wellness continuum framework.* Retrieved from http://health.afn.ca/uploads/files/24-14-1273-fn-mental-wellness-framework-en05_low.pdf

Holmes, D., Jacob, J. D., & Perron, A. (2014). *Power and the Psychiatric Apparatus: Assistance, Repression and Transformation.* Surrey, UK: Ashgate Publishing.

Jutel, A. (2010). Framing disease: the example of female hypoactive sexual desire disorder. *Social Science & Medicine, 70*(7), 1084–1090.

Kirby, M. J. (2008). Mental health in Canada: Out of the shadows forever. *Canadian Medical Association Journal, 178*(10), 1320–1322.

Kirby, M. J., & Keon, W. J. (2006). *Out of the shadows at last: Transforming mental health, mental illness and addictions services in Canada.* Ottawa, ON: Standing Senate Committee on Social Affairs, Science and Technology.

Kirmayer, L. J., Narashlah, L., Munoz, M., Rashid, M., Ryder, A., Guzder, J., . . . Canadian Collaboration for Immigrant and Refugee Health. (2011). Common mental health problems in immigrants and refugees: General approach in primary care. *Canadian Medical Association Journal, 183*(12), 959–967.

Kisely S., & Campbell, L. (2014). Compulsory community and involuntary outpatient treatment for people with severe mental disorders. *Cochrane Database of Systematic Reviews, 12.*

Kutcher, S., & McLuckie, A. (2010). *Evergreen: A child and youth mental health framework for Canada.* Calgary, AB: Mental Health Commission of Canada.

Lauder, W., Kroll, T., & Jones, M. (2007). Social determinants of mental health: The missing dimensions of mental health nursing? *Journal of Psychiatric and Mental Health Nursing, 14,* 661–669.

Lawrence, D., & Kisley, S. (2010). Inequities in healthcare provision for people with severe mental illness. *Journal of Psychopharmacology, 24*(4 Suppl.), 61–68.

Leavey, J. E. (2015). *Living recovery: Youth speak out on "owning" mental illness.* Waterloo, ON: Wilfred Laurier University Press.

LeFrançois, B., Menzies, R., & Reaume, G. (2013). *Mad matters: A critical reader in Canadian mad studies.* Toronto, ON: Canadian Scholars' Press.

Le Noury, J., Nardo, J. M., Healy, D., Jureidini, J., Raven, M., Tufanaru, C., . . . Abi-Jaoude, E. (2016). Study 329 continuation phase: Safety and efficacy of paroxetine and imipramine in extended treatment of adolescent major depression. *International Journal of Risk and Safety in Medicine, 28*(3), 143–161.

Luanaigh, C. Ò., & Lawlor, B. A. (2008). Loneliness and the health of older people. *International Journal of Geriatric Psychiatry, 23*(12), 1213–1221.

Maniglio, R. (2009). Severe mental illness and criminal victimization: A systematic review. *Acta Psychiatrica Scandinavica, 119*(3), 180–191.

McGibbon, E. (2012). *Oppression: A social determinant of health.* Winnipeg, MB: Fernwood.

Mental Health Commission of Canada (MHCC). (2012). *Changing directions, changing lives. The mental health strategy for Canada, Summary.* Calgary, AB: Mental Health Commission of Canada.

Mental Health Commission of Canada (MHCC). (2013a). *Housing and homelessness.* Retrieved from http://www.mentalhealthcommission.ca/English/issues/housing-and-homelessness

Mental Health Commission of Canada (MHCC). (2013b). *Opening minds interim report.* Used with permission of the Mental Health Commission of Canada. Retrieved from http://www.mentalhealthcommission.ca/English/system/files/private/document/opening_minds_interim_report.pdf

Mental Health Commission of Canada (MHCC). (2015a). *Guidelines for Recovery-Oriented Practice.* Ottawa, ON: Mental Health Commission of Canada.

Mental Health Commission of Canada (MHCC). (2015b). *Informing the future: Mental health indicators for Canada.* Retrieved from http://www.mentalhealthcommission.ca/English/system/files/private/document/MHCC_MentalHealthIndicators_Jan2015_ENG.pdf

Müller, V. I., Cieslik, E. C., Serbanescu, I., Laird, A. R., Fox, P. T., & Eickhoff, S. (2017). Altered brain activity in unipolar depression revisited: Meta-analyses of neuroimaging studies. *JAMA Psychiatry, 74*(1), 47–55.

National Collaborating Centre for Environmental Health and National Collaborating Centre for Determinants of Health (2017). *Environmental influences on population mental health promotion for children and youth.* Canada: National Collaborating Centres for Public Health.

Nolan, P. W. (1993). A history of the training of asylum nurses. *Journal of Advanced Nursing, 18*(8), 1193–1201.

Nunavut Bureau of Statistics. (2015, June 3). Nunavut suicides by region, sex, age group and ethnicity, 1999 to 2014. Retrieved from http://www.stats.gov.nu.ca/Publications/Historical/Deaths/Nunavut%20Suicides%20by%20Region,%20Sex,%20Age%20Group%20and%20Ethnicity,%201999%20to%202014.xlsx

Nyttingnes, O., Ruud, T., & Rugkåsa, J. (2016). "It's unbelievably humiliating"—Patients' expressions of negative effects of coercion in mental health care. *International Journal of Law and Psychiatry, 49,* 147–153.

Ogrodniczuk, J., Oliffe, J., Kuhl, D., & Gross, P. A. (2016). La santé mentale des hommes. *Canadian Family Physician, 62*(6), e284–e286.

Perreault, M., Provencher, H., Roberts, S., & Milton, D. (2012). Predictors of caregiver satisfaction with mental health services. *Journal of Community Mental Health, 48,* 232–237.

Phippen, J. W. (11 April 2016), The suicide emergency among Canada's First Nations. *The Atlantic*. Retrieved from https://www.theatlantic.com/international/archive/2016/04/canada-suicide/477684

Read, J., & Cain, A. (2013). A literature review and meta-analysis of drug company-funded mental health websites. *Acta Psychiatrica Scandinavica, 128*(6), 422–433.

Ryan-Nicholls, K. D., & Haggarty, J. M. (2007). Collaborative mental health care in rural and isolated Canada: Stakeholder feedback. *Journal of Psychosocial Nursing, 45*(12), 37–45.

Schissel, B. (2011). *About Canada: Children and youth*. Black Point, NS: Fernwood Publishing.

Shakya, Y., Khanlou, N., & Gonsalves, T. 2015. *Determinants of mental health for newcomer youth: Policy and service implications*. Retrieved from http://accessalliance.ca/wp-content/uploads/2015/03/Determinants_of_Mental_Health_for_Newcomer_YouthCdn_Issues.pdf

Sharma, T., Guski, L. S, Freund, N., & Gøtzsche, P.C. (2016). Suicidality and aggression during antidepressant treatment: Systematic review and meta-analyses based on clinical study reports. *BMJ, 352*, i65.

Shulman, M., & Tahirali, J. (11 April 2016). *Suicide among Canada's First Nations: Key numbers*. CTVNews. Retrieved from https://www.ctvnews.ca/health/suicide-among-canada-s-first-nations-key-numbers-1.2854899

Sigurdson, J. F., Undheim, A. M., Wallander, J. L., Lydersen, S., & Sund, A. M. (2015). The long-term effects of being bullied or a bully in adolescence on externalizing and internalizing mental health problems in adulthood. *Child and Adolescent Psychiatry and Mental Health, 9*, 42.

Sprooten, E., Rasgon, A., Goodman, M., Carlin, A., Leibu, E., Lee, W. H., & Frangou, S. (2017). Addressing reverse inference in psychiatric neuroimaging: Meta-analyses of task-related brain activation in common mental disorders. *Human Brain Mapping, 38*, 1846–1864.

Stall, N. (2013). Imprisoning the mentally ill. *Canadian Medical Association Journal, 19, 185*(3), 201–202.

Statistics Canada. (n.d.). *Suicides and suicide rate, by sex and by age group*. Retrieved from https://www.statcan.gc.ca/tables-tableaux/sum-som/l01/cst01/hlth66d-eng.htm

Statistics Canada (2014). *Canadian Forces mental health survey, 2013*. Retrieved from http://www.statcan.gc.ca/daily-quotidien/140811/dq140811a-eng.htm

Sussman, S. (1998). The first asylums in Canada: A response to neglectful community care and current trends. *Canadian Journal of Psychiatry, 43*, 260–264.

Swinkels, H., Pottie, K., Tugwell, P., Rashid, M., & Naraslah, L. (2011). Development of guidelines for recently arrived immigrants and refugees to Canada: Delphi consensus on selecting preventable and treatable conditions. *Canadian Medical Association Journal, 183*(12), 928–932.

Thomas, S. P., & Nandrha, H. S. (2009). Early intervention in psychosis: A retrospective analysis of clinical and social factors influencing duration of untreated psychosis. *Primary Care Companion Journal of Clinical Psychiatry, 11*(5), 212–214.

Thompson, J. M., VanTil, L. D., Zamorski, M. A., Garber, B., Dursun, S., Fikretoglu, D., . . . Pedlar, D. J. (2016). Mental health of Canadian Armed Forces Veterans: Review of population studies. *Journal of Military, Veteran and Family Health, 2*(1), 70–86.

Tonmyr, L., & Shields, M. (2017). Childhood sexual abuse and substance abuse: A gender paradox? *Child Abuse & Neglect, 63*, 284–294.

Truth and Reconciliation Commission of Canada. (2015). *The survivors speak: A report of the Truth and Reconciliation Commission of Canada*. Retrieved from http://www.trc.ca/websites/trcinstitution/File/2015/Findings/Survivors_Speak_2015_05_30_web_o.pdf

United Nations. (2017). *Special Rapporteur on the right of everyone to the enjoyment of the highest attainable standard of physical and mental. Depression: Let's talk about how we address mental health*. Retrieved from http://www.ohchr.org/EN/NewsEvents/Pages/DisplayNews.aspx?NewsID=21480&%3BLangID=E

Wakefield, J. C. (2016). Diagnostic issues and controversies in DSM-5: Return of the false positives problem. *Annual Review of Clinical Psychology, 12*, 105–32.

World Health Organization (WHO). (2004). *Prevention of mental disorders: Effective interventions and policy options*. Geneva, CH: World Health Organization.

World Health Organization (WHO). (2014). *Social determinants of mental health*. Geneva, CH: World Health Organization.

Wolke, D., & Lereya, S. T. (2015). Long-term effects of bullying. *Archives of Disease in Childhood, 100*(9), 879–885.

Zakrison, T. L., Hamel, P. A., & Hwang, S. W. (2004). Homeless people's trust and interactions with police and paramedics. *Journal of Urban Health: Bulletin of the New York Academy of Medicine, 81*(4), 596–605.

ABOUT THE AUTHORS

Amélie Perron, RN, PhD, is Associate Professor at the School of Nursing, University of Ottawa, and co-founder of the Nursing Observatory. She has worked on several research projects in psychiatry and forensic psychiatry in Canada, France, and Australia. Her research is grounded in critical theory, and her fields of interest include psychiatric nursing, forensic psychiatry, power relationships, and issues related to risk, gender, and ethics. Her clinical practice is grounded in community psychiatry and crisis intervention.

Dave Holmes, RN, PhD, formerly of the School of Nursing, University of Ottawa, is now Full Professor and Associate Dean Academic and Student Affairs at the Sue and Bill Gross School of Nursing, University of California-Irvine. He has worked several years as clinician in forensic psychiatric settings, both in closed/secured institutions and in the community. Most of his work, comments, essays, analyses, and research are based on the principles of critical social theory.

CHAPTER 24

Rural and Remote Health

Mary Ellen Labrecque and Kelley Kilpatrick

LEARNING OUTCOMES

After studying this chapter, you should be able to:

1. Describe the characteristics of rural and remote communities in a Canadian context and the impact of geographical diversity on health status.

2. Recognize health inequities associated with access to care for residents living in rural or remote communities in Canada.

3. Explain the context of nursing practice and interrelationship with the social determinants of health when caring for clients in rural and remote areas.

4. Identify challenges and rewards in the development of a nursing role in a rural or remote community and evidence-informed strategies that support role development.

5. Explore ways in which rural and remote community health nurses have a role in addressing health policy.

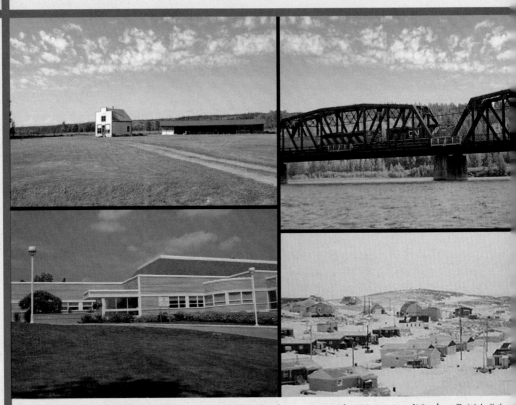

Sources: Courtesy of Mary Ellen Labrecque/University of Saskatchewan; Erin Wilson/University of Northern British Colum Erin Wilson/University of Northern British Columbia; Martha MacLeod/University of Northern British Columbia

INTRODUCTION

This chapter introduces concepts relevant to caring for clients and populations residing in rural and remote areas of Canada. The characteristics of rural and remote are delineated with an emphasis on cultural diversity, equity in distribution of health services, and the rural and remote community health nurse (CHN) role in addressing historical colonialism and health inequities. The aim of the chapter is to assist nursing students to develop an understanding of health and the role of CHNs in rural and remote geographical locations.

Descriptions of rural and remote nursing practice provided by CHNs in national surveys (MacLeod et al., 2017) include community characteristics, geographical location, health equity, human and technical resources, and nursing practice characteristics. In the chapter, the features of rural and remote CHN practice are identified and expanded to include perspectives on the increasing need for advocacy work by CHNs. Critical-thinking questions will enable students to explore the differences between rural and remote communities, rural and remote area CHN practice, health care and community services, and will encourage students to think upstream about the inequities faced by residents living in rural and remote Canada.

THE CHARACTERISTICS OF RURAL AND REMOTE CANADA

Definitions

Approximately 95% of Canada's land mass can be considered rural and remote (Moazzami, 2015). However, longstanding debate exists about the definitions of key terms that describe the geographical location of communities as **rural**, **remote**, **Northern**, and **isolated**. One of the first comprehensive reviews of the literature examining rurality highlighted that indexes reported differing methods for assessing *rural* (Minore, Hill, Pugliese, & Gauld, 2008). Some of the indices report on access to health care, population, or number of physicians as a measure of rurality. Therefore, it is important to note that there are few rurality indices that define *rural* and *remote*, and little consensus exists in the literature about the definition of remote, with the choice of index dependent on the focus of research endeavours (Kulig, Kilpatrick, Moffitt, & Zimmer, 2015). Pitblado (2005) suggested two main ways to define rural: technical and social.

Technical approaches to the definition of *rural* include locators or geographic regions, like the location of hospitals, roads, or specific political areas (i.e., provinces, counties). For example, Statistics Canada (du Plessis, Beshiri, & Bollman, 2001) examined six possible ways to define *rural*, each emphasizing different criteria, such as population size, population density, and settlement or labour market contexts. This definition of "census rural" refers to "individuals living in the countryside outside centres of 1000 or more population" (du Plessis et al., 2001, p. 6). The Canadian Institute for Health Information (CIHI) adds the notion of distance to, and relationship with, urban areas (Canadian Institute for Health Information [CIHI], 2013). The First Nations and Inuit Health Branch (FNIHB) within Health Canada (2005) defines the degrees of rurality as follows:

- *Non-isolated community* includes communities with road access of less than 90 kilometres to physician services.
- *Semi-isolated community* includes communities with road access greater than 90 kilometres to physician services.
- *Isolated community* refers to communities with good telephone service, scheduled air transportation flights, but no road access.
- *Remote, isolated community* means the communities have no scheduled air flights, minimal telephone or radio access, and no road access.

Many of the indices of rurality are old, have held only theoretical value, and have never been put into operation. Almost all of the indices have been designed with physicians—not nurses—in mind. In the analysis of the perceptions of rurality by rural registered nurses (RNs), Kulig et al. (2008) concluded that there was no benefit in developing a national numerical index of rurality based on distance to advanced health care services because of the variability of absolute distance (ranging from 20 to 1000 kilometres) and mode of travel (e.g., air or ground). In addition, most rurality models focus on deficits rather than the strengths of rural communities. The FNIHB

designations highlight the importance of access to services and the types of locally available health services while considering transportation and communication limitations as important factors in their differentiation between what isolated is and is not. A wide variety of indices of rurality exist, such as the Canadian General Practice Rurality Index (Leduc, 1997) or the Rurality Index of Ontario (Kralj, 2001).

Social approaches to defining rural refer to the nature of the rural community, including such features as specific services that are normally associated with larger population sizes (e.g., specific types of stores or restaurants) (Pitblado, 2005). Although the social nature of place in defining rural is relevant to health care service delivery, particularly the recruitment and retention of health professionals, including RNs, there has been limited work done on examination of its specific meaning or application. The definition offered by Statistics Canada identifies "rural and small town" as "individuals in towns or municipalities outside the commuting zone of larger urban centres" (du Plessis et al., 2001, p. 6). Using this definition, in 2016, 5 918 771 or approximately 17% of Canadians lived in communities with populations of less than 10 000 people (Statistics Canada, 2017a). This is the definition of rural employed in this chapter. It is selected because of its growing use in studies of rural and remote issues in Canada, including the determinants of health and the delivery of health care.

Diversity of Rural and Remote Communities

Rural and remote communities in Canada are diverse, and their economies vary by the specific geographic features. Traditionally, rural and remote economies have been dependent on the natural resources of the geographic landscape, such as oil and gas extraction, forestry, fishing, and agriculture. It is incumbent on CHNs to understand the socioeconomic context in the community where they work, given the influence of economic development on the determinants of health.

The **resource base** of a community will influence the health status of those who live in it. In rural, remote, and isolated communities where there is a heavy reliance on industries such as oil and gas, logging, mining, fishing, and agriculture, interrelated injuries and illnesses impact the individuals as well as the community at large. For example, in 2015 there were 271 935 farm operators across Canada (Statistics Canada, 2017b). Operators on medium-size farms had the highest incidence of injury because they worked the longest hours without reliance on hired help in comparison to those on the largest farms (Maltais, 2010). Farm operators are also aging, possibly contributing to the higher incidence of injury in an industry that continues to have one of the highest fatality rates. According to statistics from the Association of Workers' Compensation Boards of Canada (AWCB, 2017), in 2015, there were 3331 accepted time-loss injuries (i.e., "an injury where a worker is compensated for a loss of wages following a work-related injury") and 10 fatalities in the agriculture and related service industry across Canada. The Canadian Agricultural Injury Reporting system found that annual average number of deaths between 2003 and 2012 was 101, with 70% being machine-related and 91% of the fatalities being male (Canadian Agricultural Injury Reporting, 2016).

Other natural resource industries also employ a significant number of individuals and impact rural areas. Individuals who work in the oil and gas, logging, and mining industries may experience personal health issues such as respiratory problems from environmental exposure to reduced air and **water quality** as well as the potential for accidents on the job (Fraser Basin Council, 2012). For instance, individuals in the logging industry and specifically sawmill workers are exposed to wood dust, which can lead to acute and chronic upper and lower respiratory health conditions (Demers, 2011). In 2015, there were 1330 accepted time-loss injuries and 13 deaths in the logging and forestry industry, and 1705 accepted time-loss injuries and 52 deaths in the mining, quarrying, and oil well industries across Canada (AWCB, 2017). Events such as explosions (e.g., the Burns Lake Sawmill in 2012), oil spills, and mining accidents all have the potential to affect not just those who are directly impacted by the event but also family and friends who must deal with premature death or long-term health impacts of community members. Also of concern is the potential loss of employment and ultimately negative long-term changes in the community.

In some natural-resource-dependent areas, industrial camps are set up for varying periods of time. The local health regions may be responsible for enforcing environmental and public health regulations for camps and for helping to address health issues that may arise (Northern Health, 2012). Potential health issues involve impacts of shift work, including obesity, emotional distress, and domestic issues, all of which may be interrelated with substance abuse (Northern Health, 2012). Another issue CHNs may need to address is the perception among workers that cancer can be attributed to working in the oil and gas industry (Fraser Basin Council, 2012); this has implications for individual and community health assessments in identifying relationships and occupational trends.

The **socioeconomic status** of rural and remote communities is not static. For example, in areas where natural resources are depleted, or when global pricing and demand decreases, communities often seek alternate economic ventures, such as tourism, to sustain their economic and social viability. As the rural and remote populations change, such as communities with an increasing percentage of older adults, so too do community health needs.

Not all individuals who live rural or remote experience similar access to **employment opportunities**. Having access to local opportunities to earn a reasonable living wage, purchase healthier food options, and care for family members corresponds to a number of the social determinants of health. For example, in rural and remote areas of Canada, employment opportunities are considerably limited, particularly for women. The most recent Statistics Canada (2017a) census data analysis reported that 45.6% of rural and 44.6% of remote women were in the labour force, compared to 47.8% of the urban labour force (Status of Women, 2016). Reserve-based First Nation (FN) women's income was lower than non-Indigenous women working on reserves and Indigenous women living in rural or urban settings. Only 56% of women living in a remote community were reported to have a certificate, diploma, or degree, compared to rural (69%) or urban (78%) women. For rural Indigenous women, 41% were found to have no certificate, diploma, or degree, compared to 35% of urban-based Indigenous women. The statistics identified a strong relationship with residing in an urban area and obtaining a university education and decreasing numbers in rural areas, with the lowest rates on reserves. There is also unequal access to post-secondary education in rural and remote areas, which limits the ability for people to change their income and subsequently impacts the socioeconomic status of their communities.

Being Rural and Remote

Emphasizing such notions as a "type" of rural or remote person can lead to generalizations and inaccurate descriptions of the variety of people who live in rural and remote settings. Rural and remote residents have been the focus of a very small number of studies examining the meaning of health. A recent systematic review of literature exploring the definition of health from the perspective of rural- and remote-living people identified that there may be a difference in how health is perceived by remote, rural, and urban dwellers (Gessert et al., 2015). Findings of this review suggested a definition that included the ability to participate in work and community social events, and being independent. One important older study on the health beliefs of rural Canadians in two western provinces found that being healthy was defined as having a holistic relationship among mental, social, physical, and spiritual aspects (Harbison, Coughlan, Karabanow, & VanderPlaat, 2005). In another study, the participants defined sickness as a curable and short-term condition, whereas illness was perceived as chronic and life-threatening (Thomlinson, McDonagh, Baird, Crooks, & Lees, 2004). The limited number of studies exploring the meaning of health for rural and remote residents requires that CHNs need to explore this issue. The definition of health is diverse and has cultural and geographical elements.

Other research with rural and remote residents has focused specifically on health status—examining differences in disease patterns and occurrences. For example, one study found that a lower proportion of individuals living in small-town regions, rural regions, and northern regions rated their health as excellent. Specific conditions such as arthritis are higher than the national average among rural populations (Barnabe et al., 2017), and residents of northern regions have a higher prevalence of hypertension (Reading, 2015). Canadian studies (DesMeules et al., 2006; DesMeules et al., 2012; Lavergne & Kephart, 2017) that examined health status and health determinants among the rural population found variations of prevalence, incidence, and risk for specific diseases and compared to urban residents, as explored in the "Health Variations among Rural, Remote and Indigenous People" box.

Rural health status and rural-specific determinants of health point to the importance of disease prevention and health promotion through public health initiatives in rural and remote settings. However, what is less clear is whether conventional strategies, mostly developed by urban program planners for urban residents, are equally effective in rural and remote settings. In addressing rural health concerns, CHNs can apply the three levels of prevention: primary (reducing risks for a potential problem), secondary (providing screening and early detection and treatment), and tertiary (maintaining health). For instance, primary prevention would include providing health education for individuals in rural and remote communities to maintain the lower rates of cause-specific cancers; secondary prevention activities would include developing and implementing diabetes screening programs for women at risk for death from diabetes; and tertiary prevention would include monitoring the effectiveness of treatment for circulatory and respiratory diseases.

It is important to note that no amount of health education will change the social determinants of health of individuals and populations living in rural or remote locations. More often than not, the root causes of adverse health outcomes for a population are the result of policies, inadequate programs, a lack of infrastructure, high cost of living, and a lack of focus on the specific strengths and needs of individuals who live rurally or remotely. One population that faces noteworthy barriers to the social determinants of health is the Indigenous people of Canada, many of whom are rural and remote and face challenges related to a number of determinants, including inequities; chronic diseases; underemployment; high costs of food; housing, and hydro; and dramatically inequitable access to health care.

HEALTH VARIATIONS AMONG RURAL, REMOTE, AND INDIGENOUS PEOPLE

- Rural areas reported higher proportions of people with low income and less than secondary education level. Completion of high school was reported as highest among non-Indigenous people and lowest among Inuit peoples.

- Health-related factors, such as the prevalence of smoking and obesity, were elevated in rural Canada, while other health influences, such as dietary practices and leisure-time physical activity, were lower in rural areas. On-reserve FN populations reported higher percentages of adults with diabetes.

- Life expectancy at birth was significantly higher in urban areas and lower among Indigenous people.

- Higher overall mortality risks among rural communities appear to be driven by higher death rates from such causes as circulatory diseases, injuries, and suicide; residents of the most rural areas are often at highest risk.

- Incidence rates of most cause-specific cancers were lower in rural areas.

- Respiratory disease mortality risks were, for the most part, significantly higher among rural residents. The ratio of cases of tuberculosis is higher among Indigenous than non-Indigenous populations.

- Women living in the most-rural areas had higher risks of dying from diabetes.

Sources: Canadian Institute for Health Information (2006). Adapted and reproduced with permission from the Minister of Health, 2018.

Population Diversity in Rural and Remote Areas of Canada

In addition to unique geographic features that affect the livelihood and everyday life cycle of rural and remote residents, there is diversity in the groups of people who live in rural and remote areas. Many of these groups face challenges in being unique and living in a rural or remote environment; some may feel excluded from community life, whereas others who want to live apart prefer residing where they can co-exist with other groups but not be expected to interact. It is part of the role for CHNs to assess the rural and remote communities within which they live and work to determine the diversity, strengths, and needs that arise from such diversity. The changing face of immigration, which includes the influx of temporary foreign workers in some rural communities, adds to diversity in rural community populations (Rice & Webster, 2017) and challenges in the delivery of culturally sensitive health care services.

Identifying diversity in a rural, remote, or isolated community population is important for the development and implementation of appropriate nursing care that incorporates an intersectional approach to the social determinants of health. For example, in some rural areas of Canada, the existence of unique religious groups, including Amish, Hutterites, Mennonites, and Conservative Dutch, means that some health behaviours, such as immunization (Vandenberg, 2013), are not commonly accessed. The example highlights that it is important for CHNs to conduct community assessments that acknowledge the religious, sociohistorical, and policy contexts within which individuals, families, and groups are located. Rather than focus on describing specific groups and practices, the principle of cultural safety that is reflective of cultural awareness, sensitivity, and competence is the appropriate focus. The five principles of cultural safety are protocols (i.e., respect for cultural forms of engagement), personal knowledge (i.e., understanding one's own cultural identity), process (i.e., engaging in mutual learning), positive purpose (i.e., ensuring the process yields the right outcome for the client), and partnerships (i.e., promoting collaborative practice) (McCall & Pauly, 2012; Polaschek, 1998).

Discussions of cultural safety and CHN in a Canadian context must encompass an understanding of the historical colonial context that informs the basis of our knowledge about the development of our nation and the perpetuation of colonialism in the social and political context of the Canadian health care system. This is especially relevant for CHNs working in Indigenous communities in rural and remote areas. Chapter 22 discusses the work of the Truth and Reconciliation Commission of Canada (2015) and the calls to action, which address social determinants of health and the particular inequities stemming from oppressive anti-Indigenous policies. FN, Inuit, and Métis communities historically have been deprived of basic resources and rights for achieving optimal health and wellness. These are important elements of the work of CHNs in Indigenous rural and remote communities.

HEALTH INEQUITIES EXPERIENCED BY RESIDENTS OF RURAL AND REMOTE COMMUNITIES

Although they are known for strength, resilience, and community cohesion, residents of rural and remote Canadian communities are challenged by numerous inequities—most often reported in the literature as access to health care services, reliable **access to technologies**, poor water quality, and **food insecurity**.

Inequity in Health Care Access

Rural and remote communities by nature have fewer health care delivery options. Boom-and-bust cycles affect economic stability and availability of local services for rural and remote residents, and the resulting underemployment leads to poverty, a significant issue for rural and remote people (Rice & Webster, 2017). In rural and remote communities, poverty is a condition that has been largely "invisible" to urban dwellers. The rural and remote poor are disadvantaged because they need to travel longer distances for services. Poverty is exacerbated by the declining populations and the subsequent declining employment and economic resource opportunities in rural and remote communities.

Economic resources, employment opportunities, and poverty have impacts on health status in general and in particular on mental health services. For example, in communities that are dependent on oil and gas extraction, many single men or young families have few supports, which increases levels of stress and needs for mental health resources. Although research has demonstrated that rural and remote prevalence rates of mental health concerns do not differ from that in urban communities, there is a lack of access to local resources in communities. Regionally accessible providers are more apt to be utilized given the perception of a lack of anonymity in accessing local mental health services (Smith, Humphreys, & Wilson, 2008). Many of the inequities in rural and remote mental health services impact all rural people; however, effects of colonization, legislation, policy, reserve conditions, resources, and residential schools contribute additional layers of concern for Indigenous peoples.

In remote Indigenous communities, health and education programs and services are primarily served by non-Indigenous individuals or groups, which affects the level of cultural sensitivity in the provision of these activities. CHN practice needs to specifically address the historical and political context of each rural and remote community, particularly in Indigenous communities. CHNs need to advocate for the inclusion of Indigenous healers and local knowledge keepers in health program design and delivery. Further, one of the high priorities for the delivery of health care in Indigenous communities is the education of community members as nurses and other health care providers (Canadian Nurses Association [CNA], 2014). This is particularly important in

terms of the communication of health prevention and promotion being offered in the language of the community, exploring concepts of health from a traditional knowledge perspective, and integrating new health care technologies into culturally appropriate practices that address local health care priorities.

Inequity and Technology

Technology includes services such as internet connectivity, health informatics, and telehealth. One large area of inequity for rural and remote communities is access to reliable internet service. In 2018, the Canadian Radio-television and Telecommunications Commission announced new funding for broadband projects aimed at improving internet access and mobile wireless network access for underserved areas, including rural and remote regions of Canada (Canadian Radio-television and Telecommunications Commission, 2017). Where internet connectivity was intermittent or severely limited, Melvin and colleagues (Melvin, Bunt, Oduor, & Neustaedter, 2015) found that family communication was hindered and social isolation increased. This may also impact reserve-based Indigenous people as well as those living in rural and remote communities.

Inequitable access to technology impacts health care delivery, including the need for strengthened health informatics. Access to health informatics represents the bringing together of data, information, knowledge, and technologies to support decision making by patients, consumers, physicians, nurses, and other stakeholders (Mancuso & Myneni, 2016). Important considerations for nurses to have their voices heard are the extent to which different perspectives are represented in technologies. Such steps can facilitate the accurate measurement and representation of nursing activities and patient-centred care (Tai-Seale et al., 2014) as well as inform decisions about care quality (Kelley, Brandon, & Docherty, 2011).

For example, some rural and remote communities have access to technologies such as telehealth. This virtual environment allows for health education, such as prenatal teaching or online support programs for individuals with chronic illnesses. Rural- and remote-based CHNs need to become familiar with using e-health initiatives in order to positively impact their clients' health (Nagel & Penner, 2016) and for their own continuing professional education (Kulig et al., 2015).

Inequity, Water Quality, and Food Insecurity

The Canadian Nurses Association (CNA) recently updated a position statement on the role of nurses in addressing indoor and outdoor environments as linked to the determinants of health (CNA, 2017). The CNA supports nurses to assess community hazards, advocate for change, engage in interdisciplinary collaboration to address hazards, decrease exposure, and reduce harm to people and the environment. One of the most basic needs for human health is clean drinkable water. However, near the end of 2015, "there were 138 Drinking Water Advisories (DWA) in effect in 94 FN communities across Canada, excluding British Columbia" (Bradford, Bharadwaj, Okpalauwaekwe, & Waldner, 2016). Although DWAs occur in non-Indigenous communities, they are typically treated as emergencies and resolved in a matter of days. Conversely, many FN communities have been on DWA for years—sometimes decades.

Bradford and colleagues (Bradford et al., 2016) conducted a scoping review of the literature surrounding water quality and effect on the health status of Indigenous people. The research identified concerns related to government policies and data collection as barriers to addressing safe water resources in Northern and isolated communities. The most often cited health concerns in the literature were gastrointestinal illnesses and skin problems. From the perspective of health challenges, researchers need to develop collaborations with health care providers to add to the evidence linking water quality and health concerns. Researchers are also encouraged to approach investigations about water quality from a decolonized view, considering humankind's relationship and responsibility to water as more than a physical requirement for health. Traditionally, women are the caretakers of the water. Tending to this role is inclusive of a spiritual connection to all life.

Water quality and food insecurity are two inter-related inequities linked to the health of rural and remote populations. A discussion paper by Food Secure Canada (2013) presents issues for rural and remote communities in securing local access to nutritious food for health. Of concern for rural communities is the higher cost of food the farther communities are located from larger urban centres, where the cost of food includes transportation to the community, and poverty limits food choices to less expensive and often less nutritious options. Rural communities may be more agriculture-based than remote communities, although the production of food products from agricultural sources is mostly centred in urban areas that can support food production and distribution businesses. Isolated communities, particularly in the North, face food insecurity due to exorbitant transportation costs to bring in fresh foods, potentiating a dependence on processed foods known to be obesogenic and nutrient-lacking.

In many remote Indigenous communities, hunting and fishing increase the self-sufficiency of access to food (Food Secure Canada, 2013). There has been a movement toward the development of food products from traditional fish and game sources in remote communities, but regulatory policies for food packaging and inspection hinder innovation and economic development. Further, the lack of cost-effective transportation sources to get Northern packaged foods to market impacts the cost to urban consumers and affects the sustainability of reciprocal food distribution from remote to rural and urban markets. Until the issues related to food costs, transportation, and production are addressed, little change will occur related to food security for rural and remote communities.

YES, BUT WHY?

Pregnancy and the Rural and Remote Family Unit

What?

For decades, federal and provincial health policies have required expectant mothers to travel long distances to urban communities to deliver their babies (Health Canada, 2017). The policies support the provision of a high level of specialized care and safety for both mother and child during delivery, as few surgical and anesthesia resources are available in remote communities to support cesarean births. Given the unpredictable nature of deliveries, all rural and remote expectant mothers are requested to travel to be near a medical centre with obstetrical services at 38 weeks gestation.

In remote areas of the country, prenatal and postnatal care is provided by local family physicians, nurse practitioners, midwives, and CHNs. Although the level of care may be comparable to that provided in urban settings, access to ultrasound and specialty obstetrical services requires travel to a larger centre. Telehealth technologies are beginning to address local access to prenatal and postnatal care, specialist consultations, and diagnostic ultrasounds in remote communities, decreasing some of the need for travel.

So What?

The challenge for rural and remote Indigenous and non-Indigenous people has been the disruption to family caused by travel to a large urban centre at the end of a pregnancy for delivery. The CIHI (2013) identified that from 2008–2012, 67% of expectant rural mothers delivered their children in urban hospitals. The frequency of births in hospitals by rural mothers was highest in Nunavut (where there are no large urban care facilities), Saskatchewan, Manitoba, and Newfoundland (where there are few northern facilities equipped for obstetrical care). Of the rural deliveries in hospitals, 65.8% were vaginal births and 25.6% were C-sections, compared to 60.8% and 28.6% for urban women (CIHI, 2013).

There is some evidence that travel of over two hours to a rural or urban hospital for delivery has effects on birth outcomes (CIHI, 2013; Grybowski, Stoll, & Komelsen, 2011). Moreover, these studies reported that increasing travel time had negative emotional and financial consequences related to time off work, travel expenses, and separation from family (Komelsen, Stoll, & Gyrbowski, 2011). The stress caused by the travel over 100 kilometres was likely to be rated as moderate to severe.

Policies for expectant Northern and remote Indigenous mothers changed in 2017 to allow for a medical escort (Health Canada, 2018). Previous to this time, maternal travel to urban centres most often did not include a support person. In high-risk pregnancies, women are most often transported to large urban communities that are commonly a far distance from their home community. In low-risk pregnancies, women might be able to deliver in a rural community hospital, presumably closer to home. The choice of facility appears reasonable given the potential for risk to the woman and her unborn child, and the ability to have a companion for travel should decrease the emotional stress on the expectant mother. The lack of access to local obstetrical care represents a form of colonialism and breaches the rights of Indigenous women.

Now What?

Although federal policies pertaining to escorted travel will persist, the development of birthing centres in the Canadian North holds promise for expectant mothers to share the birth of their children with their significant other and family members. There has been ongoing lobbying for expanding the development of birthing centres in rural and remote areas, which may help to address the stress that happens with travel to large urban centres and post-colonial traditions and celebrations around childbirth and maintaining the family unit. The recent change to include escorted travel for an expectant mother is an example of inequitable health policies and hopefully prompts a review of other health services policies that effect all people in remote and rural locations across the country.

Standards of Practice Fulfilled

#1 Health Promotion
 – Considers the determinants of health, the social and political context, and systemic structures in collaboration with the client to determine action

#6 Health Equity
 – Advocates for healthy public policy and social justice by participating in legislative and policy-making activities that influence determinants of health and access to services (Community Health Nurses of Canada [CHNC], 2019, revised).

CHNs IN RURAL AND REMOTE COMMUNITIES

As a cornerstone of Canada's health care system, primary health care is the focus of intensive renewal efforts (Kates et al., 2012). In rural and remote communities, CHNs provide primary care services or work as part of a team providing primary health care. The roles and responsibilities of CHNs in primary health care vary based on the needs and services of the community (MacLeod et al., 2008) as well as the complexity of the community setting and surrounding area.

Regardless of practice setting, all rural and remote CHNs are faced with addressing issues in clinical practice, leadership, and the work environment. Rural and remote nursing practice is shaped by the context of communities, with their limited transportation, communications, and other resources. Within small communities, CHNs provide care to clients who also may be friends and neighbours with a wide range of conditions. Rural nurses experience practice as being multifaceted and complex, with considerable decision-making challenges and little backup (MacLeod et al., 2008). Rural and remote practice demands significant knowledge and skills to be responsive to community needs (CARRN, 2008). For

example, CHNs in northern British Columbia found they could be more responsive to high-risk and vulnerable families when they focused on creating working relationships with families instead of on "home visiting" protocols, because their services to families happened in many locations in the community, including the grocery store (Moules, MacLeod, Hanlon, & Thirsk, 2009).

Innovations that reflect changes to rural and remote nursing roles, settings, and modes of practice are of particular interest as health systems transition toward a primary care model of service provision and delivery (Banner, MacLeod, & Johnston, 2010). It is important to be aware of successful examples of health care innovation in these settings (Wakerman & Humphreys, 2011). For example, recognizing collaboration between rural and remote stakeholders supports the spread of innovation and represents a step forward in improving the health of rural and remote populations (Canadian Foundation for Healthcare Improvement, 2013).

CHNs in rural and remote settings may practise in acute, chronic, tertiary, mental health, or occupational health care. The CHN role often identified with nursing practice in Northern communities blends specialized knowledge for performing activities related to public health, home care, emergency care, palliative care, and management of episodic and chronic conditions. Given the breadth of CHN practice, these nurses have the capacity to effectively collaborate and lead interprofessional teams to improve health outcomes for rural and remote populations (Canadian Health Services Research Foundation, 2012).

Nursing practice, as part of an interprofessional primary-care team, may appear very different from the practice of urban-based teams. A rural or remote team may include only one or two CHNs and a community health worker (Mills et al., 2010) collaborating with a nurse practitioner, physician, or itinerant specialist (e.g., dentists, pediatricians) via telephone, telehealth, or other electronic means. In urban settings, all team members typically can interact daily in a face-to-face manner. As such, the scope, autonomy, and tools for practice of rural or remote CHNs may go beyond that of an urban colleague, depending on the focus of the team and the client's health concerns.

The vast physical distances that can separate team members necessitate deliberate consideration for professional and collegial communication in order to ensure interprofessional collaboration (Bainbridge, Nasmith, Orchard, & Wood, 2010) and to provide high-quality comprehensive primary-care services. Telehealth is one technology that has been successfully implemented in some locations and is used to complement primary-care services. In Takla Landing, a remote Indigenous community in northern British Columbia, the CHNs are able to use telehealth to consult with off-site health care providers (Mah, 2013) supporting patients to optimize management of acute and chronic health conditions without leaving their community; this reduces the stress experienced by patients and families while also saving patients and the health care system money. Telehealth initiatives currently offer several medical specialties in Takla Landing, including general surgery, infectious disease, dermatology, and addictions. CHNs manage and support the patient on-site, and patients receive the same specialist care as their urban counterparts.

Technologies such as telehealth are increasingly considered as a resource to improve access and comprehensiveness of care (Gibson et al., 2011; Taylor, Stone, & Huijbregts, 2012), although not yet operationalized in all rural and remote communities. Rural and remote CHNs often work in settings of chronic resource shortages of equipment, other providers, and services (Forbes & Edge, 2009; Kulig et al., 2008). Given that CHNs are front-line providers working at significant distances from tertiary-care settings, rural and remote nursing practice requires a broad knowledge base (Jackman, Myrick, & Yonge, 2012) and advanced educational preparation (Cant, Birks, Porter, Jacob, & Cooper, 2011). In an analysis of responses from a national nursing survey, the most common reason nurses reported intent to leave their position was to undertake further nursing education (Stewart et al., 2011).

Rural and remote CHNs working in primary care assume multiple roles that may not be captured by a formal job description (Mitton, Dionne, Masacci, Wong, & Law, 2011). Program planning and evaluation, well-woman clinics and immunization clinics, quality-assurance initiatives such as practice audits, and extended periods of time

on call are all activities that a rural- and remote-area nurse may be expected to perform in addition to being competent in direct patient care, illness prevention, health promotion, and emergency care. The demands of providing primary care in rural and remote communities are challenging, and turnover rates can be high in some circumstances (Tarlier, Johnson, Browne, & Sheps, 2013). A rural or remote CHN's intent to leave a position is influenced by interrelated individual, workplace, and community factors (Stewart et al., 2011). Increasingly, and particularly in remote communities, primary care is provided by relief nurses who stay only short periods of time in the communities (Minore et al., 2005). When primary health care service provision is fragmented, continuity of care and health outcomes may worsen for populations already enduring significant health disparities (Tarlier et al., 2013).

Rural and remote CHNs are resourceful and innovative. Rural health care environments may be open to trying things differently (CFHI, 2013), and CHNs can enjoy and take pride in accepting the challenge of providing best practices in rural and remote communities. Rural and remote CHNs providing

---

CASE STUDY

The Gibbons family lives on their family farm 90 kilometres east of a small city (population 68 000). After completing high school, Nancy and John were married in the Anglican church. Nancy is now 45, and John is 46. Nancy has been an active mother, raising their three sons while also volunteering in the community. John and his son Peter work on the farm together, which has been in the family for two generations. The two older sons, Jack and Ian, live and work in cities that are three to five hours from the family farm. Both Jack and Ian are married and have children. Their jobs, family life, and other responsibilities mean that they are not able to visit the farm very often.

Nancy has had an uneventful health history that includes regular physical examinations, three normal pregnancies, and a hysterectomy. From a health perspective, she was expecting to enjoy retirement with her husband and their sons, daughters-in-law, and grandchildren. About a year ago, Nancy began to feel "unwell." She was tired, shaky, and having difficulties sleeping. Four months ago, tests revealed that she had amyotrophic lateral sclerosis (ALS), a terminal condition for which there is no cure.

She was referred to home care for assessment, but John refused to have them in the home and instead has provided all of Nancy's care. The ALS Society was notified by home care about Nancy's diagnosis and has called to offer visits and assist in any way possible. John would agree only after Peter convinced his mother and father that it could be helpful. While the ALS Society was at the home, John expressed his frustration at his wife's deteriorating condition and related he was unsure if he could continue providing care by himself. Nancy is now dependent upon John to bathe

her, assist her with feeding, and transfer her to the toilet. She is also frequently in pain and, due to the muscle weakness, is at risk for falls. Depression has set in, and Nancy has said that "life is not worth living." At the same time, she wants to die peacefully at the farm and does not want to be moved into the city hospital. John is increasingly upset about his wife's condition and appears overwhelmed and bewildered; he realizes that he needs support to continue to care for Nancy in their home.

It takes some time but John finally agrees to have a home care nurse return, do another assessment, and set up equipment resources such as oxygen and personal care aides on a routine basis. The home care nurse also refers the family to the palliative care nurse. Peter calls his brothers and asks that they come home to visit their mother as soon as possible.

Discussion Questions

1. What are the challenges that arise for CHNs in addressing the mental health needs and supports for this family?

2. Identify three factors related to living in a rural setting that provide challenges in the delivery of nursing care for Nancy Gibbons. Identify how a home care nurse could address these factors.

3. Identify three rural community resources that could provide assistance to the Gibbons family. Identify how a palliative care nurse could incorporate these factors into a care plan for Nancy.

Source: This case study is a modified version from the Nursing Education in Southern Alberta curriculum used by the collaborative partners, the University of Lethbridge, and Lethbridge College.

primary care services must be adaptable, perseverant, critical thinkers who are willing to listen and learn (Martin-Misener et al., 2008).

In the first national study of rural and remote nursing practice in Canada, almost all nurses identified issues related to nursing leadership (MacLeod et al., 2008). Issues included finding ways of working through conflicting priorities, coping with having leaders at a distance, and creating support networks. Leadership was more effective when leaders set up possibilities for quality practice, even in situations of few resources. When leaders planned for the realities of rural and remote practice, CHNs felt supported. For nursing leaders, providing the appropriate support at a distance was a challenge; for CHNs, seeking and accepting that support was equally challenging. Both nursing managers and CHNs needed to work creatively within organizations that did not always understand the realities of their practice.

Creating quality work environments in rural and remote nursing practice settings is particularly challenging. A central challenge is that many nurses in rural and remote settings work alone much of the time (Andrews et al., 2005). A strategy for developing quality work environments in rural or remote CHN practice includes developing consistent expectations and approaches among managers and nurses to address practice issues at the site level. This includes relevant rural and remote practice standards; policies and practices that support rural CHNs' scope of practice; practice-driven, rural- and remote-focused nursing education programs; rural and remote reality-based preceptorship and mentorship programs; and the development of sustained processes for direct rural and remote nursing involvement in local and regional planning (Martin-Misener et al., 2008; Stewart et al., 2011).

RURAL AND REMOTE COMMUNITY HEALTH NURSING PRACTICE

Analyses of the Nurses Database reveal that there were 28 799 RNs working in rural and remote Canada in 2010 (Pitblado et al., 2013). Of those rural and remote RNs, 22.9%, worked in community settings, most were women and working full time. Nurse-to-population ratios vary by region, but on average there were half as many nurses per 100 000 people in rural and remote Canada compared to urban Canada. There is also an east-to-west trend, with higher nurse-to-population ratios in eastern Canada. Rural and remote RNs were found to have a lower level of education at entry to practice than their urban counterparts, but there has been a significant positive change in the percentage of rural and remote RNs with a baccalaureate degree: 32.5% of rural and remote RNs had achieved a baccalaureate degree as their highest level of education by 2010, compared to 18.5% in 2003 (Pitblado et al., 2013). Despite this improvement, limited access to continuing nursing education remains a concern for rural- and remote-living RNs.

CANADIAN RESEARCH 24.1

Experiences of Disasters among Rural and Remote Nurses in Canada. (Kulig et al., 2017) Copyright © 2017 by Elsevier Ltd. Used by permission of Elsevier Ltd. doi: 10.1016/j.aenj.2017.04.003.

There has been a notable rise in disasters around the globe, highlighting the role of rural and remote CHNs in disaster mitigation, response, and recovery. This study explored the experiences of rural- and remote-area nurses in responding to disaster events in their communities. The analysis of the data from this study was discussed within each of the World Health Organization/International Council of Nurses' disaster nursing competency frameworks to emphasize the relevance for rural and remote nursing practice and education. The findings indicated that nurses between 50–59 years of age working in a remote community, and having worked in more than four rural or remote communities, were more likely to have assisted with a disaster in the previous five years. The most common types of disasters were reported as floods, wildfires, and other weather events.

Rural and remote nurses' intimate knowledge of their communities makes them ideal members of disaster planning teams as well as advocates for their rural communities during all phases of the disaster. One important challenge for nurses who work in small communities is the provision of care to people who may be known to them personally, and their personal and professional recovery needs. Preparation of nursing students to act in this role and ongoing training for rural and remote nurses are essential to assist communities to recover after traumatic events.

Discussion Questions

1. What initiatives can nursing organizations take to support nurses who work in rural and remote settings?

2. What is the responsibility of health regions in preparing rural- and remote-area nurses to address disasters?

3. Given the geographic isolation of many rural- and remote-area nurses, what is the best way to ensure ongoing training in disaster preparation and recovery?

A DAY IN THE LIFE

Although all graduates of nursing programs in Canada are prepared for generalist practice, working in rural and remote communities stretches the meaning of being a generalist nurse. The generalist practice of a rural and remote CHN differs by setting and across regions in Canada. The following instances of "a day in the life" of CHNs in various settings are meant to illustrate the diversity in nursing practice in rural, remote, and isolated communities. The descriptions that follow combine elements of practice and do not represent a particular CHN in a specific location.

Rural

Sandra lives on a farm in rural British Columbia. She is married with two school-age children. Her husband manages their mixed-farming operation while Sandra leaves home each day and commutes 50 kilometres to the next community, where she is employed full-time as a home care nurse. For Sandra, the only typical part of her day is leaving home and travelling to work. The commute for Sandra to begin her workday changes depending on weather and road conditions. The first 20 kilometres are a gravel road that leads to the highway, which makes driving a challenge on stormy winter mornings.

Sandra's workday begins at her office, planning her route to client homes within and outside of the small town. Like her urban colleagues, Sandra provides wound-care and chronic-care services to her clients. Unlike her urban colleagues, she knows most of her clients and their families outside the context of her job, even though they are in the next community, as this is where her family also does their shopping and her children go to school. Sandra finds that knowing her clients well is sometimes positive. It helps her to focus quickly on what might be affecting their quality of life. It also might be negative when they withhold information because they are concerned about potential breaches of confidentiality due to Sandra's dual role as nurse and neighbour. This embeddedness in the community adds to Sandra's ethical responsibility for confidentiality.

Remote

CHNs in remote and isolated communities often practise in clinics, but the distance from other services may expand the scope of practice. Daniel, a community health nurse practitioner (NP) working in a northern Ontario nursing station, begins his day walking down the hall from his apartment to the attached clinic. The close proximity of work and home can be a benefit to clients, as they know Daniel is there, and they feel free to come to the clinic at any time of day for treatment. But it can be a challenge for nurses, as there is little separation between work and home life, and it can pose an ethical issue regarding professional boundaries. Daniel also finds that it can be difficult living in accommodations attached to his workplace, as he lives and works with his co-workers over a long period of time.

The typical day for Daniel, as an NP in a remote community, includes primary-care and health-promotion activities. On this typical day, Daniel finds himself applying primary prevention through immunizing infants, children, and adults. Secondary prevention occurs through collecting, ordering, and reviewing client laboratory results; assessing and treating common medical conditions; and monitoring and referring chronic care and prenatal clients. Tertiary prevention occurs through caring for wounds and suturing lacerations. In remote communities, an NP like Daniel might also provide care to clients in emergency situations, such as status epilepticus or trauma from a motor vehicle collision.

Isolated

Carol works in the far North. Her practice is much the same as Daniel's in her remote setting. Carol may have more technologies available to her that help to bridge the gap between her location and the urban health centre that she accesses for client consultations or emergency treatment supports. Canadian communities that might be considered more isolated include small-island Northern and Arctic communities where road access is not available and planes arrive infrequently.

A typical day for Carol may involve taking a picture of a wound and emailing the picture to a dermatologist in the south for assessment and treatment advice. She offers a chronic-care clinic in the afternoon that includes connecting via telehealth to a specialist for client follow-up appointments. In the evening when a client comes in with a severe traumatic injury, Carol connects with ER physicians over telehealth. They support Carol, in real time, with assessment and treatment prior to air ambulance personnel arriving and transporting the client to a larger facility.

Although nursing practice in the previous descriptions use the word *typical*, most CHNs practising in these settings will suggest that although there are common elements in their day, little is typical. All CHNs in these settings experience a high demand for ongoing flexibility and openness to changes in routine. The attraction to rural practice for CHNs like Sandra, Daniel, and Carol includes the challenging nature of the work and the chance to live and work in a rural community setting that is or may become their home.

HEALTH POLICIES AND SUPPORT FOR CHN PRACTICE

Rural and remote CHNs in Canada have been described as a marginalized group within health care and are often excluded from key policy decisions (Jackman et al., 2010). Most policies in Canada, with health policies being no exception, are based on an urban perspective with little consideration of their applicability in rural and remote environments. To best address the health care needs of rural and remote patients, nurses have argued that they are best situated to advocate as they have the greatest contact with patients (Cole, Wellard, & Mummery, 2014). Although well-intentioned, such perspectives may place nurses in a paternalistic role that compromises patients' autonomous abilities to make decisions. Others have argued that there is a "thin line" between advocacy and paternalism for nurses and other health professionals. A critical analysis of the literature by Kalaitzidis and Jewel (2015) highlighted that advocacy was an essential part of the nurse's professional role, but there is limited consensus on how to implement advocacy. More specifically for nurses working in rural and remote communities, advocacy is informed by adapting nurses' practice to the local contexts, engaging in personal and relational actions that ensure safety, and addressing systemic health inequities (MacKinnon & Moffitt, 2014).

The following key issues need to be addressed to promote the CHN's involvement in rural and remote health policies.

- Federal and provincial nursing associations need to ensure the profession is meeting responsibilities and acknowledging our colonial history, and work to address the Truth and Reconciliation Commission's calls to action.
- Ongoing research supports for rural remote nursing research chairs in Canada continue to address the unique situations experienced by rural and remote residents, particularly around access to care.
- Few CHNs are educationally prepared for work in the policy arena, and although nurse educators include information about health policy in curriculum, CHNs need to be encouraged to embrace the strength of their political voice.
- Relevant information about the nature of rural, remote, and Indigenous communities, including the number and location of residents and their health issues, is not readily available to inform health policy and health human resource decisions.
- The perspectives of rural, remote, and Indigenous residents and their involvement in setting policy and health service agendas, even at the local level, need to be acknowledged and respected as a key component of rural and remote community development.

CONCLUSION

This chapter focused on the health of rural and remote populations as well as the unique roles of the rural and remote CHN in Canada. Many diverse practice settings in rural and remote regions of Canada offer opportunities for a rewarding nursing practice. Rural nurses characterize their work as a wonderful opportunity to affect change by being deeply immersed in the community in order to see, feel, and know it. The requisite creativity required, as well as the autonomy, ability to enact all skills, and opportunity to work downstream, midstream, and upstream all in the same day, keep rural and remote CHNs in the field.

Research with rural and remote CHNs commonly reports high levels of work satisfaction and community engagement. Working in rural and remote communities that are diverse requires the application of principles associated with cultural safety and reflective practice. It is important for all CHNs to remember that rural and remote residents demonstrate resilience and connectedness to the land and history of their communities. These characteristics offset the management of unique challenges such as inequitable local access to health care services, advanced education, food and water security, and stable local employment.

In moving forward to address health care delivery and provision of nursing care, CHNs must critically evaluate, respond to, and become involved in research and policy development about health inequities that present as areas in need of change. It is important for all CHNs who work in rural, remote, and isolated communities to partner with diverse populations and to engage in the delivery of strong, culturally safe health care.

Although the integration of technologies into rural, remote, and isolated community care practices may increase access to services, tailoring services to meet the unique context and diversity of communities will require CHNs to become involved at local, provincial, and federal policy levels to effect positive changes that will be acceptable to local communities.

KEY TERMS

access to technologies (p. 448)
employment opportunities (p. 446)
food insecurity (p. 448)
isolated (p. 445)
Northern (p. 445)
remote (p. 445)
resource base (p. 445)
rural (p. 445)
social approaches (p. 445)
socioeconomic status (p. 446)
technical approaches (p. 445)
water quality (p. 446)

STUDY QUESTIONS

1. Identify what CHNs working in remote settings can do to generate information about the communities they work in.
2. Identify four concepts that would be discussed in a rural and remote nursing course.
3. Identify four challenges experienced by nurses working in a Northern community.
4. Maria is a 35-year-old Low German Mennonite woman who has just had her fifth child. She was diagnosed with gestational diabetes and requires follow-up to monitor her health. How would you apply the principles of cultural safety in the care of Maria?
5. Timothy has been working as a public health nurse in an Indigenous community for the past four years. Over a year ago the community experienced the loss of several family members in a house fire. Identify the levels of prevention and specific strategies that Timothy can address in collaboration with community members to deal with the loss and prevent such tragedies in the future.

INDIVIDUAL CRITICAL-THINKING EXERCISES

1. Examine the provincial or territorial nursing standards related to professional boundaries, and identify three challenges in the provision of care in rural and remote communities. As a professional RN, how would you address the challenges without jeopardizing ethical standards and professional boundaries?
2. You work in a public health office in a large agricultural area that includes established farm families and feedlot operators. Over the past few years, there has been an increase in migrant farm workers from Mexico that has added to the diverse mix of the area, which includes conservative

religious groups who also work in the agricultural industry. Locating and communicating with these groups has become increasingly challenging, and ensuring routine public health programs such as immunizations has become even more difficult due to varied beliefs and practices. What are three barriers that need to be addressed? Who can you turn to for guidance and support? What actions on your part might facilitate collaboration? What are short- and long-term goals in this situation?

3. You work in collaboration with a long-term care facility that has just developed a support group for rural families caring for a relative with dementia, which is most commonly caused by Alzheimer's disease. After the first six months of the service, only three family members have attended the group, even though you are sure that many others could benefit from the support. What issues could make families reluctant to participate in this service? In what ways can technology (e.g., Skype, telehealth) be used to facilitate participation?

GROUP CRITICAL-THINKING EXERCISES

1. You work part time as a CHN in a two-nurse office in a remote community. The other nurse works full time. You are both responsible for implementing the full range of public health programs. Because of the difficulty in finding casual replacements over the last two months, you deferred your vacation and have worked more than full time. You have just received a call that the full-time nurse has gone on sick leave. As your manager, who works 500 kilometres away, tells you this, she adds that the medical health officer has identified two tuberculosis cases in your community. Your manager asks you to work overtime again, and you are debating what your answer should be. As a group, identify the following:

   • Personal and professional concerns you would face in this situation

   • Dilemmas being faced by the public health administration

   • Potential impacts on client and community safety

   • Strategies, including ones that reflect interprofessional practice, to address the previous concerns

2. You are the new CHN in an outpost setting on a community-based Indigenous reserve. Two other nurses are stationed at the centre, but they are from the community and live with their spouses away from the station. You are the only nurse who works at the outpost accommodation. This particular community, with a population of 545, is fly-in only with interruptions of flight service due to inclement weather. As a group with your classmates, identify the following:

   • Priorities you would engage in as the new nurse

   • The process you would use to assess the community

   • How you would develop a relationship with the other nurses and community residents

3. You have been a home care nurse working in several eastern coastal communities for five years. It is a job you love mostly because of the people you care for and the diversity within your everyday work. You are currently mentoring an undergraduate nursing student from an urban-based nursing program. The student has made it clear that it was not her choice to come to a rural area or to do home care. As a group, identify how you will address the student's issues in a productive manner. Identify ways in which you can encourage the student to see the benefits of her practicum experience in rural communities.

REFERENCES

Andrews, M. E., Stewart, N. J., Pitblado, J. R., Morgan, D. G., Forbes, D., & D'Arcy, C. (2005). Registered nurses working alone in rural and remote Canada. *Canadian Journal of Nursing Research, 37*(1), 14–33.

Association of Workers' Compensation Boards of Canada. (2017). *2016 lost time claims in Canada.* Toronto, ON: Author. Retrieved from http://awcbc.org/?page_id=14

Bainbridge, L., Nasmith, L., Orchard, C., & Wood, V. (2010). Competencies for interprofessional collaboration. *Journal of Physical Therapy Education, 24*(1), 6–11.

Banner, D., MacLeod, M. L. P., & Johnston, S. (2010). Role transition in rural and remote primary health care nursing: A scoping literature review. *Canadian Journal of Nursing Research, 42*(4), 40–57.

Barnabe, C., Jones, A., Bernatsky, S., Peschken, C., Voaklander, D., Homik, J., . . . Hemmelgarn, B. (2017). Inflammatory arthritis prevalence and health services use in First Nations and non-First Nations populations of Alberta, Canada. *Arthritis Care & Research, 69*(4), 467–474.

Bradford, L. E. A., Bharadwaj, L. A., Okpalauwaekwe, U., & Waldner, C. L. (2016). Drinking water quality in Indigenous communities in Canada and health outcomes: A scoping review. *International Journal of Circumpolar Health, 75*(1). Retrieved from https://www.ncbi.nlm.nih.gov/pmc/articles/PMC4967713/pdf/IJCH-75-32336.pdf

Canadian Agricultural Injury Reporting. (2016). *Canadian agricultural injury reporting: Agriculture-related fatalities in Canada.* Retrieved from http://www.cair-sbac.ca

Canadian Association of Rural and Remote Nurses (CARRN). (2008). *Rural and remote nursing practice parameters: Discussion document.* Unpublished document: Author.

Canadian Foundation for Healthcare Improvement. (2013). *Northern, rural and remote pan-provincial collaboration.* Ottawa, ON: Author. Retrieved from http://www.cfhi-fcass.ca/WhatWeDo/Collaborations/NorthernRuralRemote.aspx

Canadian Health Services Research Foundation. (2012). *Evidence synthesis for the effectiveness of interprofessional teams in primary care.* Ottawa, ON: Author.

Canadian Institute for Health Information (CIHI). (2006). *How healthy are rural Canadians? An assessment of their health status and health determinants.* Ottawa, ON: Author.

Canadian Institute for Health Information (CIHI). (2013). *Hospital births in Canada: A focus on women living in rural and remote areas.* Ottawa, ON: Author.

Canadian Nurses Association (CNA), (2014). *Aboriginal health nursing and Aboriginal health: Charting policy direction for nursing in Canada*. Ottawa, ON: Author.

Canadian Nurses Association (CNA), (2017). *Nurses and environmental health: A position statement*. Ottawa, ON: Author.

Canadian Radio-television and Communications Commission. (2017). *Closing the broadband gap*. Retrieved from https://crtc.gc.ca/eng/internet/internet.htm

Cant, R., Birks, M., Porter, J., Jacob, E., & Cooper, S. (2011). Developing advanced rural nursing practice: A whole new scope of responsibility. *Collegian: Journal of the Royal College of Nursing Australia, 18*(4), 177–182. doi:10.1016/j.colegn.2011.08.001

Cole, C., Wellard, S., & Mummery, J. (2014). Problematising autonomy and advocacy in nursing. *Nursing Ethics, 21*(5), 576–582.

Community Health Nurses of Canada. (2019, revised). *Canadian community health nursing: Professional practice model & standards of practice*. Ottawa, ON: Author.

Demers, P. (2011). Disease and injury patterns: Lumber industry. In P. Demers & K. Teschke, (Eds.), *Encyclopedia of Occupational Health and Safety*. Geneva, CH: International Labor Organization.

DesMeules, M., Pong, R. W., Guernsey, J. R., Want, F., Luo, W., & Dressler, M. P. (2012). Rural health status and determinants in Canada. In J. Kulig & A. M. Williams, (Eds.). *Health in rural Canada* (pp. 23–43). Vancouver, BC: UBC Press.

DesMeules, M., Pong, R., Lagacé, C., Heng, D., Manuel, D., Pitblado, R. J., & Koren, I. (2006). *How healthy are rural Canadians? An assessment of their health status and health determinants*. Ottawa, ON: Canadian Population Initiative, Canadian Institute for Health Information.

du Plessis, V., Beshiri, R., & Bollman, R. (2001). Definitions of rural. *Rural and Small Town Analysis Bulletin, 3*(3), 1–17. #21-006-XIE. Ottawa, ON: Statistics Canada. Available at http://statcan.gc.ca

Food Secure Canada. (2013). *Food sovereignty in rural and remote communities*. Discussion paper retrieved from https://foodsecurecanada.org/resources-news/newsletters/2-food-sovereignty-rural-and-remote-communities

Forbes, D. A., & Edge, D. S. (2009). Canadian home care policy and practice in rural and remote settings: Challenges and solutions. *Journal of Agromedicine, 14*(2), 119–124. doi:10.1080/10599240902724135

Fraser Basin Council. (2012). *Identifying health concerns relating to oil and gas development in northeastern BC*. Victoria, BC: BC Ministry of Health.

Gessert, C., Waring, S., Bailey-Davis, L., Conway, P., Roberts, M., & VanWormer, J. (2015). Rural definition of health: A systematic review. *BMC Public Health, 15*, 378–392.

Gibson, K., Coulson, H., Miles, R., Kakekakekung, C., Daniels, E., & O'Donnell, S. (2011). Conversations on telemental health: Listening to remote and rural First Nations communities. *Rural and Remote Health, 11*. Retrieved from http://www.rrh.org.au/publishedarticles/article_print_1656.pdf

Grybowski, S., Stoll, K., & Komelsen, J. (2011). Is rural maternity care sustainable without general practitioner surgeons? *Canadian Journal of Rural Medicine, 11*(3), 218–220.

Harbison, J., Coughlan, S., Karabanow, J., & VanderPlaat, M. (2005). A clash of cultures: Rural values and service delivery to mistreated and neglected older people in Eastern Canada. *Practice: Social Work in Action, 17*(4), 229–246. doi:10.1080/09503150500425091

Health Canada. (2005). *Ten years of health transfer First Nation and Inuit control*. First Nations and Inuit Health Branch. Adapted and reproduced with permission from the Minister of Health, 2018.

Health Canada. (2017, November). *Medical transportation benefits information*. Retrieved from https://www.canada.ca/en/health-canada/services/first-nations-inuit-health/non-insured-health-benefits/benefits-information/medical-transportation-benefits-information-first-nations-inuit-health.html

Health Canada. (2018, January). *Non-Insured Health Benefits (NIHB) Medical transportation policy framework (interim)*. Retrieved from https://www.canada.ca/en/health-canada/services/first-nations-inuit-health/reports-publications/non-insured-health-benefits/non-insured-health-benefits-nihb-medical-transportation-policy-framework-july-2005-first-nations-inuit-health.html

Jackman, D., Myrick, F., & Yonge, O. J. (2012). Rural nursing in Canada: A voice unheard. *Online Journal of Rural Nursing and Health Care, 10*(1), 60–69.

Kalaitzidis, E., & Jewel, P. (2014). The concept of advocacy in nursing: A critical analysis. *Health Care Management, 34*(3), 308–315.

Kates, N., Hutchison, B., O'Brien, P., Fraser, B., Wheeler, S., & Chapman, C. (2012). Framework for advancing improvement in primary care. *Healthcare Papers, 12*(2), 8–21.

Kelley, T., Brandon, D., & Docherty, S. (2011). Electronic nursing documentation as a strategy to improve quality of patient care. *Journal of Nursing Scholarship, 43*(2), 154–162.

Komelsen, J., Stoll, K., & Gyrbowski, S. (2011). Stress and anxiety associated with lack of access to maternity services for rural parturient women. *Australian Journal of Rural Health, 19*(1), 9–14.

Kralj, B. (2001). Measuring "rurality" for purposes of healthcare planning: An empirical measure for Ontario. *Ontario Medical Review, 67*(9), 33–52.

Kulig, J., Andrews, M. E., Stewart, N., Pitblado, R., MacLeod, M., Bentham, D., & Smith, B. (2008). How do registered nurses define rurality? *Australian Journal of Rural Health, 16*(1), 28–32. doi:10.1111/j.1440-1584.2007.00947.x

Kulig, J., Kilpatrick, K., Moffitt, P., & Zimmer, L. (2015). Recruitment and retention in rural nursing: It's still an issue. *Journal of Nursing Leadership, 28*(2), 40–50.

Kulig, J., Penz, K., Karunanayake, C., MacLeod, M., Jahner, S., & Andrews, M. E. (2017). Experiences of disasters among rural and remote nurses in Canada. *Australasian Emergency Nursing Journal, 20*(2), 98–106. Copyright © 2017 by Elsevier Ltd. Used by permission of Elsevier Ltd. doi: 10.1016/j.aenj.2017.04.003.

Lavergne, M. R., & Kephart, G. (2012). Examining variations in health within rural Canada. *International Electronic Journal of Rural and Remote Health Research, Education, Practice and Policy, 12*(1), 1848. Retrieved from https://www.rrh.org.au/journal/article/1848

Leduc, E. (1997). Defining rurality: A general practice rurality index for Canada. *Canadian Journal of Rural Health, 2*(2), 125.

MacLeod, M. L. P., Martin-Misener, R., Banks, C., Morton, M., Vogt, C., & Bentham, D. (2008). "I'm a different kind of nurse": Advice from nurses in rural and remote Canada. *Canadian Journal of Nursing Leadership, 21*(3), 24–37.

MacLeod, M. L. P., Stewart, N. J., Kulig, J. C., Anguish, P., Andrews, M. E., Banner, D., . . . Zimmer, L. (2017). Nurses who work in rural and remote communities in Canada: A national survey. *Human Resources for Health, 15*, 34. DOI 10.1186/s12960-017-0209-0

MacKinnon, K., & Moffitt, P. (2014). Informed advocacy: Rural, remote, and northern nursing praxis. *Advances in Nursing Science, 37*(2), 161–173.

Mah, S. (2013). Telehealth in northern B.C. *Canadian Health Care Technology, 18*(7), 4.

Maltais, V. (2010). *Risk factors associated with farm injuries in Canada.* 2010 catalogue #21-601-MWE. From the Agriculture and Rural Working Paper Series. Retrieved from http://www.statcan.gc.ca/bsolc/olc-cel/olc-cel?catno=21-601-MWE&lang=eng

Mancuso, P. J., & Myneni, S. (2016). Empowered consumers and the health care team: A dynamic model of health informatics. *Advances in Nursing Science, 39*(1), 26–37.

Martin-Misener, R., MacLeod, M. L. P., Vogt, C., Morton, M., Banks, C., & Bentham, D. (2008). "There's rural and then there's rural": Advice from nurses providing health care in northern remote communities. *Canadian Journal of Nursing Leadership, 30*(7), 785–800.

McCall, J., & Pauly, B. (2012). Providing a safe place: Adopting a cultural safety perspective in the care of Aboriginal Women living with HIV/AIDS. *Canadian Journal of Nursing Research, 44*(2), 130–145.

Melvin, R. M., Bunt, A., Oduor, E., & Neustaedter, C. (2015). The effect of signal expense and dependability on family communication in rural and northern Canada. *Proceedings of the 33rd Annual ACM Conference on Human Factors in Computing Systems*, pp. 717–726. doi: 10.1145/2702123.2702301

Mills, J. E., Francis, K., Birks, M., Coyle, M., Henderson, S., & Jones, J. (2010). Registered nurses as members of interprofessional primary health care teams in remote or isolated areas of Queensland: Collaboration, communication and partnerships in practice. *Journal of Interprofessional Care, 24*(5), 587–596. doi:10.3109/13561821003624630

Ministry of Health (2016). *Health status of Canadians.* Ottawa, ON: Health Canada.

Minore, B., Boone, M., Katt, M., Kinch, P., Birch, S., & Mushquash, C. (2005). The effects of nursing turnover on continuity of care in isolated First Nation communities. *Canadian Journal of Nursing Research, 37*(1), 87–100.

Minore, B., Hill, M. E., Pugliese, I., & Gauld, T. (2008, February). *Rurality literature review.* Thunder Bay, ON: Centre for Rural and Northern Health Research, Lakehead University.

Mitton, C., Dionne, F., Masucci, L., Wong, S., & Law, S. (2011). Innovations in health service organization and delivery in northern and rural and remote regions: A review of the literature. *International Journal of Circumpolar Health, 70*(5), 460–472. doi:http://dx.doi.org/10.3402/ijch.v70i5.17859

Moazzami, B. (2015). *Strengthening rural Canada: fewer and older: Population and demographic challenges across rural Canada.* Toronto, ON: Essential Skills Ontario.

Moules, N. J., MacLeod, M. L. P., Hanlon, N., & Thirsk, L. (2009). "And then you'll see her in the grocery store": The working relationships of community health nurses and high priority families in rural and northern Canadian communities. *Journal of Pediatric Nursing, 25*(5), 327–334. doi:10.1016/j.pedn/2008.12.003

Nagel, D. A., & Penner, J. L. (2016). Conceptualizing telehealth in nursing practice: Advancing a conceptual model to fill a virtual gap. *Journal of Holistic Nursing, 34*(1), 91–104.

Northern Health. (2012). *Understanding the state of industrial camps in northern BC.* Prince George, BC: Northern Health.

Pitblado, J. R. (2005). So, what do we mean by "rural," "remote," and "northern"? *Canadian Journal of Nursing Research, 37*(1), 163–168.

Pitblado, R., Koren, I., MacLeod, M., Place, J., Kulig, J., & Stewart, N. (2013). *Characteristics and distribution of the regulated nursing workforce in rural and small town Canada, 2003 and 2010.* Prince George, BC: Author.

Polaschek, N. R. (1998). Cultural safety: A new concept in nursing people of different ethnicities. *Journal of Advanced Nursing, 27*, 452–457. doi:10.1046/j.1365–2648.1998.00547.x

Reading, J. (2015). Confronting the growing crisis of cardiovascular disease and heart health among Aboriginal peoples in Canada. *Canadian Journal of Cardiology, 31*, 1077–1080.

Rice, K., & Webster, F. (2017). Care interrupted: Poverty, immigration, and primary care in rural resource towns. *Social Science & Medicine, 191*, 77–83.

Smith, K., Humphreys, J., & Wilson, M. (2008). Addressing the health disadvantage of rural populations: How does epidemiological evidence inform rural health policies and research? *Australian Journal of Rural Health, 16*, 56–66.

Statistics Canada. (2017a). *Focus on geography series, 2016 census.* Statistics Canada Catalogue no. 98-404-X2016001. Ottawa, ON. Data products, 2016 Census.

Statistics Canada. (2017b). *A portrait of Canadian farms.* Retrieved from http://www.statcan.gc.ca/pub/11-627-m/11-627-m2017010-eng.htm

Status of Women. (2016). A profile of Canadian women in rural, remote and northern *communities.* Retrieved from http://www.swc-cfc.gc.ca/initiatives/wnc-fcn/profile-en.html

Stewart, N. J., D'Arcy, C., Kosteniuk, J., Andrews, M. E., Morgan, D., Forbes, D., . . . Pitblado, J. R. (2011). Moving on: Predictors of intention to leave among rural and remote RNs in Canada. *Journal of Rural Health, 27*(1), 103–113.

Tai-Seale, M., Wilson, C. J., Panattoni, L., Kohli, N., Stone, A., Hung, D., & Chung, S. (2014). Leveraging electronic health records to develop measurements for processes of care. *Health Services Research, 49*(2), 628–644.

Tarlier, D. S., Johnson, J. L., Browne, A. J., & Sheps, S. (2013). Maternal-infant health outcomes and nursing practice in a remote First Nations community in northern Canada. *Canadian Journal of Nursing Research, 45*(2), 76–100.

Taylor, D., Stone, S., & Huijbregts, M. (2012). Remote participants' experiences with a group-based stroke self-management program using videoconference technology. *Rural and Remote Health, 12, 1947*. Retrieved from http://www.rrh.org.au

Thomlinson, E., McDonagh, M., Baird Crooks, K., & Lees, M. (2004). Health beliefs of rural Canadians: Implications for rural practice. *Australian Journal of Rural Health*, 12, 258–263. doi:10.1111/j.1440-1854.2004.00627.x

Truth and Reconciliation Commission of Canada (2015). *Truth and Reconciliation Commission of Canada: Calls to Action*. Winnipeg, MB: Author.

Vandenberg, S., (2013). *Saying no to childhood immunization: Perceptions of mothers and health care professionals in southern Alberta*. Lethbridge, AB: University of Lethbridge.

Wakerman, J., & Humphreys, J. S. (2011). Sustainable primary health care services in rural and remote areas: Innovation and evidence. *Australian Journal of Rural Health, 19*(3), 118–124. doi: 10.1111/j.1440-1584.2010. 01180.x

ABOUT THE AUTHORS

Mary Ellen Labrecque, RN(NP), PhD (University of Saskatchewan), is Assistant Professor in the College of Nursing, University of Saskatchewan, and director of the Nurse Practitioner programs. She refers to her nursing experiences as "my adventures in nursing." Her background includes working in rural and urban acute care settings and in Northern outpost and mining settings in Manitoba, Saskatchewan, Alberta, NWT, and Nunavut. Research interests include rural and remote nursing, the delivery of primary health care that addresses the unique determinants of health for a population, and the integration of technologies into practice. Mary Ellen is a member of the study "The Nature of Nursing Practice in Rural and Remote Canada, II."

Kelley Kilpatrick, RN, PhD (McGill University), is Assistant Professor with the Faculty of Nursing at the Université de Montréal, a researcher with the Maisonneuve-Rosemont Hospital Research Centre, and an affiliate faculty member with the Canadian Centre for Advanced Practice Nursing Research. She completed a postdoctoral fellowship at McMaster University (2011). She also received junior researcher awards from the Fonds de recherche du Québec-Santé (2013–2021). Kelley's research interests include nurse practitioner and clinical nurse specialist roles, boundary work activities, perceptions of team effectiveness, acute and primary care, and the effects of health care service delivery on patients and families. She is a member of the study "The Nature of Nursing Practice in Rural and Remote Canada, II." Kelley has used different approaches, including mixed methods, case study, surveys, systematic reviews, and qualitative description, to answer her research questions.

Chronic Care, Long-Term Care, and Palliative Care

Lorraine Holtslander and Shelley Peacock

chapter 25

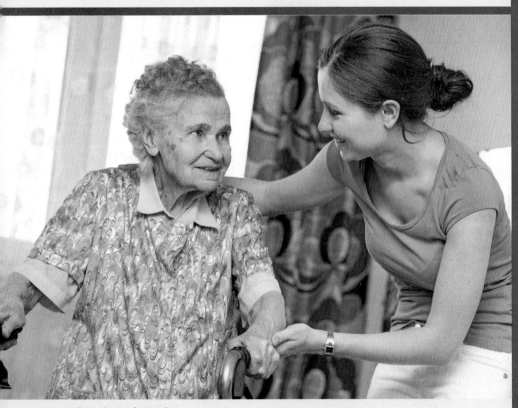

Source: Alexander Raths/Fotolia

INTRODUCTION

The number of Canadians living with and dying from chronic diseases is steadily increasing. Often negatively described as a "tsunami" of aging, this global phenomenon is expected to occur over the next 20 to 30 years. The role of the community health nurse (CHN) to promote health and strive for positive outcomes at all levels, including palliation, will be greatly impacted. Each year the number of deaths in Canada increases due to the country's growing and aging population. Cancer and heart disease were the two leading causes of death in Canada in 2015 (Statistics Canada, 2018a). The overall goal of this chapter is to introduce important considerations for the role of the CHN as they relate to providing excellent care for people living and dying with chronic conditions. An emphasis on supporting the essential role of the family caregiver is mandated by international and national guidelines within a continuum of care.

Chronic care, long-term care, and palliative care are interconnected and overlapping concepts. The relationship among the terms is often difficult to explain, and they are becoming even more linked in our current health care system. Although palliative

LEARNING OUTCOMES

After studying this chapter, you should be able to:

1. Assess the current trends in populations and diseases that will affect health care needs, resources and specific services needed in the community, while considering the impact of health inequities.

2. Describe the concept of chronic care and its relevance to the care of people living with one or more chronic conditions.

3. Through a quality-of-life lens, understand the role of long-term care homes in the community and their importance to the people who live and die in them.

4. Evaluate the goals, standards, and principles for providing palliative care in a community setting, including the need for continuity of care that extends into bereavement.

5. Explore incorporating a "palliative approach" to meet the needs of various populations with life-limiting conditions in the community.

6. Analyze the current situation of Canadian family caregivers, considering the inequities faced by various groups as well as the consequences, coping skills, and costs of caring.

care models and programs have historically focused on the cancer-care trajectory, current trends in the numbers of aging adults living longer with serious chronic illnesses and other life-limiting conditions have made it imperative that a new approach is sought. The concept of a "palliative approach," advocated by the Canadian Hospice Palliative Care Association (CHPCA) (2014), integrates the principles and values of palliative care into nursing care in any setting, such as acute care, residential, and home care (Sawatsky et al., 2017). The emphasis is on patient-centred care, symptom management, quality of life, and open communication with patients and families on appropriate goals of care in order to meet their needs in a holistic way. Interdisciplinary teams are essential, as is partnering with all care providers. Access and support for this approach across all health care sectors requires an even greater need for coordination, accessibility, and continuing care focused on prevention and health promotion.

Health inequities are of increasing concern, including among rural and remote populations; immigrant peoples; and First Nations, Inuit, and Metis communities, who are underrepresented in palliative care research (Williams, Gott et al., 2017). Diverse approaches involving community engagement are needed to understand and address local issues and priorities.

CHRONIC CARE: DEFINITION AND MODELS OF CARE

Many Canadians live with one or more chronic conditions that can lead to ill health, impaired functioning, and being unable to live independently (Hollander, Liu, & Chappell, 2009). It is challenging to define what is meant by chronic disease, and limiting classification of chronic health to individual diseases is inadequate, as indicated by the Canadian Academy of Health Sciences (2010). For our purposes, **chronic conditions** may be broadly defined as persistent conditions that require ongoing medical management over many years (Goodman, Posner, Huang, Parekh, & Koh, 2013). Common chronic conditions include arthritis, diabetes, cardiovascular disease, dementia, and chronic obstructive pulmonary disease, as well as infectious diseases such as HIV/AIDS and hepatitis. Each condition imposes different physical and psychological needs on patients and, as such, requires different health care and informal services. For example, 2.4 million Canadians over the age of 20 live with diabetes (Public Health Agency of Canada, 2011). In 2016, 564 000 Canadians lived with some form of dementia (Alzheimer Society of Canada, 2016). Patients with chronic conditions require and should have access to comprehensive, coordinated health care services from knowledgeable health care professionals; this is known as **chronic care**. Given the complexity of chronic care, it is important that a critical social theory lens be used to evaluate the delivery of health care services so that the intersection of variables (i.e., societal structures such as socioeconomic status) be considered in order to address oppressive conditions that exist within health care systems.

Advances in medicine and the aging population have resulted in an increase in the prevalence of chronic conditions. Many Canadians lead normal lives despite having a chronic condition; others experience considerable disruption due to more complex or multiple conditions that may be sometimes manageable and other times acute. Although chronic conditions exist across all stages of life, the majority occur in adults older than 65. It is important to note that despite the perception that as an individual ages, his or her health declines, as many as 50% of older adults up to the age of 85 years indicate they are in good health (Statistics Canada, 2011). Patients living with chronic conditions have diverse experiences, and all require care and support from health care and informal systems (CAHS, 2010; Goodman et al., 2013). Chronic care must address how chronic conditions are managed in the community to improve patient outcomes and quality of life (Coleman, Austin, Brach, & Wagner, 2009). Further, chronic care must address and consider the sociopolitical conditions that influence how this important care is delivered.

All over the world, countries are recognizing the need for a comprehensive approach to the provision of appropriate care for patients with chronic conditions (CAHS, 2010). This is challenging because, in general, health care is attuned to curing and managing acute-care illnesses. To manage chronic conditions or illnesses requires a shift in perspective to emphasize *care*, particularly with the needs and perspective of the client at the forefront, rather than the disease being the focus. This means a move away from an ambulatory visit to an individual family physician who assesses and evaluates the needs of a passive client and toward a **comprehensive care model** made up of an interprofessional team that engages with an informed, activated client to arrive at appropriate clinical outcomes marked by client satisfaction (Bowen et al., 2010). It is the client who is at the centre of the comprehensive care model and as such should be considered in light of what is important to that individual and their values and beliefs about health care.

Integrated comprehensive care models that have their foundation in a population-oriented primary-care approach are being established internationally (CAHS, 2010). The best-known comprehensive model to address chronic care needs of clients is the **chronic care model (CCM)**, a primary care-based framework aimed at supporting the complex needs of clients in the community living with one or more chronic conditions (Marcelli et al., 2017; Tsai, Morton, Mangione, & Keeler, 2005). The CCM is a multicomponent intervention that includes "self-management support, decision support, delivery system design, clinical information systems, health-care organization, and community resources" (Coleman et al., 2009, p. 76). Having informed, activated clients working with a proactive team of health care professionals is essential to the success of the CCM.

The **expanded chronic care model (ECCM)** was developed in Canada to broaden the clinical focus of the CCM to include elements of population health promotion with the

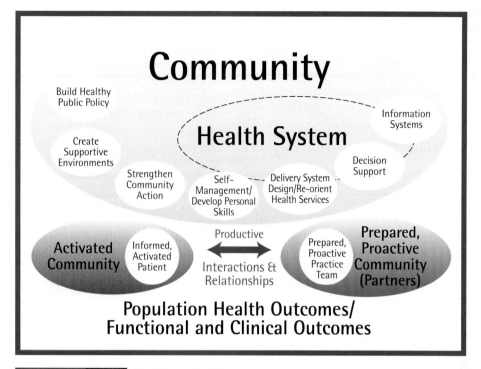

FIGURE 25.1 The Expanded Chronic Care Model

Source: Created by V. Barr, S. Robinson, B. Marin-Link, L. Underhill, A. Dotts, & D. Ravensdale. (2002). Adapted from Glasgow, R., Orleans, C., Wagner, E., Curry, S., & Solberg, L. (2001). Does the chronic care model also serve as a template for improving prevention? *The Milbank Quarterly, 79*(4), and World Health Organization, Health and Welfare Canada, and Canadian Public Health Association (1986). Ottawa Charter of Health Promotion.

aim to improve prevention of illness and enhance community participation (Barr et al., 2003). The ECCM acknowledges the association between health care and communities (see Figure 25.1). As a result, individual functional and clinical outcomes are enhanced, with the addition of measures for population health outcomes. The major aim of the ECCM is to combine population health promotion with improved treatment of conditions to provide the best option for improved health care outcomes in the long run. As an example, Alberta Health has successfully incorporated the ECCM in the province's approach to chronic disease management (Delon & MacKinnon, 2009).

In recent decades, management and treatment of chronic conditions has advanced, yet deficiencies continue to exist; this is cause for concern, owing to the increasing prevalence of chronic conditions globally (Tsai et al., 2005; World Health Organization [WHO], 2002a). There must be a continued effort to develop effective strategies to promote health and prevent and manage chronic conditions. With the support of an effective chronic care model, many patients can and do manage their chronic conditions. When this is no longer the case, there is often a shift to long-term care, where chronic care is further aligned with essential support from family or other unpaid caregivers. As illustrated in Canadian Research 25.1, the care of people living with (multiple) chronic conditions is complex, and the health and well-being of family caregivers is essential to the ongoing challenges people living with chronic conditions face.

CANADIAN RESEARCH 25.1

What influences the quality of life of family caregivers to persons living with multiple chronic conditions? (Duggleby et al., 2016)

This study is a secondary analysis of data that came from a mixed methods repeated-measures study with 194 family caregivers of individuals with multiple chronic conditions (MCCs) in Alberta and Ontario. To be included in the study, participants had to be an active informal caregiver to an older adult with two or more MCCs living in the community. The purpose of this analysis was to examine the relationships over a six-month period in health-related quality of life (e.g., physical and mental health) of family caregivers of persons with MCCs on (a) demographic variables, (b) gender identity, (c) general self-efficacy, and (d) caregiver burden. Participants completed questionnaires and various scales and tools to measure if there were any (hypothesized) changes in the variables over time.

Interestingly, participants were caring for relatives with an average of six chronic conditions, evidence of the complex reality of these family caregivers. The majority of participants were female and over the age of 65. Results for the six-month period indicated that there were no significant differences in physical health related to any of the variables. Yet participants with positive increases in mental health reported lower burden and higher self-efficacy, and were found to demonstrate masculine personality traits (e.g., assertiveness). These results highlight the important role of health care providers in supporting family caregivers to maintain their mental health and increase their confidence as they provide care. Far more research is needed to explore ways to support family caregivers in the complex situation of caring for a relative with MCCs.

Discussion Questions

1. Which variables identified in the study are most important for the CHN to consider to improve health outcomes of family caregivers of individuals living with MCCs?

2. What strategies could policy makers address to better support family caregivers?

3. How might you design a community-based social support group for family caregivers of persons living with MCCs? What content would be important to address?

LONG-TERM CARE: OVER THE CONTINUUM

Long-term care is an umbrella term that encompasses a variety of services necessary for the physical and psychological needs of clients who are no longer able to function independently. "By definition chronic care is long-term care" (Levine, Halper, Peist, & Gould, 2010, p. 117). In the 1960s the term *long-term care* tended to refer to nursing homes that provided care to people who could no longer live in their own homes (Miller, 2012). Although the notion of institutional care is strongly associated with the concept of long-term care, it is important to note that long-term care services are also provided in the community. It is useful to consider long-term care across a continuum that includes living at home with minimal assistance at one end of the spectrum versus requiring 24-hour care provided in a skilled facility at the other end (Kramer-Kile & Osuji, 2014).

Long-term care may be inevitable as the vast majority of chronic conditions have no cure, and clients live with and manage them for the rest of their lives. The transition over the spectrum of long-term care develops as a person ages and chronic conditions progress, resulting in increased dependence and reliance on others to accomplish activities of daily living. A variety of services are available over the long-term care continuum.

Community-Based Long-Term Care

The provision of **community-based long-term care** is intended as a seamless transition among various types of interventions and services (i.e., preventative, acute, rehabilitative, and supportive) based on the needs of clients. Ideally, long-term care services are put in place to enable people to remain in their own home for as long as possible (Levine et al., 2010). In Canada, the types and amount of long-term care services available in the community vary with each province and territory (Kramer-Kile & Osuji, 2014). The types of services offered in most parts of Canada include (a) nursing care; (b) personal support such as self-directed care, housekeeping,

or meal preparation; (c) respite or day programs; (d) palliative care; (e) rehabilitative care, such as occupational or physical therapy; and (f) providing necessary medical equipment and supplies (MacAdam, 2009).

The largest component of community-based long-term care in Canada is home care. The demand for home care services is increasing. To meet this demand, home care services have shifted to clients with more pressing needs of post-acute or short-term care, leaving fewer resources for long-term clients (Forbes et al., 2003; Levine et al., 2010). The result of this shift has meant that family caregivers and other unpaid caregivers are increasingly responsible for providing long-term care in the community. Family caregivers are discussed in detail later in the chapter. Home- and community-based services are intended to be utilized for individuals who do not yet qualify for admission to a long-term care facility, often with the intent to delay this admission for as long as possible (see Chapter 5). The following Case Study illustrates a common situation for many older adults and their families who face increasing care needs.

CASE STUDY

Mrs. Helen Anderson is an 82-year-old widow who was recently moved to a private care home. She was given a probable diagnosis of Alzheimer's disease more than three years ago; she also has a 20-year history with diabetes (currently receiving insulin injections twice daily) and mild hypertension, well controlled with a low dose of lasix/furosemide. She uses Gravol nightly to help her sleep. Helen had required more and more assistance with care, and her daughter, who lives in the same city, was becoming concerned for her mother's safety and thus moved her into the private care home. This move was possible because Helen and her husband had saved sufficient funds in planning for their life after retirement. However, Helen's daughter pays out-of-pocket for services not offered by the private care home; for example, foot care, hair dressing, and transportation to medical appointments.

Since the move, the private care home staff have told the home care nurse (who administers the insulin injections) that Helen has been unable to settle into the home's routine. She is reluctant to shower, is beginning to hide food (e.g., crackers and cookies) in the dresser of her bedroom, and often calls out at night for "David." During the day Helen is in constant motion as if she is looking for something and frequently asks for her coat because she states, "It's time I left." She is easily re-directed if given something to do with her hands.

Discussion Questions

1. As the home care nurse, how would you share information about Helen with her daughter and primary care physician?

2. What recommendations would you make to the staff to support Helen and her daughter in the new home?

3. What other kinds of community-based services may benefit Helen?

Facility-Based Long-Term Care

Long-term care services provided in a residential setting are the most intense type of service delivery on the long-term care continuum. According to the 2016 census, 6.8% of Canadians aged 65 years or older live in an older adult residence (Statistics Canada, 2018b). The most common older adult residences are assisted living centres, nursing homes, and chronic and long-term care hospitals. The three main components of **facility-based long-term care** include providing accommodations, hospitality services, and health services (Canadian Healthcare Association, 2009). The decision to move from one's own home to a collective dwelling can be made for a variety of reasons. Lack of availability of willing family caregivers, declining health, frailty, and concerns for safety are all motivating factors for admitting older adults to facilities that are able to provide 24-hour supportive services (Kramer-Kile & Osuji, 2014).

Residents in long-term care homes require a great deal of assistance with physical care that is usually provided by unregulated health care providers (Canadian Healthcare Association, 2009). Unfortunately, the cognitive and psychological needs of residents may be considered less important. In Canada, the titles of these health care providers vary among provinces and territories, and their work is supervised by registered nurses or licensed practical nurses (Canadian Healthcare Association, 2009). Nurses have a significant leadership role in long-term care facilities; this is particularly important with the increasing complex care that is now required in many facilities (Miller, 2012).

It is important to consider that persons living (and dying) in long-term care facilities tend to be individuals who are more vulnerable compared to community-dwelling patients (Seitz, Purandare, & Conn, 2010). For example, individuals with dementia often present with severe functional limitations, marked cognitive impairment, and problematic behaviours that are challenging for family caregivers and that precipitate the need for long-term care home admission. Approximately 45% of people aged 45 and older in long-term residential care had a diagnosis of dementia (Statistics Canada, 2016); for those aged 80 or older, this number increased to 56%.

YES, BUT WHY?

Resident-to-Resident Violence in Long-Term Care Homes

What?

It is imperative for CHNs to be aware of issues in long-term care, including staffing levels (McGregor et al., 2010) or ethical issues around provision of end-of-life care (Coventry, Grande, Richards, & Todd, 2005; Peacock, 2008). CHNs must be politically active in advocating for clients who require and receive care, including those who live in long-term care homes. One such issue in long-term care is the abuse of older adults. Sadly, it is not uncommon for media reports to expose concerns related to older adult abuse in long-term care homes (Long-term Care Task Force Ontario, 2012). Older adult abuse is generally categorized according to five types: physical, psychological/emotional, sexual, financial exploitation, and neglect

(Wangmo, Nordstrom, & Kressig, 2017). Resident-to-resident violence is defined as the abuse of one resident by another in a long-term care home (Castle, Ferguson-Rome, & Teresi, 2015).

So What?

Older adults are at risk for abuse from other residents in long-term care homes when there is a culture of overlooking such abuse and a lack of adequate supervision of residents who may be the abuser or the receiver of abuse. This includes residents living with dementia or other mental health problems, individuals who display aggressive or violent behaviours, and those who may be overly demanding (Long-term Care Task Force Ontario, 2012). The rate of violence between long-term care residents is on the rise and is now considered more common than abuse by formal care providers (Lachs & Pillemer, 2015). The consequences of resident-to-resident violence are far-reaching and not limited to immediate injury. Research demonstrates that older adults who experience abuse are at an increased risk of death, have decreased physical health, and have higher rates of depression and anxiety (Castle, Ferguson-Rome, & Teresi, 2015; Lachs & Pillemer, 2015). Further, it can be challenging to recognize abuse of older adults as the resident may be unable to verbalize that abuse is occurring. In addition, physical signs of abuse may be attributable to other concerns, or staff may feel uncomfortable and unprepared to evaluate if abuse is occurring. Long-term care homes are essential to the care of vulnerable, frail older adults with complex health conditions, and they have a responsibility to make resident safety a top priority.

Now What?

No single intervention can address the issue of resident-to-resident violence. Instead, appropriate interventions require the work of interprofessional collaborations, need to be tailored to the specific circumstances, and need adequate resources to support recognition of abuse (Lachs & Pillmer, 2015). CHNs working in or with long-term care homes need to be active in the education of all levels of staff on how to recognize, report, and decrease instances of resident-to-resident violence. It is essential for CHNs to advocate for necessary services and minimum staffing levels for people who live in long-term care homes. As our population ages and people live with more and complex health conditions, it is necessary for CHNs to be socially active and take the lead in all aspects that promote quality long-term care (Registered Nurses Association of Ontario [RNAO], 2016).

Standards of Practice Fulfilled:

#6 Health Equity

- Advocates for healthy public policy and social justice by participating in legislative and policy-making activities that influence determinants of health and access to services.

#8 Professional Responsibility and Accountability

- Assesses and identifies unsafe, unethical, illegal or socially unacceptable circumstances and takes preventive or corrective action to protect the client.
- Works collaboratively in determining the best course of action when responding to ethical dilemmas (Community Health Nurses of Canada [CHNC], 2019, revised).

PALLIATIVE CARE IN THE COMMUNITY: GOALS, STANDARDS, AND PRINCIPLES

The terms **palliative care**, **hospice care**, and **end-of-life care** are difficult to define and vary by country and context. However, all have a common goal of quality end-of-life care in any setting. The movement to relieve the suffering of dying patients, originally called hospice, was officially started in London, England, by Dame Cicely Saunders (Saunders & Sykes, 1993). Dame Saunders was a nurse, social worker, and physician who opened St. Christopher's Hospice in 1967 and hospice home care services in 1969; the movement found its way to North America shortly after. At a grassroots level, it took hold and flourished where there were strong advocates who believed in the importance of meeting the needs of the dying and their families (Ferris et al., 2002). The term "hospice" is often used interchangeably with "palliative care," a term first proposed in 1974 by a Canadian surgeon, Dr. Balfour Mount (Mount, 1997). The CHPCA has adopted the term **hospice palliative care** to recognize the convergence of hospice and palliative care into one movement that has the same principles and norms of practice (CHPCA, 2013a). Recently, the CHPCA has led the way by introducing a **palliative approach** to care (CHPCA, 2013b). This concept can be applied throughout the course of any life-threatening illness trajectory in any setting of care, with the goal of relieving suffering and improving quality of life.

The goals, standards, and principles for palliative care programs and services developed by the WHO in 2002 are an international standard for developing and evaluating palliative care programs and systems of care (WHO, 2002b). Although it was initially established as an essential aspect of the continuum of cancer care, current directions by the WHO are to include all patients with life-threatening illnesses as both needing and benefitting from palliative care. Specifically, a focus on pain and distress management, support, and integration of palliative care across disease groups and levels of care is needed. The WHO has prioritized palliative care as a global public health problem (Sepúlveda, Marlin, Yoshida, & Ullrich, 2002) requiring a community-based approach (see the box titled "Palliative Care").

The WHO guidelines have been widely adopted across the world, including by the CHPCA, which describes the values driving hospice palliative care as integrity, dignity, and autonomy. Creating a plan of care is guided by quality of life as defined by the individual, and hospice palliative care is only provided when the person and family are prepared to accept it. The CHPCA has developed a definition to guide hospice palliative care norms and practice in Canada (see box titled "Hospice Palliative Care") (CHPCA, 2013a, p. 6).

PALLIATIVE CARE

The WHO defines palliative care as an approach focused on improving quality of life for both the patient faced with a life-threatening illness and their family (WHO, 2002b).

Palliative care:

- provides relief from pain and other distressing symptoms
- affirms life and regards dying as a normal process
- intends neither to hasten nor postpone death
- integrates the psychological and spiritual aspects of patient care
- offers a support system to help patients live as actively as possible until death
- offers a support system to help the family cope during the patient's illness and in their own bereavement
- uses a team approach to address the needs of patients and their families, including bereavement counselling, if indicated
- will enhance quality of life and may also positively influence the course of illness
- is applicable early in the course of illness, in conjunction with other therapies that are intended to prolong life, such as chemotherapy or radiation therapy, and includes investigations needed to better understand and manage distressing clinical complications

---

HOSPICE PALLIATIVE CARE

Hospice palliative care aims to relieve suffering and improve the quality of living and dying. Hospice palliative care strives to help individuals and families

- address physical, psychological, social, spiritual, and practical issues, and their associated expectations, needs, hopes, and fears;
- prepare for and manage self-determined life closure and the dying process; and
- cope with loss and grief during the illness and bereavement experience.

Hospice palliative care aims to:

- treat all active issues;
- prevent new issues from occurring; and
- promote opportunities for meaningful and valuable experiences, personal and spiritual growth, and self-actualization.

Hospice palliative care is appropriate for any person or family living with, or at risk of, developing a life-threatening illness due to any diagnosis, with any prognosis, regardless of age, and at any time they have unmet expectations or needs and are prepared to accept care.

Hospice palliative care may complement and enhance disease-modifying therapy, or it may become the total focus of care.

The CHPCA advocates for a community response to unique needs. Community action will support and strengthen the community by responding to suffering in appropriate, collaborative, and community-driven approaches. For example, at the end of life, many Indigenous people focus on "preparing their spirit" with the support of kin and the community yet often face significant barriers within current health care systems (Duggleby et al., 2015). Children living in the lowest income areas or farthest from treatment centres are significantly less likely to receive specialized palliative care (Widger et al., 2018). Recognizing unique and diverse sociocultural contexts—such as rural settings, urban settings, negative socioeconomic conditions, uncertain access to services and supports, and populations experiencing health inequities—is essential in the role of the CHN to provide a socioenvironmental approach to health promotion.

CHN Standards: Promoting Health and Providing Accessible Palliative Care

The role of the CHN (as described in Chapter 3) is to promote health at all levels, including palliation, building individual and community capacity through strong relationships, and facilitating access and equity. It is important that the CHN evaluate the integration of services and supports for patients and families facing end-of-life care, including accessibility and referrals, identifying gaps, and providing care and support in the home setting. In a recent survey of 283 older adults in Saskatchewan, only 25% had a written advance care plan, suggesting the need for nurses to provide education to promote the autonomy of older adults in the community based on their readiness to participate (Goodridge, 2013). Following the model in Figure 25.2, the CHN would focus on the illness trajectory. Active treatment often continues while therapy to relieve suffering begins with a focus on improving quality of life. This mix of therapies will depend on the patient's and family's issues, goals, and treatment priorities. Care continues for the family after the person's death to support positive bereavement outcomes.

Evidence-Based Practice for Supporting Patients and Families Requiring Palliative Care

Nurses are in an optimal position to identify individuals and families facing end-of-life care needs and concerns, based on an understanding of expected end-of-life trajectories for various chronic conditions (Lunney, Lynn, Foley, Lipson, & Guralnik, 2003). Nurses begin by completing a comprehensive and holistic assessment of individuals and families based on the CHPCA's domains of care. Included in the domains are the following: disease management; physical, psychological, spiritual, social, and practical support; end-of-life care and death management; loss; and grief. Best practice guidelines have been developed to provide evidence-based recommendations for nurses caring for individuals and families facing the end of life (RNAO, 2011). It is important for CHNs to be aware of their own feelings and attitudes about death as they provide critical information, support, and practical assistance to individuals and families going through this experience.

Health Promotion Through the Levels of Prevention

Providing palliative care services requires a continuum of care, across any setting, and includes support into bereavement. A primordial prevention approach would promote health by the prevention of risk factors such as genderized roles and culturized expectations. For example, older women are expected to provide end-of-life care even when experiencing considerable burden (Williams, Giddings, Bellamy, & Gott, 2017).

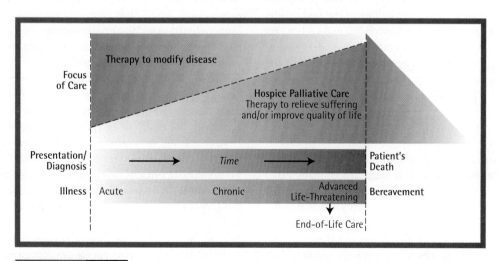

FIGURE 25.2 The Role of Hospice Palliative Care Throughout the Illness Trajectory

Source: Canadian Hospice Palliative Care Association (2013a).

Primary prevention of negative caregiver outcomes such as strain, burden, or role breakdown includes preparing and supporting family caregivers in their role. Careful assessment and intervention through providing information and support, conducting family meetings to discuss goals of care, and identifying concerns and questions will promote a positive caregiver experience (Hudson & Aranda, 2013).

Secondary prevention involves screening patients and families most at risk of deleterious outcomes. Most palliative care patients are heavily reliant on the support of family caregivers in order to remain in their homes and communities. It is essential to provide supports for the caregiver, such as offering respite, teaching self-care, and introducing cognitive-behavioural approaches that increase hope and quality of life, such as the "Living with Hope Program," a self-administered intervention. This intervention was tested with rural women caregivers of persons with advanced cancer and was found to increase hope and self-efficacy while decreasing grief (Duggleby et al., 2013).

Tertiary prevention focuses on providing excellent palliative care with the goal of a comfortable dying process and excellent support from both formal and informal care providers. In a recent study of 402 patient deaths from cancer in Toronto, better quality of dying and death scores were associated with home death that was usually accompanied by better symptom control and an extensive support network (Hales et al., 2014).

Quaternary prevention would serve to protect patients and families who face over-treatment and untested approaches (Vollman, Anderson, & McFarlane, 2017). Family caregivers bear the burden of difficult decisions made about care of the patient at the end of life into their bereavement (Holtslander et al., 2017), even more so when they have had negative interactions with health care services and providers.

What Is a Palliative Approach?

A palliative approach to support people and families with life-limiting conditions, who may be facing the end of life, has arisen from a need for improved access to end-of-life care across all settings and circumstances (Stajduhar, 2011). Integrating and applying the principles of continuity of care, community capacity building, and promoting access and equity underpin a palliative approach. It is a seamless integration of palliative care services across all health care settings for patients with life-limiting conditions and their families (CHPCA, 2012).

Although integration of palliative care is an expected practice in cancer care, it has been neglected in many other situations, such as the care of patients with severe heart disease (Lauck et al., 2014) and a host of other chronic diseases (CHPCA, 2012). There is growing evidence that integrating a palliative approach earlier in the course of a disease, combined with ongoing disease treatment and management, leads to better outcomes for patients and their families. Improved outcomes include better symptom management and quality of life, more appropriate and timely referrals, and less use of futile interventions (Smith et al., 2012). Patients and families need open information about their disease and prognosis, coordination of care, and symptom management, as well as holistic support. Interestingly, a recent survey of 2976 Canadians, conducted in 2013 through "The Way Forward" initiative of the CHPCA (2013b), revealed great support for hospice palliative care, coupled with a general reluctance to talk about death or have a discussion with someone about it. The result is that many Canadians, even those with severe, chronic, life-limiting conditions, may not be benefitting from end-of-life planning and appropriate services, information, and support.

Primary palliative care comprises an important set of skills for all clinicians, while **specialist palliative care** for managing more complex and difficult cases can be an optimal solution to meet the growing demand for widespread palliative care services (Quill & Abernethy, 2013). Expanding the role of palliative care so that it is introduced earlier in the course of an illness requires that all health care professionals provide expert pain and symptom management and are comfortable engaging in discussions with patients and families about prognosis and goals of care. Referral to the specialist in palliative care is reserved for times of very difficult distress and symptom management, and for conflict resolution regarding goals of treatment within families and among treatment teams. The application of a palliative approach has numerous implications for current health care systems, and attention is needed on providing care for caregivers in order to sustain and support them.

FAMILY CAREGIVERS: CONSEQUENCES, COPING, AND COST

As of 2012, there were 4.5 million family caregivers in Canada, an increase of 20% over the previous five years (Sinha, 2013). Over time the number of family caregivers will continue to increase, with the aging of the population, longer life expectancies, and a shift from institutionalized care to community-based care. Women outnumber men as caregivers and tend to provide more of the hands-on personal care, medical treatments, and housework, and they also spend more time caregiving when compared to male caregivers, who typically engage in home maintenance activities and transportation duties (Sinha, 2013). Many key health determinants combine to impact the health of caregivers, such as gender, age, location, education, environment, social support, access to health services, socioeconomic status, and culture. The type of caregiving greatly impacts caregiver burden and negative impact experienced (Williams, Wang, & Kitchen, 2014). Canadian caregivers require more support than they currently receive and often experience a negative impact on their quality of life due to unmet needs, loss of employment, and a further negative impact on their future opportunities; close to 50% of family caregivers manage their own chronic conditions, and less than 20% receive help from community groups (Williams, Wang, & Kitchen, 2016).

A **family caregiver** has been defined as a "relative, friend, or partner who has a significant personal relationship and provides assistance to a person . . . these individuals may be primary or secondary family caregivers and may or may not reside with the person receiving care" (Hudson et al., 2010, p. 40). Given the care that family caregivers provide, often people do not recognize their role as that of a *caregiver*; it is important to bear in mind that a caregiver is a person who provides care because the care recipient is not able to carry out particular activities independently (e.g., preparing meals, getting dressed, or managing finances). Being a caregiver is associated with both rewards and challenges (Peacock et al., 2010), yet stress is frequently significant, including physical, mental, emotional, social, and financial consequences. Often caregivers have higher rates of depression and illness and tend to be socially isolated. The quality of life for family caregivers is an immense public health issue.

Caregivers face economic costs such as employment consequences, time spent caregiving, and reduced disposable income that may jeopardize some family caregivers' current or future economic security (Fast, Keating, Lero, Eales, & Duncan, 2013). A conservative estimate of the value of unpaid care provided by family caregivers to older adults in Canada is $25 billion annually (Chappell & Hollander, 2011). Without support and preventative care for this population, family caregiver health is at risk and can result in even greater demands on the health care system. Family caregivers play a crucial role in community-based care, affecting workplaces and government policy in ways that must be acknowledged, incorporated, assessed, supported, and documented.

Of course, there are many positive aspects of being a caregiver; for instance, the reward of a reciprocal relationship, feeling closer to the care receiver, and finding meaning or a sense of personal growth in the work. It is these positive aspects that may sustain a family caregiver in his or her role for longer than would be expected. It is important to note that the rewards of caregiving should not be exploited as a way of coercing family caregivers to pick up the slack when health care services (e.g., community or facility-based care) are reduced or withdrawn (Levine et al., 2010). In a recent Canadian study, caregivers providing end-of-life care described a struggle for survival while hiding their true feelings of isolation, guilt, self-deprecation, sadness, and anger (Ward-Griffin, McWilliam, & Oudshoorn, 2012). Nurses need to build relationships with family caregivers, acknowledging their need for respite and emotional support.

Family caregivers also experience the illness and death of the person they are caring for and must embark on a healing transition through their **bereavement** experience (CHPCA, 2013a). For example, very little research has addressed the needs of family caregivers of persons with dementia at the end of life (Peacock, 2013), and the evidence needed for providing the most effective bereavement support remains lacking (Holtslander, 2008). Bereavement itself has a significant negative effect on the morbidity and mortality of caregivers (Stroebe, Schut, & Stroebe, 2007), including risk of depression (Holtslander & McMillan, 2011), loneliness, substance abuse, and physical and emotional illnesses (Schulz, Hebert, & Boerner, 2008).

Caregivers' experiences during active caregiving will affect them into bereavement, and although each experience is unique, there is a need to develop supports and interventions that improve the effectiveness of the community and the health care system to support family caregivers (Holtslander et al., 2017).

CONCLUSION

Nurses are well positioned to lead the way by improving current health care systems; engaging in necessary conversations with patients, families, and communities; and striving to relieve suffering and improve quality of life, based on a holistic person- and family-centred approach that includes a community health focus. Goals for care are shared across a spectrum of care—chronic, long term, and palliative—that aims to support patients and families with open information about their condition(s) and prognosis, the coordination of comprehensive services, symptom management, and holistic support.

KEY TERMS

bereavement (p. 467)
chronic care (p. 460)
chronic care model (CCM) (p. 460)
chronic conditions (p. 460)
community-based long-term care (p. 462)
comprehensive care model (p. 460)
end-of-life care (p. 464)
expanded chronic care model (ECCM) (p. 460)
facility-based long-term care (p. 463)
family caregiver (p. 467)
hospice care (p. 464)
hospice palliative care (p. 464)
long-term care (p. 462)
palliative approach (p. 464)
palliative care (p. 464)
specialist palliative care (p. 466)

STUDY QUESTIONS

1. What are the major differences between the expanded chronic care model and the chronic care model?

2. Which specific services are included within long-term care?

3. How can transitions between the community and acute care settings become more seamless and better integrated?

4. Which populations would benefit most from referrals to palliative care services?

5. What is the difference between generalist and specialist palliative care?

INDIVIDUAL CRITICAL-THINKING EXERCISES

1. Given the notion of an informed or activated patient being essential to chronic care, how can the CHN support and engage patients in managing their chronic conditions?

2. How do your own cultural beliefs affect your work with others?

3. What experiences of caregiving have you had? How do these experiences shape your work as a nurse?

4. Have you had family who received palliative care services? What was your experience?

GROUP CRITICAL-THINKING EXERCISES

1. In what ways do social, cultural, and environmental factors affect health, and how can they be addressed and acknowledged in the context of chronic care?

2. Considering the scarcity of health care resources, how should funding be allocated among acute, long-term, and palliative care?

3. Who should manage palliative care needs in the community setting?

4. What are the challenges and opportunities in implementing a consistent palliative approach to care across Canada?

5. What are your own feelings about death? Your experiences within your own family? How will these experiences impact your work in the community?

REFERENCES

Alzheimer Society of Canada. (2016). *Prevalence and monetary costs of dementia in Canada.* Retrieved from http://www.alzheimer.ca/~/media/Files/national/Statistics/PrevalenceandCostsofDementia_EN.pdf

Barr, V., Robinson, S., Marin-Link, B., Underhill, L., Dotts, A., Ravensdale, D., & Salivaras, S. (2003). The expanded chronic care model: An integration of concepts and strategies from population health promotion and the chronic care model. *Hospital Quarterly, 7*(1), 73–82.

Bowen, J., Stevens, D., Sixta, C., Provost, L., Johnson, J., Woods, D., & Wagner, E. (2010). Developing measures of educational change for academic health care teams implementing the chronic care model in teaching practices. *Journal of General Internal Medicine, 25*(Suppl. 4), 586–592.

Canadian Academy of Health Sciences (CAHS). (2010). *Transforming care for Canadians with chronic health conditions: Put people first, expect the best, manage for results.* Retrieved from http://www.cahs-acss.ca/wp-content/uploads/2011/09/cdm-final-English.pdf

Canadian Healthcare Association. (2009). *New directions for facility-based long-term care.* Ottawa, ON: Author.

Canadian Hospice Palliative Care Association (CHPCA). (2012). *Integrating a palliative approach into the management of chronic, life-threatening diseases: Who, how and when. The Way Forward integration initiative.* Retrieved from http://hpcintegration.ca/media/36315/TWF-integrating-palliative-approach-report-Eng_final3.pdf

Canadian Hospice Palliative Care Association (CHPCA). (2013a). *A model to guide hospice palliative care. Based on national principles and norms of practice—Revised and condensed edition: 2013.* Used by permission of Canadian Hospice Palliative Care Association. Retrieved from http://www.chpca.net/media/319547/norms-of-practice-eng-web.pdf

Canadian Hospice Palliative Care Association (CHPCA). (2013b). *What Canadians say: The Way Forward survey draft report.* Retrieved from http://www.hpcintegration.ca/media/51032/The%20Way%20Forward%20-%20What%20Canadians%20Say%20-%20Survey%20Report%20Final%20Dec%202013.pdf

Canadian Hospice Palliative Care Association (CHPCA). (2014). *Fact sheet: Hospice palliative care in Canada.* Retrieved from http://www.chpca.net/media/330558/Fact_Sheet_HPC_in_Canada%20Spring%202014%20Final.pdf

Castle, N., Ferguson-Rome, J., & Teresi, J. (2015). Elder abuse in residential long-term care: An update to the 2003 National Research Council report. *Journal of Applied Gerontology, 34*(4), 407–443.

Chappell, N., & Hollander, M. (2011). An evidence-based policy prescription for an aging population. *Healthcare Papers, 11*(1), 8–18.

Coleman, K., Austin, B., Brach, C., & Wagner, E. (2009). Evidence on the chronic care model in the new millennium. *Health Affairs, 28*(1), 75–85.

Community Health Nurses of Canada. (2019, revised). *Canadian community health nursing. professional practice model & standards of practice.* Retrieved from https://www.chnc.ca/standards-of-practice

Coventry, P., Grande, G., Richards, D., & Todd, C. (2005). Prediction of appropriate timing of palliative care for older adults with non-malignant life-threatening disease: A systematic review. *Age and Ageing, 34*, 218–227.

Delon, S., & MacKinnon, B. (2009). Alberta's systems approach to chronic disease management and prevention utilizing the expanded chronic care model. *Healthcare Quarterly, 13*(Special Issue), 98–104.

Duggleby, W., Williams, A., Holtslander, L., Cooper, D., Ghosh, S., Hallstrom, L., . . . Hampton, M. (2013). Evaluation of the living with hope program for rural women caregivers of persons with advanced cancer. *BMC Palliative Care, 12*(1), 1–11. doi:10.1186/1472-684x-12-36

Duggleby, W., Kuchera, S., MacLeod, R., Holyoke, P., Scott, T., Holtslander, L., . . . Chambers, T. (2015). Indigenous people's experiences at the end of life. *Palliative and Supportive Care, 13*(6), 1721–1733. doi:10.1017/S147895151500070X

Duggleby, W., Williams, A., Ghosh, S., Moquin, H., Ploeg, J., Markle-Reid, M., & Peacock, S. (2016). Factors influencing changes in health related quality of life of caregivers of persons with multiple chronic conditions. *Health and Quality of Life Outcomes, 14*, 81. doi:10.1186.s12955-016-0486-7

Fast, J., Keating, N., Lero, D. S., Eales, J., & Duncan, K. (2013). *The economic costs of care to family/friend caregivers: A synthesis of findings.* Retrieved from http://www.rapp.ualberta.ca/en/~/media/rapp/Publications/Documents/SynthesisCaregiversEconomicCosts_2013Dec.pdf

Ferris, F., Balfour, H., Bowan, K., Farley, J., Hardwick, M., Lamontagne, C., . . . West, P. (2002). *A model to guide hospice palliative care.* Ottawa, ON: Canadian Hospice Palliative Care Association. Retrieved from http://www.chpca.net/marketplace/national_norms/A+Model+to+Guide+Hospice+Palliative+Care+2002-URLUpdate-August2005.pdf

Forbes, D., Stewart, N., Morgan, D., Anderson, M., Parent, K., & Janzen, B. (2003). Determinants of home care nursing and home support services. *Canadian Journal of Nursing Research, 35*(4), 14–36.

Goodman, R., Posner, S., Huang, E., Parekh, A., & Koh, H. (2013). Defining and measuring chronic conditions: Imperatives for research, policy, program, and practice. *Preventing Chronic Disease, 10*:120239. http://dx.doi.org/10.5888/pcd10.120239

Goodridge, D. (2013). Planning for serious illness amongst community-dwelling older adults. *Nursing Research and Practice, 2013,* 1–7. http://dx.doi.org/10.1155/2013/427917

Hales, S., Chiu, A., Husain, A., Braun, M., Rydall, A., Gagliese, L., . . . & Rodin, G. (2014). The quality of dying and death in cancer and its relationship to palliative care and place of death. *Journal of Pain and Symptom Management, 48*(5), 839–851.

Hollander, M., Liu, G., & Chappell, N. (2009). Who cares and how much? The imputed economic contribution to the Canadian healthcare system of middle aged and older unpaid caregivers providing care to the elderly. *Healthcare Quarterly, 12*(2), 42–49.

Holtslander, L. (2008). Caring for bereaved family caregivers: Analyzing the context of care. *Clinical Journal of Oncology Nursing, 12*(3), 501–506.

Holtslander, L. F., & McMillan, S. (2011). Depressive symptoms, grief and complicated grief among bereaved family caregivers of advanced cancer patients. *Oncology Nursing Forum, 38*(1), 60–65. doi:10.1188/11.ONF.60-65

Holtslander, L., Baxter, S., Mills, K., Bocking, S., Dadgostari, T., Duggleby, . . . Peacock, S. (2017). Honoring the voices of bereaved caregivers: A metasummary of qualitative research. *BMC Palliative Care, 16*(1), 48. https://doi.org/10.1186/s12904-017-0231-y

Hudson, P., & Aranda, S. (2013). The Melbourne Family Support Program: Evidence-based strategies that prepare family caregivers for supporting palliative care patients. *BMJ: Supportive and Palliative Care, 4,* 231–2377. doi:10.1136/bmjspcare-2013-000500

Hudson, P., Remedios, C., Zordan, R., Thomas, K., Clifton, D., Crewdson, M., . . . Clarke, D. (2010). *Clinical practice guidelines for the psychosocial and bereavement support of family caregivers of palliative care patients.* Melbourne, Australia: Centre for Palliative Care.

Kramer-Kile, M., & Osuji, J. (Eds.). (2014). *Chronic illness in Canada: Impact and intervention.* Burlington, MA: Jones and Bartlett Learning.

Lachs, M., & Pillemer, K. (2015). Elder abuse. *New England Journal of Medicine, 373*(20), 1947–1956.

Lauck, S., Garland, E., Achtem, L., Forman, J., Baumbusch, J., Boone, R., . . . Webb, J. (2014). Integrating a palliative approach in a transcatheter heart valve program: Bridging innovations in the management of severe aortic stenosis and best end-of-life practice. *European Journal of Cardiovascular Nursing,* 1–8. doi:10.1177/1474515114520770

Levine, C., Halper, D., Peist, A., & Gould, D. (2010). Bridging troubled waters: Family caregivers, transitions, and long-term care. *Health Affairs, 29*(1), 116–124.

Long-term Care Task Force Ontario. (2012). *Long-term care task force on resident care and safety.* Retrieved from www.elderabuseontario.com/wp-content/uploads/2015/01/LTCFTReportEnglish.pdf

Lunney, J. R., Lynn, J., Foley, D. J., Lipson, S., & Guralnik, J. M. (2003). Patterns of functional decline at the end of life. *Journal of American Medical Association, 289*(18), 2387–2392.

MacAdam, M. (2009). *Moving toward health service integration: Provincial progress in system change for seniors.* Ottawa, ON: Canadian Policy Research Networks. Retrieved from http://www.cprn.org/documents/51302_EN.pdf

Marcelli, S., Gatti, C., Ricchi, R., Troiani, S., Di Tuccio, S., Giuli, C., . . . Santarellei, A. (2017). Chronic care model and cost reduction in initial health: A new approach for satisfaction and improvement of chronicity. *Geriatric Care, 3*(3), 1–7.

McGregor, M., Tate, R., Ronald, L., McGrail, K., Cox, M., Berta, W., & Broemeling, A. (2010). Trends in long-term care staffing by facility ownership in British Columbia, 1996 to 2006. *Health Reports, 21*(4), 1–7.

Miller, C. A. (2012). *Nursing for wellness in older adults* (6th ed.). New York, NY: Lippincott Williams and Wilkins.

Mount, B. (1997). The Royal Victoria Hospital palliative care service: A Canadian experience. In C. Saunders & R. K. Astenbaum (Eds.), *Hospice care on the international scene* (pp. 73–85). New York, NY: Springer Publishing.

Peacock, S. (2008). The moral issues involved in palliative end-of-life dementia care. *Canadian Nursing Home, 19*(2), 1–5.

Peacock, S. (2013). The experience of providing end-of-life care to a relative with advanced dementia: An integrative review. *Palliative & Supportive Care, 11*(2), 155–168.

Peacock, S., Forbes, D., Markle-Reid, M., Hawranik, P., Morgan, D., Jansen, L., . . . Leipert, B. (2010). The positive aspects of the caregiving journey with dementia: Using a strengths-based perspective to reveal opportunities. *Journal of Applied Gerontology, 29,* 640–659.

Public Health Agency of Canada. (2011). *Diabetes in Canada: Facts and figures from a public health perspective.* Retrieved from http://www.phac-aspc.gc.ca/cd-mc/publications/diabetes-diabete/facts-figures-faits-chiffres-2011/pdf/facts-figures-faits-chiffres-eng.pdf

Quill, T. E., & Abernethy, A. P. (2013). Generalist plus specialist palliative care—Creating a more sustainable model. *New England Journal of Medicine, 368*(13), 1173–1175. doi:10.1056/NEJMp1215620

Registered Nurses Association of Ontario (RNAO). (2011). *End-of-life care during the last days and hours.* Retrieved from http://rnao.ca/sites/rnao-ca/files/End-of-Life_Care_During_the_Last_Days_and_Hours.pdf

Registered Nurses Association of Ontario (RNAO). (2016). *Long-term care best practices initiative.* Retrieved from http://rnao.ca/bpg/initiatives/longterm-care-best-practices-initiative

Saunders, C., & Sykes, N. (Eds.). (1993). *The management of terminal malignant disease.* London, UK: Edward Arnold.

Sawatzky, R., Porterfield, P., Roberts, D., Lee, J., Liang, L., Reimer-Kirkham, S., . . . Baumbusch, J. (2017). Embedding a palliative approach in nursing care delivery: An integrated knowledge synthesis. *Advances in Nursing Science, 40*(3), 263–279. doi:10.1097/ANS.0000000000000163

Schulz, R., Hebert, R., & Boerner, K. (2008). Bereavement after caregiving. *Geriatrics, 63*(1), 20–22.

Seitz, D., Purandare, N., & Conn, D. (2010). Prevalence of psychiatric disorder among older adults in long-term care homes: A systematic review. *International Psychogeriatrics, 22*(7), 1025–1039.

Sepúlveda, C., Marlin, A., Yoshida, T., & Ullrich, A. (2002). Palliative care: The World Health Organization's global perspective. *Journal of Pain and Symptom Management, 24*(2), 91–96.

Sinha, M. (2013). *Portrait of caregivers, 2012.* Ottawa, ON: Statistics Canada Catalogue no. 89-652-X—No. 001. Retrieved from http://www.statcan.gc.ca/pub/89-652-x/89-652-x2013001-eng.pdf

Smith, T. J., Temin, S., Alesi, E. R., Abernethy, T. A., Balboni, T. A., Basch, E. M., . . . Von Roenn, J. H. (2012). American Society of Clinical Oncology provisional clinical opinion: The integration of palliative care into standard oncology care. *Journal of Clinical Oncology, 30*(8), 880–887.

Stajduhar, K. I. (2011). Chronic illness, palliative care, and the problematic nature of dying. *Canadian Journal of Nursing Research, 43*(3), 7–15.

Statistics Canada. (2011). *Canada year book 2011.* Retrieved from http://www.statcan.gc.ca/pub/11-402-x/2011000/pdf/seniors-aines-eng.pdf

Statistics Canada. (2016). *Health Reports: Alzheimer's disease and other dementias in Canada.* Retrieved from https://www150.statcan.gc.ca/n1/pub/82-003-x/2016005/article/14613-eng.htm

Statistics Canada. (2018a). *Deaths and causes of death, 2015.* Retrieved from https://www150.statcan.gc.ca/n1/en/daily-quotidien/180223/dq180223c-eng.pdf?st=zymAv8xo

Statistics Canada. (2018b). *Transitions to long-term care and residential care among older Canadians.* Retrieved from https://www150.statcan.gc.ca/n1/pub/82-003-x/2018005/article/54966-eng.htm

Stroebe, M., Schut, H., & Stroebe, W. (2007). Health outcomes of bereavement. *The Lancet, 370,* 1960–1973.

Tsai, A., Morton, S., Mangione, C., & Keeler, E. (2005). A meta-analysis of interventions to improve care for chronic illnesses. *American Journal of Managed Care, 11*(8), 478–488.

Wangmo, T., Nordstrom, K., & Kressig, R. (2017). Preventing elder abuse and neglect in geriatric institutions: Solutions from nursing care providers. *Geriatric Nursing, 38,* 383–392.

Ward-Griffin, C., McWilliam, C., & Oudshoorn, A. (2012). Relational experiences of family caregivers providing home-based end-of-life care. *Journal of Family Nursing, 18*(4), 491–516.

Widger, K., Sutradhar, R., Rapoport, A., Vadeboncoeur, C., Zelcer, S., Kassam, A., . . . & Pole, J. D. (2018). Predictors of specialized pediatric palliative care involvement and impact on patterns of end-of-life care in children with cancer. *Journal of Clinical Oncology, 36*(8), 801–807.

Williams, A., Wang, L., & Kitchen, P. (2014). Differential impacts of caregiving across three caregiver groups in Canada: End-of-life care, long-term care, and short-term care. *Health and Social Care in the Community, 22*(2), 187–196. doi:10.1111.hsc.12075

Williams, A., Wang, L., & Kitchen, P. (2016). Impacts of caregiving and sources of support: A comparison of end-of-life and non end-of-life caregivers in Canada. *Health and Social Care in the Community, 24*(2), 214–224.

Williams, L., Gott, M., Moeke-Maxwell, T., Black, S., Kothari, S., Pearson, S., . . . & Hansen, W. W. (2017). Can digital stories go where palliative care research has never gone before? A descriptive qualitative study exploring the application of an emerging public health research method in an Indigenous palliative care context. *BMC Palliative Care, 16*(1), 46.

Williams, L. A., Giddings, L. S., Bellamy, G., & Gott, M. (2017). "Because it's the wife who has to look after the man": A descriptive qualitative study of older women and the intersection of gender and the provision of family caregiving at the end of life. *Palliative Medicine, 31*(3), 223–230.

World Health Organization (WHO). (2002a). *Ethical choices in long-term care: What does justice require?* Retrieved from http://www.who.int/chp/knowledge/publications/ethical_choices.pdf?ua=1

World Health Organization (WHO). (2002b). *WHO definition of palliative care.* Reprinted with permission from World Health Organization. Retrieved from http://www.who.int/cancer/palliative/definition/en

Vollman, A. R., Anderson, E. T., & McFarlane, J. (2017). *Canadian community as partner: Theory and multidisciplinary practice* (4th ed.). Philadelphia, PA: Wolters Kluwer.

ABOUT THE AUTHORS

Lorraine Holtslander, RN, PhD, CHPCN(C) (University of Saskatchewan), is Professor in the College of Nursing in Saskatoon. She teaches family nursing to undergraduate students and an interdisciplinary course in qualitative research methods at the graduate level. Her clinical area of community nursing practice was as a palliative home care nurse for more than 20 years. The focus of her research is in palliative care, grief and loss, and supporting family caregivers during bereavement.

Shelley Peacock, RN, BSc, PhD (University of Alberta), is Associate Professor with the College of Nursing, University of Saskatchewan, Saskatoon. Currently, she teaches assessment and components of nursing care to undergraduate students. Her area of interest is with older adults, particularly those with dementia, and their family caregivers. Recent research using qualitative methods has involved exploring the experience of bereaved dementia family caregivers.

Correctional Health

Cindy Peternelj-Taylor and Phil Woods

CHAPTER 26

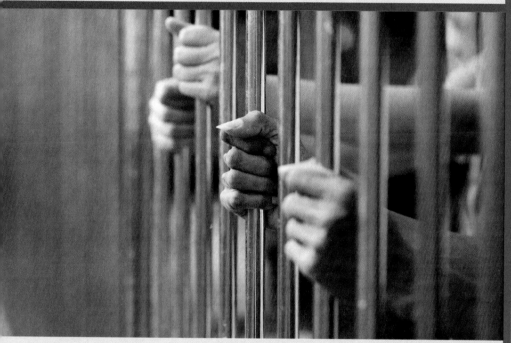

Source: Sakhorn/Shutterstock

LEARNING OUTCOMES

After studying this chapter, you should be able to:

1. Identify and discuss the roles and responsibilities of the nurse working with incarcerated persons in correctional health.

2. Describe the population of incarcerated persons in Canada.

3. Examine common health challenges encountered in correctional settings.

4. Analyze professional challenges and ethical responsibilities experienced by nurses in correctional environments.

5. Illustrate the importance of correctional nurses collaborating with community partners.

6. Reflect on ongoing education, research, advocacy, and practice developments unique to nursing in correctional settings.

INTRODUCTION

As per the United Nations Standard Minimum Rules for the Treatment of Prisoners, first published in 1957 and revised and renamed in honour of Nelson Mandela in 2015 (United Nations General Assembly [UNGA], 2016), incarcerated persons in Canadian correctional facilities are entitled to physical and mental health care in accordance with professional and community standards. The Mandela Rules, considered the international health services standards for prisons, underpin the health care directives embedded in the Corrections and Conditional Release Act (CCRA) and various provincial and territorial corrections acts responsible for the care of incarcerated persons.

Throughout history, Canadian nurses have provided care to some of the most vulnerable populations in society, including individuals who are impoverished, marginalized, and subject to discrimination and stigmatization. Indeed, this is the calling for nurses who work with incarcerated persons. Timely identification, treatment, and management of health care concerns not only contributes to the health and safety of the incarcerated population but also contributes to the health and safety of facility staff and the community at large. Nurses represent the largest group of health care professionals working with incarcerated persons, and as such they have a significant role to play.

Correctional nursing is defined as "the protection, promotion, and optimization of health and abilities; prevention of illness and injury; alleviation of suffering through the diagnosis and treatment of human response; **advocacy** for and delivery of health care to individuals, families, communities, and populations under the jurisdiction of the criminal justice system" (American Nurses Association [ANA], 2013, p. 1). In Canada, nurses practising in the criminal justice system primarily work in institutional settings, including jails, detention centres, prisons, healing lodges, correctional centres, youth custody facilities, community correctional centres, and halfway houses. The daily practice of correctional nurses "taps the knowledge and skills base of occupational health, emergency room, acute care, community health, maternity care, psychiatric care, geriatrics, and end-of-life nursing domains" (Shelton, Weiskopf, & Nicholson, 2010, p. 299). Through their use of clinical assessment and triage skills, they engage in primary, secondary, and tertiary intervention strategies when caring for incarcerated persons (see "Levels of Prevention in Correctional Health").

LEVELS OF PREVENTION IN CORRECTIONAL HEALTH

Primary Prevention

Health Promotion

- Provision of education and information
- Self-help and self-care educational strategies
- Health literacy

Illness and Injury Prevention

- Control of communicable diseases
- Case finding
- Immunization
- Suicide prevention
- Violence prevention

Classification of stressors
Advocacy
Political involvement

Secondary Prevention

- Health screening
- Pregnancy screening
- Risk-based screening for communicable diseases
- Suicide risk assessment and management
- Dementia and cognitive impairment screening

Assessment, evaluation, diagnosis, and treatment of acute and chronic health care challenges

- Acute inpatient psychiatric nursing
- Medication administration and management
- First aid, emergency, and trauma assessment and intervention
- Chronic disease management
- Crisis intervention
- Trauma-informed care

Program planning and implementation

- Creation and maintenance of a therapeutic milieu
- Substance misuse treatment

- Sex offender treatment
- Life and social skills training

Short-term therapy, counselling, psychotherapy, therapeutic groups
Appropriate referrals

Tertiary Intervention

Prevention and management of acute and chronic health care challenges
Rehabilitation and Recovery Services

- Case management
- Release planning, after-care services, community reintegration
- Vocational training
- Relapse prevention of physical and mental health care challenges
- End-of-life care
- Palliative care
- Compassionate release
- Spiritual care

Correctional facilities are not generally considered part of the traditional health care system; by default, they are responsible for the provision of health care services to large and diverse populations of incarcerated persons who have come into conflict with the law, including individuals remanded in custody while awaiting trial or sentencing (charged but not yet sentenced) and those found guilty and sentenced by the courts to various periods of time in custody. Federal, provincial, and territorial governments share the administration of correctional services in Canada. Generally, individuals receiving a sentence of two years less a day are the responsibility of either provincial or territorial correctional systems, and those sentenced to two years or longer serve their sentences within the federal system operated by Correctional Service Canada (CSC).

In the report titled "Adult Correctional Statistics in Canada, 2015–2016," Reitano (2017) notes that on an average day in 2015–2016, there were 40 100 adults in custody. Of this group, approximately 24 800 were in sentenced custody, roughly 14 700 were under federal jurisdiction, and 10 100 were in provincial or territorial custody. During the same time period, another 104 300 persons were under some form of community supervision (probation, conditional sentences, or parole). Additionally, in provincial and territorial correctional facilities, the number of individuals on remand exceeded those in sentenced custody (i.e., about 14 900 persons on remand versus about 10 100 in sentenced custody). Moreover, the majority of individuals in custody are men; women accounted for 16% of the people admitted to correctional services in 2015–2016; and young adults under the age of 35 represent more than half (58%) of admitted individuals, even though they represent only 28% of the Canadian population aged 18 and over. On any given day in 2015–2016, there were five youth in custody for every 10 000 youth in the general population. This number represents a decline of 5% from the previous year and 27% less than in 2011–2012 (Malakieh, 2017). Given the rolling cycle of admissions and releases on any given day, the total number of people affected is vastly underestimated.

HEALTH CARE OF CORRECTIONAL POPULATIONS

Historically, incarcerated individuals experienced limited and inconsistent exposure to regular health care services prior to incarceration. Although they may experience many of the same age- and gender-specific health care concerns common to the general population, morbidity and mortality data suggest higher rates of disease, disability, and death when compared to nonincarcerated populations (ANA, 2013; Kouyoumdjian, Schuler, Matheson, & Hwang, 2016). In particular, incarcerated persons in Canada experience a higher burden of chronic illness, mental illness, communicable disease, substance use, and traumatic brain injury. Coupled with early adverse events and trauma in childhood, and traumatic injuries in adulthood (Kouyoumdjian et al., 2016), the health and psychosocial issues experienced by this large marginalized group are extremely complex and contribute to treatment challenges during incarceration and upon release from custody. For many incarcerated individuals, health care received while incarcerated may be their first real opportunity to address their health care needs. Numerous opportunities exist for correctional nurses to provide leadership in the provision of health promotion and illness prevention, to advocate for policy changes directed and administered by health care as opposed to corrections (Punch, 2016), and to provide compassionate culturally safe trauma-informed care in an effort to improve the overall health and well-being of incarcerated persons in their care.

The correctional system provides care for incarcerated individuals with all types of acute and chronic illnesses. The lifestyle of many in this population includes substance misuse, which gives rise to various drug and alcohol withdrawal syndromes, diverse infectious diseases, and the need for long-term treatment interventions. Crowded living conditions can result in higher exposure to infectious diseases, a concern of public health officials worldwide, as most incarcerated individuals eventually return to the community (Kouyoumdjian et al., 2016). Furthermore, the "deinstitutionalization movement" that began in Canada in the 1960s has frequently been blamed for the **criminalization of the mentally ill** (Chaimowitz, 2012). The Mental Health Commission of Canada (MHCC) (2012) concluded that prisons have become the "'asylums' of the 21st century" (p. 60), even though they were never designed to meet the needs of those requiring treatment for mental illness. Finally, it is not uncommon for correctional nurses to care for persons who have intellectual disabilities, including fetal alcohol spectrum disorder, as well as those who have experienced multiple traumas such as sexual assaults, stabbings, beatings, and traumatic brain injuries (Peternelj-Taylor & Woods, 2019).

Special Populations in Correctional Settings

The unique needs of incarcerated individuals who experience mental illness, are aging, are women or youth, and are from diverse ethnic and gender backgrounds are highlighted here to draw attention to the health care concerns and the overall health inequities experienced by criminal justice–involved populations.

Incarcerated Persons with Mental Illness It is estimated that the number of persons with mental illness in federal corrections has increased by 60–70% since 1997 (MHCC, 2012). Studies of incarcerated populations report a high prevalence of mental health concerns, often with two or more coexisting disorders, and higher rates of psychosis, depression, anxiety, and personality disorder when compared to the Canadian population. According to Canada's Office of the Correctional Investigator [OCI] (2012), 13% of men and 29% of women are identified on admission as presenting with mental health problems. In addition, of those incarcerated, 15% of men and 30% of women had been previously hospitalized because of a psychiatric disorder. In the 2014–2015 annual report, approximately 28% of the federal incarcerated population had mental health needs (OCI, 2016). In a study of mental illness in a sample of incarcerated persons in Ontario correctional facilities, Green, Foran, and Kouyoumdjian (2016) found the self-reported prevalence of schizophrenia was 4.8%, depression 41.6%, and bipolar disorder, mania, manic depression, or dysthymia 20.8%.

It is important to note, however, that a distinction is not always made between "mental health problems" and diagnosed "mental illness"; instead, severity of symptoms is often presented. For example, it is estimated that 41.1% of incarcerated individuals in Ontario will have at least one current, severe symptom of a mental health problem; 13% of this group will experience two or more symptoms, contributing to the presence of a diagnosis of a mental disorder requiring mental health care treatment (Brown, Hirdes, & Fries, 2015). High prevalence rates are consistently reported in other countries. In a report published by the Vera Institute of Justice, Sabramanian, Delaney, Roberts, Fishman, and McGarry (2015) noted that the rate of serious mental illness in men and women in jail is four to six times higher than in the general American population. In a systematic review and meta-analysis of severe mental illness in prisoners worldwide, Fazel and Seewald (2012) found pooled prevalence of psychosis was 3.6% for men and 3.9% for women, and for major depression, 10.2% for men and 14.1% for women. When compared to their nonincarcerated counterparts, from a global perspective, incarcerated persons are more likely to be diagnosed with serious mental illness and substance use disorder (Fazel, Hayes, Bartellas, Clerici, & Trestman, 2016).

Correctional facilities are hard-pressed to provide mental health care at the same standard as that found in community mental health systems. Indeed, the OCI (OCI, 2012, 2013, 2014) has repeatedly emphasized that mental health treatment in federal facilities warrants further development when

KEY ELEMENTS OF THE MENTAL HEALTH STRATEGY FOR CORRECTIONS IN CANADA

Part I

1. Mental health promotion
2. Screening and assessment
3. Treatment, services, and supports
4. Suicide and self-injury prevention and management
5. Transitional services and supports
6. Staff education, training, and support
7. Community supports and partnerships

Source: Mental Health Strategy for Corrections in Canada, A Federal-Provincial-Territorial Partnership, Correctional Service Canada, 2011. Reproduced with the permission of the Minister of Public Works and Government Services Canada, 2015.

compared to the community standard. Promoting a mental health agenda in a correctional setting is challenging at best, as the environment is coercive by definition. The MHCC (2012) has observed that without access to appropriate treatment, incarcerated persons with serious and complex mental health needs "can get caught up in a vicious cycle of isolation, restraint, and segregation" (p. 47). Recognizing the need for more proactive mental health approaches (rather than reactive, crisis-oriented services), a collaborative venture of the MHCC and federal, provincial, and territorial correctional jurisdictions has resulted in a mental health strategy for corrections in Canada. Priority areas include knowledge generation and sharing, enhanced service delivery, improved human resource management, and building community supports and partnerships.

All incarcerated persons are assessed for suicidal thoughts and plans on admission and reassessed throughout their incarceration as necessary. For many, suicide may be viewed as the only way to cope with their charges or sentences, family responsibilities that cannot be met, fear of assault by fellow incarcerated persons, and the overall living conditions within the correctional facility. Overcrowding, isolation, and long sentences for violent crimes, coupled with a history of psychiatric disorders and substance misuse, are identified risk factors. Incarcerated persons may be placed on a suicide watch if assessment indicates and referred to a psychiatrist for further assessment, medication, other treatments, or admission to hospital as necessary. Power and Riley (2010), in a retrospective review of suicides in federal custody, found that suicides were more likely to occur on the weekends, by ligature, in cells in the general population. Nurses should be especially concerned with appropriate discharge planning, as the days following release represent a very high-risk period. The key components of a suicide prevention program as outlined by the World Health Organization (2007) include staff training in suicide prevention programs, intake screening of all incarcerated persons, post-intake observation and monitoring, and sufficient mental health treatment.

Some incarcerated individuals will present with overt signs of mental health problems upon admission, and others will develop mental health problems while incarcerated. Separation from family, friends, and community, and the ever-present potential for violence, result in an extremely high-stress environment (MHCC, 2012). Correctional nurses require highly developed assessment and communication skills to elicit data necessary to identify individuals experiencing mental health problems and to ensure their safety. Mental illness is highly stigmatized, and individuals with mental illness are especially vulnerable due to the pecking order that exists in the prison subculture. It is critical that individuals with psychosis, or who have decompensated, are housed in an area where they can be protected from predatory incarcerated persons; individuals with mental illness can be victimized and "muscled" (i.e., physically bullied) for their medications, canteen items, or other personal belongings.

Although policies vary across the country and across jurisdictions, individuals presenting with mental illness at the time of remand require an advocate to ensure that they move through the justice system as quickly as possible and that appropriate transitional discharge plans are in place. The role of the advocate often falls to the correctional nurse. There is a great opportunity for nurses to work with external community-based organizations in order to meet the treatment and release needs of this vulnerable group. By collaborating with various community agencies, correctional nurses can gain their assistance with the provision of mental health services while the person is in custody, and these same agencies can provide the link to their home communities upon release. Increasingly, through the administration of community-based treatment and support services, **diversion programs** and policies (alternatives to incarceration) have been implemented as a way of redirecting persons with mental illness and addiction who come into conflict with the law from the criminal justice system to appropriate community-based mental health and addiction services (Clark, Dolan, & Frabee, 2017). In general, several types of diversion are practised in Canada: pre-arrest and pre-booking diversion, court diversion, mental health courts, and restorative justice initiatives. Such schemes hold promise for humane treatment and reduced recidivism among this population, but they can work only if there are community-based services, treatments, and resources to support individuals who have been diverted (MHCC, 2012).

In most settings, incarcerated persons experiencing mental health problems are generally supervised 24 hours per day by correctional staff. Training and experience varies among this group, and minimal training in mental health theory and practice is often the norm. Even though correctional staff are primarily responsible for containment and security, the OCI (2014) has recommended that suitable educational programs should be an integral part of their training in order to ensure timely identification and referral of individuals with mental health problems to health care and to provide appropriate supervision. However, correctional officers cannot, and should not, replace registered nurses. Correctional nurses should be advocating for mental health care that is consistent with the MHCC's Mental Health Strategy (MHCC, 2012). Regrettably, correctional staff may see mental illness, including suicidal or self-harming behaviour, in incarcerated persons through a security or disciplinary lens and default to seclusion or segregation, which can be particularly detrimental to the overall well-being of incarcerated individuals and put them at greater risk for decompensation and suicide. In recent years, prisoners' advocates have been critical of correctional administrations for the use and abuse of segregation or solitary confinement as a way of managing challenging behaviours of incarcerated persons (OCI, 2016, 2017; Registered Nurses Association of Ontario [RNAO], 2016). The Mandela Rules (UNGA, 2016) purport that such measures should be "prohibited in the case of prisoners with mental or physical disabilities when their conditions would be exacerbated by such measures." Furthermore, to be consistent with the Mandela Rules, incarcerated individuals should not be placed in segregation for more than 15 days, and indefinite solitary confinement must be abolished. Nurses and other health care practitioners should not be a part of such harmful practices (OCI, 2017).

The Aging Incarcerated Person For an increasing number of Canadians, growing old in prison is a harsh reality, a trend also experienced in other Western countries (Hayes, Burns, Turnbull, & Shaw, 2012; Human Rights Watch [HRW], 2012). In 2015–2016 individuals aged 50 and over accounted for approximately 16% of federal and 11% of provincial admissions to custody (Reitano, 2017). This group is among the fastest-growing subgroup found within correctional environments. When compared with the previous five years for this age group, Reitman (2017) reported that custody admissions were up 22% federally and 7% provincially/territorially. The OCI (2016) reported that one in four federally incarcerated individuals was age 50 or older. Of central interest to correctional nurses is the fact that on average, incarcerated persons are thought to be 10 to 12 years older physiologically when compared to their chronological age (Uzoaba, 1998). These data challenge nurses, other health care professionals, and correctional staff to work collaboratively in the early identification and provision of health care required by this aging population. Prisons and correctional facilities were never intended for an aging and infirm population; subsequently, as a result of this "silver tsunami" (HRW, 2012), significant improvements in accommodation planning, program development, palliative care, and reintegration options are required (OCI, 2013, 2014). "Life in prison can challenge anyone but it can be particularly hard for people whose bodies and minds are being whittled away by age" (HRW, 2012, p. 4).

Physical health care needs experienced by this population include chronic physical diseases such as cardiovascular disease, pulmonary disorders, diabetes, arthritis, cancer, and liver disease (Hayes et al., 2012; OCI, 2014; Williams, Stern, Mellow, Safer, & Greifinger, 2012). Mental health concerns experienced by this group include stress, social isolation, depression and suicide. Increasingly, older incarcerated persons either present with neurocognitive disorders such as dementias and cognitive disorders at the time of admission, or they develop dementia during their incarceration experience (Gaston, 2017; Williams et al., 2012). Peacock, Hodson, MacRae, and Peternelj-Taylor (2018) have concluded that very few interventions are cited in the research literature regarding the effectiveness of programming for incarcerated individuals living with dementia. As such, research is required to guide the development and maintenance of relevant evidence-informed dementia programs and services.

For many older adult and infirm incarcerated individuals, the fear of dying while imprisoned is a terse reality (Loeb, Penrod, McGhan, Kitt-Lewis, & Hollenbeak, 2014). Prison models of palliative care, although still very much in their infancy, are based on community-based professional practice standards. Managing terminally ill incarcerated persons within the prison milieu is a time-consuming, resource-intense, exhausting endeavour, one that is fraught with perplexing practical and moral dilemmas not commonly encountered in traditional health care settings (Burles, Peternelj-Taylor, & Holtslander, 2016). Although legislation provides for parole or release by exception, also known as Royal Prerogative of Mercy, for individuals whose release will not "pose an undue risk to society" (OCI, 2014), it is rarely utilized or granted due to ongoing fears about community safety, acute bed shortages in long-term care, and the stigma associated with criminals and incarceration. In general, the public is not interested in having convicted "criminals" residing in long-term care facilities or community-based palliative care facilities, regardless of their health status. Between 2008–2009 and 2012–2013, a total of 11 requests for compassionate release were made to the National Parole Board; seven were granted, and four were denied. Six persons died before their applications were completed (OCI, 2014). Likewise, during 2014–2015, all 28 requests for Royal Prerogative of Mercy were denied by the Parole Board of Canada, with the Office of the Correctional Investigator once again calling for answers and policy direction (OCI, 2016).

Transfer of incarcerated persons from prison to long-term care requires thorough release planning; nurses are key players in promoting the successful transition to community-based long-term care facilities (Loeb, 2013). Supporting and promoting compassionate release initiatives not only contributes to decreased health care costs for this population, it is also morally and ethically the right thing to do. A round table including scholars in medicine, nursing, and human rights was convened in New York in 2011 to address prison health care, geriatrics, and palliative medicine in an effort to set priority areas for a new policy agenda (Williams et al., 2012). To the best of our knowledge to date, similar approaches to setting a policy agenda for older prisoner health care have not been explored in Canada.

Health Care Issues Unique to Incarcerated Women Women most likely to be incarcerated have grown up in poor communities, have limited education and job skills, have experienced a multitude of barriers preventing healthy lifestyles, have significant trauma histories, including violence (including sexual and physical abuse), are victims as well as perpetrators of crime, and are the primary caregivers for dependent children (Blanchette & Brown, 2006; Fisher & Hatton, 2009; van den Bergh, Gatherer, Fraser, & Moller, 2011). And, like "free" women, they are likely to experience multiple roles, such as mother, daughter, wife, sister, and friend, and to be responsible for the emotional maintenance of the family unit, even when they are not with their families (Brennan, 2014). Unfortunately, women are frequently imprisoned far from their home communities, and the fear of losing custody of their children is an ever-present reality (van den Bergh et al., 2011).

Women who are incarcerated have significant trauma histories and report physical and sexual abuse, often both as children and as adults (Mollard & Hudson, 2016; van den Bergh et al., 2011). The result is that many if not most incarcerated women require a **trauma-informed approach** to their care. Common health concerns experienced by incarcerated women include substance misuse and related sequelae; infectious diseases, including HIV, AIDS, and hepatitis B (HBV) and C (HCV); pregnancy-related concerns; gynecological problems; urinary incontinence (especially within the aging population); obesity; and chronic health disorders such as asthma, hypertension, heart disease, and diabetes (Fisher & Hatton, 2009; Nolan & Stewart, 2017; van den Bergh et al., 2011). Blanchette and Brown (2006) report that the mental health needs of women are quantitatively and qualitatively different from their male counterparts, in part due to unresolved trauma histories. In particular, women experience higher levels of anxiety disorders, post-traumatic stress disorder, depression, psychopathy, and borderline personality disorder (including nonsuicidal self-injury), serious mental illness (e.g., schizophrenia and depression), and chronic health disorders.

The problem of nonsuicidal self-injurious behaviour in women has become a critical issue in correctional facilities. Caring for female incarcerated individuals who engage in self-harming behaviours (e.g., cutting) is particularly challenging and can readily split correctional and health care staff. Power, Brown, and Usher (2013) found that women engage in self-injurious behaviour for a variety of reasons, including coping with negative emotions (e.g., anger, depression, and anxiety) and interpersonal conflict. Such behaviours are often followed by feelings of relief and regret. Although a trauma-informed correctional nurse understands this, for many prison guards, it is interpreted as posing a threat to prison safety and is approached with disdain. Effective treatment of women who engage in self-injurious behaviours needs to focus on the individual's unique experience and treatment needs.

Reproductive issues require considerable attention for women who are pregnant and incarcerated, and nurses are often thrust into a counselling role regarding women's decision making surrounding pregnancy. Given the aforementioned history of substantive trauma and related substance misuse, incarcerated pregnant women with an opioid addiction present a unique and pressing issue for corrections nurses. This population needs to have methadone maintenance treatment (MMT) initiated or continued, thereby reducing the risk of fetal complications from opiate withdrawal (Kelsey, Medel, Mullins, Dallaire, & Forestell [2017]). Nurse-to-nurse collaboration with community health and local hospitals is critical, as labour and delivery nurses are often unaware of the extra security precautions that are required during medical transfers. For example, they are not generally accustomed to working with women who are in shackles and accompanied by correctional officers (Ferszt, Hickey, & Seleyman, 2013). Following delivery, special provisions must be made so the woman has contact with her child in order to facilitate mother–child bonding and in some cases breastfeeding for the first few weeks (Brennan, 2014;

Ferszt et al., 2013). The CSC (2018) has a comprehensive institutional mother-child program, which includes an innovative project entitled CHILD LINK that allows incarcerated women to visit with their children (who live at a distance) via video conferencing. Preliminary results suggest that the pilot is successful in developing and maintaining the bond between mother and child. Nurses are often the ones involved in establishing and evaluating such innovative programming within correctional environments. Incarcerated mothers may require help with parenting skills, and nurses in consultation with community agencies can assist with these skills while the mother is in custody and again upon release. If there is a prior history of child abuse or neglect, the newborn may be taken into care as per the authority of provincial or territorial child protection services. In such cases, women may need additional support in relation to grieving over the loss of their child.

Women who are incarcerated are often interested in learning more about their health, including family planning services. It is not uncommon for correctional nurses to work with community partners in developing programs that focus on the needs of women related to prenatal, birth, and postpartum issues. Furthermore, nurses have been actively involved in the development and implementation of a number of programs, including programs related to self-harming behaviours (Roth & Pressé, 2003), trauma-informed correctional care for women (Mollard & Hudson, 2016), the use of storytelling to enhance health promotion among Indigenous women (Rowan, Auger, Toto, Simpson, & McNab, 2004), and the use of health promotion body maps with criminalized women (Donelle & Hall, 2016) (see the "Yes, But Why?" box).

YES, BUT WHY?

Women Are among the Fastest-Growing Incarcerated Population

What?

Although the number of women who come into conflict with the law is relatively small compared to their male counterparts, women now represent 16% of the incarcerated population (Reitano, 2017) and have become the fastest-growing population in Canadian corrections (OCI, 2017). Between 2007–2008 and 2016–2017, the number of federally incarcerated women increased by 29.7%; Indigenous women's incarceration increased by 60% during this same period (OCI, 2017).

So What?

The Elizabeth Fry Society (2013) declared in an advocacy poster "Women don't belong in prison: Prisons are the real crime." Unfortunately, correctional facilities in Canada, as in other parts of the world, have become in many ways society's answer to poverty, homelessness, mental illness, and addiction, while the cumulative impact of foster care; interpersonal violence, including sexual abuse (often endured at an early age); physical abuse; and intimate partner violence is minimized. When the ongoing needs of women in relation to their exposure to trauma remains untouched, drug and alcohol use and criminality soar; substance use and misuse is a common self-medicating response to trauma. As a result, women cycle through criminal justice systems, while their children cycle through social services and foster care (Marotto, 2017; Mollard & Hudson, 2016), which puts them at risk of following in their mothers' footsteps. A columnist with *The Star* recently observed that the state of women's corrections in Canada is akin to holding "a mirror and a magnifying glass to the failures of Canada's social safety net" (Mochama, 2018).

Now What?

Community health nurses in partnership with correctional nurses and advocates from community-based organizations need to work collaboratively to address this disturbing trend. Clearly, good correctional health care is good public health. Working with women and families in the community through the provision of appropriate mental health and substance misuse services, addressing poverty and homelessness, and combatting violence as a public health priority represent beginning steps in preventing the next generation of criminally involved persons. This requires both interdisciplinary and inter-sectoral collaborations such as the critical integration of re-entry programs, physical and mental health care, housing, parenting, education, and employment services (Fisher & Hatton, 2009; Mollard & Hudson, 2016; van den Bergh et al., 2016). Moreover, "One of the best preventive strategies for reducing mental illness in the correctional system is to increase access to mental health care outside of the correctional centers" (Mollard & Hudson, 2016, p. 228). Alternative measures, such as community-based sentences and drug and mental health courts for nonviolent convictions (where there is no undue risk to the public), also need to be explored. Moreover, providing safe nursing care to women who are incarcerated requires gender-sensitive, culturally appropriate, trauma-informed strategies that consider the complexities inherent in their vulnerability.

Standards of Practice Fulfilled

#2 Prevention and Health Protection
- Engages in collaborative, interdisciplinary and inter-sectoral partnerships in the delivery of preventive and protective services with particular attention to populations who are marginalized.

#4 Professional Relationships
- Respects and supports the client in identifying their health priorities and making decisions to address them while being responsive to power dynamics.

#6 Health Equity
- Collaborates with community partners to coordinate and deliver comprehensive client services with the goal of reducing service gaps and fragmentation (CHNC, 2019, revised).

Concerns Unique to Youth Youth in custody represent a significant portion of the population that is medically underserved; they experience substantial physical and mental health care challenges, and many are involved with a child protection agency at the time of their arrest. Compared to nonincarcerated populations, incarcerated youth experience significant trauma histories (including high rates of physical, sexual, and emotional abuse), higher rates of chronic health diagnoses (such as asthma and type II diabetes), complex substance misuse issues, significant mental health concerns (Perry & Morris, 2014), and greater rates of fetal alcohol spectrum disorder (Green, Cook, Stewart, & Salmon, 2016). Furthermore, they often present with histories of risky sexual health behaviours that may result in unplanned pregnancies and increase their chances of contracting HIV, hepatitis, and other sexually transmitted infections (STIs). These higher rates are often attributed to underdeveloped coping skills among this age group (Griel & Loeb, 2009; Perry & Morris, 2014).

Youth in custody frequently present with a variety of symptoms consistent with schizophrenia, anxiety disorders, depression, attention deficit hyperactivity disorder, and suicidality, although they may never have been formally diagnosed (Perry & Morris, 2014). A suicide assessment of every youth is necessary and includes previous suicidal attempts, lack of social support and stable relationships, social drift, and social impairment. The risk of suicide is greater in youth experiencing a first episode of psychosis. Given the positive and negative symptoms associated with schizophrenia (e.g., delusions, hallucinations, and social withdrawal) and high rates of substance misuse common in this population (Ventriglio et al., 2016), it is essential that correctional nurses cultivate finely tuned psychiatric and mental health assessment and intervention skills.

Twelve- to 17-year-olds residing in youth centres and youth and adult shared facilities are sentenced under the authority of the Youth Criminal Justice Act (Malakieh, 2017). In the report titled "Youth Correctional Statistics in Canada, 2015/2016," Malakieh (2017) noted a 7% reduction in admissions to correctional services from the previous year. Indigenous youth, however, continue to be overrepresented when compared to their non-Indigenous counterparts. During 2015–2016, from data supplied by nine jurisdictions, Indigenous youth accounted for 35% of all youth correctional admissions (an increase of 6% from the previous year), whereas only 7% of the youth population on average were Indigenous in these same jurisdictions. Female Indigenous youth accounted for 43% of all female youth admissions, and Indigenous boys represented 31% of all male youth admissions. Corrado, Kuehn, and Margaritescu (2014) conclude the ongoing legacy of colonialism, residential school systems, and cultural collision and assimilation further contribute to conflict with the criminal justice system among Indigenous youth.

Clearly, a focus on health promotion and prevention of illness is critical for all youth in this age group. Correctional nurses are in key positions to advocate for timely access to services, treatment as necessary, and social supports in the community. Keeping youth out of the criminal justice system through alternative measures and restorative justice initiatives with victims, their families, and communities (e.g., victim-offender reconciliation, family group conferencing, healing circles, and sentencing circles) is critical to long-term investment with this group (MHCC, 2012). For Indigenous youth specifically, courts must consider their personal circumstances and provide alternatives to custody (Malakieh, 2017). Correctional nurses, in collaboration with other health care professionals across a number of community-based sectors, can make a significant difference in the lives of those at risk of involvement with the criminal justice system through prevention efforts, early intervention strategies, and supporting successful community reintegration.

Diversity of Incarcerated Persons The cultural diversity of Canada as a whole is reflected in the demographic profile of Canadian correctional facilities. Between 2007 and 2012, the foreign-born federal incarcerated population represented 13% of the total incarcerated population, with 18% made up of visible minorities. To illustrate further, in 2011–2012, the demographic breakdown of persons under federal jurisdiction was 62.3% Caucasian, 19.3% Indigenous, 8.6% Black, 5.4% Asian, 0.9% Hispanic, and 3.4% other visible minorities (OCI, 2013). As in other Western societies, visual minorities are overrepresented in Canadian correctional systems.

Overrepresentation of Indigenous Populations Historically, Indigenous people have been disproportionately represented in provincial, territorial, and federal correctional systems when compared to their representation in the overall population. In 2016, the OCI highlighted that one in four federally incarcerated persons was Indigenous; the latest report (OCI, 2017) highlights that over the last 30 years, each year has seen an increase in the Indigenous incarceration rate. Between 2007 and 2016, although the overall prison population increased by less than 5%, the Indigenous prison population increased by 39% (OCI, 2017, p. 48). On a national level in 2015–2016, Indigenous adults accounted for 26% of all adult admissions to provincial and territorial correctional services, and 28% of all custodial admissions to federal facilities, even though they represented less than 5% of Canada's adult population (Reitano, 2017). Throughout Canada there is marked variation in the representation of Indigenous adults admitted, with the highest rates in Saskatchewan, Manitoba, Yukon, Northwest Territories, and Nunavut. Indigenous women are overrepresented in sentenced custody admissions when compared to Indigenous men (38% versus 26% provincial and territorial; 31% versus 23% federally) (Reitano, 2017). Moreover, incarcerated Indigenous persons are more likely to serve more time in custody, be classified as maximum security, spend more time in segregation, and have their parole suspended or revoked (OCI, 2016, 2017). Given this disconcerting information, it is difficult not to wonder about the role that racial bias and systemic discrimination play in their overrepresentation.

The overrepresentation of Indigenous persons in the criminal justice system has been attributed to the commingling of a number of complex factors, including rapid culture change, cultural oppression, marginalization, and the legacy of the residential school systems (Corrado et al., 2014; Hyatt, 2013; Kirmayer, Brass, & Tait, 2000), which together have contributed to high rates of poverty, substance misuse, and victimization within families and communities of origin. The

OCI (2014, 2017) continues to be critical of the federal government's response to Indigenous incarceration rates, as better use of provisions in the CCRA could be utilized that allow Indigenous communities to oversee the care and custody of Indigenous persons. Issues of cultural competence related to health promotion, peer education, and employment opportunities must be further enhanced. In the final report of the Truth and Reconciliation Commission of Canada, recommendation 30 calls "upon the federal, provincial, and territorial governments to commit to eliminating the overrepresentation of Aboriginal people in custody over the next decade, and to issue detailed annual reports that monitor and evaluate progress in doing so" (Truth and Reconciliation Commission of Canada, 2015, p. 3).

There has been growing awareness in recent years of the need to provide culturally competent and culturally safe care in all areas of health care; the same can be said for correctional systems. Increasingly, specific cultural practices are incorporated into programming offered within correctional facilities. For example, in collaboration with First Nation, Inuit, and Métis community leaders, as part of the rehabilitation process, Elders, healers, and community support facilitators offer traditional activities such as smudging ceremonies, sweat lodges, and talking circles. Mason (2010) notes that it is important to continue to engage Indigenous peoples in collaborative dialogue around correctional programming. Clearly, "increased understanding of the culture of incarceration as well as the pre-prison cultural lives of imprisoned [men and women] can serve as a means of establishing relationships and providing culturally congruent care" (Christensen, 2014, p. 230). The OCI (2017) has once again highlighted that "CSC has yet to develop tools to assess how culturally specific correctional interventions for Indigenous incarcerated persons, such as Elder services, Healing Lodges, Pathways Initiatives and partnerships with community groups and organizations contribute to an offender's progress toward successful reintegration" (p. 49).

Gender Identity in Corrections In recent years, correctional authorities and governments have been challenged regarding their treatment of transgender persons who have been incarcerated in institutions based upon their assigned sex at birth. In 2015, Ontario was the first province to house transgender persons in institutions based on their gender identity; this was followed a few months later by provincial correctional authorities in British Columbia. Federally, the CSC's gender dysphoria policy, which did not allow for placement based on gender identity, was not revised until Prime Minister Trudeau declared at a town hall meeting that he vowed to promote gender equality for all Canadians, including those who were incarcerated (OCI, 2017). Federally, the CBC reported on the first transgender offender to be transferred to a women's institution in July 2017 (Harris, 2017). Regrettably, the OCI (2017) continues to express concern that in contrast to provincial jurisdictions, "federal corrections appears mired, if not stuck, in conventional attitudes and assumptions" (p. 17). Correctional nurses can assume leadership and advocacy in this area by increasing their knowledge and by role modelling respect and sensitivity in relation to gender identity and gender expression.

COMMON HEALTH CHALLENGES

For many incarcerated persons, health care received while incarcerated may be the first real opportunity they have had to address their health care needs. Immeasurable opportunities exist for correctional nurses to provide leadership in the provision of health promotion and illness prevention, especially when individuals in their care are motivated to make lifestyle changes that would improve their overall health status.

Substance Misuse and Addiction

Substance misuse and addiction, including alcohol, nicotine, cocaine, opioids, benzodiazepines, cannabis products, and hallucinogens, is a major problem in correctional systems worldwide, and this problem is no different in Canada, although different levels of the problem are reported. Public Safety Canada (2015) reports that 75% of incarcerated individuals in Canadian federal prisons present with a substance misuse problem. For this group there is a direct link between their substance misuse and their criminal behaviours. In a review of the health of incarcerated persons in Canada, Kouyoumdjian and colleagues (2016) found that initiation of alcohol and drug use began at an early age, alcohol use and binge drinking was common, and recent drug use was typical at the time of admission. Substance misuse among this population is common, and the severity of withdrawal syndromes varies, requiring nurses to be astute in their assessments and observations regarding how withdrawal is manifested. Furthermore, nurses need to be able to differentiate individuals who are drug-seeking from those who legitimately require medications for health-related problems.

Harm Reduction Strategies Harm reduction, including opioid agonist treatments such as MMT and buprenorphine/naloxone and **prison needle and syringe programs (PNSPs)**, is the most widely accepted approach for dealing with substance misuse in correctional institutions worldwide. These strategies are not only controversial but also generally misunderstood by correctional administrators and health care professionals alike. From a public health perspective, such programs are both morally and fiscally responsible, and contribute to the protection of the community at large (Canadian HIV/AIDS Legal Network, 2008, 2010; Canadian Nurses Association [CNA], 2016; van der Meulen et al., 2016; van der Meulen, Claivaz-Loranger, Clarke, Ollner, & Watson, 2016). Still, less than 1% of prisons and correctional facilities worldwide (i.e., only 60 prisons in 10 countries) have adopted a PNSP (van der Meulen et al., 2016). Despite pleas from advocacy groups such as the Canadian HIV/AIDS Legal Network and the Prisoners HIV/AIDS Support Action Network, and professional groups such as the CNA (2016) and the PNSP Nursing Coalition (CNA, 2017), Canadian correctional authorities are loath to implement PNSPs, even though they represent an evidence-based approach to reducing blood-borne infections. Needle exchange programs, however, are readily available in communities across the country, further illustrating the discrepancies that exist

between community and correctional health care programs. In the interim, bleach kits for the purposes of decontaminating injection equipment are available in some jurisdictions. However, bleach is at best considered a second-line strategy in the absence of clean needles and syringes, as disinfection alone does not kill all viruses, such as HBV and HCV (Canadian HIV/AIDS Legal Network, 2010). Of note, a meeting funded by the Canadian Institutes of Health Research was held in 2014 for the purpose of developing PNSP implementation guidelines. A 12-month research consultation project, funded by the Ontario HIV network, that garnered the input of former prisoners and health care staff resulted in a comprehensive report entitled "On Point: Recommendations for Prison-Based Needle and Syringe Programs in Canada," published in 2016 (van der Meulen et al., 2016). To the surprise of advocates, health care professionals, and correctional authorities, on May 14, 2018, the federal government announced it will introduce a PNSP in one male and one female correctional institution as part of a phased approach prior to a full national rollout in all federal correctional facilities (Government of Canada, 2018). It will be interesting to see if provincial correctional facilities follow suit.

As of 2002, most Canadian correctional facilities had adopted policies that allowed for the continuation of MMT for individuals placed in custody while in treatment. Although full access to MMT programs (including initiation and maintenance) has been recommended by both professional and advocacy groups (Canadian HIV/AIDS Legal Network, 2008; RNAO, 2009), many jurisdictions do not allow for the initiation of MMT for individuals already in custody. MMT, like other harm-reduction strategies, is controversial. As of May 2012, 789 persons under federal custody (5.3% of the incarcerated population) were enrolled in an MMT (OCI, 2014). Unfortunately, the lack of understanding among many correctional staff members contributes to the belief that methadone administration simply replaces the illicit drug(s) taken prior to arrest. Correctional officers' concerns often stem from the fact that methadone is a highly valued commodity within correctional systems, which can lead to drug diversion attempts and to bullying for it. Consequently, the procedure for administration of methadone is tightly supervised, time consuming, and resource intense (OCI, 2014).

The RNAO (2009) outlines common MMT-related issues that are specific to correctional environments in its clinical best-practice guideline *Supporting Clients on Methadone Maintenance Treatment*. Correctional nurses are often challenged with balancing the goals of harm reduction and MMT with the goals of custody, and as such, this best-practice guideline is particularly noteworthy as it offers information related to the myths and perceptions regarding methadone, administration of methadone, discharge or release planning, and related issues specific to correctional environments. In a Canadian retrospective study designed to assess the impact of MMT on post-release recidivism among male federally incarcerated persons, MacSwain, Farrell-MacDonald, Cheverie, and Fischer (2014) found that persons who initiated MMT while incarcerated, and who continued with MMT as part of their transition to the community, had a 36% lower risk of returning to custody when compared to the other groups in the study (i.e., those who discontinued

MMT upon release, and a non-treated MMT control group). Such findings underscore the importance of correctional nurses collaborating with community-based partners to promote the successful reintegration of opioid-dependent persons upon release from custody. Community reintegration strategies, including intensive case management, may be required to facilitate positive treatment outcomes and successful reintegration.

There is no such thing as a drug-free prison (Independent Review of Corrections, 2017); correctional facilities are not immune to drug-related morbidity and mortality, and the fentanyl crisis (and fentanyl analogues) in correctional facilities continues to exert a heavy toll. Moreover, for incarcerated individuals and correctional staff alike, consumption of unknown strength and exposure of fentanyl (often laced with other harmful substances) during searches and emergency response can be deadly. Most Canadian correctional institutions are now equipped with nasal naloxone spray or injectable naloxone kits for emergency response. However, as late as November 2017, naloxone was not available in provincial correctional facilities in Manitoba, Quebec, and New Brunswick (Canadian Pharmacists Association, 2017). Since 2013, take-home naloxone kits have been provided free of charge for at-risk persons released from provincial custody through the Ontario Naloxone Program (Independent Review of Corrections, 2017). Following the success of a take-home naloxone pilot project for persons released from provincial correctional facilities in Alberta, a province-wide rollout has been implemented under the auspices of Alberta Health Services (Pijl, Bourque, Marens, & Cherniwchan, 2017). Correctional nurses and other health care professionals, together with community-based nonprofit organizations, can work collaboratively to provide awareness campaigns for incarcerated persons, including the dangers of lowered opioid tolerance and using drugs of unknown strength, particularly during the high-risk period following release from custody.

Infectious Diseases

The prevalence of blood-borne infections, STIs, and tuberculosis among offender populations is a real concern for correctional authorities. The prevalence of blood-borne infections such as HIV, HBV, and HCV are higher in the incarcerated population, primarily as a result of the high-risk behaviours engaged in before and during incarceration, such as non-sterile tattooing and piercing, intravenous drug use, and risky sexual activity. In comparison to nonincarcerated populations, HIV is estimated to be at least 10 times higher in incarcerated populations, while rates of HCV are at least 30 times higher. The picture is even more disconcerting for Indigenous women, where more than one in 10 women incarcerated in the federal system are living with HIV, and almost one in two live with HCV (van der Meulen & Ka Hon Chu, 2015). Treatment costs associated with HCV are staggering, yet the ethical and public health consequences of not treating are even more alarming and contribute to higher rates in the community upon eventual release. Although some progress has been made regarding PNSPs in

federal institutions, the rejection of harm-reduction strategies in general remains disconcerting. Harm-reduction programs, although endorsed by the health care community and advocacy groups, continue to be deemed controversial and subject to the political whim of governments, as was illustrated in the Conservative government's cancellation of the safe tattooing project that had been piloted in six federal correctional facilities. Re-instating safe tattooing as a national harm-reduction initiative in federal prisons is recommended in the most recent report of the OCI (2017). While other harm-reduction strategies such as condoms, dental dams, water-based lubricants, and bleach are generally available by request, sexual activity between incarcerated persons can result in a citation for misconduct. Consequently, many are ambivalent about requesting these products. On the one hand, they are being responsible by using coping mechanisms to prevent spread of disease; on the other hand, by merely requesting these products, they are risking misconduct. This is another example where correctional policies (e.g., custody) and health care interventions (e.g., caring) often collide.

CSC (2012a) reported that in 2007 and 2008, the number of reported infections of hepatitis B in federal facilities was 18 and 9, respectively. This corresponded to a 0.13% prevalence rate in 2007 and a 0.07% prevalence rate in 2008. In 2014, the prevalence of HCV in Canadian federal penitentiaries was 18.2%, a slight decrease from 2000, when the rate was 20.1%. The 2014 prevalence rate represented 96 persons who were diagnosed upon admission and another 63 who were diagnosed during their incarceration. HCV prevalence continues to be higher in adult women, a trend that has been previously reported. In 2015, 266 incarcerated individuals under federal jurisdiction started treatment for HCV (CSC, 2016a). HIV prevalence rates in federal facilities was 1.19% in 2014 (CSC, 2016b) and 1.2% in 2017 (Government of Canada, 2018). Similar to previous years, women had higher 2014 prevalence rates (1.14% for men and 2.49% for women). In 2014, 10 incarcerated persons under federal jurisdiction were HIV positive; five were newly diagnosed upon admission, and another five were diagnosed from the general incarcerated population (CSC, 2016b). However, as in the Canadian population, true prevalence rates are unknown because screening for HIV and other blood-borne infections is voluntary. Only 37% of new admissions in 2000 participated in testing for blood-borne illnesses, but by 2017, 96% were voluntarily tested (Government of Canada, 2018). Screening on admission and throughout incarceration represents a significant public health function, with personal health and treatment benefits upon diagnosis (Ha, Totten, Pogany, Wu, & Gale-Rowe, 2016).

CSC (2012a) released statistics on tuberculosis (TB) infection in its penitentiaries. In summary, participation in TB assessment is high (for a nine-year period, between 76.9% and 82% among incarcerated persons). The conversion rate for the TB skin test from a previous negative result consistently remained low over this same period—conversion rates were 1.49% in 2007 and 1.15% in 2008. The latent TB infection rate reduced to a rate of 16.6% in 2007 and 15.9% in 2008. Rates in men have been consistently higher over the years, as are rates in Indigenous and foreign-born incarcerated persons.

While the number of incarcerated individuals with latent TB infection has reduced over the years, the number of those on active treatment has increased. Between 1998 and 2014, 45 cases of active TB were reported (ranging from zero to six cases per year). In the latest report published by CSC, only three individuals had active TB disease in 2014 (CSC, 2017). TB in crowded correctional settings represents a public health challenge worldwide, and concerns regarding tuberculin skin test conversion among incarcerated persons and staff are of concern for provincial, territorial, and federal correctional authorities.

Nurses are often the first health care providers to assess incarcerated individuals for infectious diseases. This assessment is important in case finding and subsequent treatment. Nurses also implement infection control precautions to prevent subsequent infection of staff and other incarcerated individuals. Health education for incarcerated persons and all correctional employees on the prevention of infection transmission is a good example of a primary prevention strategy. Managing influenza outbreaks can be particularly challenging, and incarcerated individuals are especially vulnerable given conditions of overcrowding, coupled with the layering of acute and chronic health challenges. Besney and colleagues (2017) outlined the prevention, identification, and response to an influenza outbreak that occurred in a 2000-bed remand centre in Alberta that employed 900 staff members. By implementing control measures such as "enhanced isolation precautions, restricting admissions to affected living units, targeted vaccination and antiviral prophylaxis" (Besney et al., 2017, p. 1), the outbreak was restricted to six confirmed cases. Likewise, Sunil, Holt, Dixon, Dignman, and Noseworthy (2013) reported on a norovirus-like outbreak that occurred in a correctional facility in central east Ontario and illustrated the collaborative coordinated responses of the facility health and correctional staff and the local and provincial public health authorities.

Correctional nurses and infectious diseases nurses function within a very narrow margin when addressing staff members' "need to know" and incarcerated persons' right to confidentiality. Nurses cannot provide confidential information regarding diagnoses; however, they must educate and inform correctional staff of infection control and other health care procedures. The pressure from staff for confidential health care information will continue, as will the need for nurses to protect that confidentiality. In such cases, correctional nurses walk a thin and precarious line. Most nurses do find a way to provide health education to correctional staff and alleviate some of their work-related stress. For example, nurses can instruct correctional officers regarding the principles of harm reduction; the use of universal precautions; standard practices; airborne, droplet, and direct-contact isolation procedures; and the need for confidentiality in health-related matters.

PRACTICE SETTING

The impact of the correctional environment on both incarcerated persons and correctional nurses can be particularly severe given the interpersonal climate, organizational culture, and social context, which can severely impact the health status and quality of life for both. Power, control, and implicit authority are manifested in the physical and interpersonal environments of correctional systems and can be incompatible with the achievement of health-related treatment goals (Lazzaretto-Green et al., 2011). In order to develop therapeutic relationships and provide professional and ethical care, correctional nurses often are faced with confronting their own reactions to the alleged offences for which incarcerated persons have been charged or sentenced. It is important for nurses to see the person in their care as a person, and not the crime that was committed. It is also critical that they not get caught up in the sensationalism that surrounds a particular high-profile person (often dominating news programming) or the setting in which nursing practice takes place.

Nurses working with clients who are incarcerated "face significant challenges in regard to their ability to care in this **culture of incarceration**" (Christensen, 2014, p. 230). Access to clients can be difficult, depending on the mandate of the institution and the clients' specific health care needs. For instance, in many correctional facilities, individuals who are incarcerated are housed in units with two-person cells with a common day area; it is not uncommon, however, for areas of a facility to be repurposed as dormitories as a means to addressing overcrowding. Depending on the institution, incarcerated persons may be allowed out of their cells for up to 12 hours per day, and health care must be provided within this time frame. Assessment of health concerns and provision of minor interventions is often provided in the living unit and more complex care provided in a centralized ambulatory health care clinic within the institution. Correctional officers accompany and supervise nurses during their interactions with incarcerated persons, and officers must maintain visual contact at all times. Such security regulations, although appreciated, often result in nurses walking a fine line between maintaining client confidentiality, eliciting health-related information, and providing ethical nursing care.

The priorities of the correctional system focus on confinement and security, and matters of security will often take precedence over nursing care; it is not uncommon for nurses to have to wait while officers complete security-related tasks. As employees of correctional facilities, nurses must abide by the correctional policies that govern all correctional employees. As such, correctional nurses often find themselves in a "Catch-22" position as they face the competing tensions enmeshed in their collective responsibilities. Not only are they responsible to the incarcerated person, who is their client; they are also responsible to their profession, to the correctional system that is their employer, and to the community at large (Storch & Peternelj-Taylor, 2009). Although health care is often overshadowed by security and custodial concerns, as per the Mandela Rules, all health care professionals must be provided with "full clinical and professional independence" (UNGA, 2016). Consequently, correctional authorities must not interfere with or override the decisions of the health care team. Navigating such divergent responsibilities can be especially challenging for nurses who also depend on correctional staff for their personal safety should something untoward happen.

While professional autonomy in practice has often been described as a factor related to job satisfaction in correctional nurses in general (Punch, 2016), in practice this often means working alone, and professional isolation is a concern for correctional nurses. In some instances, there may only be one registered nurse on the day and evening shifts responsible for as many as 200 incarcerated persons. In a study exploring work-life issues experienced by nurses working in provincial correctional facilities in Ontario, Almost and colleagues (2013) found that, like nurses in other sectors, correctional nurses valued work environments that provided support for continuing education, positive work relationships, autonomy, control over nursing practice, and adequate staffing. Disconcertingly, they also reported that inadequate staffing, heavy workloads, limited control over their practice and scope of practice, limited resources, and challenging workplace relationships prevailed, which impacted their professional role development. These concerns also align with conclusions drawn from the Independent Review of Ontario Corrections (2017), specifically the importance of developing a sustainable, appropriately resourced, professional health care workforce that is prepared to meet the layered health care needs of incarcerated persons within institutions where competing tensions between health care and security often exist.

Regardless of the setting, the therapeutic treatment needs of incarcerated individuals must always be considered within the context of maintaining security; "the importance of balancing the need for safe custody on the one hand, and care and rehabilitation on the other" (Fraser, 2014, p. 185) cannot be underscored. For instance, nurses need to be ever vigilant regarding security awareness. This includes **static security**, the structural environmental features common to correctional facilities (e.g., video monitoring, internal barriers, perimeter fences or walls, personal protection alarms, staffing patterns, policies related to counts, and counting equipment), and **dynamic security**, which addresses such things as institutional policies and procedures related to interpersonal security (e.g., developing professional relationships, managing professional boundaries, "knowing" the client in one's care, and methods of operation). In order to practise safely in correctional settings, nurses need to be attentive to issues of both custody *and* caring. Nurses working in other community settings certainly understand the need for innovation; nurses working in correctional settings require similar "thinking outside the box."

COMMUNITY CONNECTIONS AND COLLABORATIONS

Increasingly, correctional facilities are being identified as a "public health opportunity." Yet the "very existence and continual expansion of correctional institutions is a striking example of society's failure to address complex health and social issues and to protect its most vulnerable members" (Peternelj-Taylor, 2003, p. 4). From a public health perspective, the health of the incarcerated population is a reflection of the state of health of the community at large. Incarcerated persons come to prison from the community, and they will return to the community

upon their release; in short, correctional health affects public health (Goshin, Colbert, & Carey, 2018). Correctional systems have a profound and complex effect on the health of families and communities, and effective partnerships can have a significant public health impact. Attending to the comprehensive needs of this population requires interdisciplinary and intersectoral collaboration between health care, criminal justice, education, social services, non-governmental organizations, and the voluntary sector. Furthermore, correctional nurses are in key positions to collaborate with staff in community-based residential facilities to ensure a safe release for incarcerated persons transitioning to the community. Organizations such as the St. Leonard's Society of Canada (and its affiliate members) and other not-for-profit charitable organizations such as the Mennonite Central Committee's Community Reintegration Project are excellent partners for correctional nurses as they work with preparing incarcerated persons for release into the community. Such partnerships need to be established, nurtured, and evaluated.

An important component of establishing community connections is listening to the voices of persons with the lived experience of being incarcerated. **Prisoner rights** groups in Canada such as the John Howard Society, Elizabeth Fry Society, West Coast Prison Justice Society, and Justice for Girls offer difficult yet crucial information about what life is like for incarcerated persons from their point of view. By being open to the critiques of a system they are working within, correctional nurses demonstrate their commitment to social justice. Recently, in an article in *Maclean's*, Canada's prisons were compared to residential schools for Indigenous peoples (Macdonald, 2016). Although this is an example of a difficult critique to process for correctional nurses, one of the most important contributions that correctional nurses can make is to think upstream by "tapping into [their] full potential to drive change for the most vulnerable" (Butterfield, 2017, p. 9) while being mindful of the factors that contribute to incarceration in the first place.

PROFESSIONAL DEVELOPMENT, ADVOCACY, AND RESEARCH IN CORRECTIONAL NURSING

Recognition of correctional nursing as a specialized area of nursing practice is critical to the ongoing growth and development of this specialty area. Prior to the 1960s very few nurses considered a career in correctional nursing. Since then, nurses have slowly and methodically pursued professional nursing practice in the correctional milieu, resulting in significant transformations in professional development. Correctional environments epitomize rich and fertile learning experiences, and the next generations of correctional nurses are increasingly being introduced to correctional nursing as students during their community health or mental health practicum placements. The essential role of nurses in the provision of health care in Canadian correctional systems underscores the importance of understanding their professional roles, responsibilities, and learning needs. (Refer to Canadian Research 26.1.)

CANADIAN RESEARCH 26.1

Saskatchewan Provincial Correctional Nurses: Roles, Responsibilities, and Learning Needs.
(Peternelj-Taylor & Woods, 2019)

The authors reported the results from a self-administered online survey that used two questionnaires to gain insight into the roles, responsibilities, and learning needs of nurses practicing in provincial correctional facilities in Saskatchewan. The study had four related research objectives:

- Describe the profile of Saskatchewan provincial correctional nurses (i.e., who they are).
- Explore their professional roles and responsibilities (i.e., what they do).
- Identify their unique learning needs required for continuing competence (i.e., what they need).
- Identify the contextual factors that influence their ability to work to their full scope of practice in providing evidence-informed care (i.e., what factors influence their professional roles).

Thirty-three respondents completed the questionnaires, for a 34.7% response rate. The nurses surveyed were highly experienced in nursing and correctional nursing. Respondents identified a number of learning needs that are aligned with their correctional nursing role and practice. Particularly important for professional development were mental health and disorder-related care issues such as assessment of self-harm, suicide, and mental health assessment more generally. Respondents also completed a 45-item questionnaire that targeted five skill sets relevant to their clinical practice: to (1) promote and implement principles that underpin effectiveness, quality, and practice; (2) assess, develop, implement, and improve programs of care for individuals; (3) create and maintain environments and relationships with individuals that value them as people and support their therapeutic roles; (4) provide and improve resources and services that facilitate organizational functioning; and (5) develop the knowledge, competency, and practice of self and other. Nurses were asked to rate their involvement and the importance of the skill set to their professional role; all nursing interventions were considered important to varying degrees. Finally, nurses talked about the importance of continuing education to their professional role development, yet due to fiscal restraints, they simply were expected "to do more with less." Findings from this study provide a strong foundation for continuing education, practice, and future research in correctional nursing.

Discussion Questions

1. Why are the learning needs identified in the study important for correctional nursing practice?
2. How might correctional nurses incorporate interventions from the five skill sets into their everyday practice as a way of supporting ongoing practice development?
3. Based on these findings, what areas for further research should be explored?

In 2005, the RNAO Correctional Nurses Interest Group, the first such group in Canada, was established by correctional nurses. In 2007, the Forensic Nurses Society of Canada was approved as an emerging special interest group of the CNA, representing all forensic nursing specialties, including correctional nursing. However, unlike the ANA (2013), which published *Corrections Nursing: Scope and Standards of Practice*, and the Royal College of Nursing (2009), which published *Health and Nursing Care in the Criminal Justice Service* and *Supporting Nursing Staff Caring for Patients from Places of Detention* (Royal College of Nursing, 2017), comparable nursing documents and standards to guide and direct nurses working in Canadian correctional facilities are nonexistent.

Correctional nurses, like all nurses, have a critical yet necessary role when it comes to advocating for criminal justice–involved populations—incarcerated individuals, their families, and communities. In general, the public has a less-than-sympathetic view of individuals who come into conflict with the law, and a "lock the door and throw away the key" mentality frequently prevails. Rarely is the context of a person's life truly taken into consideration in public conversations regarding crime and criminality. Instead, misguided beliefs equating imprisonment with community safety dominate contemporary discourse. As highlighted throughout this chapter, Canadian correctional nurses and their professional associations actively advocate for this highly vulnerable population through their contributions to matters of concern, including a detailed written submission to the segregation review conducted by the Ministry of Community Safety and Correctional Services (MCSCS) (RNAO, 2016a) and a letter to the Minister of the MCSCS regarding the urgent nursing shortage within corrections, including concerns regarding the ministry's ability to meet its fundamental responsibilities (RNAO, 2016b). In 2017, the RNAO and the Ontario Correctional Nurses' Interest Group participated in the MCSCS round table on corrections reform legislation and the exploration of other models of governance for correctional health care (RNAO, 2017). Correctional nurses' voices matter, and their contributions to healthy public policy extend well beyond prison walls.

The ongoing evolution of correctional nursing as a specialty is further dependent on the establishment of a nursing culture that supports and nurtures the development of nursing research. Nursing has a pivotal role to play in the translation and interpretation of research relevant to incarcerated populations and in the identification of emergent research questions from practice. Conducting research in correctional facilities, however, can be particularly challenging. There are unique issues to be considered when conducting research with incarcerated individuals; for example, ensuring that consent is free, informed, and given without expectation of special favours. Guidelines are in place that clearly prevent the offer of privileges, early release, or favourable parole assessments in return for participation in a research study while incarcerated (Peternelj-Taylor, 2005). Although correctional nursing has undergone significant transformations in professional role development in recent years, and a goldmine of research opportunities exist, the professional literature remains largely anecdotal, as correctional environments have attracted very few nurse researchers. An integrative review by Goshin and colleagues (2018) concluded that nurse-authored research is making important contributions to the identification and management of health disparities among criminal justice–involved people. However, gaps remain, particularly in the areas of alternatives to incarceration, transition programming, reproductive health and trauma-informed care, and explicitly connecting this important work with its human rights implications.

Since 1989, the College of Nursing, University of Saskatchewan, in collaboration with the Regional Psychiatric Centre (Prairies), CSC, has sponsored a biennial nursing conference that showcases the unique contributions nurses make to health care within criminal justice systems. This international forum provides opportunities for clinical practitioners, educators, administrators, researchers, and policy makers to learn about matters unique to correctional nursing, including innovative health care practices and the advancement of a nursing research agenda.

CASE STUDY

A 55-year-old male was transferred to a regional treatment centre of a federal penitentiary with end-stage liver failure. His family lives in another province and visit when they can. His pain needs are marginally addressed by the use of a fentanyl patch, which often "disappears" before the next patch change. His family indicated that they saw a news report on "compassionate release" of incarcerated persons in the United States and wondered if such options were available in Canada. Visiting has become a real hardship for the family, and they would like to care for him at home.

Discussion Questions

1. What are your thoughts, feelings, and beliefs about providing palliative care within the correctional milieu? What challenges might be encountered?
2. What barriers might be faced when an application for compassionate release is made?
3. What community-based resources are available in your area to assist with providing care for this person?

CONCLUSION

Correctional nursing, as a specialty area of practice, has undergone significant transformation in role development in recent years. Correctional nurses experience challenges unique to their roles, the persons for whom they provide care, and the environments in which they practise. Accepting the challenge to provide nursing care where health care delivery is not the primary goal can lead to a myriad of personal and professional issues for nurses. To be successful, nurses need to clearly understand their purpose—to provide competent nursing care—ever mindful of their ethical responsibilities. At the same time, they need to be cognizant of the security implications inherent in their professional roles and resist being co-opted by the custodial mandate inherent in correctional institutions. It is within this context

that the moral climate is shaped and embraced by correctional nurses. Custody and caring can co-exist, and nurses learn to traverse these competing demands. Correctional nursing is collaborative and interdisciplinary by its very nature; addressing the comprehensive needs of persons who find themselves enmeshed within the criminal justice system requires the enduring conviction that caring for incarcerated individuals is morally and professionally the right thing to do.

KEY TERMS

advocacy   (p. 471)
correctional nursing   (p. 471)
criminalization of the mentally ill   (p. 473)
culture of incarceration   (p. 481)
diversion programs   (p. 474)
dynamic security   (p. 482)
prison needle and syringe programs (PNSPs)   (p. 479)
prisoner rights   (p. 482)
static security   (p. 482)
trauma-informed approach   (p. 476)

STUDY QUESTIONS

1. What are the nursing implications associated with the implementation of a methadone maintenance treatment program within a correctional facility?
2. Discuss the reasons why correctional nurses often find themselves in a Catch-22 position when working with incarcerated persons in correctional settings.
3. What knowledge, skills, and abilities do nurses need to possess to be successful in their work in secure environments?
4. Increasingly, correctional facilities are being identified as a "public health opportunity." Discuss.
5. What issues need to be considered when implementing harm-reduction strategies in correctional facilities?

INDIVIDUAL CRITICAL-THINKING EXERCISES

1. Define "vulnerability" within the context of nursing research. How is this definition relevant to individuals who are incarcerated? What guidelines exist to protect incarcerated persons as research participants?
2. What would be the advantage of having standards for practice for Canadian nurses who work in correctional facilities?
3. If you were a correctional nurse in your community, what community-based organizations and resources would you collaborate with in meeting the needs of clients in your care?

GROUP CRITICAL-THINKING EXERCISES

1. Nurses who chose to work in correctional environments are often asked the following questions: "Why would you want to work there?" "How can you stand working with those

criminals?" "Aren't you afraid of getting hurt?" What are your initial thoughts about these questions? What do you think is behind such questions?

2. In comparison to other Western countries, Canadian statistics regarding youth incarceration, especially First Nation, Inuit, and Métis youth, are particularly alarming. What factors contribute to this phenomenon in Canada?

3. How would you describe contemporary public opinion regarding crime, criminality, and criminals?

REFERENCES

American Nurses Association. (2013). *Correctional nursing: Scope and standards of practice* (2nd ed.). Silver Spring, MD: Author.

Almost, J., Doran, D., Ogilvie, L., Miller, C., Kennedy, S., Timmings, C., . . . Bookey-Basset, S. (2013). Exploring work-life issues in provincial corrections settings. *Journal of Forensic Nursing, 9*, 3–13. doi: 10.1097/JFN.0b013e31827a5613

Besney, J., Moreau, D., Jacobs, A., Woods, D., Pyne, D., Joffe, A.M., & Ahmed, R. (2017). Influenza outbreak in a Canadian correctional facility. *Journal of Infection Prevention, 18*(4), 193–198. doi: 10.1177/1757177416689725

Blanchette, K., & Brown, S. L. (2006). *The assessment and treatment of women offenders: An integrative perspective.* Chichester, UK: John Wiley & Sons.

Brennan, S. (2014). Canada's mother-child program: Examining its emergence, usage, and current state. *Canadian Graduate Journal of Sociology & Criminology, 3*(1), 1–33. doi: http://dx.doi.org/10.15353/cgjsc-rcessc.v3il.84

Brown. G. P., Hirdes, J. P., & Fries, B. E. (2015). Measuring the prevalence of current, severe symptoms of mental health problems in a Canadian correctional population. *International Journal of Offender Therapy Comparative Criminology, 59*(1), 27–50. doi: 10.1177/0306624X13507040.

Burles, M., Peternelj-Taylor, C., & Holtslander, L. (2016). A "good death" for all? Examining issues for palliative care in correctional settings. *Mortality, 21*(2), 93–111. doi:10.1080/13576275.2015.1098602

Butterfield, P. G. (2017). Thinking upstream: A 25-year retrospective and conceptual model aimed at reducing health inequities. *Advances in Nursing Science, 40*(1), 2–11. doi: 10.1097/ANS0000000000000161

Canadian HIV/AIDS Legal Network. (2008). *Opioid substitution therapy in prisons: Reviewing the evidence.* Retrieved from http://www.aidslaw.ca/site/wp-content/uploads/2013/04/OST_brief_08-EN.pdf

Canadian HIV/AIDS Legal Network. (2010). *Under the skin: A people's case for prison needle and syringe programs.* Retrieved from http://www.pasan.org/Toolkits/Under_the_Skin.pdf

Canadian HIV/AIDS Legal Network. (2018, May 14). *Statement: Advocates welcome major concessions in Government of Canada's prison needle exchange announcement.* Retrieved from http://www.aidslaw.ca/site/advocates-welcome-major-concessions-in-government-of-canadas-prison-needle-exchange-announcement/?lang=en

Canadian Nurses Association (CNA). (2016). *Focus on harm reduction for injection drug use in Canadian prisons: A supplement to CNA's harm reduction discussion paper.* Retrieved from https://www.cna-aiic.ca/~/media/cna/page-content/pdf-en/cna-harm-reduction-in-canadas-prisons-a-companion-document.pdf?la=en

Canadian Nurses Association (CNA). (2017, January 5). *Nursing coalition granted intervener status in Superior Court case to support clean needle programs in prisons.* Retrieved from https://www.cna-aiic.ca/en/news-room/news-releases/2017/nursing-coalition-granted-intervener-status-in-superior-court-case-to-support-clean-needle-programs-in-prisons

Canadian Pharmacists Association. (2017). *Environmental scan: Access to naloxone across Canada.* Ottawa, ON: Author.

Chaimowitz, G. (2012). Position Paper: The criminalization of people with mental illness. *The Canadian Journal of Psychiatry, 57*(2), Insert 1–6.

Christensen, S. (2014). Enhancing nurses' ability to care within the culture of incarceration. *Journal of Transcultural Nursing, 25*(3), 223–231. doi:10.1177/1043659613515276

Clark, N., Dolan, K., & Farabee, D. (2017). Public health alternatives to incarceration for drug offenders. *Eastern Mediterranean Health Journal, 23*(3), 222–230.

Community Health Nurses of Canada. (2019, revised). *Canadian community health nursing. Professional practice model & standards of practice.* St. John's, NL: Author.

Corrado, R. R., Kuehn, S., & Margaritescu, I. (2014). Policy issues regarding the over-representation of incarcerated Aboriginal young offenders in a Canadian context. *Youth Justice, 14*(1), 40–62. doi:10.1177/1473225413520361

Correctional Service Canada. (2012a). *Infectious diseases surveillance in Canadian federal penitentiaries 2007–2008.* Retrieved from http://www.csc-scc.gc.ca/publications/005007-7602-eng.shtml

Correctional Service Canada. (2012b). *Mental health strategy for corrections in Canada: Federal-Provincial-Territorial Partnership.* Retrieved from http://www.csc-scc.gc.ca/health/092/MH-strategy-eng.pdf

Correctional Service Canada. (2016a). *Infectious diseases surveillance 2014: Hepatitis C Virus (HCV).* Ottawa, ON: Author. Retrieved from http://www.csc-scc.gc.ca/publications/092/005007-3038-eng.pdf

Correctional Service Canada. (2016b). *Infectious diseases surveillance 2014: Human immunodeficiency virus (HIV).* Ottawa, ON: Author. Retrieved from http://www.csc-scc.gc.ca/publications/092/005007-3035-eng.pdf

Correctional Service Canada. (2017). *Infectious diseases surveillance 2014: Active tuberculosis.* Ottawa, ON: Author. Retrieved from http://www.csc-scc.gc.ca/publications/092/005007-3040-eng.pdf

Correctional Service Canada. (2018). *Institutional mother-child program.* Retrieved from http://www.csc-scc.gc.ca/politiques-et-lois/768-cd-eng.shtml

Donelle, L., & Hall, J. (2016). Health promotion body maps of criminalized women. *Journal of Correctional Health Care, 22*(4), 331–341. doi: 10.1177/1078345816669963.

Elizabeth Fry Society. (2013). *Women don't belong in cages.* Retrieved from http://www.caefs.ca/wp-content/uploads/2013/04/poster.jpg

Fazel, S., Hayes, A. J., Bartellas, K., Clerici, M., & Trestman, R. (2016). Mental health of prisoners: Prevalence, adverse outcomes, and interventions. *Lancet Psychiatry, 3*(9), 871–881. doi: 10.1016/S2215-0366(16)30142-0

Fazel, S., & Seewald, K. (2012). Severe mental illness in 33,588 prisoners worldwide: Systematic review and meta-regression analysis. *British Journal of Psychiatry, 200*(5), 364–373. doi:10.1192/bjp.bp.111.096370

Ferszt, G. G., Hickey, J. E., & Seleyman, K. (2013). Advocating for pregnant women in prison: The role of the correctional nurse. *Journal of Forensic Nursing, 9*(2), 108–110. doi:10.1097/JFN.0b013e318281056b

Fisher, A. A., & Hatton, D. C. (2009). Women prisoners: Health issues and nursing implications. *Nursing Clinics of North America, 44*(3), 365–373. doi:10.1016/j.cnur.2009.06.010

Fraser, A. (2014). Staff health and well-being in prisons: Leadership and training. In S. Enggist, L. Møller, G. Galea, & C. Udesen (Eds.) *Prisons and health* (pp. 185–189). Copenhagen, Denmark: World Health Organization. Retrieved from http://www.euro.who.int/__data/assets/pdf_file/0005/249188/Prisons-and-Health.pdf.

Gaston, S. (2017). Vulnerable prisoners: Dementia and the impact on prisoners, staff and the correctional setting. *Collegian*, http://dx.doi.org/10.1016/j.colegn.2017.05.004

Goshin L. S., Colbert, A. M., & Carey, J. F. (2018). An integrative review of nurse-authored research to improve health equity and human rights for criminal justice involved people. *Journal of Forensic Nursing, 14*(2), 53–60. doi: 10.1097/JFN0000000000000193

Government of Canada. (2018, May 14). *Backgrounder: Correctional Service Canada Prison Needle Exchange Program.* Retrieved from https://www.canada.ca/en/correctional-service/news/2018/05/backgrounder-correctional-service-canada-prison-needle-exchange-program.html

Green, C. R., Cook, J. L., Stewart, M., & Salmon, A. (2016). *FASD and the criminal justice system.* Canada FASD Research Network. Retrieved from http://canfasd.ca/wp-content/uploads/sites/35/2016/05/FASD-and-Justice-Nov-16.pdf

Green, S., Foran, J., & Kouyoumdjian, F. G. (2016). Access to primary care in a provincial correctional facility in Ontario, *BMC Research Notes, 9*, 131. doi: 10.1186/s13104-016-1935-4

Griel, L. C., & Loeb, S. J. (2009). Health issues faced by adolescents incarcerated in the juvenile justice system. *Journal of Forensic Nursing, 5*, 162–179. doi: 10.1111/j.1939-3938.2009.01049.x

Ha, S., Totten, S., Pogany, L., Wu, J., & Gale-Rowe, M. (2016). Hepatitis C in Canada and the importance of risk-based screening. *Canadian Communicable Disease Report, 42*, 57–62.

Harris, K. (2017, July 21). In historic 1st, transgender inmate wins transfer to women's prison. Canadian Broadcasting Corporation. Retrieved from http://www.cbc.ca/news/politics/fallon-aubee-transgender-inmate-1.4215594.

Hayes, A. J., Burns, A., Turnbull, P., & Shaw, J. J. (2012). The health and social needs of older male prisoners. *International Journal of Geriatric Psychiatry, 217*, 1155–1162. doi: 10.1002/gps.3761

Human Rights Watch. (2012). *Old behind bars: The aging prison population in the United States.* Retrieved from http://www.hrw.org/sites/default/files/reports/usprisons0112webw-cover_0.pdf

Hyatt, A. (2013). Healing through culture for incarcerated Aboriginal people. *First Peoples Child & Family Review: An Interdisciplinary Journal, 8*(2), 40–53.

Independent Review of Ontario Corrections. (2017). *Corrections in Ontario: Directions for reform.* Retrieved from https://www.mccs.jus.gov.on.ca/sites/default/files/content/mcscs/docs/Corrections%20in%20Ontario%2C%20Directions%20for%20Reform.pdf

Kelsey, C. M., Medel, N., Mullins, C., Dallaire, D., & Froestell, C. (2017). An examination of care practices of pregnant women incarcerated in jail facilities in the United States. *Maternal Child Health Journal, 21,* 1260–1266. doi: 10.1007/s10995-016-2224-5

Kirmayer, L. J., Brass, G. M., & Tait, C. L. (2000). The mental health of Aboriginal peoples: Transformations of identity and community. *Canadian Journal of Psychiatry, 45*(7), 607–616.

Kouyoumdjian, F., Schuler, A., Matheson, F. I., & Hwang, S. W. (2016). Health status of prisoners in Canada. *Canadian Family Physician, 62*, 215–222.

Lazzaretto-Green, D., Austin, W., Goble, E., Buys, L., Gorman, T., & Rankel, M. (2011). Walking a fine line: Forensic mental health practitioners' experience of working with correctional officers. *Journal of Forensic Nursing, 7*, 109–119. doi: 10.111/j.1939-3938.2011.01107.x

Loeb, S. J. (2013). Shifting institutions. Preparing for transfers from prison to long-term care facilities. *Journal of Gerontological Nursing, 39*(6), 2–3. doi:3928/00989134-20130318-01

Loeb, S. J., Penrod, J., McGhan, G., Kitt-Lewis, E., & Hollenbeak, C. (2014). Who wants to die in here?: Perspectives of prisoners with chronic conditions. *Journal of Hospice & Palliative Care Nursing, 16*(3), 173–181. doi: 10.1097/NJH.0000000000000044

Macdonald, N. (2016, February 18). Canada's prisons are the new "residential schools." *Maclean's.* Retrieved from http://www.macleans.ca/news/canada/canadas-prisons-are-the-new-residential-schools.

MacSwain, M. A., Farrell-MacDonald, S., Cheverie, M., & Fischer, B. (2014). Assessing the impact of methadone maintenance on post-release recidivism among male federal correctional inmates in Canada. *Criminal Justice and Behaviour, 41*(3), 380–394. doi:10.1177/0093854813501495

Malakieh, J. (2017). Youth correctional statistics in Canada, 2015/2016. *Juristat* (No. 85-002-X). Ottawa, ON: Canadian Centre for Justice Statistics.

Marotta, P. L. (2017). Childhood adversities and substance misuse among the incarcerated: Implications for treatment and practice in correctional settings. *Substance Use & Misuse, 52*(6), 717–733.

Mason, R. (2010, March). Aboriginal correctional programs. *Let's Talk, 34*(2), 10.

Mental Health Commission of Canada. (2012). *Changing directions, changing lives: The mental health strategy for Canada.* Retrieved from https://www.mentalhealthcommission.ca/sites/default/files/mhstrategy_strategy_eng.pdf

Mochama, V. (2018, January 4). Treatment of women in Canadian prisons a human rights travesty. *The Star.* Retrieved from https://www.thestar.com/opinion/star-columnists/2018/01/04/treatment-of-women-in-canadian-prisons-a-human-rights-travesty.html

Mollard, E., & Hudson, D. B. (2016). Nurse-led trauma-informed correctional care for women. *Perspectives in Psychiatric Care, 52*, 224–230. doi: 10.1111/ppc.12122

Nolan, A. M., & Stewart, L. A. (2017). Chronic health conditions among incoming Canadian federally sentenced women. *Journal of Correctional Health Care, 23*(1), 93–103. doi: 10.1177/10783458|6685707

Office of the Correctional Investigator. (2012). *Annual report of the Office of the Correctional Investigator 2011–2012.* (No. PS100-2012E-PDF). Ottawa, ON: Her Majesty the Queen in Right of Canada.

Office of the Correctional Investigator. (2013). *Annual report of the Office of the Correctional Investigator 2012–2013.* (No. PS100-2013E-PDF). Ottawa, ON: Her Majesty the Queen in Right of Canada.

Office of the Correctional Investigator. (2014). *Annual report of the Office of the Correctional Investigator 2013–2014.* (No. PS100-2014E-PDF). Ottawa, ON: Her Majesty the Queen in Right of Canada.

Office of the Correctional Investigator. (2016). *Annual report of the Office of the Correctional Investigator 2015–2016.* (No. PS100E-PDF). Ottawa, ON: Her Majesty the Queen in Right of Canada.

Office of the Correctional Investigator. (2017). *Annual report of the Office of the Correctional Investigator 2016–2017,* No. PS100. Ottawa, ON: Her Majesty the Queen in Right of Canada.

Peacock, S., Hodson, A., MacRae, R., & Peternelj-Taylor, C. (2018). Living with dementia in correctional settings. *Journal of Forensic Nursing, 14*(3), 180–184.

Perry, C. W., & Morris, R. E. (2014). Health care for youth involved with the correctional system. *Primary Care, 41*(3), 691–705. doi:10.1016/j.pop.2014.05.007

Peternelj-Taylor, C. (2003). Incarceration of vulnerable populations. *Journal of Psychosocial Nursing and Mental Health Services, 41*(9), 4–5.

Peternelj-Taylor, C. (2005). Conceptualizing nursing research with offenders: Another look at vulnerability. *International Journal of Law and Psychiatry, 28,* 348–359.

Peternelj-Taylor, C., & Woods, P. (2019, in press). Saskatchewan provincial correctional nurses: Roles, responsibilities, and learning needs. *Journal of Correctional Health Care, 25*(2).

Pijl, E. M., Bourque, S., Martens, M., & Cherniwchan, A. (2017). Take home naloxone kit distribution: A pilot project involving people who use drugs and who are newly released from a correctional facility. *Canadian Journal of Criminology and Criminal Justice, 59*(4), 559–571. doi: 10.3138/cjccj.2017.0001.R2

Power, J., & Riley, D. (2010). A comparative review of suicide and self-injury investigative reports in a Canadian federal correctional population. *Research at a Glance.* Retrieved from http://www.csc-scc.gc.ca/005/008/092/005008-0221-eng.pdf

Power, J., Brown, S. L., & Usher, A. M. (2013). Non-suicidal self-injury in women offenders: Motivations, emotions, and precipitating events. *International Journal of Forensic Mental Health, 12*(3), 192–204. doi:10.1080/14999013.2013.832442

Public Safety Canada. (2015). *Substance abuse.* Retrieved from https://www.publicsafety.gc.ca/cnt/cntrng-crm/crrctns/sbstnc-bs-en.aspx

Punch, D. (2016). Better health behind bars. *Registered Nurse Journal, 28*(3), 10–13, 26.

Registered Nurses' Association of Ontario. (2009). *Supporting clients on methadone maintenance treatment.* Toronto, ON: Author.

Registered Nurses' Association of Ontario, (2016a, February 22). *Transforming Ontario's correctional services: Starting, but not stopping, with segregation. Written Submission to the Segregation Review conducted by the Ministry of Community Safety and Correctional Services.* Retrieved from http://rnao.ca/sites/rnao-ca/files/RNAO_submission_segregation_Feb_22_2016.pdf

Registered Nurses Association of Ontario. (2016b, December 22). *Addressing urgent nursing staffing shortages within corrections.* Retrieved from http://rnao.ca/policy/letters/addressing-nursing-staffing-shortages-within-correction

Registered Nurses Association of Ontario. (2017, July 28). *RNAO's feedback on strengthening legislation to enable correctional reform.* Toronto, ON: Author.

Reitano, J. (2017). Adult correctional statistics in Canada, 2015/2016. *Juristat* (No. 85-002-X). Ottawa, ON: Canadian Centre for Justice Statistics.

Roth, B., & Pressé, L. (2003). Nursing interventions for para-suicidal behaviors in female offenders. *Journal of Psychosocial Nursing and Mental Health Services, 41*(9), 20–29.

Rowan, J., Auger, S., Toto, H., Simpson, S., & McNab, C. (2004). The use of stories for healing interventions with women. *Forum on Corrections Research, 16*(1), 42–44.

Royal College of Nursing. (2009). *Health and nursing care in the criminal justice service.* London, UK: Author.

Royal College of Nursing. (2017). *Supporting nursing staff caring for patients from places of detention.* London, UK: Author.

Sabramanian, R., Delaney, R., Roberts, S., Fishman, N., & McGarry, P. (2015). *Incarceration's front door: The misuse of jails in America.* New York, NY: Vera Institute of Justice.

Shelton, D., Weiskopf, C., & Nicholson, M. (2010). Correctional nursing competency development in the Connecticut Correctional Managed Health Care Program. *Journal of Correctional Health Care, 16*(4), 299–309. doi:10.1177/1078345810378498

Storch, J., & Peternelj-Taylor, C. (2009). Ethics for health care providers: Codes as guidance for practice in prisons. In D. Hatton & A. Fisher (Eds.), *Women prisoners and health justice* (pp. 109–116). Oxford, UK: Radcliffe.

Sunil, V., Holt, A. M., Dixon, R., Dingman, D., & Noseworthy, A. L. (2013). Norovirus-like virus outbreak in a correctional facility in Haliburton Kawartha Pine Ridge District Health Unit, March to April 2008. *Journal of Correctional Healthcare, 19,* 269–277. doi:10.1177/1078345813499311

Truth and Reconciliation Commission of Canada. (2015). *Truth and Reconciliation Commission of Canada: Calls to action.* Retrieved from http://www.trc.ca/websites/trcinstitution/File/2015/Findings/Calls_to_Action_English2.pdf.

United Nations General Assembly. (2016). *Resolution adopted by the General Assembly on 17 December 2015. United Nations standard minimum rules for the treatment of prisoners (the Nelson Mandela Rules).* Retrieved from https://www.penalreform.org/wp-content/uploads/1957/06/ENG.pdf

Uzoaba, J. H. E. (1998). Managing older offenders: Where do we stand? Correctional Service Canada. Retrieved from http://www.csc-scc.gc.ca/research/092/r70_e.pdf

van den Bergh, B. J., Gatherer, A., Fraser, A., & Moller, L. (2011). Imprisonment and women's health: Concerns about gender sensitivity, human rights and public health. *Bulletin of the World Health Organization, 89*(9), 889–994.

van der Meulen, E., & Ka Hon Chu, S. (2015). Harm reduction behind bars: Prison based needle and syringe programs. *CATIE: Canada's Source for HIV and Hepatitis C Information.* Retrieved from http://www.catie.ca/en/pif/spring-2015/harm-reduction-behind-bars-prison-based-needle-and-syringe-programs

van der Meulen, E., Claivaz-Loranger, S., Clarke, S., Ollner, A., & Watson, T. M. (2016). *On point: Recommendations for prison-based needle and syringe programs in Canada.* Toronto, ON. Retrieved from http://www.aidslaw.ca/site/download/13446

Ventriglio, A., Gentile, A., Bonfitto, I., Stella, E., Mari, M., Steardo, L., & Bellomo, A. (2016). Suicide in the early stage of schizophrenia. *Frontiers in Psychiatry, 7,* 116. doi:10.3389/fpsyt.2016.00116

Williams, B. A., Stern, M. F., Mellow, J., Safer, M., & Greifinger, R. B. (2012). Aging in correctional custody: Setting a policy agenda for older prisoner health care. *American Journal of Public Health, 102*(8), 1475–1481. doi:10.2105/AJPH.2012.300704

World Health Organization. (2007). *Preventing suicide in jails and prisons.* Retrieved from http://www.who.int/mental_health/prevention/suicide/resource_jails_prisons.pdf

ABOUT THE AUTHORS

Cindy Peternelj-Taylor, RN, BScN, MSc (University of Saskatchewan), is a professor with the College of Nursing, University of Saskatchewan; a Distinguished Fellow—International Association of Forensic Nurses; and Editor-in-Chief, *Journal of Forensic Nursing.* Much of Cindy's career has focused on professional and ethical role development for nurses who work with vulnerable populations in forensic psychiatric and correctional settings.

Phil Woods, RPN, PhD (Anglia Polytechnic University), is a professor and associate dean with the College of Nursing, University of Saskatchewan. He trained as a mental health nurse in the United Kingdom and is a registered psychiatric nurse in Saskatchewan. Phil's portfolio of research on risk assessment and management, violence prediction, and developing mental health and forensic mental health practice can be found in related journals and books.

Ecological Determinants of Health and Environmental Health Inequities

Andrea Chircop

CHAPTER 27

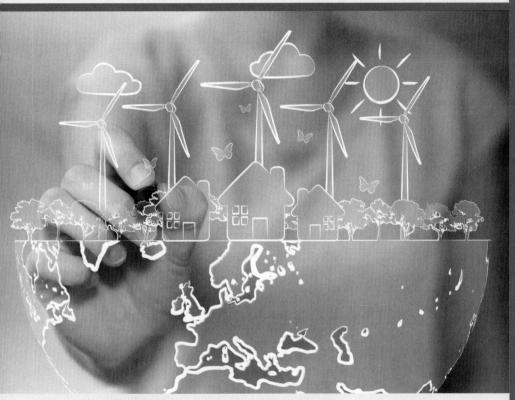

Source: Sdecoret/Shutterstock

INTRODUCTION

The **ecological determinants of health** are necessary to sustain all life forms on Earth. Simply put, without clean air, water, and soil to grow food, humans and other forms of life are not viable. Today, we understand the ecological determinants of health to include resources and ecological processes that are fundamental to all life. Leading scholars agree we have entered the age of the Anthropocene, a period in Earth's evolution that has seen the significant impact of human activity on the environment to such an extent that some of the ecological determinants are threatened (EcoWatch, 2016; Myers, 2017). The good news is we have also witnessed some positive change; for example, some rivers, including the Thames in London, England, that were heavily polluted, have been cleaned up (Hardach, 2015). Grassroots community action has been successful in cleaning up toxic sites. One example of a cleanup initiative is the Sydney tar ponds in Cape Breton, Nova Scotia (CBC, 2013). Another is the hole in the ozone, which has shrunk to its smallest size since 1988, largely by banning ozone-depleting chemicals (NASA, 2017; Ripple et al., 2017).

LEARNING OUTCOMES

After studying this chapter, you should be able to:

1. Recognize how ecological determinants of health are fundamental to all life on the planet.

2. Explain how social and geopolitical locations can contribute to environmental health inequities.

3. Identify major issues of global change.

4. Identify frameworks for approaches to planetary health and environmental health equity.

5. Describe primordial, primary, secondary, tertiary, and quaternary prevention roles of community health nurses as they relate to the ecological determinants of health and environmental health equity.

In Canada we have inspiring models of how our relationship as humans with non-human life can be respectful and sustainable in the rich histories and philosophies of traditional Indigenous wisdom. It is important to recognize that the environment does not affect all human and other life equally. Rather, much of the unequal distribution of resources for healthy living has been socially created and facilitated by a logic of domination—a logic that falsely legitimizes oppression and exploitation of nature and marginalizes people, politically and economically, at the same time (Chircop, 2008; Warren, 2000). As health care professionals, we need to recognize the relationships between powerful and dominant groups in society that have contributed to, and benefit from, environmental exploitation and social inequities. Moreover, it is a matter of intergenerational justice that community health nurses (CHNs) collaborate with other health care professionals and communities to provide stewardship for the preservation and protection of the ecological determinants of health for future generations.

The aim of this chapter is to introduce ecological determinants of health by highlighting some pressing issues of **global change** and, through a social justice lens, to identify concerns of **environmental health inequities**. Selected frameworks that offer explanations for conceptualizing our interactions with the ecological determinants of health are suggested, and nursing practice examples are highlighted.

THE ECOLOGICAL DETERMINANTS OF HEALTH

The ecological determinants of health comprise interacting ecosystems of Earth's atmosphere, oceans, and terrestrial surfaces, or the "natural goods and services" that are essential for life on our planet. In addition to oxygen, clean water, and soil, we depend on resources for energy and materials for shelter. We depend on ecological systems, including the ozone layer, to protect us from harmful ultraviolet rays; clean oceans and marine systems to provide food; natural systems to detoxify waste; and a stable climate that can sustain life globally (Hancock et al., 2015; Myers, 2017). The ecological determinants of health are non-negotiable (Parks, 2011).

The Lancet Commission on pollution and health (Landrigan et al., 2017) recognizes the interconnections between pollution-related global change and the attainment of the United Nations Sustainable Development Goals, in that pollution control will help alleviate poverty. The Commission states:

> Environmental injustice is the inequitable exposure of poor, minority, and disenfranchised populations to toxic chemicals, contaminated air and water, unsafe workplaces and other forms of pollution, and the consequent disproportionate burden among these populations of pollution-related diseases, often in violation of their human rights. (Landrigan et al., 2017, p. 27)

Indigenous Traditional Knowledge about ecosystems is closely linked to land and place of community, and as such it is diverse and reflects the diversity of Indigenous people around the world (Hatcher, Bartlett, Marshall, &

Marshall, 2009). The ancestral relationship with the land has given Indigenous peoples unique insights called **Traditional Ecological Knowledge and Wisdom (TEKW)** based on beliefs and traditional practices in relation to the natural environment (Turner, Boelscher Ignace, & Ignace, 2000). This dynamic, embodied knowledge has been handed down through oral tradition for generations and acquired through life experiences by being part of an ecosystem while observing, feeling, tasting, breathing, and listening (Lefale, 2010). TEKW has been recognized and acknowledged by several international organizations, including the United Nations, for its importance in understanding and interacting with our environment. Global change, however, threatens the survival of TEKW, due to displacement of Indigenous peoples and animals and to global warming in the Arctic and Pacific (Lafale, 2010; Turner et al., 2000).

ENVIRONMENTAL HEALTH INEQUITIES

Our planet's ecological systems are threatened by human action, brought about by unprecedented forces, including **climate change**, **pollution**, **resource depletion**, **marine degradation**, and **population growth** (Hancock et al., 2015). It is estimated that nearly 25% of the global disease burden is attributable to **environmental risks** such as air and water pollution (Prüss-Ustün et al., 2016). Not all people and societies have contributed equally to global change, and not everyone is equally affected. In Canada it is recognized that children, older adults, and First Nation, Metis, and Inuit communities are particularly vulnerable to environmental health inequities (Assembly of First Nations, 2009; Health Canada, 2017). For example, children are more susceptible to residential use of pesticide exposure than adults; older adults are more vulnerable to weather events such as heat waves; and Indigenous communities are vulnerable due to inadequate housing that can expose them to overcrowding, mould, or unsafe drinking water.

Global change phenomena, including climate change, pollution, resource depletion, marine degradation, and overpopulation, are interconnected with the social determinants of health through governance and upstream decisions that perpetuate the exploitation of natural resources and the oppression and domination of less powerful groups in society, leading to environmental health inequities. The environment affects people differently depending in part on geographic and geopolitical location, and social location along axes of gender, race and ethnicity, socioeconomic status, occupation, and developmental stage.

Geographic and Geopolitical Location

People living in the Arctic, the Niagara region, the Rocky Mountains, or coastal communities of the Pacific and Atlantic oceans are exposed to vastly different physical environments and climates. Different geographic locations provide different contexts for everyday life, including variations in temperature, seasons, water supplies, vegetation, agricultural, fishing and foraging opportunities, air quality, wildlife, and plant ecosystems.

Differences also exist depending on geopolitical location—whether people live in countries that have adopted progressive climate change policies or environmental policies that aim to prevent the extinction of endangered species, that adhere to environmental impact assessments, that set stringent standards for the chemical industry and consumer health protection. People are exposed to different political environments that aim to regulate environmental and social policies for the benefit of human and non-human life. For example, some policies regulate air pollution from the burning of fossil fuels, or soil and water pollution from mining industries. Other regulations deal with the application of pesticides on agricultural products. Today, the most heavily polluted regions on Earth are Southeast Asia and the western Pacific (Landrigan et al., 2017). Both regions have emerging global economies with a growing new middle-class that aspires to a Western lifestyle of consumerism that is very resource and energy intensive and as such will contribute to increased greenhouse gas emissions (World Economic Outlook, 2008). Ironically, post-industrial countries like Canada and other G7 countries that were historically the major polluters during the industrial period managed to reduce their greenhouse gas emissions from industry and automobile traffic to varying degrees (Aden, 2016; Eurostat, 2017). This is due in part to international agreements (Climate Action Tracker, 2017) that lead to the adoption of more stringent environmental policies for emission controls, facilitated by new technologies and a change in consumer practices (European Commission, 2017; Eurostat, 2017). However, there may have also been a relocation of greenhouse gas–emitting industries from post-industrial to industrial countries (Aden, 2016).

Further, political boundaries do not always align with natural or ecosystem boundaries. For example, natural ecosystems such as the Arctic or the Great Lakes regions in North America are divided by the political boundary between Canada and the United States, two countries with different environmental and social policies. Yet certain species, such as the North Atlantic right whale, may have their habitat in areas that span national borders that do not align with ecosystem boundaries. The unequal causes and effects of climate change and pollution are further illustrations of how geopolitical boundaries are not synchronized with ecosystems. For example, Inuit in the Arctic are negatively affected by climate change because the melting of ice caps and permafrost interferes with their livelihoods, preventing them from travelling over the ice for hunting and fishing; yet they have not benefitted equally from industries farther south that have contributed to climate change (McClymont Peace & Myers, 2012). In addition, **persistent organic pollutants (POPs)**, harmful chemicals produced by industries around the Great Lakes region of North America, have been found in the breastmilk of Inuit women (Kristensen et al., 2016). "POPs are chemicals of global concern due to their potential for long-range transport, persistence in the environment, ability to bio-magnify and bio-accumulate in ecosystems, as well as their significant

negative effects on human health and the environment" (World Health Organization [WHO], 2017a, p. 1).

In general, people do not or cannot always choose where to grow up and live, and clearly their location geographically and geopolitically has an impact on their health and well-being. As social human beings, we are always exposed to both the physical and social environment at the same time, and mechanisms underlying environmental health inequities are complex and often related to social location and the intersections of gender, race and ethnicity, and socioeconomic status.

Social Location

Social location refers to your place or position in society and has an impact on your access to a clean environment and how much, if any, control you have over that environment. Whether you identify as woman, man, LGBTQ2S, a child, or an older adult, or as a member of a certain ethnic or religious group will have an impact on your location of power and privilege within a given society and your access to the ecological determinants of health. Norms and expectations about the roles of women and men in society differ around the globe. Globally, however, health inequities for women persist, particularly for women disadvantaged by various forms of oppression (Morrow, Hankivsky, & Varcoe, 2007). Child rearing, childcare, and care of older adults largely remain roles for women in most societies.

Women take on different social roles and responsibilities that expose them to different environments, potentially leading to negative health outcomes. For example, responsibilities for child and older adult care may confine women to a domestic environment with higher exposure to various indoor air pollutants from cooking with woodstoves, particularly in resource-poor countries, or chemical cleaning products. In many regions of the world, domestic roles are carried out by women and girls, including the carrying of fresh water from wells to homes, which can take up considerable time that could otherwise be spent on schoolwork (WHO, 2010). Personal hygiene is a significant factor for many girls and women in resource-poor countries without proper toilets or running water, which is particularly challenging during menstruation, keeping women and girls confined to the home (WHO, 2010).

As much as poverty has been recognized as a leading determinant of health inequities (Raphael, 2016), it can also operate as a determinant of environmental health inequities, particularly as it intersects with gender and race or ethnicity (Chircop, 2008, 2012). Pollution-related diseases are much higher among the poor and contribute to the perpetuation of intergenerational poverty (Landrigan et al., 2017). People who live in poverty have less material resources to enable them to avoid harmful environmental exposure. In Canada, poverty is concentrated in certain geographic locations, and evidence suggests that people in some neighbourhoods are healthier than others. From a population health perspective, in Canada the majority of people living in poverty are women, specifically single-parenting mothers and their children (Statistics Canada, 2017). When ethnicity or race and socioeconomic status intersect with gender, the negative health outcomes worsen (Employment and Social Development Canada, 2017). Low-income neighborhoods can expose residents to inadequate housing, leading to negative health outcomes such as depression and exposure to lead, pesticides, moulds, noise, and unintentional injuries (Chircop, 2012; WHO, 2010).

Indigenous peoples in Canada are among the most affected by environmental injustice due to structural racism that exposes their communities disproportionately to pollution-related morbidity, in addition to the pollution of their land and waters, which are crucial to maintaining their traditional ways of life and the protection of natural ecosystems (Downing & Cuerrier, 2011; Landrigan et al., 2017). For decades, several First Nation communities in Canada have not had clean and safe drinking water, unlike most non-Indigenous communities (Bradford, Okpalauwaekwe, Waldner, & Bharadwaj, 2016; Sarkar, Hanrahan, & Hudson, 2015). Health concerns related to unsafe drinking water include gastrointestinal infections, birth defects, cancer, and mental stress (Bradford et al., 2016).

The contamination of traditional food sources with POPs caused by distant industries farther south is a prime example of environmental injustice. For centuries, Inuit and Northern First Nation communities used their local wildlife and fish as traditional food sources, which kept them healthy for generations. By continuing to eat traditional food that is contaminated with pollutants, these communities risk serious illness, birth defects, disability, and early mortality on the one hand; but on the other hand, by turning to processed food imported from the South, they risk malnutrition and chronic diseases, especially diabetes (Public Health Agency of Canada, 2015; Watt-Cloutier, 2016).

Occupational roles expose workers to different environments such as office buildings, factories, or construction sites, and occupational practices can expose workers to harmful physical, chemical, and biological agents. *The Lancet* Commission on pollution and health lists several occupational carcinogens, including asbestos, arsenic, benzene, cadmium, and formaldehyde, and states that 40% of all deaths caused by occupational carcinogens are due to asbestos (Landrigan et al., 2017, p. 19). Other occupation-related diseases are bladder cancer, leukemia, and lung cancer.

The increasing use of neurotoxicants in pesticides are of alarming concern due to their effects on brain development. Epidemiological studies indicate associations between developmental neurotoxicants and prenatal exposure of children, resulting in cognitive impairment, learning disabilities, attention deficit and hyperactivity disorders, dyslexia, and autism (Landrigan et al., 2017, p. 19). Some health risks are specific to women's exposure to occupational toxicants. For example, women who work in the cosmetics industry are exposed to fumes from nail polish, perfume, shampoos, and hair dye—all products that potentially contain endocrine disruptors. These chemicals have been linked to autistic behaviour in children and anomalies in boys' reproductive organs (Landrigan et al., 2017, p. 20). Our roles and responsibilities place us in different physical environments that often prove more harmful to particular social groups, including women, girls, the poor, and Indigenous communities.

Developmental Stage

Children and older adults are particularly vulnerable to environmental exposure. This is due in part to children's underdeveloped protective mechanisms during early stages of development and to a weakening of protective defence mechanisms in older adults. For example, recent studies indicate a link between air pollution and detrimental effects on the developing brain through a process of neuroinflammation (Brockmeyer & D'Angiulli, 2016). Windows of opportunity during several stages of development from fetus to young adult create conditions for harmful exposure to pollutants that interfere with normal processes of development. As mentioned, POPs and synthetic chemicals such as neurotoxicants and xenoestrogens have been linked to cancer, neurologic and cognitive disorders, and reproductive interference with both male and female sex organs. According to the Assembly of First Nations (2009), the lifelong exposure of Indigenous older adults to pollutants in their traditional diets results in a disproportionately higher accumulation of toxins in their system. Further, children's and older adults' exposure to unsafe sanitary conditions as a result of poor housing infrastructure, armed conflict, or environmental disasters makes them more vulnerable to morbidity and mortality due to their limited abilities to cope with resulting infectious diseases and injuries (WHO, 2017b). In addition, children and older adults alike are vulnerable to extreme weather events such as heat waves (Health Canada, 2017). In order to recognize the potential for environmental health inequities, it is necessary then to differentiate between geographic location, social location, and developmental stage across the lifespan.

THE ECOLOGICAL DETERMINANTS OF HEALTH AND GLOBAL CHANGE

The following section will highlight select key issues of global change and how some ecological determinants of health intersect with social determinants of health with the potential to produce environmental health inequities. Among the pressing issues with significant health implications introduced are climate change, pollution, and sociopolitical trends, and from a positive perspective, the salutogenic or health-enhancing and -producing effects of the environment.

Climate Change

Leading scientists have concluded that our climate is changing, that humans are largely responsible for global warming, and that the changes are happening faster than previously anticipated (Wuebbles et al., 2017). The last 100 years have been the warmest in the history of human civilization, largely attributed to a rise in greenhouse gases. Particularly CO_2, or carbon dioxide from burning of fossil fuels such as oil, gas, and coal, is the major driver of global warming. Higher temperatures are causing sea levels to rise due to melting of sea ice; in fact, sea levels have risen more since 1900 than during any other period over the last 2800 years.

The rise in temperature is also thought to contribute to the melting of permafrost in the Arctic, meaning the ground upon which Inuit communities are built, especially along receding shorelines, will disappear (Downing & Cuerrier, 2011). Weather events will become more intense, even extreme. For example, heavy rainfall will cause floods and threaten important infrastructures of roads, railways, and bridges. In addition, heat waves contribute to forest fires with implications for human safety, drinking water, air quality, agricultural production, and ecosystem functioning (Wuebbles et al., 2017). Global warming already contributes to the spread of vector-borne diseases, such as the Zika virus, into northern regions of the planet that previously only occurred in tropical regions (Watts et al., 2015).

Climate change continues to have devastating effects on Indigenous peoples worldwide. In Canada, Inuit communities in the Arctic have relied for centuries on their TEKW to survive. Through observation, they have been able to predict weather conditions suitable for hunting and fishing, and ice conditions suitable for travel and movement. Changing weather patterns and ice conditions, however, are making it increasingly difficult to predict animal movement and when it is safe to hunt and travel (Downing & Cuerrier, 2011; Watt-Cloutier, 2016). Climate change clearly has an effect on the physical environment and is impacting Indigenous cultures, identities, food security, and health on a global scale.

Pollution

Pollution and climate change are closely related in that air pollution, specifically the increase in CO_2, is a major driver of climate change, at the same time causing respiratory and cardiovascular diseases. In addition to air pollution, we are also concerned about the contamination of freshwater ecosystems, including rivers, estuaries, lakes, and oceans. Equally concerning is soil contamination with metals and synthetic chemicals that affect food supplies and agricultural products. "Diseases caused by pollution were responsible for an estimated 9 million premature deaths in 2015—16% of all deaths worldwide—three times more deaths than from AIDS, tuberculosis, and malaria combined, and 15 times more than from all wars and other forms of violence. In the most severely affected countries, pollution-related disease is responsible for more than one death in four" (Landrigan et al., 2017, p. 1). Pollution is a major threat to planetary health, which in turn affects ecosystems and human health worldwide.

The overwhelming majority of deaths due to pollution occur in populations rendered vulnerable, including children and the poor. During different stages of development, children and expectant mothers are especially susceptible to pollutants that interfere with normal growth and development (Landrigan

et al., 2017). Women, due to their childbearing responsibilities, are affected by the environment in different ways from men. Baby girls are born with a complete set of ovaries, and daughters potentially can be affected by their grandmother's environmental exposure to contaminants during pregnancy because organic pollutants have been found in human ovarian follicular fluid (Jarrell et al., 1993). Furthermore, women have proportionately more adipose tissue than men, and several harmful chemicals are lipophilic, meaning they accumulate in fatty tissue. Therefore, women tend to be at greater risk for accumulating potentially harmful chemicals. Male infertility due to environmental toxicants is of global concern (Wong & Cheng, 2011). Low sperm count has been related to exposure to human-made chemicals that mimic hormones, called xenoestrogens (Manfo, Nantia, & Mathur, 2014).

Ecotoxicity and loss of biodiversity are interconnected with pollution. Ecotoxicity is concerned with the accumulation and impact of toxins on ecosystems and natural detoxifying mechanisms. The introduction of synthetic chemicals into the environment has not only contributed to changing ecosystems and loss of species but also act like a boomerang that comes back to harm human life (Landrigan et al., 2017). For example, the accumulation of POPs in wildlife and our food chain contributes to a lifelong body burden of multiple chemicals with health consequences yet unknown (Hancock et al., 2015; Landrigan et al., 2017). Air, soil, and water pollution are ubiquitous and do not stop at national borders, which makes pollution a global health threat. Of particular concern is the intergenerational perpetuation of poverty related to pollution (Landrigan et al., 2017). People who live in poverty often live in unhealthy environments, near polluting factories or toxic waste sites. Again, the social and ecological determinants of health are fundamentally interconnected. (See Figure 27.1.)

CASE STUDY

Ecological Footprint: Creating Your Personal Case Study

Many of us are not aware of how much energy and natural resources we use daily. Often, we take for granted: the shower we have in the morning, our car drive to work, the electronic devices we use for our work or entertainment, and the access we have to fresh produce, meat, and dairy products. Yet all these practices take up energy and natural resources. The ecological footprint calculator can help you find out how much of the world's energy and resources you consume. This helps you understand the amount of land that would be required to maintain your lifestyle.

Go to www.footprintcalculator.org and follow the guidelines to determine your own ecological footprint.

Discussion Questions

1. Discuss the insights you have gained and what are you going to do about them?
2. How can CHNs use this tool in their practice?

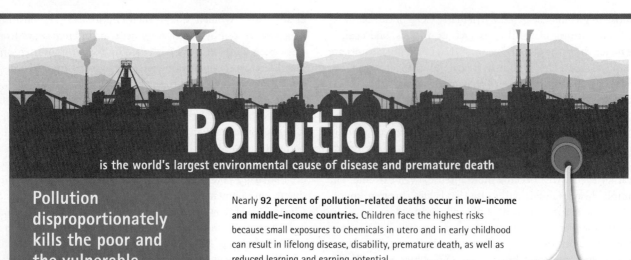

Pollution

is the world's largest environmental cause of disease and premature death

Pollution disproportionately kills the poor and the vulnerable.

Nearly **92 percent of pollution-related deaths occur in low-income and middle-income countries.** Children face the highest risks because small exposures to chemicals in utero and in early childhood can result in lifelong disease, disability, premature death, as well as reduced learning and earning potential.

In 2015, diseases caused by pollution were responsible for

9 million premature deaths.
That is 16 percent of all global deaths.

Exposures to contaminated air, water and soil kill more people than a high-sodium diet, obesity, alcohol, road accidents, or child and maternal malnutrition. They are also responsible for three times as many deaths as AIDS, tuberculosis, and malaria combined, and for nearly 15 times as many deaths as war and all forms of violence.

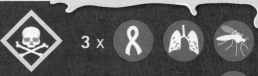

Air pollution and climate change are closely linked and share common solutions.

Fossil fuel combustion in higher-income countries and the burning of biomass in lower-income countries accounts for 85 percent of airborne particulate pollution.

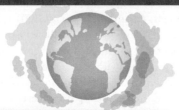

Major emitters of carbon dioxide are coal-fired power plants, chemical producers, mining operations, and vehicles. Accelerating the switch to cleaner sources of energy will reduce air pollution and improve human and planetary health.

The cost of inaction is high, while solutions yield enormous economic gains.

Welfare losses due to pollution are estimated at **$4.6 trillion per year— 6.2 percent of global economic output.** In the United States, investment in pollution control has returned $200 billion each year since 1980 ($6 trillion total). The claim that pollution control stifles economic growth and that poor countries must pollute to grow is false.

Pollution is neglected by funding agencies worldwide.

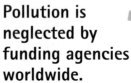

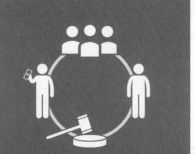

We can all help to make a difference.

Governments can integrate pollution challenges and control strategies into planning processes. Ask for support from development assistance agencies. Design and implement programs that reduce pollution, and save lives. End government subsidies and tax breaks for polluting industries.

International donors, foundations, health professionals, and individuals should prioritize funding for pollution planning, interventions, and research.

People affected by pollution can review data related to toxic exposures in their neighborhood and connect with help by visiting **www.pollution.org**

Infographic © 2017 Mount Sinai Health System

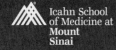 Icahn School of Medicine at **Mount Sinai**

THE LANCET

GAHP
GLOBAL ALLIANCE ON
HEALTH AND POLLUTION

FIGURE 27.1 Pollution: What Can We Do About It?

Source: From Landrigan, P. J., Fuller, R., Acosta, N. J. R., Adeyi, O., Arnold, R., Basu, N., . . . Zhong, M. (2017). *The Lancet* Commission on pollution and health, © 2017. Reprinted with permission from Elsevier.

YES, BUT WHY?

Plastic and Health

What?

Plastic products have become a major source of pollution and pose a threat to human and non-human health. Only a fraction of plastic products is recycled, and the bulk ends up in landfill sites, rivers, and oceans. Over time, plastic products break down into microplastics that have been found in seafood and drinking water sources around the world (*The Lancet*, 2017).

So What?

Most concerning, we don't know much about the health effects of microplastics on humans (Carbery, O'Connor, & Thavamani, 2018). During manufacturing processes, certain chemicals, including polychlorinated bisphenols (PCBs), cadmium, and lead, are introduced into plastic. These chemicals have been implicated as potential threats to human health and have been linked to cancer and cognitive impairment. The scientific community is calling for rigorous studies to understand their effects on human health and the ecosystem (Carbery et al., 2018; *The Lancet*, 2017).

Now What?

CHNs can intervene by collaborating in research studies to generate the evidence required for advocacy action. Advocacy can take the form of lobbying government through the Canadian Nurses Association to introduce legislation to ban or reduce certain plastic consumer products. Similar efforts have been undertaken in the European Union (European Commission, 2018), where a plastic ban is in effect for products that can be produced with alternative materials, including plastic cutlery, plates, and straws. CHNs can also participate by raising awareness through public education about the need to reduce the use of plastic products and their safe disposal.

Standards of Practice Fulfilled

#6 Health Equity
- Engages with the client using critical social theory and intersectional approach from a foundation of equity and social justice
- Advocates for healthy public policy and social justice by participating in legislative and policy-making activities that influence determinants of health and access to services.

#7 Evidence Informed Practice
- Uses professional expertise in considering best available research evidence, and other factors such as client context and preferences, and available resources to determine nursing actions (CHNC, 2019, revised).

Sociopolitical Trends

In addition to climate change and pollution, significant sociopolitical trends drive global change. Among them are increasing urbanization and displacement, with related food and housing insecurity.

It is estimated that by 2030, two-thirds of the world's population will live in urban areas (Jowell, Zhou, & Barry, 2017). The health impacts of megacities include malnutrition from food shortages and an increase in obesity due to sedentary lifestyles. Higher population densities can lead to increased sexual violence against women, contributing to higher incidence of sexually transmitted infections. Negative health outcomes of air pollution include chronic obstructive pulmonary disease and lung cancer, and the creation of heat islands in urban environments can lead to dehydration, stroke, and cardiovascular and respiratory diseases (Jowell et al., 2017).

An estimated 26 million people globally have already been displaced by climate change (Downing & Cuerrier, 2011, p. 57). Displacement of Indigenous communities in Canada as a result of colonialism has already had devastating consequences on their health and well-being. Because Indigenous peoples are traditionally connected to their land, any further displacement due to climate change would mean further loss of identity, culture, health, and livelihood (Watt-Cloutier, 2016). Involuntary human migration has complex roots, and events such as civil conflicts can result in crop failure and famine (Myers, 2017; Watts et al., 2017). Among the populations forced to leave their homes are the poor, who have least access to resources. The resulting mental health implications of displacement, whether directly or indirectly related to the effects of climate change, are significant and include chronic anxiety, depression, post-traumatic stress disorder, and suicide (Myers, 2017; Watts et al., 2017).

According to *The Lancet* Commission, Canadian municipalities and provinces have generated a positive track record on climate change action (Watts et al., 2017). Governance at this level can have several significant impacts on public health, including sanitation and fresh water supply, transport, waste management, and housing. Mayors of the world's largest cities have created influential networks to benefit climate change action. For example, New York City has implemented energy-efficient building policies. For CHNs, action on climate change may seem too daunting; however, at the municipal level, CHNs and public health nurses have ample opportunities to get involved and to collaborate on the health benefits of climate change action.

Salutogenic Effects of Nature

On a positive note, it is important to acknowledge the therapeutic effect of nature on human health. **Salutogenic**, or health-enhancing, environments are supported by scientific evidence. Salutogenesis is regarded as an alternative approach to pathogenesis (Lindström & Eriksson, 2005); where pathogenesis aims to discover the causes and pathways to illness, salutogenesis aims to look for the pathways to health and healing. As such, it is a valuable tool for health promotion and encourages exposure to non-human nature as a way to enhance health. Exposure to and interaction with green spaces are associated with psychosocial well-being (Beute & deKort, 2017; Crouse et al., 2017), women's health (Thomas, 2015), and a decrease in cardiovascular mortality rates (Gascon et al., 2016).

Human interaction and relationships with animals also have been shown to support overall health and well-being. Canine companionship and service dogs for veterans with post-traumatic stress disorder are beneficial for rehabilitation (Woodward, Jamison, Gala, & Holmes, 2017). There is also evidence that human–animal relations support a consciousness of "being with nature" (Gorman, 2017). Whether through exposure to the natural environment or relationships with non-human beings, CHNs can tap into these resources and can provide stewardship to protect and preserve them for current and future generations. It is critical that we ensure equal opportunities to access clean nature, with particular consideration for the urban poor, Indigenous populations, and displaced individuals.

CANADIAN RESEARCH 27.1

Food for thought: The value of nature-based initiatives.
(Little, Hansen-Ketchum, & Purcell, 2015)

This study illustrates the potential effectiveness of utilizing school gardens as a tool to promote the health and development of children and youth. An edible school garden project can enable children and youth to work in partnership with public health workers, school staff, and community members to share knowledge and resources for the development, implementation, and evaluation of the initiative. A group of students at the school known as the "Green Team" worked with the public health nurse, school administrators, community members, and organizations to facilitate a school vegetable garden project. The project is youth-driven, with students having a high level of involvement in the decision-making process. Students prepare raised beds with compost from a local waste management facility and plant seeds and fruit trees, with funding provided by a community health board and other local and provincial sponsors.

The researchers concluded that it is time for a better balance in the health system and public sector with joint efforts for more equitable access to conditions and programs that support health and subsequently prevent disease. Resources are needed to enable access to healthy outdoor environments. These resources must be sustained through community involvement and multi-sector partnership alongside engagement between young people and older adults to create the collective hands-on work needed to grow, harvest, and share the bounty.

Discussion Questions

1. How might the actions in this study contribute to co-benefits for humans and the environment?

2. How might CHNs ensure that populations rendered vulnerable have equal access to projects like this?

3. What values can a project like this teach children and future generations?

THREE ENVIRONMENTAL FRAMEWORKS

When issues are as complex as the ones discussed in this chapter, it is difficult to point to one overarching theoretical framework that captures all the necessary concepts. In this section, three different environmental frameworks are presented: Indigenous perspectives on health and the environment, intersectional ecological-feminist approaches, and planetary health approaches.

Indigenous Perspectives on Health and the Environment

Recurring patterns of **Indigenous perspectives on health and the environment** can be seen in Indigenous people's relationships to the land, which are characterized as having deep respect, humility, and responsibility to protect the environment and preserve it for the benefit of future generations (Hatcher et al., 2009; Hunt, 2015; Parks, 2011). This holistic understanding has been developed over millennia and reflects the core principles that ought to guide our relationship as humans with non-human life on Earth. This insight, then, ought to be the starting point for our engagement with environmental health. As health care professionals, we purport to be reflective practitioners, beginning with our own positions and relationships with nature.

Leading scientists have come to realize that in order to move into a better future for all on this planet, Western scientific knowledge alone will not suffice to lead the way. As Samuel Myers (2017), a senior scientist with the Rockefeller Foundation, eloquently stated during a recent lecture about planetary health,

> In the end, achieving planetary health will require a renaissance in how we define our place in the world. A new narrative will reject the one streaming into our homes—that happiness comes from relentlessly acquiring more things—and embrace what we know: that what truly makes us happy is time spent with those we love, connection to place and community, feeling connected to something greater than ourselves, taking care of each other. (p. 8)

Ultimately, in addition to rational intelligence and the use of scientific evidence, we need emotional intelligence to guide our decisions and practices. The simultaneous use of scientific knowledge and Indigenous traditional knowledge has been proposed by Mi'kmaq Elder Albert Marshall of the First Nation of Unama'ki (Cape Breton, Nova Scotia) with the concept of Two-Eyed Seeing (National Collaborating Centre for Aboriginal Health, 2016). **Two-Eyed Seeing**, as a holistic concept, helps overcome the prevailing Western dualistic thinking and instead opens possibilities for a re-imagination of our relationship with the environment as being part of it rather than having dominion over it.

Intersectional Ecological-Feminist Approaches

Emotional intelligence requires the skill of empathy, which is central to nursing practice. Empathy is a sensibility to understand another's emotions and situation, and is a prerequisite to emotional intelligence and caring. The notion of a care-sensitive ethic (Warren, 2000), particularly for policy and decision making, includes valuing caring work done in society for children, the sick, older adults, and the environment.

Necessary for a holistic understanding of our relationship with the environment, according to **intersectional ecological-feminist approaches**, is refraining from two approaches: (a) value dualism, which is used to establish opposition and exclusiveness; for example, when reason (which in Western society is often associated with the masculine) is regarded as the opposite of emotion (which in Western society is often associated with the feminine); and (b) value-hierarchical thinking, which is used to establish a hierarchy to justify domination—in other words, the exploitation and pollution of natural resources by humans and the simultaneous oppression of populations rendered vulnerable by those with more economic and political power (Chircop, 2008; Warren, 2000). Any framework that facilitates this explication has to have a component to make oppressive relations visible in order to re-negotiate and re-construct a more viable society and sustainable future.

Planetary Health Approaches

Planetary health is concerned with the unprecedented impact of human activity on Earth's ecological systems in the atmosphere, in oceans, and on land and its consequences for human health. Instead of looking at the environment as something dangerous and to be feared, planetary health recognizes that we can achieve and sustain the health of future generations by taking care of our planet's natural systems (Myers, 2017). The framework of planetary health depicted in Figure 27.2 illustrates how human activities in the form of consumerism, overpopulation, and environmentally damaging technologies are the underlying drivers of ecological change.

This change negatively impacts air quality, food production, infectious disease exposure, fresh water access, and natural phenomena. Socially mediating factors contribute to negative health outcomes, including malnutrition, infectious diseases, non-communicable diseases, displacement and conflict, and mental health. The mediating factors of public policies, decision making in governance, and advances in technology can also contribute to positive health outcomes. This framework attempts to explain the forces currently driving global change and at the same time suggests where and how social action could lead to positive health outcomes.

This framework depicts a mechanism of how humans are harming their own health by harming life-sustaining ecosystems. To be consistent with this chapter's approach to environmental health equity and Indigenous traditional knowledges, the planetary health framework could be complemented with insights and wisdom from Indigenous ecological knowledges to re-imagine our relationship with nature as a starting point. In addition, insights from intersectional ecological-feminist approaches offered above could be integrated into the mediating factors of the planetary health framework to make explicit the sociocultural, economic, gender, and political power imbalances that lead to oppression in the form of resource depletion, exploitation of the environment, and environmental health inequities.

COMMUNITY HEALTH NURSING PRACTICE

The following examples of nursing practice at the five levels of prevention incorporate the theoretical approaches just discussed. Each example serves as an illustration for nursing practice by being mindful that meaningful and effective approaches

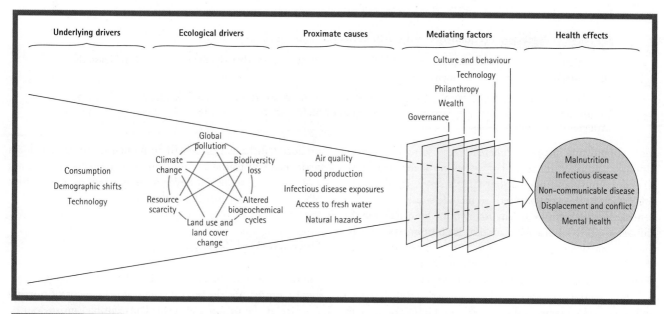

FIGURE 27.2 Impacts of Anthropogenic Change on Human Health

Source: Myers, S. S. (2017). Planetary health: Protecting human health on a rapidly changing planet. *The Lancet, 390*(10114), 2860–2868. Reprinted with permission.

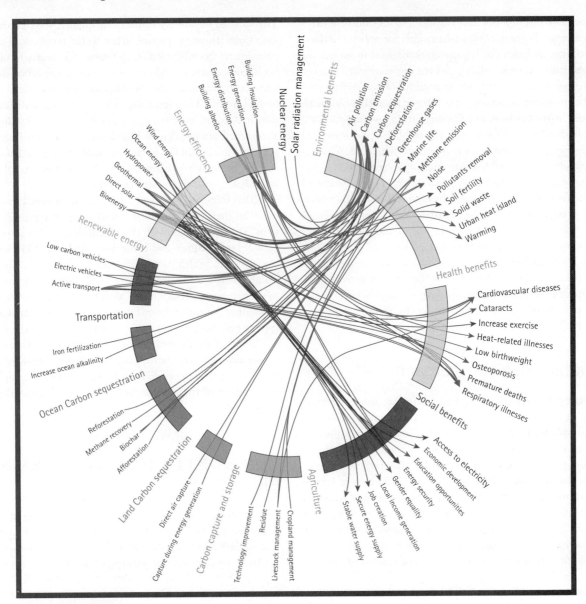

FIGURE **27.3** Frequently Cited Co-Benefits of Major Mitigation Techniques

Note: Red arrows between a mitigation technology and an effect indicate that the technology will increase the effect; green arrows indicate an opposite trend.

Source: From Watts, N., Adger, W. N., Agnolucci, P., Blackstock, J., Byass, P., Cai, W., & Costello, A. et. al. (2015). Health and climate change: policy responses to protect public health. *The Lancet, 386,* 1861–1914. © 2015. Reprinted with permission from Elsevier..

for environmental justice are inherently intersectoral, interdisciplinary, and interprofessional as well as in collaboration with the community and populations CHNs serve. Importantly, prevention in this context needs to include strategies for preventing further harm to the environment by human action. In this sense, CHNs must focus on health **co-benefits**, that is, nursing practice to promote action to the co-benefit of both the environment/nature and human health (Watts et al., 2015). Figure 27.3 depicts several of these co-benefits.

An important consideration is to ensure that well-intended and -designed co-benefits do not exclude certain populations such that inequities are created or reinforced. Unintended consequences can arise when prevention strategies are designed without a health equity lens. For example, promoting organic

produce will have a co-benefit to human health as it reduces toxic load and to the environment as it protects biodiversity and other ecosystems. However, we need to ensure accessibility of organic produce for all populations.

Primordial Prevention

International, national, provincial, and municipal policies that aim at protecting the environment are the focus of nursing practice at the primordial level. For example, nurses can be familiar with the precautionary principle, which "denotes a duty to prevent harm, when it is within our power to do so, *even when all the evidence is not in*" (Canadian Environmental Law

Association, 2017). Instead of allowing a potentially harmful activity to proceed until evidence of its impact on the environment and human health is collected, this principle supports a preventative approach. By making use of the precautionary principle to support advocacy action with communities during environmental impact and health-equity impact assessments, nurses can be effective collaborators for positive change. As an example, at the national level, Canada signed the Stockholm Convention of Persistent Organic Pollutants in 2001, which aims to restrict or eliminate the production and use of POPs (Government of Canada, 2017).

Primary Prevention

Nursing practice in primary prevention could include the initiation of discussions with new parents on how they can facilitate healthy environments. Parents want the best possible future for their children, and this is an opportune time to have discussions about our relationship with the environment to ensure healthy development and future lives.

Another example with co-benefits is Ontario's one-health model (Panning, Lem, & Bateman, 2016). This model is a collaboration between public health and veterinary medicine. People who are homeless are among the most vulnerable and hard-to-reach populations, and they often have dogs as companions. The one-health outreach service provides free veterinary care alongside human health services such as immunization for the homeless pet owner. The objectives of the one-health model are "to 1) improve access to veterinary and human health resources for an at-risk population, and 2) leverage the human-animal bond to increase human health resource uptake" (Panning et al., 2016, p. e222).

Secondary Prevention

Secondary prevention involves screening. The purpose is to detect a harmful occurrence before it can cause more harm. In keeping with the co-benefit approach, an example of secondary prevention would be a collaboration with an interdisciplinary team to ascertain if newly proposed policies will have a negative impact on the environment and health equity outcomes. For instance, if a new subdivision is proposed by urban developers, an interdisciplinary team that includes nurses and environmental experts could collaborate with planners and municipal decision makers to screen the subdivision proposal for potential harmful effects to the natural environment or to ensure sufficient green spaces are included. At the same time, the proposal could be screened for health equity outcomes for residents, such as affordability, access to transportation, and other public services.

Tertiary Prevention

Tertiary prevention aims to prevent further deterioration of an already existing condition. Nova Scotia has an environmental health clinic in Fall River, near Halifax, to treat patients with a variety of conditions, including multiple chemical sensitivities (Nova Scotia Health Authority, 2017). In this clinic, registered nurses and nurse practitioners work in collaboration with an interprofessional health care team. A population health co-benefit approach would include advocating with the client community on issues such as pesticide-free lawns and gardens to protect humans and non-human nature, such as bees, from harmful chemicals.

Quaternary Prevention

The definition for quaternary prevention is "Action taken to identify a patient or a population at risk of over-medicalization, to protect them from invasive medical interventions, and provide them with care procedures which are ethically acceptable" (Primary Health Care Classification Consortium, 2016). Clear linkages exist between over-medicalization of humans and ecosystem health. There is concern about the occurrence of pharmaceutical compounds in freshwater and saltwater marine species (Landrigan et al., 2017). These chemicals make their way into fish and other species via discharge from pharmaceutical industries and hospitals into urban wastewater discharge and include antibiotics, estrogens, and chemotherapy drugs (Landrigan et al., 2017). Nursing practice at the level of quaternary prevention would include advocating with patients for a prudent selection of only the most necessary drugs to be prescribed by physicians and nurse practitioners.

CONCLUSION

Clearly, the issues of global change related to the ecological determinants and their population health implications are of tremendous proportion and complexity, and they require imminent action. For health care professionals, it is an ethical imperative to join interdisciplinary efforts to engage at all levels of governance, from local to regional, national, and international efforts toward mitigation and progress for a clean environment. Public understanding and engagement for a cleaner, healthier, and more just society is necessary and requires support from community leaders. The nursing profession is one of the most trusted in society, and this trust comes with a responsibility to work for social and ecological justice for current and future populations. Much has already been accomplished to combat global change, sustainable development, and social justice. However, much work remains to be done! A good starting point to curb pollution and reduce greenhouse gas emissions for a healthy, viable, just, and sustainable future begins with each and every person reflecting and asking, "What can I do today to contribute?"

KEY TERMS

climate change   (p. 490)
co-benefits   (p. 498)
ecotoxicity   (p. 493)
ecological determinants of health   (p. 489)
environmental health inequities   (p. 490)
environmental risks   (p. 490)
global change   (p. 490)
Indigenous Traditional Knowledge   (p. 490)

STUDY QUESTIONS

1. Identify three ecological determinants of health.

2. Which populations are most vulnerable to environmental health inequities?

3. Identify three key messages from the *Climate Science Special Report* (Wuebbles et al., 2017).

4. What is meant by the concept of "Two-Eyed Seeing"?

5. Identify examples of health co-benefits at the level of primary prevention.

INDIVIDUAL CRITICAL-THINKING EXERCISES

1. Reflect on your daily personal practices related to carbon-generating energy consumption, and identify one co-benefit of reduced consumption.

2. Reflect on how much waste your daily personal and nursing practices generate and how you can reduce it.

3. Take a position and discuss why you agree or disagree with the argument that in order to make progress for a clean, just, and sustainable future, we need to address resource depletion and environmental degradation while we also address oppression and exploitation of vulnerable and marginalized populations.

GROUP CRITICAL-THINKING EXERCISES

1. Discuss how your personal responsibility and professional nursing obligations to become a steward for the ecological determinants of health and environmental health equity overlap and support each other.

2. Discuss how you can incorporate the proposed framework and concepts for planetary health into your daily nursing practice at the individual, family, community, and population levels.

3. Draft a policy brief to the prime minister of Canada for his next visit to an international climate change conference on the importance of reducing global warming to protect, in particular, Northern First Nation and Inuit health.

REFERENCES

Aden, N. (2016). The roads to decoupling: 21 countries are reducing carbon emissions while growing GDP. Retrieved from http://www.wri.org/blog/2016/04/roads-decoupling-21-countries-are-reducing-carbon-emissions-while-growing-gdp

Assembly of First Nations. (2009). Environmental health older adults and seniors (Elders). Retrieved from http://www.afn.ca/uploads/files/rpenviro_health_and_older_adults_and_seniors.pdf

Beute, F., & deKort, Y. A. W. (2017). The natural context of wellbeing: Ecological momentary assessment of the influence of nature and daylight on affect and stress for individuals with depression levels varying from none to clinical. *Health and Place, 17*(49), 7–18. doi:10.1016/j.healthplace.2017.11.005

Bradford, L. E., Okpalauwaekwe, U., Waldner, C. L., & Bharadwaj, L. A. (2016). Drinking water quality in Indigenous communities in Canada and health outcomes: A scoping review. *International Journal of Circumpolar Health, 75*(1), 32336.

Brockmeyer, S., & D'Angiulli, A. (2016). How air pollution alters brain development: The role of neuroinflammation. *Translational Neuroscience, 7*(1), 24–30. doi:10.1515/tnsci-2016-0005

Canadian Environmental Law Association. (2017). *The precautionary principle.* Retrieved from http://www.cela.ca/collections/pollution/precautionary-principle

Carbery, M., O'Connor, W., & Thavamani, P. (2018). Trophic transfer of microplastics and mixed contaminants in the marine food web and implications for human health. *Environment International, 115*, 400–409. doi.org/10.1016/j.envint.2018.03.007

CBC. (2013). Remediated Sydney tar ponds unveiled as green space. Retrieved from http://www.cbc.ca/news/canada/nova-scotia/remediated-sydney-tar-ponds-unveiled-as-green-space-1.1304232

Chircop, A. (2008). An ecofeminist conceptual framework to explore gendered environmental health inequities in urban settings and to inform healthy public policy. *Nursing Inquiry, 15*(2), 135–147.

Chircop, A. (2012). Public policy analysis to redress urban environmental health inequities. *Policy, Politics & Nursing Practice, 12*(4), 245–53. doi:10.1177/1527154411429198.

Climate Action Tracker. (2017). *Improvement warming outlook India and China move ahead Paris agreement gap still looms large.* Retrieved from https://climateactiontracker.org/publications/improvement-warming-outlook-india-and-china-move-ahead-paris-agreement-gap-still-looms-large

Community Health Nurses of Canada (CHNC). (2019, revised). *Canadian community health nursing standards of practice.* Retrieved from http://www.chnc.ca/nursing-standards-of-practice.cfm

Crouse, D. L., Pinault, L., Balram, A., Hystad, P., Peters, P. A., Chen, H., . . . Villeneuve, P. J. (2017). Urban greenness and mortality in Canada's largest cities: National cohort study. *Lancet Planet Health,* (1), e289–97.

Downing, A., & Cuerrier, A. (2011). A synthesis of the impact of climate change on the First Nations and Inuit of Canada. *Indian Journal of Traditional Knowledge, 10*(1), 57–70.

EcoWatch. (2016). *It's official: The Anthropocene epoch is here.* Retrieved from http://www.ecowatch.com/anthropocene-1991220147.html

Employment and Social Development Canada. (2017). *Snapshot of racialized poverty in Canada.* Retrieved from https://www.canada.ca/en/employment-social-development/programs/communities/reports/poverty-profile-snapshot.html

European Commission. (2017). *Climate action.* Retrieved from https://ec.europa.eu/clima/news/articles/news_2012102402_en

European Commission. (2018). *Single-use plastics: New EU rules to reduce marine litter.* Retrieved from http://europa.eu/rapid/press-release_IP-18-3927_en.htm

Eurostat (2017). *Greenhouse gas emission statistic.* Retrieved from http://ec.europa.eu/eurostat/statistics-explained/index.php/Greenhouse_gas_emission_statistics

Gascon, M., Triguero-Mas, M., Martinez, D., Dadvand, P., Rojas-Rueda, D., Plasencia, A., & Nieuwenhuijsen, M. J. (2016). Residential green spaces and mortality: A systematic review. *Environment International, 86*, 60–67. doi:10.1016/j.envint.2015.10.013

Gorman, R. (2017). Thinking critically about health and human-animal relations: Therapeutic affect within spaces of care farming. *Social Science and Medicine.* In press. https://doi-org.ezproxy.library.dal.ca/10.1016/j.socscimed.2017.11.047

Government of Canada. (2017). Persistent organic pollutants: Stockholm Convention. Retrieved from https://www.canada.ca/en/environment-climate-change/corporate/international-affairs/partnerships-organizations/persistent-organic-pollutants-stockholm-convention.html

Hancock, T., Spady, D. W., & Soskolne, C. L. (Eds.). Allison, S., Chircop, A., Harper, S., McKibbon, G., Parkes, M., Poland, B. (Contributing Authors). (2015). *Global change and public health: Addressing the ecological determinants of health. The report in brief.* Retrieved from http://www.cpha.ca/uploads/policy/edh-brief.pdf

Hardach, S. (2015). How the river Thames was brought back from the dead. Retrieved from http://www.bbc.com/earth/story/20151111-how-the-river-thames-was-brought-back-from-the-dead

Hatcher, A., Bartlett, C., Marchall, A., & Marshall, M. (2009). Two-Eyed Seeing in the classroom environment: Concepts, approaches, and challenges. *Canadian Journal of Sciences, Mathematics and Technology Education, 9*(3), 141–153.

Health Canada. (2017). Heat waves. Retrieved from https://www.canada.ca/en/sr.html?cdn=canada&st=s&num=10&langs=en&st1rt=1&s5bm3ts21rch=x&q=heat+waves&_charset_=UTF-8&wb-srch-sub=

Hunt, S. (2015). *Review of core competencies for public health: An Aboriginal health perspective.* National Collaborating Centre for Aboriginal Health.

Jarrell, J. F., Villeneuve, D., Franklin, C., Bartlett, S., Wrixon, W., Kohut, J., & Zouves, C. G. (1993). Contamination of human ovarian follicular fluid and serum by chlorinated organic compounds in three Canadian cities. *Canadian Medical Association Journal, 148*(8), 1321–1327.

Jowell, A., Zhou, B., & Barry, M. (2017). The impact of megacities on health: preparing for a resilient future. *The Lancet, 1*, e176–e178. Retrieved from http://www.thelancet.com/planetary-health

Kristensen, S. L., Ramlau-Hansen, C. H., Ernst, E., Olsen, S. F., Bonde, J. P., Vested, A., . . . Toft, G. (2016). Reproductive function in young adulthood. *Environment International, 92*(93), 366–372.

Landrigan, P. J., Fuller, R., Acosta, N. J. R., Adeyi, O., Arnold, R., Basu, N., . . . Zhong, M. (2017). *The Lancet* Commission on pollution and health. *The Lancet,* Published online. http://dx.doi.org/10.1016/S0140-6736(17)32345-0

Lefale, P. F. (2010). Ua 'afa le Aso Stormy weather today: Traditional ecological knowledge of weather and climate. The Samoa experience. *Climatic Change, 100*(2), 317–335.

Lindström, B., & Eriksson, M. (2005). Salutogenesis. *Journal of Epidemiology & Community Health, 59*(6), 440–442.

Little, V., Hansen-Ketchum, P., & Purcell, L. (2015). Food for thought: The value of nature-based initiatives. *CRNNS Connections.* Retrieved from http://crnns.ca/newsletters/connections-september-2015/weather and climate

Manfo, F. P., Nantia, E. A., & Mathur, P. P. (2014). Effect of environmental contaminants on mammalian testis. *Current Molecular Pharmacology, 7*(2),119–35.

McClymont Peace, D., & Myers, E. (2012). Community-based participatory process—Climate change and health adaptation program for northern First Nations and Inuit in Canada. *International Journal of Circumpolar Health, 71,* 18412. http://dx.doi.org/10.3402/ijch.v71i0.18412

Morrow, M., Hankivsky, O., & Varcoe, C. (2007). *Women's health in Canada: Critical perspectives on theory and policy.* Toronto, ON: University of Toronto Press Inc.

Myers, S. S. (2017). Planetary health: Protecting human health on a rapidly changing planet. *The Lancet, 390*(10114), 2860–2868.

NASA. (2017). *Warm air helped make 2017 ozone hole smallest since 1988.* Retrieved from https://www.nasa.gov/feature/goddard/2017/warm-air-helped-make-2017-ozone-hole-smallest-since-1988

National Collaborating Centre for Aboriginal Health. (2016). *Transforming our realities: The determinants of health and Indigenous peoples.* Prince George, BC: Author.

Nova Scotia Health Authority. (2017). *Integrated chronic care service.* Retrieved from http://www.nshealth.ca/content/integrated-chronic-care-service-iccs

Panning, C., Lem, M., & Bateman, S. (2016). Profiling a one-health model for priority populations. *Canadian Journal of Public Health, 107*(3), e222–e223. doi:10.17269/CJPH.107.5463

Parks, M. (2011). *Ecohealth and Aboriginal health. A review of common ground.* National Collaborating Centre for Aboriginal Health. Retrieved from https://www.ccnsa-nccah.ca/495/Ecohealth_and_Aboriginal_health__A_review_of_common_ground_.nccah?id=49

Primary Health Care Classification Consortium. (2016). *Quaternary prevention.* Retrieved from http://www.ph3c.org/4daction/w3_CatVisu/en?wCatIDAdmin=1128

Prüss-Ustün, A., Wolf, J., Corvalán, C., Neville, T., Bos, R., & Neira, M. (2016). Diseases due to unhealthy environments: An updated estimate of the global burden of disease attributable to environmental determinants of health. *Journal of Public Health, 39*(3), 464–475.

Public Health Agency of Canada. (2015). *Chronic diseases.* Retrieved from https://www.canada.ca/en/public-health/services/chronic-diseases/reports-publications/diabetes/

diabetes-canada-facts-figures-a-public-health-perspective/chapter-6.html

Raphael, D. (Ed.). (2016). *Social determinants of health. Canadian perspectives*. Toronto, ON: Canadian Scholars' Press Inc.

Ripple, W. J., Wolf, C., Newsome, T. M., Galetti, M., Alamgir, M., Crist, E., . . . & 15,364 scientist signatories from 184 countries. (2017). World scientists' warning to humanity: A second notice. *BioScience, 67*(12), 1026–1028.

Sarkar, A., Hanrahan, M., & Hudson, A. (2015). Water insecurity in Canadian Indigenous communities: Some inconvenient truths. *Rural Remote Health, 15*(4), 3354.

Statistics Canada. (2017). *Children living in low income households*. Catalogue no. 98-200-X2016012. Retrieved from http://www12.statcan.gc.ca/census-recensement/2016/as-sa/98-200-x/2016012/98-200-x2016012-eng.pdf

The Lancet. (2017). Microplastics and human health—an urgent problem. *The Lancet Planetary Health, 1*, e254. Retrieved from http://www.thelancet.com/planetary-health

Thomas, F. (2015). The role of natural environments within women's everyday health and wellbeing in Copenhagen, Denmark. *Health Place, 35*, 187–195. doi:10.1016/j.healthplace.2014.11.005

Turner, N. J., Boelscher Ingnace, M., & Ignace, R. (2000). Traditional ecological knowledge and wisdom of Aboriginal peoples in British Columbia. *Ecological Applications, 10*(5), 1275–1287.

Warren, K. J. (2000). *Ecofeminist philosophy. A Western perspective on what it is and why it matters*. Oxford, UK: Rowman & Littlefield Publishers Inc.

Watt-Cloutier, S. (2016). *The right to be cold*. Toronto, ON: Penguin.

Watts, N., Adger, W. N., Agnolucci, P., Blackstock, J., Byass, P., Cai, W., . . . Costello, A. (2015). Health and climate change: policy responses to protect public health. *The Lancet, 386*, 1861–1914.

World Health Organization (WHO). (2010). *Social and gender inequalities in environment and health*. Retrieved from http://www.euro.who.int/__data/assets/pdf_file/0010/76519/Parma_EH_Conf_pb1.pdf

World Health Organization (WHO). (2017a). *Food safety: Persistent organic pollutants*. Retrieved from http://www.who.int/foodsafety/areas_work/chemical-risks/pops/en

World Health Organization (WHO). (2017b). *10 facts on children's environmental health*. Retrieved from http://who.int/features/factfiles/children_environmental_health/en

Wong, E. W. P., & Cheng, C. Y. (2011). Impacts of environmental toxicants on male reproductive dysfunction. *Trends in Pharmacological Science, 32*(5), 290–299. doi:10.1016/j.tips.2011.01.001

Woodward, S. H., Jamison, A. L., Gala, S., & Holmes, T. H. (2017). Canine companionship is associated with modification of attention bias in post-traumatic stress disorder. *PloS One, 12*(10), e 0179912. doi:10.1371/journal.pone.0179912

World Economic Outlook. (2008, April). *Climate change and the global economy*. IMF. Retrieved from http://www.imf.org

Wuebbles, D. J., Fahey, D. W., Hibbard, K. A., DeAngelo, B., Doherty, S., Hayhoe, K., . . . Weaver, C. P. (2017). *Climate science special report: Fourth national climate assessment, Volume 1*. U.S. Washington, DC: Global Change Research Program, 12–34. doi:10.7930/J0DJ5CTG.

ABOUT THE AUTHOR

Dr. Andrea Chircop is an assistant professor at the School of Nursing, Dalhousie University. Her program of research is focused on health equity, the social and ecological determinants of health, and healthy public policy. Her research methodologies are informed by intersectional ecological-feminist approaches and include urban and institutional ethnography, case studies, and mixed methods. Her areas of teaching are community/population and public health nursing for undergraduate students and supervision of graduate studies.

Violence and Health

Elizabeth McGibbon, Annette Bailey, Sionnach Lukeman

CHAPTER
28

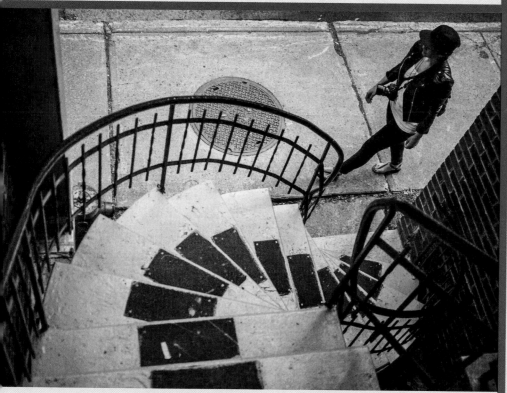

Source: © *Riley Smith Photography*

LEARNING OUTCOMES

After studying this chapter, you should be able to:

1. Discuss what is meant by root or structural causes of violence.

2. Apply the People, Poverty, Power Model to a case study about community-based violence.

3. Discuss the following forms of violence: systemic forms of violence such as colonialism, racism and sexism, family violence, interpersonal violence, stalking, cyberbullying, and human trafficking. Pay particular attention to incidence, community health nursing roles, and structural or root causes.

4. Discuss how power and control are involved in individual, family, and community violence; and structural violence.

5. Describe how trauma and violence-informed practice and atraumatic care apply to community health nursing.

INTRODUCTION

This chapter focuses on the root, or structural, causes of societal violence. Compassionate, upstream-minded short- and long-term community health nursing intervention is much more likely when nurses tackle these **root causes** of violence. We describe the **People, Poverty, Power (3P) Model** (Bailey, 2018) to provide an overarching way for community health nurses (CHNs) to understand and intervene, and to act for social change to address violence and its economic, psychological, spiritual, and physical health impacts. We specifically explore areas of violence that are integral to community health nursing, including community-based violence and violence against key groups such as women and girls, older adults, and lesbian, gay, bisexual, transgender, questioning, or Two-Spirited (LGBTQ2S) people. These forms of violence heavily impact Canadians and are central in the roles and responsibilities of CHN.

Our discussion is grounded in **trauma and violence-informed care (TVIC)**. We integrate the many forms of **traumatic stress** that are associated with violence, including **vicarious trauma** or secondary traumatic stress and their impacts of violence on CHNs. **Atraumatic care** is also emphasized in CHN practice in the context of violence. The **Power and Control Wheel** (Pence & Paymar, 1993) is applied to describe micro (e.g., individual and family), meso (e.g., public health systems, health care institutions), and macro (e.g., colonialism, patriarchy) violence and health interventions—from individual and family intervention to social change for addressing violence. Rather than a separate section about implications for CHNs, we have woven ideas about CHN roles and responsibilities throughout the chapter. We further explore important processes and forms of violence such as **intimate partner violence (IPV)**; **sexualized violence**; **family violence**; **bullying**, **cyberbullying**, and **sexting**; and **human trafficking**. Although statistical data provide a great deal of information about violence against women, children, and men, there is growing recognition of the limitations of using only binary (male, female) gender categories in data collection and reporting.

OVERVIEW OF VIOLENCE AND HEALTH

Violence is an integral aspect of life for all of us, whether or not we experience it directly. For example, we are all impacted by media images of war and related crimes. Mass rape of women and girls is a well-documented weapon of war (United Nations [UN], 2015b). Sexualized violence is endemic in Western cultures, and sexualized images have become an everyday part of our lives through corporate marketing of everything from video games to clothing. The microaggressions associated with ageism, genderism, heterosexism, sexism, and racism are also common and insidious forms of violence. For example, a large Canadian study found that abuse of LGBT youth was prevalent in all Canadian provinces and that verbal homophobic abuse often preceded physical abuse (Peter, Taylor, & Chamberland, 2015). In Canada, the violence of genocide, including cultural genocide against First Nations, Inuit, and Métis peoples, is also a well-documented form of violence that heavily impacts Indigenous peoples and the country as a whole.

Violence is a complex social and public health problem that is strongly associated with the distribution of the social and structural determinants of health. It is also related to historical and contemporary patterns of thought, perspectives, attitudes, and behaviours influenced by an array of forces. Diverse patterns of violence are deeply rooted in cultural, political, and economic contexts and trends, such as the influences of mass media and mass communication on the ways we perceive different forms of violence (Carll, 2003). In the foreword of the World Report on Violence and Health, the late Nelson Mandela wrote that "many who live with violence day in and day out assume that it is an intrinsic part of the human condition. But this is not so. Violence can be prevented . . . Governments, communities and individuals can make a difference" (Krug, Dahlberg, Mercy, Zwi, & Lozano, 2002, para. 3).

The World Health Organization (WHO) defines violence as the intentional use of physical force or power against yourself, another person, or a group or community. This violence can be threatened or actual, and results in or is likely to result in injury, death, psychological harm, maldevelopment, or

deprivation (Krug et al., 2002). The word *power* and the phrase *use of physical force* are included in the definition to expand our conventional understanding of violence so we can identify violent acts that result from a power relationship, including threats and intimidation (Krug et al., 2002).

Violence contributes to lifelong ill health and early death, and it also costs the health, criminal justice, social and welfare, and economic sectors billions of dollars each year (World Health Organization [WHO], 2014). In conflict-affected regions, such as those experiencing war and other kinds of military-induced unrest, concentrated violence can perpetuate crime, stigma, and discriminatory patterns of thought and behaviours, and exacerbate societal divisions, which can restrict reduction, recovery, and other efforts (WHO, 2014). The social and psychological impact of violence on individuals, families, communities, and the global community is extensive and requires urgent attention across many disciplines. Nursing has a unique role in community health to lobby for policy change at the population level. This approach means that knowledge about how public policy operates (e.g., the policy cycle) is a core tool for CHNs. Collaborative efforts will foster capacity building across disciplines (e.g., nursing, anthropology, sociology, medicine, information science) and sectors (e.g., health, education, law).

Adoption and dissemination of evidence-based strategies for violence prevention are foundational considerations in community health nursing (Sleet et al., 2011). The CHN plays a pivotal role in violence prevention, as outlined in the Community Health Nurses of Canada's standards of practice (Community Health Nurses of Canada [CHNC], 2011, revised). These include screening and early detection of violence, prevention at all levels, and expanded collaboration across sectors to provide early intervention. The type of collaborative and prevention-focused approach described by the WHO is consistent with the collaborative public health approach well known to CHNs, who can work with community partners to intervene at all levels of prevention and health promotion. Specifically, our ethical foundations mean that we actively and reflectively practise with a knowledge base of the cycle of oppression (described more fully in Chapter 9) and specifically engage in anti-racist, anti-oppressive practice.

Data available to support evidence-based strategies, especially with respect to family violence and violence against women, is often hidden and difficult to capture because it relies on individual incidents reported to police. It is widely recognized that people are reluctant to report incidents of family violence because of concerns about personal and children's safety, stigma, and not being believed (Public Health Agency of Canada [PHAC], 2016). Women; children; First Nations, Inuit, and Métis peoples; people with disabilities; and people who identify as LGBTQ2S are under greater threat of experiencing family violence (PHAC, 2016). Based on a combination of police reports and population surveys in Canada, it is estimated that, in 2014, over 323,000 Canadians were victims of a violent crime, and for 85,000 of those victims, the perpetrators were family members (Perreault, 2015). Two-thirds of victims of intimate partner and family-related homicide are women (UN, 2015b).

It is also known that one in three Canadians report having experienced abuse before the age of 15. Although it is challenging to determine the true scope of violence against children, it is estimated that globally, during childhood, 25% of adults experienced physical abuse as children, and 20% of women and 8% of men experienced sexual abuse (WHO, 2016). According to Statistics Canada (2018), in 2016 there were approximately 54 900 children and youth who lived with family violence (aged 17 and younger). Approximately 16 200 (30%) were victims of family violence perpetrated by a parent, sibling, spouse, or other family member. The majority (59%) of children and youth were abused by their parents. Abuse by a parent decreased with age—it was most common when children were under age one (87%) and least common among youth (aged 12 to 17; 49%) (Statistics Canada, 2018). From 2011 to 2016, rates of family-related sexual assault against children and youth remained between four and five times higher among female victims, where one in three girls experience sexual violence before the age of 18 (Statistics Canada, 2018). When children have a physical or mental disability, they are at an even greater threat of experiencing physical and psychological abuse (Svensson, Bornehag, & Janson, 2011) and sexual abuse (Child Welfare Information Gateway, 2004). These threats include coercion or arbitrary deprivation of liberty, whether in public or in private life (UN, 1993). Health and social impacts are substantial. (See Figure 28.1.)

Women, children, and older adults are disproportionately impacted by nonfatal physical, sexual, and psychological abuse (WHO, 2014). According to Statistics Canada (2018), Canadian rates of older adult abuse are consistent with these findings. In 2016, more than 10 300 seniors (65 years and older) were victims of police-reported violent crime in Canada. Fifty-eight percent were women, with a rate 19% higher than that of older adult men. Overall, older adult victims of police-reported family violence were most likely to have been victimized by their child (32%), a spouse (27%), or another family member other than their child, spouse, or

sibling (29%). Examples of violence against women include IPV, nonpartner sexualized violence, and human trafficking. Violence against women is a broad term, defined by the UN as any act of gender-based violence that results in, or is likely to result in, physical, sexual, or mental harm or suffering to women. IPV is defined as any behaviour that causes physical, sexual, or psychological harm. This type of violence includes perpetration by current and former spouses as well as other intimate partners (WHO, 2013).

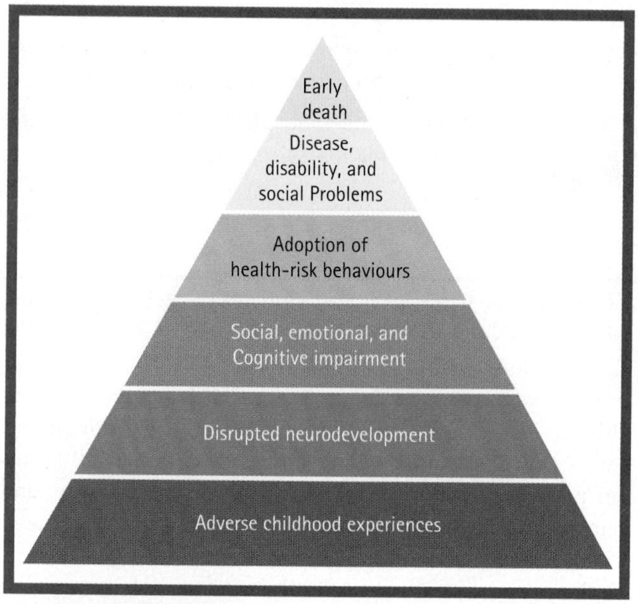

ROOT OR STRUCTURAL CAUSES OF SOCIETAL VIOLENCE

When we think of violence from a health field perspective, we most often think at the micro, or individual, level—individual or family causes and corresponding interventions. Although CHNs can and do intervene in these complex situations, it is important to consistently link these individual actions and reactions to the root causes of violence—the larger systemic power structures. They are called structural because "they are part of the political, economic, and social structure of society and of the culture that informs them" (Navarro, 2007, p. 2). When we consider violence from a structural perspective, we are thinking about the role of systemic processes in the creation and perpetuation of violence, such as the ways that violence is framed and organized by the health care system, the legal system, and many other societal systems and institutions. For this reason, **structural violence** is also called systemic violence. **Privilege**, further described in this chapter, happens in tandem with power. Some examples are white privilege, settler privilege, heterosexual privilege, male privilege, and class privilege. These are some of the underlying structures that create and sustain the many forms of violence.

For example, if you think of a wharf, the platform or walkway on top of the wharf is mostly what you see (Photo 28.1). Underneath this surface, multiple wooden and metal supports

FIGURE 28.1 The ACE Pyramid and Outcomes of Adverse Childhood Experiences

Source: National Center for Disease Prevention and Control (2016). *The Ace Pyramid.* Atlanta, Georgia: Centers for Disease Control.

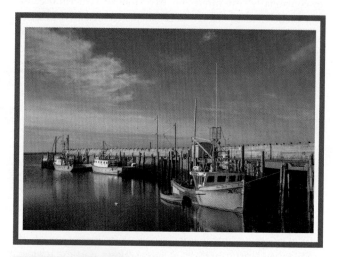

PHOTO 28.1 Understanding Structural Violence: A Seaside Wharf

Source: © Riley Smith Photography

provide the foundational structures that underpin the walking platform. In terms of violence and health, on the platform are all the aspects of violence you can "see," such as the statistical incidence of violence, the physical results of violence, and the human and environmental impacts of war, to name a few. However, you do not see the root causes because they are hidden below the surface in the systemic structures. **Systemic oppressions**, such as heterosexism, racism, and sexism, are examples of these societal structures (further described in Chapter 9). Systemic oppression is a broad term that describes racism and other systemic injustices that intersect and impede people's aspirations, progression, and quality of life.

The language used to describe violence provides insight into how to think and analyze at the structural level. For example, when we discuss individuals, families, and communities who are struggling with violence and inequities in the social determinants of health, we most often think in terms of vulnerable populations in an attempt to identify individuals who are particularly "at risk." However, since community health nursing is about tackling root, or structural, systemic causes of violence and inequities, and oppression-related health outcomes, it is very important to reframe vulnerable people as people under threat. The language of vulnerability implies that an individual or community is somehow more prone to experiencing health inequities, in much the same way as one might be prone to catching a cold (McGibbon, 2012).

The concept of vulnerability worked well when it first came into common usage because it allowed us to name the people who are most oppressed and thereby attempt to influence public policy in the direction of social justice. However, the term is not ultimately effective in decreasing physical, spiritual, and psychological suffering caused by injustice because it reinforces the idea of a vague force that is somehow causing violence and ill health. CHNs can help to shift this language to explicitly identify the structural threats that are causing ill health: colonization, re-colonization, post-colonialism, and imbalances in systemic power and privilege, to name a few (McGibbon, 2017). The interesting challenge for CHNs is to continually search out and "see" root or structural causes of violence and to engage in social-justice oriented practice. Canadian Research 28.1 describes how these structural contexts create violent attitudes and actions that impact health and quality of life for trans people.

CANADIAN RESEARCH 28.1

Negotiating violence in the context of transphobia and criminalization: The experiences of trans sex workers in Vancouver, Canada (Lyons et al., 2017).

Recent international evidence reports that trans sex workers are at greater risk of experiencing violence. The objective of this study was to examine how macro, structural contexts shape trans sex workers' experiences of violence. Thirty-three trans sex workers participated in semi-structured interviews in Vancouver. Qualitative analysis revealed three overarching themes: (1) transphobic violence, (2) clients' discovery of participants' gender identity, and (3) negative police responses to experiences of violence. In keeping with the emphasis on a structural approach to understanding violence in communities as outlined in this chapter, the authors describe trans sex workers' experience with violence within systemic social, political, and legal contexts. The intersection of poverty and gender with trans sex workers can lead to health inequities and violence. Further, 69.7% of participants were First Nations, Inuit, and Métis, which highlights the layer of racism and colonialism and their impacts on health.

Violence was a common and expected experience for trans sex workers in this setting and was shaped by the intersections of discrimination based on gender identity, gender expression, and the criminalization of sex work. Many participants discussed violence in terms of fear for their safety if clients discovered their gender identity. Police inaction to violence against trans sex workers reinforced participants' feelings of "deserving violence," which led to an adaption of their gender expression as a way to manage the violence they experience from their sex trade clients. The dominant relationship police have over trans sex workers, as demonstrated by inaction, is an example of the perpetuation of structural violence. The criminalization of sex work increases trans sex workers' vulnerability because it prevents them from reporting incidents. For First Nations, Métis, and Inuit participants, criminalization is intertwined with historical colonization and an overrepresentation of Indigenous people in Canadian jails and prisons (Correctional Investigator, 2014).

Discussion Questions

1. What are the intersecting macro, structural elements that First Nations, Inuit, and Métis trans sex workers might experience?

2. How would the decriminalization of sex work promote trans sex workers' occupational health and safety?

3. What are some of the root, structural interventions that address transphobia (e.g., health-related public policy)?

Given the many ways that violence impacts health, what can the CHN do in order to initiate meaningful change? The UN's 17 Sustainable Development Goals (SDGs) are a key example of a specific framework for CHNs to take action to initiate change. The SDGs have four goals: "eliminate all forms violence against women and girls; eliminate all harmful practices such as child, early and forced marriage, and female genital mutilation; significantly reduce all forms of violence and related death rates everywhere; and end abuse, exploitation, trafficking and all forms of violence against children" (UN, 2015a). There is potential for the SDGs to be a powerful violence prevention agenda, and CHNs can use many of these specific targets as a starting point when identifying priorities for action and interventions with their partnering communities.

THE PEOPLE, POVERTY, POWER MODEL: GIVING VOICE TO STRUCTURAL POWER AND PRIVILEGE

People, poverty, and power all intersect and overlap in the context of violence. These intersections are at the core of understanding the complexities of community-based violence. The People, Poverty, Power (3P) Model (Figure 28.2) demonstrates that violence involves more than individual behaviour. It is also a result of interactions between oppressive societal structures and social conditions such as poverty. These interactions create, and eventually increase, the prevalence of violence in Canada.

Many forms of violence are linked to privilege and power differentials. Privilege is a systematic or "institutional (rather than personal) set of benefits" that gives certain groups of people access to unearned power more than others (Kendell, 2002). Privilege is very difficult to see, especially for those who were born with, and live with, ready access to power and resources such as money, education, and freedom from worry about housing, food, or heat insecurity (Kendell, 2002). Power imbalances operate in many ways, particularly through decisions that create persisting and unjust disadvantages for some people and groups more than others. How individuals and groups view and understand power imbalances informs how they see their value and position in the world. For example, the meanings that individuals and groups make about differences in power and privilege influence their coping methods as well as their adaptive and responsive actions. Imbalances in power and privilege are evident in conditions of systemic oppression.

Central to the 3P Model is trauma, indicating that trauma is also central to violence. Trauma results from peoples' cumulative stressful experiences. In a root cause or structural perspective, we see how the stress of poverty is a result of inequities in the social determinants of health rather than laziness or lack of ambition. It is important to note that trauma is different from stress—trauma is long-term and has a greater physiological, psychological, and spiritual impact. Trauma also makes people especially sensitive to anything they interpret to be a risk. Different kinds of traumas intersect and compound to impact peoples' perspectives, behaviours, and views of the world and self. When people grapple with these traumas, their ways of thinking about the world around them become shifted, altering their self-identity. The result may be what is called a trauma-altered identity, which in some instances results in perpetrating acts of violence.

Poverty is now understood to be central to experiences of community violence. Conditions of poverty are related to a range of factors and conditions commonly found in poor neighbourhoods. As shown in the 3P Model, trauma is directly and indirectly connected to structural oppression, which intersects directly with poverty. Therefore, power and poverty are supporting foundations in peoples' trauma. Importantly, poverty leading to violence is not only a result of economic or monetary limits. People can also experience **social poverty** as a result of social inequities, such as lack of resources related to social support, social connection, family and community support, and access to culturally safe health and social services. Social poverty feeds violence because it makes people feel less worthy, and it can often stir bitterness.

Violence, as shown in the 3P Model, is not only an output or outcome but also an input. In other words, violence begets violence. For example, the encounters of Black youth with poverty, mistreatment in schools, and police profiling and hostility are forms of violence. These forms of violence look different from others, especially through the eyes of the person who is marginalized. The 3P Model allows us to pay attention to the way violence manifests not only on the person but also through the intersections of poverty and power. Poverty, privilege, and oppression lead to violence and are also acts of violence themselves.

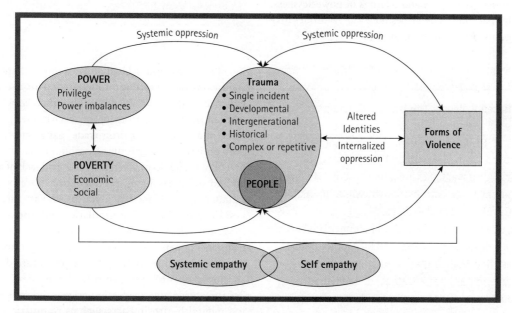

FIGURE 28.2 Community-based Violence: The People, Poverty, Power Model

The 3P Model highlights the importance of empathy in approaches to both address and prevent violence. A stance of empathy directs us to ask questions related to "how" and "why" a person commits violent acts. **Systemic empathy** and **self-empathy** are important foundations for preventing violence. Systemic empathy is an inherent understanding embedded in societal systems, such as the judicial, health care, and education systems, of the importance of striving for structural changes and community liberation. Systemic empathic approaches consider questions such as: Is there a way to measure the impact of trauma among people under threat? How and why is the intensity of the trauma endured by people a legitimate factor in their violent experiences? How can trauma and violence-informed public policy create specific interventions for addressing systemic violence, such as gun violence?

Self-empathy may be defined as actualized self-forgiveness by people experiencing poverty and oppression, and it is a key to building resilience. However, social poverty, and imbalances in power and privilege, can hinder peoples' efforts toward self-empathy. When both forms of empathy intersect or act together, as seen in the 3P Model, the process can strongly facilitate peoples' understanding of the roots of their trauma and therefore can serve to prevent violence. Systemic empathy, and self-empathy in persons who experience violence, are the foundation for necessary system change and related leadership in nursing practice, policy making, and research.

The intersections in systemic violence are like threads well woven into a sweater, where each thread becomes indistinguishable. The sweater is not woven with isolated attention to each thread but to the whole. Although the 3P Model is a somewhat linear depiction of this complex process, it helps CHNs focus on common reasons that surface when we ask "why" and "how" in situations of violence. CHNs can then analyze the root causes of struggles people encounter across the lifespan and how these struggles contribute to traumatization and violence. The 3P Model highlights the forces people have to navigate that, without the right tools, can result in hopelessness. This hopelessness perpetuates trauma experiences and feelings of powerlessness. The Case Study that follows describes how the 3P Model may be applied to gun violence in communities.

receive counselling. Husbands told the court that on the day of the shooting, while in a shopping mall, he saw two of the men who were involved in brutally beating him. Believing they were there to kill him, he retaliated out of fear, firing his gun at them 14 times.

The two assailants were killed, and five others were injured. Husbands also recounted an incident when he was 12 years old that impacted his trajectory in life. He was asked by one of his teachers to speak at a town hall held at his school on policing and violence. On his way to the school, he was stopped by Toronto Police. He was questioned, aggressively thrown against a wall, and threatened by police. In a CBC interview, his teacher recalled that he arrived at the town hall late and vividly shaken. When it was his turn to speak, he took the mic and stated, "My name is Christopher. I'm from Regent Park. My question is why isn't there a police hotline or a place for kids, where kids could go and speak out that are being targeted?"

These experiences were followed by a series of behavioural issues in school and criminal charges with a jail term. Husbands admitted in court that at the time of the shooting, he reacted out of a state of shock, traumatized from the brutal beating he'd encountered a few months earlier. Husbands was sentenced to life in prison, eligible for parole in 30 years. His teacher remarked. "To look at them [young Black men] and think that it's a one-dimensional thing is a mistake as a society. These young men did not need to end up in this situation—dead or in jail for the rest of their lives. It's not predestined, and there are lots of things we could do to make it better."

Discussion Questions

1. Why and how did Christopher Husbands become involved in violent acts in his community?

2. In what ways can CHNs take action to decrease gun violence in communities?

Author Generated

CASE STUDY

Community-Based Violence: The Story of Christopher Husbands

At the age of 11, Christopher Husbands, a young Black man, moved from Guyana to Regent Park, one of Toronto's most disadvantaged neighbourhoods. He lived in a single-parent home with his father, while his mother remained in Guyana, addicted to drugs. At age 12, Husbands fell into drug dealing. In June 2012, Christopher Husbands opened fire in a crowded shopping mall in Toronto, Canada. Husbands testified that in the months leading up to the shooting, he was brutally beaten, stabbed, and left to die by a group of young men. Following this incident, he struggled with fear, paranoia, and severe trauma, for which he did not

The Christopher Husbands example demonstrates that conditions of poverty are fundamental to the prevalence of violence in disadvantaged neighbourhoods, which are often marked by poor distribution of services and programs, existence of a local gun or drug trade, gang activity, exposure to over-policing, and stigma. Compounding these factors are neighbourhood decay, overcrowding, and lack of access to mental and social resources, producing or exacerbating immense trauma, especially for Black youth, who are further marginalized by race. With the accumulation and intersections of these factors, Black youth such as Husbands become witnesses and recipients of neighbourhood crime, racial profiling, and police hostility as well as the impacts of premature death of friends and loved ones to community violence. Many of these youth feel threatened, deprived, stigmatized, and trapped, with ensuing mental health impacts such as traumatic stress, anxiety, depression, fear, a sense of hopelessness, anger, and aggression.

Poverty among the most impoverished Black and First Nations, Inuit, and Métis communities in Canada is linked to the brutality of colonial histories of oppression. Stories of these oppressions are passed down through generations and are lived out through feelings of unworthiness, which grow as seeds in an oppressed mind (Jones, 2000). The meanings that come from historical reminders are compelling. For example, in some Black youth, these reminders play out in families and in community interactions that inform how they see themselves in this world, how they interact, and the value they ascribe to themselves. Public narratives of them further solidify their negative self-identity. Historic oppression can be painful, and when it continues to live in present-day social inequities, the impact is traumatic. Racialized and marginalized groups, including Black Canadians, are living two oppressive realities—historical and present. History informs their lived experiences and shapes their self-value, and present day impacts of these realities reinforce pain, resentment, and trauma. Systemic oppression does not target an individual. It targets the identities that are associated with who we are—age, culture, gender identity, race, sexual orientation, social class, and religion, to name a few. Early intervention is important to frame young people's vision of themselves and the world. As depicted in the 3P Model, when these early interventions are missing, it is necessary to implement system interventions rooted in empathy to take guns out of their hands.

MORE FORMS OF STRUCTURAL POWER, PRIVILEGE, AND VIOLENCE

In this chapter we have discussed a number of forms of violence and applied the 3P Model to help CHNs understand how violence is about power and privilege. In the following sections, we continue to talk about violence, with more examples of societal violence and how it is connected to systemic power.

Sexualized Violence, Family Violence, and Interpersonal Violence

Sexualized violence, including sexual harassment and sexual assault, disproportionately impacts women, and it is an example of violence that is rooted in gender inequity. Sexualized violence is defined as "any sexual act, attempt to obtain a sexual act, unwanted sexual comments or advances, or acts to traffic, or otherwise directed against a person's sexuality, using coercion, by any person regardless of their relationship to the victim, in any setting, including, but not limited to, home and work" (Jewkes, Sen, & Garcia-Moreno, 2002). In 2014 there were more than 635 000 incidents of sexual assault reported by Canadians (Conroy & Cotter, 2017). Sexual assault is a subcategory of sexualized violence that "includes the use of physical or other force to obtain or attempt sexual penetration" (WHO, 2013). Seventy-one percent of incidents of sexual assault in Canada included unwanted sexual touching, 20% were sexual attacks, and 9% involved sexual assault where the victim was unable to consent due to drugs, intoxication, or manipulation (Conroy & Cotter, 2017).

The rate of self-reported sexual assault was unchanged in Canada from 2004 to 2014. In all other forms of violence and nonviolent crime measured by the same survey, the rates of crime declined significantly. Although self-reported rates were unchanged, it is important to note that police-reported sexual assault declined by 20%. Police-reported data can underestimate the extent of sexual assault—some of the reasons for not reporting include not wanting to deal with police, not considering the incident important enough, feeling that there is a lack of evidence, or believing the offender will not be adequately punished. Rates of sexual assault are highest among the following women: single; First Nations, Inuit, and Métis; individuals who rate their mental health as fair or poor; students; individuals who self-identify as gay, lesbian or bisexual; and women aged 15–24 (Conroy & Cotter, 2017).

YES, BUT WHY?

Sexual and Psychological Non-Fatal Physical Violence Disproportionately Impacts Women

What?

Substantial evidence tells us that violence against women is a common feature in the lives of Canadian women. It is vital to connect this violence with the persistent violence against women in all countries. Globally, one in five women have been sexually abused as children. (See Figure 28.3.) Further, one in three women was a victim of physical or sexual violence by an intimate partner at some point in her lifetime (WHO, 2014). Though these rates are similar for women in Canada, First Nations, Inuit, and Métis women are more than two times as likely as non-First Nations, Inuit, and Métis women to experience intimate partner violence (Statistics Canada, 2015). Women are also more likely to be killed by an intimate partner (PHAC, 2016). Sexualized violence, including sexual harassment and assault, disproportionately affect women—women are far more likely to be stabbed, murdered, beaten, or otherwise abused than men. Although it is crucially important to identify men who are under threat (e.g., boys, youth, older adult men, trans men, men with disabilities, LGBTQ2S people), women and girls bear the brunt of these forms of violence.

So What?

It is difficult to understand and, for some, to believe, that violence against women is so common. However, the facts are clear, whether we use evidence from Statistics Canada, the UN, or the WHO. The causes of these differences are the unequal distribution of financial, economic, and cultural power. Violence against women is rooted in the structural determinants of health: patriarchy, colonialism, and persistent economic and sociopolitical inequities and injustices. Consider the following statistics: women make up less than 10% of world leaders (Geiger & Kent, 2017); Canadian women earn an average of $0.87 for every $1 a man earns (Flexhaug, 2017); racialized women and women with disabilities earn even less; only 6.4% of CEOs of Fortune 500 companies are women (Fortune Editors, 2017); and women represent 40% of the world's labour force but hold just 1% of the world's wealth (World Bank, 2018). Statistics such as these can form the foundation of CHNs' understanding of the persistence of violence against the women in their communities. When women lack economic and political power, their power to control their lives is diminished, which places them under more threat of abuse, including violence.

Now What?

CHNs have a key role in turning the lens inward and educating themselves about the breadth and depth of violence against women. This path will inevitably lead to a feminist analysis of gender and power. Nursing students can seek out and enroll in women's and gender studies courses. CHNs can engage in continued learning such as community-based education and online courses. Both students and registered nurses can specifically seek out public presentations and forums about violence against women, especially first-voice accounts that analyze sexualized violence, including systematic violence against First Nations, Inuit, and Métis women in Canada. However, education is not enough. An advocacy role is the ethical next step, where students and CHNs themselves create forums to educate others about violence against women, building community capacity to take action. Nursing students can work collaboratively with other students to organize town hall meetings and debates about violence on university campuses. They can familiarize themselves with Wijeyesinghe, Griffin, and Love's (2010) Social Change Continuum, where educating themselves and others leads to social justice strategies for prevention at the individual, family, and community levels, as well as in systemic or public policy realms.

Standards of Practice Fulfilled

#1 Health Promotion
- Considers the determinants of health, the social and political context, and systemic structures in collaboration with the client to determine action.

#6 Health Equity
- Advocates for healthy public policy and social justice by participating in legislative and policy-making activities that influence determinants of health and access to services.
- Understands historical injustices, inequitable power relations, institutionalized and interpersonal racism and their impacts on health and health care and provides culturally safe care (Community Health Nurses of Canada [CHNC], 2019, revised).

The phrase #MeToo was coined in 2006 by Tarana Burke, a woman who had experienced sexual assault and wanted to prevent other incidents against African American women (Johnson & Hawbaker, 2018). In the last decade, #MeToo has become the slogan for the anti-sexual harassment movement.

Initially, the goal of this Twitter campaign was to give the public a sense of the magnitude of the issues surrounding sexual harassment, but the movement developed into worldwide social media activism (Gilbert, 2017). Examples include the recent (2017–2018) women's marches focused on disapproval of American administration and policies related to sexual violence, as well as the establishment of the anti-harassment coalition called Time's Up, a legal defence fund to provide subsidized support for women and men who have experienced sexual violence in the workplace (Stevens, 2018).

The #MeToo movement has sparked conversations and dialogue that are creating pressure to influence policy in Canada, as shown in the 2018 federal budget and the new Royal Canadian Mounted Police (RCMP) task force to address supposedly "unfounded" cases of sexual assault. Unfounded, a 20-month long project spearheaded by *Globe and Mail* reporter Robyn Doolittle (2017), investigated the way the Canadian police handle sexual-assault complaints. Using data gathered from hundreds of police services across the country, Doolittle demonstrated that sexual-assault complaints are twice as likely to be dismissed as unfounded than complaints in other assault cases. Through public pressure, the investigation caused law-enforcement agencies to review more than 37 000 cases, and some agencies pledged to revamp their approach to policing sexual violence. This policy intervention is an excellent example of public pressure to build healthy public policy, one of the main public health principles in the Ottawa Charter (WHO, 1986).

A recent report released by the Chief Public Health Officer in Canada (PHAC, 2016) focused on family violence. Family violence was defined as violence, abuse, unhealthy conflict, or neglect by a family member toward another family member that has the potential to lead to ill health, and intimate partners were included in the broader category of family members. Some common types of family violence include physical, sexual, emotional, and financial abuse, as well as neglect and exposure to intimate partner violence, such as when children witness their father's violence toward their mother. In addition to women, children, older adults, and First Nations, Inuit, and Métis peoples, people living with disabilities and members of the LGBTQ2S community were found to be under greater threat of experiencing family violence (PHAC, 2016). For First Nations, Inuit, and Métis peoples, family violence has its historical roots in the impacts of intergenerational trauma related to the Indian residential schools as well as historical and political contexts that have contributed to generations of oppression (PHAC, 2016). Of particular concern to the CHN is self-reported data from the 2014 General Social Survey on Canadians' Safety (Victimization) showing that 70% of persons subjected to spousal violence, and 93% of children who were physically or sexually abused, never spoke to authorities about their experiences (Burczycka & Ibrahim, 2016). Figure 28.4 illustrates how family violence leads to health impacts.

Physical impacts of IPV and family violence are compounded by chronic stress and responses used to cope with chronic stress (Statistics Canada, 2015). Women are more likely than men to experience the health impacts of IPV (PHAC, 2016). Women, men, and children who experience family

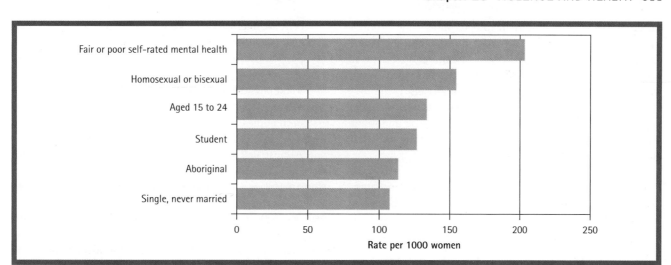

violence are also more likely to have negative impacts on their mental health (PHAC, 2016). Social impacts of family violence include the person's diminished capacity to have healthy social relationships, poor academic performance in school, and missing work or being less productive at work. These factors can lead to unemployment and financial instability (PHAC, 2016). From 2009–2014, self-reported Statistics Canada survey data showed that 4% of Canadians aged 15 and older experienced violence by

a current or former spouse or common-law partner—about 760 000 individuals (Burczycka & Ibrahim, 2016; Statistics Canada, 2018). The same survey reported that women are more likely to experience the most severe forms of spousal violence (including sexual assault and being beaten or choked), have injuries, and suffer long-term psychological consequences, such as those associated with post-traumatic stress disorder.

Given the troubling statistics regarding women's experiences of violence, CHNs have an important role and responsibility in caring for women who are experiencing IPV. Universal screening for IPV is recommended as best practice for all girls and women above the age of 12 (Registered Nurses Association of Ontario [RNAO], 2012). It is also imperative to identify boys and men who are particularly under threat of experiencing violence (IPV, family violence, sexual and physical assault), such as trans men and LGBTQ2S men; young people, regardless of gender, who work in the sex trade, often engaging in survival sex to pay for food and shelter; and older adult men. This comprehensive screening also includes assessment and intervention across diverse personal and family contexts, including LGBTQ2S relationships. In addition to universal screening, CHNs are also responsible for creating a practice environment that supports disclosure, which requires that they ask key questions about IPV and respond appropriately. This critical role requires nurses to engage in reflective practice to examine their own values and beliefs, the ever-present systemic and political contexts of violence, and the core importance of trauma.

In Canada there are no mandatory obligations for the nurse to report IPV unless the person experiencing violence decides that this is what they would like to do. For children between 12 and 14 years of age, the exceptions to this law include instances where the age difference between the two people engaging in sexual activity is more than two years or the other person is in a position of trust or authority. For young people between the ages of 14 to 16, the nurse has a duty to report if the age difference is more than five years or the other person is in a position of trust or authority. If IPV is occurring in a home with

FIGURE 28.4 How Family Violence Leads to Health Impacts

children present, it is important to determine if the children have been exposed emotionally, verbally, or physically. Prior to reporting to the local department of children's services, it is important that the nurse talk with the person experiencing violence and advise them of this obligation. Because each province and territory has different acts that describe obligations for reporting to the department of child services, it is important that nurses be familiar with their local legislation and legal obligations (RNAO, 2012).

When asking people about IPV, it is important to do so in a private location when they are alone. The following questions illustrate some examples of ways to ask women about IPV (RNAO, 2012, Appendix D):

- "Because violence against women is so common in many people's lives, I now ask all my clients about it. May I ask you a couple of questions?"
- "Many of the women I see are dealing with abuse in their relationships. Some are too afraid and uncomfortable to bring it up themselves, so I've started asking about it routinely. May I ask you a couple of questions?"
- "Have you ever been emotionally, physically, or sexually abused by your partner or someone important to you?"

If the woman says no, do not explore further. If the woman responds yes, ask more specific questions in the context of trauma and violence-informed care, discussed in detail later in this chapter.

There is no one single cause of family violence and IPV, and there is a strong association between these forms of violence and the social determinants of health. The chronic stress of housing, food, and heat insecurity places a remarkable burden on individuals, families, and communities over time. Prevention should be targeted at multiple levels, and CHNs can consider the principles of population health, where systemic factors, such as housing policies and policies to support a living wage, impact the threat of family violence and IPV.

Stalking, Cyberbullying, and Human Trafficking

Innovations in information technology, such as the use of the internet for violent or abusive means, are increasingly damaging the health of Canadians. Stalking, cyberbullying, and human trafficking often integrate many forms of violence, including sexualized violence and IPV. **Stalking** is an increasingly prevalent form of IPV in Canada. Text and social media stalking has particularly increased since 2004. According to the 2014 General Social Survey (Statistics Canada, 2018, p. 4):

> Stalking is defined as repeated and unwanted attention that causes a person to fear for their personal safety or for the safety of someone they know, a definition which qualifies as criminal harassment under the Criminal Code of Canada (s. 264).1, 2 While stalking, by definition, makes someone feel unsafe, it can take the form of actions that do not include overt threats of physical violence. Examples include threats to divulge sensitive

personal information and unwanted romantic advances that make the person feel unsafe, despite not including threats of physical harm. Stalking can encompass a range of behaviours, such as someone waiting outside a person's home, school or work, physical or electronic surveillance, damage to property and various kinds of unwanted communication, as further outlined in the Criminal Code (ss. 372(2) and (3)).

Almost half of people who were subjected to stalking were between 15 and 34 years of age (48%), and most were women (62%) (Statistics Canada, 2018). Although most stalkers were male, the proportion who were female increased between 2004 and 2014 (15%–19%). Stalking took the form of threats or intimidation against someone else they knew (reported by 39%); repeated, obscene, or silent phone calls (31%); and unwanted emails, texts, or social media messages (28%) (Statistics Canada, 2018). One-third of people who were stalked endured physical intimidation or threats of violence consistent with Criminal Code definitions of assault (32%), and one in five (18%) experienced actual physical violence. Half of those who were stalked reported that their stalker was someone they knew, other than an intimate partner (49%), and 27% were stalked by strangers. Twenty-one percent of stalkers were current or former intimate partners (Statistics Canada, 2018). Certain populations, including First Nations, Inuit, and Métis individuals and those identifying as gay, lesbian, or bisexual, were overrepresented among people who are stalked. In intimate partner stalking, women are significantly more likely to be stalked, and there was a greater association with violence and higher levels of reporting to police (Statistics Canada, 2018).

Bullying is the exertion of power and control over another, typically by using vulnerabilities of others to control them. Bullying may take many forms: direct (physical or verbal aggression, intimidation), and indirect (social isolation or exclusion, spreading lies) (Craig & McCuaig, 2012). It may include sexual harassment or discrimination related to any of the isms (e.g., ableism, ageism, genderism, heterosexism, racism, sexism). Bullying through the internet is cyberbullying—harassment over social media or other platforms, including sexting explicit pictures or content. Approximately 40% of adolescents in a Canadian study reported having been both the bully and the victim (Craig & McCuaig, 2012). The most frequent incidence was in the younger grades, decreasing by grade six, until approximately grade nine or ten, when bullying became relatively less frequent. Over half of the bullying was through indirect means or teasing.

Boys were more often victims of physical bullying than girls; sexual harassment and cyberbullying was experienced at a far greater rate for girls in all grades (Lamb, Pepler, & Craig, 2009). Disruption in relationships with parents has been found to place young people under more threat of being bullies or of being bullied (Lereya, Muthanna, & Wolke, 2013). Bullies are also more likely to have experienced abuse before entering school. Warm, affectionate relationships with parents, parental involvement, and supervision were protective factors that decreased chances of being bullied. Cyberbullying has been linked to many serious consequences, including academic dropout, mental health struggles, gang involvement, and suicide (Notar, Padgett, & Roden, 2013). CHN interventions to address bullying include strategies to promote empathy and prosocial behaviour and to reduce peer reinforcement of bullying behaviour (Lamb et al., 2009).

Fifty-nine percent of trans youth from the Atlantic provinces who participated in an online study reported having been bullied once or more in the past year, with 33% reporting they had been bullied between one and three times in the past year (Gahagan, Ferguson, Saewyc, Frohard-Dourlent, & Veale, 2018). Thirty percent of younger trans youth said they had been bullied through the internet in the past year, and 65% of older trans youth reported having been threatened or received aggressive emails or instant messages in the past year (Gahagan et al., 2018). Some CHN interventions to address violence against trans youth include creating safer schools through designing and implementing gender-inclusive school policies; positive space training for teachers, administrators, and counsellors on gender identity and gender affirming approaches; awareness campaigns and education for students; and gender-neutral washrooms and change rooms. In order to provide knowledgeable and accessible health care services, CHNs require discipline-specific training, which would include education about gender identity and protocols for addressing trans youth health concerns. CHNs can also advocate for healthy public policy that prevents barriers in accessing care. A pivotal component to addressing issues for trans youth is engaging them in a meaningful way because they are the experts in their own experiences of access barriers.

Another pervasive form of violence, human trafficking, is an extremely lucrative transnational business, reaching as far as, and generating the same amount of money as, drugs and firearms trafficking. Profit is mostly created through sex trade exploitation (Government of Canada, 2016). Human trafficking relies on controlling and exploiting people to generate ongoing income, and people are often pushed or lured into trafficking through conditions of extreme poverty, disadvantage, lack of education, and civil unrest such as war. The majority of persons who are trafficked are women, and they are recruited through threats, coercion, abduction, fraud, or use of power to gain control (WHO, 2012). Drug and alcohol use (forced or coerced) is used as a means to control individuals (or as a coping mechanism by people who are trafficked), as are financial exploitation and control of their means of economic survival (WHO, 2012). Although human trafficking is perhaps seen as something happening elsewhere, the statistics concerning girls in Canada are disturbing, with the majority of these girls being Canadian citizens or permanent residents of Canada (Royal Canadian Mounted Police [RCMP], 2014).

The average age for exploitation is 13 to 15 years (Government of Canada, 2016). Individuals most under threat of human trafficking include First Nations, Inuit, and Métis youth, who make up 30–50% of exploited youth; lesbian, gay, and bisexual youth; previously exploited and abused youth (25%); homeless youth; migrants; and children in protective care (RCMP, 2014). Non-Canadian victims were found to be most often from Asia (Thailand, Cambodia, Malaysia, and Vietnam) and eastern European countries. Some women are brought to Canada to work as live-in domestics and are subsequently trafficked (RCMP, 2014).

CHNs have a key role and responsibility in early identification of people who have been or are being trafficked. Important indicators include repeat visits for sexually transmitted infections, unexplained injuries, fearful behaviour, and perhaps language barriers (Crane & Moreno, 2011). Research has shown that almost half of people who are trafficked sought health care for various reasons, and yet they were not asked about safety, why they had so many infections, or if they were ever expected to have sexual intercourse when they did not want it (Konstantanopoulos et al., 2013). They may not initially disclose, but studies have shown that individuals would have eventually done so if asked (Konstantanopoulos et al., 2013). Once identified, the next step is for the CHN to assist people in accessing relevant resources. Toronto and Vancouver have been active centres in developing guidelines for trafficking recognition and interventions, as have the RCMP and Status of Women Canada. Some initiatives include training for groups most under threat, such as First Nations, Inuit, and Métis communities and refugee communities, training of law enforcement and community service agencies, development of trafficking laws in the Canadian Criminal Code, provision of temporary immigration status and work permits for rescued foreign victims, and international partnerships with police and border service agencies (Government of Canada, 2016).

REVISITING POWER AND VIOLENCE: THE POWER AND CONTROL WHEEL

The Power and Control Wheel (Pence & Paymar, 1993) is a key tool for CHNs to assess and intervene in violence. The wheel (Figure 28.5) specifically describes the ways interpersonal power can operate. Coercion and threats, intimidation, emotional abuse, isolations, and minimizing, denying, and blaming are some of the well-known forms of physical and sexualized violence that occur in interpersonal relationships. Other forms may be less acknowledged, including using children, using male privilege, and economic abuse. The following case application activity explores how CHNs can apply the Power and Control Wheel in assessing and intervening in abuse of people 65 and over.

POWER AND CONTROL WHEEL CASE APPLICATION ACTIVITY: ABUSE OF PEOPLE 65 AND OVER

Goal: This Power and Control Wheel activity is designed to help you think about the many forms of violence and how they operate in the everyday lives of people in your communities and in your nursing practice. Specifically, you will gain a deeper understanding of the violence and health struggles of older adults and communities with whom you provide nursing care.

Instructions:

1) Divide yourselves into groups of no more than eight people.
2) Each group makes up a brief case study involving an older adult. The case study should include at least the following information about the individual or family: name, age (65+), gender, sexual orientation, race, socioeconomic status, and living situation. You are encouraged to be creative and inclusive. Also include the community-based nursing care setting (e.g., community health center, long-term care, public health).
3) Choose at least three of the forms of violence in the wheel, and integrate them into your case study. Collectively reflect about and describe how these forms of violence would actually play out in the life of the individual.
4) Each group shares its case study.

Questions for Personal Reflection, Group Discussion and Debate, and Nursing Action

1. In each group, describe what it was like to construct the case studies. What thoughts and emotions were present? Which areas of abuse were more (or less) difficult to integrate?
2. Using your case study as an example, what are some barriers the person or her or his family might experience in attempting to seek intervention?
3. Make a list of the resources in your area (title of agency, location, contact information) that would be most appropriate to recommend for the person in your case study. Include considerations regarding to barriers accessibility (e.g., disability, lack of cultural safety, lack of services in rural areas).

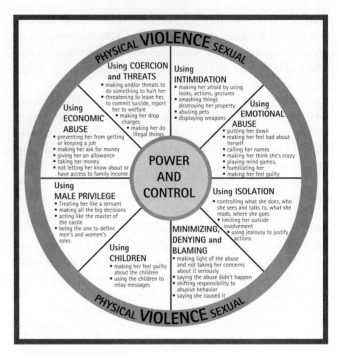

FIGURE 28.5 The Power and Control Wheel

Source: Registered Nurses' Association of Ontario. (2005). Woman abuse: Screening, identification and initial response. Toronto, Canada: Registered Nurses' Association of Ontario. Original Diagram from Pence & Paymar, 1993.

Canadian government power to act, or not act, on the Commission's recommendations. Lack of government action reflected overall Canadian minimizing, denying, and blaming related to the realities of ongoing discrimination of First Nations, Métis, and Inuit women (Jacobs, 2010).

TRAUMA AND VIOLENCE–INFORMED CARE

We are most familiar with power and control in IPV and family violence. However, power and control also occur at the systemic level. The Christopher Husbands case study of community-based violence in this chapter provides a detailed explanation about how individual acts of violence are connected to macro structural issues involving poverty and power. Structural power and control are also illustrated in the Unfounded Project described earlier in the chapter, where police administration and police officers together used many of the forms of power and control depicted in the Power and Control Wheel: minimizing, denying, and blaming; emotional abuse; intimidation; and male privilege. Another important example of how the wheel operates at the systemic level involves the missing and murdered First Nations, Inuit, and Métis women and girls in Canada. In 2017 the Native Women's Association of Canada released its report card assessing the progress of the Commission for the National Inquiry into the Missing and Murdered Indigenous Women and Girls (Native Women's Association of Canada, 2017). The Canadian government, through the commissioners, received a failing grade on 10 of 15 assessment areas and no passing grades on the remaining five areas—a troubling example of power imbalances, in this case, the dominance of

Violence inscribes deep physical, spiritual, and psychological wounds caused by processes such as the misogyny inherent in violence against women and girls, the hatred of LGBTQ2S people, the legacy of slavery in the United States and Canada, and the historical injustices of colonialism against First Nations, Inuit, and Métis peoples and peoples in the African diaspora. Trauma is, by its nature, deeply embedded in the soul, psyche, and cognitive schema of individuals who are traumatized (McGibbon, 2017). The world may become reframed as a dangerous place, and continued survival often involves feelings of detachment or numbing. Recurring images and nightmares of traumatic experiences create a persistent reliving of the trauma(s) (Herman, 1997). Poverty and biologically induced traumas—such as hunger or prolonged malnutrition, inadequate and crowded shelter, inadequate medical care, unemployment, underemployment, or employment in temporary jobs without medical, dental, and eye-care benefits—all cause severe mental health consequences over time. These trauma-related impacts can cause parental insecurity; overwork, fatigue, and accompanying irritability; limited availability of parents to children due to overwork, fatigue, tension, and illness; and chronic ongoing threats to security and well-being for parents and their children (Kira, 2001). The 3P Model described how trauma can impact individuals, families, and communities over time.

Trauma is an everyday aspect of community-based nursing. It may involve single incident trauma, where the person experiences one trauma experience (e.g., physical/sexual assault, motor vehicle accident), developmental trauma (e.g., experiencing or witnessing early ongoing or repetitive trauma), intergenerational trauma (e.g., family experiences of gun and gang violence), historic trauma (e.g., Holocaust, slavery, and experiences of long-term physical, spiritual, and cultural assaults of Indian Residential Schools), and complex or repetitive trauma (e.g., domestic violence, war, ongoing betrayal). The overlapping circles in Figure 28.6 illustrate that these forms of trauma can and do happen at the same time in any one individual, family, and community.

Intergenerational trauma transmission and historic trauma are often a key piece to the puzzle of community-based traumas, where CHNs assess and intervene with families and communities. The centrality of cultural, spiritual, and material loss is a cornerstone of intergenerational trauma transmission among oppressed peoples. In intergenerational family trauma transmission, adults' traumatic experiences and their effects are transmitted within a family system across generations. For example, according to Mi'kmaq Elder and historian Dr. Daniel Paul, abuses in residential schools severely impacted Indigenous peoples' adult lives and their parenting over time (Paul, 2007), thus creating the context for family trauma transmission. There is no doubt that the way many Indigenous people remember their past, and interpret those traumatic events as individuals and as a people, contributes to contemporary social problems in Indigenous communities (Wesley-Esquimaux & Smolewski, 2004).

When CHNs practise TVIC, they assume the very real possibility of trauma experiences in the individuals, families, and communities with whom they practise—regardless of practice area. Our engagement, assessment, intervention, and follow-up care are all guided by knowledge of the process of traumatic stress and its impacts. Trauma-informed care may also involve the need to respond to an individual's intersecting experiences of trauma, mental health struggles, and substance use concerns (Arthur et al., 2013).

Trauma and violence-informed care (practice, policy making, leadership) is care that integrates the importance and implication of trauma with the inevitable traumatic outcomes of violence. This integration is very important because "people who have experienced trauma likely have experienced boundary violations and abuses of power" (EQUIP Health Care, 2017, p. 1). CHNs can play a central role in creating a space where people feel as physically and emotionally safe as possible, especially since they may currently be in unsafe relationships with ongoing violence, and they may live in unsafe conditions, such as racism and poverty (EQUIP Health Care, 2017). According to EQUIP Health Care (EQUIP Health Care, 2017, pp. 2–3), there are four key ways to practise trauma and violence-informed care:

1. Build awareness among staff and clients. All services taking a trauma and violence-informed approach begin with building awareness among staff and clients: Organizations must ensure that training about trauma, violence and TVIC is accessible to staff—meaning that it is available, and they are supported to complete it both in terms of time and costs;

2. Emphasize safety and trust: It is not necessary to know an individual's history of trauma and violence in order to provide TVIC. Everyone should receive respectful, safe care;

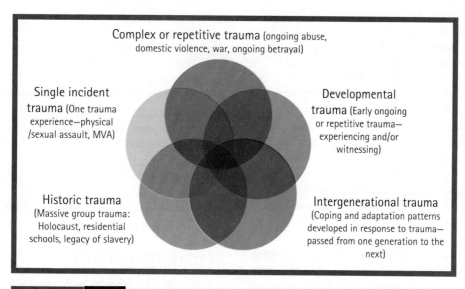

FIGURE | **28.6** Connections Among the Different Forms of Trauma

Source: Based on Arthur et al., 2013.

3. Adapt your language: Organizations can model non-stigmatizing language everywhere, from signage to EMR systems to how clients' situations are discussed by staff;

4. Consider trauma a risk factor: Women exposed to interpersonal violence have increased risks of chronic physical health problems.

A closely related aspect of TVIC is engaging in atraumatic care. The concept of atraumatic care, introduced by Dr. Donna Wong, a pediatric intensive care nurse, is defined as "care that minimizes the psychologic and physical stress that health promotion and illness can inflict" (Hockenberry & Wilson, 2015). Wong further explains that nurses are often desensitized regarding the ways that health care intervention may be difficult for those who seek care, including their families and communities. Most importantly, atraumatic nursing care involves continuously setting a mindful stance to minimize the occurrence of additional trauma inflicted by clinicians and the health care system in the course of care. Some examples of atraumatic care for CHNs include meticulous attention to physical, emotional, and spiritual privacy, and deliberately creating a physical and emotional environment that is compassionate and welcoming, including practising in a culturally safe way.

Vicarious Trauma and Secondary Traumatic Stress: Nurses' Responses to Violence

Psychological and spiritual trauma are directly associated with violence, whether it is IPV, violence witnessed by children in the home, community-based violence, or systemic violence such as homophobic hatred or lack of systemic economic support to prevent individuals and families from living in poverty. As CHNs, we bear witness to all these forms of violence, honouring the complex pathways that lead people to become violent toward each other and the inevitable trauma that results. The everyday practice of nursing is replete with the witnessing of traumatic experiences. For example, CHNs observe the profound struggles of homeless people or the intergenerational impacts of violence in the family home. Trauma is foundational to the engagement of nursing, and nurses often experience vicarious trauma (VT) as a result of their engagement in practice (McGibbon, 2004). VT is the phenomenon of changes in cognition and worldview that result from empathic response and repeated exposure to narratives of trauma (Raunick, Lindell, Morris, & Backman, 2017). VT involves the transmission of emotionally laden trauma stories and witnessing of the results of psychological, spiritual, and physical traumas of people, families, and communities in the course of practice. CHNs can also experience significant VT in their social justice work to ensure that individuals and families have access to food, heat, and shelter, as well as health care access (Austin & Holdt, 2017).

Responses to VT involve the same experiences as post-traumatic stress, including nightmares, fearful thoughts, and intrusive images. Practitioners who experience VT may also become more cynical and distrustful, and may experience increased thoughts and images associated with personal vulnerability,

such as loved ones being in a car accident (McCann & Pearlman, 1990). Clark and Gioro (1998) conducted one of the first studies about VT in nursing, reporting that nurses experienced emotional numbing, nightmares, irritability, distancing and withdrawal, and spiritual and moral suffering as a result of their trauma work. As this discussion attests, nurses' responses to violence intervention can have immediate and long-lasting impacts. Although few nursing education programs, or even continuing education programs, integrate this inevitable aspect of practice, secondary or VT is nonetheless an inevitable and predictable aspect of our practice. In the context of violence and health, it is centrally important for CHNs to openly discuss and debrief about their experiences of secondary or VT.

CONCLUSION

Violence is endemic, all the way from local communities to global communities. Whether it encompasses violent acts in family homes or more visible violence in the community, its origins are in the structural underpinnings of our social, political, economic, and cultural structures. These structures remain largely invisible to CHNs unless we commit to educating ourselves to "see" the way society creates and sustains violence in our communities. CHNs are front and centre in numerous successful initiatives across Canada that create and apply solutions to homelessness, refugee settlement, gun violence, violence against LGBTQ2S people, and violence against women and girls. Successes in making structural injustices visible and advocating to challenge and decrease these social injustices continue to provide the foundational inspiration for community health nursing.

KEY TERMS

atraumatic care (p. 503)
bullying (p. 504)
cyberbullying (p. 504)
family violence (p. 504)
human trafficking (p. 504)
intimate partner violence (IPV) (p. 504)
People, Poverty, Power (3P) Model (p. 503)
Power and Control Wheel (p. 504)
privilege (p. 505)
root causes (p. 503)
self-empathy (p. 508)
stalking (p. 512)
systemic empathy (p. 508)
systemic oppressions (p. 506)
sexting (p. 504)
sexualized violence (p. 504)
social poverty (p. 507)
structural violence (p. 505)
trauma and violence informed care (TVIC) (p. 503)
vicarious trauma (p. 503)

STUDY QUESTIONS

1. Caitlin is a 15-year-old high school student. She has come to the community health clinic looking for the "morning-after pill" (emergency contraception). You explore with her

what circumstances led to her requiring this, and she reveals that her 19-year-old boyfriend raped her. She doesn't want her parents or police to know. She doesn't think it is sexual assault, since they have had sex before. Which of the following statements is correct?

   a. This must be reported to police as it is outside the close-in-age exception.

   b. She requires her parents' permission to have the emergency contraception.

   c. It is her choice whether or not to report, and her parents cannot be told.

   d. If they have had sex before, it is not considered sexual assault.

2. Which of the following is *not* an example of a biomedical approach to addressing violence?

   a. Educate young adolescent girls about ways they can protect themselves from violence when they are alone in public.

   b. Create an awareness campaign for young children about the dangers of talking to strangers.

   c. Work to engage youth in the development and implementation of a local poverty reduction action plan.

   d. Implement a self-defence program at a university for young women who are at risk of being sexually assaulted.

3. Which of the following is *not* a main principal of trauma and violence-informed care?

   a. Emphasis on safety and trustworthiness

   b. Opportunity for choice, collaboration, and connection

   c. Report all forms of violence and trauma to the RCMP

   d. Trauma awareness

4. Which of the following was the only violent or nonviolent crime that went unchanged (did not decrease) in terms of rates from 2004–2014?

   a. Homicides

   b. Self-reported sexual assault

   c. Assault with a weapon

   d. Impaired driving

5. Which of the following is *not* a recommended intervention to reduce transphobia in youth?

   a. Requiring students to disclose their gender identity at the beginning of the school year

   b. Training for teachers and administrators on gender identity and gender affirming approaches

   c. Awareness campaigns and education for students

   d. Providing gender-neutral washrooms and change rooms

INDIVIDUAL CRITICAL-THINKING EXERCISES

1. Critically examine the difference between using the terms *people under threat* and *vulnerable populations* to describe populations that are more likely to experience violence.

2. A fellow student came to you and revealed she was sexually assaulted. She didn't want to have an examination as she was worried the police would be called. It was someone from

her dormitory, and she saw him often. She was worried the school would become involved if she spoke out and that her education would be affected.

   a) What could you tell her?

   b) What resources are available to you?

   c) How would you know if she needed further assistance?

3. What is the CHN's role in caring for a woman who is experiencing IPV?

4. Identify the key targets from the UN's SDG that address the risk factors for violence. As a CHN, identify interventions at the macro, community, and intrapersonal levels that would be priority interventions for action on preventing violence in your community.

GROUP CRITICAL-THINKING EXERCISES

1. Discuss as a group the role of social media in perpetuating, addressing, and preventing sexual violence. How can CHNs embrace the positive attributes of social media while also mitigating the risk?

2. You have been invited to a local high school to help work on a violence prevention program for grade 10 girls. So far you are the only professional who has been invited to set this up.

   a) What types of messages would you want to convey, and why?

   b) What types of activities might you have for the program, and why?

   c) Who else should be involved in the program? Why?

3. The provincial government is trying to establish a family violence prevention network. It has asked for representatives from various sectors to become involved, and you are representing CHNs on the advisory group. There are lawyers, policy makers, health services administrators, police, and social workers in attendance.

   a) If you only were able to start with one type of violence or age group to develop interventions, what would be important for your community, and why?

   b) What types of funding, laws, or policies do you think would be needed at the provincial level to support the violence prevention efforts?

   c) How could you disseminate the information so the public and other professionals will be aware of the efforts? (Consider the age group, community, and existing services in your area.)

REFERENCES

Arthur, E., Seymour, A., Dartnall, M., Beltgens, P., Poole, N., Smylie, D., . . . Schmidt, R. (2013). *Trauma informed practice guide*. Vancouver: BC Provincial Mental Health and Substance Use Planning Council.

Austin, J., & Holdt, S. (2017). Responding to the support needs of front-line public health nurses who work with vulnerable families and children: a qualitative study. *Contemporary Nurse, 57*(5), 524–535.

Bailey, A. (2018). *A people, poverty, power model for understanding and preventing community-based violence.* Toronto, ON: Ryerson University.

Burczycka, M., & Ibrahim, D. (2016). Family violence in Canada: A statistical profile, 2015. *Juristat.* Statistics Canada Catalogue no. 85-002-X.

Carll, E. (2003). News portrayal of violence and women: Implications for public policy. *American Behavioural Scientist, 46*(12), 1601–1610.

Child Welfare Information Gateway. (2004). *Risk and protective factors for child abuse and neglect.* Washington, DC: CWIG.

Clark, M., & Gioro, S. (1998). Nurses, indirect trauma, and prevention. *Image: Journal of Nursing Scholarship, 30*(1), 85–87.

Community Health Nurses of Canada (CHNC). (2019, revised). *Canadian community health nursing: Professional practice model & standards of practice.* St. John's, NL: Author. Retrieved from https://www.chnc.ca/documents/CHNCProfessionalPracticeModel-EN/index.html

Conroy, S., & Cotter, A. (2017). Self-reported sexual assault in Canada, 2014. *Juristat.* Statistics Canada. Catalogue no. 85-002-X.

Correctional Investigator (2014). *Annual report of the office of the correctional investigator 2013–2014.* Ottawa, ON: Government of Canada. Retrieved from http://www.oci-bec.gc.ca/cnt/rpt/annrpt/annrpt20132014-eng.aspx

Craig, W., & McCuaig, H. (2012). *Bullying and fighting.* Ottawa, ON: Public Health Agency of Canada. Retrieved from http://www.phac-aspc.gc.ca/hp-ps/dca-dea/publications/hbsc-mental-mentale/bullying-intimidation-eng.php.

Crane, P., & Moreno, M. (2011). Human Trafficking: What is the role of the health care provider? *Journal of Applied Research on Children: Informing Policy on Children at Risk, 2*(1), Article 7.

Doolittle, R. (2017). Unfounded: Why police dismiss 1 in 5 sexual assault claims as baseless. *Globe and Mail* (February 3). Retrieved from https://www.theglobeandmail.com/news/investigations/unfounded-sexual-assault-canada-main/article33891309

EQUIP Health Care (2017). *Trauma-and-violence-informed Care (TVIC): A tool for health & social service organizations and providers.* Vancouver, BC. Retrieved from http://www.equiphealthcare.ca

Flexhaug, D. (2017). Challenging the wage gap: Canadian women still earn less than men. *Global News,* July 17.

Fortune Editors. (2017). Fortune 500 companies with female CEOs. *Fortune,* June 7. Retrieved from fortune.com

Gahagan, J., Ferguson, M., Saewyc, E., Frohard-Dourlent, H., & Veale, J. (2018). *Being safe, being me in the Atlantic provinces: Results of the Canadian trans youth health survey.* Vancouver, BC: School of Nursing, University of British Columbia.

Geiger, A., & Kent, L. (2017). *Number of women leaders around the world has grown, but they're still a small group.* Washington, DC: Pew Research Center.

Gilbert, S. (2017). The movement of #MeToo: How a hashtag got its power. *The Atlantic.* Retrieved from https://www.theatlantic.com/entertainment/archive/2017/10/the-movement-of-metoo/542979

Government of Canada. (2016). *National action plan to combat human trafficking.* Ottawa, ON: Government of Canada. Retrieved from http://www.publicsafety.gc.ca/cnt/rsrcs/pblctns/ntnl-ctn-pln-cmbt/index-eng.aspx

Herman, J. (1997). *Trauma and recovery: The aftermath of violence—from domestic abuse to political terror* (2nd ed.). New York, NY: Basic Books.

Hockenberry, M. J., & Wilson, D. (2015). *Wong's nursing care of infants and children* (10th ed.). Maryland Heights, MO: Mosby.

Jacobs, B. (2010). *Environmental racism on Indigenous lands and territories.* Paper presented at the Canadian Political Science Association Conference, May 20, 2010.

Jewkes, R., Sen, P., & Garcia-Moreno, C. (2002). Sexual violence. In E. G. Krug et al. (Eds.), *World report on violence and health,* pp. 149–181. Geneva, CH: World Health Organization.

Johnson, C. A., & Hawbaker, K. T. (2018). #MeToo: A timeline of events. *Chicago Tribune.* Retrieved from http://www.chicagotribune.com/lifestyles/ct-me-too-timeline-20171208-htmlstory.html

Jones, C. P. (2000). Levels of racism: A theoretical framework and a Gardener's Tale. American Journal of Public Health, 90:1212–1215.

Kendell, F. E. (2002). *Understanding white privilege.* Albany, CA. Retrieved from https://www.cpt.org/files/Undoing%20Racism%20-%20Understanding%20White%20Privilege%20-%20Kendall.pdf

Kira, I. (2001). A taxonomy of trauma and trauma assessment. *Traumatology: An International Journal, 2,* 1–14.

Konstantanopoulos, W., Ahn, R., Alpert, E., Cafferty, E., McGahan, A., Williams, T., & Burke, T. (2013). An international comparative public health analysis of sex trafficking of women and girls in eight cities: Achieving a more effective health sector response. *Journal of Urban Health: Bulletin of the New York Academy of Medicine, 90*(6), 1194–1204.

Krug, E., Dahlberg, L., Mercy, J., Zwi, A., & Lozano, R. (Eds.). (2002). *World report on violence and health.* (2002). Geneva, CH: World Health Organization.

Lamb, J., Pepler, D., & Craig, W. (2009). Approach to bullying and victimization. *Canadian Family Physician Medecin de Famille Canadien, 55,* 356–360.

Lereya, S., Muthanna, S., & Wolke, D. (2013). Parenting behaviour and the risk of becoming a victim and a bully/victim: A meta-analysis study. *Child Abuse & Neglect, 37*(12), 1091–1108.

Lyons, T., Krusi, A., Pierre, L., Kerr, T., Small, W., & Shannon, K. (2017). Negotiating violence in the context of transphobia and criminalization: The experiences of trans sex workers in Vancouver, Canada. *Qualitative Health Research, 27*(2), 182–190.

McCann, I., & Pearlman, L. (1990). Vicarious traumatization: A contextual model for understanding the effects of trauma on helpers. *Journal of Traumatic Stress, 3*(1), 131–149.

McGibbon, E. (2004). *Reformulating the nature of stress in nursing: An institutional ethnography.* Doctoral Dissertation. Toronto, ON: University of Toronto.

McGibbon, E. (2012). People under threat: Health outcomes and oppression. In E. McGibbon (Ed.), *Oppression: A social determinant of health*. Halifax, NS: Fernwood Publishing.

McGibbon, E. (2017). The social determinants of health: Embodied oppression across the lifecourse. In W. Antony & J. Antony (Eds.), *Power and resistance: Critical thinking about Canadian social issues*. 6th edition. Halifax, NS: Fernwood Publishing.

National Center for Disease Prevention and Control. (2016). *The ace pyramid*. Atlanta, GA: Centers for Disease Control.

Native Women's Association of Canada. (2017). *The national inquiry into missing and murdered Aboriginal women and girls*. Retrieved from http://indigenousfoundations.web.arts.ubc.ca/marginalization_of_aboriginal_women

Navarro, V. (2007). What is national health policy? *International Journal of Health Services, 37*(1), 1–14.

Notar, C. E., Padgett, S., & Rodern, J. (2013). Cyberbullying: A review of the literature. *Universal Journal of Educational Research, 1*(1), 1–9.

Paul, D. N. (2007). *We were not the savages: Collision between European and Native American civilizations*. Halifax, NS: Fernwood Publishing.

Pence, E., & Paymar, M. (1993). *Education groups for men who batter: The Duluth Model*. New York, NY: Springer.

Perreault, S. (2015). *Criminal victimization in Canada, 2014*. Statistics Canada. Retrieved from https://www.statcan.gc.ca/pub/85-002-x/2015001/article/14241-eng.htm

Peter, T., Taylor, C., & Chamberland, L. (2015). A queer day in Canada: Examining Canadian high school students' experiences with school-based homophobia in two largescale studies. *Journal of Homosexuality, 62*, 186–206.

Public Health Agency of Canada (PHAC). (2016). *The chief public health officer's report on the state of public health in Canada: A focus on family violence in Canada*. Ottawa: PHAC. Retrieved from https://www.canada.ca/content/dam/canada/public-health/migration/publications/department-ministere/state-public-health-family-violence-2016-etat-sante-publique-violence-familiale/alt/pdf-eng.pdf

Raunick, C. B., Lindell, D. F., Morris, D., & Backman, T. (2017). Vicarious trauma among sexual assault nurse examiners. *Journal of Forensic Nursing, 11*(3), 123–128.

Registered Nurses Association of Ontario (RNAO). (2012). *Woman abuse: Screening identification and initial response. Guideline Supplement*. Toronto, ON: RNAO. Retrieved from http://rnao.ca/sites/rnao-ca/files/BPG_Women_Abuse_Supplement_Only.pdf

Royal Canadian Mounted Police (RCMP). (2014). *Missing and murdered Aboriginal women: A national operational overview*. Ottawa. ON: Royal Canadian Mounted Police. Retrieved from http://www.rcmp-grc.gc.ca/pubs/mmaw-faapd-eng.pdf

Sleet, D., Dahlberg, L., Basavaraju, S., Mercy, J., McGuire, L., & Greenspan, A. (2011). Injury prevention, violence prevention, and trauma care: Building the scientific base. *Morbidity and Mortality Weekly Report. Surveillance Summaries*. Washington, DC: 60 Suppl. 4, 78–85.

Statistics Canada. (2015). *Snapshot of family violence in Canada*. Ottawa, ON: Government of Canada. Retrieved from https://www.canada.ca/content/dam/phac-aspc/migration/phac-aspc/sfv-avf/assets/pdf/infographi-eng.pdf

Statistics Canada. (2018). *Family violence in Canada: A statistical profile, 2016*. Ottawa Government of Canada. Catalogue no. 85-002-X. Retrieved from https://www150.statcan.gc.ca/n1/pub/85-002-x/2018001/article/54893-eng.pdf

Stevens, H. (2018). Hollywood heavyweights team up to declare time's up on sexual harassment. *The Chicago Tribune*. Retrieved from http://www.chicagotribune.com/lifestyles/stevens/ct-life-stevens-times-up-sex-harassment-0102-story.html

Svensson, B., Bornehag, C.-G., & Janson, S. (2011). Chronic conditions in children increase the risk for physical abuse—but vary with socio-economic circumstances. *Acta Paediatrica, 100*(3), 407–412. doi:10.1111/j.16512227.2010.02029.x

United Nations (UN). (1993). *Declaration on the elimination of violence against women*. Geneva, CH: UN General Assembly. Retrieved from http://www.un.org/documents/ga/res/48/a48r104.htm

United Nations (2015a). *Resolution adopted by the General Assembly on 25 September 2015*. Geneva, CH: UN General Assembly. Retrieved from http://www.un.org/ga/search/view_doc.asp?symbol=A/RES/70/1&Lang=E

United Nations (2015b). *The world's women 2015: Trends and statistics*. Geneva, CH: United Nations Statistics Division. Retrieved from https://unstats.un.org/UNSD/gender/worldswomen.html

Wesley-Esquimaux, C. C., & Smolewski, M. (2004). *Historic trauma and aboriginal healing*. Winnipeg, MB: Aboriginal Healing Foundation.

Wijeyesinghe, C., Griffin, P., & Love, B. (1997). Racism and curriculum design. In M. Adams, L. Bell, & P. Griffin (Eds.). *Teaching for diversity and social justice: A sourcebook*. New York, NY: Routledge.

World Bank (2018). *World development report 2018: Learning to realize education's promise*. Washington, DC: World Bank.

World Health Organization (WHO). (1986). *The Ottawa Charter for Health Promotion*. Geneva, CH: WHO.

World Health Organization (WHO). (2012). *Human trafficking*. Geneva, CH: WHO. Retrieved from http://apps.who.int/iris/bitstream/10665/77394/1/WHO_RHR_12.42_eng.pdf

World Health Organization (WHO). (2013). *Responding to intimate partner violence and sexual violence against women: WHO clinical and policy guidelines*. Geneva, CH: WHO. Retrieved from http://apps.who.int/iris/bitstream/handle/10665/85240/9789241548595_eng.pdf?sequence=1

World Health Organization (WHO). (2014). *Global status report on violence prevention*. Geneva, CH: WHO.

World Health Organization (WHO). (2009). *World report on violence and health*. Chapter 1: *Violence: A global public health problem*. Geneva, CH: WHO. Retrieved from http://apps.who.int/iris/bitstream/handle/10665/77936/9789241500845_eng.pdf;jsessionid=A7BA34EE424A3B68F380681201ED0C62?sequence=1

World Health Organization (WHO). (2016). *Child maltreatment*. Fact Sheet. No. 150. Geneva, CH: WHO.

ABOUT THE AUTHORS

Dr. Elizabeth McGibbon, RN, MN, PhD, is a professor in the Rankin School of Nursing, St. Francis Xavier University, Nova Scotia. Her teaching, research, and publications focus on embodied oppression, access to health care, health equity and public policy, and the political economy of health. She leads a SSHRC-funded project, *Mapping Health Equity in Canadian Public Policy*, and is a co-researcher with *Debwewin: The Truth of our Hearts*, a study aiming to diversify our dialogue and understanding of heart health in Manitoban First Nations peoples (CIHR; Lead, Dr. A. Schultz). Books include *Anti-racist Health Care Practice* (with Dr. J. Etowa), and *Oppression: A Social Determinant of Health* (Edited Volume). An invited chapter author in four multiple-edition books about critical perspectives on health and society, Elizabeth's work is informed by two decades of clinical practice at the pointy edges of injustice in health care. She was one of three leads in establishment of the National Collaborating Centre, Determinants of Health (NCCDH). Along with social justice colleagues, her awards include recognition from the Nova Scotia Human Rights Commission (anti-racism community action) and the Canadian Armed Forces (refugee humanitarian work).

Dr. Annette Bailey, RN, BScN, MSN, PhD, is Associate Professor and Associate Director in the Collaborative Degree Program of the Daphne Cockwell School of Nursing, Ryerson University. She has worked in acute and community health nursing settings. Much of her work in community health nursing has focused on inter-agency collaboration to address key determinants of health for diverse populations in Toronto. Annette completed her PhD in Public Health Science with a specialization in health promotion and education. Her research examines traumatic stress and resilience among survivors of community and interpersonal violence. Her research interests span violence prevention, violence and trauma, trauma and resilience, homicide loss, resilience, and grief. One of the outcomes of her research is her ongoing development of a model that aims to help public policy makers, health professionals, and leaders in the health fields grasp and intervene in the complex areas of violence, trauma, and power. Her most recent research projects focus on traumatic stress and resilience among Black women who have lost a child to gun violence in Toronto.

Sionnach Lukeman, RN, MScN, is Assistant Professor in the Rankin School of Nursing, St. Francis Xavier University, Nova Scotia. Her research program involves three disciplines: public health services and systems, political economy of health, and building supportive environments for health. Her work is informed by a clinical specialty in perinatal nursing from the British Columbia Institute of Technology and later a leadership role in the development, monitoring, and evaluation of programs focusing on healthy development and youth health in public health. She is also the president and co-founder of the nonprofit organization BaBE (Building a Breastfeeding Environment), focused on engaging communities and stakeholders to support women to breastfeed "anytime, anywhere."

Poverty, Homelessness, and Food Insecurity

Kathryn Hardill

chapter 29

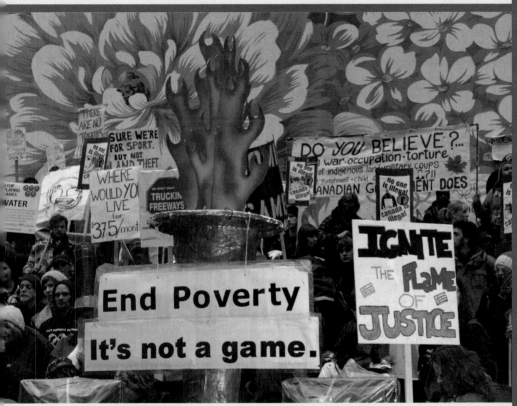

Source: Sergei Bachlakov/Shutterstock

LEARNING OUTCOMES

After studying this chapter, you should be able to:

1. Use social determinants of health and health equity lenses to assess the influence of poverty on the health of individuals and families.

2. Discuss the major issues, including root causes, related to poverty in Canada and their impact on the health of different populations and groups.

3. Explain the impact of homelessness on the health and mortality of specific populations and groups in Canada.

4. Describe the concept of food insecurity and how it may affect the health of individuals and families.

5. Describe the community health nurse role in upstream political advocacy for groups and populations affected by poverty, homelessness, and food insecurity.

INTRODUCTION

"All diseases have two causes, one pathological, the other political."

(Virchow, 1859)

Nineteenth-century German pathologist Rudolph Virchow (1821–1902) aptly characterizes disease through the lenses of the **social determinants of health (SDOH)**, healthy equity, and critical social theories introduced in earlier chapters. Using these lenses allows community health nurses (CHNs) to meaningfully understand and, more importantly, meaningfully intervene to improve the health of individuals and families made vulnerable by poverty, homelessness, and food insecurity. Nursing is often situated **downstream** and includes treating injuries and illnesses and supporting recovery and rehabilitation. But so often it is far **upstream** that we find the tools needed for primordial and primary prevention of the interrelated issues of poverty, homelessness, and food insecurity.

What we see depends on how we look at it. Do we see a mother living on low income who relies on a food bank because she has not learned how to budget appropriately? Or do we see a woman living on social assistance who is good at budgeting, who knows precisely, to the penny, where every single dollar goes every month and exactly how many days into the month she will be out of funds? In this chapter we examine some of the lenses through which to view the social context of health, which may lead us to different ways of seeing poverty, homelessness, and food insecurity.

POVERTY, HOMELESSNESS, AND THE SOCIAL DETERMINANTS OF HEALTH

The World Health Organization (2015) describes the SDOH as "the conditions in which people are born, grow, live, work and age. These circumstances are shaped by the distribution of money, power, and resources at global, national, and local levels. The social determinants of health are mostly responsible for health inequities—the unfair and avoidable differences in health status seen within and between countries" (para. 1). In Canada, Mikkonen and Raphael (2010) describe fourteen determinants of health, including income distribution, race, gender, housing, disability, social exclusion, and Indigenous identity. They argue that each of these exerts a stronger impact on the health of Canadians than "behaviours such as diet, physical activity, and even tobacco and excessive alcohol use" (p. 9). The SDOH are discussed in detail in Chapter 8.

CHNs who have worked for many years with people living on low income have accumulated multiple galvanizing experiences that inform our nursing practice and the way we see health. One of mine is exemplified in Photo 29.1, an image of me and my colleague Cathie Simpson doing nursing outreach to address the twin fundamentals of clean drinking water and sanitation. As you can probably tell by our clothing, not to mention Toronto's CN Tower in the background, we are not on a medical mission in a developing country. We are distributing bottled water and toilet paper to Canadians living in an area of Toronto's waterfront—among the most expensive real estate in the richest city in Canada and the site of a large encampment of homeless people known as Toronto's Tent City.

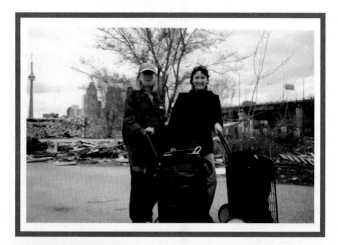

PHOTO 29.1 Health promotion nursing in Canada in the early 21st century.

Source: Courtesy of Kathy Hardill

Health Is Political: The Impact of Neoliberalism on Health

An ideological concept important to our understanding of the intersecting factors that contribute to poverty, homelessness, and food insecurity—the *etiology* of these health problems—is the political and economic ideology known as **neoliberalism**. Arising in the 1970s and coinciding with the world debt crisis, the International Monetary Fund and the World Bank gave loans to heavily indebted countries on the condition that they make changes in taxation and tariffs to facilitate globalization of trade. Central to these policy changes were reductions in social spending by governments, which led to global increases in poverty and inequality, with Canada being no exception. Loosening of regulations on financial markets led to the 2008 financial crisis, which justified the promotion of ongoing austerity measures to reduce public debt and boost economic recoveries (Labonte & Stuckler, 2016).

The health care consequences of neoliberal policies have been far-reaching and include rising poverty rates, increased homelessness, rising unemployment, and increased consumption of "obesogenic" food as food costs rise (Labonte & Stuckler, 2016, p. 314). Ongoing austerity-driven budgets in Canada have led to growing inequity in the distribution of the SDOH (Ruckert & Labonte, 2016). Nurses have argued that neoliberal globalization is responsible for a growing gap in health and wealth within rich Western nations such as Canada (Tang, Browne, Mussell, Smye, & Rodney, 2015). They argue that urban poverty ought to be understood as symptomatic of global capitalism and its neoliberal policies, which are responsible for the substandard housing, poverty, lack of affordable housing, and other conditions of social inequity.

An important feature of neoliberal thought is the idea that individuals freely make choices in their lives. This means they are also by extension to blame for unhealthy choices. It assumes an egalitarian "level playing field" environment where everyone has equal opportunities. It renders invisible the effects of poverty, homelessness, and food insecurity, or focuses responsibility for these issues directly on affected persons and away from the upstream contributors.

We have seen the rise in health promotion campaigns endorsing "healthy lifestyles" that encourage people to quit smoking, reduce saturated fat intake, exercise more, and follow guidelines for low-risk alcohol consumption. In a public health care system influenced by neoliberal beliefs, if a person is constrained by social or economic structures such as high unemployment or low wages, the goal of far too many health care professionals, including some CHNs, focuses on supporting how people cope with those constraints or assisting them to make healthier choices (Reimer-Kirkham & Browne, 2006), even if these goals fail to take into account the structural inequities that make them impossible to achieve. When CHNs view health through the lenses of SDOH and health equity, we know that individualizing systemic and structural problems is unethical. It places blame on individuals for issues that are not within their control. It is not only ineffective but also unjust for CHNs to teach people how to cope with the inequities they face and not address the upstream root causes.

An important consequence of **individualization** of blame for health problems is that the focus of attention and interventions are aimed at individuals and not at the upstream barriers and structures that create those problems in the first place. For example, a person who needs to work two or three part-time jobs with no benefits may be able to afford only "obesogenic" foods (Labonte & Stuckler, 2016, p. 314) and have no time to exercise—but may problematically be counselled to manage his type 2 diabetes using "lifestyle changes." A homeless woman who has a venous stasis ulcer that will not heal may be advised to keep her leg elevated as much as possible, which would only be a realistic intervention if she had somewhere to be able to do so.

Neoliberal policies perform double duty by contributing to increased rates of poverty, homelessness, and food insecurity at the same time as they focus the responsibility for those circumstances on the individuals experiencing them and away from the political and structural causes that create them.

POVERTY IN CANADA

About one in seven Canadians—4.8 million people in Canada—live in poverty (Canada Without Poverty/Canada Sans Pauvrete, 2018). They struggle to meet their basic needs on a daily basis: to pay rent, purchase nutritious food, buy clothes, pay for a telephone, pay for transportation, or pay for electricity. As the following table shows, Canadians more likely to live in poverty include people with disabilities, lone-parent families, youth, older adults, and people from racialized communities.

WHO IS MOST LIKELY TO EXPERIENCE POVERTY IN CANADA?

Some members of society are particularly susceptible to the effects of poverty. These statistics suggest groups who are particularly likely to experience poverty.

- People living with different abilities (both mental and physical) are twice as likely to live below the poverty line.
- Nearly 15% of people with disabilities live in poverty, 59% of whom are women.
- Estimates place the number of homeless individuals living with a disability or mental illness as high as 45% of the overall homeless population.
- Children with disabilities are twice as likely to live in households relying on social assistance.
- 21% of single mothers in Canada raise their children while living in poverty; 7% of single fathers raise their children in poverty.
- Women parenting on their own enter shelters at twice the rate of two-parent families.
- First Nation, Métis, and Inuit peoples are overrepresented among the homeless population in virtually all urban centres in Canada.
- 28–34% of shelter users are Indigenous.

- One in five racialized families lives in poverty in Canada, as opposed to one in 20 nonracialized families.
- Racialized women living in poverty are almost twice as likely to work in manufacturing jobs than other women living in poverty.
- Overall, racialized women earn 32% less at work.
- Nearly 15% of single older adults live in poverty.
- Nearly 2 million seniors receive the Guaranteed Income Supplement and live on about $17 000 per year. However, the most basic standard of living in Canada is calculated at $18 000 per year for a single person.

Source: Canada Without Poverty/Canada Sans Pauvrete. (2018). *Just the Facts.* Retrieved from http://www.cwp-csp.ca/poverty/just-the-facts/. Used with permission.

Poverty Definitions

Multiple definitions of poverty exist. Statistics Canada (2015) provides three definitions of low income:

- **Low income cut-off**: A relative measure based on income thresholds calculated before and after tax, below which a family will be required to spend 20% more of its income than the average family on food, shelter, and clothing. Levels vary by family and community size.
- **Low income measure**: A relative measure based on 50% of the adjusted median national income of the number of individuals in a given household; calculated annually; useful for international comparisons.
- **Market basket measure**: An absolute measure of the income level required for a family of two adults and two children to afford to purchase a defined set of goods and services, including nutritious food, clothing, shelter, transportation, and basic household supplies; calculated for different communities and community sizes across Canada; originally devised by Human Resources Development Canada (now Employment and Social Development Canada).

Poverty and Racialized Populations

Poverty does not equally affect all groups of people. **Racialized** populations are more likely than nonracialized populations to be poor. Statistics Canada (2012) defines *racialized* as "persons, other than Aboriginal peoples, who are non-Caucasian in race or non-white in colour" (p. 1). The racialization of poverty is "a phenomenon where poverty becomes disproportionately concentrated and reproduced among racialized group members" (p. 16). The 2006 census showed the overall poverty rate in Canada to be 11%, but for racialized persons it was 22%, compared to 9% for nonracialized persons (p. 1). It is important to note that the term *racialized* is used to acknowledge "race as a social construct," with racialization being characterized as "the process through which groups come to be designated as different and on that basis subjected to differential and unequal treatment" (Block & Galabuzi, 2011, p. 19). Block and Galabuzi argue that racialized Canadians are subject to wage disparities compared to nonracialized people. Analyzing data from the 2006 long form census survey, these authors point to the disproportionate concentration and entrenchment of poverty among racialized group members, often linked to precarious work.

YES, BUT WHY?

Racialized Families Are More Likely to Live in Poverty

What?

According to Canada Without Poverty (2018), one in five racialized families lives in poverty in Canada. Racialized Canadians experience wage disparities and are more likely to work in low-paying, precarious jobs linked to historical racial discrimination in Canadian labour markets (Block & Galabuzi, 2011). Indigenous peoples experience grossly disproportionate levels of poverty, and as a result Indigenous children lag behind other children on almost all measures of well-being (Macdonald & Wilson, 2013).

So What?

In a country many would consider as offering equality of opportunity regardless of race, CHNs must question why race is so robustly linked to poverty. Why is there discrepancy in access to the SDOH? In a country boasting universal access to health care, CHNs must question why we lack universal access to the social determinants of health, which arguably have a greater impact on health than does access to health care.

Now What?

CHNs must understand their role in health promotion related to health equity in their practice settings. The Community Health Nurses of Canada (CHNC) (2019, revised, p. 4) Standards of Practice calls on CHNs to "consider and address the impact of the determinants of health within the political, cultural and environmental context of health" and to "advocate and engage in political action and health public policy options to facilitate healthy living."

In 1999, RN Carolyn Acker had a vision. As the executive director of Regent Park Community Health Centre, located in Canada's oldest public housing complex in inner city Toronto, she became increasingly concerned about the low rates of high school completion among the largely racialized youth in Regent Park. In many cases, their families were newcomers who sometimes were quite accomplished in their home countries but lacked sufficient proficiency in English to help their children with schoolwork. The parents' poverty often required them to work several low-paying, precarious jobs. Students themselves had to work to afford bus fare to get to school.

Acker became convinced that with the right supports, the children of the largely impoverished community could become the doctors, nurses, and administrators of the health centre and within the broader community. In 2001 she and other community leaders began to build a program utilizing broad community networks to provide an innovative set of practical supports to enable racialized youth to have scholastic success, complete high school, and go on to post-secondary education. Known as Pathways to Education, this innovative program provided every young person in the community with the opportunity to enroll and obtain financial support to finish high school, tutoring, mentoring, and student/parent support workers who liaised with students, parents, schools, and the broader community. Ten years after its inception, the high school drop-out rate had decreased 70%, and the high school completion rate had risen from 20% to 80% for participants. Since then, the Pathways to Education program has expanded across Canada, with programs in 20 communities in nine provinces (Pathways to Education, 2018).

Standards of Practice Fulfilled

#4 Professional Relationships
- Recognizes own personal beliefs, attitudes, assumptions, feelings and values including racism and stereotypes and their potential impact on nursing practice.
- Builds a network of relationships and partnerships with a wide variety of individuals, families, groups, communities, and systems to address health issues and promote healthy public policy to advance health equity.

#6 Health Equity
- Understands historical injustices, inequitable power relations, institutionalized and interpersonal racism and their impacts on health and health care and provides culturally safe care (CHNC, 2018, revised)

Poverty and Indigenous Peoples

Canadian census data show that First Nation, Inuit, and Métis people experience persistent and pervasive inequitable access to the SDOH, including income, employment, housing, food security, and education (Statistics Canada, 2008). Astonishing levels of poverty exist for racialized children in Canada, with Indigenous children being the most profoundly affected. Macdonald and Wilson (2013) describe three tiers of poverty among Canadian children. The first tier reveals a poverty rate of 12%, excluding racialized, immigrant, and Indigenous children. The second-tier poverty rate that includes racialized children is 22%; the rate that includes Métis, Inuit, and non-status First Nation children is 27%; and the rate that includes immigrant children is 33%. The third tier shows that 50% of status First Nation children live below the poverty line. This percentage is even higher in Manitoba and Saskatchewan (62% and 64%, respectively) (p. 6). Not only do Indigenous children in Canada experience higher levels of poverty than non-Indigenous children, but also they lag behind other children on almost every measure of well-being, including educational attainment, poor housing, poor water quality, infant mortality, food security, prevalence of health issues, and suicide (p. 19). Considered through a historical contextual lens, the structural drivers of Indigenous child poverty (and indeed, poverty in general) can be traced back to the dawn of colonialism and the origins of Canada (Brittain & Blackstock, 2015).

Not only do Indigenous people bear a higher burden of poverty and resultant morbidity and mortality, it is also probable that accurate data on the health of Indigenous people in Canada are lacking. Indigenous health researchers point out that culturally relevant, meaningful population health data for urban Indigenous populations are "almost nonexistent" related to methodological limitations in census data collection and other population health research (Firestone, Smylie, Maracle, Spiller, & O'Campo, 2014). Using respondent-driven sampling that capitalizes on existing social networks and relationships, Firestone and colleagues conducted community-based research among urban Indigenous people living in Hamilton, Ontario, which is located on traditional Haudenosaunee and Anishinaabeg territory. Their research, which they argue may be a more representative income profile than the 2006 census data, found shocking levels of poverty, with more than 70% of the cohort (n = 554 adults) in the lowest income quintile, compared to 25% of the general Hamilton population and 20% of the Ontario population (p. 12).

Child and Family Poverty

Although some speak of child poverty as if such a thing existed in a vacuum, it is encouraging to see the evolution of understanding informing discussions on poverty in which child poverty is not truncated from the poverty of the families in which they reside. The national advocacy group Campaign 2000 has created an astute infographic "road map" to eradicating child and family poverty that juxtaposes issues with their upstream solutions (Campaign 2000, 2016). (See Figure 29.1.)

Poverty in Rural Canada

CHNs work in rural communities and witness the different ways in which inequities impact individuals and families living outside urban areas. Rural poverty has been characterized as different from the more commonly studied urban poverty. It is often more isolated, is less visible, and has few social safety net supports (Milbourne, 2010). Considering the impacts of neoliberalism on rural economies, Riser and Halseth (2017) argue that neoliberal globalization has adversely affected natural resource sectors that have historically provided the economic foundations for many rural communities. Reliance on one or two resource-related economies that cannot be sustained can result in pervasive and persistent poverty in rural communities. Further, large geographic distances and low population densities limit employment opportunities and access to supportive infrastructures, which can prolong unemployment and the duration of poverty (Halseth & Riser, 2010).

One compelling way of considering Northern poverty using a contextual lens is through the creation of a "Northern equivalence scale," which Daley, Burton, and Phipps (2015) devised to estimate the additional income required by families living in Yukon, Northwest Territories, and Nunavut to devote the same

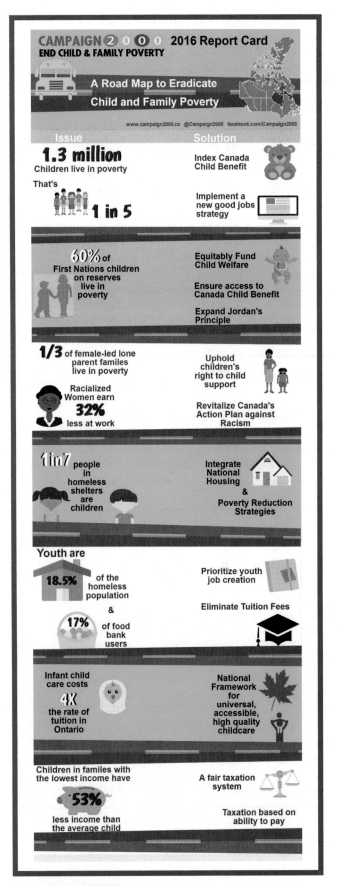

FIGURE 29.1 Campaign 2000 to End Child and Family Poverty: 2016 Report Card

Source: Reprint with permission from Campaign 2000. (2017).

proportion of their income to necessities as families living in southern Canada. They concluded that the cost of living in the North is 1.46 times higher, requiring a comparable increase in income for Northern families. Findings indicated a much higher incidence of poverty in the North, with 31.1% of families with children living in poverty, compared to 9.9% in the South.

Poverty and Illness

Canadian CHNs must be mindful of the robust links between poverty and adverse health outcomes. Low income is a risk factor for higher prevalence of many health issues, including type 2 diabetes, hypertension, osteoarthritis, chronic obstructive pulmonary disease, and asthma, as well as an increased likelihood of having more than one chronic condition (Bierman et al., 2009; Lightman, Mitchell, & Wilson, 2009). Individuals living below the poverty line experience depression at a rate 58% higher than the Canadian average (Smith, Matheson, Moineddin, & Glazier, 2007) and cardiovascular disease at a rate 17% higher than the Canadian average (Lightman, Mitchell, & Wilson, 2008). Low-income people sustain higher rates of lung, oral, and cervical cancers (Conway et al., 2008). The relationship between income and illness is linear: as poverty increases, so do morbidity and mortality (Bierman et al., 2009; Conway et al., 2008).

Complicating matters, poverty adversely affects the ability of low-income Canadians to manage illnesses such as type 2 diabetes, even when they have access to excellent health care services (Raphael et al., 2012). Tang and colleagues (2015) argue that, contrary to the taken-for-granted notion of universal health care in Canada, emerging evidence suggests that racialized and low-income people face discrimination and other access barriers. Further, they argue that health care is not only clinical space but also social space, within which "unequal power relations along the intersecting axes of 'race' and class are negotiated" (p. 698).

Addressing Victim-Blaming and Individualization of Blame

If CHNs view poverty through a critical social theory lens, we can see the upstream causes of illness rather than focusing blame on individuals. Some researchers, such as Medvedyuk, Ali, and Raphael (2017), have begun to critique traditional assumptions about health and illness, advocating for the development of interventions that focus less on changing individual factors and more on improving access to the SDOH. Using the example of obesity, they argue that epidemiologic links between obesity and illness are overstated, that the "anti-obesity" perspective deflects attention away from the primary causes of adverse health outcomes (i.e., inequitable access to the SDOH caused by problematic public policy), and that this perspective worsens health through stigmatization and blaming overweight people for their health problems.

Using these lenses to consider the example of type 2 diabetes mellitus, we can readily see how every level of prevention is informed by the sociopolitical context of health.

EXAMPLES OF PRIMORDIAL, PRIMARY, SECONDARY, TERTIARY, AND QUATERNARY PREVENTION: DIABETES MELLITUS TYPE 2

- Primordial prevention: Advocating for national policies that reduce the cost of nutritious foods and ensure adequate basic income for all.
- Primary prevention: Advocating for provincial and territorial governments to increase social assistance rates to the levels of the low-income cut-offs or Market Basket Measures.
- Secondary prevention: Implementing early screening for type 2 diabetes among low-income populations. (See one such clinical tool at Centre for Effective Practice, 2015.)
- Tertiary prevention: Implementing programming for low-income people with type 2 diabetes that provides access to no-cost exercise programs and peer support.
- Quaternary prevention: Avoiding overemphasis on medical interventions for type 2 diabetes rather than increasing access to affordable, nutritious food and exercise and healthy weight programs.

HOMELESSNESS

"Did the weather cause Canada's mass homelessness?" University of Toronto professor David Hulchanski posed this tongue-in-cheek question in 2000. Correctly, he concluded that mass homelessness began in the 1980s in Canada due to "homeless making processes" (Hulchanski, 2000, p. 1) because certain individuals, corporations, and governments benefitted from it. Further, these "homeless makers" (p. 2) aggressively promoted the notion that homelessness results from individual failings and poor choices and deflects responsibility away from those who allow homelessness to continue. Additionally, the unmistakeable influence of neoliberalism can be seen in federal government decisions to cut funding for housing and social spending. Gaetz, Dej, Richter, and Redman (2016) suggest that mass homelessness emerged in Canada in the 1980s as a result of dramatically reduced federal investment in affordable housing, structural economic shifts, and reduced spending on social safety nets.

Definitions of Homelessness

The Canadian Observatory on Homelessness (2012) created a definition of homelessness that describes a range of circumstances:

- **Unsheltered**, or absolutely homeless and living on the streets or in places not intended for human habitation
- **Emergency sheltered**, including individuals staying in overnight shelters for the homeless and for those impacted by family violence
- **Provisionally accommodated**, referring to individuals whose accommodation is temporary or lacks security of tenure

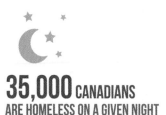

35,000 CANADIANS
ARE HOMELESS ON A GIVEN NIGHT

at least
235,000
CANADIANS EXPERIENCE
HOMELESSNESS IN A YEAR

27.3%
ARE WOMEN

18.7%
ARE YOUTH

THE NUMBER OF
**OLDER ADULTS (50-64)
AND SENIORS (65+)**
EXPERIENCING HOMELESSNESS IS GROWING

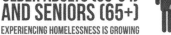

making up a combined
24.4% OF SHELTER USERS

28-34% OF THE
SHELTER POPULATION
IS INDIGENOUS

4.3% OF CANADIANS
ARE INDGENOUS

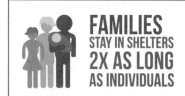

FAMILIES
STAY IN SHELTERS
2X AS LONG
AS INDIVIDUALS

approximately
2,950 VETERANS
EXPERIENCE HOMELESSNESS

2.2% OF SHELTER POPULATION

*Historically, individuals experiencing homelessness
in Canada were older, single men. The homelessness
crisis we see today is much more diverse. More
women, families and youth are experiencing
homelessness than in the past.*

FIGURE 29.2 Who Is Homeless in Canada?

Source: Gaetz, Dej, Richter, & Redman (2016), p. 5.

- **At risk of homelessness**, referring to people who are not homeless but whose current economic or housing situation is precarious or does not meet public health and safety standards

What Do We Know about Homelessness in Canada?

Quantifying homelessness in Canada, as in other jurisdictions, is challenging because only the most visibly homeless people are available for enumeration—that is, individuals living in shelters. Individuals who live outdoors or stay with relatives and friends may never be recognized as homeless and thus not captured in homelessness data collection efforts. The Canadian federal Homelessness Partnering Secretariat estimates that about 150 000 Canadians use shelters every year across Canada (Government of Canada, 2016b). Gaetz and colleagues (2016) suggest that at least 235 000 Canadians experience homelessness in a year. The Homeless Hub (2017), a Canadian homelessness research network housed at York University, suggests as a rough estimate that 28 500 individuals are homeless on any given night in Canada, with as many as 50 000 homeless people "hidden."

The Canadian National Shelter Study 2005–2014 analyzed emergency shelter use data and revealed the following information (Government of Canada, 2016a):

- Shelter use is decreasing; number of bed nights is increasing.

- Adults aged 25 to 49 make up the largest group of shelter users (52%).
- Women make up 27.3% of shelter users.
- Indigenous people are vastly overrepresented among shelter users at between 27.7% and 33.5% (while comprising less than 5% of the general population).
- Approximately 2950 military veterans make up 2.2% of the shelter population.
- On average, families stay in shelters twice as long as individuals.
- 89% of homeless families are headed by women with an average age of 34.
- Older adults aged 65 and over as well as older adults aged 50 to 64 comprise the age groups for whom shelter use has increased over the last 10 years.

What Do We Know about Homelessness in Small Urban and Rural Communities?

Although often stereotyped as a problem of large urban centres, CHNs working in small urban and rural settings will see homelessness wherever they practice. Rural homelessness is different in several important ways. Services such as shelters or soup kitchens often do not exist in rural communities.

Rather, rural homeless people tend to be much less visible. The rural homeless population includes individuals forced to live with friends or relatives, individuals who remain in abusive relationships in order to avoid homelessness, and individuals who live in temporary rental accommodations such as motels or abandoned outbuildings (Woods, 2005).

A review of literature and research in Canada found that rural homelessness is largely hidden, with rural homeless individuals often staying temporarily with friends or family or living in structures that are unsafe or inadequate for habitation or year-round habitation (such as structures in poor repair or seasonal cottages and recreational trailers). Challenges specific to rural homelessness include the lack of social services, lack of affordable housing, lower incomes in many rural areas coupled with higher costs for food and other necessities such as fuel, lack of emergency housing for women fleeing intimate partner violence, and physical deterioration of housing such as mobile homes. Although rural homelessness appears to be pervasive, much remains unknown about it.

Rural homelessness looks quite different from urban homelessness. Rural homeless people can be found sleeping rough in cars, ATMs, post office buildings, and parks, particularly in milder weather in communities such as Estevan, Saskatchewan; New Glasgow, Nova Scotia; Pointe-a-la-Croix, Quebec; Kenora, Ontario; Happy Valley/Goose Bay, Labrador; Old Crow, Yukon; and Smithers, British Columbia (Waegemakers, Schiff, & Turner, 2014). In Camrose, Alberta, high housing costs and low rental vacancy rates have led to low-income workers living out of their vehicles or resorting to makeshift shelters. In Revelstoke, BC, increased tourism has led to out-of-town people purchasing local real estate, resulting in some low-income workers moving into low-quality, unsafe former worker trailers. Rocky Mountain House, Alberta, has year-round campgrounds housing "hundreds of people" (p. 20).

Indigenous Homelessness

Inuit, First Nations, and Métis are grossly overrepresented in homeless populations across Canada. Anderson and Collins (2014) found in a scoping review of urban **Indigenous homelessness** that Indigenous people were overrepresented in all 13 Canadian cities they studied and, in all but three cases, were at least five times more prevalent in the homeless population than in the general population. Inadequate and insufficient housing is a critical problem for Indigenous people across the country, and it has been identified that in rural and remote regions, if family members did not open their homes to relatives in need, "the issue of 'overcrowding' would be identified as an issue of homelessness" (Richmond & Cook, 2016, p. 6). Thistle (2017) developed a definition of Indigenous homelessness in consultation with Indigenous scholars, community members, knowledge keepers, and Elders across Canada. (See Figure 29.3.) This definition is based on the idea that Indigenous homelessness is "best understood as the outcome of historically constructed and ongoing settler colonization and racism that have displaced and dispossessed First Nations, Métis and Inuit Peoples from their traditional governance systems and laws, territories, histories, worldviews, ancestors and stories" (p. 6). It provides

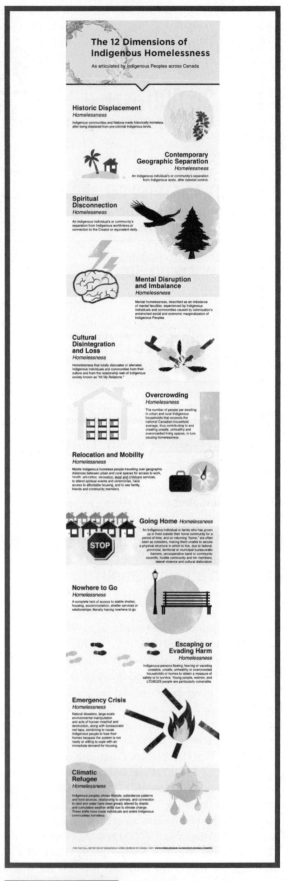

FIGURE 29.3 The 12 Dimensions of Indigenous Homelessness

Source: Reprinted with permission from Thistle, J. (2017).

an unblinking appraisal of the sociopolitical antecedents of Indigenous homelessness in colonialism, racism, discriminatory narratives about Indigenous people; cultural genocide; the destruction of Indigenous languages; chronic underfunding by governments; forced relocation to "marginal geographic spaces" (p. 8); racist policies and laws, such as the Indian Act; unfulfilled treaties; and land loss.

These 12 dimensions of Indigenous homelessness intersect in tandem, in clusters, or in constellations to cause, compound, and entrench Indigenous homelessness in Canada. The 12 dimensions also intersect with the four kinds of settler homelessness, as defined in the Canadian definition, to create the problem of Indigenous homelessness in Canada. It is worth noting that the experiences of homelessness among Indigenous people as identified by the 12 dimensions are not limited to individuals who are without shelter. The 12 dimensions underscore the loss of relationships endured by Indigenous peoples through the processes of Canadian colonization and the disconnection from the Indigenous understanding of home as "all my relations." (Thistle, 2017, p. 39)

Youth Homelessness

Over the last 20 years, Canadian research on youth homelessness has found that homeless youth typically become homeless as they seek to escape difficult and traumatic environments, including problematic child welfare placements. Despite the fact that homeless youth often characterize their lives as difficult, unhealthy, dangerous, lonely, and exploitative, homelessness is seen by many as the best option in their lives (Karabanow & Kidd, 2014). Common health concerns include mental health issues, which is not surprising given the prevalence of early life trauma; sexual health issues; HIV and hepatitis C infection; and unplanned pregnancy (Schwartz, James, Wagner, & Hart, 2014). Recent Canadian research involved asking 114 youth with experience of homelessness across the country what would prevent youth homelessness in Canada. Participants identified structural issues such as poverty, lack of affordable housing, and colonization; system failures such as child welfare and criminal justice systems; and individual and relational issues such as family conflict and social exclusion; and they suggested strategies in each area. Importantly, the voices of homeless youth are woven through this research.

A youth from Edmonton suggested early intervention: "It's more of changing what people think is 'the time' to help . . . Maybe you should help them when they are on the verge of becoming homeless, or they're well on the way, and they're seeking the help beforehand. Instead of, like, when their bank account is zero and they're on the street, and *then* you help them. Why didn't you do it when they had a few dollars and a couple of days left? Why couldn't you do it then?" (Schwan et al., 2018, p. 14). A Vancouver youth pointed out that qualifying for housing perversely required prolonging homelessness: "To access BC housing or any youth rent subsidies, you have to be homeless for a minimum of six months before they'll even look at you. Six months is a long time. And there's no need for any youth to go through that just to get a house. Cause some of them can make it through that time period, but some can't" (p. 6).

Homeless Women and Families

Homeless women are often estimated to make up just under 30% of homeless people in Canada but are more likely to be less visible or hidden (Gaetz et al., 2016). Using an upstream lens, Canadian researchers created a framework for ending women's homelessness that incorporates contextual understandings of the role of women's poverty, violence against women, trauma, discrimination, and a flawed justice system, among other factors (Yeo et al., 2015). Women are more likely to head families experiencing homelessness, who typically stay in shelters twice as long as single adults. Some groups are disproportionately represented among homeless families, including racialized people, Indigenous people, newcomer families, and families having a parent with a disability (Gaetz et al., 2016).

CANADIAN RESEARCH 29.1

Delivering care to women who are homeless: A narrative inquiry into the experience of health care providers in an obstetrical unit. (Based on Richter, Caine, Kubota, Chaw-Kant, & Danko, 2017)

As homelessness increases, CHNs and other health care providers must develop the skills and knowledge to care for homeless people. This includes understanding the ways homelessness confers health risks and intersecting barriers to care.

Richter and colleagues (2017) used narrative inquiry to explore providers' personal and professional experiences providing care to homeless pregnant women in an obstetrical unit in a large western Canadian hospital. They determined that health care providers, including nurses, have inadequate clinical knowledge for working with vulnerable populations. They argued that education must be guided by the concepts of health equity, social justice practice, and an understanding of the SDOH. These authors found a "misalignment" between what nurses and other health care providers think their patients need and what the system allows, and they point out that providers must understand that every interaction with marginalized people shapes their experiences and may have a negative impact on their willingness to seek health care in the future.

Participants identified gaps between institutional needs and care practices such as allowing homeless family members to stay overnight or sleep in a hospital bed during the day, or "sneaking" food to visitors who were hungry. Pressure to discharge patients before adequate supports were in place occurred, which some participants found distressing. The researchers noted that some providers held stereotypes and discriminatory attitudes toward patients who were homeless and that learning how to work with pregnant homeless women was often informal and imbued with "derogatory jokes and judgmental comments" (Richter et al., 2017, p. 125). One nurse participant identified that it was difficult to have conversational spaces to address stereotypes or discriminatory attitudes, in part because doing so might cause being ostracized from other staff.

Analysis of the results indicated four connected threads:

- Shaping and being shaped by institutional mandates
- The importance of conversational spaces
- The lack of inter-professional interactions
- Living with conflicted views about their practice

The research results led to several recommendations:

- Education needs to be guided by health equity, social justice, and understanding of the SDOH.
- Meaningfully involving clients who have experienced inequities in the education of health care providers could help health care providers better understand the lived experience of poverty.
- Education needs to offer more direct opportunities to engage with vulnerable populations.
- Hidden or "secret" practices created by policies need to be made visible and challenged.

Discussion Questions

1. What are some of the ways you, as a CHN, could advocate for appropriate postpartum discharge planning for a homeless pregnant patient?

2. You and your CHN colleagues have begun to notice a pattern of discriminatory attitudes in nurses being reported by homeless pregnant women admitted to the labour and delivery unit at a local hospital. What are some strategies you and your colleagues could employ to improve access to appropriate, compassionate, nonjudgmental care for these patients?

3. Stereotyping and discriminatory attitudes toward people who are homeless or living on low income are common in both acute care and community care settings. What are some of the ways you could support the creation of "conversational spaces" for discussion and learning in a community health nursing setting?

Health and Homelessness: Homelessness Is Life-Threatening

Morbidity and mortality are higher in homeless populations compared to the general population (Fazel, Geddes, & Kushel, 2014). Excess mortality is caused by infectious diseases such as HIV and tuberculosis, ischemic heart disease, substance use, unintentional injuries, and suicide. Toronto Public Health has begun tracking homeless mortality. Data for the first nine months of 2017 indicated an average of 1.8 deaths every week with a median age of 48 (Toronto Public Health, 2017). That means that nearly two people in their forties, perhaps the age of some of your parents, die every week in Toronto due to homelessness.

The Street Health Report 2007 was conducted by a community nursing organization in Toronto. Three hundred and sixty-eight homeless adults were interviewed about their health and access to care (Khandor & Mason, 2007). Astonishing findings included the following:

- One in ten had attempted suicide in the past year.
- One in three had been physically assaulted in the past year.

- One in eight had been physically assaulted by police in the past year.
- One in five women had been raped or sexually assaulted in the past year.
- 75% had at least one chronic condition.

Further, respondents were more likely to have the following health issues than the general population:

- 29 times more likely to have hepatitis C
- 20 times more likely to have epilepsy
- 5 times more likely to have heart disease
- Twice as likely to have diabetes

Access to dental care is challenging for all low-income people in the absence of publicly funded dental care for adults in Canada. Homeless individuals often have high rates of untreated dental problems, low rates of having received dental care, and high rates of using an emergency room for dental care (Figueiredo, Dempster, Quinonez, & Hwang, 2016).

Access to Health Care

Complicating homeless people's higher morbidity is their inequitable access to health care. More than half of the Street Health sample reported not having a family physician; more than one-quarter had been refused health care because they lacked a health insurance card; more than one-third felt they had been treated unfairly or without respect by a health care provider in the past year; and one in five reported a negative experience with hospital security (Khandor & Mason, 2007). Overwhelming unmet health care needs, such as mental health and addictions, chronic disease management, and urgent care issues, are challenging to address in the context of numerous barriers to receiving care. These barriers include patient mistrust of providers, competing survival priorities, financial barriers that may lead to issues with transportation and inability to afford medications, and structural problems such as lack of government identification (Campbell, O'Neill, Gibson, & Thurston, 2015). Pervasive experiences of stigmatization and discrimination often characterize heath care encounters by homeless people (Pauly, 2014).

End of Life Considerations for Homeless People

Given the excess burden of morbidity and mortality associated with homelessness, the issue of end-of-life care is significant. From the literature, it is clear that some homeless people have specific fears related to dying alone, to not being treated respectfully, and to having their wishes disregarded (Guirguis-Younger & McNeil, 2014b). Other issues include palliative-care service gaps as well as barriers like substance use, which may prove challenging to accommodate in traditional end of life settings. Shelter-based palliative-care options can reduce hospitalization costs and improve satisfaction among homeless people (Guirguis-Younger & McNeil, 2014b; Page, Thurston, & Mahoney, 2012).

FOOD INSECURITY

Food insecurity can be described as "inadequate or insecure access to food because of financial restraints" (Tarasuk, Mitchell, & Dachner, 2016, p. 2). In Canadian regions measuring food insecurity (Alberta, Saskatchewan, Ontario, Quebec, New Brunswick, Nova Scotia, Prince Edward Island, the Northwest Territories, and Nunavut), 12% of households experienced some level of food insecurity during 2014. This represents 1.3 million households, or 3.2 million individuals, including nearly 1 million children under the age of 18. More than one in six children under 18 lived in households that experienced food insecurity. Further, as might be expected, 60.9% of families reliant on social assistance were food insecure, but almost two-thirds (62.2%) of food-insecure households received income from salaries or wages (p. 3).

Food insecurity in Canada is worsening. According to McIntyre and Rondeau (2009, p. 24), "a very brief social history of food insecurity in Canada would read simply: Poverty increased, then it deepened. Food insecurity emerged, then it increased in severity." The researchers drew the connections between food insecurity and poor health, noting that food-insecure individuals are more likely to rate their health as fair or poor, are 80% more likely to report having diabetes, and are 60% more likely to report having hypertension. In addition, children from food-insecure families are more likely to experience a range of behavioural, psychological, and academic issues than children in food-secure households (p. 27). Food insecurity is strongly linked to poor mental health, and the relationship is proportional: the more severe an individual's food insecurity is, the greater impacts on mental health. Children who experience hunger as a result of food insecurity are more likely to have depression and suicidality in adolescence and young adulthood (PROOF, 2017).

Health Canada's Healthy Eating Strategy (Government of Canada, 2018) aims to improve nutritional labelling, improve nutritional food quality, reduce marketing of unhealthy foods

HOUSEHOLD FOOD INSECURITY AND FOOD BANK USE IN CANADA

- Residents in Nunavut spend twice as much on food as the rest of the country on average ($14,800 v. $7,300 annually).
- 4 million people in Canada experience food insecurity.
- 1 in 8 Canadian households struggle to put food on the table.
- In 2014, the majority of food insecure households —62.2%—were reliant on wages or salary from employment.
- 8 out of 10 provinces saw an increase in food bank usage in 2016.
- 62% of children living in the North are food insecure.
- 2 out of every 5 Northern households are food insecure.
- Food bank usage across Canada is 3% higher than 2015 and 28% higher than it was in 2008.
- 7 of 10 Inuit preschoolers live in food insecure households.
- Food bank usage has increased in all provinces since 2008, apart from Newfoundland and Labrador.
- 2% of food bank users are Indigenous.

Source: Canada Without Poverty/Canada Sans Pauvrete. (2018). *Just the Facts.* Retrieved from http://www.cwp-csp.ca/poverty/just-the-facts/. Used with permission.

HOUSEHOLD FOOD INSECURITY IN CANADA

- 24.5% of rented households experienced food insecurity, versus 6.2% of homeowners.
- The prevalence of food insecurity among households where the respondent was a recent immigrant to Canada (less than five years) was 15.2%, but the rate for households where the respondent had immigrated to the country five or more years ago was 12%, similar to the rate for Canadian-born respondents (11.8%).
- Households where the respondent was Indigenous or Black had an elevated rate of food insecurity at 25.7% and 29.4%, respectively.
- Households in rural areas experienced a rate of food insecurity slightly lower than that of households in population centres (10.3% versus 12.4%), but this difference was not statistically significant.

Source: Based on Tarasuk, Mitchell, & Dachner, 2016

to children, and support access to nutritious foods through its Nutrition North Canada program. This program provides a retail subsidy to increase affordability of food in Northern communities but has come under criticism for not actually making food affordable and not reflecting the diet of Northerners (Skura, 2016).

There appears to be nothing in the federal healthy eating strategy to address food insecurity, rendering the program largely irrelevant for the 3.2 million people who experience food insecurity in Canada.

According to Food Banks Canada (2014), 841 191 Canadians are forced to rely on food banks every month.

Northern and Indigenous Food Insecurity

Food insecurity is most pronounced in Northern Canada and the Maritime provinces. In Nunavut and the Northwest Territories, food insecurity prevalence rates were a staggering 46.8% and 24.2%, respectively (Tarasuk, Mitchell, & Dachner, 2016, p. 2). Food Banks Canada (2014) describes food insecurity in the Canadian North as a public health emergency related to high poverty, high unemployment, and the exorbitant cost of food. The organization notes that one in every five households in Canada's territories skips meals because of lack of food or eats poor quality food because of diminished access to country (traditional) foods or expensive alternatives. The disproportionate impact on First Nation, Métis, and Inuit populations can be attributed to disappearing or unhealthy game, resulting in an increased reliance on store-bought foods (Food Banks Canada, 2016). Pegg (2016) notes the disproportionate risk of food insecurity experienced by Indigenous people, particularly in Northern Canada, including the Yukon, Northwest Territories, Nunavut, Nunavik (northern Quebec), and Nunatsiavut (northern Labrador), attributed to pervasive poverty, high food costs, and the intergenerational effects of residential schools, causing the loss of traditional knowledge and practices combined with the effects of climate change on wild animal availability and other organic harvestable foods.

Responses to Food Insecurity

Numerous Canadian researchers have called for upstream responses to food insecurity (Pegg, 2016; Tarasuk, Mitchell, & Dachner, 2016). Pettes, Dachner, Gaetz, and Tarasuk (2016) reported that charitable meal programs in Canada typically struggle to provide services and are often reliant on donations and volunteer labour, and demand often exceeds resources. The researchers call for advances in research and policy to improve the way hunger and food insecurity are managed at the community level. Upstream interventions to improve food security include advocating for increased minimum wage rates, increased social assistance rates, and affordable housing and childcare (McIntyre & Rondeau, 2009).

CASE STUDY

You are a CHN working in a rural primary care clinic. You are facilitating a prenatal and postnatal group for low-income mothers on social assistance that offers education, breastfeeding and parenting support, and food vouchers to all participants. You serve a nutritious snack as well. You notice that attendance at your group fluctuates depending on the time of month, with mothers who live out of town hardly ever attending during the second half of the month. The in-town mothers tell you they are virtually out of food during the second half of the month, and the out-of-town mothers tell you they cannot afford transportation or gas money to get to the group during the same time period. Some of the children who attend appear pale, and you suspect iron deficiency anemia may be to blame. You decide to have one session that focuses on anemia and good dietary sources of iron.

During group discussion, numerous women express financial concerns in terms of having to rely on food banks, falling further and further behind in rent each month, not having money for gas, and going without food in order to feed their children. Several mothers disclose that they have to decide which bills to pay each month in order to have some money for food, and even still they often run out of money by the third week of the month. One woman says, "If the politicians think they could live on what I get every month, I'd just like to see them try. I'll bet they never have

to think about what bill they're gonna skip so their kid can go on a field trip with her schoolmates. Boy oh boy, I could sure give them an earful."

1. Working with the interdisciplinary team of providers at your clinic, such as the registered dietitian and social worker, what are some strategies you could devise to make the program more accessible for all the women in the group?

2. What are some strategies you and your colleagues could develop to increase access to the SDOH for the families in the group?

3. What are some upstream interventions you could use in this situation to reduce the impacts of health inequities related to food insecurity, lack of transportation, and lack of affordable housing?

ROLE OF THE COMMUNITY HEALTH NURSE

Recall the upstream/downstream analogy outlined in the first part of the chapter. What ought to be the role of the CHN in addressing poverty, homelessness, and food insecurity? How can CHNs tackle these issues from primordial, primary, secondary, tertiary, and quaternary prevention levels? We must question why having social justice as a practice goal is ethically necessary.

Working Downstream: Clinical Practice

CHNs caring for individuals and families who are living on low income, are food insecure, or are homeless must ensure they have accurate, up-to-date clinical knowledge to provide optimal care. The Centre for Effective Practice (2015) in Ontario developed a clinical guidelines tool that provides evidence-based screening questions and interventions for people living in poverty. For example, simply asking the question, "Do you ever have difficulty making ends meet at the end of the month?" can assist CHNs to identify people living on low income who may be at higher risk for some conditions.

Implementing innovative models of care with a health equity focus is another downstream strategy CHNs can use or advocate for to improve clinical care to low-income people. Pauly (2014, p. 211) argues that nurses are "uniquely positioned" to facilitate access to care for people who have barriers and excess morbidity. Her ethnographic research exploring homeless people's access to care found that "forging a chain of trust" was key and consisted of interpersonal organization and systemic linkages (p. 212). Important nursing strategies for improving access include building trusting relationships over time, preserving respect, acknowledging client concerns as important, being sensitive to people's life circumstances, using a harm reduction philosophy to meet people where they are, and meeting people on their "turf" using **outreach models of care**. Davy, Harfield, McArther, Munn, and Brown (2016) suggest that providing material resources that enable access to care is important, including provision of transportation to and from appointments. The emerging approach known as **inclusion health** aims to target interventions to populations traditionally excluded from mainstream society, such as homeless individuals (Luchenski et al., 2017). Interventions include case management, harm-reduction strategies, options for short-term recuperative care for homeless individuals, and addressing housing and the SDOH.

CHNs are frequently in an excellent position to identify connections between issues for individual patients and issues affecting specific populations. Imagine you are working in an inner-city community health centre located in a neighbourhood with a large population of homeless people and low-income rooming house and boarding home tenants. Over the past several years, you have noticed more people coming into your clinic with respiratory and cardiac problems during heat waves. One older adult client of your clinic died last summer in her third-floor room of respiratory problems apparently exacerbated by extreme hot weather and poor air quality. Imagine you are working in a heat wave during which the temperature is predicted to be 40 degrees Celsius with no end in sight for the next three days. On your way into the clinic, you notice several homeless people seeking refuge under the trees in the local park, and you see public works staff asking them to move along. You and your colleagues could devise interventions at several levels of prevention to lessen the risks of heat-related illness for vulnerable clients and community members:

- Develop an easy-to-read pamphlet on heat-related illness and practical strategies people can use to stay cool (e.g., drink lots of water even if you don't feel thirsty, do errands before 10:00 a.m., avoid drinking too much alcohol, signs and symptoms of heat stroke) and distribute it to appropriate locations.
- Consider organizing an information session at the local community centre on recognizing heat-related illness for staff and clients.
- Organize a brainstorming meeting of local agencies that serve low-income people to assess the feasibility of opening an air-conditioned community centre during extreme heat days or distributing bottled water to homeless people.
- Approach local businesses to see if they would donate funds to purchase refillable water bottles to give out to homeless people during hot weather.
- Consider designating one or two staff to do outreach to vulnerable clients during extreme hot weather in outdoor locations or rooming houses, which often have poor ventilation and no air conditioning.

Example of Working Upstream: Research and Political Advocacy

An important example of nursing political advocacy is found in the Canadian nurse-led organization Street Health, which conducted research on the health of homeless adults in Toronto (Khandor & Mason, 2007). What makes Street Health's community nursing research different from most is that its explicit intent was to create a tool for upstream political advocacy. The report included 13 recommendations for action that target the SDOH. As well as recommendations for more affordable housing and increased social assistance rates, the report called for an end to police violence against homeless people through reporting of incidents through a safe third party and through police officers undergoing mandatory training around homelessness and nonviolent de-escalation (p. 54) after finding that one in eight survey respondents had been assaulted by police the year before the survey (p. 4). The work of Street Health provides a useful blueprint for CHNs seeking to work upstream on structural issues that create health inequities.

CONCLUSION

In this chapter we reviewed the most current data on three serious and completely preventable health issues that affect far too many people in Canada: poverty, homelessness, and food insecurity. We saw how a critical social theory lens requires CHNs to consider the social context of health when implementing clinical practice interventions and to "think upstream" to consider broader interventions that increase access to the social determinants of health to prevent morbidity and mortality in the first place. Health is political, and few areas of nursing practice so vividly exemplify this truth as community practice settings in which individuals and families experience the effects of poverty, homelessness, and food insecurity.

No matter where CHNs work, whether in a large urban inner city or a rural community, in public health or visiting nursing or primary health care, the health impacts of poverty are unmistakable and ubiquitous. When we are situated downstream, as we so often are, it is crucial to think about what is happening for people upstream and to weave this perspective into our nursing practice every day.

KEY TERMS

at risk of homelessness   (p. 527)
downstream   (p. 521)
emergency sheltered   (p. 526)
food insecurity   (p. 531)
inclusion health   (p. 533)
Indigenous homelessness   (p. 528)
individualization   (p. 523)
low income cut-off   (p. 523)
low income measure   (p. 523)
market basket measure   (p. 523)
neoliberalism   (p. 522)
outreach models of care   (p. 532)
provisionally accommodated   (p. 526)
racialized   (p. 523)
social determinants of health (SDOH)   (p. 521)
unsheltered   (p. 526)
upstream   (p. 521)

STUDY QUESTIONS

1. What is the relevance of the social determinants of health to community health nursing practice with individuals and families affected by poverty, homelessness, and food insecurity?

2. Why are First Nations, Métis, and Inuit populations over-represented among Canadians living in poverty and experiencing food insecurity?

3. How would you explain the role of neoliberalism in creating conditions that generate poverty, homelessness, and food insecurity to your CHN colleagues who are not familiar with this concept?

4. Canada is a wealthy country. Why does homelessness exist here?

5. What is the relationship between food insecurity and health or mental health?

INDIVIDUAL CRITICAL-THINKING EXERCISES

1. What does it mean to consider that health is political in the context of understanding poverty, homelessness, and food insecurity in a wealthy country like Canada?

2. How does looking through a critical social theory lens help CHNs to provide ethical nursing care to people living in poverty?

3. Indigenous people are disproportionately overrepresented among homeless populations in Canada. What is the link between Indigenous homelessness and colonization?

GROUP CRITICAL-THINKING EXERCISES

1. You and your colleagues decide, with the support of your primary-care clinic manager, to make deputations to city council about the need to augment the affordable housing program in your municipality. Does political advocacy of this type increase the professional reputations and credibility of CHNs, or does it jeopardize it? Is the answer contingent on the particular constituency—for example, other health care professionals? Homeless individuals in your community? The general public?

2. Homeless health care providers have created strategies to provide end-of-life care for homeless people with life-limiting illnesses, such as palliative care provision in a shelter. Which is the more appropriate strategy for CHNs: providing end of life care that maintains homelessness until death in a setting familiar to someone, or advocating upstream for immediate housing for all homeless people diagnosed with a life-limiting illness?

3. Are food banks an appropriate response to food insecurity in Canada? Why or why not? What are some alternatives to food banks and other charitable responses to poverty?

REFERENCES

Anderson, J. T., & Collins, D. (2014). Prevalence and causes of urban homelessness among Indigenous peoples: A three-country scoping review. *Housing Studies, 29*(7), 959–976. doi: http://dx.doi.org/10.1080/02673037.2014.923091

Bierman, A. S., Ahmad, F., Angus, J., Glazier, R. H., Vahabi, M., Damba, C., . . . Manuel, D. (2009). Burden of illness. In A. S. Bierman, (Ed.). *Project for an Ontario women's health evidence-based report: Volume 1: Echo—Improving women's health in Ontario.* 1–143. Retrieved from http://powerstudy.ca/wp-content/uploads/downloads/2013/01/Chapter3-BurdenofIllness.pdf

Block, S., & Galabuzi, G-E. (2011). *Canada's colour-coded labour market: The gap for racialized workers.* Retrieved from http://www.wellesleyinstitute.com/wp-content/uploads/2011/03/Colour_Coded_Labour_MarketFINAL.pdf

Brittain, M., & Blackstock, C. (2015). *First Nations child poverty: A literature review and analysis.* Retrieved from https://fncaringsociety.com/sites/default/files/First%20Nations%20Child%20Poverty%20-%20A%20Literature%20Review%20and%20Analysis%202015-3.pdf

Campaign 2000. (2017). *2016 report card—A roadmap to eradicate child and family poverty.* Retrieved from http://campaign2000.ca/wp-content/uploads/2016/11/National-C2000Infographic2016.pdf

Campbell, D. J. T., O'Neill, B. G., Gibson, K., & Thurston, W. E. (2015). Primary healthcare needs and barriers to care among Calgary's homeless populations. *BMC Family Practice, 16*(139), 1–10. doi: 0.1186/s12875-015-0361-3

Canadian Observatory on Homelessness. (2012.) *Canadian definition of homelessness.* Toronto: Canadian Observatory on Homelessness Press. www.homelesshub.ca/homelessdefinition

Canada Without Poverty/Canada Sans Pauvrete. (2018). *Just the facts.* Retrieved from http://www.cwp-csp.ca/poverty/just-the-facts

Centre for Effective Practice. (2015). *Poverty: A clinical tool for primary care providers.* Retrieved from https://thewellhealth.ca/wp-content/uploads/2016/07/Poverty_flow-Tool-May1.pdf

Community Health Nurses of Canada (CHNC). (2019, revised). *Canadian community health nursing: Professional practice model & standards of practice.* St. John's, NL.

Conway, D. I., Petticrew. M., Marlborough, H., Berthiller, J., Hashibe, M., & Macpherson, L. M. D. (2008). Socioeconomic inequalities and oral cancer risk: a systematic review and meta-analysis of case-control studies. *International Journal of Cancer, 122*: 2811–2819.

Daley, A., Burton, P., & Phipps, S. (2015). Measuring poverty and inequality in northern Canada. *Journal of Children and Poverty, 21*(2), 89–110. doi: http://dx.doi.org/10.1080/10796126.2015.1089147

Davy, C., Harfield, S., McArther, A., Munn, Z., & Brown, A. (2016). Access to primary health care services for Indigenous peoples: A framework synthesis. *International Journal of Equity Health, 15*(1), 163.

Fazel, S., Geddes, J. R., & Kushel, M. (2015). The health of homeless people in high-income countries: Descriptive epidemiology, health consequences, and clinical and policy recommendations. *Lancet, 384*(9953), 1529–1540. doi: 10.1016/S0140-6736(14)61132-6

Figueiredo, R., Dempster, L., Quinonez, C., & Hwang, S. W. (2016). Emergency department use for dental problems among homeless individuals: A population-based cohort study. *Journal of Health Care for the Poor and Underserved, 27*, 860–868.

Firestone, M., Smylie, J., Maracle, S., Spiller, M., & O'Campo, P. (2014). *Unmasking health determinants and health outcomes for urban First Nations using respondent driven sampling.* Retrieved from http://www.welllivinghouse.com/wp-content/uploads/2014/04/unmasking-health-determinants-outcomes.pdf

Food Banks Canada. (2014). *Hunger count 2014: A comprehensive report on hunger and food bank use in Canada, and recommendations for change.* Retrieved from https://www.foodbankscanada.ca/getmedia/7739cdff-72d5-4cee-85e9-54d456669564/HungerCount_2014_EN.pdf.aspx?ext=.pdf

Food Banks Canada. (2016). *Hunger in the North.* Retrieved from https://www.foodbankscanada.ca/Hunger-in-Canada/Hunger-in-the-North.aspx

Gaetz, S., Dej, E., Richter, T., & Redman, M. (2016). *The state of homelessness in Canada 2016.* Toronto: Canadian Observatory on Homelessness Press. Used with permission.

Government of Canada. (2016a). *Highlights of the National Shelter Study 2005–2014.* Retrieved from https://www.canada.ca/en/employment-social-development/programs/communities/homelessness/reports-shelter-2014.html

Government of Canada. (2016b). *Understanding homelessness and the strategy.* Retrieved from https://www.canada.ca/en/employment-social-development/programs/communities/homelessness/understanding.html#s4

Government of Canada. (2018). *Health Canada's healthy eating strategy.* Retrieved from https://www.canada.ca/en/services/health/campaigns/vision-healthy-canada/healthy-eating.html

Guirguis-Younger, M., & McNeil, R. (2014b). The development and operational context of an emergency shelter-based hospice in Ottawa, Ontario: A qualitative study. In M. Guirgus-Younger, R. McNeil, & S. W. Hwang. (2014). *Homelessness and health in Canada.* Ottawa, ON: University of Ottawa Press. Retrieved from https://press.uottawa.ca/homelessness-health-in-canada.html

Halseth, G., & Riser, L. (2010). *A primer for understanding issues around rural poverty.* Retrieved from https://www.unbc.ca/assets/community_development_institute/publications/a_primer_for_understanding_issues_around_rural_poverty.pdf

Homeless Hub. (2017). *Homelessness 101: How many people are homeless in Canada?* Retrieved from http://homelesshub.ca/about-homelessness/homelessness-101/how-many-people-are-homeless-canada

Hulchanski, D. (2002). *Did the weather cause Canada's mass homelessness? Homeless-making processes and Canada's homeless-makers.* Toronto Disaster Relief Committee Research Department. Retrieved from http://www.urbancentre.utoronto.ca/pdfs/researchassociates/2000_Hulchanski_TDRC-Homeless-Makers-Canada_Discussion-pape.pdf

Karabanow, J., & Kidd, S. (2014). Being young and homeless: Addressing youth homelessness from drop-in to drafting policy. In M. Guirgus-Younger, R. McNeil, & S. W. Hwang. (2014). *Homelessness and health in Canada.* Ottawa, ON: University of Ottawa Press. Retrieved from https://press.uottawa.ca/homelessness-health-in-canada.html

Khandor, E., & Mason, K. (2007). *The street health report 2007.* Retrieved from http://www.streethealth.ca/downloads/the-street-health-report-2007.pdf

Labonte, R., & Stuckler, D. (2016). The rise of neoliberalism: How bad economics imperils health and what to do about it. *Journal of Epidemiology and Community Health, 70*, 312–318. doi: 10.1136/jech-2015-206295

Lightman, E., Mitchell, A., & Wilson, B. (2008). *Poverty is making us sick: A comprehensive survey of income and health in Canada.* Toronto, ON: Wellesley Institute. Retrieved from http://www.wellesleyinstitute.com/wp-content/uploads/2011/11/povertyismakingussick.pdf

Lightman, E., Mitchell, A., & Wilson, B. (2009). Sick and tired: *The compromised health of social assistance recipients and the working poor in Ontario.* Toronto, ON: Wellesley Institute. Retrieved from http://www.wellesleyinstitute.com/wp-content/uploads/2011/11/sickandtiredfinal.pdf

Luchenski, S., Maguire, N., Aldridge R. W., Hayward, A., Story, A., Perri, P., . . . Hewett, N. (2017). What works in inclusion health: Overview of effective interventions for marginalised and excluded populations. *The Lancet* (November 11). doi: http://dx/doi.org/10.1016/S0140-673617)31959-1

Macdonald, D., & Wilson, D. (2013). *Poverty or prosperity: Indigenous children in Canada.* Retrieved from https://www.policyalternatives.ca/sites/default/files/uploads/publications/National%20Office/2013/06/Poverty_or_Prosperity_Indigenous_Children.pdf

McIntyre, L., & Rondeau, K. (2009). Food insecurity in Canada. In D. Raphael (Ed.), *Social determinants of health: Canadian perspectives.* 2nd edition (pp. 188–204). Toronto, ON: Canadian Scholars' Press. Retrieved from http://thecanadianfacts.org/The_Canadian_Facts.pdf

Medvedyuk, S., Ali, A., & Raphael, D. (2017). Ideology, obesity and the social determinants of health: A critical analysis of the obesity and health relationship. *Critical Public Health.* doi: 10.1080/09581596.2017.1356910

Mikkonen, J., & Raphael, D. (2010). *Social determinants of health: The Canadian facts.* Toronto, ON: York University School of Health Policy and Management. Retrieved from http://thecanadianfacts.org/The_Canadian_Facts.pdf

Milbourne, P. (2010). The geographies of poverty and welfare. *Geography Compass, 4*(2), 158–171.

Page, S. A., Thurston, W. E., & Mahoney, C. E. (2012). Causes of death among an urban homeless population considered by the medical examiner. *Journal of Social Work in End-of-Life & Palliative Care, 8*, 265–271. doi: 10.1080/15524256.2012.708111

Pathways to Education. (2018). *Building a graduation nation.* Retrieved from https://www.pathwaystoeducation.ca

Pauly, B. (2014). Close to the street: Nursing practice with people marginalized by homelessness and substance use. In M. Guirgus-Younger, R. McNeil, & S. W. Hwang. (2014). *Homelessness and health in Canada.* Ottawa, ON: University of Ottawa Press. Retrieved from https://press.uottawa.ca/homelessness-health-in-canada.html

Pegg, S. (2016). *What will it take to make real progress on Northern food security? A Food Banks Canada report.* Retrieved from https://www.foodbankscanada.ca/getmedia/f6ce7d1e-849a-416c-b04b-9fbd6c5e46fb/Northern-Food-Security-EN-FINAL.pdf.aspx?ext=.pdf

Pettes, T., Dacjmer. M., Gaetz. S., & Tarasuk, V. (2016). An examination of charitable meal programs in five Canadian cites. *Journal of Health Care for the Poor and Underserved, 27,* 1303–1315.

PROOF. (2017). *Food insecurity and mental health.* Toronto, ON: University of Toronto. Retrieved from http://proof.utoronto.ca/resources/fact-sheets/#mentalhealth

Raphael, D., Daiski, I., Pilkington, B., Bryant, T., Dinca-Panaitescu, M., & Dinca-Panaitescu, S. (2012). A toxic combination of poor social policies and programmes, unfair economic arrangements and bad politics: The experiences of poor Canadians with type 2 diabetes. *Critical Public Health. 22*(2), 127–145. doi: oi.org/10.1080/09581596.2011.607797

Reimer Kirkham, S., & Browne, A. (2006). Toward a critical theoretical interpretation of social justice discourses in nursing. *Advances in Nursing Science, 29*(4), 324–339.

Richmond, C. A. M., & Cook, C. (2016). Creating conditions for Canadian Aboriginal health equity: The promise of healthy public policy. *Public Health Reviews, 37*(2), 1–16. doi: 10.1186/s40985-016-0016-5

Richter, S., Caine, V., Kubota, H., Chaw-Kant, J., & Danko, M. (2017). Delivering care to women who are homeless: A narrative inquiry into the experience of health care providers in an obstetrical unit. *Diversity and Equality in Health and Care, 14*(3), 122–129.

Riser, L., & Halseth, G. (2017). Opportunities and challenges to address poverty in rural regions: A case study from Northern BC. *Journal of Poverty, 21*(2), 120–141.

Ruckert, A., & Labonte, R. (2016). The first federal budget under Prime Minister Justin Trudeau: Addressing social determinants of health? *Canadian Journal of Public Health, 107*(2), e212–e214. doi: 10.17269/CJPH.107.5662

Schwan, K., Gaetz, S., French, D., Redman, M., Thistle, J., & Dej, E. (2018). *What would it take? Youth across Canada speak out on youth homelessness prevention.* Toronto, ON: Canadian Observatory on Homelessness Press.

Schwartz, D. R., James, C. A., Wagner, A. C., & Hart, T. A. (2014). Sexual risk behaviours and sexual health outcomes among homeless youth in Canada. In M. Guirgus-Younger, R. McNeil, & S. W. Hwang. (2014). *Homelessness and health in Canada.* Ottawa, ON: University of Ottawa Press. Retrieved from https://press.uottawa.ca/homelessness-health-in-canada.html

Skura, E., (2016). Nutritious to who? Northerners say food subsidy program needs overhaul. *CBC News* (September 27). Retrieved from http://www.cbc.ca/news/canada/north/nutrition-north-public-consultation-iqaluit-1.3780190

Smith, K. L., Matheson, F. I., Moineddin, R., & Glazier, R. H. (2007). Gender, income and immigration differences in depression in Canadian urban centres. *Canadian Journal of Public Health, 98,* Mar–Apr (2): 149–153.

Statistics Canada. (2008). *Aboriginal peoples in Canada in 2006: Inuit, Métis and First Nations, 2006 Census.* Retrieved from http://www12.statcan.ca/census-recensement/2006/as-sa/97-558/pdf/97-558-XIe2006001.pdf

Statistics Canada. (2012). Poverty profile: *Special edition— A snapshot of racialized poverty in Canada.* Retrieved from https://www.canada.ca/content/dam/esdc-edsc/migration/documents/eng/communities/reports/poverty_profile/snapshot.pdf

Statistics Canada. (2015). *Low-income lines, 2013–2014: Update.* Retrieved from https://www.statcan.gc.ca/pub/75f0002m/2015002/lico-sfr-eng.htm

Tang, S., Browne, A., Mussell, B., Smye, V. L., & Rodney, P. (2015). "Underclassism" and access to healthcare in urban centres. *Sociology of Health & Illness, 37*(5), 698–714. doi: 10.1111/1467-9566.12236

Tarasuk, V., Mitchell, A., & Dachner, N. (2016). *Household food insecurity in Canada: 2014.* Toronto, ON: Research to identify policy options to reduce food insecurity (PROOF). Retrieved from http://proof.utoronto.ca

Thistle, J. (2017.) *Indigenous definition of homelessness in Canada.* Toronto: Canadian Observatory on Homelessness Press. http://www.homelesshub.ca/sites/default/files/COHIndigenousHomelessnessDefinition.pdf

Toronto Public Health. (2017). *Monitoring deaths of homeless people.* Retrieved from https://www1.toronto.ca/wps/portal/contentonly?vgnextoid=13fbd47f61059510VgnVCM10000071d60f89RCRD

Virchow, RLK (1859). Cellular Pathology. Special Edition, 204-207. London: John Churchill; 1978.

Waegemakers Schiff, J., & Turner, A. (2014). *Housing first in rural Canada: Rural homelessness and housing first feasibility across 22 Canadian communities.* Retrieved from http://www.homelesshub.ca/sites/default/files/Rural_Homelessness_in_Canada_2014.pdf

Woods, M. (20015). *Rural geography.* London, UK: Sage Publishing.

World Health Organization. (2015). *The social determinants of health.* Retrieved from http://www.who.int/social_determinants/sdh_definition/en. © 2015

Yeo, S., Ratnam, C., Paradis, E., Oudshoorn, A., Nessa, B., Mosher, J., . . . Aguila, K. (2015). *A framework for ending women's and girls' homelessness.* Retrieved from http://www.abeoudshoorn.com/wp-content/uploads/2015/08/A-Framework-for-Ending-Womens-and-Girls-Homelessness.pdf

ABOUT THE AUTHOR

Kathy Hardill, RN(EC), MScN, is a white settler of Irish and English ancestry. She is the Executive Director/Nurse Practitioner Lead of the Peterborough 360 Degree Nurse Practitioner-Led Clinic in Nogojiwanong (Peterborough, Ontario). Her areas of expertise are in health and homelessness, in the primary care of individuals with significant health vulnerabilities, and in harm reduction and primary care. Her master's research explored the experience of health care for people who use illicit opioids in small cities and rural communities. She is convinced that health is political and has worked both upstream and downstream for the past 30 years. She is a founding member of the Street Nurses' Network and Health Providers Against Poverty—Ontario.

Substance Use

Abe Oudshoorn and Victoria Smye

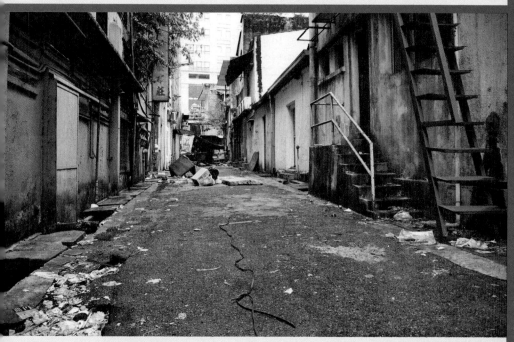

Source: 1000 Words/Shutterstock

INTRODUCTION

The purpose of this chapter is to provide the community health nurse (CHN) with knowledge and tools regarding substance use that can be utilized in community health nursing. This knowledge will assist CHNs in the prevention and minimization of harm associated with problematic substance use. For CHNs to develop and engage in health-promoting practice, they must understand the dynamics, social and health effects, and root causes of substance use. People from all walks of life can experience problematic substance use. Conversely, it cannot be assumed people who experience multiple disadvantages will inherently use substances.

Critical theoretical perspectives are taken up as a lens in this chapter to inform social justice and equity-oriented community health nursing practice. In keeping with the perspectives of Kagan, Smith, and Chinn (2014), we advocate for nursing practice that creates and embraces social justice, what Kagan et al. refer to as "praxis," meaning practice intentionally aimed at achieving social justice goals and outcomes that improve health experiences and conditions of individuals, their communities, and society. This approach takes into account structural inequities and power relations that shape health and well-being. For example, the CHN needs to understand the structural inequities that shape problematic substance use. A praxis approach is socially actionable; the CHN is expected to engage in authentic relationships with community to disrupt structural inequities (Varcoe, Browne, & Cender, 2014).

LEARNING OUTCOMES

After studying this chapter, you will be able to:

1. Differentiate among substance use, problematic substance use, dependency, and addiction.

2. Describe the Canadian context of substance use, shifting priorities, and implications.

3. Examine the relationship between problematic substance use and varying social locations.

4. Describe the intersecting relationships among trauma, violence, problematic substance use, and chronic pain.

5. Examine the relationship between problematic substance use and health inequities.

6. Recognize stigma related to substance use.

7. Understand the harmful consequences of problematic substance use and harm reduction.

8. Discuss the public health levels of prevention and how these relate to reducing problematic substance use.

9. Reflect on the role of the community health nurse in addressing problematic substance use.

REFLECT ON YOUR ATTITUDE ABOUT SUBSTANCE USE

1. Consider your personal experiences with using substances. Do you smoke, drink wine, or consume other alcoholic beverages? Do you use marijuana, or have you ever? What has impacted which substances you have used? Why do you choose to use some substances? Why do you choose not to use some substances?

2. Reflect on your thoughts, reactions, and responses to people with problematic substance use. What are your thoughts and reactions to medical marijuana? Many of us have people in our lives who have or are experiencing problematic substance use, or perhaps we have our own experiences. How does this make you feel?

3. Some substance use has no negative impact on people's lives, and other substance use can be highly problematic. What do you see as the root causes of problematic substance use versus non-problematic substance use?

To begin to engage with praxis, it is helpful to think about your own ideas, habits, values, and actions (Kagan et al., 2014) as they pertain to problematic substance use.

Problematic substance use is a complex public health issue that spans the life cycle and can have severe and permanent consequences for individuals, families, and communities. The overall cost of substance use, including alcohol, tobacco, and **illicit drugs**, to Canadians is estimated at approximately $40 billion, with tobacco and alcohol accounting for almost 80% of the total (Rehm et al., 2006). The recent surge in the problematic use of prescription opioid pain relievers can cost up to $50 billion a year, according to the Canadian Centre on Substance Use and Addition (CCSA, 2013). As such, substance use has a significant and direct impact on our health care, social service, and judicial systems. Substance use is a significant risk factor for a number of chronic health conditions, such as HIV/AIDs, several types of cancers, as well as acute problems related to injuries, violence, and suicide. Considerable non-monetary costs to Canadian society also exist, such as the pain, suffering, and bereavement experienced by families, friends, and victims, which can have profound and lasting effects that cannot be measured in dollars.

Evidence from various fields of inquiry suggests that problematic substance use is multi-factorial—that familial, genetic, psychological, socioeconomic, and historical factors are all determinants of problematic use. Other factors that may influence substance use patterns include gender, education, income, and employment status. The CHN should therefore understand the social context of problematic substance use and the social conditions that can influence the initiation of use. It also is essential for CHNs to recognize patterns of ongoing use, cessation, abstinence, and relapse (Galea, Nandi, & Vlahov, 2004). Using a socioenvironmental perspective calls for the development of comprehensive community health nursing interventions that acknowledge the interdependence among the person, the substance, and the environment. CHNs often see firsthand the impact of problematic substance use on the individual or collective. Traditionally, nurses have been described as sentinels on the riverbanks, responding to a problem occurring upstream (Butterfield, 1997). This chapter is therefore intended to challenge you to make those critical connections to what is happening upstream in your community and the reasons people use substances.

SUBSTANCE USE, ADDICTION, AND DEPENDENCE

Language is a powerful tool in framing how we understand the world. This is evident as we discuss and understand substances, the use of substances, use that is deemed as problematic, and "addiction." In 2017, the Office of National Drug Policy in the United States recommended that all departments and agencies stop using the term *substance abuse* due to the negative judgments attached to this language. Rather, it recommend using language from the *Diagnostic and Statistical Manual of Mental Disorders* (*DSM-5*; American Psychiatric Association [APA], 2013), which refers to "substance use disorders," defined as mild, moderate, or severe, which is determined by the number of diagnostic criteria met by an individual. Substance use disorders occur when the recurrent use of alcohol or drugs causes clinically and functionally significant impairment, such as health problems, disability, and failure to meet major responsibilities at work, school, or home. According to the *DSM-5*, a diagnosis of substance use disorder is based on evidence of impaired control, social impairment, risky use, and pharmacological criteria. However, this language can be contested as well, with "disorder" having a connotation as pathologizing behaviours that may or may not be problematic. The other challenge is that the language of "substance use disorders" covers only substances, while there are other addictive activities such as gambling, shopping, or sex. These other activities, when problematic, are often referred to as **process addictions** or behavioural addictions.

The terms *substance use, substance abuse, substance use disorder, addiction,* and *dependence* are sometimes erroneously used interchangeably. Some of these terms are more derogatory than others; the term *addiction* carries the greatest **stigma** and is perhaps the most overused. The term *addiction* is often equated with physical dependence, but it also is used to define non-substance-related behavioural addictions like a gambling disorder (APA, 2013).

Addiction itself has been removed from medical diagnoses, as it is both hard to define and has strong negative connotations. Consider the impact of labelling a person an "addict"; there is strong stigma attached to the term both within health care and in Canadian society in general. The language of addiction also exposes cultural norms regarding what is considered acceptable and what is not. Individuals may, for example, joke about a "caffeine addiction," speaking to a degree of coffee consumption with no negative health or social impacts, while simultaneously referring to someone who daily consumes large quantities of alcohol as "a partier." Conversely, friends may label someone who uses cocaine very occasionally as an addict due to stigma around harder substances, while refusing to consider the presence of addiction in the case of an individual who compulsively shops online and is unable to stop in spite of relationship loss and financial hardship. It is the stigma attached to substance use that makes the language nurses use so important.

In this chapter, we use the term **substance use** generically recognizing that humans consume all kinds of substances, legal and illegal, natural and pharmaceutical, prescribed and purchased. We want to avoid binary language that implies that substances are good or bad and that use is good or bad, but rather understand the complexity of substance use as interconnected with societal understandings and attitudes, which are fluid over time. However, we also want to be clear that some substance use can be objectively or subjectively problematic, and for that we will use the terminology **problematic substance use**. Problematic use is that which leads to adverse physical, psychological, legal, social, or interpersonal consequences, which may or may not involve dependence. **Dependence** is progressive in nature and affects the physiological, cognitive, behavioural, and psychological dimensions of a person's health. It is manifested by continuous use despite the presence of problems caused by use. Dependence results in tolerance, withdrawal, and compulsive substance-taking behaviour (APA, 2013). **Physical dependence** occurs when an individual's body reacts to the absence of a drug with withdrawal symptoms. **Psychological dependence** occurs when drug use becomes central to a person's thoughts and emotions.

The *DSM-5* (APA, 2013) criteria for substance use disorders are illustrative in understanding when substance use might become problematic.

In reviewing this list you should note that what substance or what behaviour and at what quantity becomes problematic is both individual and cultural. For example, where consuming alcohol during a working lunch in some settings may be deemed socially problematic, in other work contexts it would be seen as normal. Or an individual may have a high tolerance to opioid medications due to severe pain related to an injury and may experience withdrawal upon completing the course of treatment. However, this experience would relate to very different social or legal risks related to whether the opioids were prescribed or purchased illegally.

Although in this chapter we will use the less stigmatized language of "substances," common terminology both within the general public and within the health care system is the use of the word "drug." The term *drug* refers to a **psychoactive substance** that affects a person's physiological or psychological state or behaviour. Drugs can be substances consumed for medicinal and non-medicinal purposes, legally or illegally. Licit drugs (legal drugs) are drugs that are used for medicinal purposes. Licit drugs are available by prescription or sold over the counter to relieve common symptoms such as pain, anxiety, or insomnia. Some of these drugs are regulated by the Controlled Drugs and Substances Act 1996 (CA). Although the substance itself is legal, it may still be used in ways that are problematic. Illicit drugs, or illegal drugs, include phencyclidines (PCP, ketamine), hallucinogens (LSD, mescaline,

---

THE *DSM-5* CRITERIA FOR SUBSTANCE USE DISORDERS

- Substance often taken in larger amounts or over a longer period of time than intended
- A persistent desire or unsuccessful efforts to cut down or control use
- A great deal of time spent in activities necessary to obtain the substance, use it, or recover from its effects
- Craving, or a strong desire or urge to use
- Recurrent use resulting in failure to fulfill major role obligations at work, school, or home
- Continued use despite having persistent or recurrent social or interpersonal problems caused or exacerbated by use
- Important social, occupational, or recreational activities given up or reduced because of use
- Recurrent use in situations that are physically hazardous
- Use is continued despite knowledge of having a persistent or recurrent physical or psychological problem likely to have been caused or exacerbated by use
- Tolerance: the need for markedly increased amounts of substance to achieve intoxication or desired effect, or a markedly diminished effect with continued use of same amount
- Withdrawal: a characteristic syndrome, or use to relieve or avoid withdrawal

Source: APA (2013).

---

psilocybin, MDA), stimulants other than caffeine and nicotine (amphetamines, cocaine, crack), depressants (barbiturates, methaqualone, benzodiazepine), and opiates (heroin, morphine, methadone, codeine). In the next section we explore the history of legislation related to substances in order to better understand why some substances are illegal and some are legal, and why this changes over time.

THE CANADIAN CONTEXT OF SUBSTANCE USE: CHANGING PRIORITIES AND THE IMPACT ON HEALTH AND WELL-BEING

Prior to the early 1900s, substances in Canada and across the Western world were unregulated. Although concerns related to alcohol consumption and suggestions of prohibition in the United Kingdom date to the 1800s, substance laws at the national level were not introduced until 1908 in Canada, 1914 in the United States, and 1916 in the United Kingdom. Canada's first substance-related legislation was the Opium Act, 1908. It is worth noting that while this Act prohibited the importation, manufacture, and sale of opium, it included a clause stating "for other than the medicinal purpose" (Library of Parliament, 1908). The other point to note, in considering the evolution of cultural perspectives over time, is that debate at the time was focused on opium as a moral issue, frequently condemning it as "evil" and noting that it was being made illegal "throughout the Christian world" (Library of Parliament, 1908, p. 1550). This was a period when the Christian religion and the politics of Canada were deeply intertwined. This Act was expanded in 1911 in the Opium and Narcotic Drug Act with the introduction of other opiate substances.

The national prohibition of alcohol in Canada from 1918 to 1920 is illustrative of the philosophies underlying considerations of dealing with substances at the time. The key contributor to prohibition, the making of distribution and consumption of alcohol illegal, was the Temperance Movement, or Christian Temperance Movement (*The Canadian Encyclopedia*, 2015). The movement was a national and international collaboration of "temperance societies" situated in lodges or churches that perceived societal ills as caused primarily by alcohol, or alcohol as a morally corruptive substance, at odds with the goals of religion. Prohibition in Canada is now considered a failed legislative strategy that distorted the alcohol market, actually increasing alcohol use and leading to a significant increase in organized crime (*The Canadian Encyclopedia*, 2015). Although this lesson has more impact today on drug policy, influencing more well-rounded strategies such as the "Four Pillars Approach" (described below), it had little impact on the direction of drug strategy at the time, with cannabis added to prohibited substances in 1923 and continual increases of harsher sentences and more enforcement (Cherry, Dillon, & Rugh, 2002).

This approach of harsh punishments, mandatory sentences, significant enforcement, and use as primarily a concern of the criminal justice system has often been termed the "war on drugs." This terminology has different connotations in different contexts, with some politicians declaring that they will engage in a war on drugs to appeal to a voter base who wants to see more enforcement, where other citizens use it insultingly to refer to a policy approach that is very costly while having limited demonstrable effect on rates of substance use. Critics also have highlighted how an enforcement approach disproportionately affects populations experiencing inequities, such as racialized youth, Indigenous peoples, or women who are trafficked.

It was not until the early 2000s that we began to see a shift in substance use legislation in Canada. In 2001, Health Canada began to authorize the use of marijuana for medical purposes, and around the same time local communities began adopting a "Four Pillars Approach" to problematic substance use. Recognizing that a wide range of tools and solutions are needed, experts in Canada developed a framework that combines the elements of health promotion with enforcement. These elements were coined the "pillars" of Canada's Federal Drug Strategy, which recognizes the need for a balanced approach to address these problems. The four pillars are harm reduction, prevention, treatment, and enforcement (MacPherson & Rowley, 2001). While this approach still includes enforcement, it also includes a recognition that enforcement alone does not solve problematic substance use, and more upstream support and prevention will decrease both use and the need for enforcement. Unfortunately, in 2007, Canada's Drug Strategy was renamed the National Anti-Drug Strategy with a focus on only three pillars: preventing illicit drug use, treating illicit drug dependency, and combatting the production and distribution of illicit drugs. Harm reduction was removed as a pillar at that time. In light of an international shift toward public health and harm-reduction approaches, critics at this time described Canada's national policy as regressive, with an overemphasis on enforcement strategies to combat the production and distribution of illicit drugs.

Most recently, we have again seen a shift back to a comprehensive four pillar approach, one that is both upstream and downstream in focus. Although significant stigma continues to be attached to certain substances and to the idea of addiction, recent legislative changes parallel a shift in attitudes toward substances and in how we respond to problematic substance use. Most recently, the proposed October 17, 2018, legalization of marijuana is already being followed by debates on decriminalization of all substances (Félix, Portugal, & Tavares, 2017).

SUBSTANCE USE: AN INTERSECTIONAL ANALYSIS

As noted, stigma and discrimination accompany substance use. However, there are intersecting dimensions of oppression, dominance, and prejudice often associated with mental illness, substance use, poverty, gender, race, and sexuality in every part of society, including the delivery of health care. These intersecting forces create more or less disadvantage and impact health and well-being. Research findings suggest that people's experiences, although similar across some dimensions, are differentiated by the disadvantages (and advantages) posed by their location across dimensions. For example, a study conducted with various Indigenous people accessing mental health services, Smye, Browne, Varcoe, and Josewski (2011) found that although the lives of the Indigenous men and women with mental health illness on methadone maintenance treatment (MMT) who were living in poverty resembled those of other people living in poverty, the intersection of poverty, race, substance use, mental illness, HIV/AIDS, hepatitis C, and gender (as examples) brought with them special sets of circumstances and challenges to successful harm reduction. "Racialization" was relevant to all experiences; race-based oppression was present in the everyday reality of people's lives, including the experiences of accessing and delivering MMT. Yet "'[r]ace' could not be neatly shifted apart from processes of racialization, issues of gender, class relations, and other social relations that structured peoples' lives such as their education level, employment status, health, and well-being" (p. 2/12).

The CHN needs to recognize and understand these intersections to provide a comprehensive and effective approach to problematic substance use. As Weber and Parra-Medina (2003) note, inequities are often obscured when models of practice focus on individual bodies and behaviour rather than taking into account "the social structural context as the locus of a population's health" (p. 187). "Grounded in critical feminist theoretical perspectives, intersectional analyses are useful in drawing attention to the dynamics of the intersections between problematic substance use, other aspects of social identity and different forms of oppression that can guide us in addressing the multiple inequities and stigmas associated with [substance] use" (Smye et al., 2011, p. 2/12).

VIOLENCE, TRAUMA, MENTAL HEALTH, AND SUBSTANCE USE

An estimated 50% of Canadian women and 33% of Canadian men have experienced at least one incidence of sexual or physical violence over their lifetime (Ad Hoc Working Group on Women Mental Health Mental Illness and Addictions, as cited in BC Provincial Mental Health and Substance Use Planning Council, 2013). As noted in Chapter 28, here are differences in experiences of violence across gender, age, race, and sexual orientation. Interpersonal violence such as intimate partner violence (IPV), child abuse, and sexual assault has been associated with negative health effects, including problematic substance use and mental health challenges (Mason, Wolf, O'Rinn, & Ene, 2017). These effects must be understood in the context of cumulative lifetime abuse rather than as a consequence of one type of violence (Scott-Storey, 2011). For example, research has demonstrated a strong relationship between adverse childhood experiences (ACEs), problematic substance use (e.g., Dube et al., 2003), persistent pain (e.g., Haskell & Randall, 2009), and behavioural problems.

The extent of violence and trauma in the Canadian population and its strong association with negative health effects, including problematic substance use and mental health challenges, necessitates that CHNs understand violence as a possibility in the lives of any person seen in a health care or community context. The association among violence against women, substance use, and mental health has been studied extensively, showing that women who have experienced violence have significantly higher rates of substance use and mental health concerns compared to women who have not (Canadian Women's Foundation, 2011). Problematic substance use and mental health issues are consistently linked; therefore, they cannot be considered separately. A **concurrent disorder** refers to one or more co-occurring mental health challenges simultaneously with problematic substance use within the same person. Looking at the root causes of substance use, such as trauma, experiences of violence, social isolation, homelessness, and poverty, you should note significant overlap with root causes of mental health challenges. Community health nursing practice needs to reflect the understanding that problematic substance use sometimes overlaps with violence and mental health issues, and those problems need to be seen within the context of social and structural determinants of health to ensure the provision of integrated care (Poole, 2007; Salmon et al., 2006).

Chronic Pain

Pain is an incredibly complex, contextual, and subjective experience (Melzack, 2005; Winterowd, Beck, Aaron, & Gruener, 2003), thus every patient will respond to treatments differently (Negron, 2012). This complexity is emphasized by our understanding of pain as produced and processed within the brain (Melzack, 2005). As noted, trauma and violence can actually have a marked impact on structures and processes in the brain that mediate pain response. However, it is not uncommon for persons experiencing problematic substance use to encounter resistance from health professionals to their request for pain management. Clinicians may be overly suspicious of drug-seeking behaviour when considering opioids for pain management, particularly when dealing with populations rendered vulnerable (Weiner et al., 2013). However, Hwang et al. (2011) note that concerns regarding the prescription of narcotics to homeless people are not reasons to avoid addressing chronic pain management. In addition, Douglas, Gourlay, Heit, and Almahrezi (2005) note that although opioids should not routinely be considered the first choice of treatment for chronic pain, neither should opioids be a last attempt. Furthermore, the stress of living in shelters, poor sleeping conditions, and financial barriers to accessing over-the-counter medications negatively affect the experience of chronic pain in people experiencing homelessness (Hwang et al., 2011).

The CHN has an important role to play in the management of chronic pain with persons experiencing problematic substance use. We know a person-centred, empathic approach reduces health inequity (Browne et al., 2015; Drwecki, Moore, Ward, & Prkachin, 2010). The individual practitioner and their relationship with the patient influence treatment outcomes (Otis, Keane, Kerns, Monson, & Scioli, 2009; White et al., 2012; Winterowd et al., 2003) and the patient's beliefs about pain, health, and health care (Bennett & Closs, 2010). Pain education should include evidence-based information about the expected course and outcomes and effective self-care (Chou et al., 2007). However, education must be done in a way that respects a patient's underlying belief system (Pauly, Reist, Belle-Isle, & Schactman, 2013). The evidence regarding pain treatments is vast and diverse; most complementary and non-pharmacological treatments are understood as moderately effective in some cases. The highly subjective nature of pain and the influence of beliefs and relationships mean that establishing reliable evidence of efficacy and effectiveness is uniquely difficult (Bennett & Closs, 2010). In general, a multidisciplinary and multimodal approach to pain is the gold standard in care (Charlton, 2005; EQUIP Healthcare, 2014; Jessop, 2006).

The concept of **cultural safety** is consistent with the principles of patient-centred pain management; there is an emphasis on the need for health care professionals to be self-reflexive, a recognition that the client may experience the world differently, and acknowledgement that clients' values and experiences are valid and significant aspects of their health and well-being (Pauly et al., 2013). The lens of cultural safety can assist health care professionals dealing with client pain to respect differences, support client agency, and appreciate the impact of historical factors, including, for many people, multiple traumas. As noted, patient histories of violence and trauma are often inextricably linked with chronic and acute pain. Trauma- and violence-informed care refers to care that reflects an understanding of the impact of violence and trauma on an individual; this knowledge is essential to holistically and sustainably deal with problematic substance use not only to ensure the creation of a trusting provider–patient relationship but also to reduce the risk of re-traumatization and guarantee that each component of pain management is consistent with recovery from traumatic experiences (Elliott, Bjelajac, Fallt, Markoff, & Reed, 2005).

SUBSTANCE USE, HEALTH, AND SOCIAL INEQUITY

A recent report released by the Conference Board of Canada and funded by Health Canada offered more evidence that tobacco use is a significant burden on all Canadians, costing society $16.2 billion in 2012—$466 for every Canadian (Government of Canada, 2017). An estimated 45 464 deaths were attributable to smoking in Canada in 2012. To address tobacco use, the Government of Canada has announced its commitment to reduce tobacco use to less than 5% by 2035 with programs such as Picking up the Pace, a lifestyle-change-focused intervention. Lifestyle-change programs have been a central feature of tobacco cessation programs, but most fail to address the "cause of the causes." As CHNs it is important to remember tobacco use is declining dramatically in Canada, except among low-income populations. This factor reflects the stress of living in poverty, limited options for dealing with stress, limited access to tobacco-reduction supports, and health education strategies related to tobacco cessation that are not necessarily appropriate or relevant to this population (often focused on lifestyle changes).

As noted in the World Health Organization (WHO, 2008) report, "inequities in health, avoidable health inequalities, arise because of the circumstances in which people grow, live, work, and age, and the systems put in place to deal with illness. The conditions in which people live and die are, in turn, shaped by political, social, and economic forces" (p. i). For example, historical legacies of racism, **structural violence**, and dehumanization (e.g., residential schools and boarding schools) have led to health inequities for Indigenous peoples, forcing consequences such as substance use and its effects. Recent studies confirm the alarmingly high rates of injection drug use among urban Indigenous youth in Canada, especially women (Miller et al., 2011). The rate of problematic prescription drug use is two to three times higher among urban Indigenous youth than among non-Indigenous youth (Webster, 2012). According to the Government of Canada (2006), the proportion of alcohol use by Indigenous peoples is lower than that of non-Indigenous populations in Canada (66% versus 76%, respectively); however, there is a tendency for more binge drinking for some First Nation, Inuit, and Métis people, highlighting the effect of varying histories, geographies, and social conditions of Indigenous communities. Please refer to Chapter 22 for a more detailed discussion regarding Indigenous health. In their study with lesbian, gay, and bisexual people, Chow et al. (2013) found that inadequate housing increased the likelihood of crack cocaine use, highlighting the critical intersections of heterosexism, class, and other social structures in the lived realities of substance use.

The National Advisory Committee on Prescription Drug Misuse (2013) reports that certain populations in Canada, such as women, youth, older adults, First Nations, and Inuit, can have higher rates of "prescription drug use or abuse" or experience greater related harms than the general population. Further research is needed to confirm prevalence rates and related harms. A number of other groups also may be at risk for problematic prescription drug use, including military personnel and veterans, people who have experience incarceration, homeless people, individuals with concurrent disorders, and health care professionals.

As you can see, the harmful consequences of substance use extend far beyond the individual using substances. It is both a response to social breakdown and an important factor in worsening the inequities of an individual's health (WHO, 2003). Substance use can have lasting effects on individuals, families, and communities, impacting their health, safety, and quality of life. The WHO (2003) recommends that we address the complexities of the social circumstances and contexts that are responsible for problematic substance use. As such, the response to substance use problems in a community must be broad and include different interventions at the most appropriate levels of action.

Drawing on research at two primary health care (PHC) centres in Canada with explicit mandates to provide services to populations marginalized by social and structural inequity, Browne et al. (2012) identified strategies for operationalizing key dimensions of equity-oriented care at the patient-provider, organizational, and system levels. Four key dimensions provide a framework for understanding the essential elements of equity-oriented PHC services when working with populations that have been marginalized by social and structural inequity. The dimensions are interrelated and overlapping, and include the following:

- *Inequity-Responsive Care:* Explicitly addressing the social determinants of health as legitimate and routine aspects of health care, often as the main priority.
- *Trauma- and Violence-Informed Care:* Recognizing that most people affected by systemic inequities and structural violence have experienced, and often continue to experience, varying forms of violence with traumatic impact. Such care consists of respectful empowerment practices informed by understanding the pervasiveness and effects of trauma and violence, rather than "trauma treatment" such as psychotherapy.
- *Contextually Tailored Care:* Expanding the concept of patient-centred care to include services that are explicitly tailored to the populations served and local contexts. This may include organizational tailoring to address the local population demographics and social trends (e.g., programs or services addressing HIV, older adults, women's or men's issues, and support for new immigrants).
- *Culturally Safe Care:* Taking into account not only the cultural meaning of health and illness but also, equally importantly, people's experiences of racism, discrimination, and marginalization, and the ways those experiences shape health, life opportunities, access to health care, and quality of life. (p. 5/15)

Follow-up research to study the contextual factors shaping the implementation, uptake, and impact of a tailored intervention (EQUIP) took place within four diverse PHC settings. The EQUIP intervention illustrates the complexities involved in enhancing the PHC sector's capacity to provide equity-oriented care in real-world clinical contexts. One of the findings of the study was the need to add *harm reduction approaches* to the key dimensions of equity-oriented care (Browne et al., 2015). The findings of these studies point to the need for CHNs to use equity-oriented approaches in the context of health care delivery for people living with problematic substance use (Browne et al., 2015). It is suggested CHNs access the eight EQUIP modules and tools created from the EQUIP research to assist them in the delivery of equity-oriented care, for themselves and for the organization in which they practice.

YES, BUT WHY?

Confronting Stigma

What?

The issue of stigma is a highly pertinent concept intersecting with, or contributing to, the harms associated with problematic substance use (Reist, 2010). According to Goffman (1963), stigma is as an attribute associated with "difference" that is deemed to be a less desirable difference by one person (the stigmatizer) in relation to another person (the stigmatized)—a difference that, at its extreme, might deem the person as bad, dangerous, or weak (stereotyping).

So What?

Building on Goffman's earlier work, Link and Phelan (2001, 2006) present stigma as created through five interrelated and converging social processes. For example, in the case of drug use:

i) Labelling of the person with problematic substance use as different, e.g., the "drug addict" or "junkie"
ii) Negative stereotyping by linking "difference" with undesirable characteristics and fears such as drug users as "dangerous"
iii) "Othering" by creating "them" (the labelled person) and "us" categories
iv) Status loss, blame, and discrimination of the labelled person
v) Creation of power dynamics in which power is experienced by the labelled person's ability to access to key resources, such as money and social networks or institutions (Anstice, Strike, & Brands, 2009; Benoit, Shumka, & Barlee, 2010; Smye et al., 2011)

Thus, problematic substance use as a category of difference often leads to stigmatization based on the beliefs that underpin its perceived origins and an experience of and the ability of the labelled person to resist stigma (or not) dependent on their social location and perceived power.

Now What?

Although public attitudes vary toward people with problematic substance use, and many people acknowledge that people with substance use issues often come from difficult circumstances, i.e., that there are social and structural issues influencing use, there remains a strongly held view that "drug addicts" are to blame for their drug use (Lloyd, 2010). Lloyd notes that in our society, the identity as "addict, tends to take centre stage to the obscuration of all other facets of identity and personality" (p. 13). For example, as Ross, Berry, Smye, and Goldner (2017) found, nurses' problematic substance use is a response, in large part, to emotional distress and physical pain associated with the workplace—a fact well understood by nurses themselves (Bugle, 1996; Hutchinson, 1986; Lillibridge, Cox, & Cross, 2002; Tipliski, 1993). Yet nurses have viewed problematic substance use among their own as "willful misconduct" (Monroe, 2009, p. 273; Ross et al., 2017). Nurses experiencing problematic substance use also are acutely aware of the stigmatizing attitudes that other nurses generally hold toward their colleagues so affected. These are particularly evident when nurses in treatment for problematic substance use encounter harsh and demeaning attitudes and comments upon their return to work (Brewer & Nelms, 1998; College of Registered Nurses of Nova Scotia, 2008; Darbro, 2005; Howard & Chung, 2000; Lillibridge et al., 2002; as cited in Ross et al., 2017). Nurses' attitudes are shaped by societal norms; they are a reflection of the conversations in our social world. It is crucial to effective safe practice that CHNs reflect on their own prejudices, biases, and assumptions regarding illicit and problematic substance use to support the enactment of destigmatizing approaches.

Standards of Practice Fulfilled

#1 Health Promotion
- Considers the determinants of health, the social and political context, and systemic structures in collaboration with the client to determine action.

#2 Prevention and Health Protection
- Uses harm reduction principles grounded in social justice and health equity perspectives to identify and reduce risks, and increase protective factors.

#4 Professional Relationships
- Recognizes own personal beliefs, attitudes, assumptions, feelings, and values including racism and stereotypes and their potential impact on nursing practice.

#6 Health Equity
- Engages with the client using critical social theory and intersectional approach from a foundation of equity and social justice.
- Assesses how the social determinants of health influence the client's health status with particular attention to clients who are marginalized (CHNC, 2019, revised).

HARMFUL CONSEQUENCES OF SUBSTANCE USE

Some substances are prescribed by nurse practitioners and physicians, and are intended to keep us healthy but may be used in ways that cause harm. Some substances are controlled by legislation and are used recreationally, such as alcohol, but they can be used in ways that cause harm. Other substances are made illegal and have high risk of harm but may be used by people in ways that don't meet the *DSM-5* criteria for a substance use disorder. As health providers, we need to be cautious in avoiding naive assertions that "all drugs are harmful," as we work in a system that prescribes and distributes the majority of substances in our society. However, we should also avoid being naive in ignoring the potential harms related to substance use. In this section we explore a number of those harms.

As discussed, although its usage has been in decline, tobacco is a substance that continues to create significant health harm in Canada. Every year in Canada, more than 37 000 people die prematurely of tobacco-related disorders (Reid, Hammond, Burkhalter, Rynard, & Ahmed, 2013), with smoking being the leading preventable cause of death in the country (Baliunas et al., 2007). Nicotine may lead to both physical and psychological dependence, and smoking is often characterized by numerous attempts to quit. Apart from the users themselves, exposure to secondhand smoke among neonates, infants, children, and adults is associated with an increased risk of a number of acute and chronic conditions.

Problematic alcohol use can cause liver damage, increase risks of injury, have negative financial and social effects, and, in cases of those who are homeless, increase the risk of death due to exposure. Although impaired driving rates have dropped over the past couple of decades, the percentage of all motor vehicle deaths caused by drinking drivers in Canada has increased (Traffic Injury Research Foundation [TIRF], 2013). Alcohol is also frequently involved in snowmobiling and boating accidents across Canada. Almost 40% of boating deaths have alcohol involvement, and at least half of all fatally injured snowmobilers in Canada were drinking (TIRF, 2009). Other associated harms of alcohol use can include an increase in crime and violent acts; relationship breakdown; accidents at home, on roadways, and at work; negligence in care of children; and workplace or school absenteeism. While alcohol is the most commonly used substance in Canada, and most people who use alcohol do not do so in a manner deemed problematic, healthy patterns of consumption need to be promoted by CHNs.

A priority population for nursing interventions is individuals who are considering pregnancy or are currently pregnant or breastfeeding. The consumption of alcohol during pregnancy can result in **fetal alcohol spectrum disorder (FASD)**, which is manifested by developmental, neurological, and behavioural delays in infants and young children that persist into adulthood (Chudley et al., 2005). Although FASD is related to the frequency and volume of an expectant mother's alcohol intake, other contributing factors include poor nutrition, age, lack of prenatal care, and the use of other drugs. Social factors, such as poverty, social isolation, or experiences of intimate partner violence, place women at greater risk,

highlighting the need for comprehensive support for moms-to-be across the determinants of health.

Apart from substances that are common in Canada from coast to coast to coast, context is important in considering potential harms; from community to community, there are different risks related to the availability of different substances. In many communities fentanyl is a concern, particularly those with large acute-care hospitals, which are often a source of fentanyl due to diversion from staff or patients. In other communities, crystal methamphetamine is a greater concern, particularly rural or near-rural communities where the substance can be manufactured with less likelihood of detection. Frequently it is the harms of a substance, such as overdose and overdose leading to death, that drive the concerns of a local community. These concerns may spark public or political action, such as declarations of an "opioid crisis," "methamphetamine crisis," or "fentanyl crisis." While these declarations often lead to more resources put into support and treatment, they don't necessarily involve a simultaneous focus on the root causes of substance use. CHNs need to ensure they are providing both reactive support on such issues as a crisis and proactive support to create long-term community change. This is presented later in the chapter in a discussion about the various levels of prevention.

Illegal substances have unique risks. One such risk worth considering is that in making a substance illegal, individuals are more likely to take risks in obtaining that substance, use the substance in an unsupervised or unsafe manner, or avoid seeking care when they experience harm from use. The social issues that are the roots of substance use can also amplify the harms of substances, such as the magnification of harm for an individual who is homeless or living in poverty (Galea et al., 2004). People who develop dependencies related to substances, illegal or legal, may choose to inject these substances in order to increase the rapidity or intensity of the effect. When people inject substances in an unsupervised context, they are at risk for blood-borne pathogens such as HIV and hepatitis B and C. Due to the stigma related to injection drug use, individuals may be unlikely to seek out clean supplies for injecting or feel that seeking treatment might create a risk related to employment, family relationships, or friendships. In the next section, we begin to explore pragmatic ways to reduce the potential harms of substance use.

The harms of illicit drug use are made worse in certain social conditions. The harmful consequences to health and well-being are magnified when an individual is homeless or living in poverty (Galea et al., 2004). In a study of illicit drug use in five Canadian cities, Fischer and colleagues (2005) found that many people who injected illicit drugs experienced increased physical and mental health problems. They also lacked permanent housing, did not have access to treatment, and experienced social marginalization (Fischer et al., 2005).

Injecting drugs carries a number of inherent risks, including overdose and suicide; contracting infections such as HIV, hepatitis C, and other blood-borne infections; developing abscesses, poor nutritional status, and endocarditis; and experiencing adverse drug interactions. Many injection drug users report a history of physical, emotional, or sexual abuse during their time of drug use. Using injection drugs may further

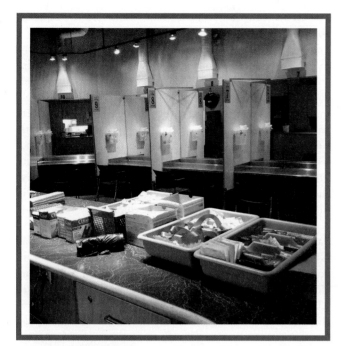

PHOTO   30.1 Safe-injection site in Vancouver

Source: Courtesy Vancouver Coastal Health

marginalize people, making it very difficult for them to access supports in the community (CCSA, 2011). As well, injection drug users may share needles and drug injection equipment, and engage in unprotected sex for money or drug exchange. Women who inject drugs face unique challenges because they may have links to the sex trade industry and become reluctant to access services for fear of having their children taken away (CCSA, 2011).

Harm Reduction

Harm reduction refers to policies, programs and practices that aim to reduce the negative health, social and economic consequences that may ensue from the use of legal and illegal psychoactive drugs, without necessarily reducing drug use. Its cornerstones are public health, human rights and social justice. It benefits people who use drugs, families and communities. (Cavalieri, 2017, para 2)

Given the complexity of problematic substance use and associated stigma, the diversity of issues that shape practices and policies associated with substance use are best understood under the pragmatic philosophy of harm reduction, a philosophy underpinned by two central values: that all life activities carry risk and that elimination of drug use is not necessarily "attainable" or *"desirable"* (emphasis added) (Pauly, 2008). Harm reduction is an approach that represents a continuum of services that embody a philosophical, pragmatic, and compassionate approach to providing care while minimizing the negative harms associated with substance use, understanding that not all people have the same ability to change, the same level of substance use, or even experience the same harms (Pauly,

Goldstone, McCall, Gold, & Payne, 2007; Smye et al., 2011). As Pauly (2008) notes, "harm reduction as a philosophy shifts the moral context in health care away from the primary goal of fixing individuals towards one of reducing harm" (p. 6).

Abstinence, on the other hand, focuses on the reduction of use with the ultimate aim of no use. Harm reduction and abstinence approaches often are conceptualized as being on a continuum with harm reduction at one end and abstinence at the other. For example, in terms of alcohol consumption, a harm reduction approach would include a focus on safe alcohol consumption, regardless of level of consumption, whereas an abstinence approach would focus on the complete cessation of alcohol use. Alcoholics Anonymous is one organization that promotes the abstinence model.

Because harm reduction is goal-oriented and humanistic, it also includes a nonjudgmental acceptance of people with problematic substance use and a person-centred approach. Health care professionals working in these programs meet clients "where they are at" (Marlatt, Blume, & Parks, 2001, p. 14) and work collaboratively with clients to establish goals and develop a plan of care (Registered Nurses of Ontario [RNAO], 2009). In keeping with this perspective, harm reduction is one aspect of a comprehensive approach to the harmful consequences of substance use, recognizing that there are many different strategies and programs of harm reduction that meet diverse clients' needs. A harm reduction approach is underpinned by a commitment to change policy or is integrated into existing health policies. However, most of these efforts deal directly with the harms that emanate from individual drug using and sexual practices, and deal less with the harms associated with the root causes of problematic substance use (violence, poverty, racism, historical trauma, and so on) and the harms associated with drug policy (such as criminalization, incarceration, and poverty). One linkage that has demonstrated promise in this regard is Housing First, a mental health strategy that focuses directly on housing people regardless of current patterns of substance use. As such, harm reduction is a key principle of Housing First (Pauly et al., 2013). CHNs' involvement in these kinds of initiatives is recommended.

Harm reduction offers a wide spectrum of opportunities for the CHN to help strengthen the capacity of individuals and communities experiencing the adverse effects of substance use. Examples of specific harm reduction strategies are supervised consumption sites, street outreach programs that target people marginalized by social and structural inequity, needle exchange programs, MMT, distribution of condoms and dental dams (all products should be freely available and offered without cost), bleach kit programs for cleaning syringes, distribution of clean crack kits, safer sex education, safer drug use and education, law-enforcement cooperation, and prescription of heroin and other drugs, among others. For more information regarding these specific harm reduction approaches, see RNAO (2009).

The need to consider harm reduction through an intersectional lens was reflected in study findings by Smye et al. (2011); for example, women and men's poverty resulted in them living in unsafe housing units in sections of the city where problematic substance use surrounded them. Their need for access to MMT and antiretroviral treatment led to confinement to particular urban settings, and their Indigenous identity further limited their housing choices in particular areas. "An intersectional lens draws attention to the disturbing ways that homelessness, poverty, substance use and racialization intersect to exacerbate peoples' experiences of social suffering, i.e., to those human conditions with roots and consequences associated with social, economic and political power—suffering that is both created by the way power is inflicted on human experience and how this power shapes the response to it" (Smye et al., 2011, p. 9/12).

As noted, harm reduction focuses on lowering the risk and severity of adverse consequences without necessarily reducing or eliminating use (International Harm Reduction Association, 2010; Pauly, 2008; RNAO, 2009). Although different, these approaches are complementary, and all have an important role in addressing substance use challenges in our communities. It is often said that harm reduction is not "what's nice, it's what works." The focus is therefore not on the use or the extent of use but on the harms associated with the use. The goal is to reduce the more immediate and tangible harms. Providing nursing care in the context of harm reduction can raise ethical questions for CHNs and community debates.

CHNs should be prepared for the controversy and debates harm reduction may elicit. Strong community stakeholder endorsement is essential, as there may be public resistance to the appropriateness of harm-reduction programs. Be aware that this can inadvertently polarize the community and shift the focus from the program's intended purpose to a debate about social, moral, or criminal issues. On the other hand, such a dialogue may be essential to produce a shift in knowledge, attitudes, and values. Harm reduction programs exist in most provinces, but generally speaking, federal political support is weak. Harm reduction approaches are still considered unconventional. They force people to move away from the comfortable but failed "just say no" approach and are therefore met with ambivalence or resistance despite being epidemiologically sound and highly effective. For example, Saskatchewan's rates of HIV/AIDS are currently the highest in Canada. Its provincial government wanted to halt unlimited needle distribution despite an earlier government-ordered review that found reductions in disease and health care costs. As such, new funding has not been offered, and the cost in harms to people and the community is severe.

Consider the highly publicized debate about the InSite facility in Vancouver. It was opened in 2003 for research purposes with a three-year exemption from the federal Controlled Drugs and Substances Act 1996 (CA), permitting users to bring illicit drugs into the centre and inject themselves while under medical supervision. The exemption was extended to 2008, at which time a new government indicated that it would not support what it considered a "failed experiment" despite the strong body of research demonstrating the success of such programs. The matter was heard by the Supreme Court of BC, which ordered the federal government to abandon its efforts to close the facility and requested an exemption be granted to protect InSite staff from prosecution for drug possession or trafficking. The government refused. The facility currently operates under a constitutional exception to the Controlled Drugs and Substances Act 1996 (CA).

Harm-reduction programs may not necessarily be available to all groups. For example, models of abstinence and prohibition in some First Nation communities may not allow moderate or reduced consumption or use, and many Indigenous treatment programs and communities adhere to models of abstinence. However, harm reduction may not be entirely incompatible in some jurisdictions that have supported harm reduction programs for Indigenous people with problematic substance use, offering abstinence as the potential but not required goal (Dell & Lyons, 2007). As with any community group, regardless of its cultural affiliation or diversity, CHNs should ensure that any harm reduction service is developed in full partnership with members of the community.

Although highly political and debated, the values of harm reduction are consistent with those of nursing (Canadian Nurses Association, 2011; RNAO, 2009). It is important for you to be aware of the controversial landscape of harm reduction, and it is equally important to consider how you will advocate for system improvements in your community or at the broader levels. Nurses have long been successful advocates for their patients.

CANADIAN RESEARCH 30.1

Sheltering risks: Implementation of harm reduction in homeless shelters during an overdose emergency.
(Wallace, Barber, & Pauly, 2018)

While harm reduction is a widely tested and acknowledged response to problematic substance use, how it is implemented is important. The goal of many services that implement a harm reduction approach, including emergency shelters, is to reduce risk of drug overdoses. There is a concern that partial implementation of harm reduction, or conflict between policies within emergency shelters, may be leading to sub-optimal implementation of harm reduction.

This research study involved eight focus groups with a mixed sample of shelter residents, shelter staff, and harm reduction workers from two emergency shelters. In total, 49 participants discussed issues around substance use in shelters, challenges related to substance use, and how harm reduction was being implemented. It is noted that both shelters were "low-barrier," meaning that individuals could access the shelter while under the influence of substances.

Participants highlighted the tension when shelters distributed safer consumption supplies while substance use on site was simultaneously prohibited. This led to fear regarding accessing these supplies as it might lead staff to be more vigilant regarding one's activities and subsequently increase risk of being banned from the shelter. Harm reduction workers noted the limited education for shelter workers regarding harm reduction principles beyond distribution of supplies. Shelter workers noted that washrooms were being used as sites for injection rather than having fully supported, clean, and supervised spaces. Although having naloxone on site led to higher rates of overdose prevention, participants did not see this as a complete solution to shelter policy concerns.

Ultimately, this study highlights the risks with partial implementation of harm reduction, focusing on distribution of supplies without also considering where and how these supplies will be utilized. The authors highlight the reality of washrooms being used as unsafe injection sites. Ultimately, they recommend that shelters consider implementation of a comprehensive harm reduction model.

Discussion Questions

1. Review the questions about your own substance use at the opening of the chapter, and reflect on your responses. After reading the case study and the chapter so far, would you change any of your answers?

2. Do you feel well-equipped to provide care within a harm reduction framework with people who use illicit substances? If so, why? If not, what would help you take the next steps in being equipped to work with people who use substances?

ETHICS AND SUBSTANCE USE: A CASE IN POINT—PREGNANCY

The use of opioid drugs during pregnancy can result in **neonatal abstinence syndrome (NAS)**. In-utero exposure to these substances results in infants born with physical dependence and withdrawal symptoms. They present with neurological, gastrointestinal, and respiratory difficulties, including a high-pitched cry, poor feeding, sleep-wake abnormalities, poor weight gain, tremors, and seizures—all of which require prolonged hospitalizations and treatment in a special-care nursery. NAS also often leads to the development of lifelong issues that may include FASD, behaviour problems, and developmental delays. Stigmatization may cause an underestimation of the prevalence of NAS; however, the Canadian Institute for Health Information has reported that its incidence more than doubled from 2004 to 2010 (Dow et al., 2012).

Pregnancy often puts women under intense scrutiny related to substance use, including alcohol, tobacco, and illicit drugs. Societal attitudes can create significant barriers that prevent women from receiving adequate prenatal care. Women may conceal substance use of any kind during pregnancy for fear of judgment, the possibility of punitive treatment of any kind, and, at worst, removal of their baby into care after birth. Associated to the fear of apprehension and other barriers to access care are many poor health outcomes and risks for the mother and child. A woman who is fearful of her child being removed many not seek prenatal care, which could result in inadequate nutrition and stress. These factors often contribute to poor obstetrical outcomes in this population. As Krausz (2010) notes, for the children of women with problematic substance use in pregnancy, environmental factors such as low socioeconomic status (SES), poor nutrition, and low quality of education have similar effects on cognitive function, mental abilities, growth, and other physical factors as illicit drugs. Researchers also have found that mothers who

have their babies apprehended at the hospital are discharged to the streets, where the cycle of poverty and homelessness begins again (Payne, 2007). Substance use often continues, and women can "recycle" via another subsequent pregnancy and child apprehension. Policies designed to protect children often have negative consequences for mothers, children, and families. There is a substantial disconnect between our knowledge, policies, and practice regarding maternal substance use during pregnancy.

CHNs working with women of childbearing age need to be attuned to these issues when screening, making referrals, and providing treatment. Often the presenting signs for substance use in pregnancy and postpartum are subtle, and they can include the following:

- Missed or inadequate prenatal care
- Recurrent somatic complaints (chronic pain, nausea, sleep)
- Psychiatric diagnosis or history or history of trauma
- Failure to gain adequate weight
- Intra-uterine growth delay
- Withdrawal signs at delivery

Problematic substance use is common in the general population, and women of childbearing age are no exception. It is imperative to build strong relationships with women with problematic substance use. Early identification and treatment, and women-centred services, have proven useful in improving retention, substance use outcomes, and psychosocial function (Kang, 2004; Payne, 2007). By reaching out to women with problematic substance use during pregnancy, the potential to provide comprehensive substance use treatment, prenatal care, social care, and unmet housing needs is significantly increased (Krausz, 2010). CHNs need to have current and factual information regarding specific substances and their effects on the fetus.

SUBSTANCE USE AND PREVENTION

Primordial Prevention

Prevention of problematic substance use at the primordial level involves nurses supporting public policy making that reduces structural inequities. For example, poverty is a significant systemic factor that increases risk related to substance use. Poverty is structural in that it is related to economic policies, employment policies, discriminatory histories and systems, access to social services, and related factors linked to public policy. Reducing poverty involves transforming this policy context, which could include the implementation of a **guaranteed annual income**, employment supports geared to refugees, or an increase in child benefits. This is congruent with the Canadian Nursing Association's position paper on nurses engaging in action for social justice. Public policy making is a complex process and usually not moved by any single individual, so it is recommended that CHNs connect with their provincial or territorial nursing associations if they have concerns about structural issues that are increasing risk related to root causes of problematic substance use.

Primary Prevention

Similar to primordial prevention, primary prevention involves preventing problematic substance use before it occurs but with more focus on the individual or community rather than broader systemic issues. In the context of substance use, this includes activities geared at preventing regular substance use from becoming problematic. An example of a primary prevention initiative is Canada's **Low-Risk Alcohol Drinking Guidelines**. These guidelines were developed to promote a culture of moderation for people who consume alcohol. The guidelines help individuals to identify what is considered a standard drink in terms of alcohol content rather than volume (see Figure 30.1). The standard drink definition is also intended to help people monitor their individual alcohol

intake against the recommended guidelines and consider when drinking alcohol becomes high-risk. This information helps Canadians in considering the balance between non-problematic and problematic substance use. It should be noted, however, that health educational interventions such as these have limited efficacy among marginalized populations if not implemented concurrently with primordial prevention that changes the context of use.

Another form of primary prevention might be to intervene with families around issues that can lead to trauma, subsequently increasing risks related to substance use. This can involve programs that support men who have been violent in changing their violent behaviours, parenting programs that provide alternative discipline options to corporal punishment, anti-racism programs in schools, or education for health and social service providers in how to be allies with people on the LGBTQ2S spectrum. In this way, programs that prevent any of the "isms"—racism, classism, sexism, ageism, ableism, colonialism, white supremacy, and homophobia—are protective against life experiences that

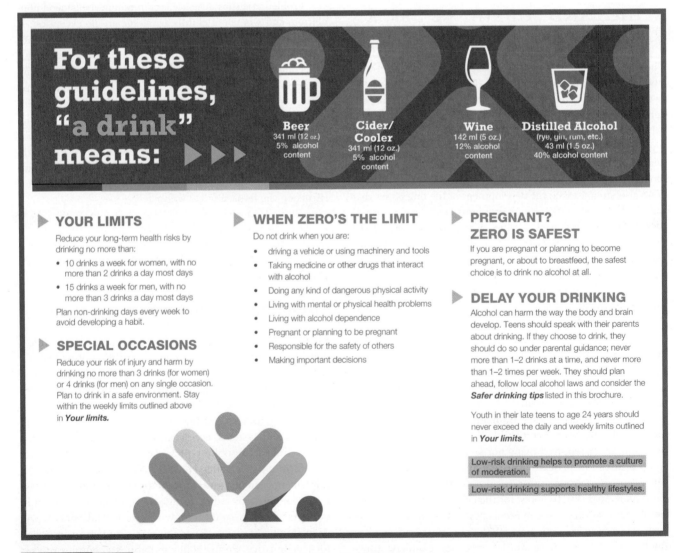

FIGURE   30.1 Canada's Low-Risk Alcohol Drinking Guidelines

Source: Reproduced with permission from Alberta Gaming, Liquor, and Cannabis. (2018).

put individuals, families, and communities at greater risk of problematic substance use.

An important principle across all levels of prevention that is well-illustrated in how a nurse might choose between the many options just discussed is working in collaboration with the population the nurse intends to support. Therefore, in considering what areas to target to prevent problematic substance use, people who use substances are the best resource. Many communities have established formal networks of substance users, such as the London Area Network of Substance Users or the Vancouver Area Network of Drug Users. Building alliances with these networks is a great step for CHNs who want to have an impact on substance use prevention in a community context.

Primary prevention includes the regulatory context of individual substance use. Policies such as tobacco by-laws, limits on the private sale of alcohol, or narcotic prescription databases are intended to reduce the risks around substances that can be problematic. They can create an environment that is conducive to healthy practices by making it easier to adopt healthy behaviours and more difficult to adopt unhealthy ones. This can go beyond substance-related policy and include policies that help to ensure healthy conditions and practices that are protective against problematic substance use. In its 2011 position paper on ending tobacco use, the Canadian Public Health Association reported that taxes imposed on tobacco help to maintain high prices, which is considered one of the most effective measures to reduce tobacco use, especially among young people who are price sensitive, and that a 10% increase in the price of tobacco products can result in a consumption drop of about 8%, with the greatest decrease among youth (Canadian Public Health Association, 2011). However, it should be noted that these policies might unintentionally privilege social groups that are less likely to experience problematic substance use (such as upper-income families) or further stigmatize individuals who use substances, such as not allowing those in acute-care hospital settings to smoke anywhere on hospital property.

Secondary Prevention

Secondary prevention involves early identification of when substance use becomes problematic and rapid support to assist the individual in addressing root causes to subsequently reduce or end substance use. This can involve substance use screening, tools, or conversations that allow for the detection of signs and symptoms of problematic use. These signs and symptoms might be the 11 criteria of substance use disorders, for example. Addressing root causes can be done through a process referred to as "treatment," the intentional process of regaining control over life after the negative effects of problematic substance use. It can occur on an inpatient or outpatient basis, be supported privately or publicly, and involve a wide variety of methods. Most methods involve some degree of individual or group counselling and a focus on moving the individual from problematic use to recovery. **Recovery** is a term used to indicate that an individual has formerly used substances problematically but is now either not using substances or using substances in a non-problematic manner.

As indicated in Canadian Research 30.1, stigma related to substance use, particularly use of illicit drugs or use of prescribed drugs in a manner other than prescribed (such as injecting prescribed oral pain medications), serves as a barrier to accessing health care supports. In the same way, this stigma serves as a barrier to implementation of secondary prevention, with individuals often facing pressure not to answer screening tools honestly or feeling uncomfortable in reaching out for treatment or even identifying as being in need to treatment support. Stigma is also not experienced equitably; research indicates, for example, that women experience different barriers to treatment services and lower rates of service access than men (Pirie, Jesseman, & National Treatment Indicators Working Group, 2013). Be aware of your own views and attitudes, and avoid falling into the "Well, they could just quit" over-simplification.

Community treatment services typically include detoxification, screening, assessment, treatment, and aftercare and follow-up. Non-residential treatment services, such as day treatment, make up the majority of all substance use treatment episodes (Pirie et al., 2013). The most common treatment services used in Canada are alcohol and drug education, problem-solving counselling, cognitive and behavioural skills training (i.e., stress management, self-control therapy), motivational interviewing and enhancement strategies, and 12-step approaches. Additionally, special programs have been designed to address the unique needs of certain population groups, such as women, youth, Indigenous peoples, people who have experienced incarceration, and people who have experienced the consequences of impaired driving and problematic drug use. Although they use some elements of coercion, diversion programs such as drug treatment courts offer alternatives to incarceration of repeat substance-involved offenders. These programs facilitate access to treatment and help reduce the harms and risk of ongoing dependence (CCSA, 2007).

A limitation on secondary prevention in the Canadian context is that the treatment and rehabilitation system in many communities is often structured as a set of individual services rather than as a continuum. Services are often not integrated or coordinated. This can create access barriers for appropriate and timely treatment, with individuals who have work insurance plans or significant personal wealth better able to access timely care. A treatment service continuum should be coordinated, provide services that are based on best practices, have medically appropriate care, provide continuity of care among programs and organizations, and meet the diverse needs of individuals, including those with concurrent disorders. Key features of an effective treatment service continuum include services that are facilitated by different means (e.g., telehealth); have standardized screening and assessment tools that respect individual considerations, including culture and language; and offer choices (National Treatment Strategy Work Group, 2008).

CHNs practising in health centres, homes, schools, and other community-based settings should be aware of the available treatment options in their communities. It is imperative that CHNs become familiar with screening and care planning in order to appropriately refer individuals who need additional support, counselling, or treatment. CHNs must have the skills to recognize the signs and symptoms of problematic substance use and be comfortable raising the topic with all clients as a matter of course. Screening can be conducted in a variety of settings, by a variety of individuals, and under a variety of conditions. In fact, health professionals such as CHNs are significantly more likely to be involved in screening than substance use specialists. Additionally, CHNs, in collaboration with professionals from other disciplines, should strive to advocate for and develop treatment options that acknowledge and integrate concurrent disorders, thus "making every door the right door" along the service continuum in their community. For this reason, it is important that CHNs understand that they can play a key role as primary screening agents in the community. Training to administer screening tools is recommended, and CHNs are encouraged to consult local substance use specialists in their community or province.

Tertiary Prevention

Tertiary prevention in the context of substance use involves reducing the harms of problematic use both for individuals who are using substances and for their families and communities. It should be noted that treatment can be included as a form of tertiary prevention as well as secondary prevention, as treatment is always an option for individuals regardless of how long substance use has been problematic in their lives. However, treatment isn't the only option, and tertiary prevention involves the realistic perspective that not everyone is ready or able to reduce their substance use in the moment.

At the individual level, our discussion on harm reduction covered much of how CHNs might engage in tertiary prevention. Clean needles, pop-up supervised consumption sites, managed alcohol programs, e-cigarettes, and naloxone distribution are all forms of tertiary prevention, reducing the harms of problematic substance use for the individual and secondarily for the community. Beyond harm reduction, CHNs also engage in tertiary prevention when they support community members through potential harmful effects of substance use such as relationship-breakdown, loss of employment, or loss of housing.

Tertiary prevention might include services for families provided through addiction support agencies, such as Al-Anon, which provides support to family members of individuals living with problematic alcohol use. Additionally, the child welfare system is intended to be a form of tertiary prevention for families, reducing the risk of harm to children whose parents are experiencing problematic substance use. We use the term "intended" purposely, as some researchers have noted challenges with the way the child welfare system is currently designed and administered in Canada, including **systemic racism**, the overrepresentation of First Nations, Métis, and Inuit children in the system (Trocmé, Knoke, & Blackstock, 2004), and the child welfare system as a pathway to homelessness (Nichols et al., 2017). CHNs, particularly those working in a primary health care context, play a key role in collaboratively supporting the health and well-being of family members living with problematic substance use.

Quaternary Prevention

Quaternary prevention in the context of substance use involves addressing the stigma around substances within the health care system and among health professionals, and ensuring that CHNs are following the lead of individuals, families, and communities in determining if substance use is problematic. Because of the complex roots of substance use in social and psychological challenges, health providers are at risk of focusing on the behaviour of substance use versus supporting the individual in addressing root causes. Labelling an individual as being an "alcoholic" or "drug addict" often leads to medically driven interventions rather than secondary prevention that focuses on trauma, marginalization, and the social determinants of health. Second, although the CHN may become aware of use that is considered to be high, or that individuals are using substances with which the nurse is uncomfortable, it is up to the individual, family, or community to determine if that use is problematic. To presume that it is, and to force interventions upon individuals, actually disempowers them and risks further marginalizing those most likely to already feel on the margins.

COMMUNITY HEALTH NURSING AND HEALTH PROMOTING PRACTICE

No single type of community intervention can resolve a community's challenges with problematic substance use. CHNs should support communities in engaging with a combination of **complementary interventions**, blending elements of all levels of prevention. Although some of the interventions outlined in the chapter come from the substance use field, they are grounded in the same principles of the population health-promotion model that is used throughout this text. The focus is not only on supporting individuals in a community context but also on addressing the policies, structural factors, cultural contexts, and system designs that frame the lives of individuals, families, communities, and populations. Developing interventions should be informed by evidence, best practices, existing community knowledge, and primarily by the insight and experiences of those affected by the issue. For example, research shows that many interventions aimed at preventing adolescents from consuming alcohol and tobacco are relatively ineffective if designed and driven by organizations without the co-leadership of youth. Interventions should integrate principles of cultural safety, as presented in Canadian Research 30.1. Additionally, CHNs should acknowledge, reflect, and act upon the structural differences and power relationships within the substance use services they provide to ensure that access is barrier-free and outcomes are achievable. Are CHNs participating in programs that discriminate against Indigenous peoples or people belonging to various ethnocultural groups, those identifying as LGBTQ2S, and people who are differently abled? To this end, health promoting practices for CHNs in the context of substance use start with the nurse examining their own perspectives as well as societal perspectives on substance use. Nurses

Reducing Harm in the Context of Chronic Problematic Alcohol Use

Daryl (a name change) came from a family that experienced extreme poverty in the context of job loss related to the collapse of the cod fishing industry in Eastern Canada. Daryl's father became a problematic user of alcohol after he became unemployed, and Daryl began drinking alcohol at the age of 13. When he was 16, Daryl left his home and came west, finding himself in Ontario and unable to manage his drinking. By the age of 33, Daryl was still drinking daily and heavily, and turned to **non-beverage alcohol** (mouthwash) as an easier means to obtain alcohol in the context of absolute poverty. At 41, he reached out to the primary health care team for support and identified as having used alcohol in a problematic manner for 25 years.

Daryl lived with many health and social consequences of his problematic drinking. He experienced liver disease, frequent bleeds throughout his gastrointestinal tract, and numerous and frequent injuries such as being struck by motor vehicles or falling. Social consequences included frequent arrests, limited social relationships, and frequent housing loss. Daryl expressed a strong desire to end his problematic drinking, but periods of recovery never lasted for more than a week, and he had tried every available treatment program multiple times.

In terms of a current system support, Daryl was spending more nights in the hospital emergency department or police cells than he was in the emergency shelter, and he often spent nights sleeping rough due to being banned from shelters for being under the influence of alcohol. He averaged more than one police contact per day, 20 paramedic contacts per month, and 12 nights in the emergency department. These services had no positive impact on his long-term health and were very costly.

For the primary health care team, Daryl's experience illustrated the need for a residential managed alcohol program. A managed alcohol program provides people who consume alcohol in a problematic manner with a consistent and controlled dose in a residential environment. This serves to concurrently minimize harm to the individual from drinking in public and spending most nights in cells or a hospital while minimizing harm to the community from theft to obtain alcohol and cost related to emergency and hospital services. Although giving alcohol to someone who has already been identified as using substances problematically seems counterintuitive, it is an effective form of tertiary prevention (Podymow, Turnball, Coyle, Yetisir, & Wells, 2006).

Discussion Questions

1. How might a CHN address community resistance to managed alcohol programs?
2. From a cost perspective, how do you think managed alcohol programs compare to usual care?
3. What do you think are some of the health consequences of long-term consumption of non-beverage alcohol? Look to the research literature to see if your guesses are accurate.

are always safest in practising competently when following the lead of the clients who they serve.

CONCLUSION

CHNs have the leadership, knowledge, and skills to influence and leverage support and resources to support people with problematic substance use and to shift policy. Doing so requires a good understanding of the interconnectedness between the use of substances and the determinants of health. Paying attention to issues that impact a community and the factors that may influence individuals who need information or professional assistance for a substance use–related problem is paramount to finding the right solution, for the right people, and at the right place and time. The application of the knowledge in this chapter can serve to guide the CHN in the advocacy and development of relevant interventions that are based on evidence; make important linkages between the individual, substance use, structures, and the environment; and reflect the values and practice standards of community health nursing.

KEY TERMS

addiction   (p. 538)
complementary interventions   (p. 550)
concurrent disorder   (p. 541)
cultural safety   (p. 541)
dependence   (p. 539)
fetal alcohol spectrum disorder   (p. 544)
guaranteed annual income   (p. 547)
harm reduction   (p. 545)
illicit drugs   (p. 538)
Low-Risk Alcohol Drinking Guidelines   (p. 548)
neonatal abstinence syndrome (NAS)   (p. 547)
non-beverage alcohol   (p. 551)
physical dependence   (p. 539)
process addictions   (p. 538)
problematic substance use   (p. 539)
psychoactive substance   (p. 539)
psychological dependence   (p. 539)
recovery   (p. 549)
structural violence   (p. 542)
stigma   (p. 538)
substance use   (p. 539)
systemic racism   (p. 550)

STUDY QUESTIONS

1. Why do people use substances?
2. What differentiates substance use from problematic substance use?
3. Why are some substances illegal, and others are legal?
4. What are some of the potential harmful consequences of substance use?
5. Explain two examples of harm reduction available in Canada.
6. Describe the four pillars of Canada's Federal Drug Strategy.

7. Describe a few community health nursing actions regarding problematic substance use at each of the five levels of prevention.

8. What are the limitations of exclusively focusing on law-enforcement interventions to deal with substance use?

INDIVIDUAL CRITICAL-THINKING EXERCISES

1. Registered nurses and other health care providers have been found to hold negative attitudes concerning people who use substances, particularly illegal drugs. Privately explore the first thing that comes to mind when you read each of the following expressions. Then explore your reactions to each expression. Do they differ from one another? If so, consider the reasons why. Did any of your reactions surprise you? If yes, reflect on how your personal values may influence your professional practice.

   - homeless alcoholic
   - needle exchange program
   - abstinence-based treatment
   - problem drinker
   - methadone treatment
   - parent with hangover
   - IV drug user
   - crack dealer
   - professor smoking marijuana
   - pregnant methadone client
   - crystal meth addict
   - chain (tobacco) smoker
   - female cocaine user
   - drunk driver
   - 20-year-old buying booze for underage sibling
   - person with HIV
   - gas sniffer
   - underage drunk
   - coffee drinker

2. Read your local newspaper or a magazine, or watch the news, a television program, or a movie. Pay attention to the images and messages about the consumption of alcohol, tobacco, and illicit or licit drugs. At whom are these messages aimed? What are they portraying? Consider the degree of influence these images and messages have on substance use patterns in society.

3. Think of a community you have lived in, and consider the factors that were attributed to that community's health status. What was the prevalence of psychoactive substances in that community? You may want to focus on one or more substances. Explore the factors that placed that community at risk and those that protected it or acted as buffers.

GROUP CRITICAL-THINKING EXERCISES

1. Select a particular issue or harm that is associated with substance use in your community (e.g., the problematic use of opioid prescription drugs, impaired driving, FASD). How would you seek to understand the issue across individual, familial, community, and societal levels?

2. For the issue identified in Question 1, have your group map your community's current capacity in terms of prevention and treatment services and programs. You may use the internet or contact local health and social service agencies. For example, you should highlight any existing screening and prevention programs, how people access general information about the issue, and, if appropriate, where people access treatment services. Make note of any service or program gaps your group observes.

3. Using the results of the mapping exercise in Question 2 and referring to the levels of prevention, discuss and analyze as a group the risk factors you believe have contributed to the development of the issue or harm identified in Question 1. Additionally, your group should explore the protective factors that have acted as buffers or that will have the capacity to create positive outcomes for your target population or for the community.

REFERENCES

Alberta Gaming, Liquor, and Cannabis. (2018). *Canada's low-risk alcohol drinking guidelines*. Retrieved from http://ccsa.ca/Resource%20Library/2012-Canada-Low-Risk-Alcohol-Drinking-Guidelines-Brochure-en.pdf

American Psychiatric Association. (2013). *Diagnostic and statistical manual of mental disorders: DSM-5* (5th ed.). Arlington, VA: American Psychiatric Association.

Anstice, S., Strike, C. J., & Brands, B. (2009). Supervised methadone consumption: Client issues and stigma. *Substance Use and Misuse, 44*(6), 794–808.

Baliunas, D., Patra, J., Rehm, J., Popova, S., Kaiserman, M., & Taylor, B. (2007). Smoking-attributable mortality and expected years of life lost in Canada 2002: Conclusions for prevention and policy. *Chronic Diseases in Canada, 27*(4), 154–162.

BC Provincial Mental Health and Substance Use Planning Council. (2013). *Trauma-informed practice (TIP) guide.* BC: Author.

Bennett, M. I., & Closs, S. J. (2010). Methodological issues in nonpharmacological trials for chronic pain. *PAIN Clinical Updates, 8*(2). International Association for the Study of Pain. Retrieved from http://www.iasp-pain.org/PublicationsNews/NewsletterIssue.aspx?ItemNumber=2091

Benoit, C., Shumka, L., & Barlee, D. (2010). *Stigma and the health of vulnerable women.* Vancouver, B.C.: Women's Health Research Network.

Brewer, M. K., & Nelms, T. P. (1998). Some recovering nurses' experiences of being labeled "impaired": A phenomenological inquiry. *Journal of Addictions Nursing, 10*(4), 172–9. Retrieved from http://www.tandf.co.uk/journals/titles/10884602.asp

Browne, A. J., Varcoe, C. M., Wong, S. T., Smye, V. L., Lavoie, J., Littlejohn, D., . . . & Fridkin, A. (2012). Closing the health equity gap: Evidence-based strategies for primary health care organizations. *International Journal for Equity in Health, 11*(1), 59. doi:10.1186/1475-9276-11-59

Browne, A. J., Varcoe, C. M., Ford-Gilboe, M., & Wathen, C. N., on behalf of the EQUIP Team. (2015). EQUIP Healthcare: An overview of a multi-component intervention to enhance equity-oriented care in primary health care settings. *International Journal for Equity in Health, 14*(1), 152. doi:10.1186/s12939-015-0271-y

Bugle, L. W. (1996). A study of drug and alcohol use among Missouri RNs. *Journal of Psychosocial Nursing & Mental Health Services, 34*(7), 41–55. Retrieved from http://www.slackinc.com

Butterfield, P. (1997). Thinking upstream: Conceptualizing health from a health population perspective. In J. Swanson & M. Nies (Eds.), *Community health nursing: Promoting the health of the aggregate* (pp. 69–92). Philadelphia, PA: W. B. Saunders.

Canadian Centre on Substance Abuse (CCSA). (2007). *Drug treatment court: Frequently asked questions.* Retrieved from http://www.ccsa.ca/Resource%20Library/ccsa-011348-2007.pdf

Canadian Centre on Substance Abuse (CCSA). (2011). Injection drug users overview.

Canadian Centre on Substance Abuse. (2013). *Prescription sedatives and tranquilizers.* Canadian Drug Summary. Retrieved from http://www.ccsa.ca/Resource%20Library/CCSA-Prescription-Sedatives-and-Tranquilizers-2013-en.pdf

Canadian Nurses Association. (2011). *Harm reduction and currently illegal drugs: Implications for nursing policy, practice, education and research discussion paper.* Ottawa, ON: Author.

Canadian Public Health Association. (2011). *The winnable battle: Ending tobacco use in Canada, a position paper.* Ottawa, ON: Author.

Canadian Women's Foundation. (2011). *Report on violence against women, mental health and substance use.* Toronto, ON: Author.

Cavalieri, W. (2017). *Harm reduction in practice.* Retrieved from http://www.canadianharmreduction.com/node/171.

Charlton, J. E. (Ed.). (2005). *Pain relief in substance abusers: Core curriculum for professional education in pain* (3rd ed.). Seattle, WA: International Association for the Study of Pain Press.

Cherry, A. L., Dillon, M. E., & Rugh, D. (Eds.). (2002). *Substance abuse: A global view.* Greenwood Publishing Group.

Chou, R., Qaseem, A., Snow, V., Casey, D., Thomas Cross, J., Shekelle, P., . . . for the Clinical Efficacy Assessment Subcommittee of the American College of Physicians and the American College of Physicians/American Pain Society Low Back Pain Guidelines Panel. (2007). Diagnosis and treatment of low back pain: A joint clinical practice guideline from the American College of Physicians and the American Pain Society. *Annals of Internal Medicine, 147*(7), 478–491.

Chow, C., Vallance, K., Stockwell, T., Macdonald, S., Martin, G., Ivsins, A., . . . & Duff, C. (2013). Sexual identity and drug use harm among high-risk, active substance users. *Culture, Health & Sexuality, 15*(3), 311–326 doi:10.1080/13691058.2012.754054

Chudley, A. E., Conry, J., Cook, J. L., Loock, C., Rosales, T., & LeBlanc, N. (2005). Fetal alcohol spectrum disorder: Canadian guidelines for diagnosis. *Canadian Medical Association Journal, 172*(5 suppl), S1–S21.

College of Registered Nurses of Nova Scotia (CRNNS). (2008). *Problematic substance use in the workplace: A resource guide for registered nurses.* Halifax, NS: Author. Retrieved from http://www.crnns.ca/documents/Problematic%20Substance%20Use%20Resource%20Guide.pdf

Community Health Nurses of Canada (CHNC). (2019, revised). *Canadian community health nursing professional practice model & standards of practice.* Toronto, ON: Author. Retrieved from http://www.chnig.org/wp-content/uploads/2016/02/chnc-standards.pdf

Darbro, N. (2005). Alternative diversion programs for nurses with impaired practice: Completers and non-completers. *Journal of Addictions Nursing, 16*(4), 169–185. Retrieved from http://www.tandf.co.uk/journals/titles/10884602.asp

Dell, C. A., & Lyons, T. (2007). *Harm reduction for special populations in Canada: Harm reduction policies and programs for persons of Aboriginal descent.* Canadian Centre on Substance Abuse. Retrieved from http://www.addictionresearchchair.ca/wp-content/uploads/Harm-Reduction-Policies-and-Programs-for-Persons-of-Aboriginal-Descent.pdf

Douglas L., Gourlay M. D., Heit, H. A., & Almahrezi, A. (2005). Universal precautions in pain medicine: A rational approach to the treatment of chronic pain. *Pain Medicine, 6*(2):107–112. Retrieved from http://onlinelibrary.wiley.com/doi/10.1111/j.1526-4637.2005.05031.x/full

Dow, K., Ordean, A., Murphy-Oikonen, J., Pereira, J., Koren, G., Roukema, H., & Turner, R. (2012). Neonatal abstinence syndrome: Clinical practice guidelines for Ontario. *Journal of Popular Clinical Therapies and Pharmacology, 19*(3), 488–506.

Drwecki, B. B., Moore, C. F., Ward, S. E., & Prkachin, K. M. (2010). Reducing racial disparities in pain treatment: The role of empathy and perspective taking. *PAIN, 152*(5), 1001–1006.

Dube, S. R., Felliti, V. J., Dong, M., Chapean, D. P., Giles, W. H. & Anda, R. F. (2003). Childhood abuse, neglect, and household dysfunction and the risk of illicit drug use: The adverse childhood experiences study. *Pediatrics, 11*(3), 564–572.

Elliott, D. E., Bjelajac, P., Fallot, R. D., Markoff, L. S., & Reed, B. G. (2005). Trauma-informed or trauma-denied: Principles and implementation of trauma-informed services for women. *Journal of Community Psychology, 33*(4), 461–477.

EQUIP Healthcare. (2014). *Non-pharmacological pain management: A literature review.* Author: BC.

Félix, S., Portugal, P., & Tavares, A. (2017). *Going after the addiction, not the addicted: The impact of drug decriminalization in Portugal* (No. 10895). IZA Discussion Papers.

Fischer, B., Rehm, J., Brissette, S., Brochu, S., Bruneau, J., El-Guebaly, N . . . . Baliunas, D. (2005). Illicit opioid use in Canada: Comparing social, health, and drug use characteristics of untreated users in five cities (OPICAN study). *Journal of Urban Health: Bulletin of the New York Academy of Medicine, 82*(2), 250–266.

Galea, S., Nandi, A., & Vlahov, D. (2004). The social epidemiology of substance use. *Epidemiological Reviews, 26*(1), 36–52.

Goffman, E. (1963). *Stigma: Notes on the management of spoiled identity.* Englewood Cliffs, NJ: Prentice-Hall.

Government of Canada. (2006). *The human face of mental health and mental illness in Canada.* Ottawa, ON: Author. Retrieved from http://www.phac-aspc.gc.ca/publicat/human-humain06/pdf/human_face_e.pdf

Government of Canada. (2017). *The cost of tobacco use in Canada, 2012*. Retrieved from https://www.canada.ca/en/health-canada/services/publications/healthy-living/costs-tobacco-use-canada-2012.html

Haskell, L., & Randall, M. (2009). Disrupted attachments: A social context complex trauma framework and the lives of Aboriginal peoples in Canada, *Journal of Aboriginal Health, 5*(3), 48–99.

Howard, M. O., & Chung, S. S. (2000). Nurses' attitudes toward substance misusers. III. Emergency room nurses' attitudes, nurses' attitudes toward impaired nurses, and studies of attitudinal change. *Substance Abuse & Misuse, 35*(9), 1227–1261. Retrieved from http://informahealthcare.com/sum

Hwang, S. W., Wilkins, E., Chambers, C., Estrabillo, E., Berends, J., & MacDonald, A. (2011). Chronic pain among homeless persons: Characteristics, treatment, and barriers to management. *BMC Family Practice, 12*(73). Retrieved from https://bmcfampract.biomedcentral.com/track/pdf/10.1186/1471-2296-12-73

Hutchinson, S. (1986). Chemically dependent nurses: The trajectory toward self-annihilation. *Nursing Research, 35*(4), 196–201. Retrieved from http://journals.lww.com/nursingresearchonline/pages/default.aspx

International Harm Reduction Association. (2010). *What is harm reduction? A position statement from the International Harm Reduction Association*. London, UK. Retrieved from http://www.ihra.net/what-is-harm-reduction

Jessop, J. (2006). *Contextual cognitive-behavioural therapy for chronic pain*. L. M. McCracken (Ed.), International Association for the Study of Pain. ISBN: 0-931092-83-3

Kagan, P. N., Smith, M. C., & Chinn, P. L. (Eds.) (2014). *Philosophies and practice of emancipatory nursing: Social justice as praxis*. New York, NY. Routledge Taylor and Francis Group.

Kang, S. (2004). Substance use disorders in pregnancy and post-partum. *Women Issue of Visions Journal, 4*. Retrieved from http://www.heretohelp.bc.ca/visions/women-vol2/substance-use-disorders-in-pregnancy-and-postpartum

Krausz, M. (2010). *Addiction in maternity: Mixed methods study on substance use during maternity, access to services and perceptions of addiction in maternity*. Centre for Health Evaluation and Outcome Sciences, University of British Columbia.

Library of Parliament. (1908). *Senate Debates*, 10th Parliament, 4th Session, Vol 2.

Link, B. G., & Phelan, J. C. (2001). Conceptualizing stigma. *Annual Review of Sociology, 27*(1), 363–385.

Link, B. G., & Phelan, J. C. (2006). Stigma and its public health implications. *Lancet, 367*(9509), 528–529.

Lloyd, C. (2010). *Sinning and sinned against: The stigmatisation of problem drug users*. London, UK: The UK Drug Policy Commission (UKDPC).

Lillibridge, J., Cox, M., & Cross, W. (2002). Uncovering the secret: Giving voice to the experiences of nurses who misuse substances. *Journal of Advanced Nursing, 39*(3), 219–229. doi:10.1046/j.1365-2648.2002.02268.x

MacPherson, D., & Rowley, M. L. (2001). *A framework for action: A four-pillar approach to drug problems in Vancouver*. Vancouver, BC: City of Vancouver.

Marlatt, G. A., Blume, A. W., & Parks, G. A. (2001). Integrating harm reduction therapy and traditional substance abuse treatment. *Journal of Psychoactive Drugs, 33*(1), 13–21.

Mason, R., Wolf, M., O'Rinn, S., & Ene, G. (2017). Making connections across silos: intimate partner violence, mental health, and substance use. *BMC Women's Health, 17*(1), 29. Retrieved from http://doi.org/10.1186/s12905-017-0372-4

Melzack, R. (2005). Evolution of the neuromatrix theory of pain: The Prithvi Raj Lecture. Presented at the Third World Congress of World Institute of Pain, Barcelona 2004. *World Institute of Pain, 5*(2), 85–94. Retrieved from https://www.researchgate.net/publication/227691901_Evolution_of_the_Neuromatrix_Theory_of_Pain_The_Prithvi_Raj_Lecture_Presented_at_the_Third_World_Congress_of_World_Institute_of_Pain_Barcelona_2004

Miller, C. L., Pearce, M. E., Moniruzzaman, A., Thomas, V., Schechter, M. T., & Spittal, P. M. (2011). The Cedar Project: Risk factors for transition to injection drug use among young, urban Aboriginal people. *Canadian Medical Association Journal, 183*(10), 1147–1154.

Monroe, T. (2009). Addressing substance abuse among nursing students: Development of a prototype alternative-to-dismissal policy. *Journal of Nursing Education, 48*(5), 272–278. Retrieved from http://www.slackinc.com

National Advisory Committee on Prescription Drug Misuse. (2013). *First do no harm: Responding to Canada's prescription drug crisis*. Ottawa, ON: Canadian Centre on Substance Misuse. Retrieved from http://www.ccsa.ca/resource%20library/canada-strategy-prescription-drug-misuse-report-en.pdf

National Treatment Strategy Working Group. (2008). *A systems approach to substance use in Canada: Recommendations for a national treatment strategy*. Ottawa, ON: National Framework for Action to Reduce the Harms Associated with Alcohol and Other Drugs and Substances in Canada. Retrieved from http://www.ccsa.ca/Resource%20Library/nts-systems-approach-substance-abuse-canada-2008-en.pdf

Negron, A. (2012). *Working with survivors of torture who suffer chronic pain: An experience*. Special Interest Group Related to Torture, Organized Violence, and War Symposia. International Association of the Study of Pain. Retrieved from: https://www.iasp-pain.org/files/Content/ContentFolders/SIGS2/TOVW/Symposia2012/Andreia_Negron_Working_with_survivors.pdf

Nichols, N., Schwan, K., Gaetz, S., Redman, M., French, D., Kidd, S., O'Grady, B. (2017). *Child welfare and youth homelessness in Canada: A proposal for action*. Toronto, ON: Canadian Observatory on Homelessness Press.

Office of National Drug Control Policy. (2017). *Changing the language of addiction*. Retrieved from https://www.whitehouse.gov/sites/whitehouse.gov/files/images/Memo%20-%20Changing%20Federal%20Terminology%20Regrading%20Substance%20Use%20and%20Substance%20Use%20Disorders.pdf

Otis, J. D., Keane, T. M., Kerns, R. D., Monson, C., & Scioli, E. (2009). The development of an integrated treatment for veterans with comorbid chronic pain and posttraumatic stress disorder. *Pain Medicine, 10*(7):1300–1311.

Pauly, B. (2008). Harm reduction through a social justice lens. *International Journal of Drug Policy, 19*(1), 4–10.

Pauly, B., Goldstone, I., McCall, J., Gold, F., & Payne, S. (2007). The ethical, legal and social context of harm reduction. *Canadian Nurse, 103*(8), 19–23.

Pauly, B., Reist, D., Belle-Isle, L., & Schactman, C. (2013). Housing and harm reduction: What is the role of harm reduction in addressing homelessness? *International Journal of Drug Policy, 24*(4), 284–290. doi:10.1016/j.drugpo.2013.03.008

Payne, S. (2007). Caring not curing: Caring for pregnant women with problematic substance use in an acute care setting: A multidisciplinary approach. In S. C. Boyd & L. Marcellus (Eds.), *With child: Substance use during pregnancy: A woman-centred approach.* Halifax, NS: Fernwood Publishing.

Pirie, T., Jesseman, R., & National Treatment Indicators Working Group. (2013). *National Treatment Indicators Report: 2010–2011 Data.* Ottawa, ON: Canadian Centre on Substance Abuse.

Podymow, T., Turnball, J., Coyle, D., Yetisir, E., & Wells, G. (2006). Shelter-based managed alcohol administration to chronically homeless people addicted to alcohol. *Canadian Medical Association Journal, 174*(1), 45–49.

Poole, N. (2007). Gender does matter: Coalescing on women and substance use. *Cross Currents.* Retrieved from http://www.camh.net/Publications/Cross_Currents/Spring%202007/genderdoesmatter_spring07crcu.html

Registered Nurses Association of Ontario (RNAO). (2009). *Supporting clients on methadone maintenance treatment: Clinical best practice guidelines.* Toronto, ON: Registered Nurses' Association of Ontario.

Rehm, J., Ballunas, D., Brochu, S., Fischer, B., Gnam, W., Patra, J., & Taylor, B. (2006). The costs of substance abuse in Canada, 2002 highlights. Retrieved from http://www.ccsa.ca/Resource%20Library/ccsa-011332-2006.pdf

Reid, J. L., Hammond, D., Burkhalter, R., Rynard, V. L., & Ahmed, R. (2013). *Tobacco use in Canada: Patterns and trends, 2013 Edition.* Waterloo, ON: Propel Centre for Population Health Impact, University of Waterloo. Retrieved from http://www.tobaccoreport.ca/2013

Reist, D. (2010). *Methadone maintenance treatment in British Columbia, 1996–2008: Analysis and recommendations.* Victoria, BC: Ministry of Healthy Living and Sport and the Centre for Addictions Research in BC, University of Victoria.

Ross, C. A., Berry, N. S., Smye, V., & Goldner, E. M. (2017). A critical review of knowledge on nurses with problematic substance use: The need to move from individual blame to awareness of structural factors. *Nursing Inquiry, 25*(2). e12215. https://doi.org/10.1111/nin.12215

Salmon, A., Poole, N., Morrow, M., Greaves, L., Ingram, R., & Pederson, A. (2006). *Improving conditions: Integrating sex and gender into federal mental health and addictions policy.* Vancouver, BC: The British Columbia Centre of Excellence for Women's Health.

Scott-Storey, K. (2011). Cumulative abuse: Do things add up? An evaluation of the conceptualization, operationalization, and methodological approaches in the study of the phenomenon of cumulative abuse. *Trauma, Violence & Abuse, 12*(3), 135–150. doi:10.1177/1524838011404253

Smye, V., Browne, A. J., Varcoe, C., & Josewski, V. (2011). Harm reduction and methadone maintenance treatment: Intersections of gender, class, race and ability. *Harm*

Reduction Journal, 8(17), 7, doi:10.1186/1477-7517-8-17. Retrieved from http://www.harmreductionjournal.com/content/8/1/17

The Canadian Encyclopedia (2015). Temperance Movement in Canada. Retrieved from http://www.thecanadianencyclopedia.ca/en/article/temperance-movement

Tipliski, V. M. (1993). The characteristics of recovering chemically-dependent Manitoba nurses. *International Journal of the Addictions, 28*(8), 711–717. Retrieved from http://www.ncbi.nlm.nih.gov/pubmed/8349388

Traffic Injury Research Foundation (TIRF). (2009). *The alcohol crash problem in Canada: 2006.* Ottawa, ON: Author.

Traffic Injury Research Foundation (TIRF). (2013). *The alcohol crash problem in Canada: 2010.* Canadian Council of Motor Transport Administrators and the Minister of Public Works and Government Services, represented by the Minister of Transport. Retrieved from http://www.tirf.ca/publications/publications_show.php?pub_id=292

Trocmé, N., Knoke, D., & Blackstock, C. (2004). Pathways to the overrepresentation of Aboriginal children in Canada's child welfare system. *Social Service Review, 78*(4), 577–600.

Varcoe, C., Browne, A. J., & Cender, L. M. (2014). Promoting social justice and equity by practicing nursing to address structural inequities and structural violence. In P. N. Kagan, M. C. Smith, & P. Chinn (Eds.). *Philosophies and practice of emancipatory nursing: Social justice as praxis* (pp. 266–284). New York, NY: Routledge Taylor and Francis Group.

Wallace, B., Barber, K., & Pauly, B. (2018). Sheltering risks: Implementation of harm reduction in homeless shelters during an overdose emergency. *International Journal of Drug Policy, 53*, 83–89.

Weber, L., & Parra-Medina, D. (2003). Intersectionality and women's health: Charting a path to eliminating disparities. *Advances in Gender Research, 7*, 181–230.

Webster, P. C. (2012). Prescription drug abuse rising among Aboriginal youths. *Canadian Medical Association Journal, 184*(12), 647–648.

Weiner, S. G., Griggs, C. A., Mitchell, P. M., Langlois, B. K., Friedman, F. D., Moore, R. L., . . . Feldman, J. A. (2013). Clinician impression versus prescription drug monitoring program criteria in the assessment of drug-seeking behaviour in the emergency department. *Annals of Emergency Medicine, 62*(4), 281–289.

White, P., Bishop, F. L., Prescott, P., Scott, C., Little, P., & Lewith, G. (2012) Practice, practitioner, or placebo? A multifactorial, mixed-methods randomized controlled trial of acupuncture. *PAIN, 153*(2), 455–462.

Winterowd, C., Beck, A., Aaron, T., & Gruener, D. (2003). *Cognitive therapy with chronic pain patients.* New York, NY: Springer Publishing.

World Health Organization. (2003). *Social determinants of health: The solid facts* (2nd ed.). R. Wilkinson & M. Marmot (Eds.). WHO: Copenhagen, Denmark.

World Health Organization (WHO). (2008). *Closing the gap in a generation: Health equity through action on the social determinants of health.* Geneva, CH: World Health Organization. Retrieved from http://apps.who.int/iris/bitstream/10665/69832/1/WHO_IER_CSDH_08.1_eng.pdf

ABOUT THE AUTHORS

Dr. Abe Oudshoorn, RN, PhD, is Assistant Professor in the Arthur Labatt Family School of Nursing, Western University. With a clinical background in primary health care with people experiencing homelessness, Dr. Oudshoorn's research is focused on issues of health, housing, and social policy in the context of homelessness. In addition to his academic role, Dr. Oudshoorn remains engaged in the community through the United Way Elgin Middlesex, the London Homeless Coalition, and the Centre for Research on Health Equity and Social Inclusion.

Dr. Victoria (Vicki) Smye, RN, PhD, is Associate Professor and Director of the Arthur Labatt Family School of Nursing, Western University. Dr. Smye began on an academic career path after over two decades in clinical practice. Her research program is located at the intersections of violence, gender, poverty, mental health, substance use, and Indigenous health. Over the past 15 years she has led several studies conducted in collaboration with other researchers, community agencies, and community members that cross these domains of practice. For example, recently Dr. Smye completed a CIHR-funded study entitled *Indigenous Men's Health Narratives: Reclaiming Our Lives.* In addition, she has been a co-investigator on several studies, for example, health equity research in primary health care (EQUIP) and a study to examine an intervention for health enhancement and living (iHeal) for women who have left an abusive partner.

Sexually Transmitted and Blood-Borne Infections

Wendi Lokanc-Diluzio and Tammy Troute-Wood

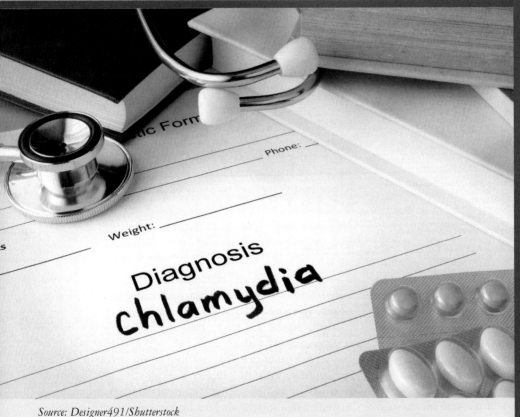

Source: Designer491/Shutterstock

INTRODUCTION

Sexually transmitted and blood-borne infections (STBBIs) are significant public health issues in Canada. STBBIs are infections that are spread through insertive and receptive sexual practices (vaginal, anal, or oral) with an infected person. Additionally, some viral STBBIs, such as genital herpes and human papillomavirus (HPV), can be transmitted by intimate skin-to-skin contact, and STBBIs such as human immunodeficiency virus (HIV) and hepatitis B are carried and transmitted by blood (Government of Alberta, 2012; Public Health Agency of Canada [PHAC], 2017a).

In Canada, some STBBIs are notifiable (or reportable) diseases. The Public Health Agency of Canada (PHAC) (PHAC, 2017a) stipulates which ones are reportable nationally, and each province or territory can add diseases to be reported in that jurisdiction. The need for partner notification, contact tracing, testing, and treatment can differ among jurisdictions.

People affected by STBBIs encounter stigmatization and discrimination and often elicit emotional reactions such as anxiety, fear, and shame. The stigma associated with STBBIs may impede people from protecting themselves as well as from seeking testing and treatment. Societal reactions of intolerance toward people at risk for contracting STBBIs, as well as those living with HIV and acquired immune deficiency syndrome (AIDS) may further marginalize populations who already experience health inequities.

In this chapter, you will learn how community health nurses (CHNs) are challenged to promote health, build capacity, and facilitate access and equity through innovative community strategies to address STBBIs. Historical and current challenges regarding the prevention of STBBIs and the development of healthy public policies are discussed. An overview of common STBBIs, their incidence, and their prevalence in Canada are presented. Prevention and risk- and harm-reduction strategies are discussed, and examples of innovative prevention strategies are offered.

HISTORY OF STBBIs AND THE IMPACT ON HEALTHY PUBLIC POLICY

Over the years, STBBIs have been labelled in different ways. The term venereal disease (VD), defined as a disease that was only transmitted by sexual intercourse (Campbell & Herten, 1981), was used for centuries (Shriver, Byer, Shainberg, & Galliano, 2002). In the 1970s the term VD was viewed as inaccurate (Shriver et al., 2002) and replaced by sexually transmitted disease (STD), which was defined as a disease that could be transmitted from person to person through sexual intercourse or intimate sexual contact with the genitals, mouth, or rectum (Campbell & Herten, 1981). In Canada, around 2006, the term **sexually transmitted infection (STI)** became preferred, as it was viewed as an encompassing term that includes infections that may be asymptomatic (Government of Canada, 2006). The term **blood-borne infection (BBI)** was used when referring to infections that could be carried and transmitted through the blood. Recently, the acronym **sexually transmitted and blood-borne infections (STBBI)** is used when referring to both STIs and BBIs. In this chapter we use the term STBBI as an umbrella term, and where applicable, STI and BBI are used as well.

Healthy public policies and guidelines are revisited and updated based on research to assist in protecting the public from the consequences of infection. Prior to the discovery of antibiotics, bacterial STBBIs were not treatable and caused serious illness. Historically, public policies were implemented to test men and women for syphilis prior to marriage. With the advent of antibiotic treatment, new policies were developed. Although no longer recommended, from the late 1800s until 2015, antibiotic eye drops were routinely given to all newborns to prevent blindness from gonorrhea (Moore & McDonald, 2015). Currently, the PHAC recommends screening for HIV, syphilis, chlamydia, gonorrhea, and hepatitis B at the first prenatal visit and recommend ongoing evaluation for new STBBIs and consideration for rescreening each trimester to prevent neonatal infection through **vertical transmission** (PHAC, 2017a).

Healthy public policies have also been developed in response to community action. The Canadian Red Cross became entrenched in public health scandal when it was discovered that over 1000 Canadians had become infected with HIV from blood transfusions. Although the medical community was aware of a new BBI in the late 1970s and early 1980s, strict HIV blood surveillance guidelines were not implemented until 1985. People infected with HIV from blood transfusions launched class actions, and other compensation programs were established. The risk of HIV transmission via blood transfusion decreased from roughly 1 in 16 000 in 1985 (PHAC, 2009) to 1 in 21.4 million in 2015 (Canadian Blood Services, 2016).

SEXUALLY TRANSMITTED AND BLOOD-BORNE INFECTIONS

STBBIs are categorized as bacterial, viral, or ectoparasitic infections. A person who has one STBBI is at risk for other STBBIs. All insertive and receptive sexual practices (oral, vaginal, anal) put people at risk for STBBIs (Government of Alberta, 2012). The following is a brief summary of the most common STBBIs in Canada.

Bacterial STIs

The most common reportable bacterial STIs are chlamydia, gonorrhea, and syphilis. **Chlamydia** and **gonorrhea** are primarily transmitted through unprotected (sex without a condom) vaginal and anal intercourse, and less often through unprotected (sex without a condom or dental dam) oral intercourse. Infections can also pass from mother to newborn baby during delivery (PHAC, 2017a). Most often, people do not have symptoms, resulting in ongoing spread of infection. Symptoms in women may include abnormal vaginal discharge or bleeding, lower abdominal pain, pain during intercourse, burning during urination, or rectal pain and discharge (PHAC, 2017a). Symptoms in males may include unusual penile discharge, burning while urinating, pain or swelling of the testes, or rectal pain and discharge. Pharyngeal infection may present as a sore throat (PHAC, 2017a). In women, untreated chlamydia and gonorrhea infections may lead to pelvic inflammatory disease (PID), an inflammation of the upper female genital tract. Complications of PID include chronic pelvic pain, infertility, and ectopic pregnancy. In men, untreated infections may lead to infections of the testicles and scrotum, infertility, and chronic pelvic pain (PHAC, 2017a).

Many people avoid STI testing because of fear of pain or embarrassment. Chlamydia and gonorrhea infections are detected via urine testing or cervical, penile, rectal, or throat swabbing. Both infections are curable with antibiotics (PHAC, 2017a). An uncomplicated chlamydia infection

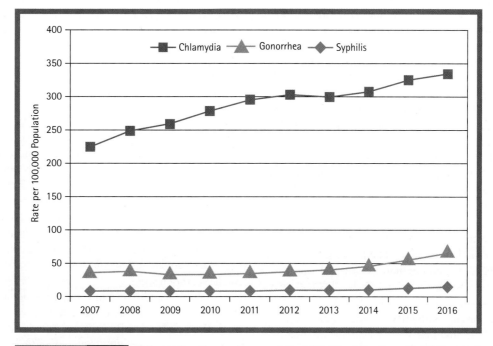

FIGURE 31.1 Chlamydia, Gonorrhea, and Syphilis Rates in Canada: 2007–2016

Source: The Public Health Agency of Canada, modified: 2018. Adapted and reproduced with permission from the Minister of Health, 2018.

is treated with azithromycin or doxycycline. In recent years, gonorrhea has become increasingly resistant to antibiotics. Preferred antibiotic treatment regimens can differ by region depending on surveillance data about antimicrobial resistance. For both types of infection, people should abstain from sexual contact until after all partners have been tested and treated (PHAC, 2017a).

In Canada, chlamydia is the most prevalent reportable STI. From 2007–2016, the chlamydia rate increased from 224.8 to 334.3 per 100 000 persons (PHAC, 2017b). A disproportionate number of youth between the ages of 15 and 24 and females are infected with chlamydia. In 2016, approximately 56% of all Canadian chlamydia cases were among youth ages 15–24, and approximately 61% of cases were among females (PHAC, 2017b). Gonorrhea is the second most prevalent reportable STI in Canada. From 2009–2016, the rate increased from 33.2 to 65.4 per 100 000 people (PHAC, 2017b). In 2016, gonorrhea was more prevalent in males (64%) compared to females (36%) (PHAC, 2017b). See Figure 31.1 for rates of chlamydia and gonorrhea in Canada.

Syphilis is transmitted via unprotected (sex without a condom or dental dam) vaginal, oral, or anal sexual contact with an infected person. The symptoms of syphilis are often overlooked because it first manifests as a painless open sore or ulcer at the site where the bacteria entered the body. Left untreated, syphilis progresses through four stages of infection: primary, secondary, latent, and tertiary (Government of Canada, 2015). Diagnosis is often delayed until later stages, when there may be damage to the central nervous or cardiovascular systems, resulting in complications such as paralysis, mental illness, or even death (PHAC, 2017a). Syphilis is diagnosed through blood tests, direct exam of lesion material with dark-field microscopy, and clinical findings (e.g., lesions or rash that

can appear anywhere, including the trunk, palms of the hands, or soles of the feet) (PHAC, 2017a). Syphilis is treated with antibiotics, and negative long-term outcomes are reduced with early diagnosis and treatment (PHAC, 2017a). Having syphilis increases the risk of getting or spreading HIV (Government of Canada, 2015). Syphilis can be passed from mother to baby during pregnancy or childbirth, resulting in congenital syphilis or even fetal death (PHAC, 2017a). There is a theoretical risk of transmission during breastfeeding if primary or secondary lesions are present. All pregnant women should be screened for syphilis during the first trimester of pregnancy. Women who are considered high risk or in an area experiencing outbreaks in heterosexual populations should be re-screened at 28–32 weeks and again at delivery (PHAC, 2017a).

In Canada, syphilis is the least common of the reportable STIs. From 2009–2016, the syphilis rate increased from 8.3 to 14.8 per 100 000 population (PHAC, 2017b). Over the past decade, there have been several syphilis outbreaks across Canada, including in Montreal, Ottawa, Toronto, Winnipeg, Calgary, Edmonton, Vancouver, Yukon, and Northwest Territories (PHAC, 2011). The majority of the outbreaks have been linked to men who have sex with men (MSM) and sex-trade worker populations (PHAC, 2017a). See Figure 31.1 for rates of infectious syphilis.

Viral STIs

Genital herpes simplex virus (HSV) and **human papillomavirus (HPV)** are highly prevalent viral STIs. These viruses spread easily, are difficult to prevent, and are non-reportable. Genital HSV and HPV are transmitted through intimate skin-to-skin sexual contact. They can also be spread from mother to baby through childbirth and can cause serious complications such as abnormal development or death (PHAC, 2017a).

HSV types 1 and 2 can cause genital infection. Genital herpes often appears as one or a group of painful, itchy, fluid-filled blisters in or around the genitals, buttocks, and/or thighs. People may experience burning during urination, fever, flu-like symptoms, and swollen glands. Some people experience only one outbreak of herpes; others may experience recurrent outbreaks. Recurrent outbreaks tend to be short-lived and less severe than first outbreaks. It is important to note that of new genital herpes infections, 60% are asymptomatic (PHAC, 2017a).

Genital HSV is diagnosed through clinical examination and culture of the fluid from a sore (PHAC, 2017a). There is no cure for genital HSV; however, outbreaks can be managed through antiviral medication. The incidence and prevalence of genital HSV is unknown; however, the PHAC (2017a) reports that genital HSV is increasing worldwide. Condom use decreases transmission by 50% (PHAC, 2017a).

Many people infected with HPV have no symptoms. There are more than 130 strains of HPV with about 40 strains affecting the anogenital tract (PHAC, 2017a). Some HPV strains cause genital warts; other carcinogenic strains cause abnormal cell changes on the cervix. This may lead to cervical cancer if left untreated. Abnormal cervical cell changes from HPV infection are detected through having cervical cancer screen tests and Pap tests on a regular basis (PHAC, 2017a). Abnormal cervical cell changes may be monitored by repeat screening or through referral for colposcopy for diagnostic testing and treatment. Genital warts appear as groups of cauliflower-like growths in the genital area. Clinical examinations and special testing are used to visualize genital warts. Freezing, burning, or laser therapies are used to treat genital warts. HPV is also linked to oral, penile, and anal cancers (PHAC, 2017a). Because HPV is non-reportable, its incidence is unknown. However, the PHAC carries out studies to assess the prevalence of the virus and the incidence of HPV types associated with cancer. It is estimated that 70% of adults will experience at least one type of HPV infection in their lifetime. This viral infection usually clears up on its own within two years; however, for some people the virus persists (PHAC, 2017a).

Ectoparasites

Ectoparasites include pubic lice (crabs) and scabies. Both can be transmitted through sexual or non-sexual (e.g., contact with infected towels or bed linens) contact. Pubic lice are most commonly found in genital and surrounding hair; however, they can also be found in chest, armpit, or facial hair (PHAC, 2017a). The adult louse lays eggs in the hair, and within 5 to 10 days they hatch. Symptoms of lice include itching and skin irritation.

Scabies are parasites that burrow under the skin, leaving red bumps that cause irritation and itchiness (PHAC, 2017a). Scabies can be found on any part of the body; however, they prefer warm, moist places such as the genital area. Both conditions, ectoparasites and scabies, are diagnosed through careful examination of infected areas and are treated with over-the-counter products containing insecticides such as permethrin (PHAC, 2017a).

Vaginal Infections

Vaginal infections are often called vaginitis. **Vaginitis** is the most common reason for gynecological visits. Depending on the etiology, they may or may not be classified as an STI. Vaginal infections are characterized by one or more of the following: vaginal discharge, rash, itching, irritation, and vaginal odour. The three most common vaginal infections are bacterial vaginosis (BV), candidiasis (yeast), and trichomoniasis (PHAC, 2017a). Treatment for the most common types of vaginitis differ according to the cause, so first-time sufferers should avoid self-diagnosis and seek medical assessment as diagnosis is based on laboratory testing.

BV and candidiasis infections are not usually sexually transmitted but are associated with increased acquisition of HIV. **Trichomoniasis** is an STI caused by the protozoa *Trichomonas vaginalis*. Trichomoniasis symptoms include foamy yellow or green vaginal discharge that may be musty or foul smelling, itching or burning around the vagina, and pain with urination or sexual intercourse. The preferred treatment is the antibiotic metronidazole. Men usually do not have symptoms or may have mild discharge or pain with urination (PHAC, 2017a).

BLOOD-BORNE INFECTIONS

BBIs such as HIV, hepatitis B, and hepatitis C need special consideration as they are not solely transmitted by sexual activity. Transmission can also occur by reusing drug, tattooing, or piercing equipment that has residual traces of infected blood, and from mother to neonate during pregnancy or birth (PHAC, 2017a). Additionally, HIV can be transmitted through breast milk, and hepatitis B and C can be transmitted by sharing razors or toothbrushes with an infected person (PHAC, 2017a).

HIV/AIDS

Advances in **human immunodeficiency virus (HIV)** treatment and antiretroviral therapies have slowed the progression of HIV to a point where the disease is accepted to be a manageable, chronic condition (PHAC, 2013a). In addition, according to the Government of Canada (2017c), there have been no new confirmed cases of HIV by sexual transmission when the person living with HIV is on continuous antiretroviral therapy with sustained viral suppression. The U=U campaign, which is undetectable equals untransmittable, raises awareness about the importance of treatment (Government of Canada, 2017a). However, in 2014, 21% of people in Canada infected with HIV were unaware of their status (PHAC, 2015a). Undiagnosed cases of HIV are a public health concern and represent a missed opportunity to improve the prognosis for people living with HIV and reduce rates of transmission. It is estimated that up to 90% of individuals infected experience primary or acute HIV symptoms, which occur two to six weeks after infection (Government of Canada, 2017b). Symptoms are generally mild and flu-like and may include sore throat, fatigue, fever, headache, rash, nausea, diarrhea, and vomiting (PHAC, 2017a). The chronic symptomatic phase occurs when the HIV weakens the immune system, and the body exhibits long-term symptoms such as swollen lymph nodes, skin lesions, fever, and diarrhea. **Acquired immune deficiency syndrome (AIDS)** is diagnosed when a person with HIV experiences one or more AIDS-defining illnesses, including opportunistic infections (e.g., recurrent bacterial pneumonia, fungal infections), malignancies (e.g., lymphomas, Kaposi's Sarcoma), or neurological diseases (e.g., AIDS dementia) (PHAC, 2017a).

HIV is diagnosed through a blood test. In Canada, testing first became available in 1985 (PHAC, 2012a). There is a period of time, or window, after acquisition of HIV infection when the person is highly infectious, but antibody tests are negative. This window period has changed as screening tests have improved and varies between types of tests (Government of Canada, 2017b). It is now recommended that HIV testing be made a component of routine medical care whenever a person requests one, has symptoms of HIV infection or weakened immune system, is pregnant or planning to be pregnant, or is the victim of sexual assault (PHAC, 2013a). Pre- and post-test discussion by CHNs can be important because it is an opportunity to engage clients, prepare them for the potential impact of test results, and raise awareness of safer sexual practices such as condom use. The minimum requirement for HIV testing is informed verbal consent and an understanding of the testing procedures and results (PHAC, 2013a). The Government of Canada (2017a) has endorsed global HIV efforts to commit to 90% of people living with HIV to be diagnosed, 90% of those people with HIV to be on treatment, and 90% of those people on treatment being virally suppressed by 2020, also referred to as 90-90-90.

In 2016 there were 2344 positive HIV tests reported in Canada, with a cumulative total of 84 409 positive HIV tests reported since 1985 (Bourgeois et al., 2017a). From 2007–2015, the HIV rate decreased from 7.3 to 5.8 per 100 000 population. In 2016 the rate increased to 6.4 per 100 000 people (Bourgeois et al., 2017a). The HIV rate that year was higher among males (9.8) than females (3.0); 44.1% of all positive adult HIV tests were identified as originating from exposure through the MSM population, 32.3% as exposure through heterosexual contact, and 15.1% as exposure through injection drug use (Bourgeois et al., 2017b). See Figure 31.2 for HIV rates in Canada. The figure shows that males have a higher rate compared to the general population and females have a lower rate compared to the general population.

Hepatitis B

Hepatitis B is a liver disease caused by the hepatitis B virus (HBV) and is spread by contact with infected body fluids, including blood, semen, and vaginal fluid. It is more infectious than HIV. Following infection, about 50% of people are asymptomatic, and 50% of people will develop symptoms of fatigue, nausea, vomiting, jaundice, decreased appetite, and arthralgia. About 95% of healthy people will clear the virus, with the remaining people becoming chronic carriers. People who have chronic HBV may eventually develop liver cancer, liver failure, or cirrhosis. Diagnosis is confirmed by blood testing. Combination antiviral drugs are available to treat HBV (PHAC, 2014).

It is estimated that fewer than 5% of Canadians show signs of past hepatitis B infection, and fewer than 1% are carriers of HBV (PHAC, 2013b). Certain sub-populations tend to be at greater risk for the virus, including individuals who were born in endemic areas, MSM, sex-trade workers, and injection drug users (PHAC, 2013b). The widespread availability of hepatitis B vaccine has assisted in prevention of the

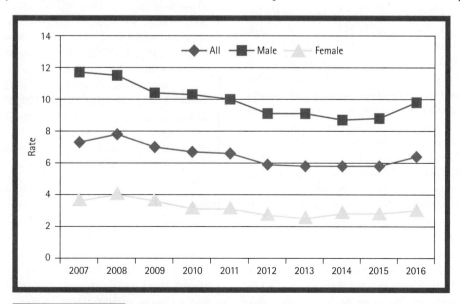

FIGURE 31.2 HIV Rates in Canada: 2007–2016

Source: Bourgeois et al. (2017a).

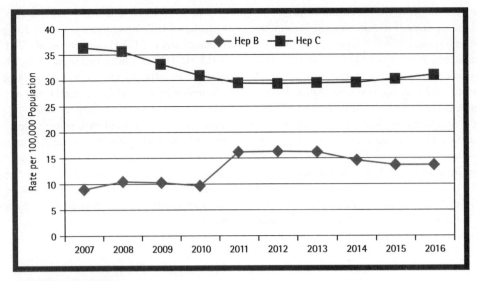

FIGURE 31.3 Hepatitis B and C Rates in Canada: 2007–2016

Source: The Public Health Agency of Canada, modified: 2018. Adapted and reproduced with permission from the Minister of Health, 2018.

infection. Publicly funded vaccination programs are offered in all Canadian provinces and territories. Hepatitis B vaccine is routinely offered to all Canadian children and adolescents. If parents are hepatitis B carriers, or they were born in endemic areas, the vaccination is offered to children during the first year of life (PHAC, 2013b).

In 2016, there were 4961 newly reported hepatitis B cases in Canada, for a rate of 13.7 per 100 000 people. Over the past decade, the hepatitis B rate has fluctuated, ranging from 9.0 to 16.3 (PHAC, 2017b). See Figure 31.3 for hepatitis B rates in Canada.

Hepatitis C

Hepatitis C is a liver disease caused by the hepatitis C virus (HCV) and is most commonly spread by percutaneous exposure with infected blood and less commonly by sexual activity or perinatal exposure. Following infection, most people are asymptomatic; about 30% of people may experience fatigue, jaundice, or arthralgia. Approximately 45% of healthy people will spontaneously clear HCV, and 55–85% of people will develop chronic infection. Diagnosis is confirmed by blood testing. Treatment is rapidly changing due to new antiviral medications and is recommended for all people with chronic infection (Ahmad, 2017). The majority of HCV cases in Canada are among people who inject drugs, accounting for 61% of new infections. HCV is recognized as a growing public health concern among people living with HIV. Co-infection with HIV and other STIs increases the risk of HCV transmission (PHAC, 2012b).

In 2016 there were 11 265 newly reported cases of HCV in Canada, a rate of 31.1 per 100 000 persons (PHAC, 2017b). From 2007–2012, the HCV rate declined from 36.4 to 29.4 per 100 000 persons (PHAC, 2017b). From 2013–2016 there were some minor rate fluctuations (PHAC, 2017b). See Figure 31.3 for hepatitis C rates.

YES, BUT WHY?

Creating Safer and Welcoming Health Care for People Who Are Sexually and Gender Diverse

What?

People who are sexually and gender diverse (LGBTQ2S) are overrepresented in their burden of STBBIs. Their experiences of real or perceived homophobia or transphobia can contribute to sexual risk behaviours and increased vulnerability to STBBI (PHAC, 2015b) and can act as a barrier against seeking care (CPHA, n.d.).

So What?

STBBIs remain a public health concern. STBBI prevention, testing, and treatment depends on the engagement of people with health care. People who are sexually and gender diverse (LGBTQ2S) have many unmet health needs and reduced likelihood of accessing routine, emergency, and preventive health services (Alberta Health Services Sexual & Reproductive Health Calgary Zone, 2018a). Canada's Human Rights Act protects people against discrimination based on sexual orientation, gender identity, and gender expression. Despite these protections, inequities exist in the burden of disease and how people access care.

Now What?

CHNs can support the creation of safer and welcoming health care for LGBTQ2S individuals. The Canadian Public Health Association (CPHA) outlined an organizational assessment tool to create inclusive health care environments. Three criteria should be met, including supportive and inclusive organizational polices, culture, and environment; providers who possess inclusive skills relevant to their roles; and service that allows people to feel comfortable, welcome, and supportive when accessing health care services (CPHA, 2017). CHNs can advocate for completing the organizational assessment, developing an improvement plan, and evaluating outcomes.

Standards of Practice Fulfilled

#1 Health Promotion
- Uses a collaborative relationship with the client and other partners to facilitate and advocate for structural system change and healthy public policy using multiple health promotion strategies.
- Considers the determinants of health, the social and political context, and systemic structures in collaboration with the client to determine action.

#2 Prevention and Health Protection
- Engages in collaborative, interdisciplinary and inter-sectoral partnerships in the delivery of preventive and protective services with particular attention to populations who are marginalized.

#4 Professional Relationships
- Builds a network of relationships and partnerships with a wide variety of individuals, families, groups, communities, and systems to address health issues and promote healthy public policy to advance health equity.

#8 Professional Responsibility and Accountability
- Advocates for effective and efficient use of community health nursing resources (Community Health Nurses of Canada [CHNC], 2019, revised).

IMPLICATIONS OF STBBIs

All STBBIs are underreported, as many Canadians neither go for testing nor know that they are infected (PHAC, 2017a). Large numbers of people live with non-reportable STBBIs, such as herpes and HPV. Rates of reportable STBBIs provide CHNs with some understanding of the scope of the problem. If STBBIs remain inadequately addressed and untreated, they can lead to ongoing spread of the infection, infertility, neonatal complications, pelvic inflammatory disease, or even death (PHAC, 2017a). STBBIs can negatively impact a person's relationships, self-esteem, mental health, coping abilities, and work productivity. Additionally, there are societal economic implications due to the medical costs associated with diagnosis and treatment (McKay, 2006), especially in the case of complications such as infertility and neonatal infection. CHNs must attempt to address not only medical issues such as testing and treatment but also social and economic issues. For example, CHNs can advocate for the development of support groups that can assist people to cope with their diagnosis of herpes or HIV while supporting them to pursue loving, sexual relationships with an understanding partner. Additionally, CHNs can raise awareness in the workplace and community to increase the funding for HIV medication, research, and alternative employment during times of intense treatment.

STBBI PREVENTION AND HARM REDUCTION

When considering the prevention of STBBIs, it is paramount to take into account all levels of prevention. Primordial prevention refers to preventing STBBI risk factors from existing (Vollman, Anderson, & McFarlane, 2017). This includes the underlying conditions that lead to the cause of STBBIs, starting with the social and economic conditions that place people at risk (Porta, 2014). Primordial prevention includes the creation of programs and policies that keep youth off the streets or advocating for access to comprehensive **sexual health education**. Sexual health education is defined as "the process of equipping individuals, couples, families, and communities with the information and motivation needed to enhance sexual health and avoid negative sexual health outcomes" (PHAC, 2008, p. 5).

Primary prevention refers to preventing the start of disease with the goal of decreasing incidence. It involves activities that are started prior to any sign of disease or injury (University of Ottawa, 2015). Important to decreasing the transmission of STBBIs is the accurate and consistent use of penile or vaginal condoms (see Photos 31.1a and 31.1b) (PHAC, 2017a). A **penile or male condom** is a disposable latex or polyurethane sheath worn on the penis. A **vaginal or female condom** is a disposable polyurethane sheath placed inside the vagina (Black et al., 2015). Condoms prevent direct contact between the genitals, inhibiting the exchange of bodily fluids such as semen, pre-ejaculate fluid, and vaginal secretions. Condoms help to protect against pregnancy and STBBIs (Black et al., 2015). It is important to note that condoms are not 100% effective in protecting against herpes or HPV (e.g., genital warts on the testicles or labia). Abstinence from all types of sexual activity (e.g., genital-to-genital contact) is the only 100% effective method of preventing these STBBIs.

Another important primary prevention strategy is vaccination. As mentioned previously, hepatitis B is prevented through vaccination. Additionally, from 2006–2015, Health Canada approved three HPV vaccines that prevent between two and nine types of HPV infections. More information on HPV vaccines is provided later in this chapter. Infection by HIV, hepatitis B, and hepatitis C are prevented by condom use *and* by other primary prevention strategies such as using clean needles and equipment for tattooing, piercing, and injecting drugs. Condoms (Photos 31.1a and 31.1b) and dental dams (Photo 31.2) should always be used for oral sex (PHAC, 2017a).

Secondary prevention refers to the early detection of disease (University of Ottawa, 2015) and involves regular testing and screening for STBBIs. STBBI testing may include blood tests, urine samples, genital examinations, and sometimes swabs (PHAC, 2017a). Tertiary prevention refers to measures aimed at decreasing the progress of a disease and controlling long-term negative consequences (Porta, 2014; Vollman et al., 2017). Tertiary prevention may involve using medications to treat an infection (e.g., chlamydia or gonorrhea), manage symptoms (e.g., genital herpes), or slow down

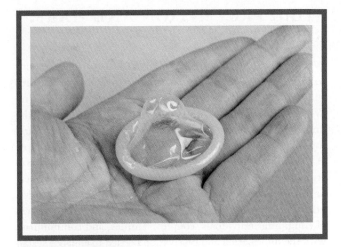

PHOTO 31.1A Penile (male) condom

Source: Xuejun li/Fotolia

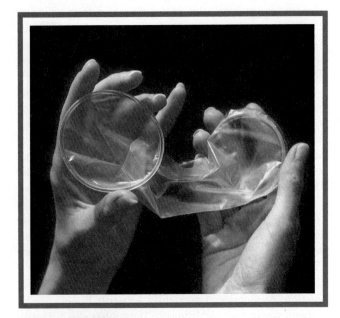

PHOTO 31.1B Vaginal (female) condom

Source: Scott Camazine/Science Source

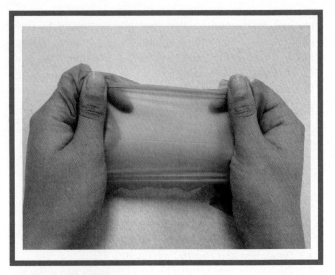

PHOTO 31.2 Dental dam

Source: TrouteWood, Tammy

the disease process (e.g., HIV). Finally, quaternary prevention involves methods to avoid results of unnecessary or excessive interventions in the health system (Porta, 2014) and protects from new procedures that are yet to be tested (Vollman et al., 2017). As new medications or treatments are developed for treating STBBIs, it is important to ensure that patients are not placed in any harm. For patients participating in drug trials, it is important that consent is obtained before participating, and participants have the ability to withdraw from the trial at any time.

Harm reduction can be defined as a strategy targeted at groups or individuals that endeavours to reduce the harms related to certain behaviours (Canadian Paediatric Society, 2008). Examples of harm reduction strategies include educating sex-trade workers about penile and vaginal condoms, and the implementation of needle exchange programs or supervised consumption sites (discussed in Chapters 8 and 30). Although these types of interventions are important, they must be timely and relevant to the target population to have an impact.

Emerging Challenges

Preventing, diagnosing, treating, and managing STBBIs is paramount (CPHA, 2017) to nurses working in the community. Nevertheless, stigma and discrimination within various health care settings thwart the efforts made by CHNs by acting as an obstruction to clients attempting to access services (CPHA, 2017). Stigma refers to the "dynamic process of devaluation that significantly discredits an individual in the eyes of others, such as when certain attributes are seized upon within particular cultures or settings and defined as discreditable or unworthy. When stigma is acted upon, the result is discrimination" (UNAIDS, 2015, p. 44). Discrimination is defined as any form of "arbitrary distinction, exclusion, or restriction affecting a person, usually (but not only) because of an inherent personal characteristic or perceived membership of a particular group" (UNAIDS, 2015, p. 44). Stigma and discrimination stem from values, beliefs, attitudes, and behaviours of individuals, as well as the culture, policies, and procedures of an organization (CPHA, 2017).

Another challenge faced by CHNs is **safer sex fatigue**, which refers to an individual's apathy regarding hearing about and complying with safer-sex messages, resulting in risky behaviour (PHAC, 2017a). Treatment optimism, on the other hand, refers to not feeling too worried about contracting HIV because of the medications available to decrease HIV-associated morbidity and mortality (Rowniak, 2009). Some research demonstrates that individuals with higher levels of safer sex fatigue and treatment optimism are more likely to participate in condomless sex (Hanif et al., 2014; Macapagal, Birkett, Janulis, Garofalo, & Mustanski, 2017).

CANADIAN RESEARCH 31.1

A focus group qualitative study of HIV stigma in the Canadian healthcare system (Wagner, McShane, Hart, & Margolese, 2016)

HIV-related stigma in the health care system has an ongoing deleterious effect on the physical, mental, and sexual health of individuals living with HIV. A power imbalance exists between patients living with HIV and their health care providers, which may cause further stigma and vulnerability. This study examined, from a critical perspective, the perception of health care providers' attitudes and beliefs regarding HIV-positive individuals.

A total of 26 participants took part in four focus groups. The groups were comprised of men (n=6) and women (n=5) living with HIV, nursing and medical students (n=9), and multidisciplinary HIV health care providers (n=6). Focus groups were 60–75 minutes in length, audiotaped and transcribed. The researchers asked four open-ended questions exploring stigma and perceived attitudes, beliefs, and actions in relation to people living with HIV. To analyze the data, the researchers used immersion/crystallization to promote theme development, which was data driven versus imposing preexisting notions of themes on the data. The analysis revealed two main thematic categories and several related theses.

Thematic Category 1: HIV-Specific Behaviours

This thematic category consisted of three themes:

- HIV is a complex and changing chronic illness that differs from person to person.
- Some health care providers had positive characteristics: nonjudgmental, thoughtful, honest, comfortable, compassionate, and advocacy.
- There is a cumulative impact on patient satisfaction. Early negative and stigmatizing experiences impacted how patients interpreted later experiences.

Thematic Category 2: Components of Stigma

This thematic category consisted of six themes:

- Discrimination: Participants identified various acts of discrimination, including "othering," which creates feelings of "us versus them."
- Stereotypes: Participants discussed stereotypes regarding who contracts HIV, particularly the modes of transmission. There are stereotypes regarding the behaviours and identity of individuals living with HIV.
- Prejudice: Participants discussed prejudice in terms of negative and emotionally charged attitudes. Anger and fear were identified as prejudicial, which in turn could lead to negative attitudes.
- The interplay of various components of stigma: Participants addressed the need to halt the interaction between prejudice, discrimination, and stereotyping.
- Institutional factors: Participants spoke to institutional practices such as policies and procedures that promote discrimination.

- Overlapping stigmas: Participants living with HIV spoke about overlapping stigmas such as injection drug use stigma and HIV stigma or homophobia and HIV stigma.

Discussion Questions

1. How can stigma impact the health of individuals living with HIV?
2. What are some institutional practices that could promote stigma?
3. How can CHNs assist in stopping the cycle of stigma?

SPECIFIC POPULATIONS AT A HIGHER RISK FOR ACQUIRING STBBIs

Individuals who may be at a higher risk for acquiring STBBIs include but are not limited to people who are sexually active between the ages of 15 and 24, report more than two new sexual partners in the past year, report the use of non-barrier methods of contraception, report unprotected (sex without a condom) anal or vaginal intercourse, report injection or other drug use, report anonymous sexual partnering, and are victims of sexual abuse or assault (Government of Alberta, 2012). Specific at-risk populations are discussed in the following sections.

Men Who Have Sex with Men

In Canada, MSM have the highest incidence of new HIV infections when compared to other sub-populations (PHAC, 2015a). In 2014, approximately 54.3%, or 1396, newly diagnosed cases of HIV were in the MSM population. This is similar to estimates in 2011, when there were 1416 new cases reported in this population. Of further public health concern is undiagnosed HIV infections, which represent the difference between the total of people living with HIV and the total of people living with HIV who have been diagnosed. PHAC (2015a) estimates that among people living HIV who are undiagnosed, about 18% acquired it through MSM contact.

Although traditional health education messages address safer sexual practices and condom use, it is clear that certain cohorts of MSM are still not being reached with these prevention strategies. There are innovative practices to help prevent acquisition of new infection, including pre-exposure prophylaxis (PrEP) and post-exposure prophylaxis (PEP) and promoting early diagnosis and care, such as rapid or point-of-care testing (POCT). POCT gives the HIV result at one visit, usually in less than one hour. Evidence suggests that people prefer rapid testing over standard testing, and people who test positive are successfully linked to care (Canada's Source for HIV and Hepatitis C Information [CATIE], 2015).

Sex Workers

Sex workers are at increased risk for contracting and spreading STBBIs for several reasons, including stigma and discrimination (Argento et al., 2016; Lazarus et al., 2012); having a high number of sexual partners; having limited ability to access social, health, and legal services; lifestyle risks such as substance use; and limited economic resources (PHAC, 2017a). Condom use varies among sex-trade workers (Sou et al., 2015), and the choice to use condoms may be controlled by the customer (Comack & Seshia, 2010). Sexual violence is prevalent among sex workers. In a Winnipeg study, 58% of "bad date reports" included some form of sexual violence (e.g., refusal to use a condom, unwanted touching, or sexual assault) (Comack & Seshia, 2010).

CHNs working with sex workers can promote a variety of risk-reduction strategies (e.g., correct use of male or female condoms) to prevent this population from acquiring or spreading STBBIs. Since access to and the cost of condoms may deter sex workers from using them, it is paramount that condoms are available for free. Peer education strategies have proven promising in terms of increasing knowledge related to STIs and HIV and safer sex practices (PHAC, 2017a). Overall, it is important that the services developed for sex workers (e.g., peer education, hepatitis B vaccinations, STBBI testing and treatment) are delivered innovatively (e.g., from a mobile van, hotel room, community centre) with the workers' input (Deering et al., 2015; Lazarus et al., 2012; PHAC, 2017a). Finally, it is of utmost importance that the services provided to sex workers are culturally safe and non-stigmatizing (Sou et al., 2015).

Street-Involved Youth

Street-involved youth have been rendered extremely vulnerable. For many, addressing the basic necessities of life is of greater priority than preventing or addressing potential health risks (Lokanc-Diluzio & Reilly, 2016). Furthermore, due to the multiple and intersecting stigmas they face (e.g., risky sexual practices, drug use, gender stereotypes), they may be less likely to access health care services such as STBBI testing (Karamouzian et al., 2017).

Canadian research shows that street-involved youth do not always take effective action in preventing STBBIs. In an Ottawa study, street youth aged 15 to 24 reported inconsistent use of condoms. For example, approximately 50% of street youth reported use of condoms during their last vaginal or anal sexual encounter, and 15% stated they used condoms for their last oral sexual encounter (Ottawa Public Health, 2011). Another factor that impacts STBBIs in street youth is their use of alcohol and drugs. In qualitative interviews, youth indicated alcohol and other substances impacted their ability to make decisions (Lokanc-Diluzio, 2014; Lokanc-Diluzio & Reilly, 2016). Furthermore, 93% of Ottawa street youth reported use of non-injection drugs, and 19% reported use of injection drugs (Ottawa Public Health, 2011).

STBBIs are higher among street youth in comparison to mainstream youth. In the Ottawa study, 8.8% of youth were infected with chlamydia, and 0.59% were infected with gonorrhea. Among non-injection drug users, 5% were infected with hepatitis C, and 2% were infected with HIV. Among youth who used injection drugs, 24% were infected with hepatitis C, and 4% were infected with HIV (Ottawa Public Health, 2011). Resources must be allocated for both sufficient outreach with this population and comprehensive programming that entails prevention, screening, and treatment services. Furthermore, creating interventions that target CHNs and other health care providers that aim to decrease attitudes and behaviours that are stigmatizing may help this population to seek STBBI testing and sexual health services (Karamouzian et al., 2017).

Injection Drug Users

Injection drug users represent a growing concern for CHNs, as the craving for "another hit" overrides the importance of using a clean needle to prevent the transmission of HIV, hepatitis B, or hepatitis C. Offering better access to condoms and clean needles or drug equipment via needle exchange programs and supervised injection sites are harm reduction strategies that may help these populations lower their risk of contracting STBBIs while they search for effective treatment (PHAC, 2017a).

Ethnocultural Communities

In 2011, about 6.3 million people in Canada, or about 19.1% of the population identified as people of color (PHAC, 2015b). Although there are differences within and between ethnocultural groups, the PHAC (2015b) states that ethnocultural communities are disproportionately affected by STBBIs. The new HIV infection rate is estimated to be nine times higher among people where HIV is endemic compared to other Canadians. The majority of HIV infection is acquired by heterosexual contact among people who self-identify as Black. Many immigrants and refugees come from countries with a high prevalence of hepatitis C and account for about 35% of infections in Canada. As Canada becomes increasingly diverse, it is important to address the health needs of these communities, including access to STBBI prevention, screening, and treatment services (PHAC, 2015b).

Citizenship and Immigration Canada requires mandatory syphilis and HIV testing for immigrants and refugees over the age of 15 seeking Canadian citizenship. HIV testing is also required for children born to a mother infected with HIV, those with blood or blood product exposure, or those who may be an international adoptee. Hepatitis B and C testing in not required (PHAC, 2017a). Language, cultural, socioeconomic, and educational barriers may deter certain immigrant subpopulations from seeking health services (PHAC, 2017a). New immigrants and refugees are overwhelmed with adapting to new cultural and health care practices. Many come from countries where HIV, hepatitis, and other STIs are more prevalent and treatment is inaccessible (PHAC, 2017a). Cultural beliefs may also influence a person's motivation to access health services. Some may try a variety of herbs or culturally accepted medications before seeking medical treatment for an STI or

HIV. Many Canadian provinces lack services and resources that are translated, culturally safe, and accessible to newcomers. It is important that CHNs be attentive to the stressful and complex issues faced by immigrants and refugees as they integrate into Canadian culture (PHAC, 2017a).

Unwilling or Unable Population

There are some HIV-positive individuals who are recalcitrant or "unwilling or unable" to prevent the spread of HIV (Government of Alberta, 2015). Unable refers to "an HIV-positive individual who does not have the capacity to prevent HIV transmission for physical, mental, or environmental reasons" (Government of Alberta, 2015, p. 4). Unwilling, on the other hand, refers to HIV-positive individuals who intentionally participate in behaviours that can transmit HIV when they know the risks and have the ability to prevent transmission (Government of Alberta, 2015). These individuals represent a very small portion of HIV-positive individuals but require a substantial amount of resources as they pose a considerable risk to other people and typically have numerous other personal, health, and social issues. For example, they may be homeless, socially isolated, and have lower self-esteem. Additionally, they may be substance users or have mental illness. When working with this population, it is paramount to consider who is unable to prevent HIV transmission versus able. It is often challenging, however, to determine who falls under which category (Government of Alberta, 2015). Health regions across Canada are addressing this issue in different ways, ranging from implementing comprehensive referral systems to providing housing and treatment.

People in Correctional Facilities

People in Canada's correctional facilities have disproportionately high rates of STBBIs, including HIV, hepatitis B, and hepatitis C (PHAC, 2013c; PHAC, 2017a). People in corrections facilities may participate in high-risk behaviours such as injection drug use, other substance abuse, and unprotected (sex without a condom or dental dam) sex. Also, people in correctional facilities who have consensual or non-consensual sexual contact, or participate in practices such as injection drug use or tattooing or piercing while incarcerated, are at risk for becoming infected and contributing to disease transmission (PHAC, 2017a).

A study of 500 males who were incarcerated at an Ontario correctional facility, revealed study participants reported high levels of drug use and risky sexual behaviours. The overall prevalence of chlamydia and gonorrhea was 2.9% and 0.6%, respectively (Kouyoumdjian, Main, Calzavara, & Kiefer, 2011). A qualitative study of Canadian females who were incarcerated revealed that there were numerous barriers to access health services that in turn resulted in negative health consequences, interruption of treatment, poor physical and mental health, and health disempowerment (Ahmed et al., 2016).

The time of incarceration represents a public health opportunity. Upon admission and during the period of incarceration,

Correctional Services Canada offers voluntary infectious disease testing, pre- and post-test counselling, treatment, and access to medical specialists. STBBI prevention programs offering education, voluntary testing and counselling, drug-dependence treatment, and harm-reduction strategies (distribution of condoms and clean needles) have been proven to reduce STBBI risk in prisons (PHAC, 2017a).

The Sexual & Reproductive Health Program in Calgary provides education services to individuals in correctional facilities. After completing a 90-minute education session on male sexual health, pre- and post-test findings revealed that knowledge increased by 17%. Furthermore, when participants (n=33) were asked about their perceived benefits of the class, 97% agreed or strongly agreed that because of the class, they knew more about how to lower sexual risk (Alberta Health Services Sexual & Reproductive Health Calgary Zone, 2018b).

Indigenous Peoples

First Nations, Inuit, and Métis peoples have disproportionately high rates of HIV compared to non-Indigenous Canadians (PHAC, 2014). In 2014, compared to other ethnicities, Indigenous people were 2.7 times more likely to get HIV (Canadian Aboriginal AIDS Network, 2018). Furthermore, in 2011 this population accounted for about 12% of all new Canadian HIV infections and approximately 9% of all HIV-positive persons (PHAC, 2014). The use of injection drugs is a significant risk factor for HIV transmission among First Nation, Inuit, and Métis people. In 2011, the estimated percentage of new HIV infections attributed to injection drug use exposure was higher among Indigenous people (58%) compared to all Canadians (14%) (PHAC, 2014). Indigenous individuals diagnosed with HIV infection are younger than infected non-Indigenous people. As reported, from 1998–2012, 32% of Indigenous individuals diagnosed with HIV were less than 30 years old, compared to 22% of people from other ethnicities (PHAC, 2014).

Traditional strategies to prevent STBBIs within Indigenous contexts could benefit from recent insights and interest surrounding syndemics. **Syndemics** is defined as "a conceptual framework for understanding diseases or health conditions, and how these are exacerbated by the social, economic, environmental, and political milieu in which a population is immersed" (Andermann, 2017, p. 125). Using traditional strategies to prevent and control STBBIs is not always efficacious, particularly with populations who are disadvantaged and marginalized. Andermann (2017) advocates for a broader approach, which analyzes the manner in which systems and policies prevent or support effective responses and recognizes the structural changes necessary to develop environments that are supportive while increasing resilience of the population. Regardless of the type of STBBI, it is important for CHNs to acknowledge the following: (a) the social determinants of health impact STBBI rates; (b) traditional values and strategies to control STBBIs are needed but are not enough; and (c) by using a "syndemic lens," CHNs can influence action at several levels to address the root causes of ill health and create strategies that are more effective for improving the health of Indigenous people while lessening health inequities (Andermann, 2017).

With any of the specific populations we have discussed, it is important for CHNs to forge new partnerships with the agencies these populations access. For example, to promote the health of new immigrants, CHNs can partner with cultural organizations, public health centres, community groups, or religious centres. For street-involved youth, CHNs can collaborate with sexual and reproductive health centres, mental health services, social services, detox or drug treatment programs, and community groups. Moreover, it is important to actively involve clients in the development, dissemination, and evaluation of promotion and prevention programs.

INNOVATIVE STI AND BBI PREVENTION INTERVENTIONS IN CANADA

It is vital to find innovative ways to promote the use of penile and vaginal condoms and dental dams. CHNs must think upstream and use health-promotion approaches that address the issues of their target population. CHNs can reach individuals through street outreach, counselling, and peer mentoring programs. Furthermore, CHNs can explore innovative ways to make these risk- and harm-reduction measures appealing to groups or communities through social media or poster and social marketing campaigns. CHNs can work with other sectors and multidisciplinary groups to develop healthy public policy to address STBBIs. Offering chlamydia urine testing in outreach vans and putting condom machines in schools are examples of health promotion activities resulting from healthy public policies.

The population health promotion model (Hamilton & Bhatti, 1996) provides a comprehensive tool for CHNs to utilize when planning STBBI prevention interventions with individuals, families, communities, and populations. Please refer to Chapter 8 for more information on the population health promotion model. Novel and innovative strategies are being implemented across Canada in an attempt to lower the prevalence of STBBIs.

Needle Exchange Programs and Supervised Consumption Sites

Intravenous drug use is a mounting public health concern in Canada. Individuals who participate in high-risk drug injection behaviours (e.g., sharing needles) pose a number of potential health risks to themselves and others, such as transmission of HIV/AIDS and hepatitis B and C (PHAC, 2017a). Some Canadian communities have addressed the issue of needle sharing with harm-reduction strategies such as needle-exchange programs and supervised consumption sites.

Needle exchange programs (NEPs), also called needle and syringe programs, provide injection drug users with free, sterile injecting equipment to reduce their risk of contracting and spreading infection (Elliott, Malkin, & Gold, 2002). This harm-reduction strategy is endorsed by the World Health Organization as well as health authorities across Canada. However, NEPs are considered controversial among policy makers and the general public. Werb and colleagues (2013) investigated NEPs in Vancouver from 1996–2010. During that time, the number of NEPs increased from 1 to 29. Their research suggests that as the number of NEPs increased, the proportion of injection drug users reporting cessation increased as well.

Supervised consumption sites (SCS) provide a safe location for drug users to use or inject their own drugs with clean equipment under the supervision of medically trained professionals (Small et al., 2011). Evidence suggests that SCSs are associated with a decrease in HIV infections, lower overdose deaths, and fewer ambulance calls for overdose treatment (Ng, Sutherland, & Kobler, 2017). Since 2017, SCSs have been approved in several cities across Canada (Government of Canada, 2018).

Social Marketing Campaigns

Social marketing can be defined as "a program-planning process that applies commercial marketing concepts and techniques to promote voluntary behavior change" (Grier &

CASE STUDY

I found a place that I feel OK about going to. The staff at the Healing Lodge Community Health Centre seemed happy to see me. They didn't request a health care card or home address and gave me free antibiotics to treat my arm infection. They even gave me clean needles without asking too many questions. Lately I haven't been feeling well and noticed my eyes were yellow so I went back for help. The nurse told me straight up that she thinks I might have hepatitis C and that I am at risk for HIV. They took my blood and I have to go back for the results. I'm worried about the test results, but not sure I will go back.

As a CHN, you want to improve accessibility to services for Indigenous youth by creating welcoming and non-stigmatizing health care services—a place where people will feel safe and return for ongoing care.

Discussion Questions

1. Discuss the importance of collaborating with local Indigenous groups for improving access to services.

2. What social determinants of health will the CHN need to be aware of when planning services?

3. What health promotion strategies can CHNs implement to improve accessibility?

Bryant, 2005, p. 319). In Canada, these types of campaigns are becoming more innovative as they provide blatant and, at times, provocative messages to different segments of the population. Unfortunately, many of these campaigns are not properly evaluated for their short- or long-term impact on the target population. Please refer to Chapter 8 for an in-depth discussion of social marketing.

The Fraser Health Authority in British Columbia implemented and evaluated a Cineplex TimePlay campaign called "Testing is Healthy" to address the increasing rates of STBBIs (Zhang et al., 2017). TimePlay is an interactive gaming experience that engages moviegoers prior to the start of the movie and is played via mobile application. It contains gaming elements along with a platform for advertising services and products. The target population was mainly young adults between the ages of 20–29, as they have the highest chlamydia and gonorrhea rates in BC. Prior to the start of the movie, moviegoers answered questions about STBBIs, and then they were connected to a clinic finder on the BC Centre for Disease Control Sex Smart Resource website. The campaign received more than 500 000 views and over 77 000 plays. It reached a large number of people at a relatively low cost. Furthermore, there was a correlation between the campaign and sharp increases in the unique page views for the clinic finder page of the Sex Smart Resource website (Zhang et al., 2017).

Capacity Building

As discussed in Chapter 8, capacity building is a process that increases the ability of an individual, a community, or an organization to promote health. CHNs build capacity through actively involving and working with individuals and groups. The intention is to build upon strengths, develop knowledge and skills, and encourage the ability to take action (CHNC, 2011, revised).

In one Canadian study, face-to-face and online training programs were used as a means for capacity building of service providers working with street-involved youth (Lokanc-Diluzio, 2014; Lokanc-Diluzio & Reilly, 2016). Knowledge related to STBBIs and condoms was measured three times (prior to the training programs, immediately after the training programs, and six weeks after the training programs). Participants in both training programs experienced statistically significant increases in knowledge immediately after the training programs and six weeks later. Self-reported comfort discussing STBBIs and condoms were also measured three times. The face-to-face participants experienced a statistically significant increase in comfort addressing those topics immediately after the training; however, the comfort was not sustained at six weeks later. The online participants, on the other hand, experienced statistically significant increases in comfort addressing those topics immediately after the training program and six weeks later. Six weeks after the training, approximately 46% of face-to-face participants and 72% of online participants had reportedly used their knowledge from their respective training programs.

Online Services and Websites

Online sexual health services and websites have become important in terms of health education and prevention of STBBIs as well as support for individuals living with HIV or AIDS (Shoveller Knight, Davis, Gilbert, & Ogilvie, 2012). Contemporary interventions are utilizing technology, such as the Internet, to reach populations most at risk. GetCheckedOnline (BC Centre for Disease Control, 2016) is a confidential and free STBBI testing service. In order to use the online service, clients need to create an account and a lab form, and give samples at a lab. Once test results are ready, clients receive an email. If the results are either inconclusive or positive, a nurse will contact clients about treating and testing. GetCheckedOnline offers tests for offers STBBI tests for chlamydia, gonorrhea, syphilis, HIV, and hepatitis C.

Websites can also be used to disseminate information on STBBI signs and symptoms, prevention, treatment, and referral. For example, Talking About Sexuality in Canadian Communities (TASCC) (see Photo 31.3) was developed to provide accurate, relevant, and timely resources for parents and service providers of high-risk youth and youth with different abilities. TASCC offers current information and resources that reflect best practices in sexual health promotion and education. Additionally, TASCC provides practical strategies and tools for working with high-risk youth and youth with different abilities (TASCC, 2018).

HIV Prevention: Oral Pre-Exposure Prophylaxis (PrEP) and Post-Exposure Prophylaxis (PEP)

In 2016, Health Canada approved pre-exposure prophylaxis (PrEP) for the prevention of HIV by sexual transmission. In some countries, it is also approved for prevention of HIV transmission by intravenous drug use. PrEP is a combination of two antiretroviral mediations available by prescription and can help reduce risk by more than 90%. It is taken by people who are HIV negative and are at substantial risk of HIV exposure. Good medication compliance is very important as

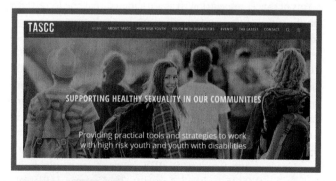

PHOTO   31.3 Website for service providers and parents of high-risk youth and youth with different abilities.

Source: Tascc.ca

PrEP is taken orally, every day. PrEP is less effective when not taken as prescribed. People wanting PrEP need ongoing care and require pre-screening for HIV, STI, hepatitis B, liver and kidney functions, and routine monitoring every few months (CATIE, 2017).

Post-exposure prophylaxis (PEP) is a combination of two or three antiretroviral mediations available by prescription only. It is taken as soon as possible and started no longer than 72 hours after high-risk or known HIV positive exposure to prevent HIV infection. Substantial risk of acquiring HIV can include condomless sex or condom breakage with partner(s) who are known HIV positive or intravenous drug users, in cases of sexual assault, and for occupational exposure. People needing PEP must consult an infectious disease specialist or health care provider experienced in HIV care (CATIE, 2011).

Human Papillomavirus Vaccination

In 2006, Health Canada approved a vaccine (**Gardasil**) that protects against four strains of HPV (National Advisory Council on Immunization [NACI], 2012). According to the National Advisory Council on Immunization (NACI), two of the strains are responsible for approximately 70% of cervical cancer cases (HPV 16 and 18), whereas the other two strains are responsible for around 90% of genital warts cases (HPV 6 and 11) (NACI, 2012; Shier & Bryson, 2007). In 2010, a second HPV vaccine, Cervarix, was approved by Health Canada (GlaxoSmithKline, 2010; NACI, 2012). Cervarix was designed to protect against two strains of HPV (HPV 16 and 18) causing cervical cancer. It also provides some protection from two additional strains (HPV 45 and 31). Together, the four strains account for 80% of cervical cancer cases (GlaxoSmithKline, 2014). Although Cervarix does not protect against genital warts, it may offer longer-term protection against HPV causing cervical cancer (GlaxoSmithKline, 2010). In 2015, a third vaccine, Gardasil 9, was approved by Health Canada. Gardasil 9 protects against nine HPV strains (HPV 6, 11, 16, 18, 31, 33, 45, 52, and 58). These nine strains cause around 80% of cervical pre-cancers, 90% of cervical cancers, 75% of HPV-related anal, vulvar, and vaginal pre-cancers and cancers, and more than 90% of genital warts (Society of Obstetricians and Gynecologists of Canada, n.d.). HPV vaccination is considered a medical milestone in terms of cancer prevention. It is anticipated that the long-term implications of the vaccine will result in a reduction of cervical cancer cases, although the need for women to have regular Pap tests will continue (Shier & Bryson, 2007). The NACI (2007, 2012) released statements on HPV immunizations in 2007 and 2012 to inform Canadian health care providers regarding appropriate use of HPV vaccines. The Society of Obstetricians and Gynaecologists of Canada's (n.d.) website (www.hpvinfo.ca) provides current HPV information for youth, adults, parents, teachers, and health professionals.

Gardasil and Gardasil 9 HPV vaccines are available for females aged 9–45 and males aged 9–26. Cervarix HPV vaccine is available for females aged 9–45 (Government of Canada, 2017c). Currently, all Canadian provinces have publicly funded vaccination strategies in place for school-aged individuals in Grades 5 to 9 (PHAC, 2017c). Some provinces also cover the cost of Gardasil 9 for transgender women and MSM aged 17 to 26 (Government of Alberta, 2017). For people who do not qualify for the publicly funded programs but are within the recommended age group, the vaccination is available for a cost for the three doses. People outside of the recommended age group should be encouraged to speak to their health care provider.

CONCLUSION

This chapter discussed the complex issues surrounding STBBIs in Canada. The history of STBBIs and how healthy public policy addresses prevention were briefly outlined. We provided a review of STBBI statistical trends and epidemiology. The needs of specific populations who may present unique challenges to CHNs related to STBBIs were illustrated. Finally, suggestions were made on how CHNs can use the PHP model to plan innovative prevention strategies.

KEY TERMS

acquired immune deficiency syndrome (AIDS)　(p. 561)
blood-borne infection (BBI)　(p. 558)
chlamydia　(p. 558)
ectoparasites　(p. 560)
Gardasil　(p. 570)
genital herpes simplex virus (HSV)　(p. 559)
gonorrhea　(p. 558)
hepatitis B　(p. 561)
hepatitis C　(p. 562)
human immunodeficiency virus (HIV)　(p. 560)
human papillomavirus (HPV)　(p. 559)
needle exchange programs (NEPs)　(p. 568)
penile or male condoms　(p. 563)
safer sex fatigue　(p. 564)
sexual health education　(p. 563)
sexually transmitted and blood-borne infections (STBBIs)　(p. 558)
sexually transmitted infection (STI)　(p. 558)
syndemics　(p. 567)
syphilis　(p. 559)
supervised consumption sites (SCS)　(p. 568)
trichomoniasis　(p. 560)
vaginitis　(p. 560)
vaginal or female condoms　(p. 563)
vertical transmission　(p. 558)

STUDY QUESTIONS

1. When developing information on STBBIs, what are the three most common bacterial STBBIs and their symptoms that would need to be included?

2. What three key messages about HIV transmission would a CHN want to include in a community presentation on "Protecting Yourself from HIV"?

3. What are three main points plus supporting evidence that a CHN could integrate into client sexual health history taking to increase safer sexual practices and potentially reduce the transmission of STBBIs?

4. What strategies can a CHN ensure are in place within primary health services to help prevent congenital syphilis?

5. How would a CHN describe supervised consumption sites when planning a community harm-reduction strategy?

INDIVIDUAL CRITICAL-THINKING EXERCISES

1. Reflect on your personal values related to sexuality. How do personal values impact sexual health education?

2. STI rates are increasing in males 15–24 years old. The PHAC states that testing and education are important to prevent STIs. Unfortunately, many youth at risk for STIs leave school early and become street involved, thus missing the benefit of sexual health education. What determinants of health could be addressed by CHNs related to the issues of street youth and STBBIs?

3. Search the Internet and find one STBBI prevention resource that can be used with teens. How can CHNs use this resource in a teen clinic?

4. The recommendation to vaccinate elementary schoolchildren against HPV has caused controversy in Canada. What can CHNs say to parents who are uncertain of whether or not to have their children vaccinated?

5. People involved in the sex work may participate in higher risk sexual behaviours (e.g., condomless sex, sex with multiple partners), placing them at risk for STBBIs. How can CHNs protect and promote the sexual health of this population?

GROUP CRITICAL-THINKING EXERCISES

1. LGBTQ2S youth often face rejection from significant support systems such as family and friends when they "come out." Some youth quit school and leave home to live on the street. Some rely on panhandling and sex work to support themselves or to pay for drugs that help them cope. High-risk activities and a lack of resources increase these youths' risk for STBBIs. How can a CHN use the Canadian Community Health Nursing Standards of Practice to plan care for these youth at a sexual health clinic?

2. To address the complications associated with STBBIs, healthy public policy has been initiated and developed by policy makers and health professionals but often with little input from the public. How can CHNs use primary health care's principle of public participation to inform the development of healthy public policy related to STBBIs?

3. Social marketing campaigns can be effective in raising awareness about public health issues.

   a) Create an idea for a social marketing campaign addressing rising rates of STBBIs.
   b) What is (are) the objective(s) of the campaign?
   c) What is the message of the campaign?
   d) How will the message be delivered?

REFERENCES

Ahmad, J. (2017). Hepatitis C. *British Medical Journal, 358.* Retrieved from: http://www.bmj.com.ahs.idm.oclc.org/content/bmj/358/bmj.j2861.full.pdf

Ahmed, R., Angel, C., Martel, R., Martel, R, Payne, D., & Keenan, L. (2016). Access to healthcare services during incarceration among female inmates. *International Journal of Prisoner Health, 12*(4), 204–215.

Alberta Health Services Sexual & Reproductive Health Calgary Zone (2018a). *Sexual orientation, gender identity & gender expression (SOGIE): An introductory toolkit for creating safer and welcoming healthcare.* Calgary, AB: Author.

Alberta Health Services Sexual & Reproductive Health Calgary Zone. (2018b). *Evaluation of sexuality education programming.* Calgary, AB: Author.

Andermann, A. (2017). Outbreaks in the age of syndemics: New insights for improving Indigenous health. *Canada Communicable Disease Report, 43*(6), 125–129.

Argento, E., Duff, P., Bingham, B., Chapman, J., Nguyen, P., Strathdee, S. A., & Shannon, K. (2016). Social cohesion among sex workers and client condom refusal in a Canadian setting: Implications for structural and community-led interventions. *AIDS and Behavior, 20*(6), 1275–1283.

BC Centre for Disease Control. (2016). *GetCheckedOnline.* Retrieved from https://getcheckedonline.com/Pages/default.aspx

Black, A., Guilbert, E., Costescu, D., Dunn, S., Fisher, W., Kives, S., . . . Whelan, A. M. (2015). Canadian contraception consensus (part 2 of 4). *Journal of Obstetrics and Gynaecology Canada, 37*(11), 1033–1035.

Bourgeois, A. C., Edmunds, M., Awan, A., Jonah, L., Varsaneux, O., & Siu, W. (2017a). *HIV in Canada—Supplementary tables, 2016.* Retrieved from https://www.canada.ca/en/public-health/services/reports-publications/canada-communicable-disease-report-ccdr/monthly-issue/2017-43/ccdr-volume-43-12-december-7-2017/hiv-2016-supplementary-tables.html

Bourgeois, A. C., Edmunds, M., Awan, A., Jonah, L., Varsaneux, O., & Siu, W. (2017b). HIV in Canada—Surveillance report, 2016. *Canada Communicable Disease Report, 43*(12), 248–256.

Campbell, C. E., & Herten, R. J. (1981). VD to STD: Redefining venereal disease. *The American Journal of Nursing, 81*(9), 1629–1635.

Canada's Source for HIV and Hepatitis C Information (CATIE). (2011). *Post-exposure prophylaxis (PEP).* Retrieved from http://www.catie.ca/en/fact-sheets/prevention/post-exposure-prophylaxis-pep

Canada's Source for HIV and Hepatitis C Information (CATIE). (2015). Rapid point-of-care HIV testing: A review of evidence. Retrieved from http://www.catie.ca/en/pif/spring-2015/rapid-point-care-hiv-testing-review-evidence

Canada's Source for HIV and Hepatitis C Information (CATIE). (2017). *Oral pre-exposure prophylaxis (PrEP).* Retrieved from http://www.catie.ca/fact-sheets/prevention/pre-exposure-prophylaxis-prep

Canadian Aboriginal AIDS Network. (2018). *HIV in Canada: A primer for service providers.* Retrieved from http://www.catie.ca/en/hiv-canada/2/2-3/2-3-4

Canadian Blood Services. (2016). *Surveillance report 2015.* Retrieved from https://blood.ca/sites/default/files/External_Surveillance_Report_2015.pdf

Canadian Paediatric Society. (2008). Harm reduction: An approach to reducing risky health behaviours in adolescents. *Paediatric Child Health, 13*(1), 53–56.

Canadian Public Health Association (CPHA). (n.d.). *Sexually transmitted infections and blood-borne infections (STBBIs) and related stigma.* Retrieved from https://www.cpha.ca/sexually-transmitted-and-blood-borne-infections-stbbis-and-related-stigma-0

Canadian Public Health Association (CPHA). (2017). *Organizational assessment tool: For sexually transmitted and blood-borne infections (STBBIs) and stigma.* Retrieved from https://www.cpha.ca/sites/default/files/uploads/resources/stbbi/orgtool_e.pdf

Comack, E., & Seshia, M. (2010). Bad dates and street hassles: Violence in the Winnipeg street sex trade. *Canadian Journal of Criminology and Criminal Justice, 52*(2) 203–214.

Community Health Nurses of Canada (CHNC). (2019, revised). *Canadian community health nursing: Professional practice model & standards of practice—Revised March 2011.* St. John's, NL: Author. Reprinted with permission. Further reproduction prohibited. Retrieved from https://www.chnc.ca/documents/CHNC-ProfessionalPracticeModel-EN/index.html

Deering, K. N., Montaner, J. S., Chettiar, J., Jia, J., Ogilvie, G., Buchner, C., . . . & Shannon, K. (2015). Successes and gaps in uptake of regular, voluntary HIV testing for hidden street-and off-street sex workers in Vancouver, Canada. *AIDS Care, 27*(4), 499–506.

Elliott, R., Malkin, I., & Gold, J. (2002). *Establishing safe injection facilities in Canada: Legal and ethical issues.* Ottawa, ON: Canadian HIV/AIDS Legal Network.

GlaxoSmithKline. (2010). *Health Canada approves Cervarix, new GSK cervical cancer vaccine.* Retrieved from http://www.gsk.ca/english/docs-pdf/FINAL_Press_Release_Cervarix_EN.pdf

GlaxoSmithKline. (2014). *Product monograph: Cervarix.* Retrieved from http://www.gsk.ca/english/docs-pdf/product-monographs/Cervarix.pdf

Grier, S., & Bryant, C. A. (2005). Social marketing in public health. *Annual Review of Public Health, 26,* 319–339.

Government of Alberta. (2012). *Alberta treatment guidelines for sexually transmitted infections (STI) in adolescents and adults.* Retrieved from https://open.alberta.ca/dataset/6880386/resource/bc4f118e-ebc7-4584-a430-27eae8b5d0a9

Government of Alberta. (2014). *Health and wellness interactive health data application.* Retrieved from http://www.ahw.gov.ab.ca/IHDA_Retrieval

Government of Alberta. (2015). *HIV-positive individuals who are unwilling or unable to prevent the spread of HIV in Alberta.* Retrieved from https://open.alberta.ca/dataset/376a4ee2-b93d-44b3-8065-478a365e1ebd/resource/5d2df284-5a61-4974-b91e-48dfccd0fcaa/download/HIV-Positive-Spread-HIV-Report-2015.pdf

Government of Alberta. (2017). *Preventing sexually transmitted infections.* Retrieved from https://www.alberta.ca/release.cfm?xID=499655A3FBA9E-B943-CECC-7FC53A8C-C2A090D5

Government of Canada. (2006). *Sexually transmitted infections.* Retrieved from https://www.canada.ca/en/health-canada/services/health-concerns/diseases-conditions/sexually-transmitted-infections.html

Government of Canada. (2015). *Syphilis.* Retrieved from https://www.canada.ca/en/public-health/services/diseases/syphilis.html

Government of Canada. (2017a). *Statement on behalf of the Council of Chief Medical Officers of Health.* Retrieved from https://www.canada.ca/en/public-health/news/2017/11/statement_on_behalfofthecouncilofchiefmedicalofficersofhealth.html

Government of Canada. (2017b). *For health professionals: HIV and AIDS.* Retrieved from https://www.canada.ca/en/public-health/services/diseases/hiv-aids/health-professionals-hiv-aids.html#s1

Government of Canada. (2017c). *Human papillomavirus (HPV).* Retrieved from https://www.canada.ca/en/public-health/services/diseases/human-papillomavirus-hpv.html?_ga=2.66221867.447107789.1516277899-379693334.1516277899

Government of Canada. (2018). *Supervised consumption sites: status of applications.* Retrieved from, https://www.canada.ca/en/health-canada/services/substance-abuse/supervised-consumption-sites/status-application.html

Hamilton, N., & Bhatti, T. (1996). *Population health promotion: An integrated model of population health and health promotion.* Ottawa, ON: Public Health Agency of Canada, Health Promotion Development Division. Retrieved from http://www.phac-aspc.gc.ca/ph-sp/php-psp/index-eng.php

Hanif, H., Bastos, F. I., Malta, M., Bertoni, N., Winch, P. J., & Kerrigan, D. (2014). Where does treatment optimism fit in? Examining factors associated with consistent condom use among people receiving antiretroviral treatment in Rio de Janeiro, Brazil. *AIDS and Behavior, 18*(10), 1945–1954.

Karamouzian, M., Shoveller, J., Dong, H., Gilbert, M., Kerr, T., & DeBeck, K. (2017). Perceived devaluation and STI testing uptake among a cohort of street-involved youth in a Canadian setting. *Archives of Sexual Behavior, 46*(7), 2165–2172.

Kouyoumdjian, F. G., Main, C., Calzavara, L. M., & Kiefer, L. (2011). Prevalence and predictors of urethral chlamydia and gonorrhea infection in male inmates in an Ontario correctional facility. *Canadian Journal of Public Health, 102*(3), 220–224.

Lazarus, L., Deering, K. N., Nabess, R., Gibson, K., Tyndall, M. W., & Shannon, K. (2012). Occupational stigma as a primary barrier to health care for street-based sex workers in Canada. *Culture, Health & Sexuality, 14*(2), 139–150.

Lokanc-Diluzio, W. (2014). A mixed methods study of service provider capacity development to protect and promote the sexual and reproductive health of street-involved youth: An evaluation of two training approaches. (Doctoral dissertation). Retrieved from http://hdl.handle.net/11023/1507

Lokanc-Diluzio, W., & Reilly, S. M. (2016). Enhancing the personal skills of service providers to promote the sexual health of street-involved youth. In A. R. Vollman, E. T. Anderson, & J. McFarlane (Eds.), *Canadian community as partner: Theory & multidisciplinary practice* (4th ed.). New York, NY: Wolters Kluwer Health.

Macapagal, K., Birkett, M., Janulis, P., Garofalo, R., & Mustanski, B. (2017). HIV prevention fatigue and HIV treatment optimism among young men who have sex with men. *AIDS Education and Prevention, 29*(4), 289–301.

McKay, A. (2006). Chlamydia screening programs: A review of the literature. Part 1: Issues in the promotion of chlamydia testing of youth by primary care physicians. *The Canadian Journal of Human Sexuality, 15,* 111.

Moore, D. L., & MacDonald, N. E. (2015). Preventing ophthalmia neonatorum. *Paediatrics & Child Health, 20*(2), 93–96.

National Advisory Council on Immunization (NACI). (2007). Statement on human papillomavirus vaccine. *Canadian Communicable Disease Report, 33*(ACS-2), 1–32.

National Advisory Council on Immunization (NACI). (2012). Update on human papillomavirus (HPV) vaccines. *Canadian Communicable Disease Report, 38*(ACS-1), 1–62. Retrieved from http://www.phac-aspc.gc.ca/publicat/ccdr-rmtc/12vol38/acs-dcc-1/index-eng.php

Ng, J., Sutherland, C., & Kolber, M. R. (2017). Does evidence support supervised injection sites? *Canadian Family Physician, 63*(11), 866.

Ottawa Public Health. (2011). *Enhanced street youth surveillance in Ottawa 2011.* Ottawa, ON: Author. Retrieved from http://ottawa.ca/calendar/ottawa/citycouncil/obh/2011/11-21/F%205788%20OPH%20E%20SYS%20Report%20Eng%20WEB%20Tagged%20Nov14-11.pdf

Porta, M. (Ed.). (2014). *A dictionary of epidemiology* (6th ed.). Oxford University Press.

Public Health Agency of Canada (PHAC). (2008). *Canadian guidelines for sexual health education.* Ottawa, ON: Author. Retrieved from http://www.phac-aspc.gc.ca/publicat/cgsheldnemss/index-eng.php

Public Health Agency of Canada (PHAC). (2009). *Transfusion transmitted injuries section: Transfusion transmitted diseases/infections.* Ottawa, ON: Author.

Public Health Agency of Canada (PHAC). (2011). *Report on sexually transmitted infections in Canada: 2009.* Ottawa, ON: Author. Retrieved from http://www.catie.ca/sites/default/files/2009%20Report%20on%20STI%20in%20Canada_EN.pdf

Public Health Agency of Canada (PHAC). (2012a). *HIV and AIDS in Canada: Surveillance report to December 31, 2011.* Ottawa, ON: Author. Retrieved from http://www.catie.ca/sites/default/files/PHAC_HIV-AIDS_2011%20Report_Eng-Fr.pdf

Public Health Agency of Canada (PHAC). (2012b). *Hepatitis C in Canada: 2005–2010 Surveillance report.* Ottawa, ON: Author. Retrieved from http://www.phac-aspc.gc.ca/sti-its-surv-epi/hepc/surv-eng.php

Public Health Agency of Canada (PHAC). (2013a). *Human immunodeficiency virus: HIV screen and testing guide.* Ottawa, ON: Author. Retrieved from http://www.phac-aspc.gc.ca/aids-sida/guide/hivstg-vihgdd-eng.php

Public Health Agency of Canada (PHAC). (2013b). *Canadian immunization guide: Evergreen edition.* Ottawa, ON: Author. Retrieved from http://www.phac-aspc.gc.ca/publicat/cig-gci/index-eng.php#toc

Public Health Agency of Canada (PHAC). (2013c). *The chief public health officer's report on the state of public health in Canada, 2013: Infectious disease—The never ending threat.* Ottawa, ON: Author. Retrieved from http://www.phac-aspc.gc.ca/cphorsphc-respcacsp/2013/index-eng.php

Public Health Agency of Canada (PHAC). (2014). *HIV/AIDS epi updates.* Chapter 8: HIV/AIDS among Aboriginal People in Canada. Retrieved from http://www.catie.ca/sites/default/files/Chapter-8-Epi-Update-Aboriginal-people-in-Canada.pdf

Public Health Agency of Canada (PHAC). (2015a). *Summary: Estimates of HIV incidence, prevalence and proportion undiagnosed in Canada, 2014.* Retrieved from http://www.catie.ca/sites/default/files/2014-HIV-Estimates-in-Canada-EN.pdf

Public Health Agency of Canada (PHAC). (2015b). *At a glance: Prevention of sexually transmitted and blood borne infections among ethnocultural communities.* Retrieved from https://www.canada.ca/content/dam/phac-aspc/migration/phac-aspc/std-mts/assets/pdf/blood_ethno_commun-sang_commun_ethno-eng.pdf

Public Health Agency of Canada (PHAC). (2017a). *Canadian guidelines on sexually transmitted infections.* Ottawa, ON: Author. Retrieved from https://www.canada.ca/en/public-health/services/infectious-diseases/sexual-health-sexually-transmitted-infections/canadian-guidelines/sexually-transmitted-infections.html

Public Health Agency of Canada (PHAC). (2017b). *Notifiable diseases on-line.* Ottawa, ON: Author. Retrieved from http://dsol-smed.phac-aspc.gc.ca/dsol-smed/ndis/index-eng.php

Rowniak, S. (2009). Safe sex fatigue, treatment optimism, and serosorting: New challenges to HIV prevention among men who have sex with men. *Journal of the Association of Nurses in AIDS Care, 20*(1), 31–38.

Shier, M., & Bryson, P. (2007). Vaccines. *Journal of Obstetrics and Gynaecology Canada, 29*(8), S51–S54.

Shriver, S. P., Byer, C. O., Shainberg, L. W., & Galliano, G. (2002). *Dimensions of human sexuality* (6th ed.). Boston, MA: McGraw-Hill.

Shoveller, J., Knight, R., Davis, W., Gilbert, M., & Ogilvie, G. (2012). Online sexual health services: Examining youth's perspectives. *Canadian Journal of Public Health, 103*(1), 14–18.

Small, W., Shoveller, J., Moore, D., Tyndall, M., Wood, E., & Kerr, T. (2011). Injection drug users' access to a supervised injection facility in Vancouver, Canada: The influence of operating policies and local drug culture. *Qualitative Health Research, 21*(6), 743–756.

Society of Obstetricians and Gynaecologists of Canada. (n.d.). *Prevention.* Retrieved from http://hpvinfo.ca/prevention

Sou, J., Shannon, K., Li, J., Nguyen, P., Strathdee, S., Shoveller, J., & Goldenberg, S. M. (2015). Structural determinants of inconsistent condom use with clients among migrant sex workers: Findings of longitudinal research in an urban Canadian setting. *Sexually Transmitted Diseases, 42*(6), 312–316. doi:10.1097/OLQ.0000000000000276

TASCC. (2018). *About TASCC.* Retrieved from https://tasccalberta.com/about-tascc

UNAIDS. (2015). *UNAIDS terminology guidelines.* Retrieved from http://www.unaids.org/sites/default/files/media_asset/2015_terminology_guidelines_en.pdf

University of Ottawa. (2015). *Categories of prevention.* Retrieved from https://www.med.uottawa.ca/sim/data/Prevention_e .htm

Vollman, A. R., Anderson, E. T., & McFarlane, J. (2017). *Canadian community as partner: Theory and multidisciplinary practice* (4th ed.). Philadelphia, PA: Wolters Kluwer.

Wagner, A. C., McShane, K. E., Hart, T. A., & Margolese, S. (2016). A focus group qualitative study of HIV stigma in the Canadian healthcare system. *The Canadian Journal of Human Sexuality, 25*(1), 61–71.

Werb, D., Kerr, T., Buxton, J., Shoveller, J., Richardson, C., Montaner, J., & Wood, E. (2013). Patterns of injection drug use cessation during an expansion of syringe exchange services in a Canadian setting. *Drug and Alcohol Dependence, 132*(3), 535–540.

Zhang, Q., Huhn, K. J., Tan, A., Douglas, R. E., Li, H.G., Murti, M., & Lee, V. (2017). "Testing is Healthy" TimePlay campaign: Evaluation of sexual health promotion gamification intervention targeting young adults. *Canadian Journal of Public Health, 108*(1), E85–E90.

ABOUT THE AUTHORS

Wendi Lokanc-Diluzio, RN, BN (University of Calgary), MN (University of Calgary), PhD (University of Calgary), has worked in public health since 1997. Since 2002, Wendi has worked as a sexual and reproductive health specialist for Alberta Health Services, where she provides leadership in the area of child and youth sexual health promotion, service provider education and training, and program evaluation. Wendi is currently a co-investigator with the University of Calgary, Faculty of Nursing, and an instructor with the University of Lethbridge and the University of Alberta.

Tammy Troute-Wood, RN, BScN (British Columbia Institute of Technology), MN (Athabasca University), has worked in the area of reproductive health since 1994. Since 2008 Tammy has worked as a sexual and reproductive health specialist for Alberta Health Services. Her passion is capacity building with health care providers for increasing knowledge and comfort for healthy sexuality, inclusive and affirming care, and transforming these skills into professional practice. Tammy volunteers as a board member for the Alberta Society for the Promotion of Sexual Health and is an instructor at the University of Lethbridge and the University of Alberta.

Emergency Preparedness and Disaster Nursing

Alana Devereaux and Claire Farella

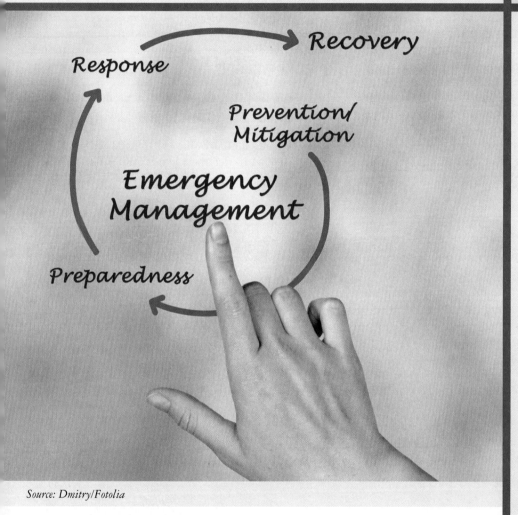

Source: Dmitry/Fotolia

LEARNING OUTCOMES

After studying this chapter, you should be able to:

1. Define disaster, the various types of disasters, and their consequences.

2. Describe national legislative frameworks and key activities involved in Canadian public safety and emergency preparedness.

3. Discuss examples of past crises in public health.

4. Explain the roles and responsibilities of the Public Health Agency of Canada in emergency preparedness using a health equity and social justice lens.

5. Identify the key functions and roles of community health organizations and community health nurses before, during, and following a public health disaster.

6. Discuss the safety of vulnerable and priority populations during and following disasters.

INTRODUCTION

In the last decade, over 2.6 billion people in more than 45 countries worldwide experienced health threats as a result of natural disasters or social and economic crises; enormous efforts were required to save lives and reduce illness and suffering (World Health Organization [WHO], 2014). Different types of disasters vary in severity, each with its own degree of death, mass injury, illness, and loss. How a disaster will impact a community depends on the community's social, cultural, economic, and health makeup. In order to respond effectively in a disaster situation, special expertise in emergency management is required.

Emergency preparedness and disaster nursing is an emerging specialty. The Canadian Nurses Association (CNA) (2014) states that registered nurses must be well prepared to respond and provide essential services to people affected by disasters with a goal to preserve health and safety. This chapter begins with a description of the different types of disasters, followed by a discussion of public safety and emergency preparedness in Canada. Different crises in public health and responses are also discussed. Last, an overview of the roles of different community health organizations and community health nurses (CHNs) in emergency planning and disaster situations is discussed.

WHAT IS A DISASTER?

Disasters typically occur suddenly and can be caused by nature, human error, biological hazards, or infectious diseases. They include earthquakes, floods, fires, hurricanes, major storms, volcanic eruptions, spills, air crashes, droughts, epidemics, food shortages, and civil strife (Landesman, 2012). Disasters often are perceived as random killers. They affect public safety and leave communities with long-term adverse socioeconomic, health, and environmental effects. Individuals at greatest risk include vulnerable or priority groups such as women, children, older adults, the poor, and people with mental and physical disabilities (Centers for Disease Control and Prevention, 2015; Statistics Canada, 2016). Life-threatening conditions brought on by disasters and their adverse health effects often result in increased mortality and morbidity.

According to the Canadian Disaster Database (Public Safety Canada, 2013a), chemical and fuel spills, floods, snowstorms, and forest fires were the most common disasters in Canada in the last decade. (See Table 32.1.)

Types of Disasters

Natural Disasters **Natural disasters** are unpredictable; they can happen very quickly or slowly. However, with advance warning, such as weather reports, impacts can sometimes be mitigated. Some examples of natural disasters include droughts, heat waves, ice storms, heavy snowfalls, earthquakes, tornadoes, floods or thunderstorms, tsunamis, volcanoes, wildfires, train derailments, and plane crashes. Recent incidents of natural disasters include the December 24, 2004, earthquake, which triggered a massive tsunami that hit Southeast Asia, leaving 280 931 dead; and the earthquake in Haiti on January 12, 2010, that left approximately 150 000 dead (Cable News Network, 2013). In 2017, wildfires in British Columbia burned 1216 350 hectares, causing 65 000 residents to flee their homes (BC Wildfire Service, 2017).

Table 32.1	**Selected Canadian Disasters**	
Date and Location	**Disaster**	**Human Consequences (Number of People)**
1918 to 1925 Canada	Spanish flu	2 million people ill, over 50 000 died
1936 Canada	Heat wave (2 weeks)	1180 died
2000 Ontario (Walkerton)	Drinking water contamination	7 died, 2300 injured
2003 Canada (Toronto)	SARS epidemic	44 died (of 438 cases)
2005 Alberta (16 communities)	Floods	2 dead, 7028 evacuated, ~40 000 homes damaged
2009 Across Canada	Biological epidemic	425 fatalities, 8582 injured/infected
2009 British Columbia	Wildfire	20 000 evacuated
2010 Newfoundland[1]	Hurricane	7000+ affected
2011 Alberta	Wildfire	12 055 evacuated
2011 Goderich, Ontario	Tornado	1 died, 37 injured
2013 Alberta	Flood	100 000+ evacuated
2013 Quebec (Lac-Mégantic)	Runaway train derailed and exploded	42 died, 5 missing
2013 Ontario (Toronto)[2]	Ice storm	230 000 affected (without power)
2016 Alberta (Fort McMurray)	Wildfires	~90 000 evacuated, 2 dead
2017 British Columbia[3]	Wildfires	~65 000 evacuated

Source: Adapted from Public Safety Canada. (2013a).

Sources: [1]CBC (2010).

[2]CBC (2013).

[3]BC Wildfire Service (2017).

Human-Made Disasters **Human-made disasters** often result in mass numbers of civilian injuries and deaths. Bioterrorism, bombings, and technical disasters, such as nuclear disasters and oil spills, are all examples of human-made disasters.

The September 11, 2001, terrorist attacks on the World Trade Center in New York and the Pentagon in Washington in the United States are among the most recent and well-watched examples of a human-made disaster. Twenty-five Canadians were among the 2977 killed when terrorists attacked the World Trade Center towers (Weinreb, 2007).

Bioterrorism is the intentional use of a micro-organism to cause infection or death. The release of smallpox or anthrax with the intent to infect humans is an example of a bioterrorist attack. Ideologically or politically inspired bombings and riots resulting in social instability are also examples of human-made disasters.

Technological malfunctions can occur in industrial sites and can be triggered by a natural disaster. Contamination of the water or food supply, the unintentional release of deadly airborne substances, such as anthrax, fires, explosions, oil spills, and exposure to hazardous materials are all conduits for technological disasters. Building or bridge collapses, transportation crashes, dam or levee failures, nuclear reactor accidents, and breaks in water, gas, deep-sea oil drilling, and sewer lines may also result in a disaster of this type (Canadian Broadcasting Cooperation [CBC], 2010; Landesman, 2012). Both human-made and natural disasters leave people injured, put emergency responders at risk, and have a lasting financial, environmental, or health impact on the communities they affect.

Epidemics An **epidemic** can occur when an infectious disease spreads rapidly, affecting a large number of individuals within a population, community, or region. This can quickly lead to an emergency situation if the right conditions exist. Conditions that to contribute to epidemic development include being exposed to a densely populated area, lack or loss of proper sanitation and hygiene practices, lack of equipment and supplies, lack of experienced professional personnel to manage the epidemic, and lack of or disrupted public health services.

The current Canadian opioid crisis is an example of an epidemic that is not caused by an infectious disease. The creation of illicit (non-prescription) opioids such as fentanyl, in uncontrolled environments, has increased the number of people overdosing, significantly impacting national morbidity and mortality rates (Canadian Public Health Association, 2016). Epidemics of any kind often lead to economic and social disruptions.

Epidemics become **pandemics** when the infection becomes widespread in different parts of the globe and affects a significantly higher proportion of the population than normal. The emergence of the 2009 H1N1 influenza A virus in humans in Mexico is an example of how a local infectious disease outbreak can spread internationally and be declared a pandemic within months (Public Health Agency of Canada, [PHAC], 2010).

PUBLIC SAFETY AND EMERGENCY PREPAREDNESS IN CANADA

Disaster preparedness and response at national and provincial or territorial levels ensures support for public health authorities and other officials who are responsible for managing the health of their community before, during, and after a disaster. Public health officials attend to prevention of infectious disease and injury. They routinely conduct surveillance for infectious disease, and they work in collaboration with other agencies within the health sector. They have governmental jurisdiction to oversee the public's health, and they use triage skills in disaster situations (PHAC, 2012).

Emergency management and preparedness responses in Canada begin at the local level. Local municipalities have the first responsibility in managing an emergency, and if their capacity is exceeded, they call on their respective province, which in turn can call on the federal government for assistance. Therefore, local emergency preparedness plans are key to the success in managing emergencies. Some countries have an opposite response chain of command in place: all responses to large-scale emergencies and disasters are initiated at the federal level.

Government Authority and Legislative Framework

Federal legislation with respect to emergencies and emergency preparedness is found in three complementary acts: the Emergencies Act, the Emergency Preparedness Act, and the Emergency Management Act. The first two legislations were enacted in 1988, at which time the Emergencies Act replaced the War Measures Act as the source of the federal government's authority to act in the event of a national emergency.

The Emergencies Act The **Emergencies Act** (Ministry of Justice, 2014a) allows the federal government to grant the use of special powers to ensure the safety and security of Canadians during a national emergency. The Emergencies Act defines a **national emergency** as "an urgent and critical situation of a temporary nature that seriously endangers the lives, health or safety of Canadians and is of such proportions or nature as to exceed the capacity or authority of a province to deal with it, or seriously threatens the ability of the Government of Canada to preserve the sovereignty, security and territorial integrity of Canada, and cannot be effectively dealt with under any other law of Canada" (p. 8).

Federal government intervention is restricted to only the most serious emergency situations, while respecting the authority of the provinces and territories to govern within their own geographical jurisdictions.

There are four categories of national emergency:

1. *public welfare emergencies*, such as a major natural disaster or accident, which are beyond the authority of the province or territory in which the disaster occurs to address;

2. *public order emergencies*, wherein there is a serious national security threat;

3. *international emergencies* arising from acts of coercion or intimidation or the serious use of force or violence, which threaten the sovereignty, security, or territorial integrity of Canada or its allies; and

4. *a state of war*, either active or imminent, involving Canada or its allies.

It is important to note that the extraordinary powers extended by the federal government must be tailored to the specific disaster and may not exceed what is necessary to deal with the situation. The Emergencies Act is not designed to justify the arbitrary or excessive use of power on the part of the federal government.

The Emergency Preparedness Act The **Emergency Preparedness Act** (Ministry of Justice, 2014c) functions as companion legislation to the Emergencies Act. While the Emergencies Act provides the authority for government action, the Emergency Preparedness Act provides a basis for the planning necessary to address disasters of all kinds. Specifically, the Emergency Preparedness Act addresses the need for cooperation between the provinces and territories at the federal level to establish responsibilities and provides structure for training and education in emergency planning.

The Emergency Management Act The **Emergency Management Act** (Ministry of Justice, 2014b) replaces parts of the Emergency Preparedness Act to strengthen the government's readiness to respond to major emergencies by defining the roles and responsibilities for all federal ministers. It also enhances information sharing between various levels of government and the private sector. It provides critical infrastructure consisting of physical and information technology facilities, networks, services, and assets that are vital to the health, safety, security, or economic well-being of Canadians and for the effective functioning of governments in Canada (Public Safety Canada, 2013b).

Emergency Management

Emergency management is an essential discipline involving a diverse group of professionals, with the ultimate responsibility resting with the government to assess and deal with risk in an effort to protect the health and safety of the public. A "crisis" or "emergency" is a threatening condition that requires urgent action. Effective emergency management action can avoid the escalation of an event into a disaster.

Hazard Identification Risk Assessment

Emergency response plans generally use an all-hazards approach where activities will be applicable to any type of emergency.

Communication and media plans, business continuity plans, employee health and safety plans, and procurement of supplies and purchasing plans are examples of strategies generic to all response plans. The Hazard Identification Risk Assessment (HIRA) is a tool used to prepare for the worst and most likely risks specific to communities. By completing a HIRA, organizations can prioritize specific threats based on risk of probability and consequence or impact. **Probability** is the likelihood of an event occurring within a given time period. **Impact** assesses the level or degree to which the hazard will affect three critical dimensions: human, physical infrastructure, and business impacts.

All levels of government as well as public health agencies and hospitals use this process. Community-level response organizations, such as public health units and hospitals, need to incorporate the individual response plans into a local coordinated community response plan. For example, a fire services agency is the lead for responding to a hazardous materials spill in the community, whereas the public health unit and the hospital would have supporting roles. In comparison, public health would be the lead in responding to a community infectious disease outbreak, and the local first-responder agencies would have supporting roles.

Stages of Emergency Management

In some provinces in Canada, such as in Ontario, emergency management programming is organized into five stages: prevention, mitigation, preparedness, response, and recovery, as outlined by the Public Health Ontario (2014). In some provinces the prevention and mitigation stages are addressed together and are continuously ongoing.

1. *Prevention* involves activities taken to prevent or avoid an emergency or disaster, before the emergency. It focuses on the hazard by promoting healthy lifestyles through public health education.

2. *Mitigation* involves actions that can reduce the impact of a disaster on the community. Influenza vaccination and infection control measures are health-specific examples of mitigation.

3. *Preparedness* programs are intended to maximize the efficiency of the response through planning and preparation. Actions taken before the emergency focus on plans to establish communication systems, conduct training, and test response plans.

4. *Response* activities are designed to address the immediate effects of an emergency. They focus on operations and include the mobilization of providers, the coordination of health care services, and the acquisition of necessary supplies.

5. *Recovery* programs are designed to return a situation to an acceptable and normal condition. Recovery is usually the longest phase and focuses on restoration. It includes

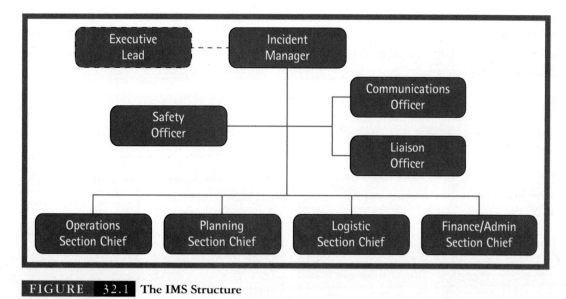

FIGURE 32.1 The IMS Structure

Source: PHO (2016).

activities to restore services, rebuild infrastructure, and care for the sick or injured. It may also include prevention or mitigation measures designed to avert future emergencies.

Organizational Structure and Chain of Command: National Incident Management System

An international system known as the **National Incident Management System (NIMS)** was developed by the Department of Homeland Security in the United States and released in March 2004. The Government of Canada adopted the NIMS structure as a framework to develop emergency response plans for different emergencies, of varying complexity, among all levels of government in Canada.

Incident Management System

The **Incident Management System (IMS)** is a standardized, function-driven model used by agencies throughout North America to manage and respond to emergencies. A similar version, the **Incident Command System (ICS)**, is used at on-site emergency scenes by first responders using a formal command approach. Public health authorities use the IMS as an operational framework for emergency preparedness and response planning. Lessons from previous complex emergencies have demonstrated the need for such a standardized incident management system to avoid confusion and enhance response (Ministry of Community Safety and Correctional Services, 2016). The benefits of the IMS are to enhance capacity, streamline resources, improve communication, and facilitate

the cooperation of activities and interoperability among organizations.

The basic IMS structure consists of five components: command, operations, planning, logistics, and finance and administration. (See Figure 32.1 and Table 32.2 on page 584.) The pertinent functional components are established only when necessary, depending on the magnitude of the emergency. Within the IMS, staff can communicate directly with other health care jurisdictions and emergency response organizations. This is done to coordinate the distribution of medical supplies from federal and provincial logistical section stockpiles the front-line local health units.

Integrated Community Emergency Preparedness

Although provincial and federal emergency preparedness and response-planning parameters can provide local community emergency planners with a variety of tools and structure, local community response mechanisms are often led by first-responder agencies, such as police, fire, and emergency medical services, to manage health or non-health emergencies. As infectious disease–related emergencies occur more often, local planners must engage all health care professionals and agencies in planning for a health-related emergency. In this instance, the health care sector becomes the lead or command agency, with emergency-response agencies having a supporting role. There needs to be consensus and collaboration regarding agency and professional roles in advance of any emergency. Public health agencies may facilitate these discussions and challenge key community stakeholders to develop, implement, and maintain a comprehensive preparation, response, and recovery plan for health emergencies.

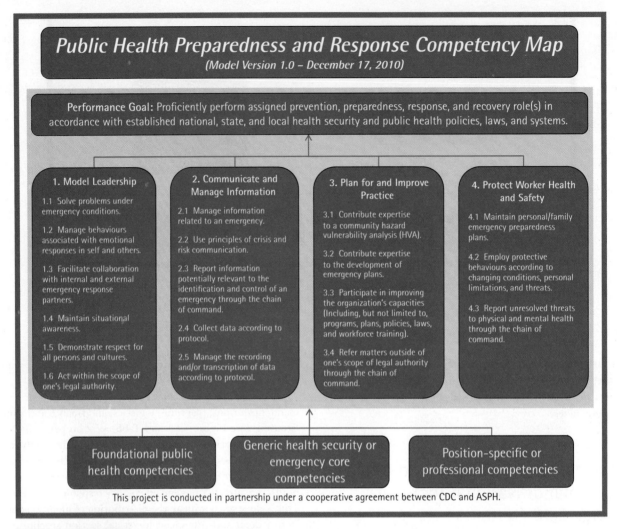

FIGURE 32.2 Public Health Preparedness and Response Competency Map

Source: Association of Schools and Programs of Public Health. (2010, December 17). *Public health preparedness and response core competency model* (p. 2). Retrieved from http://www.cdc .gov/phpr/documents/perlcPDFS/PreparednessCompetencyModelWorkforce-Version1_0.pdf

Across Canada, provincial public health units and departments have mandated requirements for fundamental public health programs and services. (See Figure 32.2.) In Ontario, a review of the 1997 Mandatory Program and Services Guidelines identified a need to add new standards and protocols. In 2008, the Emergency Preparedness Program Standard was added to the revised and newly named Ontario Public Health Standards (Ontario Ministry of Health and Long-Term Care [MOHLTC], 2008).

The goal of the Emergency Preparedness Program Standard is to enable and ensure a consistent and effective response to public health emergencies with public health impacts. The Emergency Management Guideline (MOHLTC, 2018) identifies the minimum expectations for programs and services by providing direction on how health units must operationalize specific requirements. Key components of this protocol include

- assessing the relevant hazards and risks to public health;
- developing a continuity of operations plan;

- developing an emergency response plan utilizing the IMS;
- implementing 24/7 notification protocols for communications with staff, community partners, and government bodies;
- increasing public awareness regarding emergency preparedness;
- delivering emergency preparedness and response training for health staff and officials; and
- testing the operations continuity plan, the emergency response plan, and the 24/7 notification protocols.

CRISES IN PUBLIC HEALTH

The face of emergency preparedness in Canada has been shaped by recent events that highlighted the gaps and weaknesses in the Canadian public health system and infection control capacity.

CASE STUDY

H1N1 was declared a pandemic influenza on June 11, 2009. Fortunately, immunizations were available to protect the public against the virus. However, little information existed to aid public health agencies' IMS structures in planning immunization clinics because no prior pandemic had been responded to with mass vaccinations. This was further complicated with public health nurses (PHNs) having various roles within the community and with staffing shortages (Devereaux, 2016). Canadian researcher Devereaux (2016) interviewed 23 PHNs (16 front-line immunizers, seven clinic supervisors) who worked in H1N1/09 mass vaccination clinics.

Most participants had positions in public health programs that were unrelated to vaccination and voiced feeling stress when deployed into H1N1 clinics. Those few individuals who felt equipped for H1N1/09 clinics were casual nurses who worked with regular influenza programs. Common challenges verbalized included inadequate staff training, problematic clinic locations, and the implementation of unfamiliar processes that impeded vaccination delivery (Devereaux, 2016).

Due to unfamiliarity with overall mass immunization clinics, most PHNs felt they were inadequately prepared for their roles. Despite these issues, most participants expressed personal satisfaction from working with colleagues to protect the public.

Discussion Questions

1. What type of disaster was the H1N1 influenza outbreak?

2. What did the public health agencies' IMS structures have to plan for when preparing mass vaccination clinics?

3. How can PHNs be better prepared to work in future pandemic influenza mass vaccination clinics?

The Walkerton *E. Coli* Experience

In 2000, improper execution of safe water practices in Walkerton, Ontario, led to the contamination of the town's water supply by *E. coli* O157:H7 and *Campylobacter jejuni* bacteria. One year later, the same strain of *E. coli* contaminated the drinking water in North Battleford, Saskatchewan. The Walkerton Commission of Inquiry Reports (O'Connor, 2002) highlighted the need for safe drinking water and ways to reduce the risk of infection and death.

Sudden Acute Respiratory Syndrome

In 2003, Canadians again faced the need for emergency response following the outbreak of sudden acute respiratory syndrome (SARS). SARS emerged from China in 2002 and spread quickly across the globe to Toronto (Naylor, 2003).

Following these events, there were calls for a renewal in the national public health system. All stressed the need for the federal government to provide funding support and to take stronger leadership to strengthen the public health infrastructure and health-promotion efforts in Canada (Kirby, 2003; Kirby & LeBreton, 2002).

"Learning from SARS: Renewal of Public Health in Canada: A Report of the National Advisory Committee on SARS and Public Health," known as the Naylor Report (Naylor, 2003), addressed a lack of capacity in the clinical and public health systems and epidemiological investigation of the outbreak, dysfunctional relationships between various orders of governments, absence of protocols for data or information sharing among different government levels, and inadequate business processes between and across jurisdictions for outbreak management and emergency response. The report recommended a Canadian agency for public health with a chief public health officer heading the agency and reporting to the Minister of Health, development of a national health strategy with specific health targets and benchmarks, public health partnership programs to build capacity in public health at the local or municipal level, and a national strategy to renew and sustain public health human resources (including PHNs, public health physicians, infection control practitioners, and microbiologists). The report also drew attention to the role of CHNs in emergency preparedness and noted that PHNs' contributions during the SARS outbreak received little public attention.

Listeriosis

The listeriosis outbreak in 2008 linked to deli meats produced at a Maple Leaf plant in Ontario was a significant public health event. The collective efforts of local and regional health authorities, provincial and territorial governments, and federal officials detected and contained the outbreak following three weeks of higher-than-expected case reports of listeriosis in Ontario. Eventually, seven provinces were implicated in the outbreak. Of the 56 confirmed cases (75% in Ontario) and two probable cases, there were 20 deaths across five provinces (PHAC, 2008b). Consequently, recommendations were made to improve the management of food-borne outbreaks, from clarifying the roles, responsibilities, and relationships of personnel involved to providing Public Health Agency of Canada (PHAC) staff with training and practice in outbreak response.

Pandemic H1N1 Flu Virus

Influenza, or the flu, is a common viral respiratory infection that accounts for approximately 12 200 hospitalizations and 3500 deaths annually. In the spring of 2009, H1N1 was a new strain of the influenza virus with outbreaks that started in Mexico and spread to Canada within weeks. The first Canadian cases of H1N1 were confirmed on April 26, 2009. As the H1N1 flu virus spread around the world, the World Health Organization (WHO) declared it a pandemic influenza virus (PHAC, 2014).

Influenza pandemics are difficult to predict. At the very outset of the pandemic, the PHAC called on the National Microbiology Laboratory for laboratory assistance, and five PHAC scientists helped with testing in Mexico over the course of six weeks. The PHAC was the first to characterize the entire genomic sequence of the pandemic H1N1 influenza virus; it was instrumental in making a significant contribution to international scientific understanding of this novel strain.

Canada experienced two waves of H1N1 in 2009: the first between April 12 and August 29 and the second in early November. Canada's second wave of H1N1 resulted in four to five times more hospitalizations and deaths compared with the first wave. Because H1N1 was a new strain of influenza, a large number of populations had little to no natural immunity to the virus. Those with higher rates of hospitalization and mortality were Indigenous people, pregnant women, and individuals with at least one underlying medical condition. Over 400 people in Canada died due to pandemic H1N1.

Opioid Crisis

In 2016, the opioid crisis in Canada was identified as a public health emergency. Using the epidemiological model of disease causation to illustrate, the illicit opioid is the stimulus. An individual, the host, can be impacted by a number of factors in the environment that cause the individual to engage in substance use and be negatively impacted. The growing number of overdoses and deaths caused by illicit opioids, including fentanyl, is a complex health and social issue that requires a comprehensive, collaborative, compassionate, and evidence-based response. Currently, the PHAC is enabling a pan-Canadian response to the opioid crisis that is based on the values of the Canadian drug and substance strategy. This includes a four-pillar approach focusing on prevention, harm reduction, treatment, and enforcement, which is supported by strong evidence to identify trends and best practices (Health Canada, 2017).

Provincial public health agencies take initiative and provide leadership in coordinating opioid crisis response strategies. In particular, they identify specific and targeted approaches for at-risk individuals. These include individuals living in poverty, those who have lower education, individuals with poor access to health care, and Indigenous people, who have higher reported rates of opioid abuse and related deaths (Alberta Health, 2017). All individuals at risk require strategies that are inclusive and embed a health equity and social justice lens in order to be successful.

Roles and Responsibilities for Public Health

As public health faced recent crises, such as SARS, contaminated water, food poisoning, and H1N1, various commission reports recommended that even though many emergency response organizations were using some form of the IMS, there should be one common emergency response system "to bring an orderly, consistent, and flexible chain of command and control within an emergency response" (Campbell, 2005, p. 322). Further, it was identified that the health care system needs to be properly funded in order to plan and deliver public health programs and emergency medical services. This would help build a cohesive public health model, establish infection control networks and standards, improve emergency preparedness, develop a communications infrastructure in the event of an emergency, enhance surveillance, and increase enrolment in key public health professions.

THE PUBLIC HEALTH AGENCY OF CANADA

Following the terrorist attacks of September 11, 2001, and the outbreak of SARS, Emergency Preparedness Canada was created and renamed Public Safety Canada (PS) in 2003. This was to ensure that federal departments and agencies responsible for national security and the safety of Canadians could work more closely together.

On September 24, 2004, the Government of Canada established the PHAC and appointed the first chief public health officer (CPHO) of Canada. In June 2017, Dr. Theresa Tam was named the current CPHO of Canada. The agency provides leadership in promoting health, investigating and controlling disease outbreaks, supporting public health infrastructure, and fostering collaboration across and between governments. The PHAC and PS work with the provincial and territorial governments to coordinate a unified response to any national public health emergency (PHAC, 2006). The 2006 Public Health Agency of Canada Act (Government of Canada, 2014) recognized the agency with enabling legislation and by establishing the dual role of the CPHO as head of the PHAC and lead public health professional in Canada.

PUBLIC HEALTH RESPONSE IN A DISASTER

Public health preparedness for all types of disasters, especially infectious disease emergencies, has become essential in today's world. CHNs must learn from past disasters that include infection prevention and control in mass casualty incidents, public education, internal and external communication, and building partnerships with outside agencies (Rebmann, Carrico, & English, 2008). As the largest group of health care professionals in any given jurisdiction, nurses must play pivotal advocacy and leadership roles to facilitate agency-specific and community-wide preparations for health-related emergencies and disasters. (See Canadian Research 32.1.)

CANADIAN RESEARCH 32.1

An analysis of mass casualty incidents in the setting of mass gatherings and special events (Turis, Lund, & Bowles, 2014)

This collaborative research among the School of Nursing, the Department of Emergency Medicine, and the Centre for Applied Research at the University of British Columbia analyzed the literature for mass casualty incidents (MCIs) and mass gatherings (MGs) from 1982 to 2012 to guide emergency preparedness services. Their findings revealed that of the 290 MCIs, the most frequent involved people under crowded conditions (55.9%); hazards, such as airplane crashes, pyrotechnic displays, car crashes, boat collisions (19.6%); structural failures, such as building code violations and balcony collapses (13.1%); deliberate events (9%); and toxic exposures (2.4%). These MCIs took place in North America (27%), Asia (24%), Europe (24%), Africa (17%), South America (9%), the Middle East (9%), and Australasia (1%). The researchers recommended that a centralized database be created to guide prevention efforts and minimize the effects of MCIs during MGs.

Discussion Questions

1. Give examples of at least three types of MGs.
2. Give at least three examples of categories of mass casualties or incidents.
3. What are the possible actions and implications to prevent MCIs?

ROLE OF COMMUNITY HEALTH ORGANIZATIONS IN DISASTERS

Current trends in disaster and emergency response recognize the importance of collaboration and responding using a standardized approach. The IMS provides such a model as it functions on the roles and responsibilities as assigned, not the designation of individuals assigned to those roles. Individual agencies and organizations involved in disaster and emergency response designate the most appropriate individuals to IMS roles. Depending on the type of emergency, nurses often find themselves assigned to roles such as liaison, operations, planning, and safety officer. Each has specific responsibilities that are identified in job action sheets. Tabletop scenarios are part of the preparation phase and provide the opportunity to practise the roles in relation to specific emergencies.

COMMUNITY HEALTH NURSES IN DISASTERS: THE NURSING PROCESS

Nurses play a critical role during all phases of a disaster and emergency response. They need to be knowledgeable about current emergency preparedness frameworks, structures, and responses within their own professional practice and place of employment. To effectively contribute during a disaster, CHNs must apply nursing process and be competent to respond in an emergency in areas such as leadership, communication and managing information, planning for and improving practice, and protecting worker health and safety, as outlined in Table 32.2. CHNs are accountable for having a basic understanding and knowledge of competencies related to emergency preparedness, management, and response activities.

In alignment with the emergency management structure previously identified, the role of CHNs can vary depending on the area they practise in. A PHN may focus on the health of the population, and a home health nurse may focus on the health of individuals and families. A nurse brings a unique set of skills to disaster and emergency planning, as he or she can ensure the principals of health equity and social justice are incorporated. Multisectoral collaboration informs the development of local strategies and decreases health inequities. Nurses can advocate for the opportunity to discuss the impacts of the social determinants of health on health outcomes and increased support for actions to decrease health inequities. Priority populations and First Nation, Inuit, and Métis communities need to be meaningfully engaged in planning, as this will contribute to achievable outcomes. For example, in each phase of disaster and emergency planning, consideration must be given to factors related to poverty, poor education, lack of access to health services due to geographical location, and social connectedness in order to accommodate different populations' ability to prepare as well as cope with outcomes.

The PHAC (2008a) has outlined core competencies for public health that outline the necessary knowledge, skills, and attitudes required for public health practice. The seven categories incorporate 36 competencies statements on which to base public health practice, which include preparing and responding to a disaster or emergency. The categories related to assessment, planning, partnerships and collaboration, communication, and leadership all align with the IMS structure roles and responsibilities.

The CNA provides information related to global nursing issues, including disasters. The CNA has partnered with the PHAC's Centre for Emergency Preparedness and Response to provide expertise and consultation in developing the role of nurses in a national emergency plan. The CNA (2012) articulates the integral role that the nursing profession plays in all aspects of emergencies, including prevention, mitigation, preparedness, response, and recovery. In order for an effective, coordinated community emergency response to take place, effective interprofessional collaboration and shared responsibilities among professionals in non-governmental organizations, such as the health, social services, safety, transportation, meteorology, and voluntary sectors, must be developed and nurtured before emergencies occur. Table 32.2 links the phases of a disaster to the nursing process.

The CNA (2017) also brings attention to the ethical considerations for nurses in a natural or human-made disaster, communicable disease outbreak, or pandemic. The focus is on CHNs' duty to provide care as well as what is ethically required of a nurse in the preparation and response planning phases, in particular when considering the needs of vulnerable populations.

Public health surge interventions "improve access and availability of limited health resources for the entire population"

Table 32.2	**Phases of Disaster Linked to the Nursing Process**

Examples of Each Disaster Phase Aligned with the Nursing Process

Preparedness, response, and recovery focuses on the public health infrastructure needed to monitor the environment, assess population needs, and allocate resources in times of disaster.

Based on Jakeway, Larosa, Cary, & Schoenfisch (2008).

Disaster Cycle	Definition*	Assessment	Planning	Implementation	Evaluation
Preparedness	Preparedness includes prevention, protection, and mitigation. It comprises "the capabilities necessary to avoid and/or prevent a disaster, as well as to reduce the loss of life and property by lessening the impact of disasters." Elimination of threats before a disaster strikes.	Assess the region for populations at risk for access and functional needs during times of disaster. Conduct a hazard vulnerability assessment for threats and hazards that pose the greatest risk.	Develop a care plan to address access and functional needs of populations during times of disaster. Complete this assurance function in collaboration with stakeholders to address needs such as sheltering in place, evacuation, and mass casualty surge capabilities.	Conduct training, drills, and exercises related to the care of individuals, families, and communities during disasters, focusing on populations with access and functional needs in an identified region.	Evaluate the training, drills, and exercises related to the care of populations with access and functional needs in disasters, identifying gaps and remaining needs. Evaluate operational plans for preparedness, response, and recovery for populations with access and functional needs.
Response			Collaborate with response partners to develop plans for triage algorithms that determine appropriate care and sustenance logistics for populations, based on their symptoms and co-morbid conditions (e.g., chronic disease).	Identify and place PHNs and other support personnel to provide care according to the developed algorithms. Ensure that logistics are in place to support community care during the crisis period. Conduct ongoing rapid needs assessments during the response phase in order to meet population needs.	Participate in ongoing response planning during the incident (e.g., the IMS and its Planning "P"). Participate in service planning, and provide real-time adjustment on the basis of real-time public health response evaluation. Ensure needed and necessary public health nursing care.
Recovery			Work with community stakeholders to plan for any long-term health concerns following an incident, getting ahead of the curve by identifying key resources and critical care logistics.	Participate in the reconstitution of critical services and the sustainment of the health and social infrastructure. Assist the community to find its "new normal" post-disaster.	Conduct evaluation of the long-term impact of disaster consequences on the whole community, promoting public health essential services through public health nursing.

*Definitions retrieved from www.fema.gov.

(Burkle, 2006). Mass immunization clinics during a pandemic are an example of a public health surge event. The operations of mass immunization clinics during a pandemic would overwhelm public health agencies but would have a minimal effect on hospital systems. **Medical triage** differs from public health triage in that medical triage sorts individuals to maximize the number of lives saved, and **public health triage** is the sorting or identifying of populations for priority interventions (Polivka et al., 2008). The population-based model of care used in public health practice during non-surge events needs to continue during surge events associated with public health triage. In preparation for a public health surge event related to opioid overdoses, the Ministry of Health and Long-Term Care in Ontario has given direction to public health units to develop "cluster opioid overdose response plans" to ensure communities have a coordinated approach to responding (Stewart, 2017).

SAFETY OF VULNERABLE AND PRIORITY POPULATIONS

Nursing organizations and home health nurses (HHNs) must know the types of disasters and biological agents that could occur or be released in their community to be able to provide medical management for their clients while ensuring their own personal protection when responding to an emergency. Management must provide education and training of HHNs to understand the agency emergency preparedness plan, document skill sets of each staff member, know how to answer questions, and establish a clear communication plan in an emergency response (Sawyer, 2003).

Clients receiving home care may be ventilator dependent, so their life is threatened if an electrical failure should occur. Many clients may be hearing impaired, be unable to access a telephone due to physical limitations, and have no close support from their family members who may live out of town. The Hazard Vulnerability Analysis assessment tool can be used by HHNs to determine the level of risk to their caseload of clients by focusing on "preparation" and "prevention" (Rodriguez & Long, 2006). In the event of an emergency, HHNs are in an excellent position to provide increased surveillance of those clients who make up their caseload. After assessing the client's home environment, family, social support networks, and community partners, the HHN can develop a plan to ensure communication, protect the client from death, and reduce the impact of a disaster on those most susceptible. As participants in a community emergency, HHNs can also report any suspected evidence of a biological agent, monitor and support individuals who are quarantined in their homes, and offer skills in health screening and administer vaccines at community sites.

In order to ensure that vulnerable and priority populations are protected in the event of a disaster, long-term care facilities and community-based support services must be integrated into local and regional disaster planning to provide for clear communication and appropriate response plans. Knowledge of the current and evolving health status of vulnerable and priority populations within a community will assist in the response and recovery outcomes for those affected by an emergency.

YES, BUT WHY?

Vulnerable Populations' Experiences during Disasters

What?

According to Statistics Canada (2016), a number of social, economic, and demographic characteristics have been associated with individuals exhibiting decreased levels of emergency preparedness during disasters. These individual characteristics include being a recent immigrant, a visible minority, or an older adult; having a mental health condition; and living with a decreased household income (Statistics Canada, 2016). These individuals are also more vulnerable to the negative consequences of disasters, including having limited access to community social and health services. Consequences people experience vary depending on the type of disaster that occurs. For example, unpredictable natural disasters, such as floods, might only affect localized geographical areas, whereas infectious epidemics can impact multiple regions.

So What?

It has also been found that Canadians frequently rely on their family and social connections to negate the challenges that occur during and following an emergency (Statistics Canada, 2016). However, although many Canadians have support networks, not all do. Once again, older adults, immigrants, individuals with an activity-limiting health condition, and those from lower-income households were found to have fewer existing social support connections (Statistics Canada, 2016).

Now What?

CHNs, with their skills in disaster preparedness and planning, have many different roles during emergencies, depending on the type of disaster response and how nurses are assigned within implemented IMS structures. CHNs need to become familiar with local agency emergency plans and key agency personnel, and utilize their community mobilization skills to assist in identifying and developing the required health infrastructure to ensure emergency response readiness, surge capacity, and sustainability. In particular, it is important they advocate for and assist vulnerable populations who have limited social connections. This is to ensure they have adequate and appropriate supports to manage the impacts of encountered disasters.

Standards of Practice Fulfilled

#2 Prevention and Health Protection
- Engages in collaborative, interdisciplinary and intersectoral partnerships in the delivery of preventive and protective services with particular attention to populations who are marginalized.

#4 Professional Relationships
- Builds a network of relationships and partnerships with a wide variety of individuals, families, groups, communities, and systems to address health issues and promote healthy public policy to advance health equity.

#6 Health Equity
- Assesses how the social determinants of health influence the client's health status with particular attention to clients who are marginalized (CHNC, 2019, revised).

To date, there has been limited guidance on preparedness activities addressing at-risk populations. However, efforts are being made to provide emergency-preparedness information to at-risk populations, and many innovative practices to better serve at-risk communities are being developed. The need for information exchange is significant in all phases of emergency management and particularly important for vulnerable populations. Nurses play a critical role in facilitating this exchange of knowledge and information and are often the advocacy voice for at-risk and vulnerable populations. They can also ensure that at-risk individuals and vulnerable populations are present during disaster planning discussions to influence emergency preparedness and policies, as this would allow for some of their specific needs to be identified and addressed. This is particularly important for Indigenous communities, including in rural and remote areas, who may have traditional ways of dealing with disaster that could inform the formal system plans. Health and social service agencies are starting to incorporate emergency-preparedness activities into their high-risk clients' care plans. Information and education on the contents of a 72-hour personal or family emergency-preparedness kit are provided by nurses as part of home visiting care.

CONCLUSION

This chapter has outlined the types of disasters and challenges to which the nursing profession must learn to competently respond during a disaster. It describes how the federal government works collaboratively with the provinces, territories, and individual communities from prevention to recovery of a disaster. Disaster mitigation efforts involve leadership from the PHAC; the chief public health officer; and established emergency procedures, legislation, regulations, and processes to build the current framework and legislation essential to health care delivery during any emergency.

Canadian nurses must develop an agenda that strengthens education in **disaster nursing**. An understanding of disaster training, combined with community health and public health nursing experience, as well as technological knowledge, strengthen the role of PHNs in emergency preparedness and response. New knowledge can be translated to action when nursing research is applied to emergency response practice, education, and health policy. CHNs play a vital role in emergency preparedness. They are key facilitators in the community mobilization process. Nurses contribute to the capacity to conduct surveillance; they educate health professionals, volunteers, and the public; they assess needs and allocate resources; they provide health care services; they evaluate response measures; and they make decisions about resource allocation where resources are limited (CNA, 2014).

Nurses comprise the largest group of health professionals in any given jurisdiction. CHNs who are knowledgeable and competent in emergency preparedness are necessary to meet the challenges of unpredictable threats from disaster. Further, it is essential that nurses who are experienced in emergency and disaster planning are actively involved in the development of health care policies. This will ensure future disaster responses are based on valuable nursing expertise and will help to meet the needs of vulnerable populations.

KEY TERMS

bioterrorism (p. 577)
disasters (p. 576)
disaster nursing (p. 586)
Emergencies Act (p. 577)
emergency management (p. 578)
Emergency Management Act (p. 578)
Emergency Preparedness Act (p. 578)
epidemic (p. 577)
impact (p. 578)
Incident Command System (ICS) (p. 579)
Incident Management System (IMS) (p. 579)
human-made disasters (p. 577)
medical triage (p. 585)
national emergency (p. 577)
National Incident Management System (NIMS) (p. 579)
natural disasters (p. 576)
pandemics (p. 577)
probability (p. 578)
public health surge interventions (p. 583)
public health triage (p. 585)

STUDY QUESTIONS

1. Describe the types of disasters and their consequences.

2. What are the essential elements to respond effectively in a disaster situation?

3. Distinguish among the Emergencies Act, the Emergency Preparedness Act, and the Emergency Management Act.

4. Explain the five areas of emergency management in the life-cycle process of a disaster.

5. Describe the purpose of the IMS structure in a disaster or emergency situation.

6. When nurses are participating in disaster and emergency planning, what are the unique needs of vulnerable and priority populations?

INDIVIDUAL CRITICAL-THINKING EXERCISES

1. List the community health nursing competencies and skills required in order to participate in health emergency planning, such as for an outbreak or pandemic.

2. What are the ethical issues a nurse must consider when preparing to respond to a disaster or emergency situation?

3. Discuss what CHNs must consider following a disaster.

4. How does the PHAC play a key role in emergency preparedness?

GROUP CRITICAL-THINKING EXERCISES

1. Due to flooding in a Northern Ontario reserve community, many First Nation families are unable to occupy their homes. Local politicians and emergency response planners

have declared a disaster in the area and ordered citizens to evacuate to a shelter.

    a) Utilizing a health equity and social justice lens, discuss what essential public health services are needed in this situation.

    b) How would nursing students assist in this response?

2. What special considerations need to be given when a disaster takes place in developing countries or First Nation communities?

3. Discuss what lessons were learned from disasters such as the SARS crisis for emergency preparedness planning.

REFERENCES

Alberta Health. (2017, November 6). *Opioids and substances of misuse among first nations people in Alberta.* Retrieved from https://open.alberta.ca/dataset/cb00bdd1-5d55-485a-9953-724832f373c3/resource/31c4f309-26d4-46cf-b8b23a990510077c/download/Opioids-Substances-Misuse-Report-FirstNations-2017.pdf

Association of Schools and Programs of Public Health. (2010, December 17). *Public health preparedness and response core competency model* (p. 2). Retrieved from http://www.cdc.gov/phpr/documents/perlcPDFS/PreparednessCompetency-ModelWorkforce-Version1_0.pdf

BC Wildfire Service. (2017). *Current statistics.* Retrieved from http://bcfireinfo.for.gov.bc.ca/hprScripts/WildfireNews/Statistics.asp

Burkle, F. M. (2006). Population-based triage management in response to surge-capacity requirements during a large-scale bioevent disaster. *Academic Emergency Medicine: Official Journal of the Society for Academic Emergency Medicine, 13*(11), 1118–1129.

Cable News Network. (2013, September 20). *Japan earthquake–Tsunami fast facts.* Retrieved from http://www.cnn.com/2013/07/17/world/asia/japan-earthquake—tsunami-fast-facts

Campbell, A. (2005). *The SARS Commission second interim report: SARS and public health legislation.* Retrieved from http://www.health.gov.on.ca/en/common/ministry/publications/reports/campbell05/campbell05.pdf

Canadian Broadcasting Cooperation (CBC). (2010, September 22). *Hurricane Igor attacks Newfoundland.* Retrieved from http://www.cbc.ca/news/canada/newfoundland-labrador/hurricane-igor-attacks-newfoundland-1.935880

Canadian Broadcasting Cooperation (CBC). (2013, December 23). *Toronto ice storm leaves 230,000 without power.* Retrieved from http://www.cbc.ca/news/canada/toronto/toronto-ice-storm-leaves-230-000-without-power-1.2473543

Canadian Nurses Association (CNA). (2012). *Emergency preparedness and response (Position Statement).* Ottawa, ON: Author. Retrieved from https://www.cna-aiic.ca/~/media/cna/page-content/pdf-en/ps119_emergency_preparedness_2012_e.pdf?la=en

Canadian Nurses Association (CNA). (2014). *Emergency and pandemic preparedness.* Retrieved from http://www.cna-aiic.ca/en/on-the-issues/better-health/infectious-diseases/emergency-and-pandemic-preparedness

Canadian Nurses Association (CNA). (2017). *Code of ethics.* Retrieved from https://www.cna-aiic.ca/en/on-the-issues/best-nursing/nursing-ethics

Canadian Public Health Association. (2016). *The opioid crisis in Canada: Position statement December 2016.* Retrieved from https://www.cpha.ca/sites/default/files/uploads/policy/positionstatements/opioid-positionstatement-e.pdf

Centers for Disease Control and Prevention. (2015). *Planning for an emergency: Strategies for identifying and engaging at-risk groups. A guidance document for emergency managers.* Retrieved from https://www.cdc.gov/nceh/hsb/disaster/atriskguidance.pdf

Community Health Nurses of Canada (CHNC). (2019, revised). ©Community Health Nurses of Canada. Reprinted with permission.

Devereaux, A. (2016). *Public health nurses' experiences during the H1N1/09 response* (doctoral dissertation). Retrieved from https://ruor.uottawa.ca/bitstream/10393/35260/1/Devereaux_Alana_2016_thesis.pdf

Government of Canada. (2014). Public Health Agency of Canada Act, S.S. 2006, c.5. Retrieved from http://lois-laws.justice.gc.ca/PDF/P-29.5.pdf

Health Canada. (2017, May). *Progress report on the joint statement of action to address the opioid crisis in Canada.* Retrieved from http://www.ccsa.ca/Resource%20Library/CCSA-Addressing-Opioid-Crisis-in-Canada-Summary-Report-2017-en.pdf

Jakeway, C., Larosa, G., Cary, A., & Schoenfisch, S. (2008). The role of public health nurses in emergency preparedness and response: A position paper of the association of state and territorial directors of nursing. *Public Health Nursing, 25*(4), 353–361.

Kirby, M. (2003, November). *Reforming health protection and promotion in Canada: Time to act.* The Standing Senate Committee on Social Affairs, Science and Technology. Retrieved from http://www.parl.gc.ca/Content/SEN/Committee/372/soci/rep/repfinnov03-e.htm

Kirby, M., & LeBreton, M. (2002, October). *The health of Canadians: The federal role, final report.* Vol. 6: Recommendations for Reform. The Standing Senate Committee on Social Affairs, Science and Technology. Retrieved from http://www.parl.gc.ca/37/2/parlbus/commbus/senate/com-e/soci-e/rep-e/repoct02vol6-e.htm

Landesman, L. Y. (2012). *Public health management of disasters: The practice guide* (3rd ed.). Washington, DC: American Public Health Association.

Ministry of Community Safety & Correctional Services (MCSCS). (2016). *Emergency Management Ontario incident management system in Ontario.* Retrieved from https://www.emergencymanagementontario.ca/english/emcommunity/ProvincialPrograms/IMS/Resources/ims_doctrine.html#P268_12752

Ministry of Justice. (2014a). Emergency Act. R.S.C. 1985, c. 22 (4th Supp.). Retrieved from http://laws-lois.justice.gc.cPDF/E-4.5.pdf

Ministry of Justice. (2014b). Emergency Management Act, S.C., 2007, c.15. Retrieved from http://laws-lois.justice.gc.ca/PDF/E-4.56.pdf

Ministry of Justice. (2014c). Emergency Preparedness Act, Repealed, 2007, c15, s.13. Retrieved from http://laws.justice.gc.ca/en/showtdm/cs/E-4.6

Naylor, D. (2003). *Learning from SARS: Renewal of public health in Canada: A report of the National Advisory Committee on SARS and Public Health.* Ottawa, ON: Public Health

Agency of Canada. Retrieved from http://www.phac-aspc .gc.ca/publicat/sars-sras/naylor

O'Connor, D. R. (2002). *Walkerton Commission of Inquiry reports: A strategy for safe drinking water.* Toronto, ON: Ontario Ministry of the Attorney General. Retrieved from http://www .attorneygeneral.jus.gov.on.ca/english/about/pubs/walkerton/ part1/WI_Summary

Ontario Ministry of Health and Long-Term Care (MOHLTC). (2008, revised 2014). *Ontario public health standards 2008.* Toronto, ON: Queen's Printer for Ontario. Retrieved from http://www.health.gov.on.ca/en/pro/programs/publichealth/ oph_standards/docs/ophs_2008.pdf

Ontario Ministry of Health and Long-Term Care (MOHLTC). (2018, January 1). *Emergency management guideline, 2018.* Retrieved from http://www.health.gov.on.ca/en/pro/pro- grams/publichealth/oph_standards/docs/protocols_guidelines/ Emergency_Management_Guideline_2018_en.pdf

Polivka, B. J., Stanley, S. A. R., Gordon, D., Taulbee, K., Kieffer, G., & McCorkle, S. M. (2008). Public health nursing competencies for public health surge events. *Public Health Nursing, 25*(2), 159–165.

Public Health Agency of Canada (PHAC). (2006). *Highlights from the Canadian pandemic influenza plan for the health sector.* Retrieved from http://www.icid.com/files/Marg_Pop_ Influenza/1_Canadian_Pandemic_Influenza_Plan_for_the_ Health_Sector.pdf

Public Health Agency of Canada (PHAC). (2008a). *Core competen- cies for public health.* Retrieved from http://www.phac-aspc .gc.ca/php-psp/ccph-cesp/pdfs/cc-manual-eng090407.pdf

Public Health Agency of Canada (PHAC). (2008b). *Lessons learned: Public Health Agency of Canada's response to the 2008 listeriosis outbreak.* Retrieved from http://www.phac-aspc .gc.ca/fs-sa/listeria/2008-lessons-lecons-eng.php

Public Health Agency of Canada (PHAC). (2010). *Lessons learned review: Public Health Agency of Canada and Health Canada response to the 2009 H1N1 pandemic.* Retrieved from http://www.phac-aspc.gc.ca/about_apropos/evaluation/ reports-rapports/2010-2011/h1n1/f-c-operation-eng.php

Public Health Agency of Canada (PHAC). (2012). *Emergency preparedness and response.* Retrieved from http://www.phac- aspc.gc.ca/ep-mu/index-eng.php

Public Health Agency of Canada (PHAC). (2014). *Influenza.* Retrieved from http://www.phac-aspc.gc.ca/influenza/ index-eng.php

Public Health Ontario (PHO). (2014*). Incident management sys- tem for public health training module.* Toronto, ON: Author.

Public Health Ontario (PHO). (2016). *Incident management resources.* Retrieved from http://www.publichealthontario .ca/en/BrowseByTopic/EmergencyPreparedness/Pages/IMS- Resources.aspx

Public Safety Canada. (2013a*). Canadian disaster database.* Ottawa, ON: Government of Canada. Retrieved from http://cdd.publicsafety.gc.ca

Public Safety Canada. (2013b). *Emergency management.* Retrieved from http://www.publicsafety.gc.ca/cnt/ mrgnc-mngmnt/index-eng.aspx

Rebmann, T., Carrico, R., & English, J. F. (2008). Lessons public health professionals learned from past disasters. *Pub- lic Health Nursing, 25*(4), 344–352.

Rodriguez, D., & Long, C. O. (2006). Preparedness for the home healthcare nurse. *Home Healthcare Nurse, 24*(1), 21–27.

Sawyer, P. P. (2003). Bioterrorism: Are we prepared? *Home Healthcare Nurse, 21*(4), 220–223.

Statistics Canada. (2016, March 23). *Emergency preparedness in Canada, 2014.* Retrieved from https://www150.statcan .gc.ca/n1/en/pub/85-002-x/2015001/article/14234-eng. pdf?st=aZ-lhfCw

Stewart, P. (2017). *Leeds Grenville Lanark opioid overdose cluster response plan.* Retrieved from http://www.healt- hunit.org/harmreduction/_resources/Leeds_Grenville_ Lanark_Opioid_Overdose_Cluster_Plan.pdf

Turris, S. A., Lund, A., & Bowles, R. R. (2014). An analysis of mass casualty incidents in the setting of mass gatherings and special events. *Disaster Med Public Health Prep, 16,* pp. 1–7. Retrieved from http://www.researchgate.net/publication /261741235_An_Analysis_of_Mass_Casualty_Incidents _in_the_Setting_of_Mass_Gatherings_and_Special_Events

Weinreb, A. (2007, January 24). Defence Minister acknowledges 9/11 deaths of Canadians. *Canadian Free Press.* Retrieved from http://www.canadafreepress.com/2007/weinreb012407.htm

World Health Organization (WHO). (2014). *Emergency and essential surgical care.* Retrieved from http://www.who.int/ surgery/en

ABOUT THE AUTHORS

Alana Devereaux, RN, BN (Memorial University of Newfoundland), PhD (University of Ottawa), is a nursing professor in the Faculty of Health and Human Services at Vancouver Island University. In 2016, she completed her PhD focused on public health nurses' experiences working during the 2009 H1N1 influenza pandemic. Alana was acknowledged in 2015 by the University of Toronto as an emerging scholar and has been the recipient of the Queen Elizabeth II Graduate Scholarship in Science and Technology, the Registered Nurses' Association of Ontario Community Health Nurses' Initiative Group Research Award, and the Registered Nurses' Foundation of Ontario Infection Prevention & Control Research Award.

Claire Farella RN, BScN (Ottawa), MN (Athabasca) is Manager of Infectious and Communicable Diseases in the Community Health Protection Department at the Leeds Grenville Lanark District Health Unit (Brockville, ON). She is a member of the Ontario Association of Pub- lic Health Nursing Leaders and the Registered Nurses' Association of Ontario. She has been involved in several emergency responses, including SARS, H1N1, and the opioid crisis. She is trained in emergency management using the Incident Management System and has func- tioned in a variety of roles within the incident command system. She has provided leadership in the development of multiple community emergency response plans, most recently the opioid cluster overdose response plan.

Dr. Devereaux and Mrs. Farella would like to acknowl- edge the valuable contributions of the previous authors of this chapter in past editions of this text.

Global Health

Shahirose Premji, Aliyah Dosani, and Josephine Etowa

CHAPTER 33

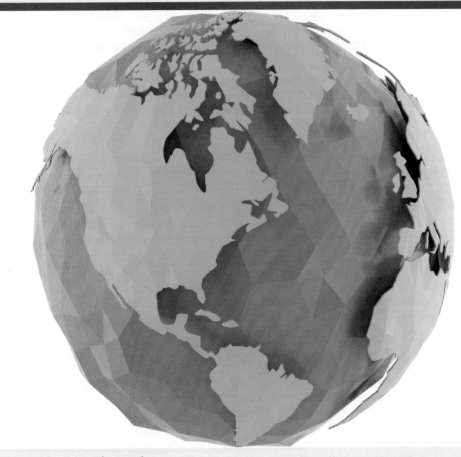

Source: Ivan Kireiev/Shutterstock

LEARNING OUTCOMES

After studying this chapter, you should be able to:

1. Define globalization and global health.

2. Describe trends in the global burden of disease.

3. Examine new and emerging infections and chronic diseases.

4. Examine maternal, newborn, and child health as markers of overall health status of families, communities, and societies.

5. Examine the implications of the United Nations Sustainable Development Goals for community health nursing.

6. Explore the roles of human rights, social justice, and the social determinants of health in global health and their implications for community health nursing.

INTRODUCTION

Working in an increasingly dynamic, diverse, and borderless world requires community health nurses (CHNs) to understand and address issues that may be vastly complex when working with individuals, families, groups, communities, and populations. Canada's multicultural society necessitates that CHNs appreciate and value various cultural and global contexts in order to work effectively and efficiently with diverse groups of people. This is significant for the Canadian context since one in five Canadians is an international migrant, making Canada one of five countries with the highest absolute number of international migrants (Cymbal & Bunjnowksi, 2010). By 2031, almost one in four Canadians will be an international migrant, given the flow of people across national borders (Cymbal & Bunjnowski, 2010; Statistics Canada, 2010). Therefore, working from a global health perspective is as much applicable to CHNs working within Canada as it is to those working abroad.

In this chapter we will provide an overview of globalization and global health. Next, we provide trends in the global burden of disease and health in the Canadian context. This is followed by a discussion of new and reemerging infections and chronic diseases in global health. We consider the evolution of global health equity policy, which includes a description of the United Nations Sustainable Development Goals (SDGs) and the associated implications for community health nursing. We describe global trends and community health nursing, including global health diplomacy, and nursing and global citizenship. The roles of human rights, social justice, and the social determinants of health in global health are explored. We have taken a social justice lens when considering these issues, with a key focus on addressing health inequities. The chapter concludes with some reflections on global health ethics for CHNs who choose to work in this exciting and developing area of practice.

GLOBALIZATION

Globalization has been defined as "a constellation of processes by which nations, businesses, and people are becoming more connected and interdependent via increased economic integration, communication exchange, and cultural diffusion" (Labonte & Togerson, 2005, p. 158). These interdependent processes have far-reaching effects, positive and negative, and, taken together, the globalization process may generate unbalanced outcomes for populations both between and within countries (Spiegel, Labonte, & Ostry, 2004). Thus far, the evidence indicates that although globalization has promoted advances in technology, science, communication, and cross-national interdependencies, it has also increased wide disparities in access to societal resources and the opportunities they afford (Taylor, 2009). Disparities in access have given rise to much discussion and debate regarding the implications of globalization for health and health for all.

GLOBAL HEALTH—WHAT IS IT?

While many definitions of global health exist, Koplan et al. (2009) provide a comprehensive explanation of the differences between global health, international health, and public health. Koplan et al. (2009) characterize **global health** as an area for study, research, and practice that places a priority on improving health and achieving equity for all people worldwide (see Table 33.1). Areas of health care that are often identified as explicitly associated with understanding and addressing the effects of globalization on health are public health, international health, and global health. Although distinctions are made between these terms, which have implications for understanding the unique primary objectives of each, public, international, and global health share a common concern for

preventing disease and promoting health for communities and whole populations. The distinctions exist in terms of geographical considerations and how people and organizations work together.

TRENDS IN GLOBAL BURDEN OF DISEASE

The impact of a health problem, or **disease burden**, relates to the number of years lost due to disease as measured by financial cost, mortality, morbidity, or other indicators. A worldwide observational epidemiological study, The **Global Burden of Disease Study**, estimated cause-specific deaths and **years of life lost (YLL)** by age, sex, geography, and year. In 2016, the 10 leading causes of total YLL were ischemic heart disease, cerebrovascular disease, lower respiratory infections, diarrheal diseases, road injuries, malaria, neonatal preterm birth complications, HIV/AIDS, chronic obstructive pulmonary disease, and neonatal encephalopathy resulting from birth asphyxia and trauma (Global Burden of Disease [GBD] 2016 Causes of Death Collaborators, 2017). The World Health Organization (WHO) estimates global burden of disease based on mortality as well as morbidity, that is, YLL due to ill health and disability, which is referred to as **disability-adjusted life year (DALY)** (WHO, 2017c). The 10 leading causes of death are presented in Figure 33.1. Worldwide, there were 128.8 million live births and 54.7 million deaths in 2016 (*The Lancet*, 2017). According to the WHO (2017c), more than half (52%) of all deaths in low-income countries in 2015 were caused by the so-called "Group I" conditions, which include communicable diseases, maternal causes, conditions arising during pregnancy and childbirth, and nutritional deficiencies. By contrast, less than 7% of deaths in high-income countries were due to such causes. Lower respiratory infections were among the leading causes of death across all income groups. Non-communicable diseases (NCDs) caused 70% of deaths globally, ranging from 37% in low-income countries to 88% in high-income countries. All but one of the 10 leading causes of death in high-income countries were NCDs.

The collective susceptibility to diseases across national boundaries calls for providers such as CHNs to understand the basic strategies for detecting, controlling, and preventing infectious disease and managing chronic diseases globally. Emerging challenges such as the Ebola and Zika viruses, which have made global headlines, exemplify how increasing global trade and travel facilitate the rapid spread of diseases worldwide. In addition to epidemic prevention and control, global health is also essential to sustainable development as illness and death are often both the cause and the result of inequities in opportunities for wealth, income, and health. Contemporary issues in global health include cost containments, lack of basic health care access, social determinants of health, and advancing innovation. Major regions of the world are expected to see health care spending increases ranging from 2.4–7.5% between 2015 and 2020 (WHO, 2017c). Shortages in funding, along with other global forces such as

Table 33.1	Comparison of Global Health, International Health, and Public Health		
	Global Health	**International Health**	**Public Health**
Geographical scope	Deals with issues that directly affect health of all people in the world including those that transcend national boundaries.	Deals with health issues of resource constrained countries rather than one's own country of residence or citizenship.	Deals with issues that shape population health of a community or entire country and within the geographic boundary of that country.
Level of collaboration and cooperation	Initiatives often require cooperation of countries around the world. In addition, collaboration occurs across various sectors within government, non-governmental organizations and the private that are involved in finding solutions to global health problems.	Various interventions that are planned and put into action usually require bi-national cooperation.	Various solutions that are planned and put into action typically do not necessitate global cooperation; interventions occur within individual countries only.
Focus on Individuals or populations	Concerned with all strategies that improve the health of all people, including health promotion and illness prevention at the population level and clinical care of individuals. Builds on national public health initiatives and institutions.	Encompasses both health promotion and illness prevention in populations and clinical care of individuals. However, the scope of solutions is limited to the countries working together	Focuses on health promotion and illness prevention programs at the population-level within a country.
Access to health	Primary objective is health equity among nations and for all people. Embraces transnational research and action that promotes the health of all people in the world. Considers underlying social, economic, political, and environmental determinants of health.	This often appears as resource-rich countries assisting resource-poor countries to improve the health of their populations, respectively.	Focuses on promoting health equity within and between communities within the geographic boundary of a country.
Areas of expertise	Promotes approaches that are highly interdisciplinary and intersectoral.	Welcomes collaboration between a few disciplines but no emphasis is placed on taking intersectoral approaches to solutions.	Promotes intersectoral collaboration, especially between those working within the health sciences and social sciences.

Sources: Beaglehole & Bonita (2010); Koplan et al. (2009).

lack of frontline providers with the expertise to properly diagnose and treat diseases, also limit health care access. Refugee crises, ongoing large-scale migration, management of fast-moving diseases (e.g., Ebola and Zika), and patterns of opioid misuse are straining health and social service systems and driving demand for more health care professionals globally.

Although many causes of early deaths have been reduced, as evident from a global shift toward deaths in older ages, YLLs have "increased globally for causes such as diabetes mellitus or some neoplasms, and in some locations for causes such as drug use disorders, and conflict and terrorism" (GBD 2016 Causes of Death Collaborators, 2017, p. 1152). In the discussion that follows, we draw from both the Global Burden of Disease Study and WHO estimates of the global burden of disease to examine trends in communicable diseases, NCDs, and maternal, newborn, and child health.

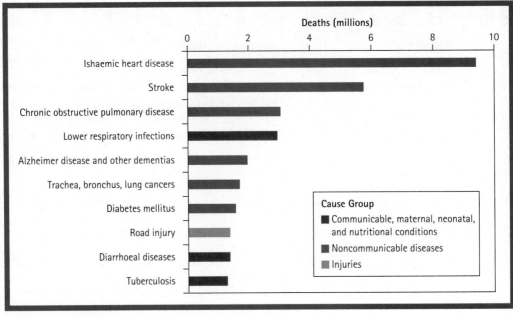

FIGURE 33.1 Top 10 Causes of Death Worldwide

Source: Reprinted from World Health Organization (WHO) (2018b)

Communicable Diseases

Over the past four decades, we have observed declining rates of communicable diseases across various countries (GBD 2016 Causes of Death Collaborators, 2017). However, the global HIV/AIDS pandemic persists. Around the world approximately 2.1 million people became infected with HIV in 2015, and at the end of that year a total of 36.7 million people were living with HIV globally (WHO, 2017f). Furthermore, tuberculosis (TB) also continues to be a major global health problem even though it is preventable, treatable, and curable (WHO, 2017f). Approximately one-third of the world's population is currently infected with TB bacteria (WHO, 2017a). In 2016 there were about 10.4 million new cases of TB worldwide, with 1.4 million TB deaths, including 0.4 million deaths resulting from TB among HIV-positive people (WHO, 2017a). Although the global burden of disease of HIV/AIDs and TB is substantial, equally concerning are the new and reemerging infections seen every year in various parts of the world. Experts anticipate that this trend will continue because of overall growth in the global population size, the increased aging population, ease of travel, urbanization, and climate change, which all produce environments that are conducive to the emergence, evolution, and spread of new pathogens (Bloom, Black, & Rappuoli, 2017).

Non-Communicable Diseases

With respect to chronic NCDs, cardiovascular disease, cancer, chronic respiratory disease, and diabetes are the world's biggest killers, accounting for a combined 40 million deaths in 2015 (WHO, 2017c). Deaths due to NCDs accounted for 70% of the 56 million deaths worldwide (WHO, 2017c). Globally, wide-ranging trends with respect to NCDs have been observed.

For example, in high-income countries, remarkable declines in both the incidence and mortality from ischemic heart disease and ischemic stroke are evident since the middle of the 20th century (Herrington, Lacey, Sherliker, Armitage, & Lewington, 2016). Most low- and middle-income countries have also reported decreases in mortality from stroke over the past few decades, but a more varied trend is observed with respect to ischemic heart disease, with some countries in Eastern Europe and Asia reporting increases (Herrington et al., 2016). Part of this global variation could be due to inequitable access to the required medication to treat and manage cardiovascular disease (Khatib et al., 2016).

Canadian Context

Although Canada ranked number eight among 149 nations as the best place to live, Canada's performance was lowest on the sub-index of health, dropping eight places due to the rising incidence of preventable illness and growing numbers of Canadians reporting more health problems (Legatum Institute, 2017). The Legatum Prosperity Index compares 104 variables categorized into nine sub-indexes—business environment, economic quality, education, governance, health, natural environment, personal freedom, safety and security, and social capital—to assess the nature and changing profile of global prosperity (Legatum Institute, 2017). Although prosperity is growing around the world, Canada experienced the lowest level of prosperity in 11 years, falling three positions from fifth to eighth place (Legatum Institute, 2017). Declining prosperity threatens the well-being of Canadians as it impacts available life chances and opportunities (Legatum Institute, 2017), particularly for people rendered most vulnerable in the nation. Canada's decline in the sub-index of personal freedom and social capital means financial help is not readily available from relatives or friends during times of need (Legatum Institute, 2017).

At the opening ceremony of the 25th Harm Reduction International Conference in Montréal in 2017, Minister of Health Jane Philpot explained that the "death toll [from opioid overdose] is worse than any other infectious epidemic in Canada, including the peak of AIDS deaths, since the Spanish flu that took the lives of 50 000 people a century ago." Canada declared a national opioid crisis in 2017 and launched a public health emergency response to deal with the 2800 opioid-related deaths in 2016. There was a 53% increase in hospitalization resulting from opioid overdose in the past decade, with 40% of this increase occurring in the past three years (Canadian Institute for Health Information, 2017; Government of Canada, 2017). The impact to the health care system is significant given the number of individuals seeking emergency hospital care. Identifying trends in mortality and morbidity for new and reemerging infectious diseases, NCDs, and drug use disorders is important. Such information can inform global decision makers and regional stakeholders about how to prioritize global health issues and make relevant decisions about which interventions to implement, which programs are working, and where progress is lagging (GBD 2016 Causes of Death Collaborators, 2017).

NEW AND REEMERGING INFECTIONS AND CHRONIC DISEASES IN GLOBAL HEALTH

Over centuries, humanity has observed and experienced several infectious disease pandemics. For example, the plague ("Black Death") that killed 50% of the European population between the 14th and 18th centuries was related to pilgrimage networks that were established to promote medieval trading (Gómez & Verdú, 2017; Spyrou et al., 2016). The smallpox pandemic was also thought to be one of the worst, spreading quickly and killing one-third of those infected (Reardon, 2014). Throughout history, smallpox affected First Nation, Inuit, and African populations disproportionately, with entire populations perishing after contracting the disease from European settlers between the 16th and 18th centuries (Reardon, 2014). Similar trends were observed in Mexico when *cocoliztli* (a type of hemorrhagic fever) appeared in 1545, and 80% of the population succumbed to the disease within three years (Acuna-Soto, Stahle, Therrell, Griffin, & Cleaveland, 2004).

Our experiences with recent pandemics, including severe acute respiratory syndrome (SARS) during 2002–2003, pandemic influenza A (H1N1) in 2009, scarlet fever in 2011, wild polio virus in 2011, Ebola virus in 2014, and Zika virus in 2015–2016, to name a few, have reminded us how ill-equipped health professionals are to address these significant global health concerns (Bloom et al., 2017; Lee, Cowling, & Lau, 2017; Rao et al., 2017). Although most of the recent new and reemerging infectious diseases have been viral, bacterial infections are also a threat to global health. For example, the cholera epidemic devastated Haiti, and the food-borne *Escherichia coli* 0104:H4 outbreak in Germany led to haemolytic uremic syndrome for 276 individuals (Bloom et al., 2017; WHO, 2017c). The most significant risk from bacteria around the world currently is antibiotic-resistant strains, such as multidrug-resistant *Staphylococcus aureus* (Bloom et al., 2017). Regardless of whether the illness is viral or bacterial, new and emerging infectious diseases are unpredictable and have the potential for spreading quickly with high morbidity, which often results in significant social consequences for the populations affected (Bloom et al., 2017; Fauci & Morens, 2012).

With the new and reemerging infectious diseases being profiled at a rapid rate, there comes a "danger of complacency and failure to appreciate the potential scope of diseases" we are encountering globally (Paules & Fauci, 2017, p. 691). For example, many questions about the most recent reemerging disease, Zika virus, remain unanswered, including the pathogenesis of the virus and the acute and long-term consequences (Paules & Fauci, 2017). Perhaps this is due to the ever-changing foci of diseases that fall into this category. However, quickly changing our foci without fully understanding the scope of the consequences of an infectious agent is hazardous to the health of the global population. Through our experiences with new and reemerging infectious diseases, recently we have recognized that the global community has a desperate need for building capacity for early detection and timely response (Rao et al., 2017). Having the capacity for early detection gives us the ability to make accurate risk assessments and results in appropriate global health interventions and recommendations. Having systems in place to respond appropriately when epidemics arise will allow the global community to fully understand diseases in their acute phases before epidemics diminish and endemicity develops (Paules & Fauci, 2017). Although there is agreement on the need for effective surveillance of new and reemerging diseases globally, there is no consensus on how best this may be achieved. One proposition that could have significant value is to strengthen the capacity of the local public health system and workforce for early detection and response to infectious diseases worldwide (Halliday et al., 2017; Laxminarayan, Kakkar, Horby, Malavige, & Basnyat, 2017).

MATERNAL, NEWBORN, AND CHILD HEALTH

Globally, the health of women and children is considered a key marker for the overall health status of families, communities, and societies, and it is upheld as an indicator for the overall health of people. Women and children around the world face barriers in acquiring even the most basic health care services. Even though some of the poorest countries in the world have improved maternal health and cut neonatal deaths by half since the mid-1990s, there is a continuing need to improve the health and well-being of women and children around the world. Women and children living in South Asia and sub-Saharan Africa continue to face the highest rates of maternal, neonatal, and child deaths.

Even though there has been a global decline in maternal mortality rates, it is alarming that nearly 830 women die every day from complications related to pregnancy and childbirth (WHO, 2018a). The inequities across the globe tell us that most maternal deaths can be prevented by access to appropriate health care during pregnancy, labour, childbirth, and the postpartum period (WHO, 2016). The largest contributors to maternal deaths worldwide are hemorrhage, hypertensive disorders, and sepsis (Say et al., 2014). Although maternal mortality decreased by 44% between 1990 and 2015, almost all maternal deaths (99%) occur in low- and middle-income countries, bringing attention to inequities in access to health services between rich and poor countries (WHO, 2016).

Significant progress has been made in decreasing childhood mortality, but child survival remains a critical global health issue (United Nations Inter-Agency Group for Child Mortality Estimation [UN IGCM], 2017). Approximately 5.6 million children under the age of five years died in 2016, of which 2.6 million deaths (almost half) occurred in the first month of life (WHO, 2017b). The leading causes of neonatal deaths are complications from preterm birth, birth asphyxia, and infections; pneumonia, diarrhea, and malaria are the main causes of death from the end of the neonatal period through the first five years (WHO, 2017b). Nearly half of all deaths in children under age five are attributable to undernutrition (Figure 33.2). Malnutrition is the underlying contributing factor that makes children more vulnerable to severe illness (WHO, 2017b). More than half of these child deaths, amounting to 15 000 child deaths per day, could have been prevented or treated with access to simple and affordable treatments (UN IGCM, 2017; WHO, 2017b). Whereas we have observed significant improvement in child survival since 1990—the global under-five mortality rate has decreased by 56% (UN IGCM, 2017; WHO, 2017b)—we are still seeing substantial global inequities between the rich and the poor when it comes to child health. Children in sub-Saharan Africa are more than 15 times more likely to die before their fifth birthday than children in high-income countries (UN IGCM, 2017; WHO, 2017b).

Women, infants, and children around the world face numerous barriers in achieving an optimal health status. In response to these inequities, in 2010, Secretary-General of the United Nations Ban Ki-moon launched the Every Woman Every Child initiative to address improving policy and financing related to maternal, infant, and child health. The Every Woman Every Child initiative takes a human rights–based approach to maternal, newborn, and child health and directs the actions of governments, nongovernmental organizations (NGOs), the private sector, and societies to address the substantial health challenges that women, infants, and children face around the world. Although access to health has long been viewed as a fundamental human right (Office of the United Nations High Commissioner for Human Rights & WHO, 2008), we have seen recent advances in highlighting maternal, newborn, and child health as a fundamental human right. Building on the momentum of Every Woman Every Child, the Global Strategy for Women's, Children's and Adolescents' Health (2016–2030) was released in 2015 emphasizing that "no woman, child, or adolescent should face a greater risk of preventable death because of where they live or who they are" (Every Woman Every Child, 2015, p. 5). Aligned with the SDGs, this global strategy has three main objectives: survive, thrive, and transform (Every Woman Every Child, 2015). These objectives will be met by creating enabling environments for health and transforming societies "so that women, children, and adolescents everywhere can realize their rights to the highest attainable standards of health and well-being" (Every Woman Every Child, 2015, p. 5).

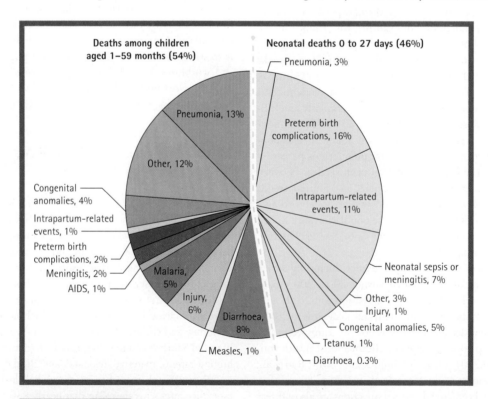

FIGURE **33.2** Global Distribution of Deaths among Children under Age Five, by Cause, 2016

Source: United Nations Inter-Agency Group for Child Mortality Estimation. (2017).

CANADIAN RESEARCH 33.1

A qualitative study of pregnancy-related anxiety among women in Tanzania. (King Rosario, Premji, Nyanza, Raffin Bouchal, & Este, 2017)

Pregnancy-related anxiety (PRA) is linked to poor maternal and infant health outcomes in many high-income countries. Little research is available about the specific phenomenon of anxiety that is directly related to pregnancy in low-income countries. The purpose of this study was to explore and understand the experiences and priorities of women living with PRA in Mwanza, Tanzania. A descriptive phenomenological approach was used. Ten women who were pregnant or postpartum who scored high on a PRA scale in a larger quantitative study were invited to participate in semi-structured interviews. As experienced by the women in the study, PRA was a state of worry and concern that caused physical symptoms. Five themes about PRA emerged from the data analysis: lack of knowledge of what is *normal* in terms of the pregnancy and taking care of the newborn, the importance of social support from partners during the pregnancy, both positive and negative interactions with the health care system, drawing on spirituality for courage and peace during times of difficulty, and fear of either having HIV/AIDS or passing the disease onto their unborn children. Although the PRA scale might be appropriate for use in high-income countries, this study indicates that it is likely not appropriate for use in all country contexts. The themes that emerged from this study represent additional areas related to the experience of PRA that also require consideration when assessing PRA in low-income countries.

Discussion Questions

1. In the context of global health and working with resource-poor populations, should you as CHN be aware of power in relationships and giving voice to at-risk populations? Explain.

2. How can CHNs, in partnership with others, support women in the perinatal period when working in another country context?

3. How can the CHN integrate culturally safe care into practice with this population?

YES, BUT WHY?

Vertical Transmission of HIV in Canada

What?

Women of childbearing age account for half of the world's HIV cases, and Black women are disproportionately affected. They make up the largest percentage of women living with HIV in Canada (54.2%) and the United States (45%). Black women represent 46% of pregnant women living with HIV in Canada. Vertical transmission of the disease through breastfeeding is estimated to be 20% (Etowa et al., 2018). In acknowledgment of mothers being the main source of HIV infection among children, there has been targeted global effort to thwart vertical or mother-to-child transmission. The WHO recommends that HIV-positive women breastfeed their infants for up to 12 months provided they strictly adhere to their antiretroviral regime during that same period. These guidelines are implemented differently in various countries.

So What?

Western countries like Canada, England, and the United States recommend exclusive formula feeding for HIV-positive women, but these countries also promote breastmilk as the best food for infants (WHO, 2017d). Breast milk has more nutritional value and provides immunity against infections (Hazemba, Ncama, & Sithole, 2016). Breastfeeding is also associated with enhanced mother–baby emotional bond (Green et al., 2015). Public health messages that promote exclusive breastfeeding as the best method of infant feeding may motivate some women who might otherwise not choose to breastfeed their infants. However, these public health education messages do not seem to recognize the sociocultural implications and realities of breastfeeding among women living with HIV (Greene et al., 2015; Odeny et al., 2016) and may unintentionally ostracize them. This creates significant tension for Black women who are faced with the cultural expectation of breastfeeding as an integral part of being a "good mother" (Etowa et al., 2018). This is particularly problematic for HIV-positive African immigrant women who have relocated to countries like the United States, Canada, or England from countries and cultures where breastfeeding is an expectation of all new mothers and where using formula is a sign of illness and disease (Kapiriri et al., 2014).

Now What?

CHNs need to understand the social determinants of infant feeding choices and practices in this sub-population and the implications of infant feeding guidelines that promote formula feeding. As Etowa (2012) asserts, childbirth and related processes such as infant feeding practices are significantly influenced by culture. Culture teaches people and creates a longing for a particular preference and ways of being, including decisions about childbirth and infant feeding practices (Etowa, 2012). Sociocultural knowledge may enhance efforts to understand the needs of African immigrant women who make infant feeding choices while living with HIV. CHNs who are knowledgeable about the cultural expectations of motherhood in this sub-population would be better positioned to develop and implement effective interventions to support women's decision to exclusively breast or formula feed their infants while living with HIV, thereby reducing the risk of vertical transmission of HIV among highly exposed infants.

Standards of Practice Fulfilled

#6 Health Equity
- Advocates for healthy public policy and social justice by participating in legislative and policy-making activities that influence determinants of health and access to services.
- Assesses how the social determinants of health influence the client's health status with particular attention to clients who are marginalized.
- Understands historical injustices, inequitable power relations, institutionalized and interpersonal racism and their impacts on health and health care and provides culturally safe care (CHNC, 2019, revised).

THE EVOLUTION OF GLOBAL HEALTH EQUITY POLICY

Health for All Movement

As discussed in Chapter 8, in 1978, WHO member states convened for an international conference on primary health care in Alma-Ata, USSR (now Almaty, Kazakhstan). The outcome was the **Declaration of Alma-Ata**, which expressed "the need for urgent action by all governments, all health and development workers, and the world community to protect and promote the health of all the people of the world" (WHO, 1978, p. 1). The declaration led to the formation of the Health for All movement, which pledged that health could be achieved for all by the year 2000. Although the original goal is yet to be achieved, the Health for All strategy set an important direction for health equity policy and health programming.

Millennium Development Goals

In September 2000, after a series of United Nations conferences and summits, world leaders convened at United Nations Headquarters in New York to accept the United Nations Millennium Declaration. This led to global partnership to address the **Millennium Development Goals (MDGs)** and identify specific health-related targets to be achieved by 2015. The eight goals were as follows:

1. Eradicate extreme hunger and poverty.
2. Achieve universal primary education.
3. Promote gender equality and empower women.
4. Reduce child mortality.
5. Improve maternal health.
6. Combat HIV/AIDS, malaria, and other diseases.
7. Ensure environmental sustainability.
8. Develop a global partnership for development. (United Nations, 2000)

The MDGs provided a framework of time-bound goals and targets using a baseline of 1990 (United Nations, 2000). However, various challenges were apparent, including persistent inequalities; food and nutrition insecurity; knowledge challenges; growing environmental footprints; conflict, violence, and insecurity; governance deficits at all levels; and shifting demographics (e.g., migration, urbanization, and aging). Although many targets were met, others demonstrated insufficient progress, no progress, or even, in some cases, a deterioration. In a few countries, there have been insufficient data available to evaluate progress made to date. This pointed to a critical need to find new approaches to promote global health equity, leading to the initiation of the SDGs (United Nations System Task Team on the Post-2015 UN Development Agenda, 2012).

Sustainable Development Goals

The outcome document of the 2010 MDG Summit (United Nations Secretary-General, 2010) requested the Secretary-General to initiate thinking on the global development agenda beyond 2015. This ultimately led to discussions at the 2012 Rio+20 Conference to devise a road map to move forward with the MDG agenda. The outcome document of the 2012 Rio+20 Conference on Sustainable Development instigated an inclusive process to develop a set of **Sustainable Development Goals (SDGs)**. The process of arriving at this new framework was member state–led, with broad participation from external stakeholders, such as civil society organizations, the private sector and businesses, and academia and scientists (United Nations Sustainable Development Solutions Network, 2013). The Sustainable Development Solutions Network has established 12 thematic groups that are *solution oriented* rather than research oriented. The goal is to stimulate governments, United Nations agencies, and the public toward discovery of practical solutions to the greatest challenges of sustainable development.

17 Sustainable Development Goals

- Goal 1. End poverty in all its forms everywhere.
- Goal 2. End hunger, achieve food security and improved nutrition, and promote sustainable agriculture.
- Goal 3. Ensure healthy lives and promote well-being for all, at all ages.
- Goal 4. Ensure inclusive and equitable quality education and promote lifelong learning opportunities for all.
- Goal 5. Achieve gender equality and empower all women and girls.
- Goal 6. Ensure availability and sustainable management of water and sanitation for all.
- Goal 7. Ensure access to affordable, reliable, sustainable, and modern energy for all.
- Goal 8. Promote sustained, inclusive, and sustainable economic growth; full and productive employment; and decent work for all.
- Goal 9. Build resilient infrastructure, promote inclusive and sustainable industrialization, and foster innovation.
- Goal 10. Reduce inequality within and among countries.
- Goal 11. Make cities and human settlements inclusive, safe, resilient, and sustainable.
- Goal 12. Ensure sustainable consumption and production patterns.
- Goal 13. Take urgent action to combat climate change and its impacts (acknowledging that the United Nations Framework Convention on Climate Change is the primary international, intergovernmental forum for negotiating the global response to climate change).
- Goal 14. Conserve and sustainably use the oceans, seas, and marine resources for sustainable development.
- Goal 15. Protect, restore, and promote sustainable use of terrestrial ecosystems; sustainably manage forests; combat desertification; and halt and reverse land degradation, and halt biodiversity loss.
- Goal 16. Promote peaceful and inclusive societies for sustainable development; provide access to justice for all; and build effective, accountable, and inclusive institutions at all levels.
- Goal 17. Strengthen the means of implementation and revitalize the global partnership for sustainable development (United Nations, 2014).

Table 33.2	New Opportunities Provided by the 2030 Agenda with Reference to Six Main Lines of Action	
	Six main lines of action	**Opportunities provided by the 2030 Agenda**
Building better systems for health	Intersectoral action by multiple stakeholders (see section 1.6)	Placing health in all sectors of policy-making; combining the strengths of multiple stakeholders
	Health systems strengthening for UHC (see section 1.2)	Disease-control programmes embedded in a comprehensive health system that provides complete coverage through fully staffed and well-managed health services, with financial risk protection
	Respect for equity and human rights (see section 1.3)	Improving health for whole populations by including all individuals ("leave no one behind") and empowering women
	Sustainable financing (see section 1.4)	Attracting new sources of funding; emphasizing domestic financing, with alignment of financial flows to avoid duplication of health system functions
Enabling factors	Scientific research and innovation (see section 1.5)	Reinforcing research and innovation as foundations for sustainable development, including a balance of research on medical, social and environmental determinants and solutions
	Monitoring and evaluation (see section 1.1)	Exploiting new technologies to manage large volumes of data, disaggregated to ascertain the needs of all individuals; tracking progress towards SDG 3 and all other health-related targets

Source: Reprinted from World Health Organization (2017e).

Health system strengthening to achieve universal health coverage is central to promoting the health and well-being of present and future generations (WHO, 2017c, 2017f). In this regard, the WHO has proposed six main lines of action (see Table 33.2) to ensure health equity toward universal health coverage consistent with the principle that "health is a fundamental right of every human being as their constitution," which appears in its constitution (WHO, 2017c, p. 2, 2017f).

The WHO monitors, in 194 member states, multi-sectoral determinants of health, as it measures 13 health targets of the SDGs, 16 health-related targets in other goals, indicators for NCDs, mental health, injuries, and three overarching indicators—life expectancy, healthy life expectancy, and number of deaths before 70 years (WHO, 2017a, 2017f). The more than 50 SDG indicators are grouped into the following seven themes: (a) reproductive, maternal, newborn, and child health; (b) infectious diseases; (c) NCDs and mental health; (d) injuries and violence; (e) universal health coverage and health systems; (f) environmental risks; and (g) health risks and disease outbreaks (WHO, 2017a, 2017f). The GBD study's analysis of country progress toward meeting SDG goal number three suggests that no countries will meet more than 13 of the 24 targets by 2030 (GBD 2016 Causes of Death Collaborators, 2017). For instance, more focused efforts are required in sub-Saharan Africa and Southeast Asia if we are to meet SGD three, target 3.2: reduce newborn mortality to at least as low as 12 per 1000 live births in every country and reduce under-five mortality to at least as low as 25 per 1000 live births in every country (WHO, 2017c).

Promoting population health and well-being is essential to achieving the SDGs and their targets (WHO, 2017c, 2017f). Public health leadership will be required for an intersectoral approach (i.e., between two or more sectors promoting physical, economic, and social environments) to align policies with health plans oriented toward modifiable determinants of health (WHO, 2017c, 2017f). *The Lancet* editorial emphasizes scrutiny of country-specific health issues, strengthening of health systems, vertical initiatives, and recognition of new risks, including ecosystem resources that impact the health and well-being of individuals and the planet and influence decision making (*The Lancet*, 2017). CHNs are uniquely positioned to embrace these recommendations and develop health-related metrics that considers the other 16 SDGs and initiate calls to action that consider policy implications.

GLOBAL TRENDS AND COMMUNITY HEALTH NURSING

Global Health Diplomacy

Determinants of health are often influenced by global forces and need to be addressed through global strategies. The challenge is to capitalize on the benefits and diminish the harm of globalization while keeping our eye on human rights and equity (Owen & Roberts, 2005). One way of challenging oppressive power relationships in the hopes of achieving social justice is global health diplomacy. Within a **global health diplomacy** framework, state and non-state actors work together to increase the prominence of health issues in foreign policy decision making (Labonte & Gagnon, 2010). Usually key actors in global health diplomacy include those working in public health, international affairs, management, law, and economics (WHO, 2013). The alliance between

A Village Developed by Sylvia Loewen and Aliyah Dosani

A village has decided it needs a hospital. The government will not pay for a hospital, so the village leaders put in a request to a local NGO working in their country. You now work for the NGO and are part of a delegation sent to work with the community. You learn the village has 100 000 people, and 50% of them are under 18 years of age. Severe vomiting and diarrhea account for much of the illness and 5–10% of infant deaths. The estimate is that 10% of the children have TB. Two years ago, five children died due to measles, and on average the community loses at least one child to tetanus each year. It is a six-hour bus ride to the nearest centre with health services. The bus arrives in the evening, and the villagers usually sleep on the sidewalk outside the public health office until it opens. The health centre vaccinates children on a first-come, first-served basis.

The community gathers together often to provide support to its members in whatever way they can. This may include sharing food, shelter, clothing, and any other basic necessities of life. A group of community women often come together to share resources as they sew clothing for their children. At times, sharing of staple food such as cornmeal may occur.

Children can attend the government school if their parents can afford a uniform, supplies, and books. One teacher offers Saturday morning basic reading and arithmetic classes free of charge to children who cannot afford school. He accepts 30 children for each term for his free classes.

About half the population lives in makeshift housing. They use back alleys to urinate, but for bowel movements they usually go up the hill to where there are trees that offer privacy. The same teacher who offers free classes on Saturdays taught the villagers to dig small holes to use as latrines to keep the area cleaner. The village gets its water from a stream that runs down from the hill and through the town. In springtime the water flows rapidly, but in late summer it is sluggish.

Discussion Questions

1. Which of the SDGs we discussed relate to this case study?

2. How would you as a CHN work with the community to identify three priority areas for action on health?

3. Suppose the priority areas identified with the stakeholders are education, sanitation, and immunization. Suggest some short-term and long-term goals in relation to these three areas.

health, foreign policy, and trade is at the "cutting edge of global health diplomacy" (WHO, 2013). The WHO has a large role to play in global health diplomacy. In this area its goals are as follows:

- to support the development of a more systematic and proactive approach to identify and understand key current and future changes impacting global public health; and

- to build capacity among member states to support the necessary collective action to take advantage of opportunities and mitigate the risks for health. (WHO, 2013)

The significance of including global health issues in the foreign policy agenda is that health affects the global dimensions of security, economics, and social justice (Kickbusch, 2011). With respect to security, global health diplomacy focuses on preventing the spread of pathogens across borders and responds to humanitarian conflicts, natural disasters, and emergencies. In the economic domain, global health diplomacy is concerned with improving the socioeconomic status of countries in efforts to improve health. Last, social justice is emphasized, reinforcing that health is a human right, supporting the United Nations' SDGs, advocating access to medicines and primary health care, and calling for investment in various global health initiatives (Kickbusch, 2011). Engaging in global health diplomacy presents both opportunities and challenges for health. In the past, nation states have focused on health and policy within their own national boundaries.

Globalization of Nursing and Global Citizenship

Worldwide there are 13 million nurses who provide front-line health care to individuals, families, and communities; thus, nurses are well positioned to reduce inequities in health outcomes as a result of globalization (International Council of Nurses, 2011). The coming together of these 13 million nurses to ensure health for all (individuals and society) is implicit in the concept "**One World, One Health**" (Premji & Hatfield, 2016). Although a new term for nurses, it appeared in the literature in 2008 with reference to the Sixth International Ministerial Conference on Avian and Pandemic Influence in Egypt (Premji & Hatfield, 2016; World Bank, 2010). According to Premji and Hatfield (2016)

> One World, One Health typifies our interconnectedness, between not only humans but nonhumans (i.e., animals) and our ecosystem and emphasizes coequal collaborations and partnerships [6], providing a privileged intersection in which the capacity of healthcare providers, regardless of geographical boundaries, is enhanced for society's well-being. (p. 2)

We, therefore, have a shared responsibility to develop a cohesive response to meet the challenges to the profession and to individual nurses to reduce inequities in health outcomes as a result of globalization to ensure health for all (Grootjans & Newman, 2013; Premji & Hatfield, 2016).

Postcolonial Feminism Postcolonialism, specifically postcolonial feminism (PCF), is a perspective that provides an opportunity for cultivating global citizenship. **Postcolonialism** may be described as a theory and political movement that challenges Western authority and its ethnocentric ideas that naturalize the current global economic and political order rather than problematize them as the consequence of centuries of colonialism (Loomba, 2005). Postcolonialism seeks to explain people's lives in places and times other than "the West," celebrate pluralism, and strongly critique any assumptions about universal knowledge. Given that nations and communities are social constructs supported by particular notions of gender, race, and class, **PCF** offers a theoretical lens through which to address the intersections of such social "locations" and to explore their corresponding forms of oppression that are inherently part of everyday experiences (Anderson et al., 2003; Loomba, 2005).

PCF sheds light on inequities in any global context and facilitates examination of the complex nature of health issues. It explicitly calls on nurses to critique current global (including Canadian) disparities in health and health care arising from such phenomena as sexism, racism, or the imposition of Eurocentric colonialist views over Indigenous, and other, knowledge and ways of understanding health and healing (Chavez, Peter, & Gastaldo, 2008). PCF represents an opportunity for nurses to acknowledge their multiple social and cultural locations as individuals and health care professionals. It challenges deeply held certainties about the "right way" to provide care and considers all knowledge as being situated with a given place and within the power relations therein. Using this perspective enables us to consider multiple perspectives on meanings of health and illness (Anderson & McCann, 2002), including economics, politics, and culture, as well as the complex issues associated with the global locations of nursing practice and caregiving.

Precision Public Health

Precision public health (PPH) involves use of advancing methods and technologies to improve our ability to promote health while reducing health disparities (Khoury, 2016). PPH interventions by CHNs informed by root causes of inequities will enable all countries to reach their targets for each SDG. PPH provides an opportunity to examine the multiple determinants of health (Khoury, 2016) to improve our ability to promote conditions or attributes that mitigate risk and enable well-being in parents, families, and communities. PPH emphasizes prediction and prevention using data from both high- and low-resourced countries (e.g., Global Health Data Exchange from 195 countries) to personalize interventions strategies (Dowell, Blazes, & Desmond-Hellmann, 2016). Finally, the key to successful PPH is the participatory approach from multiple stakeholders (Dowell et al., 2016).

Advanced Community Health Nursing Practice

In Canada, a national framework for **advanced nursing practice** characterizes advanced practice nurses as graduate-prepared nurses with advanced levels of clinical nursing practice who work collaboratively to innovate health care services to meet the complex health needs of individuals, families, groups, communities, and populations (Canadian Nurses Association, 2008). Only two roles are recognized within this framework: clinical nurse specialist and nurse practitioner. Implicit within this framework is the value placed on the care of individuals within the context of families and community, which is consistent with the historical tradition of caring for individuals in acute-care settings (Swider, Levin, & Kulbok, 2015). The

CNA's conceptualization of advance nursing practice requires a conceptual shift, as promoting population health and well-being is essential to achieving SDGs and targets through global strategies that are responsive to the global forces impacting the determinants of health. Community health nursing's social context for health is primarily at the community and population levels and involves improving overall health outcomes of populations across settings (Swider et al., 2015). CHNs with graduate education in advance practice in community health nursing will be well positioned to identify innovative solutions to (a) the complex interplay of global forces impacting health and (b) threats to nursing due to globalization.

GLOBAL HEALTH ETHICS

Community health nursing necessarily involves making ethical decisions in daily practice (see Chapter 6). Ethical theory helps to guide such decisions and has been expressed in codes of ethics and standards of practice (CHNC, 2011, revised). **Global health ethics** is a particular avenue of ethical theory that closely aligns with public health ethics, moves beyond traditional bioethical principles, draws from the philosophy of health as a human right, and acknowledges work in this area as largely involving at-risk populations (Pinto & Upshur, 2009). Benatar, Daar, and Singer (2003) argue that it is imperative to move beyond individually focused biomedical ethical principles to a more comprehensive approach that focuses on improving health globally: a shift in mindset that requires "a realization that health, human rights, economic opportunities, good governance, peace and development are all intimately linked within a complex interdependent world" (p. 108). Global health ethics can guide moral decision making in settings other than one's home community from the perspective of the nurse as global citizen. Situations involving moral dilemmas for researchers and practitioners alike in international settings are innumerable. Some examples include using the already scant resources of host agencies to become culturally familiar with primary health care practices; working through translators, which places a burden on locals who are already overworked and may impede the natural flow of care; and balancing learned local standards of care with what is drawn from one's own ethnocentric knowledge so that interventions are culturally appropriate without being problematic.

CONCLUSION

CHNs as global citizens look past the dominant emphasis on individual care (commonly disconnected from social, economic, political, and cultural contexts); engage critically and reflexively with social, historical, and political issues; and develop their capacity in identifying tensions between personal professional interests and global interests. A nurse who can exercise her or his global citizenship professionally works from the premise that people's experiences of health and illness are culturally and geographically located. In addition, it is important to recognize that the majority of the people in the world live under severe social and economic inequities and suffer from preventable or curable diseases. Unfortunately, the majority of people in this world experience an enormous amount of unnecessary human suffering. Nurses working in the global health arena should have the ability to address the health concerns of most of the world's population. Nurses, the largest group of health professionals in the world, are strategically located and needed to leverage their position to advocate for global health in this globalized world.

KEY TERMS

advanced nursing practice   (p. 599)
Declaration of Alma-Ata   (p. 596)
disability-adjusted life year (DALY)   (p. 590)
disease burden   (p. 590)
globalization   (p. 590)
Global Burden of Disease Study   (p. 590)
global health   (p. 590)
global health diplomacy   (p. 597)
global health ethics   (p. 599)
Millennium Development Goals (MDGs)   (p. 596)
One World, One Health   (p. 598)
postcolonialism   (p. 598)
precision public health (PPH)   (p. 599)
Sustainable Development Goals (SDGs)   (p. 596)
years of life lost (YLL)   (p. 590)

STUDY QUESTIONS

1. Differentiate among public health, international health, and global health.
2. Discuss efforts made to decrease inequity in health status among people around the world.
3. Why is it important for CHNs in Canada to learn about globalization and global health?
4. How can the notion of global citizenship guide your nursing practice?
5. What is global health diplomacy, and why is this important?

INDIVIDUAL CRITICAL-THINKING EXERCISES

1. Define global citizenship in your own words, and describe it using examples from your life story or that of someone close to you.
2. Imagine you are working in a First Nation community in Canada.
   a. In what ways might you see the effects of globalization on the community?
   b. How might the SDGs apply to First Nation communities in Canada?
3. As you have come to understand the role of CHNs throughout the text, how do you now understand this role specific to a global health perspective?

4. Write a brief rebuttal to the following statement: "Public health, international health, and global health are really all the same anyway, so making distinctions in language is not meaningful or useful."

GROUP CRITICAL-THINKING EXERCISES

1. "When spider webs unite, they can tie up an elephant."
   —Ethiopian proverb

   Imagine forming a web of connections among global health topics raised in this chapter that brings together the health issues, the sociopolitical global context, and corresponding concerns for nursing. Take a few minutes to individually draw a "global health and nursing" web representing what you have imagined, labelling and identifying its various strands. Share your drawing with the group, explaining the following:

   - Your identification of the central strands that give strength to the whole web (i.e., foundational ideas) and those strands that may be further out in the web (i.e., those that are important but not central)
   - Your understanding of the points where the strands connect as points where nurses may take action (i.e., how issues, context, and nursing concerns come together to direct care in global health)

2. Chen is waiting to be seen in the outpatient clinic with her granddaughter, who looks to be about 10 years old. It is about 6:30 p.m. when a primary health care nurse invites them into her office for assessment and discovers that Mrs. Chen has only recently arrived in Canada and speaks no English. The nurse does not like to use family members as interpreters, but the hospital interpreters and the Cantonese-speaking receptionist have left for the day. Not knowing what else to do, the nurse begins the interview with the help of the granddaughter acting as interpreter. In carrying out some open-ended questions, the nurse realizes Mrs. Chen may be seriously depressed. She wants to ask more focused questions to assess the risk of suicide but feels uncomfortable about posing these questions through Mrs. Chen's granddaughter. As a group, discuss the following:
   a. What global health issues arise in this situation?
   b. What are the implications for nursing practice that would reflect global citizenship?

3. Imagine you are in a remote, resource-constrained area of a majority world country, working in a health clinic staffed only by one nurse and two lay health workers. Write a letter home describing your imagined experience. Tell the person to whom you are writing about (a) situations in which your taken-for-granted assumptions have been challenged, (b) where you felt discomfort in taking action or felt great confidence, and (c) when you felt marginalized in some way. Read your letters to one another in the group, and discuss how these experiences can be understood through postcolonial feminism.

REFERENCES

Acuna-Soto, R., Stahle, D. W., Therrell, M. D., Griffin, R. D., & Cleaveland, M. K. (2004). When half of the population died: The epidemic of hemorrhagic fevers of 1576 in Mexico. *FEMS microbiology letters, 240*(1), 1–5.

Anderson, J. M., & McCann, E. K. (2002). Toward a post-colonial feminist methodology in nursing research: Exploring the convergence of post-colonial and black feminist scholarship. *Nurse Researcher, 9*(3), 7–27.

Anderson, J., Perry, J., Blue, C., Brown, A., Henderson, A., Khan, K. B., . . . Smye, V. (2003). Rewriting cultural safety within the postcolonial and postnational feminist project: Toward new epistemologies of healing. *Advances in Nursing Science, 26*(3), 196–214.

Beaglehole, R. & Bonita, R. (2010). What is global health? *Global Health Action, 3.* doi:10.3402/gha.v3i0.5142.

Benatar, S. R., Daar, A. S., & Singer, P. A. (2003). Global health ethics. The rationale for mutual caring. *International Affairs, 79*(1), 107–138.

Bloom, D. E., Black, S., & Rappuoli, R. (2017). Emerging infectious diseases: A proactive approach. *Proceedings of the National Academy of Sciences, 114*(16), 4055–4059. Retrieved from http://www.pnas.org/cgi/doi/10.1073/pnas.1701410114

Canadian Institute for Health Information. (2017). *Opioid crisis having "significant" impact on Canada's health care system.* Retrieved from https://www.cihi.ca/en/opioid-crisis-having-significant-impact-on-canadas-health-care-system

Canadian Nurses Association (CNA). (2008). *Code of ethics for registered nurses.* Ottawa, ON: Author. Retrieved from http://www.cna-aiic.ca/~/media/cna/files/en/codeofethics.pdf

Chavez, F. S., Peter, E., & Gastaldo, D. (2008). Nurses as global citizens: A global health curriculum at the University of Toronto, Canada. In V. Tschudin & A. J. Davis (Eds.), *The globalization of nursing* (pp. 175–186). Oxford, UK: Radcliffe.

Community Health Nurses of Canada (CHNC). (2019, revised). © Community Health Nurses of Canada. Reprinted with permission.

Cymbal, W., & Bunjnowski, S. (2010). Migration patterns and trends: A quantitative snapshot. *Health Policy Research Bulletin, 17.* Retrieved from http://www.hc-sc.gc.ca/sr-sr/pubs/hpr-rpms/bull/2010-health-sante-migr/index-eng.php#a6

Dowell, S. C., Blazes, D., & Desmond-Hellmann. (2016). Four steps to precision public health [comment]. *Nature, 540,* 189–191.

Etowa, J. (2012). Becoming mother: The meaning of childbirth for African Canadian women. *Contemporary Nurse, 41,* 28–40.

Etowa, J., MacDonald, S., Hannan, J., Phillips, J. C., Boadu, N. Y., & Babatunde, S. (2018). Sociocultural factors influencing infant-feeding choices among African immigrant women living with HIV: A synthesis of the literature. *Journal of the American Association of Nurse Practitioners 30*(4), 208–235.

Every Woman Every Child. (2015). *The global strategy for women's, children's, and adolescents' health (2016–2030).* Retrieved from https://data.unicef.org/wp-content/uploads/2017/02/EWEC_globalstrategyreport_200915_FINAL_WEB.pdf

Fauci, A. S., & Morens, D. M. (2012). The perpetual challenge of infectious diseases. *New England Journal of Medicine, 366*(5), 454–461.

Global Burden of Disease (GBD) 2016 Causes of Death Collaborators. (2017). Global, regional, and national age-sex specific mortality for 264 causes of death, 1980–2016: A systematic analysis for the Global Burden of Disease Study 2016. *The Lancet, 390*(10100), 1151–1210.

Gómez, J. M., & Verdú, M. (2017). Network theory may explain the vulnerability of medieval human settlements to the Black Death pandemic. *Scientific Reports, 7,* 43467. doi:10.1038/srep43467

Government of Canada. (2017). *Federal action on opioids.* Retrieved from https://www.canada.ca/en/health-canada/services/substance-abuse/prescription-drug-abuse/opioids/federal-actions.html#health_emergency_response

Greene, S., Ion, A., Elston, D., Kwaramba, G., Smith, S., Carvalhal, A., & Loutfy, M. (2015). "Why aren't you breastfeeding?": How mothers living with HIV talk about infant feeding in a "breast is best" world. *Health Care for Women International, 36,* 883–901.

Grootjans, J., & Newman, S. (2013). The relevance of globalization to nursing: A concept analysis. *International Nursing Reviews, 60,* 78–85.

Halliday, J. E., Hampson, K., Hanley, N., Lembo, T., Sharp, J. P., Haydon, D. T., & Cleaveland, S. (2017). Driving improvements in emerging disease surveillance through locally relevant capacity strengthening. *Science, 357*(6347), 146–148.

Hazemba, A. N., Ncama, B. P., & Sithole, S. L. (2016). Promotion of exclusive breastfeeding among HIV-positive mothers: An exploratory qualitative study. *International Breastfeeding Journal, 11,* 1–10.

Herrington, W., Lacey, B., Sherliker, P., Armitage, J., & Lewington, S. (2016). Epidemiology of atherosclerosis and the potential to reduce the global burden of athero-thrombotic disease. *Circulation research, 118*(4), 535–546. doi:10.1161/CIRCRESAHA.115.307611

International Council of Nurses. (2011). Nurses convene in Malta to share knowledge, discuss global health priorities. *International Nursing Review, 58*(3), 277–279. doi:10.1111/j.1466-7657.2011.00936_1.x

Kapiriri, L., Tharao, W., Muchenje, M., Masinde, K., Siegel, S., & Ongoiba, F. (2014). The experiences of making infant feeding choices by African, Caribbean and Black HIV-positive mothers in Ontario, Canada. *World Health Population, 15,* 14–22.

Khatib, R., McKee, M., Shannon, H., Chow, C., Rangarajan, S., Teo, K., . . . Kumar, R. (2016). Availability and affordability of cardiovascular disease medicines and their effect on use in high-income, middle-income, and low-income countries: An analysis of the PURE study data. *The Lancet, 387*(10013), 61–69. http://dx.doi.org/10.1016/

Khoury, M. J. (2016, September 7). *Precision public health: More precision ahead for individual and population interventions* [We log post]. Retrieved from https://blogs.cdc.gov/genomics/2016/09/07/precision_public_health

Kickbusch, I. (2011). Global health diplomacy: How foreign policy can influence health. *British Medical Journal, 342* (d3154). doi:10.1136/bmj.d3154

King Rosario, M., Premji, S. S., Nyanza, E. C., Bouchal, S. R., & Este, D. (2017). A qualitative study of pregnancy-related anxiety among women in Tanzania. *BMJ Open, 7*(8), e016072.

Koplan, J. P., Bond, T. C., Merson, M. H., Reddy, K. S., Rodriguez, M. H., Sewankambo, N. K., & Wasserheit, J. N. (2009). Towards a common definition of global health. *The Lancet, 373,* 1993–1995.

Labonte, R., & Torgerson, R. (2005). Interrogating globalization, health and development: Towards a comprehensive framework for research, policy, and political action. *Critical Public Health, 15*(2), 157–179.

Labonte, R., & Gagnon, M. L. (2010). Framing health and foreign policy: Lessons for global health diplomacy. *Globalization and Health, 6,* 14. Retrieved from http://www.globalizationandhealth.com/content/6/1/14

Laxminarayan, R., Kakkar, M., Horby, P., Malavige, G. N., & Basnyat, B. (2017). *Emerging and re-emerging infectious disease threats in South Asia: Status, vulnerability, preparedness, and outlook.* http://dx.doi.org/10.1136/bmj.j1447

Lee, C. F., Cowling, B. J., & Lau, E. H. (2017). Epidemiology of reemerging scarlet fever, Hong Kong, 2005–2015. *Emerging Infectious Diseases, 23*(10), 1707–1710. https://doi.org/10.3201/eid2310.161456

Legatum Institute. (2017). *The Legatum Prosperity Index™ 2017: Creating the pathways from poverty to prosperity. Legatum Institute Foundation.* Retrieved from http://www.prosperity.com/globe/canada

Loomba, A. (2005). *Colonialism/postcolonialism* (2nd ed.). New York, NY: Routledge.

Odeny, B. M., Pfeiffer, J., Farquhar, C., Igonya, E. K., Gatuguta, A., Kagwaini, F., . . . Bosire, R. (2016). The stigma of exclusive breastfeeding among both HIV-positive and HIV-negative women in Nairobi, Kenya. *Breastfeeding Medicine, 11,* 252–258.

Office of the United Nations High Commissioner for Human Rights & World Health Organization. (2008). *The right to health. Fact sheet. N. 31.* Geneva, CH: Author. Retrieved from http://www.ohchr.org/Documents/Publications/Factsheet31.pdf

Owen, J. W., & Roberts, O. (2005). Globalization, health and foreign policy: Emerging linkages and interests. *Globalization and Health, 1*(12). Retrieved from http://www.globalizationandhealth.com/content/pdf/1744-8603-1-12.pdf doi:10.1186/1744-8603-1-12

Paules, C. I., & Fauci, A. S. (2017). Emerging and reemerging infectious diseases: The dichotomy between acute outbreaks and chronic endemicity. *Journal of the American Medical Association, 317*(7), 691–692. doi:10.1001/jama.2016.21079

Pinto, A. D., & Upshur, R. E. (2009). Global health ethics for students. *Developing World Bioethics, 9*(1), 1–10.

Premji, S. S., & Hatfield, J. (2016). Call to action for nurses/nursing. *BioMed Research International.* doi:10.1155/2016/3127543

Rao, C. Y., Goryoka, G. W., Henao, O. L., Clarke, K. R., Salyer, S. J., & Montgomery, J. M. (2017). Global disease detection—Achievements in applied public health

research, capacity building, and public health diplomacy, 2001–2016. *Emerging Infectious Diseases, 23*(Suppl 1), S138–S146. https://doi.org/10.3201/eid2313.170859

Reardon, S. (2014). Smallpox watch. *Nature, 509*(7498), 22–24.

Say, L., Chou, D., Gemmill, A., Tunçalp, Ö., Moller, A. B., Daniels, J., . . . Alkema, L. (2014). Global causes of maternal death: A WHO systematic analysis. *The Lancet Global Health, 2*(6), e323-e333. http://dx.doi.org/10.1016/S2214-109X(14)70227-X

Spiegel, J. M., Labonte, R., & Ostry, A. S. (2004). Understanding "globalization" as a determinant of health determinants: A critical perspective. *International Journal of Occupational and Environmental Health, 10*(4), 360–367.

Spyrou, M. A., Tukhbatova, R. I., Feldman, M., Drath, J., Kacki, S., de Heredia, J. B., . . . Gazimzyanov, I. R. (2016). Historical Y. pestis genomes reveal the European black death as the source of ancient and modern plague pandemics. *Cell Host & Microbe, 19*(6), 874–881. http://dx.doi.org/10.1016/j.chom.2016.05.012

Statistics Canada. (2010). Study: Projections of the diversity of the Canadian population. *The Daily,* March 9 [cited 2010 Mar 25]. Retrieved from: http://www.statcan.gc.ca/daily-quotidien/100309/dq100309a-eng.htm

Swider, S. M., Levin, P. F., & Kulbok, P. A. (2015). Creating the future of public health nursing: A call to action. *Public Health Nursing, 32*(2), 91–93.

Taylor, S. (2009). Wealth, health and equity: Convergence to divergence in late 20th century globalisation. *British Medical Bulletin, 91*(1), 29–48.

The Lancet. (2017). Life, death, and disability in 2016. *The Lancet, 390*(10100), 1083. doi:10.1016/S0140-6736(17)32465-0

United Nations. (2000). Millennium summit (6-8 September 2000). Used with permission of United Nations. Retrieved from http://www.un.org/en/events/pastevents/millennium_summit.shtml

United Nations. (2014). *General Assembly August 12, 2014: Report of the open working group of the General Assembly on Sustainable Development Goals.* Retrieved from http://www.un.org/ga/search/view_doc.asp?symbol=A/68/970&Lang=E

United Nations Secretary-General. (2010). *Keeping the promise: A forward-looking review to promote an agreed action agenda to achieve the Millennium Development Goals by 2015.* Retrieved from http://www.un.org/en/mdg/summit2010

United Nations Sustainable Development Solutions Network. (2013). Membership. Retrieved from http://unsdsn.org/membership/about-our-network

United Nations System Task Team on the Post-2015 UN Development Agenda. (2012). *Realizing the future we want for all: Report to the Secretary-General.* Retrieved from http://www.un.org/en/development/desa/policy/untaskteam_undf/untt_report.pdf

United Nations Inter-Agency Group for Child Mortality Estimation. (2017). *Levels and trends in child mortality.* Geneva, CH: United Nations Children's Fund. Retrieved from http://childmortality.org/files_v21/download/IGME%20report%202017%20child%20mortality%20final.pdf

World Bank. (2010). *People, pathogens and our planet. Volume 1: Toward a one health approach for controlling zoonotic disease,* Washington, DC: World Bank. Retrieved from http://siteresources.worldbank.org/INTARD/Resources/PPPWeb.pdf

World Health Organization (WHO). (1978). *Declaration of Alma Alta: International conference on primary health care, Alma-Ata, USSR, 6–12*. Europe: Reprinted with permission from World Health Organization. Author. Retrieved from http://www.who.int/publications/almaata_declaration_en.pdf

World Health Organization (WHO). (2013). *Trade, foreign policy, diplomacy and health: Global health diplomacy*. Reprinted with permission from World Health Organization. Retrieved from http://www.who.int/trade/diplomacy/en

World Health Organization (WHO). (2016). *Maternal mortality*. Fact sheet N. 348. Geneva, DH: Author. Retrieved from http://www.who.int/mediacentre/factsheets/fs348/en

World Health Organization (WHO). (2017a). *10 facts about tuberculosis*. Retrieved from http://www.who.int/features/factfiles/tuberculosis/en/

World Health Organization (WHO). (2017b). *Children: Reducing mortality. Fact sheet N. 178*. Geneva, CH: Author. Retrieved from http://www.who.int/mediacentre/factsheets/fs178/en

World Health Organization (WHO). (2017c). *Health statistics and information systems: Estimates for 2000–2015*. Geneva, CH: Author. Retrieved from http://www.who.int/healthinfo/global_burden_disease/estimates/en/index2.html

World Health Organization (WHO). (2017d). *Infant and young child feeding*. Retrieved from http://www.who.int/mediacentre/factsheets/fs342/en

World Health Organization. (2017e). *Six lines of action to promote health in the 2030 agenda for sustainable development*. Retrieved from http://www.who.int/gho/publications/world_health_statistics/2017/EN_WHS2017_Part1.pdf?ua=1

World Health Organization (WHO). (2017f). *World health statistics 2017: Monitoring health for the SDGs*. Geneva, CH: Author. Retrieved from http://www.who.int/gho/publications/world_health_statistics/2017/en

World Health Organization (WHO). (2018a). *Maternal mortality: Key facts*. Retrieved from http://www.who.int/news-room/fact-sheets/detail/maternal-mortality

World Health Organization (WHO). 2018b. *The top 10 causes of death*. Retrieved from http://www.who.int/en/news-room/fact-sheets/detail/the-top-10-causes-of-death

ABOUT THE AUTHORS

Shahirose Premji, RN, BSc, BScN, MScN, PhD, FAAN, is now Director and Professor, School of Nursing, Faculty of Health at York University. She was an associate professor in the Faculty of Nursing and Adjunct Associate Professor in the Cumming School of Medicine, Department of Community Health Sciences at University of Calgary in Calgary. She holds a PhD in Clinical Health Sciences (Nursing) from McMaster University. She leads an international team on two CIHR funded projects: Pakistan and China. She is the founder and first president of the Canadian Association of Neonatal Nurses. She is the recipient of the Jeanne Mance Award, the College & Association of Registered Nurses of Alberta's Centennial Award, and the Nursing Excellence in Research Award. To mark the 150th anniversary of Canadian Confederation, the Canadian Nurses Association honored her as one of 150 nurses!

Aliyah Dosani, RN, BN, MPH, PhD, is Associate Professor in the School of Nursing and Midwifery, Faculty of Health, Community and Education at Mount Royal University in Calgary, Alberta. She is also an Adjunct Associate Professor in the Department of Community Health Sciences, Cumming School of Medicine, at University of Calgary in Calgary. She holds a PhD from the University of Calgary with a specialization in population/public health. Her nursing practice includes instructing students in the Bachelor of Nursing program, population/public health, community health nursing, and legal issues in nursing. Her work focuses on maternal, newborn, and child health. Her research interests include working on health equity and social justice issues through community-based programs and interventions. She also shares a passion for global health issues.

Josephine Etowa, RM, RN , BScN, MN, PhD, FWACN, FAAN, is a professor and Loyer-DaSilva Research Chair in Public Health Nursing at the University of Ottawa. She is a senior investigator with the Nursing Best Practice Research Centre at the University of Ottawa and a founding member and past president of the Health Association of African Canadians. Her program of research is grounded in over 25 years of clinical practice in maternal newborn and child health, and community health nursing, with projects funded by local, national, and international funding organizations. She is currently the nominated Principal Investigator for a CIHR-funded three-year-three-country study, investigating infant feeding practices among Black women living with HIV/AIDs in Ottawa (Canada), Port Harcourt (Nigeria), and Miami (United States).

CHAPTER 34

Critical Community Health Nursing: An Imperative

Aliyah Dosani, Josephine Etowa, and Cheryl van Daalen-Smith

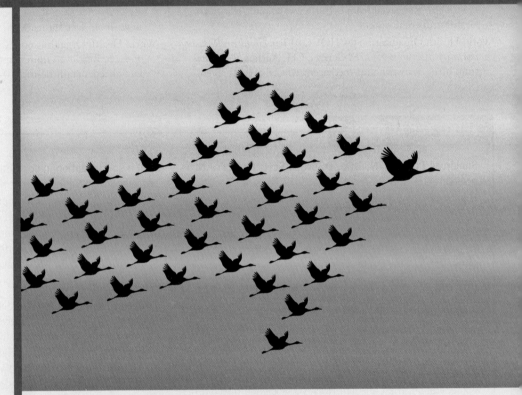

Source: Harish Marnad/Shutterstock

"Reducing health inequities is . . . an ethical imperative.
Social injustice is killing people on a grand scale."

WHO (2008, p. 40).

INTRODUCTION

Community health nurses (CHNs) work in a variety of settings where people live, work, play, worship, and learn. They attend to the diverse social determinants of health that influence the opportunity for optimal health across the lifespan, and they use collaborative actions to promote, protect, and restore the health of populations. In May 2018 a powerful report confirmed what Canada's CHNs know: There are marked health inequities still faced by numerous populations in Canada. The Public Health Agency of Canada's Key Health

Inequalities in Canada report indicates that in some cases these health inequities are actually growing (Public Health Agency of Canada [PHAC], 2018). According to this report, racialized persons in Canada, Indigenous persons, gender variant persons, and individuals left with precarious access to the social determinants of health have the poorest health and quality of life.

While studying the chapters of this text, you have come to understand how the various structural determinants of health contribute to health equity gaps for individuals, families, communities, and populations. Social issues such as poverty, homelessness, violence, and food insecurity produce both physiological and psychological stress that pose health risks to individuals across the lifespan (Garg, Sandel, Dworkin, Kahn, & Zuckerman, 2012). Although the opportunities for CHNs to influence change are limitless, it is essential that CHNs are well prepared to actively engage in critical community health nursing. It is important for CHNs to use a critical social theory lens to advance social justice and advocacy through upstream and intersectional analyses. Akin to the Canadian Nurses Association (2010), the editorial team believes that "social justice is both a means to an end, and an end in itself" (p. 1). Rather than going along with the status quo, it is our belief that Canada's CHNs seek to ameliorate health inequities in partnership with the communities they serve. Further, given the recommendations put forth by the Truth and Reconciliation Commission of Canada (2015), it is fundamental that CHNs address the legacy of colonization to promote and advocate for the well-being of Indigenous peoples in Canada. Indeed, social justice and health for all is the aim of community health nursing practice in Canada and the intended goal of this text. To that end, the previous 33 chapters are rooted in a health equity and social justice lens, crafted especially for Canada's community health nursing nurses, professors, practice instructors, and students. If community health nursing practice is to be truly critical, CHNs need to be aware of how health is impacted by trends and the pedagogy of CHN education (i.e., both content and approach). For such practice to flourish, CHNs need to enact leadership that enables transformations both in practice and in practice settings.

TRENDS IN COMMUNITY HEALTH NURSING

Canada's CHNs have a momentous legacy of speaking up because they've witnessed health inequities, and this history can be used to fuel our envisioned future. It is crucial for CHNs to be well informed of socioeconomic, political, and environmental trends (such as global warming, the opioid crisis, or forced migration) to understand the impact on the health of various communities. First, the demographics of the Canadian population are changing, as seen in an aging population, a widening gap between the rich and the poor, increasingly diverse ethnocultural and racialized communities, and the increase in Indigenous sub-populations. As stated above, there are marked health inequities still faced by numerous populations in Canada. Efforts to address health equity ought to include strategies and solutions that create an environment of empowerment for

disadvantaged communities to dismantle the forces of marginalization such as systemic discrimination (Marmot, Allen, Bell, Bloomer, & Goldblatt, 2012). A one-size-fits-all approach fails to reflect an awareness of the diversity of experiences of oppression or privilege. Strategies to improve population health will need to reflect the different groups living in Canada; as the Canadian population becomes increasingly diverse, it is CHNs' duty to know who their populations are and what their specific strengths and health needs truly are. CHNs can provide critical community health nursing care that is grounded in cultural safety and humility. This involves consideration of health equity approaches that are intersectional and rooted in social justice.

Second, with longer life expectancy for most Canadians, we are seeing rising rates of chronic diseases such as cancers, lung diseases, obesity, diabetes, heart conditions, debilitating arthritis, chronic pain, and Alzheimer's disease. These illnesses vary along ethnoracial and socioeconomic lines. There still are significant "health inequities—the differences in health status between groups resulting from social disadvantages that can be modified through policy and program intervention" (PHAC, 2018, p. 61). The PHAC report associates these differences in health within sub-groups of Canadians with "social, political, and economic advantages or disadvantages that these groups experience, which affect their chances of achieving and maintaining good health over their lifetimes" (p. 425). In response, CHNs need to be creative in using both upstream and downstream strategies to reduce inequities. Best addressed with approaches mindful of intersectional and critical social theory lenses that will dismantle barriers to accessing health, these frameworks will assist CHNs to proactively position themselves as co-creators of sustained change.

GETTING CRITICAL

Critical community health nursing practice means CHNs focus on broader and societal-level factors that impact the health of populations. It involves our ongoing involvement in higher-level initiatives that address the root causes of inequities in health status. To be critical means we ask, "Yes, but why?" when faced with staggering statistics regarding the inequities in health and quality of life of communities, especially communities rendered vulnerable by unjust structural policies and practices. We approach health promotion with a strengths-based approach in partnership with our communities, taking their lead, and with cultural humility, especially when working alongside First Nation, Inuit, and Métis populations. We are intersectional in our work, ensuring we avoid cookie-cutter approaches that are often based on Eurocentric and classist values, which can, if we are not careful, bring about more harm than good.

In being critical, Canada's CHNs seek to ameliorate inequities, using our moral courage and our standards of practice, which call on us to notice patterns, ask tough questions, and advocate for the health of all. Instead of relying solely on behavioural models of health promotion, focusing on the individual in front of us, we recognize the neoliberal assumptions underpinning uncritical community health nursing work that assumes we can health teach individuals into "right choices and behaviours." We need to challenge the right choices model that is based on assumptions that individuals are solely responsible for their health. Instead, "nurses can refer to the strong evidence that inequalities in health outcomes are about unequal access to the SDOH" and the "biologic effects of stress that result from these unequal opportunities to be healthy. CHNs can (and should) point out that trying to change behavior without changing its social context is unlikely to be successful" (Cohen, 2010, p. 48). In fact, the Key Health Inequities in Canada report explicitly states: "Public health actions that focus on individual-level behavioural determinants may inadvertently *increase* health inequalities in the absence of accompanying efforts that target 'upstream' socioeconomic, political, cultural, and environmental factors" (PHAC, 2018, p. 10). Being critical reflects an awareness that the answer to "Why are some people healthy and others not?" is often "a toxic combination . . . of poor social policies and programs, unfair economic arrangements, and bad politics" (Marmot & Bell, 2011, p. S74).

Critical and Responsive Education

Community health nursing has always been part of baccalaureate nursing curricula, with a broad-based approach that identifies individuals, families, communities, and populations as our clients. We believe that in order for CHN practice to address and prevent health inequities, community health nursing education is required to be responsive, critical, and proactive. We invite our Canadian nurse educators to broaden the discussions about community health. Our educators provide the ideal classroom space to unpack complex circumstances surrounding the health of diverse communities through intersectional and social justice lenses. Furthermore, educators oversee student placements in increasingly diverse settings so that students can learn from people's lived experiences while seeing health from various vantage points. As Canadian nursing moves toward a shared-care practice model, it is important for CHN educators to advocate for inter-professional education opportunities where community health nursing students can role model critical practice that is intersectional.

Graduate opportunities in community health are increasing in number, scope, and variety. For example, the Canadian Nurse Practitioner Initiative of the CNA worked with provincial organizations and schools of nursing to create curricula for primary health care nurse practitioner programs. Also, graduate nursing students have opportunities to tailor MN and MScN degrees to a community health specialty or to consider interdisciplinary Master of Public Health programs that are established across the country. Here also, we encourage our nursing colleagues to ensure that at the graduate level, we continue to inspire our students to ask complex questions regarding why some people are healthy and others are not, focusing on structural barriers to health and quality of life.

The Canadian Association of Schools of Nursing's (CASN) Community Health Interest Group was created after the CASN Public Health Nursing Task Force disbanded in 2015. The initial work of the Task Force was to create guidelines (Canadian Association of Schools of Nursing [CASN], 2010)

for universities when securing quality community clinical placements for students to ensure students had access to working with groups and populations. Additionally, expected qualifications for faculty advisors and preceptors were outlined. The Task Force made prodigious efforts to ensure that competencies existed to define how public health nurses should apply knowledge and skills to address the determinants of health and to build relationships with communities to achieve population health (Community Health Nurses of Canada, 2014). Additionally, to support the integration of the competencies into curricula, a public health nursing teaching strategies website was developed. The Interest Group has most recently developed national curriculum guidelines for integrating community health into baccalaureate nursing programs (CASN, 2018).

IMPLICATIONS FOR COMMUNITY HEALTH NURSING PRACTICE

When the foundation of community health nursing education is grounded in learning how to address community health issues from critical and intersectional lenses, we will have nurses who are prepared to address health equity gaps at various levels. This will subsequently have workplace implications—for critical CHN education will birth nursing graduates who will insist on a scope of practice that enables them to advocate for health equity and social justice for populations rendered vulnerable by structural or policy inequity.

Although many CHNs have been working critically for decades, current societal structures, including various work environments, may limit the scope of the CHN's practice. We hope an influx of new graduates firmly grounded in critical community health nursing practice will challenge the status quo. Community health nursing practice began in response to social injustice that was observed in early Canadian history. We ask that CHNs remember our roots and return to this form of practice where CHNs worked tirelessly to improve access to the social determinants of health. For such a shift to take place, similar changes in research and leadership practice are required.

Critical Research

Research informed by a critical social theory lens is, at its core, about the examination of power relations. This is necessary to uncover how power is implicated in health equity and in our thoughts, feelings, and actions (e.g., prejudice, stigma, discrimination, justification of inequities, and oppression). Community health nursing researchers as agents of society exercise power, which can be used positively to transform societal structures. Traditionally, community health nursing practice has been rooted in theories of behavioural psychology, biomedical science, and public administration (Potvin, Gendron, Bilodeau, & Chabot, 2005). However, the evidence on the structural determinants of health and the complexity of contemporary health service delivery calls for research that takes a critical theory approach.

Throughout this text, we have included selected Canadian nursing research studies to address various aspects of community health and nursing practice. The ultimate goal of any type of health research is to improve quality of life. Over the past decade, we have seen a welcome diversification in methods of engaging in research at the community and population levels that include participatory action research (PAR) and population health intervention research (PHIR). PAR is not new, but it has come to the forefront again as more emphasis is being placed on working *with* communities. The goal of PAR is to build capacity among community members and associated stakeholders to empower them to engage in some form of social change (MacDonald, 2012). Canada's CHNs recognize that community-based participatory research is the preferred model of engaging in research (Blumenthal, Diclemente, Braithwaite, & Smith, 2013). The use of PAR is particularly important in resource-poor communities where health-promotion work best takes place at the grassroots level.

It will be increasingly important for CHNs to be familiar with and use PHIR to inform their nursing practice. The goal of PHIR is to "produce knowledge about policy, programs, and events that have the potential to impact health at the population level" (Hawe, Di Ruggiero, & Cohen, 2012, p. e468). As such, it is imperative that CHNs advocate for developing critical research questions and using intersectional approaches during analyses of data. Such research is useful in framing prevention initiatives, including interventions to alter the underlying sociocultural and environmental risks that will ultimately decrease health inequities (Benach, Malmusi, Yasui, Marinez, & Muntaner, 2011; Rose, 1992). Hence, PHIR identifies the decisions people make, including the choice and power that individuals in decision-making positions have that ultimately result in some people being rich and others poor (Hawe et al., 2012).

Looking to the future, CHNs will need to advocate for critical empowerment-based research that gives voice to communities that are otherwise unheard or misunderstood. Ensuring the deployment of a wide variety of research approaches that accurately reflect the myriad of community health issues that need to be addressed to decrease health inequities *is* the CHN's research imperative. This means CHNs will need to excel in the research process, from conceiving research ideas that are community-derived, to data collection and analysis, and finally to disseminating the results. We know that women, racialized populations, older adults, people living in rural areas, and other marginalized populations are often underrepresented in research (Cottler et al., 2013). CHNs can find ways to use their rapport-building skills to engage various communities and population groups in the research process and as research participants. At the same time, care must be taken to avoid further marginalization of various populations that are already disadvantaged. Furthermore, in keeping with the principles of primary health care, it is important for CHNs to keep public participation at the forefront of their research initiatives, regardless of the community or setting they may be working in.

To be responsive to the needs and preferences of society in general and of diverse communities more specifically, educational institutions, health care employers, professional nursing associations, and individual CHNs need to follow developments in research. It is critical for nurse educators to be aware of the current research being undertaken at the community and population levels so that graduating nurses are prepared to engage in community health nursing practice in a meaningful way—either by being involved in the research process or by utilizing community health research results to inform their nursing practice. Educators can act as role models, helping to develop a culture of nursing research and curiosity when working with their students. Furthermore, it is vital for employers to influence working conditions so that CHNs may have various opportunities to either engage in research activities or have sufficient resources at their disposal to make informed practice decisions based on evidence. When national, provincial, and local community health nursing associations, as well as individual CHNs, incorporate such evidence into their practice, we see community voices finally being heard and community health nursing practice move forward.

Transformational Leadership

CHNs are ideally positioned to act as leaders in promoting health and advancing health care in Canadian communities. Their intimate knowledge of healthcare and community needs both at the point-of-care and population health level gives them the unique opportunity to advocate for, and lead positive systemic change. CHNs have an integral role to play in collaborating with diverse communities to prioritize and address their health needs. Transformational leadership is one way to ensure meaningful engagement of communities to address a common problem. If community health nursing practice is to be critical, transformational leadership is imperative. Transformational CHN leadership is necessary to address health equity especially as it affects historically disadvantaged communities such as Indigenous and Immigrant people. It is congruent with social justice lens which is an essential aspect of community health nursing practice. Cusack, Cohen, Mignone, Chartier, and Lutfiyya (2018) call for public nursing leaders to "actively strive to implement programs and policies based on participatory approaches that include nursing staff in decisions pertinent to their practice" (p. 1545). Creating an empowering environment for CHNs to flourish at all levels of practice requires a certain kind of authority, autonomy, and power distribution. Transformational leadership has been described as "a process of creating a vision and delivering a sense of belonging to employees" (Choi, Goh, Adam, & Tan, 2016, p. 4). It is instrumental in promoting intellectual stimulation and enhancing employee performance, trust, and commitment, which builds confidence through multiple levels of mentoring (Choi et al., 2016).

While working collaboratively with other professionals and community members, CHNs "develop leaders that are able to build a shared vision within a group/organization/community and who facilitate the distribution of leadership processes according to the group's expertise, as well as act as a catalyst for shared decision-making processes and collective actions" (Careau et al., 2014, p. 43). It is crucial for CHNs to build leadership capacity by working with multidisciplinary teams on common health issues, with a goal to achieve health outcomes that align with community needs (Careau et al., 2014). Humphreys et al. (2015) describe the importance of understanding how various models of leadership affect health disparities, conflict resolution and negotiation, and community organizing. Ultimately, the goal is to develop leadership capacity, building within community members themselves such that community empowerment can be achieved. To this end, CHNs will need to strategically place themselves at various levels of decision making within health systems and governments if we are to see significant improvements in health equity.

CONCLUSION

If our role as community health nurses is to decrease health inequities, advocate for sustained social justice in partnership with our communities and prevent health issues in the first place—*critical* CHN practice, education, research and education truly is our shared imperative. As affirmed by the WHO's Commission on the Social Determinants of Health (World Health Organization, 2008), the presence or absence of social justice can mean life or death. It is therefore imperative for Canada's CHNs to maintain social justice as our ethos and to embed it in everything we do.

This has been a most humbling experience, to work with 34 author teams so that we may bring this, our offering, to you. May this text and the way you use it be *your* call to action. Canada's CHNs have an amazing legacy of partnering with communities in order to make real change. Here's to another impactful century.

REFERENCES

Benach, J., Malmusi, D., Yasui, Y., Marinez, J. M., & Muntaner, C. (2011). Beyond Rose's strategies: A typology of scenarios of policy impact on health and health inequalities. *International Journal of Health Services, 41*(10), 1–9.

Blumenthal, D. S., Diclemente, R. J., Braithwaite, R., & Smith, S. A. (Eds.). (2013). *Community based participatory research: Issues, methods, and translation to practice* (2nd ed.). New York, NY: Springer Publishing Company, LLC.

Canadian Association of Schools of Nursing (CASN). (2010). *Guidelines for quality community health nursing clinical placements for baccalaureate nursing student.* Retrieved from http://casn.ca/vm/newvisual/attachments/856/Media/CPGuidelinesFinalMarch.pdf

Canadian Association of Schools of Nursing (CASN). (2018). *Curricular guidelines for integrating community health into baccalaureate programs of nursing.* Ottawa, ON: Community Health Education Interest Group. Retrieved from https://www.chnc.ca/en/membership/documents/loadDocument?id=1641&download=1#upload/membership/document/2018-05/community-health-guidelines-1332-.pdf

Canadian Nurses Association (CNA). (2010). *Social justice: A means to an end and an end in itself.* Retrieved from https://www.cna-aiic.ca/~/media/cna/page-content/pdf-en/social_justice_2010_e.pdf

Careau, E., Biba, G., Brander, R., van Dijk, J. P., Verma, S., Paterson, M., & Tassone, M. (2014). Health leadership education programs, best practices, and impacts on learners' knowledge, skills, attitudes, and behaviors and system change: A literature review. *Journal of Healthcare Leadership, 6*, 39–50. http://dx.doi.org/10.2147/JHL.S61127

Choi, S. L., Goh, C. F., Adam, M. B. H., & Tan, O. K. (2016). Transformational leadership, empowerment, and job satisfaction: The mediating role of employee empowerment. *Human Resources for Health, 14*(1), 73. doi:10.1186/s12960-016-0171-2

Cohen, B. (2010). From witness to social justice advocate. *Canadian Nurse, 106*(7), 48.

Community Health Nurses of Canada. (2014). *CHNC position statement: Community health nursing education.* St. John's, NL: Author. Retrieved from https://www.chnc.ca/documents/PositionStatementCHNEducationFINAL-2015March1.pdf

Cottler, L. B., McCloskey, D. J., Aguilar-Gaxiola, S., Bennett, N. M., Strelnick, H., Dwyer-White, M., . . . Evanoff, B. (2013). Community needs, concerns, and perceptions about health research: Findings from the clinical and translational science award sentinel network. *American Journal of Public Health, 103*(9), 1685–1692. doi:10.2105/AJPH.2012.300941

Cusack, C., Cohen, B., Mignone, J., Chartier, M. J., & Lutfiyya, Z. (2018). Participatory action as a research method with public health nurses. *Journal of Advanced Nursing, 74*, 1544–1553 doi:10.1111/jan.13555

Garg, A., Sandel, M., Dworkin, P. H., Kahn, R. S., & Zuckerman, B. (2012). From medical home to health neighborhood: Transforming the medical into a community-based health neighborhood. *The Journal of Pediatrics, 160*(4), 535–536. doi:10.1016/j.jpeds.2012.01.001

Hawe, P., Di Ruggiero, E., & Cohen, E. (2012). Frequently asked questions about population health intervention research. *Canadian Journal of Public Health, 103*(6), e468–e471.

Humphreys, B. P., Couse, L. J., Sonnenmeier, R. M., Kurtz, A., Russell, S. M., & Antal, P. (2015). Transforming LEND leadership training curriculum through the maternal and child health leadership competencies. *Maternal and Child Health Journal, 19*, 300–307. doi:10.1007/s10995-014-1587-8

MacDonald, C. (2012). Understanding participatory action research: A qualitative research methodology option. *Canadian Journal of Action Research, 13*(2), 34–50.

Marmot, M. G. & Bell, R. G. (2011). Improving health: Social determinants and personal choice. *American Journal of Preventive Medicine, 40*(1), S73–S77.

Marmot, M., Allen, J., Bell, R., Bloomer, E., & Goldblatt, P. (2012). WHO European review of social determinants of health and the health divide. *The Lancet, 380*(9846), 1011–1029.

Potvin, L., Gendron, S., Bilodeau, A., & Chabot, P. (2005). Integrating social theory into public health practice. *American Journal of Public Health, 95*(4), 591–595.

Public Health Agency of Canada (PHAC) (2018). *Key health inequities in Canada.* Retrieved from https://www.canada.ca/content/dam/phac-aspc/documents/services/publications/science-research/key-health-inequalities-canada-national-portrait-executive-summary/hir-full-report-eng.pdf

Rose, G. (1992). *The strategy of preventive medicine*. Oxford, UK: Oxford University Press.

Truth and Reconciliation Commission of Canada. (2015). *Truth and Reconciliation Commission of Canada: Calls to Action*. Retrieved from http://www.trc.ca/websites/trcinstitution/File/2015/Findings/Calls_to_Action_English2.pdf

World Health Organization (WHO). (2008). *Commission on the social determinants of health. Closing the gap in a generation: Health equity through action on the social determinants of health*. Full report and executive summary. Retrieved from http://www.who.int/social_determinants/thecommission/finalreport/en

ABOUT THE AUTHORS

Aliyah Dosani, RN, BN, MPH, PhD, is Associate Professor in the School of Nursing and Midwifery, Faculty of Health, Community and Education at Mount Royal University in Calgary, Alberta. She is also an Adjunct Associate Professor in the Department of Community Health Sciences, Cumming School of Medicine, at University of Calgary in Calgary. She holds a PhD from the University of Calgary with a specialization in population/public health. Her nursing practice includes instructing students in the Bachelor of Nursing program, population/public health, community health nursing, and legal issues in nursing. Her work focuses on maternal, newborn, and child health. Her research interests include working on health equity and social justice issues through community-based programs and interventions. She also shares a passion for global health issues.

Josephine Etowa, RM, RN, BScN, MN, PhD, FWACN, FAAN, is Professor and Loyer-DaSilva Research Chair in Public Health Nursing at the University of Ottawa. She is a senior investigator with the Nursing Best Practice Research Centre at the University of Ottawa and a founding member and past president of the Health Association of African Canadians. Her program of research is grounded in over 25 years of clinical practice in maternal, newborn, and child health and community health nursing with projects funded by local, national, and international funding organizations. She is currently the nominated Principal Investigator for a CIHR-funded three-year, three-country study, investigating infant feeding practices among Black women who are living with HIV/AIDs in Ottawa (Canada), Port Harcourt (Nigeria), and Miami (United States). She serves on the board of directors of the Canadian Public Health Association and the Community Health Nurses of Canada (CHNC) Research Committee, and she co-chairs the CHNC's Standards of Practice Advisory Committee.

Cheryl van Daalen-Smith, RN, PhD, is a critical public health nurse and an associate professor in the School of Nursing, Faculty of Health at York University. She is cross appointed to the School of Gender, Sexuality and Women's Studies, Critical Disability Studies, Interdisciplinary Studies, and to the Children's Studies Program, where she brings a practice-rooted upstream, critical, and intersectional lens on health and quality of life to her teaching and scholarship. In partnership with a long-serving community development worker, she is currently working with a group of young women in developing a community-owned and driven Women's Hub in the Jane-Finch core of Toronto. She has simply loved her time working with her author teams and her co-editors, Josephine and Aliyah, to bring this fifth edition to fruition.

Appendix A: The Canadian Community Health Nursing Standards of Practice

INTRODUCTION

The Canadian Community Health Nursing Standards of Practice (the Standards) represent a vision for excellence in community health nursing. The Standards define the practice of a registered nurse in the specialty area of community health nursing. They build on the generic practice expectations of registered nurses and identify the practice principles and variations specific to community health nursing in Canada. The Standards apply to community health nurses who work in the areas of practice, education, administration, and research.

PURPOSE OF STANDARDS OF PRACTICE

- Define the scope and depth of community nursing practice.
- Establish criteria and expectations for acceptable nursing practice and safe, ethical care.
- Provide criteria for measuring actual performance.
- Support ongoing development of community health nursing.
- Promote community health nursing as a specialty and provide the foundation for certification of community health nursing by the Canadian Nurses Association.
- Inspire excellence in and commitment to community nursing practice.
- Set a benchmark for new community health nurses.

USING THE STANDARDS OF PRACTICE

- Nurses in clinical practice use the standards to guide and evaluate their practice.
- Nursing educators include the standards in course curricula to prepare new graduates for practice in community settings.
- Nurse administrators use the standards to direct policy and guide performance expectations.
- Nurse researchers use the standards to guide the development of knowledge specific to community health nursing.

COMMUNITY HEALTH NURSING PRACTICE

Community health nurses value caring, principles of primary health care, multiple ways of knowing, individual and community partnerships, empowerment, and social justice.[xviii]

Community health nursing acknowledges its roots and traditions, embraces advances, and recognizes the importance of the need to continually evolve as a dynamic nursing specialty.[i] (See Figure 1, History of Community Health Nursing.)

A new nurse entering community health practice will likely need at least two years to achieve the practice expectations of these specialty Standards. Strong mentorship, leadership and peer support, as well as self-directed and guided learning all contribute to the achievement of the expertise required.

Community health nurses practise in a variety of specialty care services and work in a variety of settings. (See Appendix F–*Community Health Nursing by Area of Practice*.) Home health nursing and public health nursing are linked historically through common beliefs, values, traditions, skills and above all their unique focus on promoting and protecting community health.

Evolving from centuries of community care by laywomen and members of religious orders, community health nursing started to gain recognition as a nursing specialty in the mid-1800s. Florence Nightingale and Lillian Wald as well as organizations such as the Victorian Order of Nurses, the Henry Street Settlement, and the Canadian Red Cross Society have permanently shaped community health nursing. During the 20th century, public health and home health nursing emerged from common roots to represent the ideals of community health nursing. Community health nursing is situated on a foundation of ethical practice and caring.[i]

FIGURE 1 History of Community Health Nursing

Home health nursing and public health nursing differ in their client and program emphasis. Both Public Health Nurses[vi] and Home Health Nurses[vii] have discipline specific competencies that define the integrated knowledge, skills, and attributes required to achieve the standards. (See Appendix G for a diagram depicting the *Relationship Between Standards and Competencies*.)

Community health nurses view health as a dynamic process of physical, mental, spiritual, and social well-being. Health includes self-determination, realization of hopes and needs, and a sense of connection to the community.[i] Community health nurses consider health as a resource for everyday life that is influenced by circumstances, beliefs, and the determinants of health. The determinants of health are factors and conditions that affect health status and include social, cultural, political, economic, physical, and environmental health determinants. Additional determinants of health specific to aboriginal populations have also been identified. (See also Appendix C—*Determinants of Health*)

A *Glossary of Terms*, which further describes relevant concepts and terms related to community health nursing practice can be found at http://chnc.ca/nursing-publications.cfm

STANDARDS OF PRACTICE FOR COMMUNITY HEALTH NURSES

STANDARD 1: HEALTH PROMOTION
STANDARD 2: PREVENTION AND HEALTH PROTECTION
STANDARD 3: HEALTH MAINTENANCE, RESTORATION, AND PALLIATION
STANDARD 4: PROFESSIONAL RELATIONSHIPS
STANDARD 5: CAPACITY BUILDING
STANDARD 6: HEALTH EQUITY
STANDARD 7: EVIDENCE INFORMED PRACTICE
STANDARD 8: PROFESSIONAL RESPONSIBILITY AND ACCOUNTABILITY

Standard 1: Health Promotion

Community health nurses integrate health promotion into practice using the five Ottawa Charter health promotion strategies (build healthy public policy, create supportive environments, strengthen community actions, develop personal skills and reorient health services).[i] "Health promotion is the process of enabling people to increase control over, and to improve, their health."

The Community Health Nurse. . .

a. Applies health promotion theories and models in practice such as change theories, primary health care, population health promotion model, and social and ecological determinants of health including Aboriginal peoples'.[ii, iii]

b. Collaborates with client to do a comprehensive, evidence informed, and strength-based holistic health assessment using multiple sources and methods to identify needs, assets, inequities and resources.

c. Seeks to identify and assess the root and historical causes of illness, disease and inequities in health, acknowledges diversity and the adverse effects of colonialism on Indigenous people, and when appropriate incorporates Indigenous ways of knowing including connectedness and reciprocity to the land and all life in health promotion.

d. Considers the determinants of health, the social and political context, and systemic structures in collaboration with the client to determine action.

e. Implements appropriate communication approaches such as social marketing and media advocacy to disseminate health information and raise awareness of health issues at individual and/or societal level.

f. Includes cultural safety and cultural humility approaches in all health promotion interventions.[iv]

g. Uses a collaborative relationship with the client and other partners to facilitate and advocate for structural system change and healthy public policy using multiple health promotion strategies.

h. Evaluates and modifies health promotion activities in partnership with the client.

- Identifies the level of intervention necessary to promote health.
- Identifies which determinants of health require action or change to promote health.
- Uses a comprehensive range of strategies to address health-related issues.

FIGURE 2 Population Health Promotion Model

Standard 2: Prevention and Health Protection

Community health nurses use the socio-ecological model to integrate prevention and health protection activities into practice.[v] These actions are implemented in accordance with government legislation and nursing standards to minimize the occurrence of disease or injuries and their consequences.

The Community Health Nurse. . .

a. Participates in surveillance, recognizes trends in epidemiology data, and utilizes this data through population level actions such as health education, screening, immunization, and communicable disease control and management.

b. Uses prevention and protection approaches with the client to identify risk factors and to address issues such as communicable disease, injury, chronic disease, and physical environment (e.g. air, climate, housing, work, water, land).

c. Applies the appropriate level of prevention (primordial, primary, secondary, tertiary and quaternary)[vi, vii] to improve client health.

d. Facilitates informed decision making with the client for protective and preventive health measures.

e. Collaborates with the client to provide emergency management including prevention/mitigation, preparedness, response, and recovery.[viii]

f. Uses harm reduction principles grounded in social justice and health equity perspectives to identify and reduce risks, and increase protective factors.

g. Includes cultural safety and cultural humility approaches in all aspects of prevention and health protection interventions.[iv]

h. Engages in collaborative, interdisciplinary, and intersectoral partnerships in the delivery of preventive and protective services with particular attention to populations who are marginalized.

i. Evaluates and modifies prevention and health protection activities in partnership with the client.

Standard 3: Health Maintenance, Restoration, and Palliation

Community health nurses integrate health maintenance, restoration and palliation into their practice to maintain maximum function, improve health, and support life transitions including acute, chronic, or terminal illness, and end of life.

The Community Health Nurse. . .

a. Holistically assesses the health status, and functional competence of the client within the context of their environment, social supports, and life transitions.

b. Supports informed decision making and co-creates mutually agreed upon plans and priorities for care with the client.

c. Uses a range of intervention strategies related to health maintenance, restoration and palliation to promote self-management of disease, maximize function, and enhance quality of life.

d. Includes cultural safety and cultural humility approaches in all aspects of health maintenance, restoration and palliation interventions.[iv]

e. Facilitates maintenance of health and the healing process with the client in response to adverse health events.

f. Evaluates and modifies health maintenance, disease management, restoration and palliation interventions in partnership with the client.

Standard 4: Professional Relationships

Community health nurses work with others to establish, build and nurture professional and therapeutic relationships. These relationships include optimizing participation, and self-determination of the client.

The Community Health Nurse. . .

a. Recognizes own personal beliefs, attitudes, assumptions, feelings and values including racism and stereotypes and their potential impact on nursing practice.

b. Assesses the client's beliefs, attitudes, feelings, and values about health and the impact of these on the professional relationship and potential interventions.

c. "Acknowledges that the current state of Aboriginal health in Canada is a direct result of previous Canadian government policies" in working with Indigenous people as stated in the Truth and Reconciliation Commission of Canada: Calls to Action.[ix]

d. Respects and supports the client in identifying their health priorities and making decisions to address them while being responsive to power dynamics.

e. Uses culturally safe communication strategies in professional relationships, recognizing communication may be verbal or non-verbal, written or graphic. Communication can occur via a variety of mediums.

f. Recognizes and promotes the development of the client's social support networks as an important social determinant of health.

g. Promotes awareness of, and supports linkages to, appropriate community resources that are acceptable to the client.

h. Maintains professional boundaries in therapeutic client relationships.

i. Negotiates terminating therapeutic relationships in a professional manner.

j. Builds a network of relationships and partnerships with a wide variety of individuals, families, groups, communities, and systems to address health issues and promote healthy public policy to advance health equity.

k. Incorporates the domains from the National Interprofessional Competencies framework in working with other nurses and health care team members. Domains include 1) interprofessional communication, 2) patient/client/family/community-centered-care, 3) role clarification, 4) collaborative leadership, and 6) interprofessional conflict resolution.[x]

l. Evaluates and reflects on the nurse/client and other community relationships to ensure responsive and effective nursing practice.

Standard 5: Capacity Building

Community health nurses partner with the client to promote capacity. The focus is to recognize barriers to health and to mobilize and build on existing strengths.

The Community Health Nurse. . .

a. Uses an asset approach and facilitates action to support the priorities of the *Jakarta Declaration*.[xi] (Figure 3)

b. Enhances the client's ability to recognize their strengths[xii] their challenges, the causal factors, and the resources available that impacts their health.

c. Assists the client to make an informed decision in determining their health goals and priorities for action.

d. Uses capacity building strategies such as mutual goal setting, visioning and facilitation in planning for action.

e. Helps the client to identify and access available resources to address their health issues.

f. Supports the client to build their capacity to advocate for themselves.

g. Supports the development of an environment that enables the client to make healthy lifestyle choices, recognizing relevant cultural factors and Indigenous ways of knowing.

h. Recognizes the unique history of Indigenous people, and incorporates Indigenous ways of knowing and culturally safe engagement strategies in capacity building efforts.

i. Uses a comprehensive mix of strategies such as coalition building, inter-sectoral collaboration, community engagement and mobilization, partnerships and networking to build community capacity to take action on priority issues.

j. Supports community-based action to influence policy change in support of health.

k. Evaluates the impact of capacity building efforts including both process and outcomes in partnership with the client.

> The Jakarta Declaration identified the following priorities;
> 1. Promote social responsibility for health
> 2. Increase investments for health development
> 3. Consolidate and expand partnerships for health
> 4. Increase community capacity and empower the individual
> 5. Secure an infrastructure for health promotion

FIGURE 3 The Jakarta Declaration[xv]

Standard 6: Health Equity

Community health nurses recognize the impacts of the determinants of health, and incorporate actions into their practice such as advocating for healthy public policy. The focus is to advance health equity at an individual and societal level.

The Community Health Nurse. . .

a. Engages with the client using critical social theory and intersectional approach from a foundation of equity and social justice.[xiii, xiv]

b. Assesses how the social determinants of health influence the client's health status with particular attention to clients who are marginalized.

c. Understands how power structures, unique perspectives and expectations may contribute to the client's engagement with health promoting services.

d. Advocates for and with client to act for themselves.

e. Participates with community members and advocates for health in intersectoral policy development and implementation to reduce health equity gaps between populations.

f. Engages with clients who are marginalized in the coordinating and planning of care, services and programs that address their needs and perspectives on health and illness.

g. Refers, coordinates and facilitates client access to universal and equitable health promoting services that are acceptable and responsive to their needs across the life span.

h. Collaborates with community partners to coordinate and deliver comprehensive client services with the goal of reducing service gaps and fragmentation.

i. Understands historical injustices, inequitable power relations, institutionalized and interpersonal racism and their impacts on health and health care and provides culturally safe care.

j. Supports the client's right to choose alternate health care options, including "to recognize the value of Aboriginal healing practices and use them in the treatment of Aboriginal patients in collaboration with Aboriginal healers and Elders where requested by Aboriginal patients" as stated in the Truth and Reconciliation Commission of Canada: Calls for Action.[ix]

k. Advocates for resource allocation using a social justice lens.

l. Uses strategies such as home visits, outreach, technology and case finding to facilitate equitable access to services and health-supporting conditions for populations who are marginalized.

m. Advocates for healthy public policy and social justice by participating in legislative and policy-making activities that influence determinants of health and access to services.

n. Takes action with and for the client at the organizational, municipal, provincial, territorial and federal levels to address service gaps, inequities in health and accessibility issues.

o. Evaluates and modifies efforts to increase accessibility to health and community services, and to advance health equity.

Standard 7: Evidence Informed Practice

Community health nurses use best evidence to guide nursing practice and support clients in making informed decisions.

The Community Health Nurse. . .

a. Uses professional expertise in considering best available research evidence, and other factors such as client context and preferences, and available resources to determine nursing actions.

b. Seeks out reliable sources of available evidence from nursing and other relevant disciplines.

c. Understands and uses critical appraisal skills to determine quality of research evidence.

d. Understands and uses knowledge translation strategies to integrate high quality research into clinical practice, education, and research.

e. Uses quality evidence to inform policy advocacy, development and implementation.

f. Uses a variety of information sources including acknowledging diverse perspectives and Indigenous ways of knowing.

Standard 8: Professional Responsibility and Accountability

Community health nurses demonstrate professional responsibility and accountability as a fundamental component of their autonomous practice.

The Community Health Nurse. . .

a. Assesses and identifies unsafe, unethical, illegal or socially unacceptable circumstances and takes preventive or corrective action to protect the client.

b. Recognizes ethical dilemmas and applies ethical principles and CNA Code of Ethics.[xv]

c. Works collaboratively in determining the best course of action when responding to ethical dilemmas.

d. Provides leadership in collaboration with the community to advocate for healthy public policy based on the foundations of health equity and social justice.

e. Identifies and acts on factors which enhance or hinder the delivery of quality care.

f. Participates in the advancement of community health nursing by mentoring students and new practitioners.

g. Participates in professional development activities and opportunities to be involved in research.

h. Identifies and works proactively (individually or by participating in relevant professional organizations) to address health and nursing issues that affect the client and/or the profession.

i. Provides constructive feedback to peers as needed to enhance community health nursing practice.

j. Documents community health nursing activities in a timely and thorough manner.

k. Advocates for effective and efficient use of community health nursing resources.

l. Uses reflective practice to continually assess, and improve personal community health nursing practice including cultural safety and cultural humility.

m. Acts upon legal obligations (applicable provincial/territorial/federal legislation) to report to relevant authorities any situations involving unsafe or unethical care.

n. Uses available resources to systematically evaluate the achievement of desired outcomes for quality improvement in community health nursing practice.[xvi]

Source: Community Health Nurses Canada (2019, revised) – *Canadian Community Health Nursing Professional Practice Model & Standards of Practice.* Used by permission of Community Health Nurses Association of Canada. Retrieved from https://www.chnc.ca/documents/CHNC-ProfessionalPracticeModel-EN/index.html#/1/

Appendix B: Public Health Nursing Discipline-Specific Competencies

Public Health Nursing Competencies are the integrated knowledge, skills, judgment, and attributes required of a public health nurse to practice safely and ethically. Attributes include, but are not limited to attitudes, values, and beliefs (Canadian Nurses Association Code of Ethics, 2008).

1. PUBLIC HEALTH AND NURSING SCIENCES

This category includes key knowledge and critical thinking skills related to the public health sciences (behavioural and social sciences, biostatistics, epidemiology, environmental public health, demography, workplace health, prevention, of chronic diseases, infectious diseases, psychosocial problems, and injuries) as well as nursing theory, change theory, economics, politics, public health administration, community assessment, management theory, program planning and evaluation, population health principles, community development theory, and the history of public health. Competency in this category requires the ability to apply knowledge in practice.

A public health nurse is able to . . .

1.1 Apply knowledge about the following concepts: the health status of populations; inequities in health; the determinants of health and illness; social justice; principles of primary health care; strategies for health promotion; disease and injury prevention; health protection, as well as the factors that influence the delivery and use of health services.

1.2 Apply knowledge about the history, structure, and interaction of public health and health care services at local, provincial/territorial, national, and international levels.

1.3 Apply public health and nursing sciences to practice and synthesize knowledge from a broad range of theories, models, and frameworks.

1.4 Critically appraise knowledge gathered from a variety of sources.

1.5 Use evidence and research to inform health policies, programs, and practice:
   ■ contribute to the development and generation of evidence-based nursing
   ■ use available resources to systematically plan and evaluate public health nursing practice

1.6 Pursue lifelong learning opportunities in the field of public health that are consistent with current public health nursing practice; new and emerging issues; the changing needs of individuals, families, groups and communities; emerging research and evolving information about the impact of the determinants of health.

1.7 Integrate multiple ways of knowing into practice.

2. ASSESSMENT AND ANALYSIS

This category describes the core competencies needed to collect, assess, analyze, and apply information (including data, facts, concepts, and theories). These competencies are required to make evidence-based decisions, prepare budgets and reports, conduct investigations, and make recommendations for policy and program development. Community members are involved in identifying and reinforcing those aspects of everyday life, culture, and political activity that are conducive to health.

A public health nurse is able to . . .

2.1 Recognize that a health concern or issue exists:
   ■ apply principles of epidemiology
   ■ conduct comprehensive community assessments with individuals, families, groups, and communities using quantitative and qualitative strategies
   ■ recognize patterns and trends in epidemiological data and service delivery
   ■ assess the impact of the broad social, cultural, political, and economic determinants of health.

2.2 Identify relevant and appropriate sources of information, including community assets, resources, and values in collaboration with individuals, families, groups, communities, and stakeholders.

2.3 Collect, store, retrieve, and use accurate and appropriate information on public health issues.

2.4 Analyze information to determine appropriate implications, uses, gaps, and limitations.

2.5 Assess impact of specific issues on health such as political climate and will; values and culture; social and systemic structures; settings; as well as the individual, family, group, and community's readiness and capacity.

2.6 Assess the health status and functional competence of individuals, families, groups, communities, or populations within the context of their environmental and social supports.

2.7 Determine the meaning of information, considering the ethical, political, scientific, socio-cultural, and economic contexts:
   ■ identify attitudes, beliefs, feelings, and values about health and their effect on relationships and interventions

- support individuals, families, groups, and communities to identify risks to health and make informed choices about protective and preventive health measures
- describe the role of power in relationships by giving voice to the vulnerable
- demonstrate skill in dealing with diversity and high levels of ambiguity.

2.8 Recommend specific actions based on the analysis of information:
- identify a range of appropriate interventions including health promotion; health protection; disease and injury prevention; and clinical care using a multi-strategy and multi-target approach
- identify short- and long-term goals
- identify outcome indicators
- identify research questions

2.9 Recognize opportunities to promote social justice.

3. POLICY AND PROGRAM PLANNING, IMPLEMENTATION, AND EVALUATION

This category describes the core competencies needed to effectively choose options, and to plan, implement, and evaluate policies and/or programs in public health. This includes the management of incidents such as outbreaks and emergencies.

3(A). Policy Development

A public health nurse is able to . . .

3A.1 Describe selected policy options to address a specific public health issue.

3A.2 Describe the implications of each policy option, especially as each applies to the determinants of health, and recommend or decide on a course of action.

3A.3 Develop a plan to implement a course of action taking into account relevant evidence, legislation, emergency planning procedures, regulations, and policies.

3A.4 Implement a policy.

3A.5 Support community action to influence policy change.

3A.6 Build community capacity to improve health and address health inequities.

3A.7 Advocate for healthy public policy and services that promote and protect the health and well-being of individuals, families, groups, and communities.

3A.8 Advocate for the reduction of inequities in health through legislative and policy-making activities.

3(B). Program Planning

A public health nurse is able to . . .

3B.1 Describe selected program options to address a specific public health issue.

3B.2 Describe the implications of each option, especially as each applies to the determinants of health and recommend or decide on a course of action.

3B.3 Develop a plan in collaboration with individuals, families, groups, and communities to implement a course of action that is responsive to needs taking into account relevant evidence, legislation, emergency planning procedures, regulations, and policies.

3(C). Implementation and Intervention

A public health nurse is able to . . .

3C.1 Take action, across multiple levels, to address specific public health issues by using a comprehensive mix of public health strategies to address unique needs and to build individual, family, group, and community capacity.

3C.2 Facilitate planned change with individuals, families, groups, communities, systems, or population(s) by applying the Population Health Promotion Model, primary health care principles, and appropriate change theory.

3C.3 Demonstrate the ability to integrate relevant research and implement evidence informed practice.

3C.4 Participate in collaborative, interdisciplinary, and intersectoral partnerships to enhance the health of individuals, families, groups, communities, and populations.

3C.5 Maximize the capacity of the individual, family, group, or community to take responsibility for and to manage their health needs according to resources available and personal skills.

3C.6 Set and follow priorities and maximize outcomes based on available resources.

3C.7 Fulfill functional roles in response to a public health emergency.

3C.8 Facilitate access to services in the health sector and other sectors.

3C.9 Adapt practice in response to the changing health needs of the individual, family, group, and community and in response to the unique characteristics of the setting.

3C.10 Take action to protect individuals, families, groups, and communities from unsafe or unethical circumstances.

3C.11 Advocate in collaboration with, and on behalf of, and with individuals, families, groups, and communities on social justice–related issues.

3(D). Evaluation

A public health nurse is able to . . .

3D.1 Evaluate an action, policy, or program in a systematic and continuous manner by measuring its effect on individuals, families, groups, or communities.

3D.2 Evaluate programs in relation to determinants of health and health outcomes.

3D.3 Evaluate programs in partnership with individuals, families, groups, communities, and other stakeholders.

4. PARTNERSHIPS, COLLABORATION, AND ADVOCACY

This category captures the competencies required to influence and work with others to improve the health and well-being of the public through the pursuit of a common goal. This includes the concepts of: social justice, which is the fair distribution of society's benefits and responsibilities and their consequences (Canadian Nurses Association, Code of Ethics, 2008); partnership and collaboration, which is to optimize performance through shared resources and responsibilities; advocacy, which is to speak, write, or act in favour of a particular cause, policy, or group of people and aims to reduce inequities in health status or access to health services.

A public health nurse is able to . . .

4.1 Advocate for societal change in support of health for all:
- collaborate with partners to address public health issues and service gaps in order to achieve improved health outcomes
- build coalitions, intersectoral partnerships, and networks
- facilitate the change process to impact the determinants of health and improve health outcomes.

4.2 Use skills such as team building, negotiation, conflict management, and group facilitation to build partnerships and to support group development.

4.3 Mediate between differing interests in the pursuit of health and well-being, and advocate for appropriate resource allocation and equitable access to resources.

4.4 Advocate for healthy public policies and services that promote and protect the health and well-being of individuals and communities.

4.5 Involve individuals, families, groups, and communities as active partners to identify assets, strengths, and available resources and to take action to address health inequities, needs, deficits, and gaps.

5. DIVERSITY AND INCLUSIVENESS

This category identifies the competencies required to interact effectively with diverse individuals, families, groups, and communities in relation to others in society as well to recognize the root causes of disparities and what can be done to eliminate them (Canadian Nurses Association, Code of Ethics, 2008). It is the embodiment of attitudes and actions that result in inclusive behaviours, practices, programs, and policies.

A public health nurse is able to . . .

5.1 Recognize how the determinants of health (biological, social, cultural, economic, and physical) influence the health and well-being of specific population groups.

5.2 Address population diversity when planning, implementing, adapting, and evaluating public health programs and policies.

5.3 Apply culturally relevant and appropriate approaches with people from diverse cultural, socioeconomic, and educational backgrounds, and persons of all ages, genders, health status, sexual orientations, and abilities.

6. COMMUNICATION

Communication involves an interchange of ideas, opinions, and information. This category addresses numerous dimensions of communication including internal and external exchanges; written, verbal, non-verbal, and listening skills; computer literacy; providing appropriate information to different audiences; working with the media and social marketing techniques.

A public health nurse is able to . . .

6.1 Communicate effectively with individuals, families, groups, communities, and colleagues:
- use verbal, non-verbal, and written or graphic communication skills
- speak and write in plain language
- use multi-sensory forms of communication to address unique communication styles
- use culturally relevant communication when building relationships

6.2 Interpret information for professional, nonprofessional, and community audiences.

6.3 Mobilize individuals, families, groups, and communities by using appropriate media, community resources, and social marketing techniques.

6.4 Use current technology to communicate effectively.

7. LEADERSHIP

This category focuses on leadership competencies that build capacity, improve performance and enhance the quality of the working environment. They also enable organizations and communities to create, communicate, and apply shared visions, missions, and values.

A public health nurse is able to . . .

7.1 Describe the mission and priorities of the public health organization where one works, and apply them in practice.

7.2 Contribute to developing key values and a shared vision to assess, plan, and implement public health programs and policies in the community by actively working with health professionals and in partnership with community partners to build capacity.

7.3 Use public health and nursing ethics to manage self, others, information, and resources and practise in accordance with all relevant legislation, regulating body standards, and codes (e.g., provincial health legislation, child welfare legislation, privacy legislation, Canadian Nurses Association Code of Ethics for registered nurses).

7.4 Contribute to team and organizational learning in order to advance public health goals.

7.5 Contribute to the maintenance of organizational performance standards.

7.6 Demonstrate an ability to build capacity by sharing knowledge, tools, expertise, and experience:
- participate in professional development and practice development activities
- mentor students and orient new staff
- participate in research and quality assurance initiatives

8. PROFESSIONAL RESPONSIBILITY AND ACCOUNTABILITY

This category addresses a number of dimensions, including the recognition that nurses are accountable for their actions and are responsible for making sure they have the required knowledge and skills needed to ensure the delivery of safe, compassionate, competent, and ethical care. It includes the competencies required to maintain quality work environments and relationships needed in a professional practice. Public health nurses are responsible for initiating strategies that will address the determinants of health and generate a positive impact on people and systems. They are accountable to a variety of authorities and stakeholders as well as to the individual and community they serve. This range of accountabilities places them in a variety of situations with unique ethical dilemmas.

A public health nurse is able to . . .

8.1 Demonstrate professionalism in independent practice in multiple settings with multiple stakeholders.

8.2 Apply ethical standards and principles taking into consideration appropriate public health and nursing ethics.

8.3 Consult as needed to determine the best course of action in response to: ethical dilemmas, safety issues, risks to human rights and freedoms, new situations, and new knowledge.

8.4 Use reflective practice to continually assess and improve practice:
- examine practice in relation to personal and individual, family, group, or community attributes, existing knowledge, and context
- adapt public health nursing techniques, approaches, and procedures to the challenges in a particular community situation or setting

8.5 Advocate for effective, efficient, and responsible use of resources.

8.6 Act upon legal and professional obligations, and practises in accordance with relevant legislation.

8.7 Contribute to the quality of public health nursing work environments by identifying needs, issues, and solutions and mobilizing colleagues by actively participating in team and organizational structures and mechanisms.

Source: Community Health Nurses of Canada (2009). *Public Health Nursing Discipline Specific Competencies Version 1.0* (pp. 2–10). Reproduced by permission of Community Health Nurses Association of Canada. Retrieved from http://www.chnc.ca/members/documents/PHNCompetenciesPrintReadyFinalEnglish.pdf

Appendix C: Home Health Nursing Competencies

1. ELEMENTS OF HOME HEALTH NURSING

These elements and associated competencies focus on the nursing activities, functions, goals, and outcomes that are central to home health nursing practice.

a. Assessment, Monitoring, and Clinical Decision Making

The home health nurse is able to . . .

i. conduct comprehensive autonomous and/or collaborative health assessments to determine the health status, functional and psychosocial needs, and competence of clients and their families within the context of their environment and social supports

ii. apply critical thinking skills and creative problem-solving analysis when making clinical decisions

iii. analyze information to determine appropriate nursing actions, implications, applications, gaps, and limitations

iv. collaborate with health care team members and others who are involved with the client to determine appropriateness and availability of required services

v. incorporate a combination of basic and advanced knowledge of health and nursing across the lifespan and the health-illness continuum

vi. keep knowledge current and use evidence to inform practice to ensure optimal case management

vii. assess the safety of the home environment with the goal of optimizing client safety and taking actions to support a safe work environment for all members of the home health care team

b. Care Planning and Care Coordination

The home health nurse is able to . . .

i. plan and prioritize visits to meet the health and scheduling needs of clients

ii. use the nursing process to collaboratively develop, coordinate, and implement mutually agreed-upon care plans, negotiating priorities in care with clear treatment and outcome goals and supporting client navigation and transition through the continuum of care

iii. support clients and families to build on their strengths to attain or maintain a desired health status within available resources

iv. anticipate the need for alternative ways of providing services and use creative problem-solving skills to overcome obstacles in delivery of client care, i.e., weather, lack of resources, etc.

v. ensure discharge planning is integrated within the care plan and occurs in collaboration with the client, family, health care team, and community

vi. promote an integrated assessment and develop a unified care and treatment plan that is collaboratively carried out by team members to maximize continuity of care within a client-centred approach

vii. appreciate and understand the roles and responsibilities and the contributions of other regulated and unregulated health workers involved in the client care plan

viii. facilitate and coordinate access to other members of the multidisciplinary team such as primary care providers, specialist physician, community pharmacist, nurses, and other allied health professionals to address a specific health issue

ix. collaboratively evaluate care plan interventions through reassessment and ongoing evaluation of results and adapt them to the changing conditions of the client and the client's family

c. Health Maintenance, Restoration, and Palliation

The home health nurse is able to . . .

i. assist clients and families to maintain and/or restore health by using a comprehensive mix of strategies to address their health needs across the lifespan and illness continuum

ii. understand and/or educate clients, their families/caregivers, and colleagues in the safe and appropriate use and maintenance of various types of equipment, technology, and treatments to maintain health and assist clients and families to integrate them into their everyday life/routine

iii. communicate effectively with clients and families while supporting them through the decision-making process about end-of-life issues

iv. use basic and advanced nursing skills to perform and adapt complex procedures in the home health setting

v. recognize when specialized counselling beyond the scope of nursing is required and facilitate an appropriate referral

vi. respond to the ever-changing and evolving health care needs of the client and family by strategically revising interventions and therapies

vii. self-identify the need for assistance when not familiar with care requirements and seek support to assure continued excellence in care

d. Teaching and Education

The home health nurse is able to . . .

i. assess the knowledge, attitudes, level of motivation, values, beliefs, behaviours, practices, stage of change, and skills of the client/family

ii. consider and integrate into educational planning the factors that may impact the client/family's ability to learn. For example: environment, readiness, willingness, literacy level, educational background, socioeconomic situation, health status, etc.

iii. interpret and explain complex information for clients and families

iv. apply appropriate learning principles, teaching methods, and educational theories to educational activities

v. include family, volunteers, and caregivers in teaching and education

vi. evaluate the effectiveness of health education interventions

e. Communication

The home health nurse is able to . . .

i. use effective listening, verbal, and non-verbal communication skills to understand the client's perspective and be understood by the client, family, and other caregivers involved in the care

ii. use effective interviewing skills and strategies to engage in constructive dialogue with clients and their families

iii. use effective communication skills to engage, connect, appreciate, respond, empathize, and support the empowerment of others

iv. identify and use strategies to overcome language and communication barriers

v. maintain a focused approach amidst multiple distractions within the home environment

vi. employ negotiation and conflict-management skills

vii. use techniques that are client-centred, client-driven, and strength-based when counselling clients

viii. use documentation as an effective communication tool

ix. use technology to effectively communicate and manage client care in a confidential manner

f. Relationships

The home health nurse is able to . . .

i. optimize the health of the client and caregiver(s) by establishing and maintaining a therapeutic nurse–client relationship based on mutual trust, respect, caring, and listening within the context of being "a guest in the house"

ii. acknowledge the contribution that the family/caregiver provides to client health in a way that makes them feel valued and respected and support them to maintain relationships that support effective care

iii. work effectively and non-judgmentally in a wide range of environments with varying conditions of cleanliness

iv. use skills such as team building, negotiation, conflict management, and group facilitation to build and sustain partnerships

v. involve clients and families as active partners to identify assets, strengths, and available resources

g. Access and Equity

The home health nurse is able to . . .

i. advocate for healthy public policies and accessible, inclusive, and integrated services that promote and protect the health and well-being of all individuals and communities

ii. apply culturally relevant and appropriate approaches with people of diverse cultural, socioeconomic, and educational backgrounds, and persons of all ages, genders, health status, sexual orientations, and abilities

iii. recognize opportunities to promote social justice and advocate in collaboration with, and on behalf of, clients and families on related issues to give voice to the vulnerable

iv. optimize allocation of human, financial, and infrastructure resources in order to provide a safe and accessible health delivery system

v. advocate for the reduction of inequities in health by participating in legislative and policy-making activities

h. Building Capacity

The home health nurse is able to . . .

i. mobilize clients, families, and others to take action to address health needs, deficits, and gaps accessing and using available resources

ii. assist the client and the client's family to recognize their capacity for managing their own health needs according to available resources

iii. assist colleagues, partners, and/or clients to support and build on the capacities that are inherent in the individual, families, and the communities to influence policy change

iv. demonstrate cultural competency when addressing client care issues and when working in an environment where there may be levels of ambiguity

v. adapt and be flexible and responsive to the changing health needs of the client and family

2. FOUNDATIONS OF HOME HEALTH NURSING

These competencies focus on the core knowledge and primary health care philosophy that are central to home health nursing practice.

a. Health Promotion

The home health nurse is able to . . .

i. facilitate planned change with clients and families by applying and incorporating health promotion theory, primary health care principles, and change theory into practice

ii. recognize how the determinants of health influence the health and well-being of clients and families

iii. assess the impact specific issues may have on the client's health such as political climate; priorities, values, and culture; social and systemic structures and settings

iv. assess the readiness and capacity of the client and family to make changes to promote their health

b. Illness Prevention and Health Protection

The home health nurse is able to . . .

i. apply nursing sciences to practice and evaluate, synthesize, and apply knowledge from a broad range of theories, models, frameworks, and practice

ii. use critical thinking to consider the ethical, political, scientific, socio-cultural, and economic contexts to determine the meaning of information related to client health care needs

iii. support clients and families to identify risks to health and make informed choices about protective and preventive health measures

iv. take action to protect clients, families, and groups from unsafe or unethical circumstances

v. participate in collaborative, interdisciplinary, and intersectoral partnerships to enhance the health of clients and families

3. QUALITY AND PROFESSIONAL RESPONSIBILITY

These competencies focus on practice activities and/or strategies by which the home health nurse promotes quality of care and demonstrates professional responsibility.

a. Quality Care

The home health nurse is able to . . .

i. initiate, lead, and participate in risk management and quality improvement activities to measure effectiveness of services, cost implications, and processes

ii. initiate and participate in critical incident reviews

iii. evaluate nursing interventions in a systematic and continuous manner by measuring their effect on clients and families

iv. evaluate programs in relation to determinants of health and health outcomes

v. contribute to the quality of work environments by identifying needs, issues, and solutions and actively participating in team and organizational quality improvement processes

vi. understand the financial aspects of care and be accountable for effective, efficient, and responsible use of time and resources when delivering care to clients and families

b. Professional Responsibility

The home health nurse is able to . . .

i. demonstrate professionalism, leadership, judgment, and accountability in independent practice in multiple settings with multiple stakeholders

ii. practise independently and autonomously providing client-centred services in a wide variety of settings where nursing care and services are needed

iii. use reflective practice to continually assess and improve practice

iv. integrate multiple ways of knowing into practice

v. contribute to the development and generation of evidence-informed nursing practice

vi. pursue lifelong learning opportunities to support professional practice

vii. use nursing ethics, ethical standards and principles, and self-awareness to manage self and practise in accordance with all relevant legislation, regulatory body standards, codes, and organizational policies

viii. describe the mission, values, and priorities of the health organization where one works

ix. participate in the advancement of home health nursing by mentoring students and new practitioners

x. recognize and understand that one's attitudes, beliefs, feelings, and values about health can have an effect on relationships and interventions

Source: Community Health Nurses of Canada (2010). *Home Health Nursing Competencies Version 1.0 March 2010.* (pp. 3–9). Reproduced by permission of Community Health Nurses Association of Canada. Retrieved from https://chnc.ca/documents/HHNursingCompetenciesFINALEnglish.pdf

Index

Note: Page numbers followed by f or t represent figures or tables respectively.